WHO Classification of Tumours • 5th Edition

Endocrine and Neuroendocrine Tumours

WHO Classification of Tumours Editorial Board

International Agency for Research on Cancer

World Health Organization

Suggested citation
WHO Classification of Tumours Editorial Board. Endocrine and neuroendocrine tumours.
Lyon (France): International Agency for Research on Cancer; 2025.
(WHO classification of tumours series, 5th ed.; vol. 10).
https://publications.iarc.who.int/645.

First print run (7500 copies)

Updated corrigenda can be found at https://publications.iarc.who.int

IARC Library Cataloguing-in-Publication Data
Names: WHO Classification of Tumours Editorial Board.
Title: Endocrine and neuroendocrine tumours / edited by WHO Classification of Tumours Editorial Board.
Description: Fifth edition. | Lyon: International Agency for Research on Cancer, 2025. | Series: World Health Organization classification of tumours. | Includes bibliographical references and index.
Identifiers: ISBN 9789283245247 (pbk.) | ISBN 9789283245254 (ebook)
Subjects: MESH: Endocrine Gland Neoplasms – classification. | Neuroendocrine Tumours – classification.
Classification: NLM WK 15

The WHO classification of endocrine and neuroendocrine tumours presented in this book reflects the views of the WHO Classification of Tumours Editorial Board that convened via video conference 21–23 June 2021, as well as subsequent consultation.

The WHO Classification of Tumours Editorial Board

Expert members: Endocrine and neuroendocrine tumours

For the complete list of all contributors and their affiliations, see pages 493–498.

The WHO Classification of Tumours Editorial Board (continued)

Standing members

* Standing members marked with an asterisk also served as expert members for this volume.

For the complete list of all contributors and their affiliations, see pages 493–498.

WHO Classification of Tumours
Endocrine and Neuroendocrine Tumours

Edited by	The WHO Classification of Tumours Editorial Board
IARC Editors	Subasri Armon Ian A. Cree Anil Felix Angelo Fonseca Daphne Fonseca Gabrielle Goldman-Lévy Dilani Lokuhetty Valerie A. White Harshima Wijesinghe
Project Assistant	Asiedua Asante
Assistant	Anne-Sophie Bres
Production Editors	Jessica Cox Julia Slone-Murphy
Principal Information Assistant	Alberto Machado
Information Assistant	Catarina Marques
Layout	Meaghan Fortune
Printed by	Omnibook 74370 Argonay, France
Publisher	International Agency for Research on Cancer (IARC) 25 Av. Tony Garnier, CS 90627 69366 Lyon, CEDEX 07, France

Contents

List of abbreviations

3D	three-dimensional
AFIP	US Armed Forces Institute of Pathology
AIDS	acquired immunodeficiency syndrome
AJCC	American Joint Committee on Cancer
ALT	alternative lengthening of telomeres
AR	androgen receptor
ATA	American Thyroid Association
ATP	adenosine triphosphate
cAMP	cyclic adenosine monophosphate
CNS	central nervous system
CT	computed tomography
DNA	deoxyribonucleic acid
EBV	Epstein–Barr virus
EC cell	enterochromaffin cell
ECL cell	enterochromaffin-like cell
ER	estrogen receptor
EUS	endoscopic ultrasound
EUS-FNAB	endoscopic ultrasound–guided fine-needle aspiration biopsy
FDC	follicular dendritic cell
FDG	18F-fluorodeoxyglucose
FDOPA PET	18F-L-dihydroxyphenylalanine positron emission tomography
FIGO	International Federation of Gynecology and Obstetrics
FISH	fluorescence in situ hybridization
FNAB	fine-needle aspiration biopsy
FNAC	fine-needle aspiration cytology
GCB cell	germinal-centre B cell
GFAP	glial fibrillary acidic protein
H&E	haematoxylin and eosin stain
HBV	hepatitis B virus
HCV	hepatitis C virus
HIV	human immunodeficiency virus
HPF	high-power field
HPV	human papillomavirus
IARC	International Agency for Research on Cancer
ICD-11	International Classification of Diseases, 11th revision
ICD-O	International Classification of Diseases for Oncology
INPC	International Neuroblastoma Pathology Classification
INRGSS	International Neuroblastoma Risk Group Staging System
IQ	intelligence quotient
IRSG	Intergroup Rhabdomyosarcoma Study Group
KSHV/HHV8	Kaposi sarcoma–associated herpesvirus / human herpesvirus 8
Mb	megabase
MCPyV	Merkel cell polyomavirus
MIM number	Mendelian Inheritance in Man number
MITF	melanocyte-inducing transcription factor
MKI	mitosis-karyorrhexis index
MRI	magnetic resonance imaging
mRNA	messenger ribonucleic acid
NOS	not otherwise specified
NSE	neuron-specific enolase
OS	overall survival
PAS	periodic acid–Schiff
PASD	periodic acid–Schiff with diastase
PCR	polymerase chain reaction
PET	positron emission tomography
PR	progesterone receptor
PRRT	peptide receptor radionuclide therapy
RNA	ribonucleic acid
SEER Program	Surveillance, Epidemiology, and End Results Program
TNM	tumour, node, metastasis
UV	ultraviolet

Foreword

The WHO Classification of Tumours is a taxonomy of cancer, published as a series of books (also known as the WHO Blue Books) and now as a website (https://tumourclassification.iarc.who.int). It is an essential tool for standardizing diagnostic practice worldwide. It also serves as a vehicle for the translation of cancer research into practice. The diagnostic criteria and standards that make up the classification are underpinned by evidence evaluated and debated by experts in the field. About 200 authors and editors participate in the production of each volume, and they give their time freely to this task. We are very grateful for their help; it is a remarkable international team effort of great significance to both patients and their doctors.

This volume, like the rest of the fifth edition, has been led by the WHO Classification of Tumours Editorial Board, composed of standing and expert members. The standing members, who have been nominated by pathology organizations, are the equivalent of the series editors of previous editions. The expert members for each volume, equivalent to the volume editors of previous editions, are selected on the basis of informed bibliometric analysis and advice from the standing members. The diagnostic process is increasingly multidisciplinary, and we are delighted that several radiology and clinical experts have joined us to address specific needs.

The most conspicuous change to the format of the books in the fifth edition is that tumour types common to multiple systems are dealt with together – so there are separate chapters on mesenchymal and stromal tumours, haematolymphoid tumours, and germ cell tumours. There is also a chapter on genetic tumour syndromes associated with endocrine lesions and tumours.

We have attempted to take a more systematic approach to the multifaceted nature of tumour classification; each tumour type is described on the basis of its localization, clinical features, epidemiology, etiology, pathogenesis, histopathology, diagnostic molecular pathology, staging, and prognosis and prediction. We have also included information on macroscopic appearance and cytology, as well as essential and desirable diagnostic criteria. This standardized, modular approach makes it easier for the books to be accessible online, and it also enables us to call attention to areas in which there is little information, and where serious gaps in our knowledge remain to be addressed. Genetic disorders are of increasing importance to diagnosis in individual patients, and the study of these disorders has undoubtedly informed our understanding of tumour biology and behaviour over the past decade.

Table A Approximate number of fields per 1 mm^2 based on the field diameter and its corresponding area

Field diameter (mm)	Field area (mm^2)	Approximate number of fields per 1 mm^2
0.40	0.126	8
0.41	0.132	8
0.42	0.138	7
0.43	0.145	7
0.44	0.152	7
0.45	0.159	6
0.46	0.166	6
0.47	0.173	6
0.48	0.181	6
0.49	0.188	5
0.50	0.196	5
0.51	0.204	5
0.52	0.212	5
0.53	0.221	5
0.54	0.229	4
0.55	0.237	4
0.56	0.246	4
0.57	0.255	4
0.58	0.264	4
0.59	0.273	4
0.60	0.283	4
0.61	0.292	3
0.62	0.302	3
0.63	0.312	3
0.64	0.322	3
0.65	0.332	3
0.66	0.342	3
0.67	0.352	3
0.68	0.363	3
0.69	0.374	3

The organization of the WHO Blue Books content now follows the normal progression from benign to malignant – a break with the fourth edition, but one we hope will be welcome.

Most volumes are still organized by anatomical site (digestive system, breast, soft tissue and bone, etc.), and each tumour type is listed within a taxonomic classification that follows the format below, which helps to structure the books in a systematic manner:

Site: e.g. thyroid gland

Category: e.g. follicular cell–derived neoplasms

Family (class): e.g. malignant follicular cell–derived neoplasms

Type: e.g. papillary thyroid carcinoma

Subtype: e.g. tall cell papillary thyroid carcinoma

The issue of whether a given tumour type represents a distinct entity rather than a subtype continues to exercise pathologists, and it is the topic of many publications in the literature. We continue to deal with this issue on a case-by-case basis, but we believe there are inherent rules that can be applied. For example, tumours in which multiple histological patterns contain shared truncal mutations are clearly of the same type, despite the differences in their appearance. Equally, genetic heterogeneity within the same tumour type may have implications for treatment. A small shift in terminology in the fifth edition is that the term "variant" in reference to a specific kind of tumour has been wholly superseded by "subtype", in an effort to more clearly differentiate this meaning from that of "variant" in reference to a genetic alteration. Genetic tumour syndromes associated with endocrine lesions and tumours are addressed in a dedicated chapter at the end of the volume.

Another important change in this edition of the WHO Classification of Tumours series is the conversion of mitotic count from the traditional denominator of 10 HPF to a defined area expressed in mm^2 {943}. This serves to standardize the true area over which mitoses are enumerated, because different microscopes have high-power fields of different sizes. This change will also be helpful for anyone reporting using digital systems. The approximate number of fields per 1 mm^2 based on the field diameter and its corresponding area is presented in Table A.

We are continually working to improve the consistency and standards within the classification. In addition to having moved to the International System of Units (SI) for all mitotic counts, we have standardized genomic nomenclature by using Human Genome Variation Society (HGVS) notation. This includes the recent move in fusion gene notation to the separation of involved genes by a double colon (e.g. *BCR::ABL1*) {553}. We have also further standardized our use of units of length, adopting the convention used by the International Collaboration on Cancer Reporting (https://www.iccr-cancer.org/) and the UK Royal College of Pathologists (https://www.rcpath.org/), so that the size of tumours is now given exclusively in millimetres (mm) rather than centimetres (cm). This is clearer, in our view, and avoids the use of decimal points – a common source of medical errors.

The WHO Blue Books are much appreciated by pathologists of all types, and they are of increasing importance to practitioners of other clinical disciplines involved in cancer management, as well as to researchers. We, along with the entire editorial board, certainly hope that the series will continue to meet the need for standards in diagnosis and to facilitate the translation of diagnostic research into practice worldwide. It is particularly important that cancers continue to be classified and diagnosed according to the same standards internationally so that patients can benefit from multicentre clinical trials, as well as from the results of local trials conducted on different continents.

Dr Ian A. Cree

Former Head, WHO Classification of Tumours Programme
International Agency for Research on Cancer

Dr Dilani Lokuhetty

Head, WHO Classification of Tumours Programme
International Agency for Research on Cancer

ICD-O topographical coding of endocrine and neuroendocrine tumours

The ICD-O topography codes for the main anatomical sites covered in this volume are as follows {1442}:

C00–C14 Lip, oral cavity, and pharynx

C00 Lip
- C00.0 External upper lip
- C00.1 External lower lip
- C00.2 External lip, NOS
- C00.3 Mucosa of upper lip
- C00.4 Mucosa of lower lip
- C00.5 Mucosa of lip, NOS
- C00.6 Commissure of lip
- C00.8 Overlapping lesion of lip
- C00.9 Lip, NOS

C01 Base of tongue
- C01.9 Base of tongue, NOS

C02 Other and unspecified parts of tongue
- C02.0 Dorsal surface of tongue, NOS
- C02.1 Border of tongue
- C02.2 Ventral surface of tongue, NOS
- C02.3 Anterior two thirds of tongue, NOS
- C02.4 Lingual tonsil
- C02.8 Overlapping lesion of tongue
- C02.9 Tongue, NOS

C03 Gum
- C03.0 Upper gum
- C03.1 Lower gum
- C03.9 Gum, NOS

C04 Floor of mouth
- C04.0 Anterior floor of mouth
- C04.1 Lateral floor of mouth
- C04.8 Overlapping lesion of floor of mouth
- C04.9 Floor of mouth, NOS

C05 Palate
- C05.0 Hard palate
- C05.1 Soft palate, NOS
- C05.2 Uvula
- C05.8 Overlapping lesion of palate
- C05.9 Palate, NOS

C06 Other and unspecified parts of mouth
- C06.0 Cheek mucosa
- C06.1 Vestibule of mouth
- C06.2 Retromolar area
- C06.8 Overlapping lesion of other and unspecified parts of mouth
- C06.9 Mouth, NOS

C07 Parotid gland
- C07.9 Parotid gland

C08 Other and unspecified major salivary glands
- C08.0 Submandibular gland
- C08.1 Sublingual gland
- C08.8 Overlapping lesion of major salivary glands
- C08.9 Major salivary gland, NOS

C09 Tonsil
- C09.0 Tonsillar fossa
- C09.1 Tonsillar pillar
- C09.8 Overlapping lesion of tonsil
- C09.9 Tonsil, NOS

C10 Oropharynx
- C10.0 Vallecula
- C10.1 Anterior surface of epiglottis
- C10.2 Lateral wall of oropharynx
- C10.3 Posterior wall of oropharynx
- C10.4 Branchial cleft
- C10.8 Overlapping lesion of oropharynx
- C10.9 Oropharynx, NOS

C11 Nasopharynx
- C11.0 Superior wall of nasopharynx
- C11.1 Posterior wall of nasopharynx
- C11.2 Lateral wall of nasopharynx
- C11.3 Anterior wall of nasopharynx
- C11.8 Overlapping lesion of nasopharynx
- C11.9 Nasopharynx, NOS

C12 Piriform sinus
- C12.9 Piriform sinus

C13 Hypopharynx
- C13.0 Postcricoid region
- C13.1 Hypopharyngeal aspect of aryepiglottic fold
- C13.2 Posterior wall of hypopharynx
- C13.8 Overlapping lesion of hypopharynx
- C13.9 Hypopharynx, NOS

C14 Other and ill-defined sites in lip, oral cavity, and pharynx
- C14.0 Pharynx, NOS
- C14.2 Waldeyer ring
- C14.8 Overlapping lesion of lip, oral cavity, and pharynx

C15–C26 Digestive organs

C15 Oesophagus
- C15.0 Cervical oesophagus
- C15.1 Thoracic oesophagus
- C15.2 Abdominal oesophagus
- C15.3 Upper third of oesophagus
- C15.4 Middle third of oesophagus
- C15.5 Lower third of oesophagus
- C15.8 Overlapping lesion of oesophagus
- C15.9 Oesophagus, NOS

C16 Stomach
- C16.0 Cardia, NOS
- C16.1 Fundus of stomach
- C16.2 Body of stomach
- C16.3 Gastric antrum
- C16.4 Pylorus
- C16.5 Lesser curvature of stomach, NOS
- C16.6 Greater curvature of stomach, NOS
- C16.8 Overlapping lesion of stomach
- C16.9 Stomach, NOS

C17 Small intestine
- C17.0 Duodenum
- C17.1 Jejunum
- C17.2 Ileum
- C17.3 Meckel diverticulum
- C17.8 Overlapping lesion of small intestine
- C17.9 Small intestine, NOS

C18 Colon
- C18.0 Cecum
- C18.1 Appendix
- C18.2 Ascending colon
- C18.3 Hepatic flexure of colon
- C18.4 Transverse colon
- C18.5 Splenic flexure of colon
- C18.6 Descending colon
- C18.7 Sigmoid colon
- C18.8 Overlapping lesion of colon
- C18.9 Colon, NOS

C19 Rectosigmoid junction
- C19.9 Rectosigmoid junction

C20 Rectum
- C20.9 Rectum, NOS

C21 Anus and anal canal
- C21.0 Anus, NOS
- C21.1 Anal canal
- C21.2 Cloacogenic zone
- C21.8 Overlapping lesion of rectum, anus, and anal canal

C22 Liver and intrahepatic bile ducts
- C22.0 Liver
- C22.1 Intrahepatic bile duct

C23 Gallbladder
- C23.9 Gallbladder

C24 Other and unspecified parts of biliary tract
- C24.0 Extrahepatic bile duct
- C24.1 Ampulla of Vater
- C24.2 Distal (extrahepatic) bile duct
- C24.3 Perihilar (or proximal) bile duct
- C24.4 Cystic duct
- C24.8 Overlapping lesion of biliary tract
- C24.9 Biliary tract, NOS

C25 Pancreas
- C25.0 Head of pancreas
- C25.1 Body of pancreas
- C25.2 Tail of pancreas
- C25.3 Pancreatic duct
- C25.4 Islets of Langerhans
- C25.7 Other specified parts of pancreas
- C25.8 Overlapping lesion of pancreas
- C25.9 Pancreas, NOS

C26 Other and ill-defined digestive organs
- C26.0 Intestinal tract, NOS
- C26.8 Overlapping lesion of digestive system
- C26.9 Gastrointestinal tract, NOS

C30–C39 Respiratory system and intrathoracic organs

C30 Nasal cavity and middle ear
- C30.0 Nasal cavity
- C30.1 Middle ear

C31 Accessory sinuses
- C31.0 Maxillary sinus
- C31.1 Ethmoid sinus
- C31.2 Frontal sinus
- C31.3 Sphenoid sinus
- C31.8 Overlapping lesion of accessory sinuses
- C31.9 Accessory sinus, NOS

C32 Larynx
- C32.0 Glottis
- C32.1 Supraglottis
- C32.2 Subglottis
- C32.3 Laryngeal cartilage
- C32.8 Overlapping lesion of larynx
- C32.9 Larynx, NOS

C33 Trachea
- C33.9 Trachea

C34 Bronchus and lung
- C34.0 Main bronchus
- C34.1 Upper lobe, lung
- C34.2 Middle lobe, lung
- C34.3 Lower lobe, lung
- C34.8 Overlapping lesion of lung
- C34.9 Lung, NOS

C37 Thymus
- C37.9 Thymus

C38 Heart, mediastinum, and pleura
- C38.0 Heart
- C38.1 Anterior mediastinum
- C38.2 Posterior mediastinum
- C38.3 Mediastinum, NOS
- C38.4 Pleura, NOS
- C38.8 Overlapping lesion of heart, mediastinum, and pleura

C39 Other and ill-defined sites within respiratory system and intrathoracic organs
- C39.0 Upper respiratory tract, NOS
- C39.8 Overlapping lesion of respiratory system and intrathoracic organs
- C39.9 Ill-defined sites within respiratory system

C44 Skin
- C44.0 Skin of lip, NOS
- C44.1 Eyelid
- C44.2 External ear
- C44.3 Skin of other and unspecified parts of face
- C44.4 Skin of scalp and neck
- C44.5 Skin of trunk
- C44.6 Skin of upper limb and shoulder
- C44.7 Skin of lower limb and hip
- C44.8 Overlapping lesion of skin
- C44.9 Skin, NOS

C47 Peripheral nerves and autonomic nervous system
- C47.0 Peripheral nerves and autonomic nervous system of head, face, and neck
- C47.1 Peripheral nerves and autonomic nervous system of upper limb and shoulder
- C47.2 Peripheral nerves and autonomic nervous system of lower limb and hip
- C47.3 Peripheral nerves and autonomic nervous system of thorax
- C47.4 Peripheral nerves and autonomic nervous system of abdomen
- C47.5 Peripheral nerves and autonomic nervous system of pelvis
- C47.6 Peripheral nerves and autonomic nervous system of trunk, NOS
- C47.8 Overlapping lesion of peripheral nerves and autonomic nervous system
- C47.9 Autonomic nervous system, NOS

C48 Retroperitoneum and peritoneum
- C48.0 Retroperitoneum
- C48.1 Specified parts of peritoneum
- C48.2 Peritoneum, NOS
- C48.8 Overlapping lesion of retroperitoneum and peritoneum

C49 Connective, subcutaneous, and other soft tissues
- C49.0 Connective, subcutaneous, and other soft tissues of head, face, and neck
- C49.1 Connective, subcutaneous, and other soft tissues of upper limb and shoulder
- C49.2 Connective, subcutaneous, and other soft tissues of lower limb and hip
- C49.3 Connective, subcutaneous, and other soft tissues of thorax
- C49.4 Connective, subcutaneous, and other soft tissues of abdomen
- C49.5 Connective, subcutaneous, and other soft tissues of pelvis
- C49.6 Connective, subcutaneous, and other soft tissues of trunk, NOS
- C49.8 Overlapping lesion of connective, subcutaneous, and other soft tissues
- C49.9 Connective, subcutaneous, and other soft tissues, NOS

C50 Breast
- C50.0 Nipple
- C50.1 Central portion of breast
- C50.2 Upper-inner quadrant of breast
- C50.3 Lower-inner quadrant of breast
- C50.4 Upper-outer quadrant of breast
- C50.5 Lower-outer quadrant of breast
- C50.6 Axillary tail of breast
- C50.8 Overlapping lesion of breast
- C50.9 Breast, NOS

C51–C57 Female genital organs
C51 Vulva
- C51.0 Labium majus
- C51.1 Labium minus
- C51.2 Clitoris
- C51.8 Overlapping lesion of vulva
- C51.9 Vulva, NOS

C52 Vagina
- C52.9 Vagina, NOS

C53 Cervix uteri
- C53.0 Endocervix
- C53.1 Exocervix
- C53.8 Overlapping lesion of cervix uteri
- C53.9 Cervix uteri

C54 Corpus uteri
- C54.0 Isthmus uteri
- C54.1 Endometrium
- C54.2 Myometrium
- C54.3 Fundus uteri
- C54.8 Overlapping lesion of corpus uteri
- C54.9 Corpus uteri

C55 Uterus, NOS
- C55.9 Uterus, NOS

C56 Ovary
- C56.9 Ovary

C57 Other and unspecified female genital organs
- C57.0 Fallopian tube
- C57.1 Broad ligament
- C57.2 Round ligament
- C57.3 Parametrium
- C57.4 Uterine adnexa
- C57.7 Other specified parts of female genital organs
- C57.8 Overlapping lesion of female genital organs
- C57.9 Female genital tract, NOS

C60–C63 Male genital organs
C60 Penis
- C60.0 Prepuce
- C60.1 Glans penis
- C60.2 Body of penis
- C60.8 Overlapping lesion of penis
- C60.9 Penis, NOS

C61 Prostate gland
- C61.9 Prostate gland

C62 Testis
- C62.0 Undescended testis
- C62.1 Descended testis
- C62.9 Testis, NOS

C63 Other and unspecified male genital organs
- C63.0 Epididymis
- C63.1 Spermatic cord
- C63.2 Scrotum, NOS
- C63.7 Other specified parts of male genital organs
- C63.8 Overlapping lesion of male genital organs
- C63.9 Male genital organs, NOS

C64–C68 Urinary tract
C64 Kidney
- C64.9 Kidney, NOS

C65 Renal pelvis
- C65.9 Renal pelvis

C66 Ureter
- C66.9 Ureter

C67 Bladder
- C67.0 Trigone of bladder
- C67.1 Dome of bladder
- C67.2 Lateral wall of bladder
- C67.3 Anterior wall of bladder
- C67.4 Posterior wall of bladder
- C67.5 Bladder neck
- C67.6 Ureteric orifice
- C67.7 Urachus
- C67.8 Overlapping lesion of bladder
- C67.9 Bladder, NOS

C68 Other and unspecified urinary organs
- C68.0 Urethra
- C68.1 Paraurethral gland
- C68.8 Overlapping lesion of urinary organs
- C68.9 Urinary system, NOS

C73–C75 Thyroid and other endocrine glands

C73 Thyroid gland
- C73.9 Thyroid gland

C74 Adrenal gland
- C74.0 Cortex of adrenal gland
- C74.1 Medulla of adrenal gland
- C74.9 Adrenal gland, NOS

C75 Other endocrine glands and related structures
- C75.0 Parathyroid gland
- C75.1 Pituitary gland
- C75.2 Craniopharyngeal duct
- C75.3 Pineal gland
- C75.4 Carotid body
- C75.5 Aortic body and other paraganglia
- C75.8 Overlapping lesion of endocrine glands and related structures
- C75.9 Endocrine gland, NOS

C76 Other and ill-defined sites
- C76.0 Head, face, or neck, NOS
- C76.1 Thorax, NOS
- C76.2 Abdomen, NOS
- C76.3 Pelvis, NOS
- C76.4 Upper limb, NOS
- C76.5 Lower limb, NOS
- C76.7 Other ill-defined sites
- C76.8 Overlapping lesion of ill-defined sites

C80 Unknown primary site
- C80.9 Unknown primary site

ICD-O morphological coding: Introduction

The ICD-O coding system uses a topography (T) code and a morphology (M) code together, but these are presented in separate lists for ease of use. Behaviour is coded /0 for benign tumours; /1 for unspecified, borderline, or uncertain behaviour; /2 for carcinoma in situ and grade III intraepithelial neoplasia; /3 for malignant tumours, primary site; and /6 for malignant tumours, metastatic site. Behaviour code /6 is not generally used by cancer registries. For various reasons, the ICD-O morphology terms may not always be identical to the entity names used in the WHO classification, but they should be sufficiently similar to avoid confusion. The designation "NOS" ("not otherwise specified") is provided to make coding possible when subtypes exist but exact classification may not be possible in small biopsies or certain other scenarios. Therefore, it is usual to have "NOS" even when a more specific alternative term is listed in ICD-O.

ICD-O coding of pituitary tumours

ICD-O-3.2	ICD-O label (subtypes are indicated in grey text, with the label indented); Please note that the WHO classification of tumour types is more readily reflected in the table of contents

Anterior pituitary neuroendocrine tumours (PitNETs)

PitNETs of PIT1 lineage

8272/3*	Somatotroph PitNET/adenoma
8272/3*	Densely granulated somatotroph tumour
8272/3*	Sparsely granulated somatotroph tumour
8280/3*	Mammosomatotroph PitNET/adenoma
8271/3*	Lactotroph PitNET/adenoma
8271/3*	Sparsely granulated lactotroph tumour
8271/3*	Densely granulated lactotroph tumour
8272/3*	Thyrotroph PitNET/adenoma
8272/3*	Mature plurihormonal PIT1-lineage PitNET/adenoma
8272/3	Immature PIT1-lineage PitNET/adenoma
8280/3*	Acidophil stem cell PitNET/adenoma
8280/3*	Mixed somatotroph–lactotroph PitNET/adenoma
8280/3*	Densely granulated somatotroph and sparsely granulated lactotroph tumour
8280/3*	Sparsely granulated somatotroph and sparsely granulated lactotroph tumour

PitNETs of TPIT lineage

8272/3*	Corticotroph PitNET/adenoma
8272/3*	Densely granulated corticotroph tumour
8272/3*	Sparsely granulated corticotroph tumour
8272/3*	Crooke cell tumour

PitNETs of SF1 lineage

8272/3*	Gonadotroph PitNET/adenoma

PitNETs without distinct lineage differentiation

8272/3*	Null cell PitNET/adenoma
8272/3*	Plurihormonal PitNETs/adenomas

Multiple PitNETs

Multiple synchronous PitNETs/adenomas of distinct lineages: Code as PitNET/adenoma types

Metastatic PitNETs

8272/3	PitNET, malignant / pituitary carcinoma, NOS†

Other anterior pituitary tumours

9351/1	Adamantinomatous craniopharyngioma
9352/1	Papillary craniopharyngioma
8273/3	Pituitary blastoma

ICD-O-3.2	ICD-O label (subtypes are indicated in grey text, with the label indented); Please note that the WHO classification of tumour types is more readily reflected in the table of contents
Posterior pituitary and hypothalamic neoplasms	
Pituicyte-derived tumours	
9432/1	Pituicytoma
9582/0	Granular cell tumour of the sellar region / granular cell pituicytoma†
8290/0	Spindle cell oncocytoma / oncocytic pituicytoma†
9391/1	Ependymal pituicytoma†
Neuronal tumours	
9492/0	Gangliocytoma
9492/0	Mixed gangliocytoma–PitNET/adenoma†
9505/1	Ganglioglioma
9506/1	Sellar neurocytoma
Other sellar tumours	
9530/0	Meningioma, NOS
9531/0	Meningothelial meningioma
	Chordoma
9370/3	Conventional chordoma
9371/3	Chondroid chordoma
9370/3	Poorly differentiated chordoma
9372/3	Dedifferentiated chordoma

These morphology codes are from the International Classification of Diseases for Oncology, third edition, second revision (ICD-O-3.2) {2036}. Behaviour is coded /0 for benign tumours; /1 for unspecified, borderline, or uncertain behaviour; /2 for carcinoma in situ and grade III intraepithelial neoplasia; /3 for malignant tumours, primary site; and /6 for malignant tumours, metastatic site. Behaviour code /6 is not generally used by cancer registries.

This classification is modified from the previous WHO classification, taking into account changes in our understanding of these lesions.

n/a, not available (provisional entity).

* Codes marked with an asterisk were approved by the IARC/WHO Committee for ICD-O at its meeting in July 2022, or during subsequent consultation.

† Labels marked with a dagger have undergone a change in terminology of a previous code.

ICD-O coding of thyroid tumours

ICD-O-3.2	ICD-O label (subtypes are indicated in grey text, with the label indented); Please note that the WHO classification of tumour types is more readily reflected in the table of contents
Developmental abnormalities	
	Thyroglossal duct cyst
	Other congenital thyroid abnormalities
	Agenesis (athyreosis)
	Hypoplasia
	Hemiagenesis
	Ectopic thyroid
Follicular cell–derived neoplasms	
Benign tumours	
	Thyroid follicular nodular disease
8330/0	Follicular thyroid adenoma
8330/0	Follicular thyroid adenoma with papillary architecture†
8290/0	Oncocytic adenoma of the thyroid gland
Low-risk neoplasms	
8349/1	Non-invasive follicular thyroid neoplasm with papillary-like nuclear features
8349/1	Subcentimetre non-invasive follicular thyroid neoplasm with papillary-like nuclear features†
8349/1	Oncocytic non-invasive follicular thyroid neoplasm with papillary-like nuclear features†
	Thyroid tumours of uncertain malignant potential
8335/1	Follicular tumour of uncertain malignant potential
8348/1	Well-differentiated tumour of uncertain malignant potential
8336/1	Hyalinizing trabecular tumour
Malignant neoplasms	
8330/3	Follicular thyroid carcinoma
8335/3	Minimally invasive follicular thyroid carcinoma (capsular invasion only)
8339/3	Encapsulated angioinvasive follicular thyroid carcinoma
8330/3	Widely invasive follicular thyroid carcinoma†
8340/3	Invasive encapsulated follicular variant of papillary thyroid carcinoma
8340/3	Minimally invasive encapsulated follicular variant of papillary carcinoma (capsular invasion only)
8340/3	Encapsulated angioinvasive follicular variant of papillary carcinoma
8340/3	Widely invasive follicular variant of papillary carcinoma
8260/3	Papillary thyroid carcinoma
8340/3	Infiltrative follicular variant of papillary thyroid carcinoma†
8344/3	Columnar cell papillary thyroid carcinoma†
8342/3	Oncocytic papillary thyroid carcinoma
8260/3	Classic papillary thyroid carcinoma†
8343/3	Encapsulated classic papillary thyroid carcinoma
8350/3	Diffuse sclerosing papillary thyroid carcinoma
8260/3	Solid/trabecular papillary thyroid carcinoma†
8260/3	Warthin-like papillary thyroid carcinoma†
8260/3	Clear cell papillary thyroid carcinoma†
8260/3	Spindle cell papillary thyroid carcinoma†
8260/3	Papillary thyroid carcinoma with fibromatosis/fasciitis-like/desmoid-type stroma†
8344/3	Tall cell papillary thyroid carcinoma
8260/3	Hobnail papillary thyroid carcinoma†
8290/3	Oncocytic carcinoma of the thyroid gland
8290/3	Minimally invasive oncocytic carcinoma of the thyroid gland (capsular invasion only)†
8290/3	Encapsulated angioinvasive oncocytic carcinoma of the thyroid gland†
8290/3	Widely invasive oncocytic carcinoma of the thyroid gland†
	High-grade follicular cell–derived non-anaplastic thyroid carcinoma
8337/3	Poorly differentiated thyroid carcinoma
8337/3	High-grade differentiated thyroid carcinoma†
8020/3	Anaplastic thyroid carcinoma
Thyroid C cell–derived carcinoma	
8345/3	Medullary thyroid carcinoma
8345/3	Medullary microcarcinoma†

ICD-O-3.2	ICD-O label (subtypes are indicated in grey text, with the label indented); Please note that the WHO classification of tumour types is more readily reflected in the table of contents
Mixed medullary and follicular cell–derived carcinomas	
	Mixed medullary and follicular cell–derived thyroid carcinoma
8346/3	Mixed medullary–follicular carcinoma
8347/3	Mixed medullary–papillary carcinoma
8346/3	Mixed medullary and oncocytic carcinoma†
8346/3	Mixed medullary and poorly differentiated carcinoma†
8346/3	Mixed medullary and anaplastic carcinoma†
Salivary gland–type carcinomas of the thyroid gland	
8430/3	Mucoepidermoid carcinoma
8480/3	Mucinous carcinoma
8502/3	Secretory carcinoma
Thyroid tumours of uncertain histogenesis	
8430/3	Sclerosing mucoepidermoid carcinoma with eosinophilia†
8201/3	Cribriform morular thyroid carcinoma†
Thymic tumours within the thyroid gland	
8580/3	Thymoma, NOS
8581/3	Thymoma, type A
8582/3	Thymoma, type AB
8583/3	Thymoma, type B1
8584/3	Thymoma, type B2
8585/3	Thymoma, type B3
8580/1	Micronodular thymoma with lymphoid stroma
8580/3	Metaplastic thymoma
8588/3	Spindle epithelial tumour with thymus-like elements
8589/3	Intrathyroidal thymic carcinoma†
Embryonal thyroid neoplasms	
8970/3	Thyroblastoma†

These morphology codes are from the International Classification of Diseases for Oncology, third edition, second revision (ICD-O-3.2) {2036}. Behaviour is coded /0 for benign tumours; /1 for unspecified, borderline, or uncertain behaviour; /2 for carcinoma in situ and grade III intraepithelial neoplasia; /3 for malignant tumours, primary site; and /6 for malignant tumours, metastatic site. Behaviour code /6 is not generally used by cancer registries.

This classification is modified from the previous WHO classification, taking into account changes in our understanding of these lesions.

n/a, not available (provisional entity).

* Codes marked with an asterisk were approved by the IARC/WHO Committee for ICD-O at its meeting in July 2022, or during subsequent consultation.

† Labels marked with a dagger have undergone a change in terminology of a previous code.

ICD-O coding of parathyroid tumours

ICD-O-3.2	ICD-O label (subtypes are indicated in grey text, with the label indented); Please note that the WHO classification of tumour types is more readily reflected in the table of contents
	Parathyroid hyperplasia
	Primary hyperplasia
	Secondary hyperplasia
	Tertiary hyperplasia
8140/0	Parathyroid adenoma
8290/0	Oncocytic (oxyphil cell) parathyroid adenoma
8322/0	Water-clear cell parathyroid adenoma
8324/0	Parathyroid lipoadenoma
8140/1*	Atypical parathyroid tumour
8140/3	Parathyroid carcinoma

These morphology codes are from the International Classification of Diseases for Oncology, third edition, second revision (ICD-O-3.2) {2036}. Behaviour is coded /0 for benign tumours; /1 for unspecified, borderline, or uncertain behaviour; /2 for carcinoma in situ and grade III intraepithelial neoplasia; /3 for malignant tumours, primary site; and /6 for malignant tumours, metastatic site. Behaviour code /6 is not generally used by cancer registries.

This classification is modified from the previous WHO classification, taking into account changes in our understanding of these lesions.

n/a, not available (provisional entity).

* Codes marked with an asterisk were approved by the IARC/WHO Committee for ICD-O at its meeting in July 2022, or during subsequent consultation.

† Labels marked with a dagger have undergone a change in terminology of a previous code.

ICD-O coding of adrenal gland tumours

ICD-O-3.2	ICD-O label (subtypes are indicated in grey text, with the label indented); Please note that the WHO classification of tumour types is more readily reflected in the table of contents
Lesions in the adrenal cortex	
	Adrenal rests
	Adrenal cysts
	Endothelial (vascular) cyst
	Epithelial (mesothelial) cyst
	Parasitic cyst
	Pseudocyst
8870/0	Adrenal myelolipoma
Adrenal cortical tumours	
	Congenital adrenal hyperplasia
	21-hydroxylase deficiency (classic type and non-classic type)
	11β-hydroxylase deficiency
	17α-hydroxylase deficiency
	3β-hydroxysteroid dehydrogenase deficiency
	P450 oxidoreductase deficiency
	Congenital lipoid adrenal hyperplasia
	P450 cholesterol side-chain cleavage enzyme deficiency
	Adrenocortical nodular disease
	Sporadic nodular adrenocortical disease
	Bilateral micronodular adrenocortical disease
	Bilateral macronodular adrenocortical disease
8370/0	Adrenal cortical adenoma
8370/3	Adrenal cortical carcinoma
8370/3	Conventional adrenal cortical carcinoma†
8370/3	Oncocytic adrenal cortical carcinoma†
8370/3	Myxoid adrenal cortical carcinoma†
8370/3	Sarcomatoid adrenal cortical carcinoma†
Sex cord stromal and other tumours	
8590/1	Adrenal sex cord stromal tumour
8650/1	Leydig cell tumour
8620/3	Granulosa cell tumour
9054/0	Adenomatoid tumour, NOS
8720/3	Adrenal melanoma, NOS

These morphology codes are from the International Classification of Diseases for Oncology, third edition, second revision (ICD-O-3.2) {2036}. Behaviour is coded /0 for benign tumours; /1 for unspecified, borderline, or uncertain behaviour; /2 for carcinoma in situ and grade III intraepithelial neoplasia; /3 for malignant tumours, primary site; and /6 for malignant tumours, metastatic site. Behaviour code /6 is not generally used by cancer registries.

This classification is modified from the previous WHO classification, taking into account changes in our understanding of these lesions.

n/a, not available (provisional entity).

* Codes marked with an asterisk were approved by the IARC/WHO Committee for ICD-O at its meeting in July 2022, or during subsequent consultation.

† Labels marked with a dagger have undergone a change in terminology of a previous code.

ICD-O coding of adrenal medulla and extra-adrenal paraganglia tumours

ICD-O-3.2	ICD-O label (subtypes are indicated in grey text, with the label indented); Please note that the WHO classification of tumour types is more readily reflected in the table of contents
Neuroblastic tumours	
9500/3	Neuroblastoma
9500/3	Undifferentiated neuroblastoma†
9500/3	Poorly differentiated neuroblastoma†
9500/3	Differentiating neuroblastoma†
9490/3	Ganglioneuroblastoma, intermixed†
9490/3	Ganglioneuroblastoma, nodular†
9490/0	Ganglioneuroma
9490/0	Maturing ganglioneuroma†
9490/0	Mature ganglioneuroma†
Paraganglioma and phaeochromocytoma	
8700/3	Phaeochromocytoma
8681/3	Sympathetic paraganglioma
8693/3	Composite paraganglioma
8682/3	Parasympathetic paraganglioma (head and neck paraganglioma)
8693/3	Composite paraganglioma
Composite phaeochromocytomas and paragangliomas	
	Composite phaeochromocytoma subtypes:
8700/3	Composite phaeochromocytoma-ganglioneuroma†
8700/3	Composite phaeochromocytoma-ganglioneuroblastoma†
8700/3	Composite phaeochromocytoma-neuroblastoma†
8700/3	Composite phaeochromocytoma–malignant peripheral nerve sheath tumour†
	Composite paraganglioma subtypes:
8693/3	Composite paraganglioma-ganglioneuroma†
8693/3	Composite paraganglioma-ganglioneuroblastoma†
8693/3	Composite paraganglioma-neuroblastoma†

These morphology codes are from the International Classification of Diseases for Oncology, third edition, second revision (ICD-O-3.2) {2036}. Behaviour is coded /0 for benign tumours; /1 for unspecified, borderline, or uncertain behaviour; /2 for carcinoma in situ and grade III intraepithelial neoplasia; /3 for malignant tumours, primary site; and /6 for malignant tumours, metastatic site. Behaviour code /6 is not generally used by cancer registries.

This classification is modified from the previous WHO classification, taking into account changes in our understanding of these lesions.

n/a, not available (provisional entity).

* Codes marked with an asterisk were approved by the IARC/WHO Committee for ICD-O at its meeting in July 2022, or during subsequent consultation.

† Labels marked with a dagger have undergone a change in terminology of a previous code.

ICD-O coding of pancreatic neuroendocrine neoplasms

ICD-O-3.2	ICD-O label (subtypes are indicated in grey text, with the label indented); Please note that the WHO classification of tumour types is more readily reflected in the table of contents
Neuroendocrine neoplasms	
Neuroendocrine tumours	
8150/3	Neuroendocrine tumour, non-functioning, pancreatic
8150/3	Oncocytic non-functioning (non-syndromic) pancreatic neuroendocrine tumour
8150/3	Clear cell non-functioning (non-syndromic) pancreatic neuroendocrine tumour
8150/3	Pleomorphic non-functioning (non-syndromic) pancreatic neuroendocrine tumour
8150/3	Cystic non-functioning (non-syndromic) pancreatic neuroendocrine tumour
8150/1*	Pancreatic neuroendocrine microtumour†
8151/3	Neuroendocrine tumour, insulin-producing (insulinoma)†
8152/3	Neuroendocrine tumour, glucagon-producing (glucagonoma)†
8156/3	Neuroendocrine tumour, somatostatin-producing (somatostatinoma)†
8153/3	Neuroendocrine tumour, gastrin-producing (gastrinoma)†
8155/3	VIPoma
8241/3	Serotonin-producing tumour
Other pancreatic neuroendocrine tumours with ectopic hormone production	
8158/3	ACTH-producing tumour
8158/3	Calcitonin-producing pancreatic neuroendocrine tumour†
8158/3	CRH-producing pancreatic neuroendocrine tumour†
8158/3	Cholecystokinin-producing pancreatic neuroendocrine tumour†
8158/3	Erythropoietin-producing pancreatic neuroendocrine tumour†
8272/3	GH-producing tumour†
8158/3	GHRH-producing pancreatic neuroendocrine tumour†
8158/3	Ghrelin-producing pancreatic neuroendocrine tumour†
8272/3	Gonadotropin-producing tumour
8158/3	PTH/PTHrP-producing pancreatic neuroendocrine tumour
8158/3	Vasopressin-producing pancreatic neuroendocrine tumour
Neuroendocrine carcinomas	
8246/3	Neuroendocrine carcinoma, NOS
8041/3	Small cell neuroendocrine carcinoma
8013/3	Large cell neuroendocrine carcinoma
Mixed neuroendocrine–non-neuroendocrine neoplasms	
	Mixed ductal adenocarcinoma–neuroendocrine neoplasms
8154/3	Mixed ductal adenocarcinoma–neuroendocrine carcinoma
8244/3	Mixed ductal adenocarcinoma–neuroendocrine tumour
8154/3	Mixed acinar-neuroendocrine carcinoma

These morphology codes are from the International Classification of Diseases for Oncology, third edition, second revision (ICD-O-3.2) {2036}. Behaviour is coded /0 for benign tumours; /1 for unspecified, borderline, or uncertain behaviour; /2 for carcinoma in situ and grade III intraepithelial neoplasia; /3 for malignant tumours, primary site; and /6 for malignant tumours, metastatic site. Behaviour code /6 is not generally used by cancer registries.

This classification is modified from the previous WHO classification, taking into account changes in our understanding of these lesions.

n/a, not available (provisional entity).

* Codes marked with an asterisk were approved by the IARC/WHO Committee for ICD-O at its meeting in July 2022, or during subsequent consultation.

† Labels marked with a dagger have undergone a change in terminology of a previous code.

ICD-O coding of neuroendocrine neoplasms in non-endocrine organs

ICD-O-3.2	ICD-O label (subtypes are indicated in grey text, with the label indented); Please note that the WHO classification of tumour types is more readily reflected in the table of contents
Neuroendocrine neoplasms	
Neuroendocrine tumours	
8240/3	Neuroendocrine tumour, NOS
8240/3	Neuroendocrine tumour, grade 1
8249/3	Neuroendocrine tumour, grade 2
8249/3	Neuroendocrine tumour, grade 3
8242/3	ECL-cell neuroendocrine tumour
8156/3	D-cell neuroendocrine tumour
8153/3	G-cell neuroendocrine tumour
8241/3	EC-cell neuroendocrine tumour
8152/3	L-cell neuroendocrine tumour
9091/1	Ovarian neuroendocrine tumour
Neuroendocrine carcinomas	
8041/3	Small cell neuroendocrine carcinoma
8045/3	Combined small cell neuroendocrine carcinoma
8013/3	Large cell neuroendocrine carcinoma
8247/3	Merkel cell carcinoma
Mixed neuroendocrine neoplasms	
8154/3	Mixed neuroendocrine–non-neuroendocrine neoplasm
8013/3	Combined large cell neuroendocrine carcinoma
8045/3	Combined small cell neuroendocrine carcinoma
Paragangliomas-like neuroendocrine neoplasms	
8683/3*	Composite gangliocytoma/neuroma and neuroendocrine tumour
8693/3*	Cauda equina neuroendocrine tumour

These morphology codes are from the International Classification of Diseases for Oncology, third edition, second revision (ICD-O-3.2) {2036}. Behaviour is coded /0 for benign tumours; /1 for unspecified, borderline, or uncertain behaviour; /2 for carcinoma in situ and grade III intraepithelial neoplasia; /3 for malignant tumours, primary site; and /6 for malignant tumours, metastatic site. Behaviour code /6 is not generally used by cancer registries.

This classification is modified from the previous WHO classification, taking into account changes in our understanding of these lesions.

n/a, not available (provisional entity).

* Codes marked with an asterisk were approved by the IARC/WHO Committee for ICD-O at its meeting in July 2022, or during subsequent consultation.

† Labels marked with a dagger have undergone a change in terminology of a previous code.

ICD-O coding of mesenchymal and stromal tumours

ICD-O-3.2	ICD-O label (subtypes are indicated in grey text, with the label indented); Please note that the WHO classification of tumour types is more readily reflected in the table of contents
Lipocytic tumours	
8850/0	Lipoma, NOS
Fibrous tumours	
8815/0	Solitary fibrous tumour, benign
8815/1	Solitary fibrous tumour, NOS
8815/1	Fat-forming (lipomatous) solitary fibrous tumour
8815/1	Giant cell–rich solitary fibrous tumour
8815/3	Solitary fibrous tumour, malignant
Vascular tumours	
	Haemangiomas
9120/0	Haemangioma, NOS
9131/0	Capillary haemangioma
9131/0	Lobular capillary haemangioma
9121/0	Cavernous haemangioma
9131/0	Infantile haemangioma
9122/0	Venous haemangioma
9123/0	Arteriovenous haemangioma
9125/0	Epithelioid haemangioma
	Arteriovenous malformations
9170/0	Lymphangioma, NOS
	Lymphangiomatosis
	Papillary endothelial hyperplasia
	PEComa
8714/0	Perivascular epithelioid tumour, benign
8714/3	Perivascular epithelioid tumour, malignant
8860/0	Angiomyolipoma
8860/1	Angiomyolipoma, epithelioid
	Glomangioma and glomus tumour
8711/0	Glomus tumour, benign
8711/0	Oncocytic glomus tumour†
8711/0	Epithelioid glomus tumour†
8711/0	Myxoid glomus tumour†
8711/0	Signet-ring glomus tumour†
8711/0	Hyalinized glomus tumour†
8711/0	Symplastic glomus tumour†
8712/0	Glomangioma
8713/0	Glomangiomyoma
8711/1	Glomangiomatosis
8711/1	Glomus tumour of uncertain malignant potential
8711/3	Glomus tumour, malignant
	Glomuvenous malformation
9120/3	Angiosarcoma
Smooth muscle tumours	
8890/0	Leiomyoma, NOS
8890/3	Leiomyosarcoma, NOS

ICD-O-3.2	ICD-O label (subtypes are indicated in grey text, with the label indented); Please note that the WHO classification of tumour types is more readily reflected in the table of contents
Skeletal muscle tumours	
8900/3	Rhabdomyosarcoma, NOS
8910/3	Embryonal rhabdomyosarcoma
8920/3	Alveolar rhabdomyosarcoma
8901/3	Pleomorphic rhabdomyosarcoma
8912/3	Spindle cell / sclerosing rhabdomyosarcoma
Peripheral nerve sheath tumours	
9560/0	Schwannoma, NOS
9560/0	Ancient schwannoma
9560/0	Cellular schwannoma
9560/0	Plexiform schwannoma
9560/0	Epithelioid schwannoma
9560/0	Microcystic/reticular schwannoma
9540/0	Neurofibroma, NOS
9540/0	Ancient neurofibroma
9540/0	Cellular neurofibroma
9540/1	Atypical neurofibroma
9540/0	Plexiform neurofibroma
9580/0	Granular cell tumour, NOS
9580/3	Granular cell tumour, malignant
9540/3	Malignant peripheral nerve sheath tumour, NOS
9542/3	Epithelioid malignant peripheral nerve sheath tumour

These morphology codes are from the International Classification of Diseases for Oncology, third edition, second revision (ICD-O-3.2) {2036}. Behaviour is coded /0 for benign tumours; /1 for unspecified, borderline, or uncertain behaviour; /2 for carcinoma in situ and grade III intraepithelial neoplasia; /3 for malignant tumours, primary site; and /6 for malignant tumours, metastatic site. Behaviour code /6 is not generally used by cancer registries.

This classification is modified from the previous WHO classification, taking into account changes in our understanding of these lesions.

n/a, not available (provisional entity).

* Codes marked with an asterisk were approved by the IARC/WHO Committee for ICD-O at its meeting in July 2022, or during subsequent consultation.

† Labels marked with a dagger have undergone a change in terminology of a previous code.

ICD-O coding of haematolymphoid tumours

ICD-O-3.2	ICD-O label (subtypes are indicated in grey text, with the label indented); Please note that the WHO classification of tumour types is more readily reflected in the table of contents
9760/1	IgG4-related disease
9699/3	Extranodal marginal zone lymphoma
9680/3	Diffuse large B-cell lymphoma
9751/1	Langerhans cell histiocytosis, NOS
9751/3	Langerhans cell histiocytosis, disseminated
9749/3	Rosai–Dorfman disease
9749/3	Erdheim–Chester disease
9758/3	Follicular dendritic cell sarcoma

These morphology codes are from the International Classification of Diseases for Oncology, third edition, second revision (ICD-O-3.2) {2036}. Behaviour is coded /0 for benign tumours; /1 for unspecified, borderline, or uncertain behaviour; /2 for carcinoma in situ and grade III intraepithelial neoplasia; /3 for malignant tumours, primary site; and /6 for malignant tumours, metastatic site. Behaviour code /6 is not generally used by cancer registries.

This classification is modified from the previous WHO classification, taking into account changes in our understanding of these lesions.

n/a, not available (provisional entity).

* Codes marked with an asterisk were approved by the IARC/WHO Committee for ICD-O at its meeting in July 2022, or during subsequent consultation.

† Labels marked with a dagger have undergone a change in terminology of a previous code.

ICD-O coding of germ cell tumours

ICD-O-3.2	ICD-O label (subtypes are indicated in grey text, with the label indented); Please note that the WHO classification of tumour types is more readily reflected in the table of contents
Germ cell tumours in endocrine organs	
9080/0	Mature teratoma
9080/3	Immature teratoma
9084/3	Teratoma with somatic-type malignancy
9064/3	Germinoma
9070/3	Embryonal carcinoma
9071/3	Yolk sac tumour
9100/3	Choriocarcinoma
9085/3	Mixed germ cell tumour
Germ cell tumours with endocrine differentiation	
	Teratomas with endocrine differentiation
9090/0	Struma ovarii, NOS
9090/3	Thyroid carcinoma arising in struma ovarii†
9091/1	Ovarian neuroendocrine tumour

These morphology codes are from the International Classification of Diseases for Oncology, third edition, second revision (ICD-O-3.2) {2036}. Behaviour is coded /0 for benign tumours; /1 for unspecified, borderline, or uncertain behaviour; /2 for carcinoma in situ and grade III intraepithelial neoplasia; /3 for malignant tumours, primary site; and /6 for malignant tumours, metastatic site. Behaviour code /6 is not generally used by cancer registries.

This classification is modified from the previous WHO classification, taking into account changes in our understanding of these lesions.

n/a, not available (provisional entity).

* Codes marked with an asterisk were approved by the IARC/WHO Committee for ICD-O at its meeting in July 2022, or during subsequent consultation.

† Labels marked with a dagger have undergone a change in terminology of a previous code.

TNM staging of carcinomas of the thyroid gland

Thyroid Gland

(ICD-O-3 C73.9)

Rules for Classification

The classification applies only to carcinomas. There should be microscopic confirmation of the disease and division of cases by histological type.

The following are the procedures for assessing T, N, and M categories:

T categories	Physical examination, endoscopy, and imaging
N categories	Physical examination and imaging
M categories	Physical examination and imaging

Regional Lymph Nodes

The regional lymph nodes are the cervical and upper/superior mediastinal nodes.

TNM Clinical Classification

T – Primary Tumour*

- TX Primary tumour cannot be assessed
- T0 No evidence of primary tumour
- T1 Tumour 2 cm or less in greatest dimension, limited to the thyroid
  - T1a Tumour 1 cm or less in greatest dimension, limited to the thyroid
  - T1b Tumour more than 1 cm but not more than 2 cm in greatest dimension, limited to the thyroid
- T2 Tumour more than 2 cm but not more than 4 cm in greatest dimension, limited to the thyroid
- T3 Tumour more than 4 cm in greatest dimension, limited to the thyroid or with gross extrathyroidal extension invading only strap muscles (sternohyoid, sternothyroid, or omohyoid muscles)
  - T3a Tumour more than 4 cm in greatest dimension, limited to the thyroid
  - T3b Tumour of any size with gross extrathyroidal extension invading strap muscles (sternohyoid, sternothyroid, or omohyoid muscles)
- T4a Tumour extends beyond the thyroid capsule and invades any of the following: subcutaneous soft tissues, larynx, trachea, oesophagus, recurrent laryngeal nerve
- T4b Tumour invades prevertebral fascia, mediastinal vessels, or encases carotid artery

Note

* Including papillary, follicular, poorly differentiated, Hürthle cell and anaplastic carcinomas.

N – Regional Lymph Nodes

- NX Regional lymph nodes cannot be assessed
- N0 No regional lymph node metastasis
- N1 Regional lymph node metastasis
  - N1a Metastasis in Level VI (pretracheal, paratracheal, and prelaryngeal/Delphian lymph nodes) or upper/superior mediastinum
  - N1b Metastasis in other unilateral, bilateral or contralateral cervical (Levels I, II III, IV, or V) or retropharyngeal

M – Distant Metastasis

- M0 No distant metastasis
- M1 Distant metastasis

pTNM Pathological Classification

The pT and pN categories correspond to the T and N categories.

pN0 Histological examination of a selective neck dissection specimen will ordinarily include 6 or more lymph nodes. If the lymph nodes are negative, but the number ordinarily examined is not met, classify as pN0.

pM – Distant Metastasis*

pM1 Distant metastasis microscopically confirmed

Note

* pM0 and pMX are not valid categories.

Histopathological Types

The four major histopathological types are:

- Papillary carcinoma (including those with follicular foci)
- Follicular carcinoma (including so-called Hürthle cell carcinoma)
- Medullary carcinoma
- Anaplastic

Stage

Separate stages are recommended for papillary and follicular (differentiated), medullary, and anaplastic (undifferentiated) carcinomas:

Papillary and Follicular under 55 years*

Stage I	Any T	Any N	M0
Stage II	Any T	Any N	M1

The information presented here has been excerpted from the 2017 *TNM classification of malignant tumours*, eighth edition {532,4615}. © 2017 UICC.
A help desk for specific questions about the TNM classification is available at https://www.uicc.org/tnm-help-desk.

Papillary or Follicular 55 years and older

Stage I	T1a,T1b,T2	N0	M0
Stage II	T3	N0	M0
	T1,T2,T3	N1	M0
Stage III	T4a	Any N	M0
Stage IVA	T4b	Any N	M0
Stage IVB	Any T	Any N	M1

Medullary

Stage I	T1a,T1b	N0	M0
Stage II	T2,T3	N0	M0
Stage III	T1,T2,T3	N1a	M0
Stage IVA	T1,T2,T3	N1b	M0
	T4a	Any N	M0
Stage IVB	T4b	Any N	M0
Stage IVC	Any T	Any N	M1

Anaplastic

Stage IVA	T1,T2,T3a	N0	M0
Stage IVB	T1,T2,T3a	N1	M0
	T3b,T4a,T4b	N0,N1	M0
Stage IVC	Any T	Any N	M1

Note

* Including papillary, follicular, poorly differentiated, and Hürthle cell carcinomas.

TNM staging of carcinomas of the adrenal cortex

Adrenal Cortex

(ICD-O-3 C74.0)

Rules for Classification

This classification applies only to carcinomas of the adrenal cortex. It does not apply to tumours of the adrenal medulla or sarcomas.

The following are the procedures for assessing T, N, and M categories:

T categories Physical examination and imaging
N categories Physical examination and imaging
M categories Physical examination and imaging

Regional Lymph Nodes

The regional lymph nodes are the hilar, abdominal para-aortic, and paracaval nodes. Laterality does not affect the N categories.

TNM Clinical Classification

T – Primary Tumour

TX Primary tumour cannot be assessed
T0 No evidence of primary tumour
T1 Tumour 5 cm or less in greatest dimension, no extra-adrenal invasion
T2 Tumour greater than 5 cm, no extra-adrenal invasion
T3 Tumour of any size with local invasion, but not invading adjacent organs*
T4 Tumour of any size with invasion of adjacent organs*

Note
* Adjacent organs include kidney, diaphragm, great vessels (renal vein or vena cava), pancreas, and liver.

N – Regional Lymph Nodes

NX Regional lymph nodes cannot be assessed
N0 No regional lymph node metastasis
N1 Metastasis in regional lymph node(s)

M – Distant Metastasis

M0 No distant metastasis
M1 Distant metastasis

pTNM Pathological Classification

The pT and pN categories correspond to the T and N categories.

pM – Distant Metastasis*

pM1 Distant metastasis microscopically confirmed

Note
* pM0 and pMX are not valid categories.

Stage

Stage I	T1	N0	M0
Stage II	T2	N0	M0
Stage III	T1,T2	N1	M0
	T3,T4	N0,N1	M0
Stage IV	Any T	Any N	M1

The information presented here has been excerpted from the 2017 *TNM classification of malignant tumours*, eighth edition {532,4615}. © 2017 UICC.
A help desk for specific questions about the TNM classification is available at https://www.uicc.org/tnm-help-desk.

TNM staging of tumours of the pancreas

Pancreas

(ICD-O-3 C25)

Rules for Classification

The classification applies to carcinomas of the exocrine pancreas and/or high-grade neuroendocrine carcinomas. Well-differentiated neuroendocrine tumours of the pancreas are classified as shown on p. 24. There should be histological or cytological confirmation of the disease.

The following are the procedures for assessing T, N, and M categories:

T categories	Physical examination, imaging, and/or surgical exploration
N categories	Physical examination, imaging, and/or surgical exploration
M categories	Physical examination, imaging, and/or surgical exploration

Anatomical Subsites

C25.0 Head of pancreas[a]
C25.1 Body of pancreas[b]
C25.2 Tail of pancreas[c]
C25.3 Pancreatic duct

Notes

[a] Tumours of the head of the pancreas are those arising to the right of the left border of the superior mesenteric vein. The uncinate process is considered as part of the head.

[b] Tumours of the body are those arising between the left border of the superior mesenteric vein and left border of the aorta.

[c] Tumours of the tail are those arising between the left border of the aorta and the hilum of the spleen.

Regional Lymph Nodes

The regional lymph nodes for tumours in the head and neck of the pancreas are the lymph nodes along the common bile duct, common hepatic artery, portal vein, pyloric, infrapyloric, subpyloric, proximal mesenteric, coeliac, posterior, and anterior pancreaticoduodenal vessels, and along the superior mesenteric vein and right lateral wall of the superior mesenteric artery.

The regional lymph nodes for tumours in body and tail are the lymph nodes along the common hepatic artery, coeliac axis, splenic artery, and splenic hilum, as well as retroperitoneal nodes and lateral aortic nodes.

TNM Clinical Classification

T – Primary Tumour

TX Primary tumour cannot be assessed
T0 No evidence of primary tumour
Tis Carcinoma in situ*
T1 Tumour 2 cm or less in greatest dimension
- T1a Tumour 0.5 cm or less in greatest dimension
- T1b Tumour greater than 0.5 cm and no more than 1 cm in greatest dimension
- T1c Tumour greater than 1 cm but no more than 2 cm in greatest dimension

T2 Tumour more than 2 cm but no more than 4 cm in greatest dimension
T3 Tumour more than 4 cm in greatest dimension
T4 Tumour involves coeliac axis, superior mesenteric artery and/or common hepatic artery

Note

* Tis also includes the 'PanIN–III' classification.

N – Regional Lymph Nodes

NX Regional lymph nodes cannot be assessed
N0 No regional lymph node metastasis
N1 Metastases in 1 to 3 regional lymph node(s)
N2 Metastases in 4 or more regional lymph nodes

M – Distant Metastasis

M0 No distant metastasis
M1 Distant metastasis

pTNM Pathological Classification

The pT and pN categories correspond to the T and N categories.

pN0 Histological examination of a regional lymphadenectomy specimen will ordinarily include 12 or more lymph nodes. If the lymph nodes are negative, but the number ordinarily examined is not met, classify as pN0.

pM – Distant Metastasis*

pM1 Distant metastasis microscopically confirmed

Note

* pM0 and pMX are not valid categories.

Stage – Pancreas

Stage 0	Tis	N0	M0
Stage IA	T1	N0	M0
Stage IB	T2	N0	M0
Stage IIA	T3	N0	M0
Stage IIB	T1,T2,T3	N1	M0
Stage III	T1,T2,T3	N2	M0
	T4	Any N	M0
Stage IV	Any T	Any N	M1

The information presented here has been excerpted from the 2017 *TNM classification of malignant tumours*, eighth edition {532,4615}.
A help desk for specific questions about the TNM classification is available at https://www.uicc.org/tnm-help-desk.

TNM staging of well-differentiated neuroendocrine tumours of the gastrointestinal tract

Well-Differentiated Neuroendocrine Tumours of the Gastrointestinal Tract

Rules for Classification

This classification system applies to well-differentiated neuroendocrine tumours (carcinoid tumours and atypical carcinoid tumours) of the gastrointestinal tract, including the pancreas. Neuroendocrine tumours of the lung should be classified according to criteria for carcinoma of the lung. Merkel cell carcinoma of the skin has a separate classification.

Neuroendocrine carcinomas are excluded and should be classified according to criteria for classifying carcinomas at the respective site.

Histopathological Grading

The following grading scheme has been proposed for all gastrointestinal neuroendocrine tumours:

Grade	Mitotic count (per 2 mm^2)	Ki-67 index (%)[a]
G1	< 2	< 3
G2	2–20	3–20
G3	> 20	> 20

Notes

The final grade is the higher of the grades as determined by the mitotic count or the Ki-67 index.

[a] MIB1 antibody; % of 500–2000 tumour cells in areas of highest nuclear labelling.

Grade 3 neuroendocrine tumours are classified according to the schema for G1 and G2 neuroendocrine tumours.

Well-Differentiated Neuroendocrine Tumours (G1, G2 and G3) – Gastric, Jejunum/Ileum, Appendix, Colonic, and Rectal

Regional Lymph Nodes

The regional lymph nodes correspond to those listed under the appropriate sites for carcinoma.

TNM Clinical Classification

Stomach

T – Primary Tumour

- TX Primary tumour cannot be assessed
- T0 No evidence of primary tumour
- T1 Tumour invades mucosa or submucosa and 1 cm or less in greatest dimension
- T2 Tumour invades muscularis propria or is more than 1 cm in greatest dimension
- T3 Tumour invades subserosa
- T4 Tumour perforates visceral peritoneum (serosa) or invades other organs or adjacent structures

Note

For any T, add (m) for multiple tumours.

N – Regional Lymph Nodes

- NX Regional lymph nodes cannot be assessed
- N0 No regional lymph node metastasis
- N1 Regional lymph node metastasis

M – Distant Metastasis

- M0 No distant metastasis
- M1 Distant metastasis
  - M1a Hepatic metastasis only
  - M1b Extrahepatic metastasis only
  - M1c Hepatic and extrahepatic metastases

Stage

Stage I	T1	N0	M0
Stage II	T2,T3	N0	M0
Stage III	T4	N0	M0
	Any T	N1	M0
Stage IV	Any T	Any N	M1

The information presented here has been excerpted from the 2017 *TNM classification of malignant tumours*, eighth edition {532,4615}.
A help desk for specific questions about the TNM classification is available at https://www.uicc.org/tnm-help-desk.

TNM Clinical Classification

Duodenal/Ampullary Tumours

T – Primary Tumour

TX Primary tumour cannot be assessed
T0 No evidence of primary tumour
T1 *Duodenal:* Tumour invades mucosa or submucosa and 1 cm or less in greatest dimension
Ampullary: Tumour 1 cm or less in greatest dimension and confined within the sphincter of Oddi
T2 *Duodenal:* Tumour invades muscularis propria or is more than 1 cm in greatest dimension
Ampullary: Tumour invades through sphincter into duodenal submucosa or muscularis propria, or more than 1 cm in greatest dimension
T3 Tumour invades the pancreas or peripancreatic adipose tissue
T4 Tumour perforates visceral peritoneum (serosa) or invades other organs

Note
For any T, add (m) for multiple tumours.

N – Regional Lymph Nodes

NX Regional lymph nodes cannot be assessed
N0 No regional lymph node metastasis
N1 Regional lymph node metastasis

M – Distant Metastasis

M0 No distant metastasis
M1 Distant metastasis
M1a Hepatic metastasis only
M1b Extrahepatic metastasis only
M1c Hepatic and extrahepatic metastases

Stage

Stage I	T1	N0	M0
Stage II	T2,T3	N0	M0
Stage III	T4	N0	M0
	Any T	N1	M0
Stage IV	Any T	Any N	M1

TNM Clinical Classification

Jejunum/Ileum

T – Primary Tumour

TX Primary tumour cannot be assessed
T0 No evidence of primary tumour
T1 Tumour invades mucosa or submucosa and 1 cm or less in greatest dimension
T2 Tumour invades muscularis propria or is greater than 1 cm in greatest dimension
T3 Tumour invades through the muscularis propria into subserosal tissue without penetration of overlying serosa (jejunal or ileal)
T4 Tumour perforates visceral peritoneum (serosa) or invades other organs or adjacent structures

Note
For any T, add (m) for multiple tumours.

N – Regional Lymph Nodes

NX Regional lymph nodes cannot be assessed
N0 No regional lymph node metastasis
N1 Less than 12 regional lymph node metastasis without mesenteric mass(es) greater than 2 cm in size
N2 12 or more regional nodes and/or mesenteric mass(es) greater than 2 cm in maximum dimension

M – Distant Metastasis

M0 No distant metastasis
M1 Distant metastasis
M1a Hepatic metastasis only
M1b Extrahepatic metastasis only
M1c Hepatic and extrahepatic metastases

Stage

Stage I	T1	N0	M0
Stage II	T2,T3	N0	M0
Stage III	T4	Any N	M0
	Any T	N1,N2	M0
Stage IV	Any T	Any N	M1

TNM Clinical Classification

Appendix

T – Primary Tumour[a]

TX Primary tumour cannot be assessed
T0 No evidence of primary tumour
T1 Tumour 2 cm or less in greatest dimension
T2 Tumour more than 2 cm but not more than 4 cm in greatest dimension
T3 Tumour more than 4 cm or with subserosal invasion or involvement of the mesoappendix
T4 Tumour perforates peritoneum or invades other adjacent organs or structures, other than direct mural extension to adjacent subserosa, e.g. abdominal wall and skeletal muscle[b]

Notes
[a] High-grade neuroendocrine carcinomas, mixed adenoneuroendocrine carcinomas and goblet cell carcinoid, are excluded and should be classified according to criteria for classifying carcinomas.
[b] Tumour that is adherent to other organs or structures, macroscopically, is classified T4. However, if no tumour is present in the adhesion, microscopically, the tumour should be classified as pT1–3 as appropriate.

N – Regional Lymph Nodes

NX Regional lymph nodes cannot be assessed
N0 No regional lymph node metastasis
N1 Regional lymph node metastasis

M – Distant Metastasis

M0 No distant metastasis
M1 Distant metastasis
M1a Hepatic metastasis only
M1b Extrahepatic metastasis only
M1c Hepatic and extrahepatic metastases

The information presented here has been excerpted from the 2017 *TNM classification of malignant tumours*, eighth edition {532,4615}.
A help desk for specific questions about the TNM classification is available at https://www.uicc.org/tnm-help-desk.

pTNM Pathological Classification

The pT and pN categories correspond to the T and N categories.

pN0 Histological examination of a regional lymphadenectomy specimen will ordinarily include 12 or more lymph nodes. If the lymph nodes are negative, but the number ordinarily examined is not met, classify as pN0.

pM – Distant Metastasis*

pM1 Distant metastasis microscopically confirmed

Note
* pM0 and pMX are not valid categories.

Stage

Stage I	T1	N0	M0
Stage II	T2,T3	N0	M0
Stage III	T4	N0	M0
	Any T	N1	M0
Stage IV	Any T	Any N	M1

TNM Clinical Classification

Colon and Rectum

T – Primary Tumour

TX Primary tumour cannot be assessed
T0 No evidence of primary tumour
T1 Tumour invades lamina propria or submucosa or is no greater than 2 cm in size
 T1a Tumour less than 1 cm in size
 T1b Tumour 1 or 2 cm in size
T2 Tumour invades muscularis propria or is greater than 2 cm in size
T3 Tumour invades subserosa, or non-peritonealized pericolic or perirectal tissues
T4 Tumour perforates the visceral peritoneum or invades other organs

Note
For any T, add (m) for multiple tumours.

N – Regional Lymph Nodes

NX Regional lymph nodes cannot be assessed
N0 No regional lymph node metastasis
N1 Regional lymph node metastasis

M – Distant Metastasis

M0 No distant metastasis
M1 Distant metastasis
 M1a Hepatic metastasis only
 M1b Extrahepatic metastasis only
 M1c Hepatic and extrahepatic metastases

pTNM Pathological Classification

The pT and pN categories correspond to the T and N categories.

pM – Distant Metastasis*

pM1 Distant metastasis microscopically confirmed

Note
* pM0 and pMX are not valid categories.

Stage

Stage I	T1	N0	M0
Stage IIA	T2	N0	M0
Stage IIB	T3	N0	M0
Stage IIIA	T4	N0	M0
Stage IIIB	Any T	N1	M0
Stage IV	Any T	Any N	M1

Well-Differentiated Neuroendocrine Tumours – Pancreas (G1, G2 and G3)

Rules for Classification

This classification system applies to well-differentiated neuroendocrine tumours (carcinoid tumours and atypical carcinoid tumours) of the pancreas.

High-grade neuroendocrine carcinomas are excluded and should be classified according to criteria for classifying carcinomas of the pancreas.

Regional Lymph Nodes

The regional lymph nodes correspond to those listed under the appropriate sites for carcinoma.

TNM Clinical Classification

Pancreas

T – Primary Tumour[a]

TX	Primary tumour cannot be assessed
T0	No evidence of primary tumour
T1	Tumour limited to pancreas,[b] 2 cm or less in greatest dimension
T2	Tumour limited to pancreas,[b] more than 2 cm but less than 4 cm in greatest dimension
T3	Tumour limited to pancreas,[b] more than 4 cm in greatest dimension or tumour invading duodenum or bile duct
T4	Tumour invades adjacent organs (stomach, spleen, colon, adrenal gland) or the wall of large vessels (coeliac axis or the superior mesenteric artery)

Notes

[a] For any T, add (m) for multiple tumours.

[b] Invasion of adjacent peripancreatic adipose tissue is accepted but invasion of adjacent organs is excluded.

N – Regional Lymph Nodes

NX	Regional lymph nodes cannot be assessed
N0	No regional lymph node metastasis
N1	Regional lymph node metastasis

M – Distant Metastasis

M0	No distant metastasis	
M1	Distant metastasis	
	M1a	Hepatic metastasis only
	M1b	Extrahepatic metastasis only
	M1c	Hepatic and extrahepatic metastases

Stage

Stage I	T1	N0	M0
Stage II	T2,T3	N0	M0
Stage III	T4	N0	M0
	Any T	N1	M0
Stage IV	Any T	Any N	M1

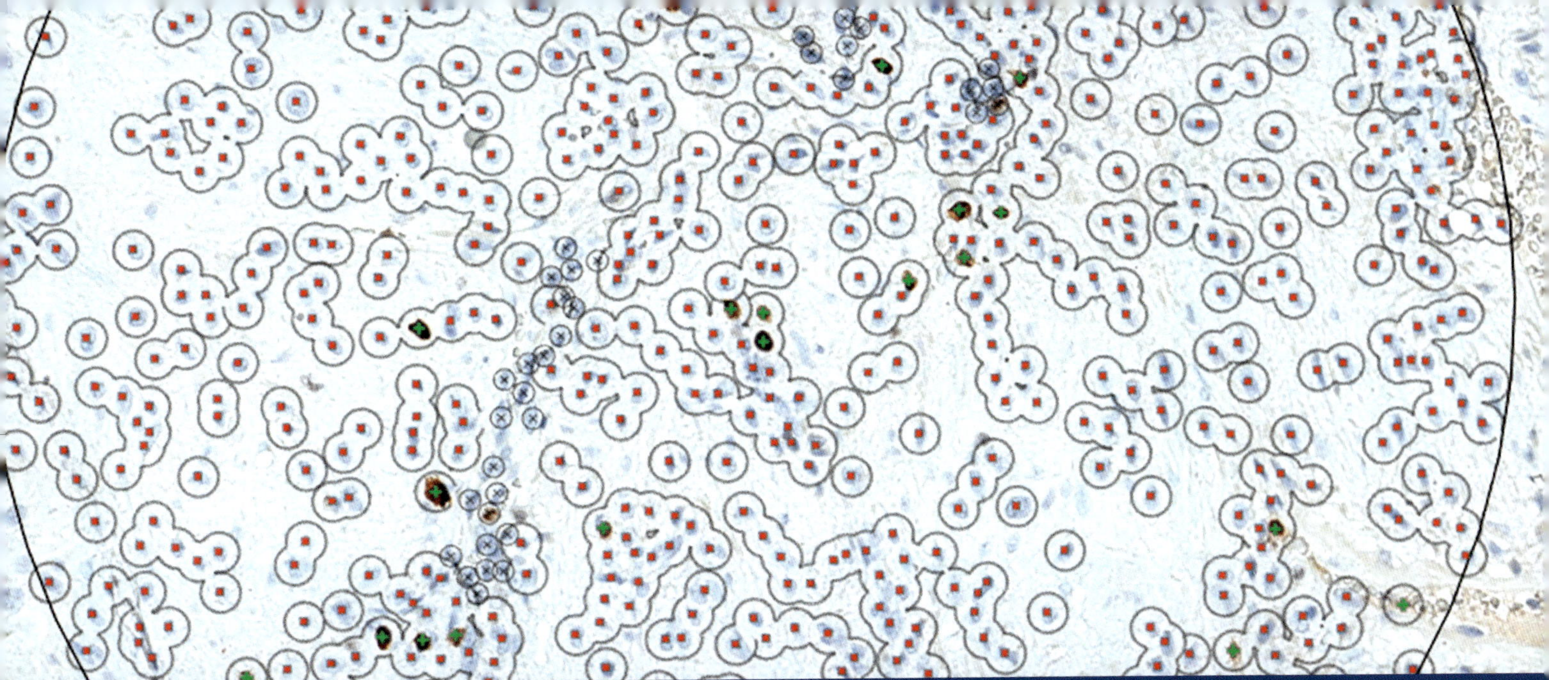

1

Introduction to endocrine and neuroendocrine tumours

Edited by: Rindi G

Introduction to endocrine and neuroendocrine tumours

Mete O
Asa SL
Baloch ZW
de Krijger RR
Erickson LA
Ghossein RA
Gill AJ
Klimstra DS
Lax SF
Lazar AJ
Nosé V
Osamura RY
Papotti M
Sobrinho-Simoes M
Tallini G

The fifth edition of the WHO classification of endocrine and neuroendocrine tumours is a timely sequel to the previous editions. It fully reflects the landscape of endocrine pathology, which is constantly evolving owing to new insights into etiology and pathogenesis and with newer methods of diagnosis, molecular and genetic testing, imaging, and management. The text incorporates not only the traditional endocrine organs but also a chapter on neuroendocrine neoplasms (NENs) in non-endocrine organs. This new WHO classification largely adopts the 2018 WHO / International Agency for Research on Cancer (IARC) terminology framework for NENs in various anatomical sites {3749}. This achieves consistency in classifying this family of endocrine tumours in a comprehensive, organized, and reproducible manner. The chapter on thyroid neoplasia has undergone extensive reorganization; and the sections on the adrenal cortex outline the advances in our understanding of steroid hormone–producing cells. The understanding of tumour syndromes is important in this field where genetic predisposition is so common.

Like in other volumes in the series, each entity has a clear and concise definition and a list of pertinent essential and desirable diagnostic criteria to ensure a unified diagnostic approach, to facilitate accurate data collection for tumour registries and further improve the quality of translational research. Special emphasis is placed on diagnostic and predictive biomarkers, including molecular analysis and immunohistochemistry.

Neuroendocrine neoplasms

NENs are derived from two main neuroendocrine cell groups: epithelial and neuronal/paraneuronal.

Pituitary NENs

The term "pituitary neuroendocrine tumour" (PitNET) is the preferred nomenclature for pituitary NENs, formerly known as pituitary adenomas {213,190}. This change is also accompanied by updated coding, aligned with other neuroendocrine tumours (NETs). PitNETs are well-differentiated NETs that reflect the cytogenesis of the various hormone-producing adenohypophysial cells. These tumours have a low frequency of metastatic spread, but they can have significant morbidity and mortality due to local invasion. When metastatic, the term "metastatic PitNET" is endorsed instead of "pituitary carcinoma". However, this edition still preserves the nomenclature of "pituitary carcinoma" and "PitNET / pituitary adenoma" as acceptable, with a view to facilitating a smooth transition to the next edition of the WHO classification where it is likely that the terms "pituitary carcinoma" and "pituitary adenoma" will be considered redundant. It also remains to be determined whether primary poorly differentiated pituitary NENs exist that would qualify for classification as neuroendocrine carcinoma (NEC) based on the WHO/IARC framework. Unlike for most NENs, there are no formal grading and staging systems applied to PitNETs. The detailed histological classification of PitNETs models the classification of NENs based on cell lineage, cell type, and related characteristics by combining the routine use of transcription factors and hormones with the use of other biomarkers, including but not limited to keratins (especially CAM5.2) and Ki-67. This approach facilitates risk stratification and also predicts the differential response to therapies among various subtypes of PitNETs {2958,1626,2961,2957,213}.

The addition of hypothalamic NENs expands the spectrum of sellar endocrine neoplasia, and the clarification of tumours such as spindle cell oncocytomas, granular cell tumours, and sellar ependymomas as subtypes of pituicytoma allows a clear distinction between neuroendocrine and glial-derived neoplasms in this region.

Parathyroid NENs

Even though parathyroid glands are neuroendocrine tissues, no effort has been made to classify parathyroid NENs as NETs, on the basis that truly benign lesions (adenomas) are very common, and biologically malignant neoplasms (parathyroid carcinomas) are very rare.

A focus of this edition has been to clarify issues in the nomenclature of hyperplasia versus neoplasia. An abnormal parathyroid gland is often enlarged and cellular, and it typically exceeds 8 mm and 60 mg {1168}; however, cellular parenchyma is not always a pathological sign. The importance of clinical, laboratory, and genetic findings in achieving accurate diagnoses of parathyroid disorders is emphasized. Traditionally, multiglandular disease has almost always been classified as "parathyroid hyperplasia". However, primary multiglandular parathyroid disease is usually due to multiple adenomas arising in the setting of a germline susceptibility syndrome, and the terminology has now been updated to reflect this. For example, multiglandular disease arising in the setting of multiple endocrine neoplasia type 1 is now classified as multiple adenomas rather than primary hyperplasia. With this approach, true hyperplasia in primary hyperparathyroidism is now an extremely uncommon manifestation that is being questioned, and true parathyroid hyperplasia is restricted to secondary hyperparathyroidism.

The diagnostic criteria of parathyroid carcinoma, which may be considered more analogous to a well-differentiated NET than a true NEC, remain unchanged. However, the role of biomarkers has been expanded. The diagnostic term "atypical parathyroid tumour" has been introduced to replace the older nomenclature of "atypical parathyroid adenoma", and it is noted that the great majority of atypical parathyroid tumours not associated with worrying clinical, molecular, or immunohistochemical features do not recur after simple excision. Practical information, including but not limited to what can simulate atypical features, is also provided, along with the crucial role of immunohistochemistry in the workup of atypical parathyroid tumours and parathyroid carcinoma.

Paragangliomas and phaeochromocytomas

Non-epithelial NENs are paragangliomas, including intra-adrenal paragangliomas known as phaeochromocytomas. Their postulated origin from neural crest–like Schwann cell precursors is new information. The occurrence of these tumours in various anatomical locations (e.g. liver, lung, pancreas, thyroid) correlates with dispersed microscopic paraganglia in close association with components of the autonomic nervous system {203}. The importance of employing immunostains for GATA3 and tyrosine hydroxylase is emphasized in the diagnosis of paragangliomas and phaeochromocytomas (PPGLs). The distinction between PPGL and epithelial NEN is of clinical significance, because the clinical management of these tumours is different. Another important feature of particular importance is the distinction of metastatic PPGLs from synchronous multifocal primary tumours that may occur due to the high frequency (≥ 40%) of germline predisposition in PPGLs. The recognition of genomic alterations {2956,2400} in subcentimetre adrenal medullary nodules supports the concept of microphaeochromocytoma {2977}; therefore, the current WHO classification restricts medullary hyperplasia only to the diffuse expansion of the adrenal medulla. The presence of diffuse medullary hyperplasia in association with (micro)phaeochromocytomas should prompt investigation of germline susceptibility (e.g. *RET*, *MAX*, *TMEM127*, and *SDHB*) {2400,1868,3790}. The routine use of molecular immunohistochemistry is encouraged in PPGLs. All PPGLs have metastatic potential, and therefore they are all considered malignant. While acknowledging them, the current WHO classification does not endorse the scoring systems that have been introduced to predict the risk of metastasis, because no single system has consistently proved to have strong predictive performance. Instead, members of the multidisciplinary endocrine oncology team are encouraged to use dynamic risk stratification and clinical correlation to estimate the recurrence risk of PPGLs. The features associated with increased risk include somatic, epigenetic, and/or germline alterations; various other factors such as anatomical tumour location, large tumour size, and immature catecholamine profiling (absence of elevated metanephrine / epinephrine [adrenaline] levels); and the Ki-67 proliferation index {546,1385,203,2120,2121,4756,2139}.

Pancreatic NENs

The classification of epithelial pancreatic NENs (PanNENs) remains largely unchanged. However, the diagnostic category of "neuroendocrine microadenoma" is being replaced with "neuroendocrine microtumour", reflecting their very low-risk metastatic potential {2470} while keeping consistency with the NEN terminology framework. Advances made in understanding the tumorigenesis of pancreatic epithelial NENs are reflected in individual entity sections. Particularly, the small indolent insulinomas are distinguished from their aggressive metastatic counterparts by ARX expression and by the alternative-lengthening-of-telomeres phenotype, *ATRX* or *DAXX* loss, and *CDKN2A* loss, similarly to non-functioning NETs {1734,5097}. In this classification, the role of immunohistochemical biomarkers has been emphasized, with a particular emphasis on keratin and hormone immunohistochemistry, and the list of functional categories now includes PPomas. The concept of NET-to-NEC progression remains to be further studied.

NENs in non-neuroendocrine organs

The topic of NENs in non-neuroendocrine tissues is addressed for the first time in this fifth edition. There is an important discussion of the various biomarkers that are used to define neuroendocrine differentiation. The use of nonspecific immunohistochemical biomarkers alone (e.g. CD56, CD57, and NSE) is discouraged. The expression of classic neuroendocrine differentiation markers (e.g. chromogranin A) may be variable in NECs {3519,1170} and in NETs with selective expression of chromogranin B (e.g. L-cell NETs of the rectum and appendix {1316, 1170}). Although negative synaptophysin expression makes the possibility of a NEN unlikely, it is not a specific marker, and the use of INSM1 (the nuclear transcription factor that regulates neuroendocrine differentiation) is useful in the diagnostic workup of neoplasms with synaptophysin and focal or absent chromogranin A expression {3808,376,2154,3188,2532}.

The arbitrary cut-off point of 30% of each component to support a diagnosis of mixed neuroendocrine–non-neuroendocrine neoplasm (MiNEN) has been challenged. Although this distinction is even more difficult in small biopsy specimens from metastases (e.g. liver core biopsies), immunohistochemically confirmed and morphologically distinct tumour components should be recognized and reported irrespective of their extent.

Advances made in the understanding of NENs with mixed epithelial and neuronal differentiation are reflected in updated terminology. The tumour formerly known as "gangliocytic paraganglioma" is now renamed "composite gangliocytoma/neuroma and neuroendocrine tumour" (CoGNET; see *Composite gangliocytoma/neuroma and neuroendocrine tumour*, p. 351), a diagnostic term better reflecting its composition and biology. Similarly, the tumours previously called "cauda equina paragangliomas" are biologically, genetically, and morphologically different from PPGLs arising elsewhere {2817,3670}. Further studies are awaited, and it is anticipated that in the future, CNS paraganglioma may be better classified as a form of NET.

Thyroid neoplasia

The data obtained from molecular studies have provided an opportunity to streamline and simplify the classification of thyroid neoplasia. There is still work to be done to elucidate the pathogenesis of the common multifocal benign proliferative lesion that is clinically known as sporadic nodular goitre but is recognized to be an admixture of hyperplastic and neoplastic proliferations. The term "thyroid follicular nodular disease" is now used to describe this entity.

Non-invasive follicular thyroid neoplasm with papillary-like nuclear features (including oncocytic and subcentimetre subtypes), thyroid tumours of uncertain malignant potential, and hyalinizing trabecular tumours are now assigned to a low-risk follicular cell–derived neoplasia category to reflect their extremely low risk of metastatic spread or structural recurrence.

At the genomic level and by their clinical behaviour, follicular thyroid carcinoma and the invasive encapsulated follicular variant of papillary thyroid carcinoma are identical malignant follicular cell–derived thyroid neoplasms with RAS-like molecular profiles. The degree of nuclear alterations varies among these tumours; however, the threshold for nuclear alterations varies

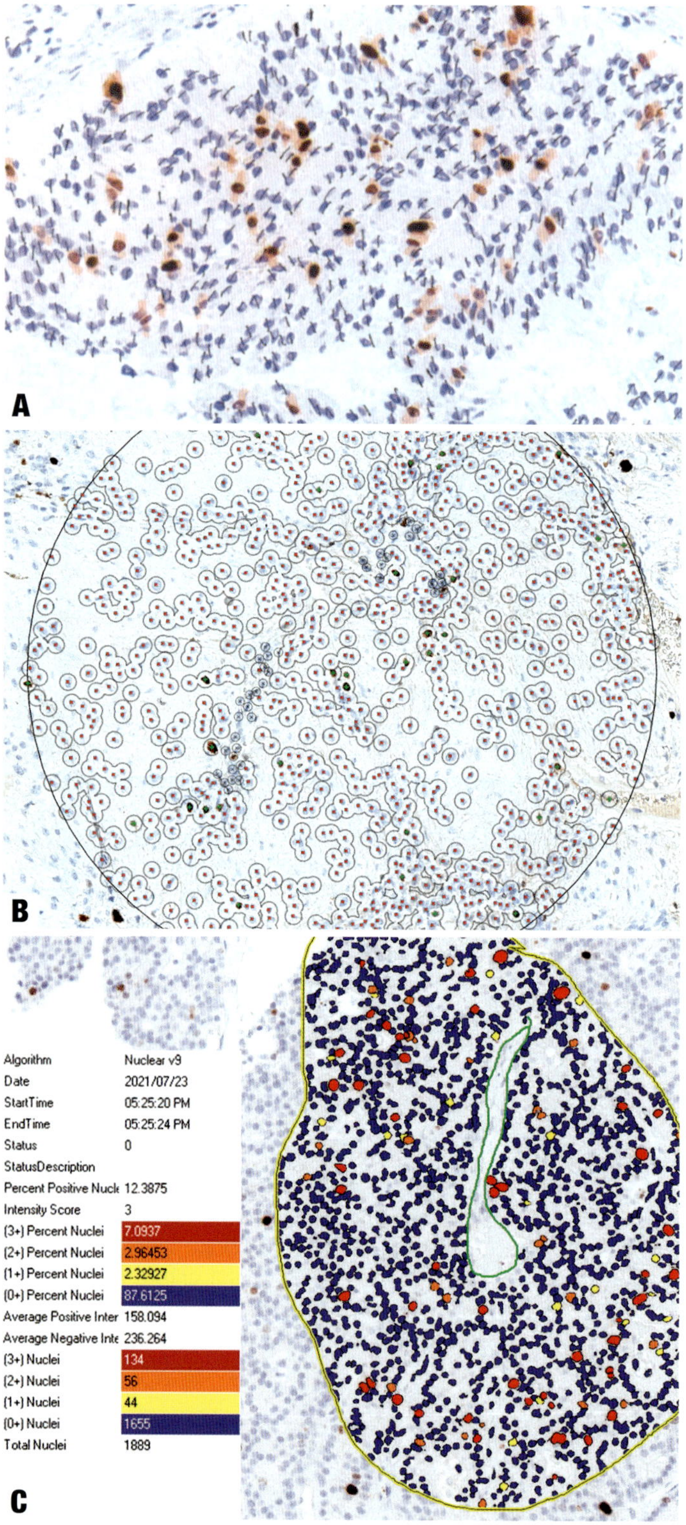

Fig. 1.01 Assessment of Ki-67 proliferation index in endocrine and neuroendocrine neoplasms. Eyeballing for Ki-67 proliferation index is not considered to be accurate. Pathologists should perform a formal manual count (**A**) or use an automated image analysis nuclear algorithm (**B,C**). **A** This image illustrates a manual count on a metastatic grade 2 (G2) neuroendocrine tumour (NET) in the liver. **B** This image shows the result of automated image analysis on a G2 NET originating from the gut. **C** This image illustrates the assessment of a parathyroid carcinoma using a different automated image analysis nuclear algorithm. The methodology used to assess the Ki-67 proliferation index should be clearly defined in pathology reports.

among experts. Therefore, the current WHO classification separates these two lesions with an expectation that in the next edition it may be possible to coalesce follicular thyroid carcinoma and encapsulated follicular variant of papillary thyroid carcinoma into a single diagnostic category of follicular-patterned differentiated thyroid carcinoma. (Although the term "variant" is now usually reserved for genetic alterations, it remains part of the entity name for invasive encapsulated follicular variant of papillary thyroid carcinoma.)

In this classification, papillary thyroid carcinoma (PTC) is defined as a class of BRAF-like neoplasms. The diagnosis still requires either papillary or solid/trabecular architecture, or infiltrative growth in follicular-patterned tumours. The various subtypes are discussed in detail and their clinical importance is reviewed. Tall cell change is defined using the rigid criterion of a height-to-weight ratio of ≥ 3:1. Papillary microcarcinomas require subtyping, similarly to PTCs exceeding 10 mm.

The term "Hürthle cell" is recognized as a misnomer, and the use of the term "oncocytic" is encouraged for tumours with this cytological alteration. The follicular cell–derived adenomas and carcinomas with extensive (> 75%) oncocytic changes are discussed separately to emphasize their specific features in terms of behaviour, molecular profile, and radioactive iodine avidity; special attention is given to recognizing the high-grade features that should prompt reclassification into a high-grade category that reflects a greater risk of adverse behaviour.

High-grade follicular cell–derived thyroid carcinoma is a new category introduced in this edition. It includes follicular cell–derived carcinomas with high-grade features based on mitotic count and tumour necrosis in the absence of anaplastic dedifferentiation. These tumours are further subtyped as high-grade differentiated thyroid carcinoma (e.g. high-grade PTC, high-grade follicular thyroid carcinoma, high-grade oncocytic carcinoma) and poorly differentiated thyroid carcinomas. The relevant message for pathologists is the importance of mitoses and necrosis even in differentiated thyroid carcinomas.

Anaplastic thyroid carcinoma remains the least common but most aggressive form of follicular cell–derived thyroid carcinomas. A particular emphasis is placed on the diagnosis of exclusion of anaplastic thyroid carcinoma from other high-grade malignancies, especially in the absence of expression of PAX8 and thyroid transcription factor 1 (TTF1). Formerly listed as a distinct tumour category, primary squamous cell carcinoma of the thyroid is now considered to be a subtype of anaplastic thyroid carcinoma.

The tumour formerly known as cribriform-morular variant of PTC is no longer classified as a subtype of PTC. It is a tumour of uncertain cytogenesis with unique morphology, genetics, and immunohistochemical features that include diffuse nuclear and cytoplasmic β-catenin expression, absence of diffuse PAX8 expression and thyroglobulin expression in the non-morular component, and a lack of TTF1 along with coexpression of CD5 and CK5 in morulae {507}. Its histogenesis awaits further clarification, therefore it has not yet joined the groups of tumours of thymic or salivary gland differentiation that also occur in the thyroid gland.

Medullary thyroid carcinoma is the classic NEN of the thyroid, and the importance of Ki-67 as well as tumour necrosis and mitotic count in this lesion is now emphasized.

In this classification, thyroblastoma is officially recognized as an extremely rare and underrecognized embryonal high-grade thyroid neoplasm that is linked to *DICER1* variants. It consists of primitive thyroid follicular cells, small cells, and primitive mesenchymal stroma {32}.

Adrenal cortical lesions

Structure, function, and morphology correlations are reflected in the classification of adrenal cortical lesions {2963,1916,2141}. CYP11B2 immunohistochemistry–based histopathology of primary aldosteronism (HISTALDO) classification {4887} is recommended in the diagnostic workup of adrenalectomy specimens with primary aldosteronism. In light of advances made in translational molecular biology, the spectrum of cortical neoplasia has been expanded to reflect sporadic nodular adrenal cortical disease and bilateral micronodular and macronodular adrenal cortical disease, because they are all composed of genetically modified cells {2963,1916,2141}. The only true adrenal cortical hyperplasia is bilateral diffuse adrenal cortical hyperplasia in the context of ACTH-dependent disease, including congenital adrenal hyperplasia.

In addition to well-established multifactorial schemes, the reticulin algorithm and Helsinki scoring systems have expanded the list of available tools to classify adrenal cortical neoplasms. The importance of venous angioinvasion stands out as a diagnostic and predictive feature of adrenal cortical carcinomas {2967}. Special emphasis is given to the role of immunohistochemical biomarkers, including paranuclear dot-like IGF2 overexpression in the distinction of adrenal cortical carcinoma from adrenal cortical adenoma {2967,2959}. In addition to mitotic tumour grading (based on the cut-off point of 20 mitoses/10 mm^2), the crucial role of Ki-67 as a diagnostic and predictive biomarker in adult and paediatric adrenal cortical carcinoma is discussed {1185,413,2967,3548,2861}. Evidence suggests that the diagnosis and prognostication of adrenal cortical carcinoma is possible using molecular diagnostics {5160}.

Endocrine tumour syndromes

The spectrum of endocrine tumour syndromes continues to grow rapidly. This edition provides important updates on the known genetic tumour syndromes as well as incorporating newly described genetic tumour syndromes. Changes include a unified terminology for succinate dehydrogenase–deficient tumour syndromes based on both clinical and molecular features. Whereas the term "Carney triad" was previously defined clinically, it is now defined by dual clinical and molecular criteria as a succinate dehydrogenase–deficient tumour syndrome where no germline SDH mutation has been identified. The use of older terminology such as "Carney–Stratakis dyad" (the clinical association of familial succinate dehydrogenase–deficient gastrointestinal stromal tumour and paraganglioma) is now discouraged in favour of nomenclature based on identification of the mutated gene {379}. *DICER1*-related disease has been significantly expanded, and the new multiple endocrine neoplasia type 5 (due to germline pathogenic *MAX* variants) and *MAFA*-related familial insulinomatosis are now defined and discussed in detail. The familial follicular cell–derived thyroid neoplasia in syndromes is well defined; however, the nonsyndromic familial follicular cell–derived thyroid carcinoma remains to be clarified.

A lack of family history and age are not reliable criteria to argue against inherited endocrine tumours / NETs, because de novo manifestations that simulate sporadic disease are not uncommon. Moreover, technical limitations in detecting pathogenic variants using next-generation sequencing panels in a small fraction of patients should be kept in mind. Whole-exome sequencing or even whole-genome sequencing can reduce the fraction of mutation-negative individuals on first-line diagnostic molecular analyses {515}.

Technical and methodological issues

Mitotic counts and the Ki-67 labelling index

In general, the fifth edition requires reporting of mitotic count (either conventional or phosphohistone H3–assisted) using mm^2 rather than HPF to provide reproducibility among practices {943}. This will also ensure a smooth transition to upcoming digital pathology practice. Eyeballing alone for the Ki-67 proliferation index is discouraged, and pathologists should normally provide the labelling index using an automated image analysis nuclear algorithm or formal manual count. The methodology used to assess mitotic count and Ki-67 proliferation index should be clearly defined in pathology reports.

Molecular immunohistochemistry

Molecular immunohistochemistry is an invaluable tool for pathologists to acquire insights into disease cytogenesis and pathogenesis. However, reliable prediction and prognostication requires technically sound methodology, accurate reagents, and rigorous validation protocols. The importance of using monoclonal antibodies has been emphasized with respect to pituitary hormones and CEA, and different antibody clones, such as those used to localize TTF1 and PAX8, can have differing sensitivities and specificities. Good immunohistochemistry can also serve as a screening tool for inherited disease when prompted by identification of precursor lesions and/or clinical features, and it is of particular value in assessing genetic variants of uncertain significance.

Angioinvasion

The subject of angioinvasion is a controversial but critical one in endocrine pathology. Endocrine organs are rich in vessels and are decorated with fenestrated endothelium, providing the basis for potential artefact. As shown in adrenal cortical carcinoma {2967}, follicular cell–derived thyroid carcinomas {2955}, medullary thyroid carcinoma {1277}, parathyroid carcinoma {1275,1276,65}, and NETs {3383,248}, angioinvasion characterized by the presence of intravascular tumour cells admixed with thrombus/platelets reliably predicts a high risk of tumour spread. The use of CD61 immunohistochemistry can assist the recognition of intravascular tumour cell–platelet aggregates by highlighting platelets when the thrombus is subtle {941}. In follicular cell–derived malignancies, the number of vessels involved has been discussed and a cut-off point of 4 vessels has been applied in some risk-stratification schemes {1554,2059,4986}; however, there is no scientific clarity or multi-institutional validation on how to count vessels and whether adjacent vessels represent a single focus or multiple foci. Furthermore, opinions vary among experts on the relevance of this requirement. Specifically in the thyroid gland, because of the lower risk of negative outcomes associated with locoregional lymph node metastasis, the distinction of vascular channels (angioinvasion) from lymphatics (lymphatic invasion) remains important.

Open questions and future vision

The endocrine system, while composed of three distinct lineages of cells with different embryogenesis, structure, and function, remains the site of some of the most indolent and some of the most aggressive neoplasms. The role of genetic predisposition and the identification of molecular subtypes of sporadic tumours has shed light on the often-unique cellular mechanisms underlying neoplastic transformation. Nonetheless, there remain many unanswered questions.

In light of current advances in the field of endocrine pathology, it is not far-fetched to anticipate that the following will be most likely addressed in the next edition of the WHO classification of endocrine and neuroendocrine tumours: (1) validation of biomarkers that truly distinguish NET from NEC, and data proving whether there is progression from NET to NEC; (2) diagnostic criteria that will distinguish MiNEN from non-neuroendocrine tumours with neuroendocrine differentiation or amphicrine features; (3) evidence of a poorly differentiated pituitary NEC; (4) development of a TNM staging system for pituitary tumours; (5) clarification as to the existence of a poorly differentiated NEC of the parathyroid gland; (6) determination of whether medullary thyroid carcinoma is better classified as a NET rather than a NEC, within the NEN terminology framework; (7) the etiology and pathogenesis of composite epithelial and neuronal tumours arising in the pituitary, duodenum, and cauda equina; and (8) the role of the environment in the epigenetic changes that are so common in endocrine tumours / NETs.

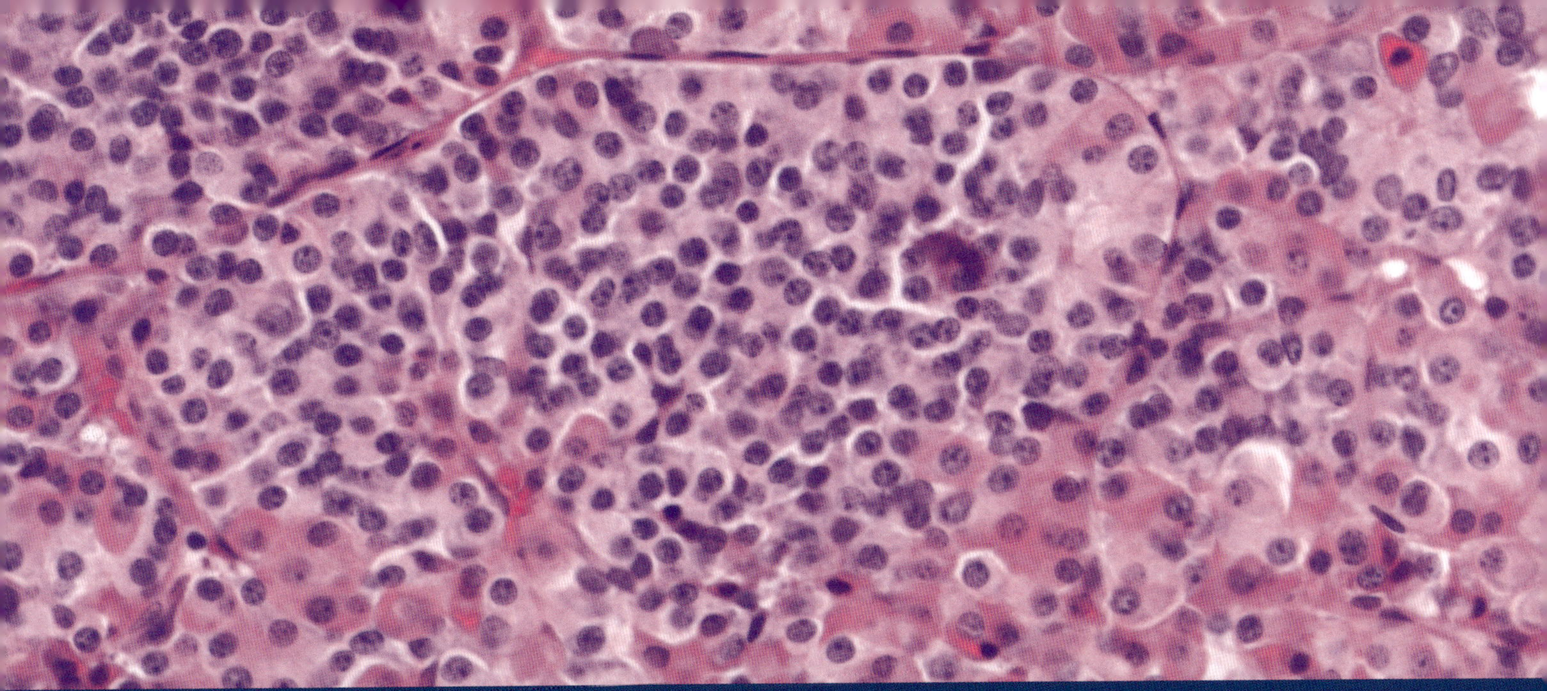

2

Pituitary tumours

Edited by: Asa SL, Mete O, Osamura RY

Pituitary tumours: Introduction

Mete O

The pituitary gland has two major components: the anterior pituitary, which is a neuroendocrine structure comprising six hormone-secreting cell types and sustentacular folliculostellate cells within a richly vascular stroma, and the posterior pituitary, which is composed of pituicytes (modified glia of hypothalamic origin) supporting the axons of hypothalamic neurons that secrete hormones into the bloodstream. The tumours that arise from this gland reflect these cell types and their embryonic origin {213,216}. Additionally, tumours in the sella turcica can arise from the meninges and stromal elements; occasional germ cell tumours and haematopoietic neoplasms involve this gland, and metastases to the pituitary occur.

Pituitary neuroendocrine tumours (PitNETs)

Evolution of the nomenclature

Tumours of adenohypophysial hormone–secreting cells have been traditionally classified as pituitary adenomas; however, these tumours may be locally invasive and can metastasize. There are no morphological features that distinguish locally aggressive and metastatic lesions from indolent ones {213}.

Adenohypophysial cells contain ultrastructural neurosecretory granules and express neuroendocrine proteins such as synaptophysin, chromogranin A, CD56, and INSM1; therefore, they are members of the family of neuroendocrine cells. Consistent with the WHO / International Agency for Research on Cancer (IARC) proposal to unify the approach to neuroendocrine tumours (NETs) {3749}, a change in nomenclature has been suggested {193}, and these neoplasms are now recognized as PitNETs {190,213}. As a transition from the fourth edition of the WHO classification of tumours of endocrine organs, in which the term "pituitary adenoma" was used, in this fifth edition, we use the term "PitNET/adenoma" to indicate that "pituitary adenomas" still can be used but "PitNET" is preferred.

This change in nomenclature is accompanied by a change in coding that aligns with other NETs. PitNETs are like well-differentiated appendiceal NETs that have a low frequency of metastatic spread, but they imply much greater morbidity and mortality. This change will obviate the need for distinguishing pituitary carcinomas on the basis of discontinuous spread or distant metastasis. It remains to be seen whether there are primary poorly differentiated high-grade malignancies that qualify for the WHO/IARC definition of neuroendocrine carcinoma (small cell [SCNEC] or large cell [LCNEC] neuroendocrine carcinomas) {3749}. The current WHO classification encourages the use of the term "metastatic PitNET" with subtype information (e.g. metastatic densely granulated corticotroph tumour) instead of "pituitary carcinoma". There is no single clinical feature, morphological parameter, or biomarker that can help accurately determine the risk of metastatic spread in PitNETs {2965,214, 213}. No widely accepted grading systems have been defined for PitNETs. The spectrum of pituitary mixed neuroendocrine–non-neuroendocrine neoplasms (MiNENs) includes PitNET in association with pituicyte-family tumours {3880} or craniopharyngiomas {5079,1383}.

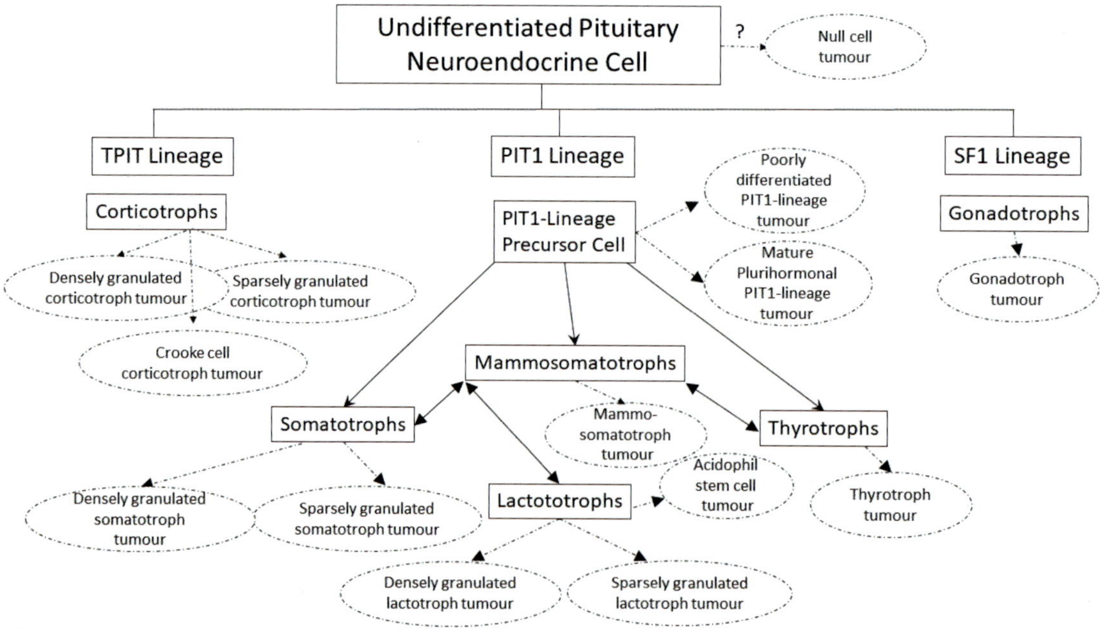

Fig. 2.01 Pituitary neuroendocrine tumour (PitNET). The classification of PitNETs reflects their derivation from six adenohypophysial cell types of three lineages, with multiple subtypes of some cell types and some tumours showing incomplete differentiation.

The new PitNET classification

PitNETs reflect their derivation from six adenohypophysial cell types with multiple morphological subtypes of each tumour type. The molecular mechanisms responsible for the differentiation of these various cells types has been carefully studied during development and tumorigenesis {217,5108,192,2518, 3377,4621,4044,201,1301,2971}. It has become clear that there are three families of cells determined by the expression of three transcription factors: PIT1, TPIT, and SF1. The PIT1 family is complex, giving rise to four terminally differentiated cell types that are known to be fluid, fluctuating from one to another in different physiological conditions. Each adenohypophysial cell type can give rise to multiple subtypes, and almost any tumour can be clinically non-functioning or may give rise to clinical and biochemical evidence of hormone excess. Some PitNETs are composed of less differentiated cells leading to an immature differentiation status as seen in immature PIT1-lineage tumours (formerly known as silent subtype 3 adenomas, then as poorly differentiated PIT1-lineage PitNETs) {2966,2972}. There are also null cell tumours that fail to demonstrate terminal differentiation

Table 2.01 Classification of pituitary neuroendocrine tumours (PitNETs)

Tumour type[a]	Transcription factor(s)	Hormone(s)	Keratin (CAM5.2 or CK18)	Tumour subtype (if applicable)	Hormone excess syndrome[b]
PIT1-lineage tumours					
Somatotroph tumours	PIT1	GH, α-subunit	Perinuclear	Densely granulated somatotroph tumour	Florid acromegaly
		GH	Fibrous bodies (> 70%)	Sparsely granulated somatotroph tumour	Subtle acromegaly
Lactotroph tumours	PIT1, ERα	Prolactin (paranuclear)	Weak or negative	Sparsely granulated lactotroph tumour	Hyperprolactinaemia[c]
		Prolactin (diffuse cytoplasmic)	Weak or negative	Densely granulated lactotroph tumour	Hyperprolactinaemia[c]
Mammosomatotroph tumour	PIT1, ERα	GH (often predominant), prolactin, α-subunit	Perinuclear		Acromegaly and hyperprolactinaemia[c]
Thyrotroph tumour	PIT1, GATA2/3[d]	α-Subunit, TSH-β	Weak or negative		Hyperthyroidism
Mature plurihormonal PIT1-lineage tumour	PIT1, ERα, GATA2/3[d]	GH (often predominant), prolactin, α-subunit, TSH-β	Perinuclear		Acromegaly, hyperprolactinaemia[c], and/or hyperthyroidism
Acidophil stem cell tumour	PIT1, ERα	Prolactin (predominant), GH (focal/variable)	Scattered fibrous bodies		Hyperprolactinaemia[c] and subclinical acromegaly
Immature PIT1-lineage tumour	PIT1, ERα, GATA2/3[d]	GH, prolactin, α-subunit, TSH-β	Focal/variable		Acromegaly, hyperprolactinaemia[c], and hyperthyroidism
TPIT-lineage tumours					
Corticotroph tumours	TPIT (TBX19), NeuroD1 (β2)	ACTH and other POMC derivatives	Strong	Densely granulated corticotroph tumour	Florid Cushing disease, often microtumour
			Variable	Sparsely granulated corticotroph tumour	Subtle Cushing disease, often macrotumour
			Intense ring-like perinuclear	Crooke cell tumour	Variable, Cushing disease
SF1-lineage tumours					
Gonadotroph tumour	SF1, ERα, GATA2/3[d]	α-Subunit, FSH-β, LH-β	Variable		Hypogonadism (virtually all) or hypergonadism (exceptional)
Tumours without distinct cell lineage					
Unclassified plurihormonal tumours	Multiple combinations	Multiple combinations	Variable		Variable
Null cell tumour	None	None	Variable		None

GH, growth hormone.

[a]Mixed tumours also occur and can constitute any combination of tumours shown; the most common is mixed somatotroph–lactotroph tumour. [b]Any tumour type can be clinically non-functioning. [c]Moderate hyperprolactinaemia can occur with any sellar mass that has suprasellar extension, interrupting hypothalamic tonic dopaminergic inhibition; however, the prolactin level rarely exceeds 150 ng/mL; lactotroph tumours usually show a characteristic correlation between tumour size and prolactin levels, whereas other prolactin-secreting tumours do not. [d]GATA2 and GATA3 are paralogues and show cross-reactivity with some available antisera.

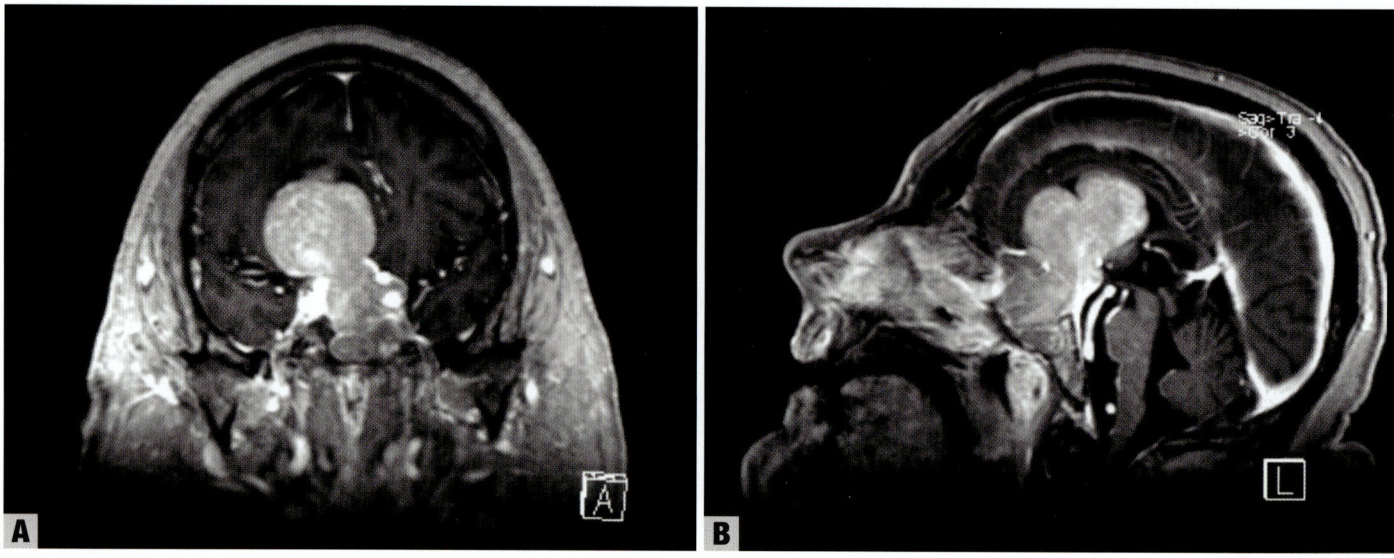

Fig. 2.02 Pituitary neuroendocrine tumour (PitNET). Coronal (**A**) and sagittal (**B**) MRI of a large invasive PitNET.

along SF1, TPIT, or PIT1 lineages {299,2961,105}. Multiple PitNETs may develop in the same gland, creating collision tumours of multiple cell lineages {2950}.

Detailed histological subtyping of a PitNET on the basis of cell lineage, cell type, and related characteristics provides critical clinical information for risk stratification, because different PitNET subtypes have different therapeutic responses {2958,1626, 2961,2957,213}. Hormone immunohistochemistry alone can sometimes be misleading because of nonspecific or diffusion-type staining, emphasizing the importance of staining for pituitary transcription factors to ensure accurate tumour characterization {2957}. The distinction of multiple synchronous PitNETs of distinct lineages absolutely requires staining for transcription factors {2950}. Therefore, the current WHO classification of PitNETs is based on routine staining for transcription factors (PIT1, SF1, TPIT, GATA3, and ERα) and antibodies against adenohypophysial hormones (ACTH, growth hormone, prolactin, TSH-β, LH-β, FSH-β, and the α-subunit of glycoprotein hormones), as well as other biomarkers including but not limited to low-molecular-weight keratins (e.g. CAM5.2, CK8/18) {2961,211,2957,213} (see Table 2.01, p. 35). Like for other NETs, the Ki-67 proliferation index should be assessed using either manual counting or automated image analysis nuclear algorithms {2961,213}. The term "PitNET NOS" can be used when pathologists do not have access to ancillary tools to enable subtyping, but such cases should be referred to centres that can perform accurate subtyping. Although routine SSTR immunohistochemistry is not required for the management of patients with PitNETs, immunoreactivity for SSTR2 and SSTR5 has been shown to predict responsiveness to somatostatin analogues {1472,3124,907}.

Epidemiology of PitNETs

Like other NETs {5045}, PitNETs that were once considered rare are increasingly diagnosed. Approximately 20% of so-called normal pituitary glands harbour an incidental radiologically detectable lesion {1239,1302}. Multiple population studies from the last 15 years have identified a prevalence of 78–116 cases per 100 000 people {974,1359,1405,48}. Central Brain Tumor Registry of the United States (CBTRUS) data from 2011–2015 estimate that surgically resected sellar tumours have an incidence of 4.12 cases per 100 000 person-years {3370}. In the Republic of Korea, the incidence in cases per 100 000 person-years was 3.5 for non-functioning pituitary tumours, 1.6 for lactotroph tumours, 0.5 for somatotroph tumours, and 0.2 for corticotroph or thyrotroph tumours {3322}. Prolactinomas causing amenorrhoea-galactorrhoea syndrome are the most common functioning PitNETs {4512,971}; these are usually sparsely granulated lactotroph tumours that are treated medically, and most are therefore not captured in cancer or surgical statistics. Surgical resection is performed for 56% of clinically diagnosed PitNETs {974}. Among those resected surgically, > 40% are hormonally inactive mass lesions of SF1 lineage {2961}, approximately 15% are of TPIT lineage, and about 30% are of PIT1 lineage, with more than half of those giving rise to growth hormone excess {3019,974,1359,2961}.

Etiology and pathogenesis of PitNETs

The pathogenesis of PitNETs remains largely enigmatic, and continued investigation is still warranted. Some cases are familial, and the genes implicated have shed some light on the development of these tumours (see Table 2.02). Sporadic tumours have, in limited cases, been shown to have mutations that affect the signalling pathways regulating hormone production (see Table 2.03, p. 38) {214}, but the majority of PitNETs have no known driver mutations {214}. Instead, epigenetic alterations are implicated in the silencing of tumour suppressor genes, mainly those involved in chromatin remodelling and cell-cycle regulation {214}.

In select cases, application of molecular immunohistochemistry tools may be used to demonstrate global loss of menin (*MEN1*), p27 (*CDKN1B*), and SDHB protein (encoded by *SDHB*) to guide further germline screening for multiple endocrine neoplasia type 1 and type 4 and succinate dehydrogenase-deficient tumour syndromes {4955,4444,1582,211,452, 3375}. The diagnosis of a sparsely granulated somatotroph tumour in a young patient should prompt genetic testing for *AIP*-related pathogenesis (familial isolated pituitary adenoma [FIPA] syndrome) {361}; however, AIP immunohistochemistry is not recommended, because it has poor sensitivity in the detection of *AIP* mutations since this protein is epigenetically downregulated in sporadic tumours {1086}. At present, it appears that the overall utility of MAX immunohistochemistry in routine clinical practice is limited, and it is not recommended as a screening test of *MAX* mutation {4047}.

Table 2.02 Genetic susceptibility to pituitary neuroendocrine tumours (PitNETs)

Syndrome/condition	Gene(s)	PitNETs	Other NETs	Other non-neuroendocrine lesions
MEN1	*MEN1*	PIT1-lineage most common All types reported	Multiglandular parathyroid adenomas (multiglandular parathyroid NETs) PanNET Duodenal NET Pulmonary NET Thymic NET	Adrenal cortical neoplasms Breast carcinoma
MEN4	*CDKN1B*	PIT1-lineage tumours (MEN1-like, often somatotroph tumours)	Parathyroid NET PanNET Small intestinal NET	Lymphoma Breast carcinoma
MEN5	*MAX*	PIT1-lineage tumours	Phaeochromocytomas and paragangliomas (including their composite forms) PanNET Multiglandular parathyroid adenomas (multiglandular parathyroid NETs)	Ganglioneuroma, neuroblastoma RCC and oncocytoma Squamous cell carcinoma Breast cancer Lung cancer Endometrial cancer
Carney complex	*PRKAR1A* Other (unknown)	Densely granulated somatotroph tumours Mammosomatotroph tumours		Pigmented nodular adrenocortical disease Testicular tumours Mucosal naevi Cardiac and other myxomas Malignant melanotic nerve sheath tumours
FIPA (isolated familial somatotropinoma)	*AIP* Other (unknown)	Sparsely granulated somatotroph tumour (most common) All types reported	PanNET Duodenal (ampullary-type) NET	Scant morphological data
SDH-related familial PGL syndromes	SDH genes	Lactotroph tumours Multiple types	Phaeochromocytomas and paragangliomas PanNET	Gastrointestinal stromal tumours RCC
Hyperparathyroidism–jaw tumour syndrome	*CDC73*	Somatotroph tumour	Parathyroid NETs	Ossifying fibromas of bone RCC Uterine tumours
***DICER1* syndrome**	*DICER1*	Pituitary blastoma		Pleuropulmonary blastoma Thyroid follicular neoplasms Sertoli–Leydig cell tumours Sarcomas
Lynch syndrome (HNPCC)	*MLH1* *MSH2* *MSH6* *PMS2*	Multiple types	PanNET	Colorectal cancer Endometrial cancer Gastric cancer Biliary and pancreatic cancer Urinary tract cancers
X-linked acrogigantism	Xq26 microduplication *GPR101*	Densely granulated somatotroph tumours Mammosomatotroph tumours		Pleuropulmonary blastoma
McCune–Albright syndrome	*GNAS*	Densely granulated somatotroph tumours Mammosomatotroph tumours		Adrenal and thyroid adenomas Polyostotic fibrous dysplasia Café-au-lait skin pigmentation Precocious puberty

FIPA, familial isolated pituitary adenoma; HNPCC, hereditary non-polyposis colorectal cancer; MEN1–5, multiple endocrine neoplasia types 1–5; NET, neuroendocrine tumour; PanNET, pancreatic neuroendocrine tumour; PGL, paraganglioma; RCC, renal cell carcinoma.

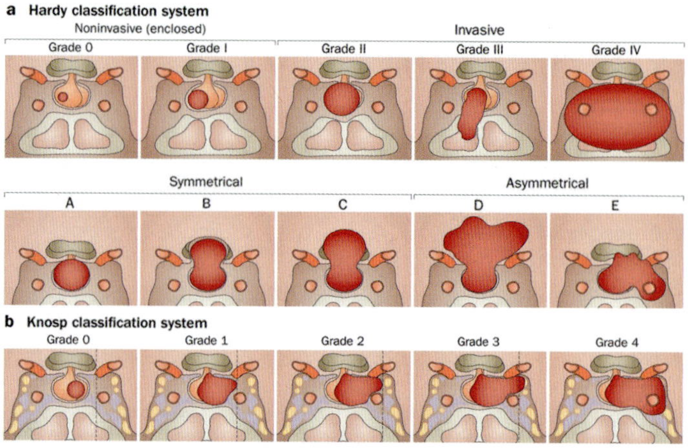

Fig. 2.03 Pituitary neuroendocrine tumour (PitNET), Hardy and Knosp staging system. Although there are no formal staging systems for pituitary tumours, the Hardy and Knosp classification defines the extension of tumours into adjacent neuroanatomical regions and forms the basis for staging that predicts a need for repeat operations, radiotherapy, and/or medical therapy.

Other anterior pituitary tumours

Craniopharyngiomas

The anterior pituitary derives from the oral ectoderm, and tumours reflecting this with squamous and adamantinomatous morphology are known as craniopharyngiomas. Molecular studies have clearly identified the basis for the morphological distinction between these two entities; papillary craniopharyngiomas harbour *BRAF* p.V600E mutations that can be detected with the monoclonal VE1 antibody, whereas adamantinomatous subtypes have *CTNNB1* mutations leading to nuclear β-catenin immunoreactivity {211,1455}.

Pituitary blastoma

Very rare primitive tumours composed of a mixture of adenohypophysial neuroendocrine cells, primitive Rathke cleft cells, and primitive folliculostellate cells are known as pituitary blastomas. These tumours are a hallmark of *DICER1* syndrome {1020,3151}.

Posterior pituitary and hypothalamic neoplasms

Pituicytomas

The tumours known as pituicytomas have long been recognized as neoplasms of pituicytes {522,3544,2973}. However, spindle cell oncocytomas {3805} and granular cell tumours were of unknown cytogenesis at the time of their initial description, and tumours with ependymal morphology were thought to be unusual ependymomas arising in the sella turcica. However, the normal posterior pituitary contains subtypes of pituicytes that correspond to these tumours: light and dark spindle cells, as well as oncocytic, granular, and ependymal pituicytes {4384}. Therefore, it is no surprise that thoughtful analyses {3995}, biomarker expression {2565,2973,3872}, and methylation profiling {641} have shown that these various neoplasms represent a spectrum of a single nosological entity and can be classified as subtypes of pituicytoma. The transition to the recognition of new terminology is proposed in this WHO classification. However, patient demographics and clinical outcomes appear to vary between these tumours, warranting their recognition as distinct subtypes despite the presence of overlapping features in some cases.

Neuronal neoplasms

The existence of gangliocytomas in the sella has been known for many years; these may be the source of adenohypophysiotropic hormones and they may be associated with PitNETs. The spectrum of neuronal tumours has recently been expanded by the recognition of hormonally active neurocytomas of hypothalamic differentiation {202,210}.

Grading and staging of primary sellar neoplasms

The prognosis of patients with sellar tumours depends on tumour type, proliferative capacity, and extent of disease. Currently there are no grading or staging systems for these tumours, but these are needed. In designing these systems, the following should be considered.

Grading

In many NETs, grade is defined by proliferative rate. However, this has not proved valuable alone in the pituitary. Instead, prognosis varies by tumour type {3943,3099,211,233,2605}, and certain tumour types are recognized as more aggressive (high-risk PitNETs), including immature PIT1-lineage tumours {1951,1264,2966}, Crooke cell tumours {1533,1112,922}, null cell tumours {105,1735,299}, and biochemically non-functioning (silent) corticotroph tumours {3992,4991}. In addition, sparsely granulated somatotroph tumours {416,277,1411,2530,2322} and acidophil stem cell tumours are often aggressive and resistant to medical therapies {1948,1949,1978}. Sparsely granulated corticotroph tumours often manifest with invasive large tumours {1126,3669}.

If complete surgical resection is not possible, the probability of recurrence and time to clinically relevant regrowth correlate

Table 2.03 Common sporadic genetic alterations in pituitary neuroendocrine tumours (PitNETs) and craniopharyngiomas

Gene(s)	PitNETs	Clinical correlates
GNAS	Densely granulated somatotroph/mammosomatotroph tumours	Florid acromegaly T2 hypointensity on MRI Somatostatin responsiveness
USP8 *USP48*	Densely granulated corticotroph tumours	Florid Cushing disease Pasireotide responsiveness
ATRX	Corticotroph tumours	Aggressive, recurrent, metastatic
CTNNB1	Adamantinomatous craniopharyngioma	
BRAF	Papillary craniopharyngioma	Targeted therapy to BRAF p.V600E

with radiological tumour doubling time {3076}. The predictive value of mitoses (conventional or phosphohistone H3–assisted count), Ki-67 labelling index, and p53 staining in this scenario remains unproven {3906,1671}.

Staging

Persistent disease after surgical resection depends on tumour size and extent of invasion {3694,2087}. Multiple efforts have been made by surgeons and radiologists to define the extension of tumours into adjacent neuroanatomical regions; namely, the Knosp classification defines the degree of lateral extension into the cavernous sinus {2354} and the Hardy classification outlines the degree of extrasellar and vertical extension into suprasellar regions {1786}. Knosp grade ≥ 3 cavernous sinus invasion predicts a need for repeat operations, radiotherapy, and/or medical therapy {4400}. Despite efforts to predict cavernous sinus invasion on MRI, the precise confirmation of invasion frequently requires surgical and/or histological examination. A pathology reporting template for pituitary tumours was introduced in 2011 {3300}, followed by the European Pituitary Pathology Group (EPPG) proposal in 2019 {4707}. There is a need to reach a multidisciplinary consensus on the staging of these tumours, so that predictive and prognostic scores can be developed and applied to individual cases.

Somatotroph PitNET/adenoma

Mete O
Ezzat S
Lopes MBS
Perry A
Yamada S

Definition

Somatotroph pituitary neuroendocrine tumour (PitNET)/adenoma is a well-differentiated PitNET composed of PIT1-lineage adenohypophysial cells with somatotroph differentiation.

ICD-O coding

8272/3 Somatotroph PitNET/adenoma
8272/3 Densely granulated somatotroph tumour
8272/3 Sparsely granulated somatotroph tumour

ICD-11 coding

2D12.Y Other specified malignant neoplasms of other endocrine glands or related structures

Related terminology

Acceptable: somatotroph tumour.
Not recommended: growth hormone–positive PitNET/adenoma; growth hormone–producing PitNET/adenoma; growth hormone–producing tumour/adenoma; growth hormone tumour/adenoma; acidophil tumour/adenoma; somatotropinoma.

Subtype(s)

Densely granulated somatotroph tumour; sparsely granulated somatotroph tumour

Localization

The majority of somatotroph tumours are located in the sellar region and show variable extension into adjacent structures including but not limited to cavernous sinuses, bone, and sinonasal mucosa. Extrasellar ectopic somatotroph tumours (e.g. clivus, sphenoidal sinus) and those arising in teratomas (e.g. ovarian teratoma) occur rarely {3038,1370,3674,3736,1917}.

Clinical features

Most somatotroph tumours are biochemically active and cause acromegaly and/or gigantism; however, rare silent forms have been reported {1547,3269}. The clinical diagnosis is often delayed; the median delay from first symptoms to diagnosis was 8 years in male patients and 2 years longer in female patients {3539}. Headache, visual field deficits, mild hyperprolactinaemia, hypopituitarism, and pituitary apoplexy have been described in invasive somatotroph macrotumours {2952,2932,3023,2230}.

Irrespective of functional status, pituitary tumours of somatotroph differentiation are divided into two clinicopathologically relevant histological subtypes on the basis of their density of growth hormone (GH)-containing secretory granules and the organization of their cytoplasmic keratin filaments using

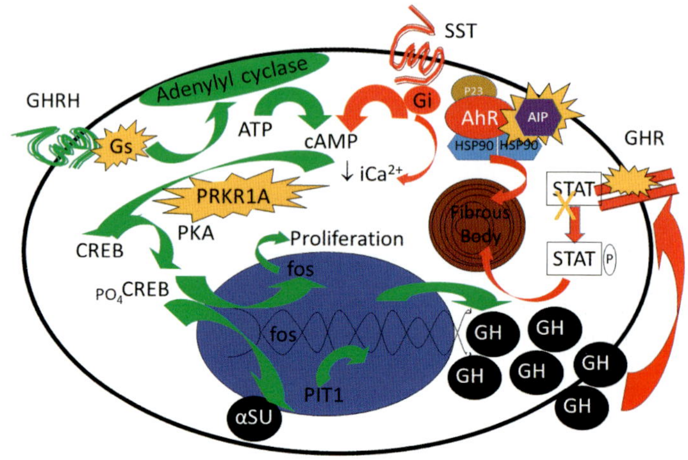

Fig. 2.04 Molecular pathogenesis of somatotroph tumours. Sporadic or germline activating mutations in *GNAS* result in the constitutive activation of $G_s\alpha$, which upregulates adenylyl cyclase, resulting in increased cAMP, causing the phosphorylation of CREB and the synthesis of growth hormone and α-subunit. In patients with Carney complex, mutations inactivating *PRKAR1A* have the same effect by enhancing CREB activation. Tumours with these alterations have a densely granulated phenotype and respond well to somatostatin analogue therapy that reduces cAMP. In contrast, changes shown on the right, including *AIP* mutation or silencing, *GHR* inactivation, or other mechanisms of reducing STAT signalling, result in sparsely granulated somatotroph tumours that have fibrous bodies.

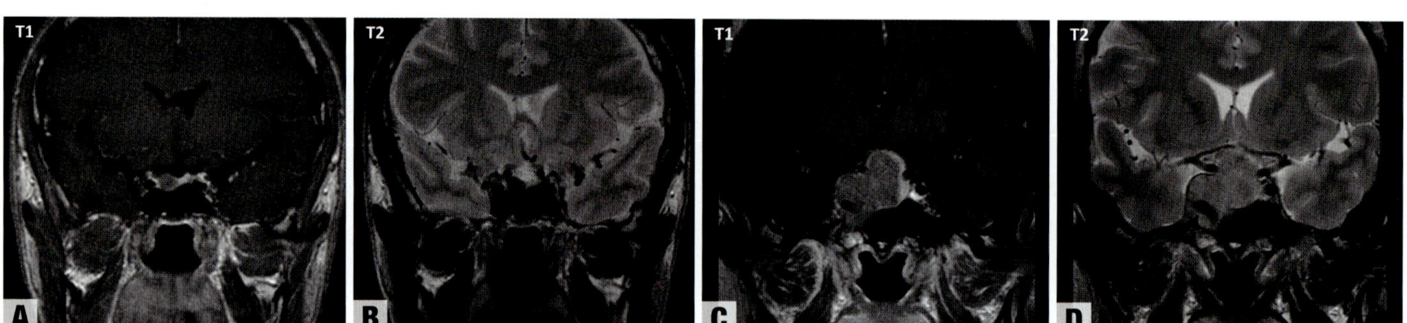

Fig. 2.05 Somatotroph PitNET/adenoma. **A** Enhanced T1-weighted MRI. Densely granulated somatotroph tumour. **B** Plain T2-weighted MRI. Densely granulated somatotroph tumours often show T2 hypointensity. **C** Enhanced T1-weighted MRI. Sparsely granulated somatotroph tumours tend to be invasive macrotumours (Knosp 4 in this case). **D** Plain T2-weighted MRI. Sparsely granulated somatotroph tumours tend to be invasive macrotumours (Knosp 4 in this case) that often show T2 hyperintensity.

low-molecular-weight cytokeratin reactivity patterns: (1) densely granulated somatotroph tumours and (2) sparsely granulated somatotroph tumours. Importantly, the size of the tumour and the age at diagnosis vary with tumour type {197}. Compared with their sparsely granulated counterparts, which are more often large and invasive at presentation, densely granulated somatotroph tumours are smaller, less frequently invade the cavernous sinus, and rarely compress the optic chiasm {3595}. On average, patients with densely granulated somatotroph tumours are 50 years of age at diagnosis, whereas those with sparsely granulated tumours present 10 years earlier {2227, 2530,2561,2322,2961}. The delay may be due to the less rapid and less aggressive growth associated with densely granulated tumours {197}.

Biochemical investigations

Virtually all patients with gigantism and/or acromegaly have increased serum GH and IGF1 levels. Serum IGF1 levels are relatively stable, whereas GH concentrations fluctuate. Oral glucose intake suppresses GH secretion in healthy individuals, but patients with functioning somatotroph tumours lack the characteristic full suppression. Therefore, the biochemical diagnosis of GH hypersecretion is based on an IGF1 level above an established age- and sex- reference range and confirmed by an oral glucose tolerance test where GH level fails to be suppressed below 0.4 µg/L {64,2230}. High IGF1 levels have been reported in pregnancy and the late adolescent period {2230}.

When an ectopic source of GHRH is suspected as the cause of acromegaly {3938,1303,1544}, plasma GHRH over the threshold of 250–300 ng/L has been shown to have excellent specificity {1502,482}. In addition, the absence of GH response to exogenous GHRH may help distinguish GHRH-related acromegaly from a primary somatotroph tumour, because there is typically no response in ectopic acromegaly {482}.

Neuroimaging

Because of the insidious nature of acromegaly, most somatotroph tumours are macrotumours (> 10 mm) at the time of diagnosis {1306,680,3595}; rarely, microtumours can be difficult to identify on conventional MRI studies {2727}. A contrast-enhanced sellar MRI study with T1- and T2-weighted sequences is important in the evaluation of acromegaly {2230}. Radiopathological correlations suggest that densely granulated tumours tend to be hypointense on T2 sequence {1411,1847,3595} and responsive to somatostatin analogues {1308,416,64,2952,2530}. In contrast, sparsely granulated somatotroph tumours are usually hyperintense on T2 sequence {1411,3595,1847,2952,4355} and tend to be resistant to first-generation somatostatin analogue therapy {1308,416,2958,1626,64}.

The normal pituitary shows physiological somatostatin uptake on functional studies (e.g. 68Ga-DOTATATE or 68Ga-DOTATOC PET-CT), complicating assessment of intrasellar tumours. In aggressive somatotroph tumours with an unresectable progressive extrasellar component that fails conventional therapies, functional imaging studies may be considered to rationalize the possibility of somatostatin-based peptide receptor radionuclide therapy (PRRT) {4762}.

A normal or bulky pituitary gland without gadolinium enhancement should prompt GHRH measurement and a search for a GHRH-secreting neoplasm, because this may indicate hyperplasia rather than neoplasia. In young patients with normal MRI and acromegaly, X-linked acrogigantism should also be considered in the differential diagnosis.

Epidemiology

The prevalence of acromegaly is 125–137 cases per 1 million population {974,1682,48}. Gigantism due to GH excess is rare and typically occurs during childhood or puberty, before the closure of the epiphyseal plate {2230,1536}. Somatotroph tumours can arise in all age groups {2961}; however, in acromegaly the median age at diagnosis is 45.2 years, with a slight predominance (54.5%) in women {3539}. As indicated above, the age at diagnosis differs between the two morphological subtypes. At the time of diagnosis, men were significantly younger than women in two series {3539,2039}.

Traditionally, somatotroph tumours were reported to account for about 10–15% of all resected PitNETs {200,88,4512}. In a large Canadian series, somatotroph tumours accounted for about 12% of surgically resected PitNETs {2961}, with almost equal numbers of densely and sparsely granulated subtypes. In several series, the incidence of GH-secreting pituitary tumours is higher (25–35%), but this figure is not limited to pure somatotroph tumours {233,3668}.

Etiology

The etiology is unknown, except for those associated with genetic syndromes (see *Pathogenesis*) {214,452}.

Pathogenesis

Most somatotroph tumours are sporadic and caused by somatic and epigenetic alterations {3208,214}. Somatic activating mutations of *GNAS* (*GNAS1*), which encodes the $G_s\alpha$ subunit of G proteins that mediate the signalling of seven-transmembrane-domain G protein–coupled receptors including GHRH, have been identified in as many as 40–60% of sporadic somatotroph tumours (traditionally called *gsp* mutations), typically in adult patients and frequently in densely granulated somatotroph tumours {5024,1411,2530}. Postzygotic mosaic somatic activating *GNAS* mutations have been also implicated in McCune–Albright syndrome–related pituitary disease {4740, 2956,3910,1626}. These mutations result in constitutive activation of the cAMP/PKA pathway that leads to increased intracytoplasmic cAMP levels, GH hypersecretion, and expression of the α-subunit of glycoprotein hormones in somatotrophs. Although the G protein–mediated high cAMP levels may explain the clinical responsiveness of densely granulated somatotroph tumours to somatostatin analogues, not all densely granulated somatotroph tumours harbour these mutations. Therefore, the histological subtype of a somatotroph tumour is considered to be a better predictor of somatostatin responsiveness than *GNAS* status {2530}. Some authors reported that differential SSTR expression between densely and sparsely granulated somatotroph tumours may also account for the response to somatostatin analogues {2900,2014}. Somatic *GHR* mutations that alter GH autoregulation and STAT signalling have been described in sparsely granulated somatotroph tumours {195,198}.

AIP-related tumours are more commonly identified in young patients and are more frequently sparsely granulated somatotroph tumours {976,361,1038,423}. Somatic *GNAS* mutations were not identified in *AIP*-related PitNETs {1871}, suggesting mutually exclusive aberrant signalling. An acromegalic patient with germline *AIP* mutation has been reported to harbour a mixed gangliocytoma and sparsely granulated somatotroph tumour {3273}.

Epigenetic alterations involving *RB1*, *DAPK1* (*DAPK*), *CDKN2A* (encoding p16), *GADD45G*, *RHBDD3* (*PTAG*), *THBS1* (*TSP1*), *RASSF1* (*RASSF1A*), *FGFR2*, *MGMT*, *CASP8*, *TP73*, and the gene(s) encoding p14 have been described in somatotroph tumours {3479}. However, most of these alterations are not specific to somatotroph tumours {3479}. Downregulation of several microRNAs targeting HMGA1, HMGA2, and E2F1 was also identified {983}. Initially isolated in rat pituitary GH4 cells {3484}, the pituitary tumour transforming gene *PTTG1* (*PTTG*) has been shown to have higher mRNA levels in somatotroph tumours than in non-functioning tumours {1997}. Subsequent studies demonstrated that PTTG expression was indeed higher in various hormone-secreting invasive PitNETs {2965}.

Transcriptome enrichment analyses identified high interferon signatures in somatotroph tumours that were also reflected in specific microRNA clusters, including but not limited to the MEG3 cluster and miR-148a {3208}. *GNAS*-driven tumours were associated with a combination of hypomethylation and chromosomal changes {3208}. Genomic imbalances were previously described at chromosomes 10q, 11q, and 13q {341,2383,1137}. Using whole-genome sequencing, no recurring mutations were seen, but an enrichment of sequence variants affecting the calcium- and ATP-related pathways, as well as chromosomal losses on chromosomes 1, 6, 13, 14, 15, 16, 18, and 22, and chromosomal gains at chromosome 12 and the X chromosome, were documented {4639}.

Dysregulation of FGFRs has been shown to play a role in the tumorigenesis of PitNETs {1311,2965,198}. Ikaros, a chromatin remodelling factor that plays an important role in the development of hypothalamic GHRH neurons {1309}, has been shown to target FGFR4 promoter activity in somatotrophs {1310}. The *FGFR4*-R388 polymorphism plays a role in the correlation between tumour size and hormone excess in somatotroph tumours {4427}.

Genetic susceptibility

About 20% of cases of childhood gigantism and 8–11% of cases of acromegaly in young individuals have been associated with mutation in *AIP*, and in at least half there is a positive family history of familial isolated pituitary adenoma (FIPA) syndrome {976,361,3608,77,1871}. At least 80% of cases of very early onset paediatric gigantism (age < 5 years at diagnosis) have been linked to X-linked acrogigantism due to a microduplication containing the gene *GPR101* {4555,2718}. Patients with pituitary GH excess may also be encountered in the setting of syndromic presentations, such as Carney complex, McCune–Albright syndrome, multiple endocrine neoplasia type 1, and multiple endocrine neoplasia type 4 {3835,452}. In contrast to lactotroph tumours, somatotroph tumours have rarely been encountered in association with germline pathogenic SDH gene variants {1038, 3866}, and they can be seen in association with paraganglioma/phaeochromocytoma {3866}. Rare examples of somatotroph tumours have been reported in association with germline *MAX* mutations (multiple endocrine neoplasia type 5) {973}. A patient with a densely granulated somatotroph tumour was reported to harbour a *TMEM127* variant (c.245-10C>G) {4956}.

Macroscopic appearance

Like other PitNETs, somatotroph tumours are white to grey and distinct from the normal pituitary gland; they are generally soft, explaining the relative preservation of normal pituitary function. Large tumours show variable degrees of invasion into adjacent anatomical structures {3267}. Tumours from patients with pituitary apoplexy exhibit haemorrhagic necrosis. Posttreatment tumours may be firm, owing to variable stromal fibrosis.

Histopathology

In both subtypes, the tumour is positive for GH (details below), diffusely positive for PIT1, and negative for other PIT1-lineage hormones such as prolactin and TSH-β, as well as other pituitary-lineage transcription factors (TPIT, SF1, ERα, GATA3, GATA2) and hormones (ACTH, FSH-β, LH-β) {2961,211}.

Rarely, somatotroph tumours occur in association with gangliocytomas {3273,2730,210}, pituitary hyperplasia, or a distinct synchronous PitNET {4358,3939,2293,2028,5185,2950}.

Densely granulated somatotroph tumours

These tumours are composed of cells that have abundant eosinophilic (acidophilic) cytoplasm, which correlates with their dense content of GH-containing secretory granules. Ultrastructurally, the tumour cells contain abundant large secretory granules measuring 400–600 nm {216}.

Immunohistochemistry

Densely granulated somatotroph tumours are positive for PIT1 (diffuse nuclear staining), GH (diffuse and strong cytoplasmic staining), and the α-subunit of glycoprotein hormones (often diffuse and strong) {2961}. Low-molecular-weight cytokeratin (CAM5.2 or CK18) usually exhibits predominant perinuclear cytoplasmic reactivity {3309,2952,2958,1626,2961,208}. These tumours are negative for CK19 and CK20 {208}.

The term "intermediate-type somatotroph tumour" has been proposed for a subset of densely granulated somatotroph tumours that display occasional (< 70% of the tumour cells and usually only scattered) fibrous bodies, which are defined as spherical juxtanuclear keratin aggregates. These fibrous bodies are usually associated with abundant cytoplasmic keratin filaments, unlike the situation in sparsely granulated tumours. Because intermediate-type somatotroph tumours were found not to be biologically different from densely granulated somatotroph tumours, most experts consider them within the morphological spectrum of densely granulated somatotroph tumours {3309,2952}.

Sparsely granulated somatotroph tumours

These tumours are composed of loosely cohesive cells with chromophobic to pale eosinophilic cytoplasm. Variable nuclear pleomorphism including multinucleated cells can be seen. One of the characteristics of these tumours is the presence of abundant fibrous bodies, which may be recognized on H&E-stained slides, as the nuclei are typically indented by these pale globular eosinophilic structures. Ultrastructurally, sparsely granulated somatotroph tumours contain only a few secretory granules, which range in size from 100 to 250 nm. Fibrous bodies are spherical aggregates of intermediate filaments with trapped secretory granules and endoplasmic reticulum {216}.

Immunohistochemistry

Consistent with the sparse granulation pattern, immunoreactivity for GH is variable and ranges from weak to focal or patchy reactivity {2961}. Unlike densely granulated tumours, these tumours lack α-subunit expression {2382,304,2952,2961}. Because the extent of GH expression can be very scarce or even absent in some sparsely granulated somatotroph tumours, the identification of diffuse fibrous bodies (see below) and the absence of α-subunit, prolactin, and TSH-β can help distinguish sparsely granulated somatotroph tumours from immature PIT1-lineage pituitary tumours.

In sparsely granulated tumours, low-molecular-weight cytokeratins reveal characteristic fibrous bodies in the vast majority (> 70%) of the tumour cells {3309,2952,1626,2961}, with scant or no cytoplasmic positivity outside these structures. A recent study of keratin profiling of PitNETs showed that CK18 expression is less intense, with more delicate staining in fibrous bodies than CAM5.2 {208}. Like all PIT1-lineage pituitary tumours, these tumours are negative for CK19 and CK20 {208}, and unlike densely granulated somatotroph tumours, they show epigenetic downregulation of E-cadherin {4981,3940,3641}, a feature that explains their discohesive growth.

In contrast to densely granulated tumours, the majority of sparsely granulated somatotroph tumours have a Ki-67 labelling index > 3% {2961}.

From a pathogenetic perspective, the application of molecular immunohistochemistry tools may be used to rationalize further germline screening in select tumours as discussed in the introduction to this chapter. Somatotroph tumours with cytoplasmic vacuoles may benefit from SDHB immunohistochemistry {4955, 1582,452}, because a loss of SDHB immunohistochemistry has been regarded as a surrogate biomarker of SDH-driven neoplasms {3375}.

The diagnosis of a sparsely granulated somatotroph tumour in a young patient should prompt genetic testing for *AIP*-related pathogenesis (FIPA syndrome) {361}; however, AIP immunohistochemistry is not recommended, because it is associated with poor sensitivity in the detection of *AIP* mutations {2078}, and this protein is epigenetically downregulated in sporadic tumours.

Although routine SSTR immunohistochemistry is not required for the management of patients with somatotroph tumours, staining for SSTR2 and SSTR5 has been shown to predict responsiveness to somatostatin analogues {1472,3124,907}.

Differential diagnosis

An important differential diagnosis in patients with acromegaly and gigantism is hyperplasia. The distinction between neoplasia and hyperplasia relies on the demonstration of a disrupted reticulin framework in tumours, whereas hyperplasia typically features an expanded but preserved reticulin framework {2952}

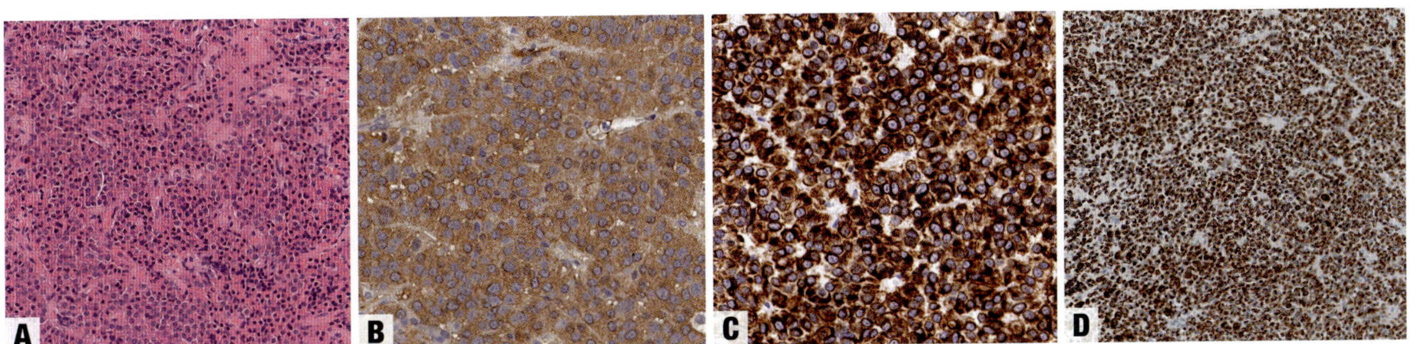

Fig. 2.06 Somatotroph PitNET/adenoma. **A** This densely granulated somatotroph tumour is composed of cells that have abundant eosinophilic (acidophilic) cytoplasm. **B** Densely granulated somatotroph tumour showing diffuse positivity for growth hormone, a finding consistent with the dense content of growth hormone–containing secretory granules in these tumours. **C** Densely granulated somatotroph tumours show predominant perinuclear reactivity for CAM5.2. **D** Scattered fibrous bodies in the background of predominant perinuclear CAM5.2 expression in a densely granulated somatotroph tumour. The term "intermediate-type somatotroph tumour" has been proposed for a subset of densely granulated somatotroph tumours that display occasional fibrous bodies. These tumours are considered within the morphological spectrum of densely granulated somatotroph tumours.

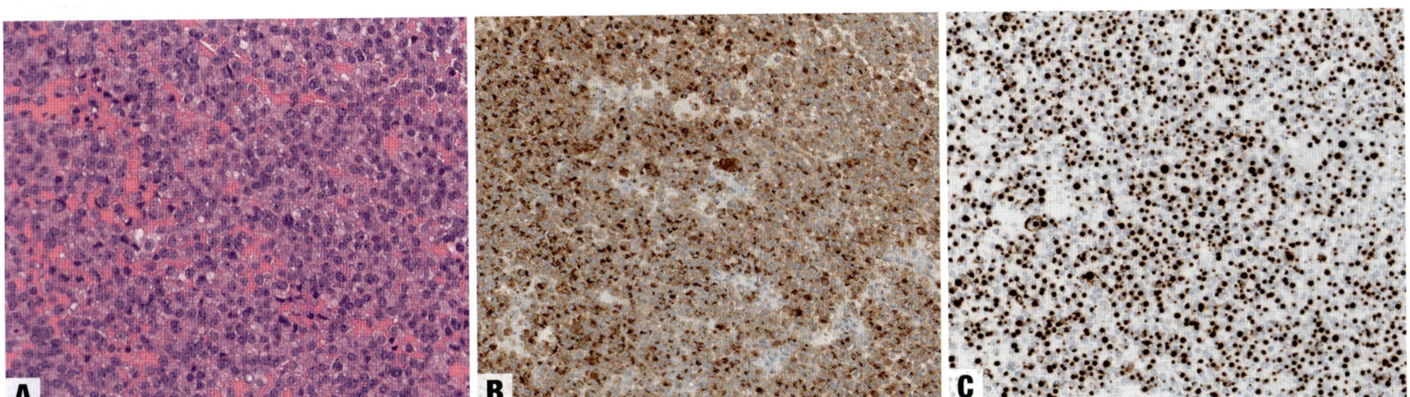

Fig. 2.07 Somatotroph PitNET/adenoma. **A** Sparsely granulated somatotroph tumours are composed of cells with chromophobic to pale eosinophilic cytoplasm. One of the characteristics of these tumours is the presence of abundant fibrous bodies. In this photomicrograph, these eosinophilic globular fibrous bodies indent the tumour nuclei. **B** Growth hormone expression is often reduced in sparsely granulated somatotroph tumours, consistent with their sparse granulation pattern. **C** Unlike in densely granulated somatotroph tumours, CAM5.2 staining shows predominant (> 70%) fibrous bodies in sparsely granulated somatotroph tumours.

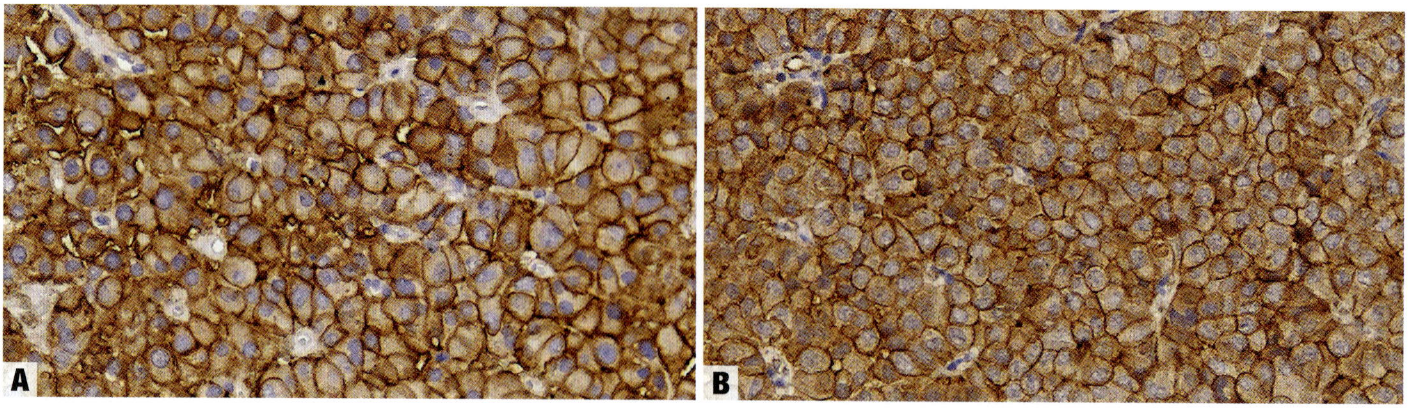

Fig. 2.08 Somatotroph PitNET/adenoma. A densely granulated somatotroph tumour showing diffuse strong reactivity for SSTR2 (**A**) and SSTR5 (**B**); this patient had a good response to first-line somatostatin analogues.

usually associated with trapped non-tumorous adenohypophysial cells of all types. The presence of somatotroph or mammosomatotroph hyperplasia in association with a neoplasm may be a harbinger of a GHRH-producing neoplasm or genetic conditions such as Carney complex, McCune–Albright syndrome {3625,4740,3917,3910,1626}, FIPA {4706}, or X-linked acrogigantism {4555}. Somatotroph hyperplasia is uncommon in patients with multiple endocrine neoplasia type 1, but when it occurs in this setting, it is frequently caused by a GHRH-producing pancreatic neuroendocrine tumour (PanNET) {4559, 219}. Nonetheless, it should be noted that hyperplasia is only rarely encountered in surgical pituitary specimens. Similarly, the association of GHRH-producing phaeochromocytoma/paraganglioma and pituitary acromegaly has been reported in a patient with germline pathogenic *MAX* variant (multiple endocrine neoplasia type 5) {4047}. A rare GHRH-producing pulmonary neuroendocrine tumour (NET) metastatic to the pituitary associated with somatotroph hyperplasia and adenomatous transformation has also been reported {3195}.

Cytology

Functioning somatotroph tumours usually do not require intraoperative consultation; however, when performed, it should be done by a smear that yields an even cellular spread. Densely granulated somatotroph tumours have abundant acidophilic granular cytoplasm; sparsely granulated somatotroph tumours have distinctive fibrous bodies identifiable on smears.

Diagnostic molecular pathology

There are no molecular tests required to diagnose somatotroph tumours. Germline screening for inherited somatotroph tumours should be considered on the basis of clinicopathological findings.

Essential and desirable diagnostic criteria

Densely granulated somatotroph tumours

Essential: PIT1 positivity; diffuse GH expression; absence of other pituitary cell differentiation; perinuclear low-molecular-weight cytokeratin staining; acidophilic cytoplasm on H&E-stained sections.

Desirable: α-subunit expression.

Sparsely granulated somatotroph tumours

Essential: PIT1 positivity; variable GH expression; absence of other pituitary cell differentiation; abundant fibrous bodies (> 70% of the tumour cells) using low-molecular-weight cytokeratin stains; absence of acidophilic cytoplasm on H&E-stained sections.

Desirable: absence of α-subunit expression.

Staging

There is no formal staging system that has been universally applied for pituitary/sellar neoplasms. A CT-era approach based on tumour size and patterns of invasion was proposed in 1973 by Hardy {1786}. Subsequently, a standardized assessment of parasellar tumour invasiveness based on MRI was published by Knosp in 1993 {2354}. There are no pathology-standardized reporting templates yet endorsed by international pathology organizations. A pathology reporting template for pituitary tumours was introduced in 2011 {3300}, followed by the European Pituitary Pathology Group (EPPG) proposal in 2019 {4707}.

Prognosis and prediction

Uncontrolled GH and/or IGF1 secretion causes significant morbidity in patients with functioning somatotroph tumours. Although the first-line treatment option for somatotroph tumours is surgical resection {3267}, cure often cannot be achieved, particularly in large tumours and those with cavernous sinus invasion {3267}. Therefore, the completeness of tumour resection and degree of extrasellar tumour extension, the histological subtype (densely granulated vs sparsely granulated somatotroph tumour), tumour growth rate (e.g. residual tumour growth on imaging studies), and response to medical therapy are all important prognostic factors {2965,2958,1626,1304,4355}.

The accurate histological subtyping of a somatotroph tumour is of clinical significance, because pharmacological GH antagonism with pegvisomant is considered in patients with sparsely granulated tumours, which often lack satisfactory responsiveness to somatostatin analogues {2958,2561,1626}. The tumour subtype on histopathology that correlates with T2 hyperintensity on MRI studies {1411,1847,3595} and the status of SSTR2/5 expression are well-recognized predictors of responsiveness to somatostatin analogues {1472,3124,907}.

Mammosomatotroph PitNET/adenoma

Mete O
Grossman AB
Perry A
Yamada S

Chapter 2

Definition
Mammosomatotroph pituitary neuroendocrine tumour (PitNET)/adenoma is a well-differentiated PitNET composed of PIT1-lineage adenohypophysial cells with mammosomatotroph differentiation.

ICD-O coding
8280/3 Mammosomatotroph PitNET/adenoma

ICD-11 coding
2D12.Y Other specified malignant neoplasms of other endocrine glands or related structures

Related terminology
Acceptable: mammosomatotroph tumour.
Not recommended: growth hormone and prolactin–positive PitNET/adenoma; growth hormone and prolactin–producing PitNET/adenoma; growth hormone and prolactin–producing tumour/adenoma.

Subtype(s)
None

Localization
These tumours are located in the sellar region and show variable extension into adjacent structures, including but not limited to the cavernous sinuses {2768}.

Clinical features
With the exception of hyperprolactinaemia, mammosomatotroph tumours often show similar clinical features to densely granulated somatotroph tumours; they manifest with macrotumours and elevated growth hormone (GH) / IGF1 levels {1944, 2768,64}. Serum prolactin levels are often lower than in mixed lactotroph and somatotroph tumours {2768}. Cystic changes may occur {4670}. Patients with mammosomatotroph tumours are significantly less likely to present with abnormal glucose metabolism than those with pure somatotroph tumours, independent of GH/IGF1 levels or tumour invasiveness {790}.

Epidemiology
Mammosomatotroph tumours account for 1.1–2% of surgically resected PitNETs {3877,2961} and represent about 7% of PIT1-lineage tumours {2961}. These tumours are more frequent in young adults and children than other PitNETs {3154,64}. The median age at diagnosis is 44 years, and there is no sex predilection {2768}.

Etiology
The etiology is unknown, except for those associated with genetic syndromes {214,452}. Mammosomatotroph tumours can occur in patients with Carney complex, familial isolated pituitary adenoma (FIPA; including patients positive for *AIP* mutation), X-linked acrogigantism, McCune–Albright syndrome, and multiple endocrine neoplasia type 1 {214,452}.

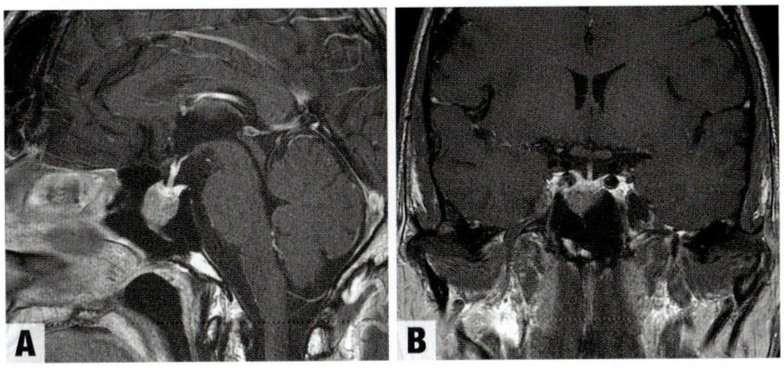

Fig. 2.09 Mammosomatotroph tumour. Preoperative T1-weighted sagittal (**A**) and coronal (**B**) MRI from a 32-year-old male patient with a microtumour that had a final pathological diagnosis of mammosomatotroph tumour.

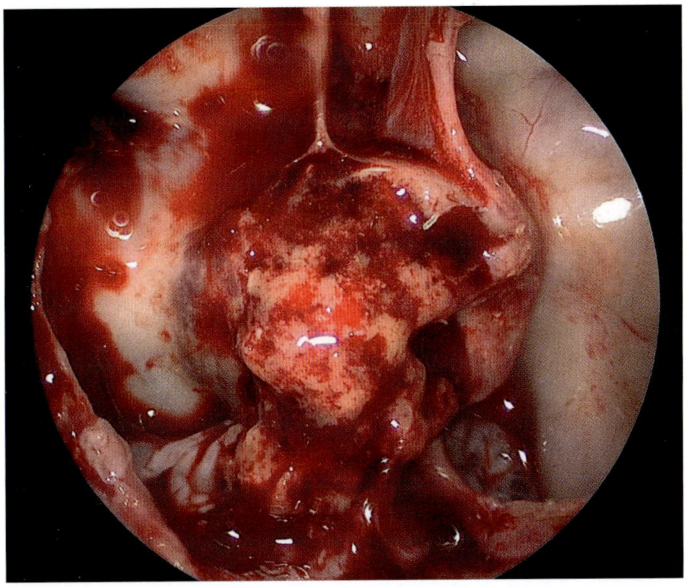

Fig. 2.10 Mammosomatotroph tumour (intraoperative gross findings). A macrotumour extending mainly into the sphenoidal sinus with dural invasion and destruction of the sellar floor, as depicted by the intraoperative photograph.

Pathogenesis
Synchronous GH/prolactin-producing tumours were clustered together with somatotroph tumours in genomic studies where the distinction of mammosomatotroph tumour was not made {3208}.

Macroscopic appearance
These tumours are soft and white to grey.

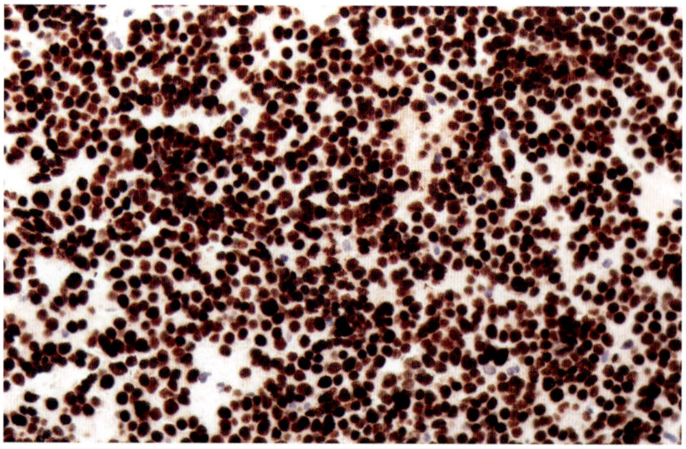

Fig. 2.11 Mammosomatotroph tumour. These tumours are diffusely positive for the transcription factor PIT1.

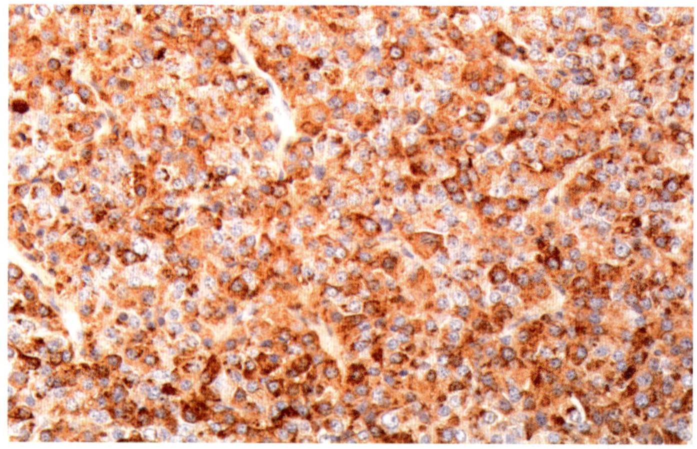

Fig. 2.12 Mammosomatotroph tumour. These tumours are composed of a single monomorphic cell population that often shows diffuse growth hormone immunoreactivity.

Histopathology

Mammosomatotroph tumours consist of a monomorphic population of cells with densely eosinophilic (acidophilic) cytoplasm packed with secretory granules containing both GH and prolactin. Ultrastructurally, these tumours show pleomorphic and heterogeneous secretory granules ranging from 150 to 1000 nm, and misplaced exocytosis {216}.

Immunohistochemistry

These tumours are positive for PIT1, ER, GH, prolactin, and α-subunit, and negative for TSH, GATA3, TPIT, SF1 and other pituitary hormones {2952,1626,2961,211,2971,197}. The extent of prolactin immunoreactivity is usually less than that of GH {3877,2972}. CAM5.2 and CK18 typically show perinuclear staining {2961,208}. The Ki-67 labelling index is variable {2768}.

Differential diagnosis

Acidophilic cytoplasm and coexpression of GH and prolactin in the same tumour cell distinguish mammosomatotroph tumours from mixed lactotroph and somatotroph tumours that are composed of two distinct tumour populations. Absence of TSH and/or GATA3 expression in mammosomatotroph tumours distinguishes these tumours from mature plurihormonal PIT1-lineage PitNETs. The cytomorphology and extent of PIT1-lineage hormone expression also distinguishes these tumours from immature plurihormonal PIT1-lineage PitNETs {2966,2972, 2957}. The lack of oncocytic cytomorphology, absence of cytoplasmic vacuoles, lack of fibrous bodies, and predominance of GH expression distinguish mammosomatotroph tumours from acidophil stem cell tumours {2972}.

Cytology

Cytologically, these tumours are indistinguishable from densely granulated somatotroph tumours and mature plurihormonal PIT1-lineage tumours.

Diagnostic molecular pathology

Molecular testing is not required for the diagnosis of mammosomatotroph tumours. Germline screening should be considered on the basis of clinicopathological findings.

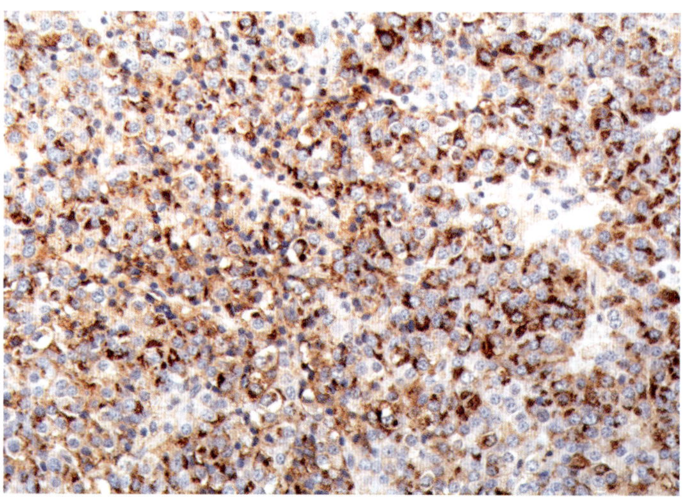

Fig. 2.13 Mammosomatotroph tumour. These tumours consist of a monomorphic cell population with both growth hormone–containing and prolactin-containing secretory granules. The extent of prolactin immunoreactivity (shown here) is usually smaller than that of growth hormone.

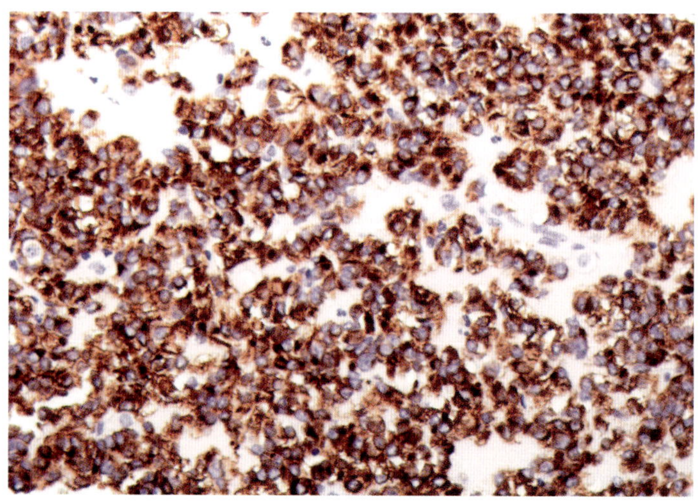

Fig. 2.14 Mammosomatotroph tumour. Similarly to densely granulated somatotroph tumours, mammosomatotroph tumours show perinuclear CAM5.2 immunoreactivity.

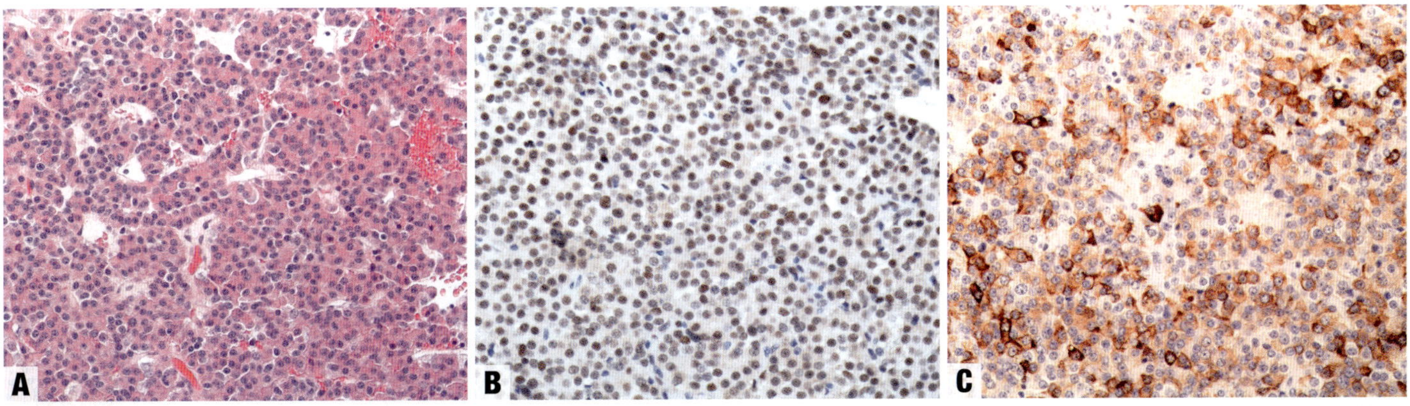

Fig. 2.15 Mammosomatotroph tumour. **A** The tumour consists of a monomorphic (single cell type) cell population with densely eosinophilic (acidophilic) cytoplasm. **B** Unlike somatotroph tumours, mammosomatotroph tumours often show near-diffuse ER expression. **C** Unlike lactotroph tumours, mammosomatotroph tumours often show α-subunit immunoreactivity.

Essential and desirable diagnostic criteria

Essential: PIT1 positivity and coexpression of GH and prolactin in the same tumour cell; monomorphic tumour cell population with acidophilic cytoplasm.

Desirable: ER and α-subunit expression; perinuclear CAM5.2 positivity.

Staging

There is no formal staging system that has been universally applied for pituitary/sellar neoplasms. A CT-era approach based on tumour size and patterns of invasion was proposed in 1973 by Hardy {1786}. Subsequently, a standardized assessment of parasellar tumour extension based on MRI was published by Knosp in 1993 {2354}.

There are no pathology-standardized reporting templates yet endorsed by international pathology organizations. A pathology reporting template for pituitary tumours was introduced in 2011 {3300}, followed by the European Pituitary Pathology Group (EPPG) proposal in 2019 {4707}.

Prognosis and prediction

Limited available data underscore that these tumours are associated with a lower frequency of Knosp grade 3–4 disease {3154,2768} and a higher frequency of gross total resection and remission {3154,2768}, especially when compared with mixed lactotroph and somatotroph tumours {2768}. The Ki-67 labelling index showed no impact on long-term remission in 1 study {2768}. Therefore, the completeness of tumour resection and response to medical therapies may be considered prognostic factors for these tumours.

Lactotroph PitNET/adenoma

Perry A
Grossman AB
Lopes MBS
Nishioka H
Uccella S

Definition

Lactotroph pituitary neuroendocrine tumour (PitNET)/adenoma is a well-differentiated PitNET composed of PIT1-lineage adenohypophysial cells with lactotroph differentiation.

ICD-O coding

8271/3 Lactotroph PitNET/adenoma
8271/3 Sparsely granulated lactotroph tumour
8271/3 Densely granulated lactotroph tumour

ICD-11 coding

2D12.Y Other specified malignant neoplasms of other endocrine glands or related structures

Related terminology

Acceptable: lactotroph tumour.

Not recommended: prolactinoma; prolactin-producing PitNET/adenoma; prolactin-secreting PitNET/adenoma; lactotroph cell PitNET/adenoma; PRLoma.

Subtype(s)

Sparsely granulated lactotroph tumour (SGLT); densely granulated lactotroph tumour (DGLT)

Localization

The majority of lactotroph tumours are intrasellar, with microtumours usually localized to the posterolateral anterior pituitary. Macrotumours are often invasive, extending to suprasellar and parasellar structures, including the cavernous and sphenoidal sinuses, and these tumours may present as a nasal mass {2004}. Ectopic examples are rare but have been reported in the sphenoidal sinus and parapharyngeal regions {3683,2276, 2713,4100}; in the clivus, middle nasal meatus, temporal bone, hypothalamus, and third ventricle {3683,2889,2332,138}; and in the parasellar/suprasellar compartments {1197,1939}. Rare examples have also arisen within ovarian teratomas {1231,79, 1720}.

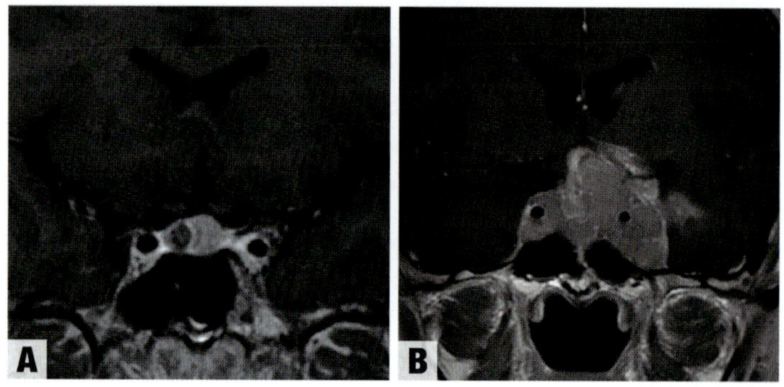

Fig. 2.16 Lactotroph PitNET/adenoma. **A** Coronal MRI showing a hypodense intrasellar microtumour from a 22-year-old woman. **B** Coronal MRI showing an aggressive macrotumour from a 49-year-old man, which initially responded well to cabergoline but then became refractory. Surgical resection revealed a sparsely granulated lactotroph tumour with an increased mitotic count and a high Ki-67 labelling index.

Clinical features

Lactotroph tumours frequently cause reproductive and sexual dysfunction, with clinical manifestations differing according to patient sex {394,4557,3268}. The most common symptoms in women with lactotroph tumours are galactorrhoea, ovulatory disorders, and amenorrhoea. In men, when symptoms are present (e.g. erectile dysfunction and decreased libido), they can be subtle, often resulting in delayed diagnosis. Men mostly present with macrotumours (> 10 mm in greatest dimension), whereas women tend to present at a younger age with microtumours that in general rarely grow, even in the absence of treatment {1072,2772}. Treatment is based on symptom control and the correction of estrogen deficiency due to hyperprolactinaemia. Lactotroph tumours are less common in men, but 80% are macrotumours, often presenting with mass effects causing visual

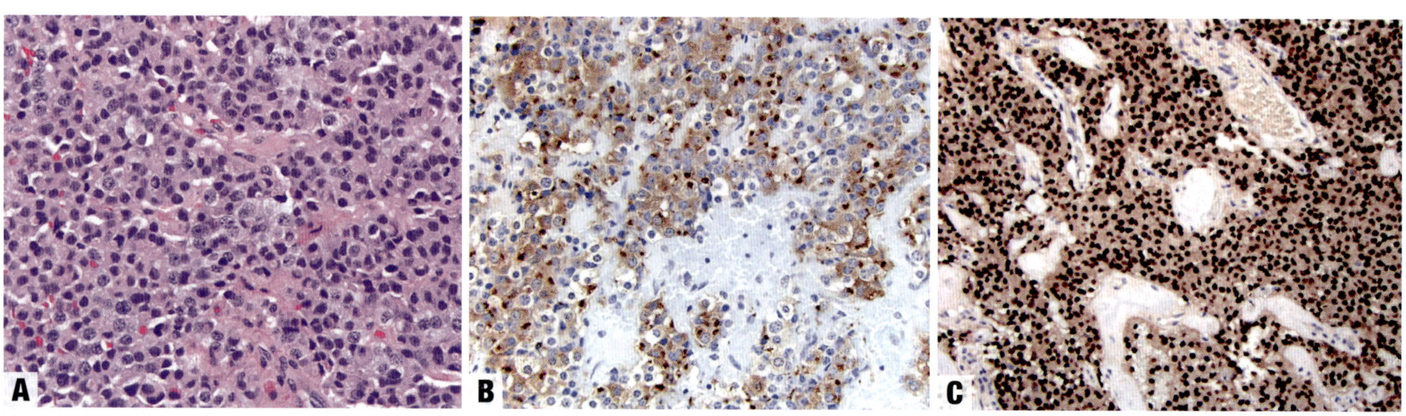

Fig. 2.17 Lactotroph PitNET/adenoma, sparsely granulated. **A** A PitNET with mostly chromophobic tumour cells, in this case arranged in sheets. **B** Prolactin immunostain showing mostly paranuclear Golgi-pattern (spherical) staining. **C** Diffuse nuclear immunoreactivity for PIT1.

field abnormalities (~45%), hypopituitarism (~35%), and/or sexual dysfunction {1072,1073}; galactorrhoea is rare. Patients with very large tumours may present with pituitary apoplexy.

Paediatric lactotroph tumours often cause primary amenorrhoea and delayed puberty. Approximately 60–80% present as macrotumours with symptoms of mass effect {2334,2026, 3909,2698,1487}, and in paediatric patients, a germline genetic tumour syndrome should always be sought.

Biochemical investigations

Serum prolactin levels are roughly proportional to tumour size, with greater pretreatment serum levels often encountered in men, due at least in part to their larger tumour sizes at presentation {3268,2772}. Patients with lactotroph microtumours (< 10 mm in greatest dimension) generally have serum prolactin levels of 100–250 ng/mL. Elevated prolactin levels (> 25 ng/mL in women and > 20 ng/mL in men) up to 100 ng/mL may be caused by drugs or stalk effect, the latter resulting from tumoural compression of the pituitary stalk, which blocks the normal dopaminergic inhibition of lactotrophs. Serum prolactin levels of > 250 ng/mL typically indicate an underlying lactotroph macrotumour. Giant lactotroph tumours (> 40 mm in greatest dimension) may yield prolactin levels of > 1000 ng/mL {2688, 2799,4124}.

Neuroimaging

Microtumours are subtle and may be difficult to diagnose on MRI. On precontrast T1-weighted sequences, they are generally hypointense relative to surrounding pituitary. After gadolinium administration, they often appear non-enhancing in the early phase but contrast-enhancing in later phases. Macrotumours may show evidence of prior haemorrhage and a suprasellar component, as well as invasion inferiorly into paranasal sinuses and adjacent structures {2004}. Microcalcification and cystic changes are also occasionally observed.

Epidemiology

Lactotroph tumours are the most common PitNETs overall, accounting for as many as half of all cases in postmortem and prevalence series {2418,974,2952,4512}. By far the most common subtype is SGLT {2952,2958}, but the incidence has diminished considerably in surgical series because of successful medical therapy with dopamine agonists. In modern surgical series, lactotroph tumours typically account for < 30% of all cases, and in 1 series it was as low as 2% {3668}. Lactotroph tumours present most often in young adult women (aged 21–40 years). In some studies, the lactotroph tumour is also the most common PitNET of childhood and adolescence, with frequencies of 41–52% {3450,2450,2698}. However, in a more recent literature review of 1284 resected paediatric pituitary tumours, a slightly lower frequency of 37% lactotroph tumours was found, with the frequency of corticotroph tumours being higher at 43% {3529}; this may again reflect the greater use of dopamine agonist therapy.

Etiology

The etiology of lactotroph PitNETs is unknown in the majority of cases. However, estrogens may play an etiological role in experimental models and during pregnancy. Additionally, a small subset arise in the setting of genetic tumour syndromes such as familial isolated pituitary adenomas (FIPAs) and others (discussed further below) {591,423,1087}.

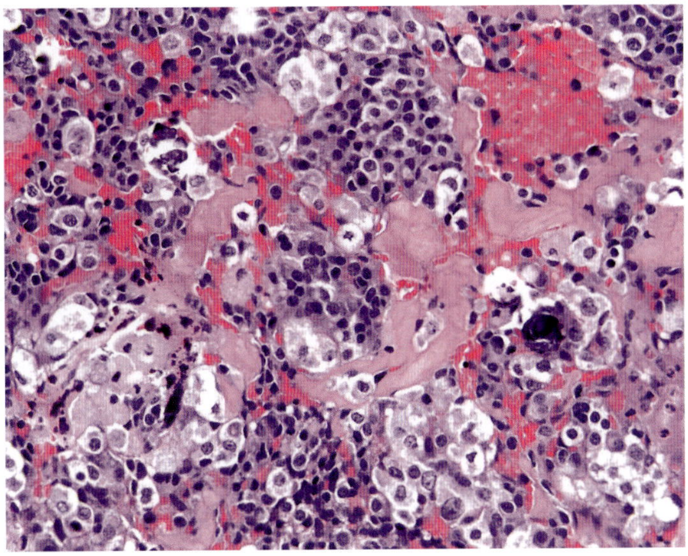

Fig. 2.18 Lactotroph PitNET/adenoma, sparsely granulated. Scattered psammoma bodies and perivascular/interstitial fibrosis.

Pathogenesis

Although recurrent somatic gene alterations are generally uncommon, *SF3B1* p.R625H hotspot mutations have recently been identified in roughly 20% of lactotroph tumours; compared with non-mutant tumours, they were associated with higher prolactin levels and shorter progression-free survival times {2627}. Rare sporadic macrotumours have also shown somatic *SDHA* mutations {1582} and *SDHD* loss of heterozygosity {3410}. Non-specific chromosomal alterations (gains more common than losses) are seen in about half of all lactotroph tumours and do not appear to be associated with aggressiveness {3208}. However, in one study, loss of chromosome 11 was reported in 2 aggressive and 3 metastatic lactotroph tumours {4878}. A large genomic study also revealed that lactotroph tumours harbour relatively unique epigenomic and transcriptional signatures, including high expression levels of MYC targets and DRD2 {3208}.

Like other PitNETs/adenomas, lactotroph tumours may also show abnormal expression of growth regulatory molecules and their receptors, intracellular signal transduction proteins, and cell-cycle regulatory molecules. A variety of etiological factors have been implicated {201,200,1301}. Epigenetic alterations involving *CDKN2A*, *RB1*, *DAPK1*, *GADD45G*, *THBS1* (*TSP1*), *RASSF1* (*RASSF1A*), *FGFR2*, *MGMT*, *CASP8*, *TP73*, and the gene(s) encoding p14 have also been described {958,3479}, but they are not considered specific to lactotroph tumours {3479}.

Familial disease

Approximately 5% of all PitNETs/adenomas arise in the setting of a germline gene variant {2854}. The syndromes include FIPA {4690,1871,423}, multiple endocrine neoplasia syndrome type 1 (where lactotroph tumours are most common) and type 4

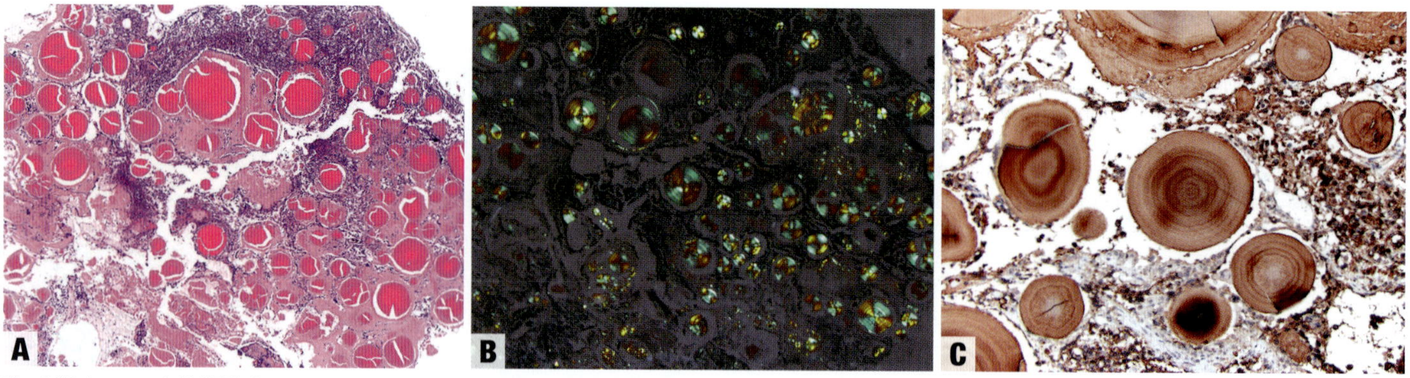

Fig. 2.19 Lactotroph PitNET/adenoma, sparsely granulated. **A** Spherical amyloid collections are seen in rare lactotroph tumours. **B** A Congo red stain with polarization highlights apple-green birefringence. **C** A prolactin immunostain highlights both the tumour cells and the amyloid.

(where lactotroph tumours are second most common), and multiple endocrine neoplasia type 5, with a germline *MAX* mutation {4559,958,4444,882,4047,1087}. More rarely, McCune–Albright syndrome, *GPR101* microduplication–related X-linked acrogigantism syndrome {363}, SDH-related syndromes {1088, 591,1087}, and Carney complex {571,975,972} are implicated {3293}. In FIPA cases due to mutations of *AIP* (~20% of all FIPAs), somatotroph and mixed somatotroph–lactotroph tumours are most common, but pure lactotroph PitNETs/adenomas account for roughly 14.5% of associated cases; in contrast to their sporadic counterparts, they tend to be large, aggressive tumours that respond poorly to dopamine agonists, are more often encountered in young patients, show a male predominance, and are more likely to undergo apoplexy {2854,423}. Considered another way, roughly 11.5% of all patients aged < 30 years with a lactotroph macrotumour harbour a germline *AIP* variant, thus emphasizing the importance of genetic screening in young patients {4495}. Lactotroph tumours are also common within the larger group of *AIP*-wildtype FIPA patients {1087}.

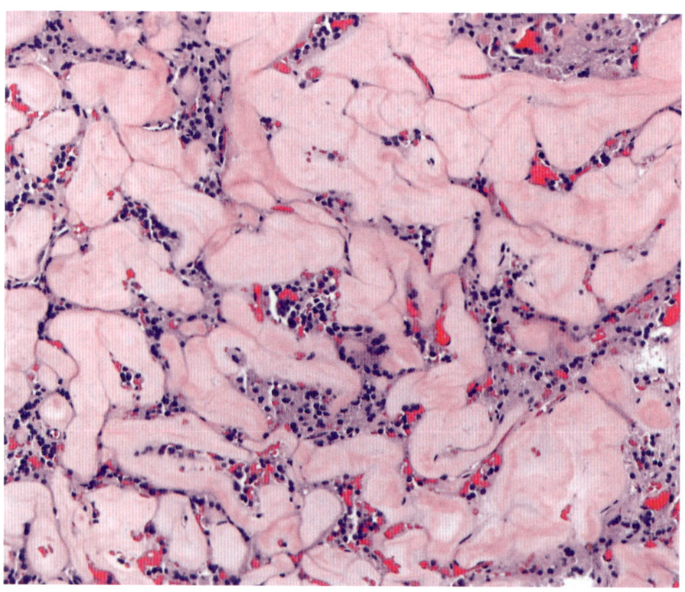

Fig. 2.20 Lactotroph PitNET/adenoma, sparsely granulated after medical therapy. This sparsely granulated lactotroph tumour that was resected after therapy with a dopamine agonist shows extensive perivascular and interstitial fibrosis, along with small cell change due to loss of tumour cytoplasm.

Macroscopic appearance

Microtumours are expansile, compressive lesions that can usually be distinguished from normal anterior pituitary by their soft consistency, red to tan appearance, and pseudocapsule. Rare examples are firm and grey to white, with an abundant collagenous and/or amyloid-rich stroma. Some have indistinct margins and a more invasive growth pattern. Macrotumours are usually widely invasive into adjacent structures. Fibrosis, cystic changes, and calcification can be seen in macrotumours, as well as in previously treated tumours {4435}.

Histopathology

Lactotroph tumours are divided into two subtypes, the common SGLT and the rare DGLT, the latter representing 1.2–10% of all lactotroph tumours in large series {2961,3874}. They must also be distinguished from the rare and aggressive acidophil stem cell tumour (see separate section). Those with apoplexy show extensive haemorrhagic necrosis, and it may be difficult to find viable tumour to assess with immunostains. Nevertheless, even in necrotic areas, a reticulin histochemical stain highlights the typical loss of the normal adenohypophysial microacinar pattern that is characteristic of a PitNET, and in most examples there is sufficient viable tumour, at least focally, to establish lactotroph differentiation with immunostains.

SGLT is composed of chromophobic tumour cells that display a large variety of growth patterns, including diffuse, solid, trabecular, papillary, and pseudopapillary architecture. Elongated cells with indistinct cell membranes can also be encountered. Nuclear pleomorphism is uncommon. Psammoma bodies are occasionally seen. Rare examples feature interstitial fibrosis or amyloid spherules that stain with Congo red and show apple-green birefringence with polarized light; the amyloidogenic hormone is also immunoreactive for prolactin {4272,1705,276, 2617}. Ultrastructurally, the tumour cells display well-developed Golgi complexes and rough endoplasmic reticulum forming concentric whorls, and sparse secretory granules measuring 150–300 nm. The hallmark ultrastructural finding in lactotroph tumours is misplaced exocytosis, characterized by extrusion of secretory granules along the lateral cell surfaces {216}.

DGLT is composed of tumour cells with densely acidophilic cytoplasm. Ultrastructurally, the tumour cells have less rough endoplasmic reticulum and more abundant secretory granules, some reaching as large as 700 nm. Misplaced exocytosis may nevertheless be seen.

Immunohistochemistry

These tumours are composed of sparsely granulated cells that resemble normal lactotrophs, and display a characteristic paranuclear globular, Golgi-type staining pattern for prolactin {200, 2952,2958,1626}. The tumour cells are also positive for PIT1 and ERα {200,2952,2958,1626}, although depending on levels of fixation and the antibody used, ERα staining may be weak or absent {2952,4558}. They are usually negative for the α-subunit of glycoprotein hormones and for cytokeratin CAM5.2. The Ki-67 proliferation index is usually low, but it can be higher in clinically more aggressive lactotroph tumours.

DGLT cells show strong and diffuse cytoplasmic prolactin expression {200,2952,2958,1626}, along with nuclear PIT1 and ER positivity.

Morphological effects of dopamine agonists

The use of dopamine agonists (e.g. bromocriptine or cabergoline) usually results in a rapid decrease in serum prolactin level followed by tumour shrinkage and variable, but often dramatic, histopathological changes. The cells can become much smaller, with minimal cytoplasm and increased N:C ratios. The nuclei are hyperchromatic. In patients on long-term treatment, extensive perivascular and interstitial fibrosis is common, as is evidence of prior haemorrhage {4272}. Single-cell necrosis is rare. Prolactin immunostaining can be greatly diminished, with some cases showing only limited positivity in scattered cells. However, other cells may appear unaltered by the therapy, and regional variability in treatment effects is common. For those with the most extensive posttherapy changes, lactotroph tumours may be mistaken for lymphoma, plasmacytoma, metastatic small cell carcinoma, or other small round cell tumours. However, the coexpression of prolactin, PIT1, and ER separates these tumours from their pathological mimics. The morphological alterations are usually rapidly reversible upon drug discontinuation, although scattered cells may retain their treatment effects long after {4272}.

Cytology

Lactotroph tumours are mostly indistinguishable from other PitNETs.

Diagnostic molecular pathology

Mutation-specific immunostains and molecular pathology studies are not routinely performed on lactotroph tumours, although germline screening may be indicated in younger patients (see *Prognosis and prediction*, below).

Essential and desirable diagnostic criteria

Essential: a PitNET with immunoreactivity for PIT1; extensive prolactin immunoreactivity; absence of other pituitary hormone staining; juxtanuclear staining for prolactin in the sparsely granulated subtype.

Desirable: immunoreactivity for ER; lack of α-subunit expression.

Staging

There is no formal staging system that has been universally applied for pituitary/sellar neoplasms. A CT-era approach based on tumour size and patterns of invasion was proposed in 1973 by Hardy {1786}. Subsequently, a standardized assessment of parasellar tumour extension based on MRI was published by Knosp in 1993 {2354}.

There are no pathology-standardized reporting templates yet endorsed by international pathology organizations. A pathology reporting template for pituitary tumours was introduced in 2011 {3300}, followed by the European Pituitary Pathology Group (EPPG) proposal in 2019 {4707}.

Prognosis and prediction

At younger ages, women tend to have microtumours, and in general these rarely grow, even in the absence of treatment. Treatment is based on symptom control and the correction of estrogen deficiency due to hyperprolactinaemia. The prognosis for lactotroph tumours is worse in men than women; this may be because the tumours are typically larger at presentation, more invasive, and generally more aggressive. This biology potentially reflects the fact that tumours in men are characterized by lower ER expression, which is generally related to higher tumour grade using the French scheme {4560}, resistance to treatment, and a worse overall prognosis {1073,2972,2694, 4877,4558}. Pharmacotherapy with dopamine agonists is the standard of care for initial treatment, with dramatic decreases

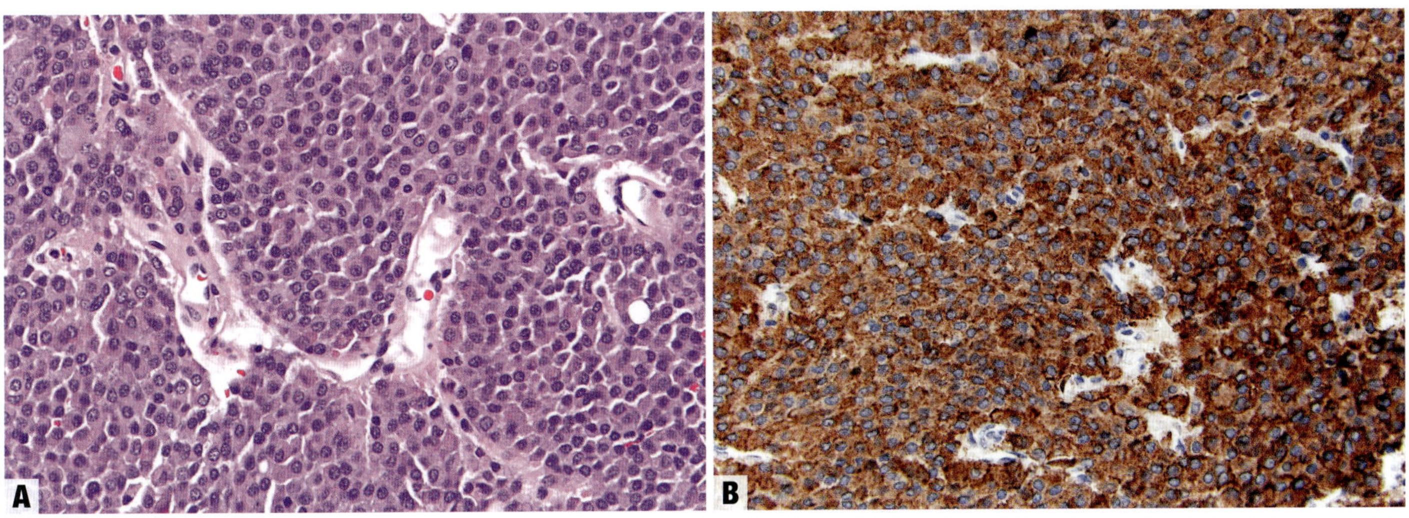

Fig. 2.21 Lactotroph PitNET/adenoma, densely granulated. **A** Acidophilic cells reflecting a densely granulated cytoplasm. **B** Extensive granular cytoplasmic immunoreactivity pattern for prolactin.

in hormone levels and subsequent tumour shrinkage typically following. Cabergoline is the main agent currently used for treating lactotroph tumours, successfully bringing prolactin levels back within the normal range in 80–90% of patients. However, because this agent merely inhibits hormone production and is cytostatic rather than cytotoxic, regrowth of tumour may resume immediately after discontinuation of medical therapy; nonetheless, there is a significant long-term permanent remission rate. Patients who have invasive macrotumours with resistance to pharmacotherapy or who are intolerant to medications may require transsphenoidal surgery {4194}. Radiotherapy or (in rare circumstances) chemotherapy with temozolomide may be considered for recurrent aggressive and invasive tumours that fail both surgical intervention and conventional drug therapies.

Genetic screening should be considered for patients with a lactotroph microtumour diagnosed before the age of 18 years or a macrotumour diagnosed before the age of 30 years; furthermore, *AIP*-mutant FIPA-associated tumours do better when diagnosed prospectively through screening, rather than when first detected from clinical symptoms; not surprisingly, the tumours detected through screening tend to be smaller, less invasive, and easier to resect {4495,2854}.

Thyrotroph PitNET/adenoma

Perry A
Grossman AB
Lopes MBS
Uccella S
Yamada S

Definition

Thyrotroph pituitary neuroendocrine tumour (PitNET)/adenoma is a well-differentiated PitNET composed of PIT1-lineage adenohypophysial cells with thyrotroph differentiation.

ICD-O coding

8272/3 Thyrotroph PitNET/adenoma

ICD-11 coding

2D12.Y Other specified malignant neoplasms of other endocrine glands or related structures

Related terminology

Acceptable: thyrotroph tumour.

Not recommended: TSH-producing PitNET/adenoma; TSH-secreting PitNET/adenoma; thyrotropin-secreting PitNET/adenoma; thyrotrope PitNET/adenoma; thyrotroph cell PitNET/adenoma; thyrotropinoma; TSHoma.

Subtype(s)

None

Localization

Most thyrotroph tumours present as macrotumours, commonly invading inferolaterally into the cavernous sinuses. Ectopic cases have been reported in the nasopharynx and sphenoidal sinus {905,4224,3363}.

Clinical features

Thyrotroph tumours may be associated with hyperthyroidism (central form), hypothyroidism, or (rarely) euthyroidism {2952}. A subset of tumours may present as non-functioning tumours with signs and symptoms of mass effect, including headaches and visual deficits {960}.

Biochemical investigations

Primary hyperthyroidism is characteristically associated with undetectable serum TSH levels, in contrast to central hyperthyroidism associated with a thyrotroph PitNET/adenoma and non-suppressible serum TSH excess called syndrome of inappropriate secretion of TSH (SITSH). In cases of longstanding primary hypothyroidism, thyrotroph hyperplasia causing increased serum TSH excess is most common; however, rare examples of

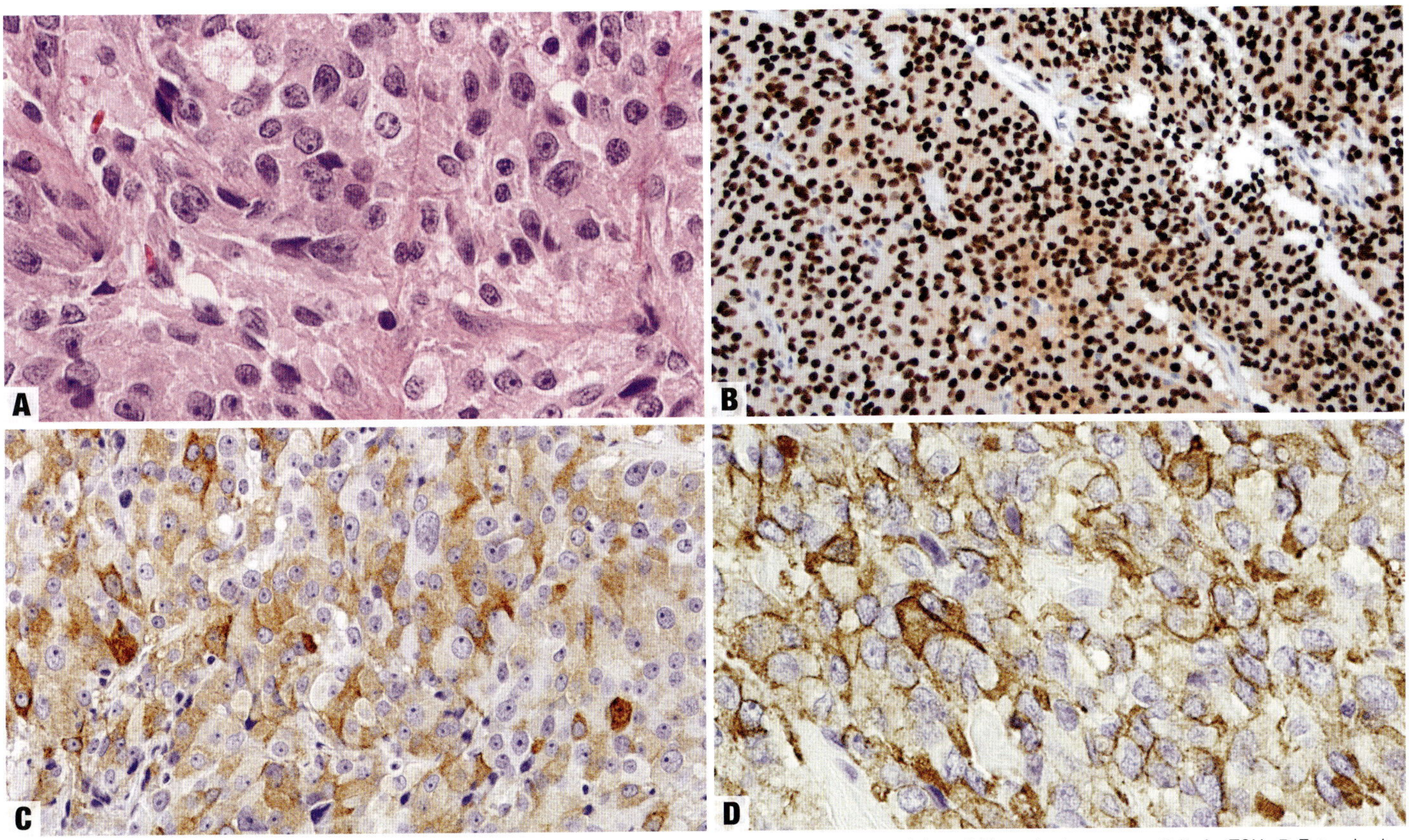

Fig. 2.22 Thyrotroph PitNET/adenoma. **A** Sheets of polygonal tumour cells. **B** Diffuse nuclear PIT1 immunostaining. **C** Extensive immunoreactivity for TSH. **D** Extensive immunoreactivity for α-subunit.

a thyrotroph PitNET/adenoma may also arise within this clinical setting. An increased ratio of serum α-subunit to TSH is also supportive of a thyrotroph tumour.

Neuroimaging

Typical neuroimaging findings include a large, invasive, contrast-enhancing tumour, often growing downward through the sellar floor and into the clivus, as well as laterally into the cavernous sinuses {2763}.

Epidemiology

Thyrotroph tumours are among the rarest pituitary tumours, accounting for < 1% of all PitNETs/adenomas {2952,4554,4513, 364}. Despite some variability among series, there is no clear male or female predominance {4554,4996,643}.

Etiology

In most cases, the etiology of these tumours is unknown, although rare examples are thought to result from chronic stimulatory feedback associated with longstanding hypothyroidism {2610,5001,410,1159}. There have also been rare reports of thyrotroph tumours encountered in tumour predisposition syndromes, such as multiple endocrine neoplasia type 1 and familial isolated pituitary adenoma (FIPA) due to germline *AIP* mutation {909,239,1087}.

Pathogenesis

Like other PIT1-lineage tumours, thyrotroph PitNETs were recently shown to have an epigenetic signature associated with diffuse DNA hypomethylation, transposable element expression, and chromosomal instability; in terms of their transcriptome, they clustered more closely with plurihormonal PIT1-lineage tumours than with somatotroph tumours {3208}.

Macroscopic appearance

The vast majority of thyrotroph tumours are large and invasive but have no distinctive macroscopic features otherwise. Variable degrees of fibrosis and calcification are seen in a subset. One series reported 74% of tumours being firm elastic or hard in consistency and 82% being macrotumours {4996}.

Histopathology

Thyrotroph tumours generally grow in diffuse and sinusoidal patterns, with variable fibrosis and (occasionally) psammomatous calcification. Tumour cells are spindled to polygonal with chromophobic cytoplasm and indistinct cell borders. Cases associated with hypothyroidism occasionally show thyrotroph hyperplasia in the adjacent non-neoplastic anterior pituitary.

Immunohistochemistry

There is diffuse PIT1 expression, and TSH positivity is extensive. The fraction of TSH-positive tumour cells often varies from case to case and regionally within the same tumour. There is variable staining for α-subunit and GATA3, as well as extensive SSTR2A expression {819,5093,2971,4465}.

Cytology

Similar features to other PitNETs

Diagnostic molecular pathology

There are no molecular tests required to diagnose these tumours. Germline screening for inherited tumour syndromes should be considered on the basis of clinicopathological findings.

Essential and desirable diagnostic criteria

Essential: a PitNET with diffuse PIT1 positivity; extensive TSH positivity; absence of other pituitary hormone staining.
Desirable: immunoreactivity for GATA3 and α-subunit.

Staging

There is no formal staging system that has been universally applied for pituitary/sellar neoplasms. A CT-era approach based on tumour size and patterns of invasion was proposed in 1973 by Hardy {1786}. Subsequently, a standardized assessment of parasellar tumour extension based on MRI was published by Knosp in 1993 {2354}.

There are no pathology-standardized reporting templates yet endorsed by international pathology organizations. A pathology reporting template for pituitary tumours was introduced in 2011 {3300}, followed by the European Pituitary Pathology Group (EPPG) proposal in 2019 {4707}.

Prognosis and prediction

Like for other large PitNETs/adenomas, surgery plays an important therapeutic role. Gross total resection was achievable in only about 45% in one series, because of the invasive tendencies of these tumours; however, all TSH-secreting PitNETs were lumped together in this study, so it is unclear if this is true in the pure thyrotroph tumours {960}. Somatostatin analogues are effective in reducing TSH secretion in > 90% of patients, although detectable tumour shrinkage is seen in only roughly one third of cases {366,367,365}.

Mature plurihormonal PIT1-lineage PitNET/adenoma

Osamura RY
Casar-Borota O
Ezzat S
Oyama K
Perry A
Tahara S

Chapter 2

Definition

Mature plurihormonal PIT1-lineage pituitary neuroendocrine tumour (PitNET)/adenoma is a well-differentiated PitNET composed of PIT1-lineage adenohypophysial cells with acidophilic cytoplasm, extensive immunoreactivity for growth hormone (GH), and variable immunoreactivity for TSH, prolactin, and α-subunit.

ICD-O coding

8272/3 Mature plurihormonal PIT1-lineage PitNET/adenoma

ICD-11 coding

2D12.Y Other specified malignant neoplasms of other endocrine glands or related structures

Related terminology

Acceptable: mature plurihormonal PIT1-lineage adenoma; mature plurihormonal PIT1-lineage neuroendocrine tumour; mature plurihormonal PIT1-lineage tumour; mature plurihormonal PIT1-positive tumour.

Not recommended: plurihormonal PitNET/adenoma of the acidophil cell line.

Subtype(s)

None

Localization

The tumours are located in the sellar region and may show variable extension into the adjacent structures {2768}.

Clinical features

Patients usually exhibit clinical features of acromegaly/gigantism with hyperthyroidism and/or hyperprolactinaemia, separately or in combination. Secondary mass effects can compromise normal pituitary function and/or vision.

Epidemiology

Mature plurihormonal PIT1-lineage PitNETs/adenomas are rare. Their exact incidence is yet to be clarified. Limited data suggest that such mature plurihormonal PIT1-lineage tumours occur in older individuals than their immature counterparts {2966,2827}.

Etiology

In most cases, the etiology is not known. However, rare examples have been reported in syndromic patients with multiple pituitary tumours {555}.

Pathogenesis

It remains unclear how multipotent plurihormonal pituitary cells become neoplastic and whether such transitions are distinct from those in their monohormonal counterparts.

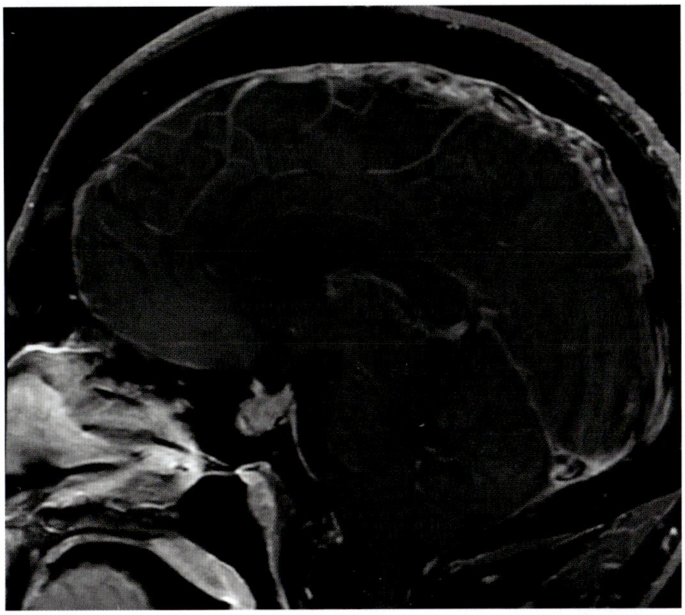

Fig. 2.23 Mature plurihormonal PIT1-lineage PitNET/adenoma. Sagittal postcontrast T1-weighted MRI reveals a modest-sized intrasellar tumour, without evidence of invasion into adjacent structures.

Macroscopic appearance

No distinctive macroscopic features have been reported for this tumour type.

Histopathology

The tumour shows a solid or sinusoidal growth pattern and is composed predominantly of acidophilic cells with interspersed chromophobes. The histological features resemble those of mammosomatotroph tumours.

Immunohistochemistry

There is diffuse nuclear immunoreactivity for PIT1 {2605} and usually extensive cytoplasmic positivity for GH, with abundant prolactin, TSH, and α-subunit, albeit in varying proportions among cases. They are also positive for ER and GATA3 {2971}.

Differential diagnosis

Mammosomatotroph tumours have a similar histological appearance; however, they produce GH and prolactin but not TSH {197}.

Immature plurihormonal PIT1-lineage tumours should be distinguished from these tumours because of their potentially more aggressive behaviour. Immature PIT1-lineage tumours are composed of epithelioid or spindle-shaped chromophobic cells with large, often pleomorphic nuclei that have prominent nucleoli and intranuclear pseudoinclusions, and they usually show only patchy expression of GH, prolactin, and TSH {2966,2827,64}.

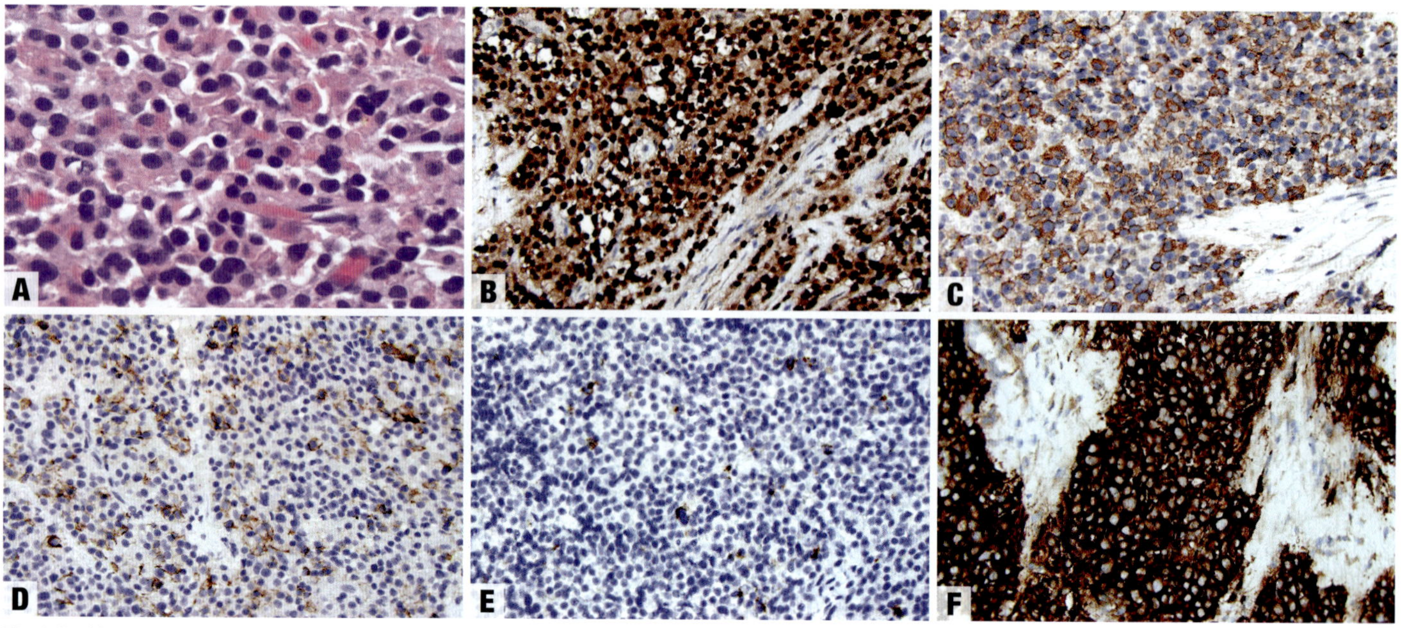

Fig. 2.24 Mature plurihormonal PIT1-lineage PitNET/adenoma. **A** Mostly acidophilic cells are seen, with scattered chromophobe cells. Clinically, this patient presented with acromegaly. **B** An immunostain for PIT1 displays diffuse nuclear positivity in tumour cells. **C** A growth hormone immunostain shows expression in most, but not all, tumour cells. **D** A prolactin stain highlights a subset of tumour cells. **E** Scattered tumour cells are immunoreactive for TSH. **F** There is strong and diffuse SSTR2A immunoreactivity in tumour cells.

Cytology

The cytology of these tumours is similar to that of other PitNETs in general.

Diagnostic molecular pathology

There are no molecular tests required to diagnose these tumours. Germline screening for inherited tumours should be considered on the basis of clinicopathological findings.

Essential and desirable diagnostic criteria

Essential: a PitNET with PIT1 immunoreactivity in all or most of the tumour cells; extensive expression of GH, with variable α-subunit, TSH, and prolactin positivity.

Desirable: GATA3 and ER expression.

Staging

There is no formal staging system that has been universally applied for pituitary/sellar neoplasms. A CT-era approach based on tumour size and patterns of invasion was proposed in 1973 by Hardy {1786}. Subsequently, a standardized assessment of parasellar tumour extension based on MRI was published by Knosp in 1993 {2354}.

There are no pathology-standardized reporting templates yet endorsed by international pathology organizations. A pathology reporting template for pituitary tumours was introduced in 2011 {3300}, followed by the European Pituitary Pathology Group (EPPG) proposal in 2019 {4707}.

Prognosis and prediction

Compared with immature plurihormonal PIT1-lineage tumours, the mature plurihormonal tumours have been reported to exhibit less aggressive behaviour {2966,1950}.

There are limited data on SSTR expression in mature plurihormonal PIT1-lineage tumours. However, it is reasonable to assume that immunohistochemical analysis of SSTRs may be of predictive value for the effectiveness of somatostatin analogues {819}.

Immature PIT1-lineage PitNET/adenoma

Perry A
Casar-Borota O
Ezzat S
Tahara S
Uccella S

Definition

Immature PIT1-lineage pituitary neuroendocrine tumour (PitNET)/adenoma is an immature PitNET composed of PIT1-lineage adenohypophysial cells with cytological atypia and limited differentiation towards thyrotroph, somatotroph, and/or lactotroph cells.

ICD-O coding

8272/3 Immature PIT1-lineage PitNET/adenoma

ICD-11 coding

2D12.Y Other specified malignant neoplasms of other endocrine glands or related structures

Related terminology

Acceptable: immature PIT1-lineage tumour, immature PIT1-positive tumour.

Not recommended: silent subtype 3 PitNET/adenoma; poorly differentiated PIT1-lineage PitNET/adenoma.

Subtype(s)

None

Localization

These intrasellar tumours often invade into surrounding anatomical structures.

Clinical features

The majority of immature PIT1-lineage tumours are clinically non-functioning, thus explaining the prior taxonomy of "silent subtype 3". However, as many as 30% show evidence of hormone excess, including hyperthyroidism, acromegaly, galactorrhoea, amenorrhoea, and/or hyperprolactinaemia {1264,2966, 197}. Symptoms of mass effect, such as headaches, visual deficits, cranial nerve palsies, hypopituitarism, and apoplexy, are encountered in roughly two thirds of patients {1264,2966}.

Neuroimaging

They are nearly always contrast-enhancing macrotumours with extensive invasion into adjacent structures. Inferolateral extension through the floor of the sella and into the sphenoidal sinus, clivus, and nasopharynx, as well as into cavernous sinuses, predominates over suprasellar growth in about 17% of cases, but combined inferolateral and suprasellar growth is most common {1264,2966}.

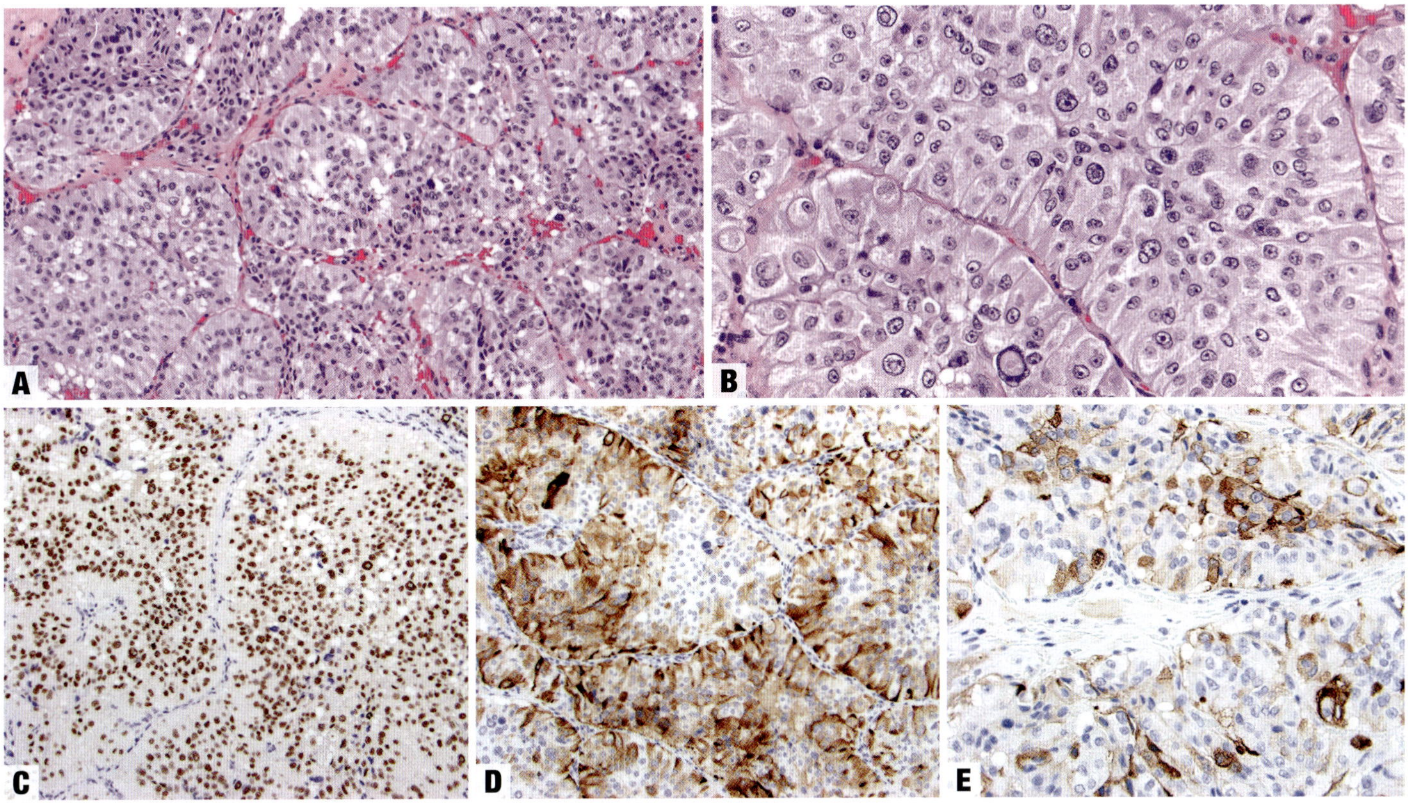

Fig. 2.25 Immature PIT1-lineage PitNET/adenoma. **A** Large pleomorphic cells forming sheets and nests. **B** Note the nuclear pseudoinclusions and large nucleoli. **C** Diffuse PIT1 immunoreactivity. **D** Patchy TSH positivity. **E** Limited prolactin positivity.

Epidemiology

Immature PIT1-lineage tumours are rare, accounting for roughly 1–3% of all PitNETs {1264,2966}. In 58 patients from two large series, the M:F ratio was close to 1:1, and the average age at presentation was about 40 years {1264,2966}.

Etiology

In most cases, the etiology is not known, although rare examples have been reported in the setting of multiple endocrine neoplasia type 1 {1264}.

Pathogenesis

Histopathological series suggest that these tumours arise from an early PIT1-lineage progenitor and partially overlap with thyrotroph tumours. In fact, a pangenomic study found that the PIT1-lineage plurihormonal tumour transcriptome most closely clusters with the thyrotroph tumours; however, the study in question did not distinguish mature from immature forms {3208}.

Macroscopic appearance

The gross appearance is similar to that of other large, invasive macrotumours.

Histopathology

Immature PIT1-lineage tumours are often diffuse to nodular proliferations of polygonal to spindle-shaped chromophobic cells with marked nuclear atypia, intranuclear cytoplasmic pseudoinclusions, and macronucleoli. Like in thyrotroph tumours, stromal fibrosis may be seen, possibly related to local production of FGF {1307}. Ultrastructurally, they partially overlap with thyrotroph cells, showing a monomorphic population of large polar cells with abundant rough endoplasmic reticulum, aggregates of smooth endoplasmic reticulum, multipolar Golgi complexes, plexiform cellular interdigitations, and sparse 100–200 nm secretory granules mostly concentrated at the cell periphery and cytoplasmic processes; a unique feature is the presence of electron-dense nuclear inclusions, known as spheridia {216, 2966}.

Immunohistochemistry

They are diffusely PIT1-immunoreactive, with variable but usually limited expression of TSH, growth hormone, and/or prolactin. Although 70–80% are plurihormonal with at least two hormones represented, rare examples express only one, or even none, of the PIT1-family hormones; in such cases, the diffuse PIT1 staining, classic cytological features, and/or ultrastructural features (see below) allow diagnostic confirmation. Most tumours also express α-subunit, ER, and GATA3, along with variable cytokeratin staining, with both perinuclear and paranuclear fibrous body patterns encountered.

Differential diagnosis

Immature PIT1-lineage tumours overlap with their mature counterparts, as well as with thyrotroph tumours and acidophil stem cell tumours. The mature PIT1-lineage tumours have much more cytological uniformity, with abundant acidophilic cytoplasm and extensive hormone immunoreactivities, and they generally lack nuclear atypia, macronucleoli, and nuclear pseudoinclusions {2827}. Thyrotroph tumours similarly lack the cytological features of immature PIT1-lineage tumours and should be monohormonal (TSH only). Acidophil stem cell tumours are oncocytic, vacuolated, and typically prolactin hormone–predominant.

Cytology

Cytological studies have not been published.

Diagnostic molecular pathology

There are no molecular tests required to diagnose these tumours. Germline screening for inherited tumours should be considered on the basis of clinicopathological findings.

Essential and desirable diagnostic criteria

Essential: diffuse PIT1 positivity, usually with patchy expression of one or more PIT1-lineage hormones (TSH, growth hormone, and/or prolactin); histology showing nuclear atypia, macronucleoli, and nuclear pseudoinclusions.

Desirable: a large invasive tumour on neuroimaging; nuclear spheridia on ultrastructural examination; variable GATA3 and ER immunoreactivity.

Staging

There is no formal staging system that has been universally applied for pituitary/sellar neoplasms. A CT-era approach based on tumour size and patterns of invasion was proposed in 1973 by Hardy {1786}. Subsequently, a standardized assessment of parasellar tumour invasiveness based on MRI was published by Knosp in 1993 {2354}.

There are no pathology-standardized reporting templates yet endorsed by international pathology organizations. A pathology reporting template for pituitary tumours was introduced in 2011 {3300}, followed by the European Pituitary Pathology Group (EPPG) proposal in 2019 {4707}.

Prognosis and prediction

This usually invasive PitNET/adenoma subtype is known for its more aggressive biology, lower rates of resectability, and a proclivity for tumour recurrence; nevertheless, some data suggest that it is sensitive to radiation therapy {1950,1951,1264,2966}. Although proliferation indexes are often higher in these tumours, they are not known to be prognostic {3513,2961,3348}. Overall, surgery has been the main therapeutic approach, and in one series, the mean time to a second operation was only 16.6 months {1264}. Another study found that nearly 80% of immature PIT1-lineage tumours are immunonegative for MGMT, suggesting that temozolomide may be an effective therapeutic strategy; however, immunohistochemistry for this marker is generally challenging, and a proof of principle for temozolomide therapy is currently lacking.

Acidophil stem cell PitNET/adenoma

Perry A
Ezzat S
Inoshita N
Mete O
Nishioka H

Definition

Acidophil stem cell pituitary neuroendocrine tumour (PitNET)/adenoma is an immature PitNET composed of PIT1-lineage adenohypophysial cells with partial lactotroph and limited somatotroph differentiation, oncocytic features, and giant mitochondria.

ICD-O coding

8280/3 Acidophil stem cell PitNET/adenoma

ICD-11 coding

2D12.Y Other specified malignant neoplasms of other endocrine glands or related structures

Related terminology

Acceptable: acidophil stem cell tumour.

Subtype(s)

None

Localization

Acidophil stem cell tumours (ASCTs) arise within the sella but frequently extend into parasellar structures.

Clinical features

ASCTs are often rapidly growing neoplasms with hyperprolactinaemia that is lower than expected for the size of the tumour, and with some phenotypic features of acromegaly despite modest biochemical evidence of it (i.e. fugitive acromegaly) {1949, 64,197}. The hyperprolactinaemia is most often associated with amenorrhoea and galactorrhoea in women and loss of libido or impotence in men. Serum growth hormone (GH) and/or IGF1 are inappropriately normal or modestly elevated. Signs and symptoms of mass effect, such as headaches, visual deficits, and cranial neuropathies, are also reported.

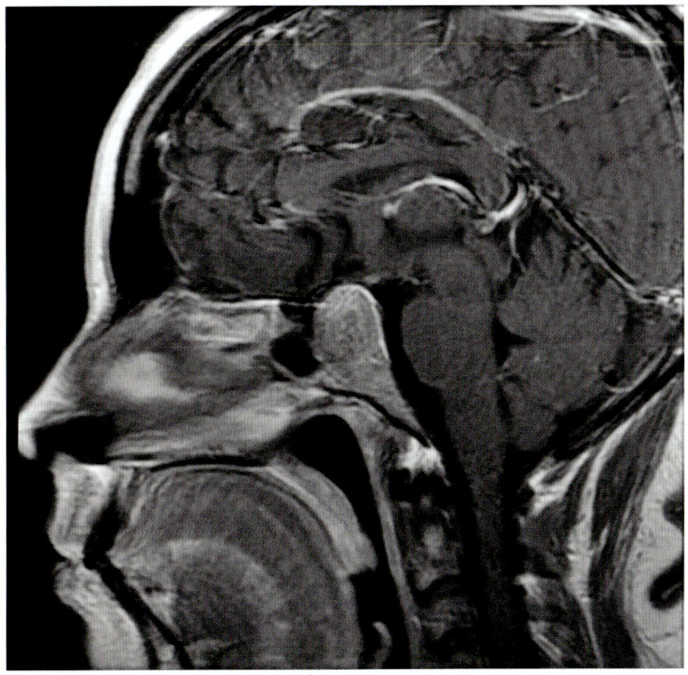

Fig. 2.26 Acidophil stem cell tumour. Postcontrast sagittal MRI showing a predominant pattern of invasion inferiorly.

Neuroimaging

The vast majority of ASCTs are large (> 10 mm), invasive tumours. On neuroimaging, an atypical, mostly inferior growth pattern is seen in roughly half of all cases, with invasion through

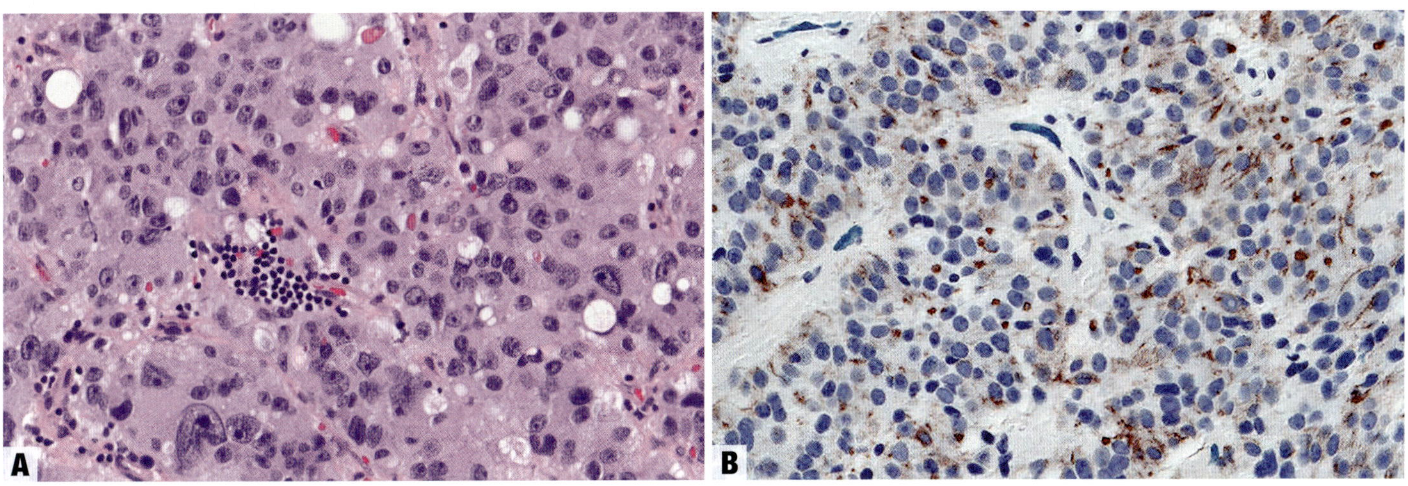

Fig. 2.27 Acidophil stem cell tumour. **A** Sheets of pleomorphic, chromophobic to slightly acidophilic cells with clear vacuoles. **B** A CAM5.2 cytokeratin immunostain highlights scattered fibrous bodies.

the sellar floor into the sphenoidal sinus and nasopharynx {1949}. Suprasellar extension is often less prominent than in other large, invasive macrotumours.

Epidemiology

ASCTs accounted for about 2% of all PitNETs and 7% of all PIT1-lineage tumours in a series of 1055 surgically resected PitNETs {2961}. In a series of 15 patients, 6 were men and 9 were women, ranging in age from 17 to 60 years (median: 42 years) {1949}.

Etiology

Not known

Pathogenesis

ASCT may arise from a mammosomatotroph precursor cell {1949,64}. Molecular studies have not been performed.

Macroscopic appearance

Like other PitNETs, ASCTs are white to grey and distinct from the normal pituitary gland; they are generally soft, explaining the relative preservation of normal pituitary function. Large tumours show variable degrees of invasion into adjacent anatomical structures.

Histopathology

ASCT usually grows in sheets and appears cytologically immature, with chromophobic to slightly acidophilic cytoplasm and variable oncocytic features due to the accumulation of mitochondria. The highly distinctive giant mitochondria that were originally described ultrastructurally manifest as variably sized clear vacuoles on routine histopathology, a useful clue to the diagnosis, particularly when prominent. On electron microscopy, the giant mitochondria retain a continuous double membrane but do not show cristae {1949}. Ultrastructural features suggest that ASCT is composed of a single immature cell type with evidence of simultaneous lactotroph and somatotroph differentiation.

Immunohistochemistry

They are diffusely PIT1-positive and show variable prolactin and ER staining, with minimal to absent GH expression; stains for TPIT, SF1, GATA3, and other pituitary hormones are negative. CAM5.2 highlights scattered paranuclear fibrous bodies in one third of these tumours {2961}. A potential immunohistochemical surrogate of ultrastructural findings is the antimitochondrial antigen stain, which variably highlights the increased number of mitochondria, as well as rimmed vacuoles suggestive of giant mitochondria.

Cytology

Not reported

Diagnostic molecular pathology

There are no molecular tests required to diagnose these tumours. Germline screening for inherited tumours should be considered on the basis of clinicopathological findings.

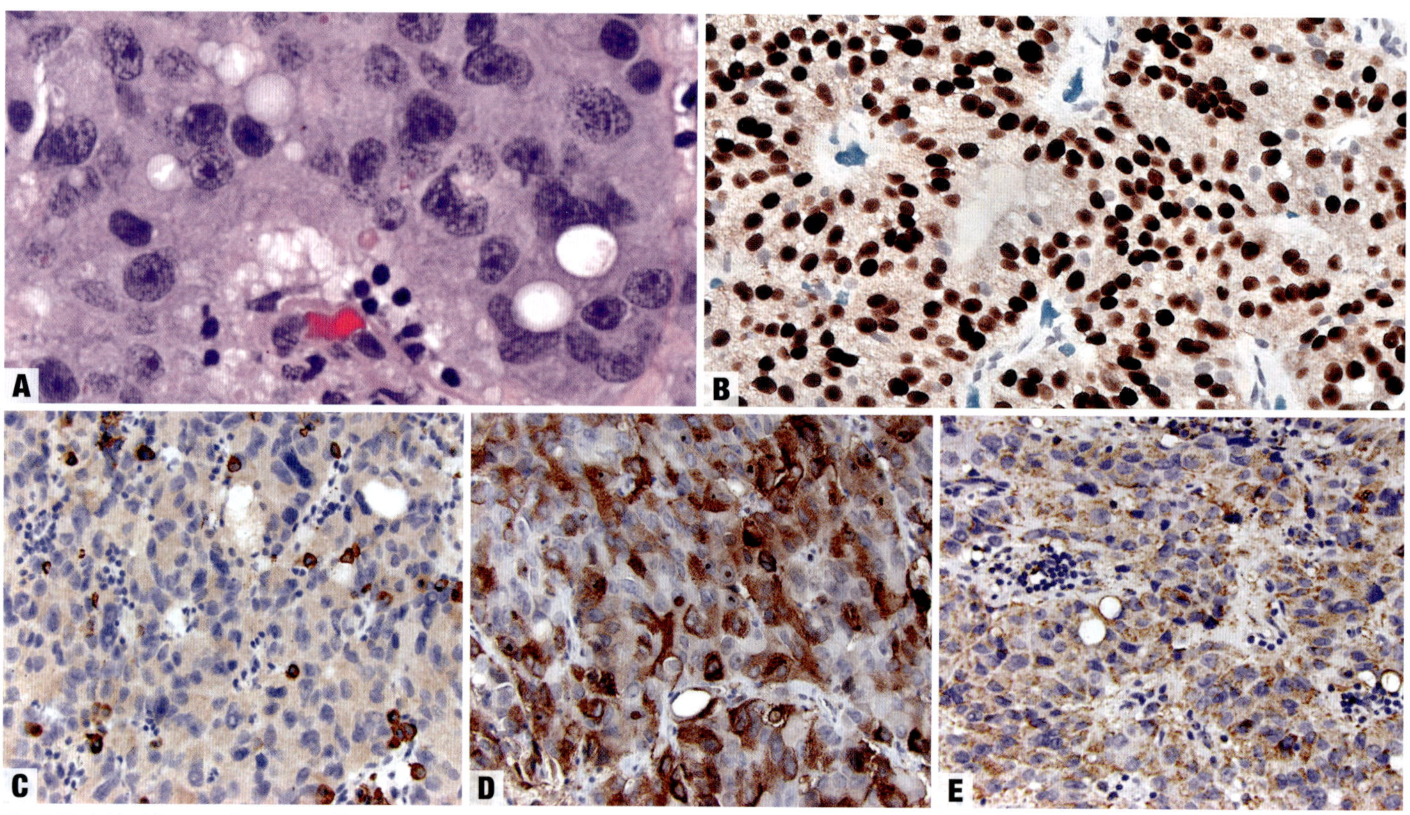

Fig. 2.28 Acidophil stem cell tumour. **A** Sheets of pleomorphic, chromophobic to slightly acidophilic cells with clear vacuoles. **B** Diffuse PIT1 immunoreactivity. **C** Focal weak positivity for growth hormone, with intense staining of entrapped non-neoplastic cells. **D** Prolactin positivity is seen in many, but not all, tumour cells. **E** An antimitochondrial antigen immunostain highlights the oncocytic changes (increased mitochondria), and the rimmed vacuoles are suggestive of giant mitochondria.

Essential and desirable diagnostic criteria

Essential: a PitNET/adenoma with diffuse PIT1 staining, variable prolactin expression, focal to absent GH, and oncocytic features.

Desirable: ER positivity; giant mitochondria; scattered GH positivity and/or cytokeratin-positive fibrous bodies; hyperprolactinaemia that is less than expected for the size of the tumour; fugitive acromegaly; downward invasion pattern.

Staging

There is no formal staging system that has been universally applied for pituitary/sellar neoplasms. A CT-era approach based on tumour size and patterns of invasion was proposed in 1973 by Hardy {1786}. Subsequently, a standardized assessment of parasellar tumour extension based on MRI was published by Knosp in 1993 {2354}.

There are no pathology-standardized reporting templates yet endorsed by international pathology organizations. A pathology reporting template for pituitary tumours was introduced in 2011 {3300}, followed by the European Pituitary Pathology Group (EPPG) proposal in 2019 {4707}.

Prognosis and prediction

Large studies have not been published, but the data thus far suggest that ASCT is an aggressive PitNET/adenoma. In contrast to lactotroph tumours, ASCTs are typically refractory to dopamine agonist therapy {1978}. Similarly, they can be somatostatin analogue–resistant, in contrast to the their more differentiated somatotroph counterparts; such therapeutic insensitivity can be the clue to the diagnosis. Therefore, other management options include surgery, radiation therapy, chemotherapy, and peptide receptor radionuclide therapy {159}.

Mixed somatotroph–lactotroph PitNET/adenoma

Lopes MBS
Inomoto C
Perry A
Uccella S

Definition

Mixed somatotroph–lactotroph pituitary neuroendocrine tumour (PitNET)/adenoma is a well-differentiated PitNET composed of PIT1-lineage adenohypophysial cells with distinct populations of somatotroph and lactotroph cells.

ICD-O coding

8280/3 Mixed somatotroph–lactotroph PitNET/adenoma
8280/3 Densely granulated somatotroph and sparsely granulated lactotroph tumour
8280/3 Sparsely granulated somatotroph and sparsely granulated lactotroph tumour

ICD-11 coding

2D12.Y Other specified malignant neoplasms of other endocrine glands or related structures

Related terminology

Acceptable: mixed somatotroph–lactotroph tumour.

Not recommended: growth hormone and prolactin-secreting PitNET/adenoma; somatotroph–mammotroph PitNET/adenoma.

Subtype(s)

Densely granulated somatotroph and sparsely granulated lactotroph tumour; sparsely granulated somatotroph and sparsely granulated lactotroph tumour

Localization

Most tumours are intrasellar with suprasellar and/or parasellar extension {2434,2768}. These can arise in ovarian teratomas {1917}.

Clinical features

Most somatotroph–lactotroph tumours are clinically functioning tumours that cause gigantism and/or acromegaly and clinical evidence of hyperprolactinaemia, including hypogonadism, amenorrhoea, or galactorrhoea due to the cosecretion of growth hormone (GH) and prolactin {2434,2561,2015}. Signs and symptoms of mass effect may also be present in patients with large tumours.

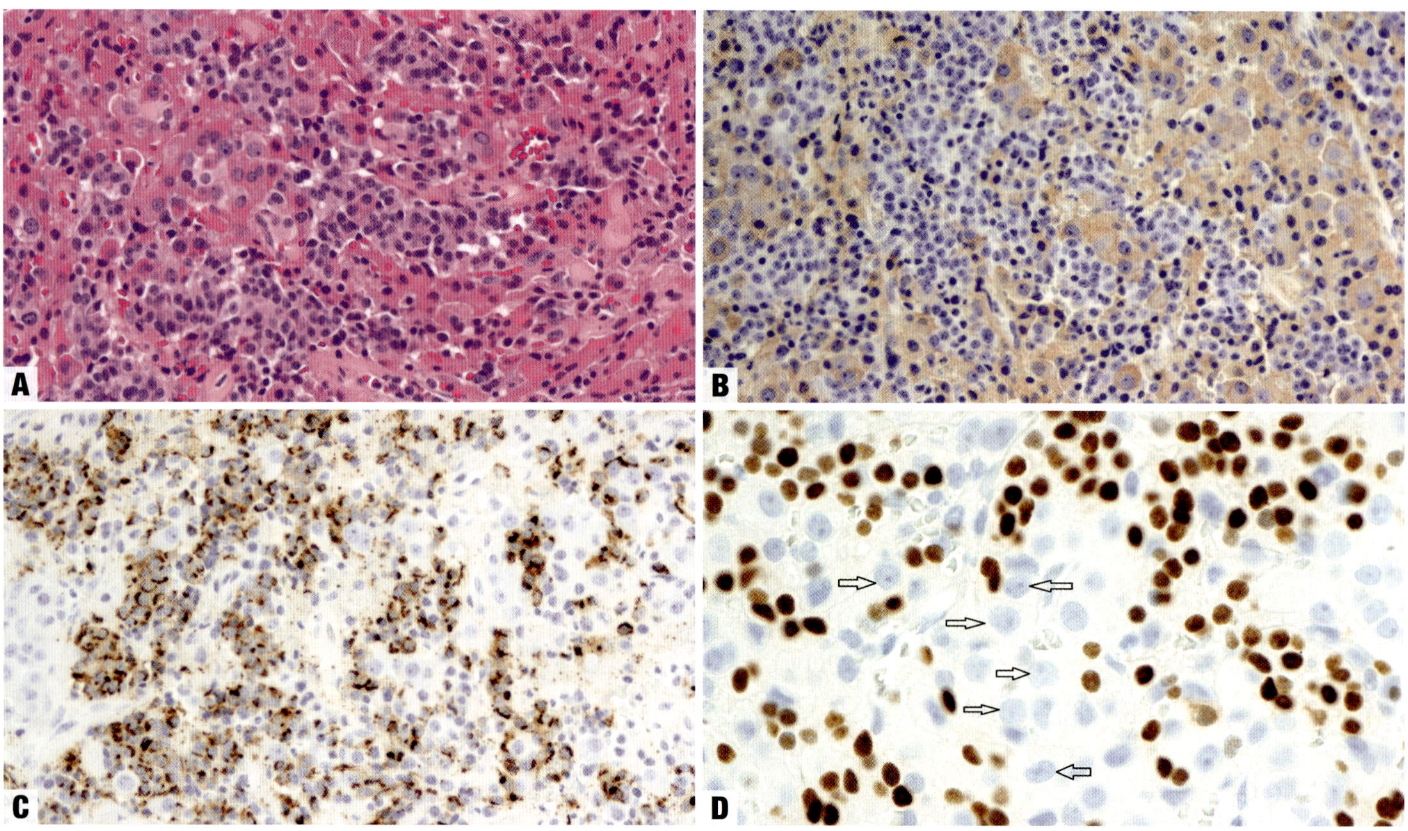

Fig. 2.29 Mixed somatotroph–lactotroph PitNET/adenoma. Such tumours consist of two cell populations of large, eosinophilic somatotroph cells intermixed with smaller, chromophobic lactotroph cells that may be distinguished by H&E (**A**). Distinct cell populations are immunoreactive for growth hormone (**B**) and for prolactin (**C**). ER immunoreactivity is observed in lactotroph cells, whereas the somatotroph cells with larger nuclei are negative (arrows) (**D**).

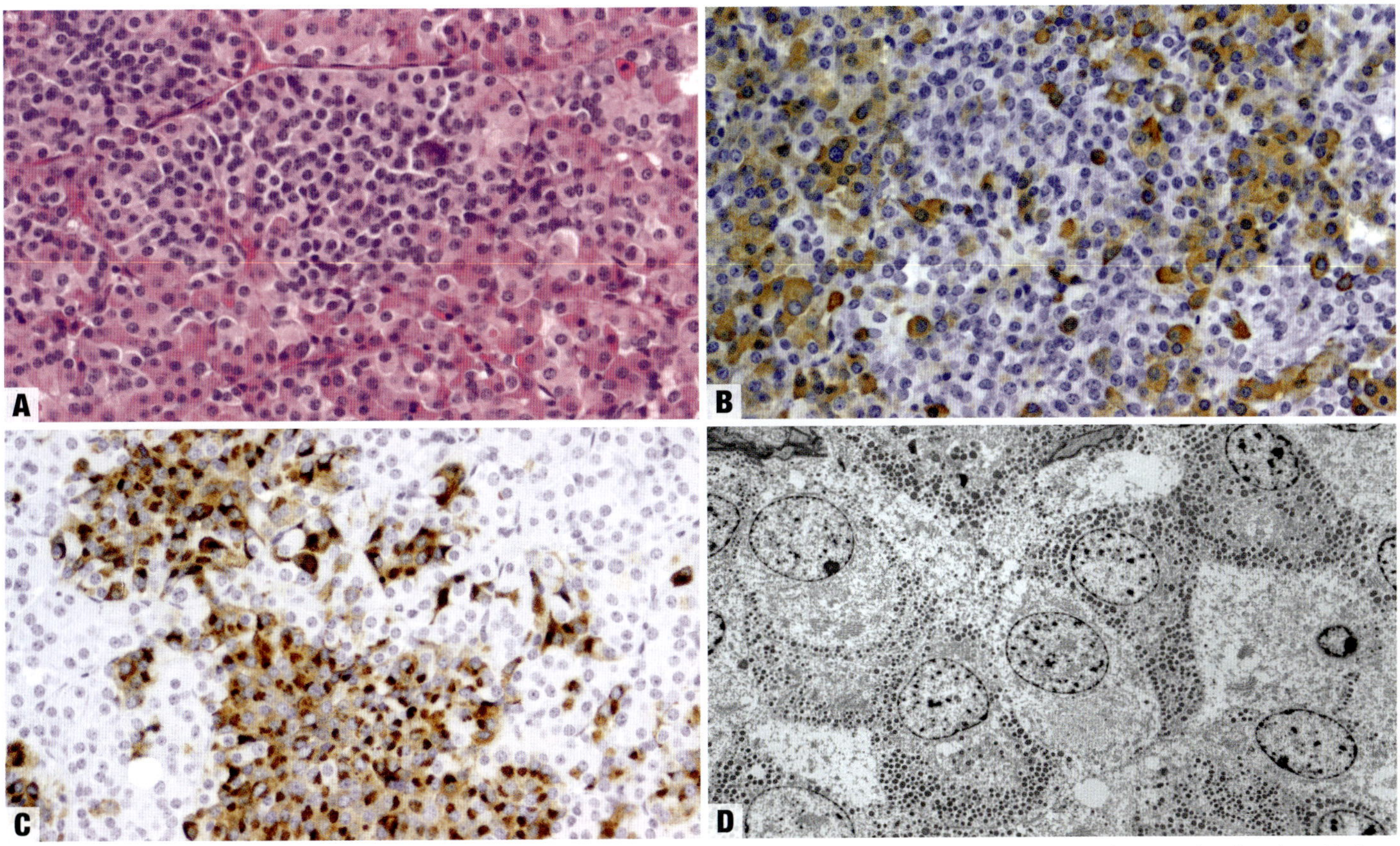

Fig. 2.30 Mixed somatotroph–lactotroph PitNET/adenoma, X-linked acrogigantism–associated. A mixed somatotroph–lactotroph adenoma in a young female patient with gigantism and a somatic *GPR101* duplication. Pathology showed a bicellular tumour with distinct somatotroph and lactotroph cells (**A**). Immunohistochemistry for growth hormone (**B**) and prolactin (**C**) is demonstrated in the different cells. Ultrastructural analysis confirmed the dual cell population of the tumour, which was composed of densely granulated somatotroph cells and sparsely granulated lactotroph cells (**D**).

Imaging

At diagnosis, these tumours are mostly macrotumours with suprasellar extension {2434,4722,2768}. Cavernous sinus invasion has been reported in as many as 38.5% of tumours {2768}.

Epidemiology

Mixed somatotroph–lactotroph tumours are rare, corresponding to 1–4% of all pituitary tumours and about 6–14% of tumours presenting with acromegaly/gigantism {2434,2561,2961,2768,3874}.

There is no reported sex predilection, and the mean age (fifth to sixth decade of life) does not differ from that of pure somatotroph tumours {2434,2561,2961,2768}, but there are insufficient detailed data in the literature separating mixed tumours from the more common pure somatotroph tumours and mammosomatotroph tumours.

Tumours in the setting of hereditary syndromes or in sporadic, non-syndromic acrogigantism (familial isolated pituitary adenomas [FIPAs], X-linked acrogigantism [X-LAG]) arise in younger patients, mostly those of prepubertal age {1536,2015,1772}. In X-LAG–associated tumours, there is a predominance of female patients {2015}.

Etiology

The etiology of mixed somatotroph–lactotroph tumours is unknown in most cases. A small subset arise in the setting of hereditary tumour syndromes, including FIPA, X-LAG, Carney complex, and McCune–Albright syndrome {2015,423,325, 1087}.

Pathogenesis

There are no specific molecular or genetic data discriminating the mixed somatotroph–lactotroph tumours from the larger population of somatotroph and mammosomatotroph tumours. Mixed somatotroph–lactotroph tumours are associated with germline or somatic mosaic duplication of *GPR101* causing X-LAG and with *AIP* mutation {2015,325}.

Macroscopic appearance

Mixed somatotroph–lactotroph tumours are soft and white to grey or red and indistinguishable from other mature PIT1-lineage tumours.

Histopathology

Mixed somatotroph–lactotroph tumours are composed of two distinct cell populations, somatotroph cells and lactotroph cells. All combinations of sparsely and/or densely granulated somatotroph and lactotroph cells have been described {2434,2961, 2768,3874}. Most typically, tumours are composed of large, eosinophilic, densely granulated somatotrophs admixed with chromophobic, sparsely granulated lactotrophs; a sparsely granulated somatotroph cell component is less frequently described {2434,2768,3874}.

Immunohistochemistry

Both tumour cellular components express PIT1. Somatotroph cells are immunoreactive for GH, and variably immunoreactive for α-subunit depending on the granularity of the cells. Lactotroph cells express prolactin and ER. A low-molecular-weight cytokeratin immunostain reveals perinuclear expression in densely granulated somatotrophs; alternatively, paranuclear fibrous bodies are present in tumours with sparsely granulated somatotrophs.

Differential diagnosis

The distinction of mixed somatotroph–lactotroph tumours from mammosomatotroph tumours may be difficult without ultrastructural analysis. Distinct cell populations of somatotroph and lactotroph cells are seen in mixed tumours, whereas mammosomatotroph tumours are composed of a monomorphic population of cells with large pleomorphic secretory granules and granular extrusions (misplaced exocytosis) {912,1945}. Another tool for the distinction of these two entities is the analysis of the pattern of ER immunoexpression that correlates with lactotroph cells and is clearly absent in somatotroph cells of mixed tumours {1440,5108,2714}.

Cytology

The cytology of mixed somatotroph–lactotroph tumours is indistinguishable from that of PitNETs/adenomas with large cells; tumours with sparsely granulated somatotrophs may be recognized by the presence of fibrous bodies.

Diagnostic molecular pathology

There are no molecular tests required to diagnose mixed somatotroph–lactotroph tumours. Genetic screening for germline and/or sporadic mutations has been recommended in young patients (aged ≤ 30 years) with acromegaly/gigantism {4495, 958,4287,2015,2855}.

Essential and desirable diagnostic criteria

Essential: a PitNET composed of two PIT1-immunopositive cell populations separately expressing GH and prolactin.

Desirable: ER immunoreactivity (for better definition of the lactotrophs); absence of the α-subunit of glycoprotein hormones in the lactotroph component; low-molecular-weight cytokeratin (for better definition of the somatotrophs).

Staging

There is no formal staging system that has been universally applied for pituitary/sellar neoplasms. A CT-era approach based on tumour size and patterns of invasion was proposed in 1973 by Hardy {1786}. Subsequently, a standardized assessment of parasellar tumour extension based on MRI was published by Knosp in 1993 {2354}.

There are no pathology-standardized reporting templates yet endorsed by international pathology organizations. A pathology reporting template for pituitary tumours was introduced in 2011 {3300}, followed by the European Pituitary Pathology Group (EPPG) proposal in 2019 {4707}.

Prognosis and prediction

Although data on this separate entity from the overall population of GH-producing tumours are very sparse, two studies have shown that patients with mixed somatotroph–lactotroph tumours have lower disease remission rates than patients with tumours in the other tumour categories including somatotroph (densely and sparsely granulated) and mammosomatotroph tumours {2434,2768}.

Corticotroph PitNET/adenoma

Mete O
Casar-Borota O
Grossman AB
Yamada S

Definition

Corticotroph pituitary neuroendocrine tumour (PitNET)/adenoma is a well-differentiated PitNET composed of TPIT-lineage adenohypophysial cells with corticotroph differentiation.

ICD-O coding

8272/3 Corticotroph PitNET/adenoma
8272/3 Densely granulated corticotroph tumour
8272/3 Sparsely granulated corticotroph tumour
8272/3 Crooke cell tumour

ICD-11 coding

2D12.Y Other specified malignant neoplasms of other endocrine glands or related structures

Related terminology

Acceptable: corticotroph tumour.

Not recommended: ACTH-positive PitNET/adenoma; ACTH-producing PitNET/adenoma; ACTH-producing tumour/adenoma; ACTH tumour/adenoma; ACTHoma; corticotropinoma.

Subtype(s)

Densely granulated corticotroph tumour; sparsely granulated corticotroph tumour; Crooke cell tumour

Localization

Most corticotroph tumours are located in the pituitary gland. Ectopic manifestations may rarely occur in the nasal cavity, sphenoidal sinus, cavernous sinus, orbit, clivus, and suprasellar region {4080,1718,2130,4061}. Corticotroph tumours can extremely rarely occur in teratomas {623,4857}.

Clinical features

Cushing syndrome is the constellation of symptoms and signs related to cortisol excess {3240}. If the syndrome is caused by a corticotroph tumour (or very rarely hyperplasia), it is classified as Cushing disease {1167,3240}. Most corticotroph tumours are biochemically functioning; however, some corticotroph tumours lack clinical and biochemical evidence of ACTH and cortisol excess, and are called silent corticotroph tumours {1946,3992,74,906,1626,213}. These silent corticotroph tumours account for 3–6% of all pituitary tumours, 10–20% of silent pituitary tumours, and about 40% of all corticotroph tumours {1157}. Silent corticotroph tumours may more frequently present with neurological or ophthalmic symptoms, including pituitary apoplexy {2732,74,2952,1626}.

The diagnosis of Cushing disease is challenging. Many symptoms and signs, including insulin resistance and diabetes mellitus, depression, obesity, and hypertension, are common in the general population, whereas Cushing disease is relatively rare. In children, weight gain with growth failure, due in part to inhibition of growth hormone release, is characteristic {1167}. Cyclic Cushing syndrome may be a feature of any form of Cushing disease {2952}. Complicating the diagnosis further, there are pseudo-Cushing states (e.g. morbid obesity, depression, anxiety, alcoholism, pregnancy, and certain medication effects) that are associated with variable degrees of hypercortisolism, simulating Cushing syndrome {2952,1167,3240}. Severe

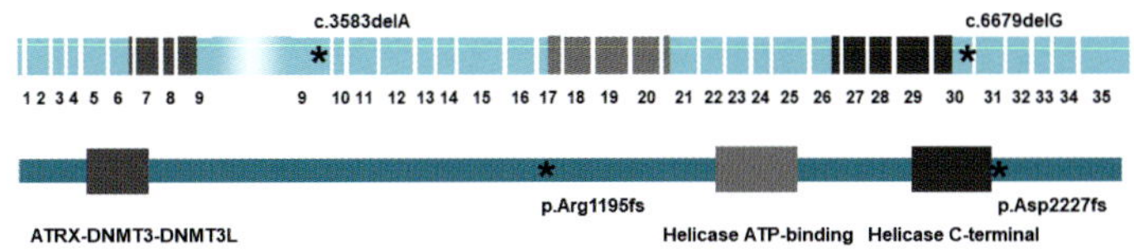

Fig. 2.31 Corticotroph PitNET, metastatic, *ATRX*-mutated. Diagram showing *ATRX* frameshift mutations in a patient with a metastatic corticotroph PitNET causing Cushing disease. The positions of the frameshift (fs) mutations c.3583delA and c.6679delG in exons 9 and 30 of *ATRX* are denoted with asterisks in this exon diagram of *ATRX*, where exon 9 is compressed for simplicity. ATRX domains are highlighted with grey shading.

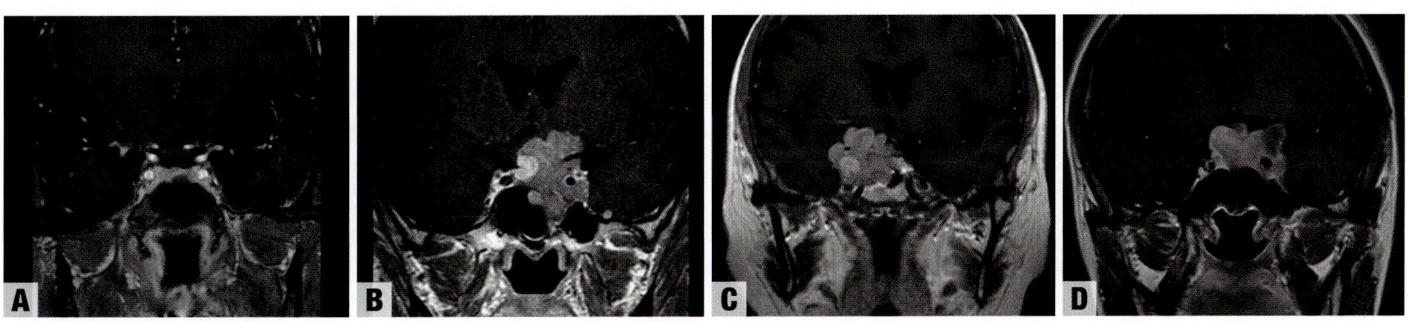

Fig. 2.32 Corticotroph PitNET. Most densely granulated corticotroph tumours are microtumours. **A** Enhanced T1-weighted coronal MRI shows a microtumour in the centre of the pituitary gland on spoiled-gradient echo. **B–D** Unlike densely granulated corticotroph tumours, sparsely granulated corticotroph tumours (**B**), Crooke cell tumours (**C**), and silent corticotroph tumours (**D**) are often associated with macrotumours with invasive growth. **B** Enhanced T1-weighted coronal MRI from a patient with a sparsely granulated corticotroph tumour shows a macrotumour invading the cavernous sinus (Knosp 4) on the left side. **C** Enhanced T1-weighted coronal MRI from a patient with a Crooke cell tumour shows a macrotumour with multilobular suprasellar extension and cavernous sinus invasion (Knosp 4), both on the right side. **D** Enhanced T1-weighted coronal MRI from a patient with a silent corticotroph tumour shows a macrotumour invading the cavernous sinus (Knosp 4) on the left side and displacing the normal pituitary to the right side.

Cushing disease and Nelson syndrome (rapid enlargement of a corticotroph tumour after bilateral adrenalectomy) may cause hyperpigmentation due to an overproduction of POMC-derived peptides.

Biochemical investigations

The principal diagnostic tests rely on the autonomous nature of cortisol release in Cushing syndrome, assessment of normal feedback, and loss of circadian rhythmicity. The most reliable tests evaluate resistance to dexamethasone feedback, including the overnight test (1 mg dexamethasone given at midnight, serum cortisol measured at 09:00 the following morning) and the 2-day Liddle test (0.5 mg given every 6 h for 48 h, serum cortisol measured at 09:00 at the 48 h mark). The loss of the circadian rhythm may be demonstrated by elevated late-night serum or salivary cortisol. If the disorder is ACTH-dependent, it is usually due to pituitary-dependent Cushing syndrome (Cushing disease). The diagnosis requires confirmation using imaging studies.

Neuroimaging

Most patients with Cushing disease have a solitary microtumour, and about 5–10% have a macrotumour {4929}. About 10% of patients with Cushing disease have no visible pituitary mass on MRI, even using high-definition 3 Tesla MRI and dynamic imaging software {4997}. In this situation, bilateral inferior petrosal sinus sampling can verify a central source of ACTH. Recent studies have suggested a possible role for 11C-methionine PET-CT or 68Ga CRH PET-CT imaging in the localization of pituitary microtumours {2412,4761}.

Densely granulated corticotroph tumours are mainly microtumours, whereas silent corticotroph tumours, sparsely granulated corticotroph tumours, and Crooke cell tumours often manifest as macrotumours {1533,1126,216}. Sparsely granulated corticotroph tumours are frequently hyperintense on T2-weighted MRI {1127}. Silent corticotroph tumours tend to present as large tumours invading the cavernous sinuses {4998,74,2079,906}.

Epidemiology

The annual incidence of pituitary Cushing disease is 3–10 cases per 1 million population {4527}. This may well be an underestimate, because patients with mild, subclinical Cushing disease may go undiagnosed, and these cases have often been misclassified as silent corticotroph tumours {2732}. Corticotroph tumours account for 15–17% of all PitNETs in surgical series {2961,3668,1687}. The peak incidence is at age 30–50 years. There is a male predominance among prepubertal patients, whereas a female preponderance is seen in adults {2788,4291, 4292,2961,1687}. Corticotroph tumours account for approximately 55% of PitNETs in children aged < 11 years {2450} and 75% of cases of Cushing syndrome in children aged > 5 years {4292,1375}. The most common histological subtype is densely granulated corticotroph tumour, followed by sparsely granulated tumours; Crooke cell tumours are rare {2961}.

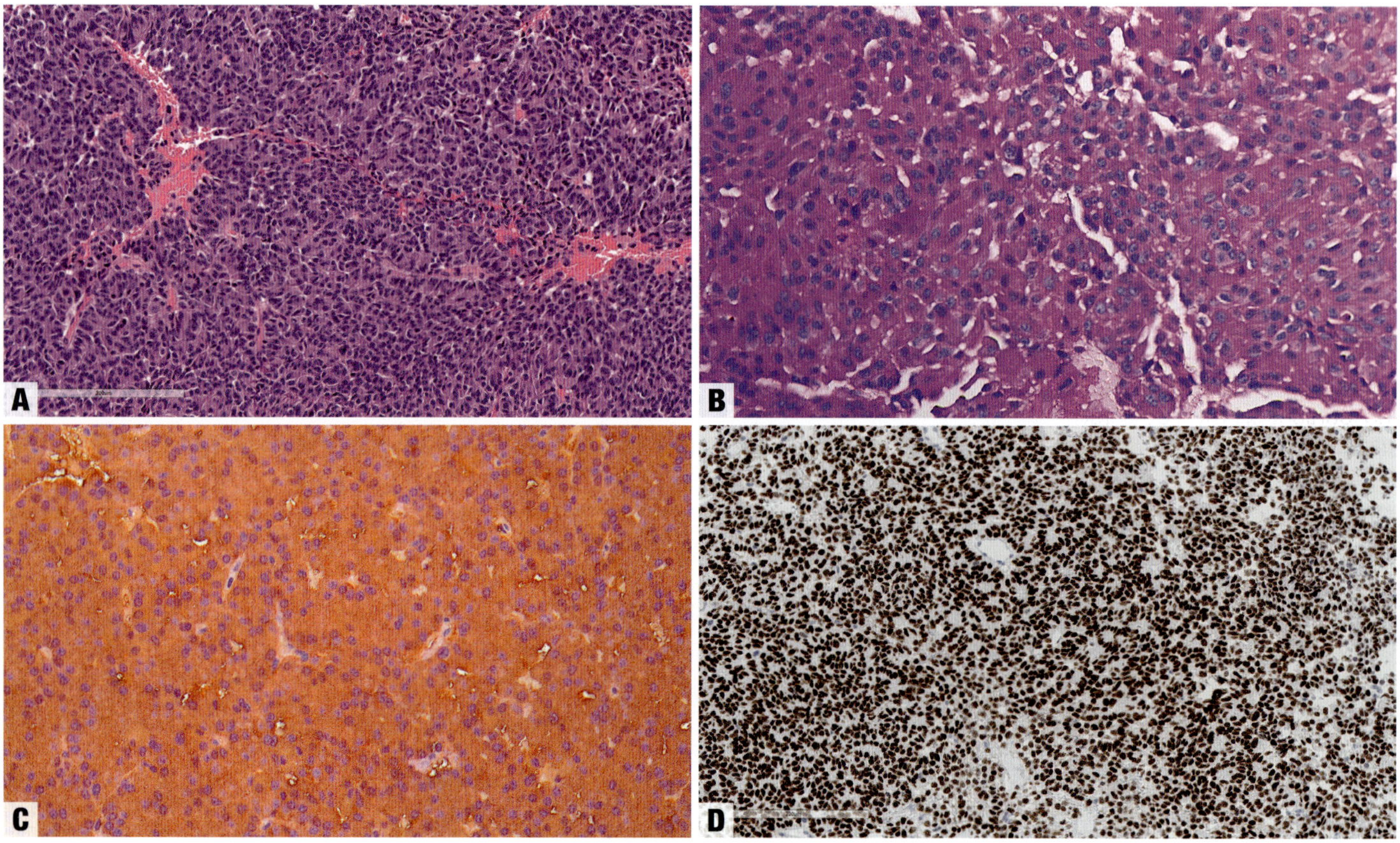

Fig. 2.33 Corticotroph PitNET, densely granulated. Densely granulated corticotroph tumours have a basophilic appearance (**A**). These tumours have abundant secretory granules, which correlate with their diffuse and strong expression of PAS (**B**) and ACTH (**C**). Like other corticotroph PitNETs, these tumours are diffusely positive for TPIT (**D**).

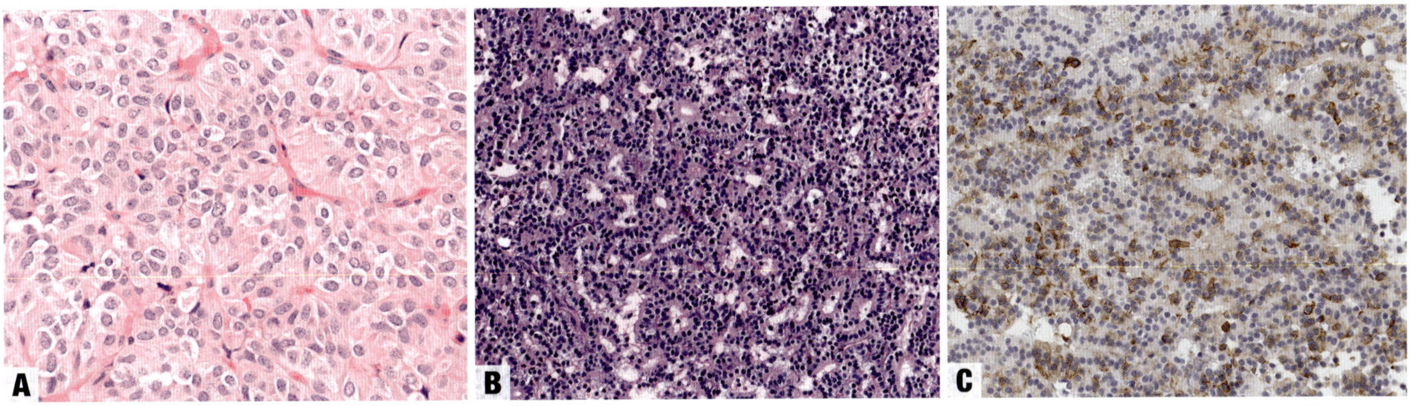

Fig. 2.34 Corticotroph PitNET, sparsely granulated. Sparsely granulated corticotroph PitNETs are composed of faintly basophilic or chromophobic tumour cells (**A**) that have variable secretory granules, which correlate with their variable and weak reactivity for PAS (**B**) and ACTH (**C**).

Etiology

Genetic and epigenetic factors, abnormal hormonal stimulation, and dysregulation of growth factors and their receptors contribute to the tumorigenesis of corticotroph tumours.

Pathogenesis

Most somatic gene alterations described in corticotroph tumours are not specific to that tumour type {1196,4060,214}. However, activating somatic *USP8* mutations are found in about 25–60% of corticotroph tumours {3716,2775,3520,1830,1342, 2736,4816,559,2860}; they are associated with increased POMC mRNA levels and increased EGFR (HER1) expression {3716,2775,3520,4453}. *USP8* mutations are most often found in functioning densely granulated corticotroph tumours and are usually absent in silent corticotroph tumours {2775,3520, 3742}. *USP8* mutation–driven corticotroph tumours have higher expression levels of SSTR5 and MGMT than *USP8*-wildtype tumours {1830}, suggesting possible responsiveness to pasireotide {1830}. *USP48* {777,3973} and *BRAF* mutations have also been reported in corticotroph tumours {777}. *TP53* alterations have been identified in a subset of *USP8*-wildtype corticotroph tumours in one series {3974,4632}, and in association with *ATRX* mutations in aggressive and metastatic corticotroph tumours {687}.

DAXX-related and/or *ATRX*-related alternative lengthening of telomeres is a feature of recurrent/aggressive mostly functioning corticotroph tumours {688,687,1843}. Increased *LGALS3*/galectin-3 expression was reported in aggressive corticotroph tumours {3745}. Invasive corticotroph tumours and Crooke cell tumours are associated with increased expression of miR-106b~25 cluster and its host gene *MCM7* on 7q22 {1500}. MCM7 protein expression is also higher in invasive corticotroph tumours {889}.

Corticotroph tumours often show normal expression of stimulatory CRH and vasopressin (antidiuretic hormone) receptors, normal glucocorticoid receptor expression, and slightly diminished ACTH feedback receptor expression, with no frequent mutations commonly found; the ratio of 11β-dehydrogenase isozymes 1 and 2 is altered, resulting in disrupted cortisol feedback, but this is not specific to corticotroph tumours. The expression of cyclins, CDKs, and their regulators is altered; the specific alterations in corticotroph tumours are the greatly reduced expression of p27 and the increased expression of cyclin E, and there are also changes in the feedback transcription factors SMARCA4 and HDAC2 {426}. Like other pituitary tumours, corticotroph tumours show increased activity of the pro-proliferative signalling pathways based on PI3K/mTOR and MAPK {1196,4953}. A recent study suggested miR-182-5p as a candidate circulating biomarker of Cushing disease {4694}.

Transcriptome analyses of a small series identified overrepresentation of genes related to endoplasmic reticulum processing in functioning corticotroph tumours {1208}. Silent corticotroph tumours have a specific pattern of expression of adhesion molecules, which differs from that in functioning tumours and is suggested to play a role in their aggressiveness {1208}. The latter would be in line with the differential expression of biomarkers related to cell invasion, motility, and migration in silent corticotroph tumours as compared with gonadotroph tumours {2969}. In addition, loss of membranous E-cadherin expression, a hallmark of epithelial–mesenchymal transition, has been correlated with larger and more invasive corticotroph tumours {1292}. Methylome studies also showed distinct signatures between functioning and silent corticotroph tumours {3742}, and exclusive GATA3 expression in silent corticotroph tumours {3742}. Epigenetic silencing of p27 has been reported to be mediated by *Skp2*-regulated degradation in corticotroph tumours {2693}, but this is disputed {3145}.

FGFR4 polymorphisms have been shown to play a role in tumour growth and sensitivity to glucocorticoid hormone negative feedback through STAT3 signalling; patients homozygous for the *FGFR4*-R388 variant have a higher frequency of silent corticotroph macrotumours than those with *FGFR4*-G388, who were more likely to have small but hormonally active microtumours {3168}.

Genetic susceptibility

Only very few cases of Cushing disease have been reported in familial isolated pituitary adenoma (FIPA) {4301}, multiple endocrine neoplasia type 1 (*MEN1*) {4155}, or multiple endocrine neoplasia type 4 (*CDKN1B*) {4953}. Pathogenic germline *USP8* variants can cause paediatric Cushing disease {881}. There have been rare case reports of corticotroph tumours in patients with tuberous sclerosis (*TSC1/TSC2*) {4497,3184}, multiple endocrine neoplasia type 2 {3201}, and Lynch syndrome {4624, 384}, and glucocorticoid resistance syndrome due to germline *NR3C1* mutations {2206}. Germline pathogenic *CABLES1* variants were reported in corticotroph tumours {1872}. Although pathogenic germline *DICER1* mutations are characteristics of pituitary blastomas (see *Pituitary blastoma*, p. 89), rare examples of missense germline *DICER1* variants have been reported in *USP8*-wildtype paediatric corticotroph tumours; however, at the somatic level, none of these had loss of heterozygosity for the *DICER1* variants {2859}.

Macroscopic appearance

Corticotroph tumours are often soft and white to greyish-red.

Histopathology

Corticotroph tumours are composed of neuroendocrine cells with variable amounts of basophilic secretory granules that are highlighted using PAS staining and ACTH immunohistochemistry. Corticotroph tumours typically have a sheet-like architecture, but they may also show papillary-like patterns such as perivascular pseudorosettes. The interface with normal gland may be indistinct, with infiltration of adjacent intact normal parenchymal elements by the tumour cells in small groups or singly. Morphologically, corticotroph tumours have been divided into three histological subtypes on the basis of their density of secretory granules and organization of their cytoplasmic keratin filaments using low-molecular-weight cytokeratin reactivity patterns. These include (1) densely granulated corticotroph tumours, (2) sparsely granulated corticotroph tumours, and (3) Crooke cell tumours. Most corticotroph tumours fall into one of these histological subtypes; however, occasional tumours have both sparsely and densely granulated components, and some have focal Crooke cell change {2961}. The term "silent corticotroph tumour" is not a histological subtype; these tumours can feature all morphological subtypes of corticotroph tumours {3992,3804,74,2952,1600}. Most corticotroph tumours are solitary neoplasms; rarely, however, they may represent a component of a double PitNET {1300,2930,2939}, or they may occur in combination with a gangliocytoma {3626,3879} or (extremely rarely) an adrenocortical choristoma {886,87,2974,1882,4586}.

Immunohistochemistry

Corticotroph tumours are positive for ACTH, TPIT, and NeuroD1, and they are negative for PIT1, SF1, and hormones of PIT1 lineage (growth hormone, prolactin, and TSH) and of SF1 lineage (gonadotropins) {2952,2958,1626,2961}. Rarely, corticotroph tumours can express GATA2/GATA3 and α-subunit {4349,2971, 4592}. ACTH staining may be weak or absent in some cases, emphasizing the importance of pituitary transcription factors for correct classification {4174,2957}. Corticotroph tumours usually have diffuse strong cytoplasmic keratin expression using CAM5.2 {2952,1626,2961,208}. The concentric pattern of keratin staining in Crooke cells is distinctive {208}. The proliferative activity of corticotroph tumours is variable {2961,1687}. Loss of p27 (encoded by *CDKN1B*) is a frequent finding in corticotroph tumours {965,2372,2693,4060,2961}, and a more common in functioning corticotroph tumours than in silent corticotroph tumours {2961}.

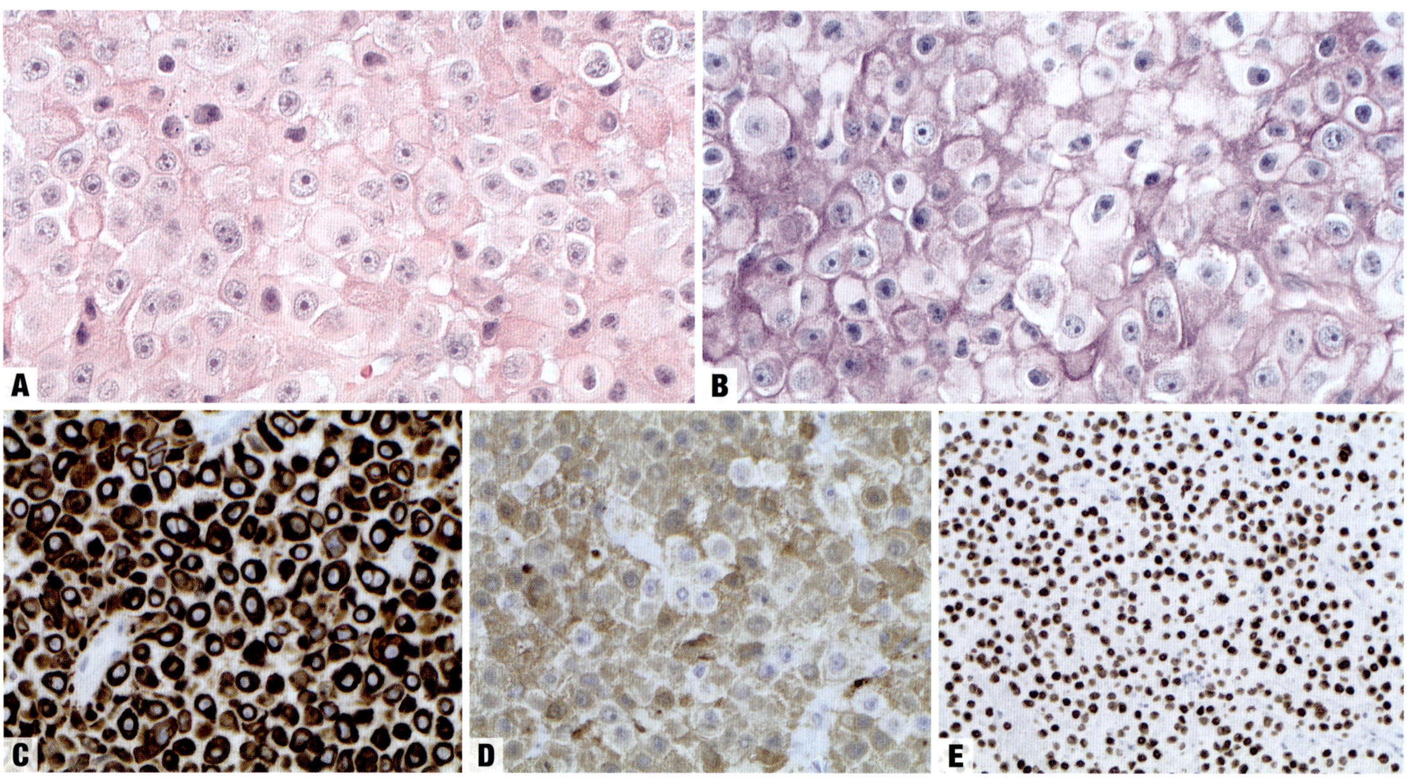

Fig. 2.35 Corticotroph PitNET. **A** Crooke cell tumour in a patient with a clinically non-functioning PitNET. Crooke hyaline change is present in a majority of the tumour cells. **B** Perinuclear hyaline material in the tumour cells of Crooke cell PitNET is PAS-negative. **C** Strong perinuclear and ring-like expression of the low-molecular-weight cytokeratin CAM5.2 corresponding to hyaline material accumulation in tumour cells of Crooke cell PitNET. **D** There is a lack of ACTH expression in the perinuclear and ring-like hyaline aggregates in tumour cells with Crooke hyaline change. ACTH immunolabelling is diffusely present in the cytoplasm of tumour cells without Crooke hyaline change or dislocated to the cell periphery in the tumour cells demonstrating Crooke hyaline change. **E** Strong nuclear expression of TPIT in tumour cells of the Crooke cell PitNET.

Densely granulated corticotroph tumours have a basophilic appearance on H&E-stained sections. The tumour cells have abundant secretory granules, which correlate with their diffuse and strong staining for PAS and ACTH {2952,2958,1626}.

Sparsely granulated corticotroph tumours are composed of faintly basophilic or chromophobic PAS-positive tumour cells with weak or patchy positivity for ACTH, consistent with the scant, small secretory granules seen ultrastructurally {2952, 2958,1626,3269}. Rarely, ACTH can be negative, and diffuse TPIT positivity confirms corticotroph differentiation {3269}.

Crooke cell tumours are composed of neuroendocrine cells with Crooke hyaline change. Ring-like cytokeratin expression is typical of these neoplasms {2952,2958,1626,211}. Positivity for PAS and ACTH is dislocated to the cell periphery and juxtanuclear region. Earlier studies suggested CK20 as a marker of corticotroph and Crooke cells {903,1281}; however, a recent study failed to reproduce this finding {208}, instead confirming CAM5.2, CK18, and AE1/AE3 as appropriate keratins to highlight Crooke hyaline change {208}.

Differential diagnosis

Corticotroph hyperplasia is an extremely rare cause of Cushing disease {3277}, but it is often not identified in surgical pathology practice; however, it has been reported in the setting of ectopic CRH-secreting tumours {3311,355,3984,1133,1413,2956} or untreated Addison disease {1326,2956,4899}.

The assessment of the surrounding anterior pituitary is critical for identifying Crooke hyaline change in non-tumorous corticotrophs. This morphological biomarker of glucocorticoid excess occurs in about 80% of patients with functioning corticotroph tumours {3346,66} and is not seen in patients with pseudo-Cushing states or silent corticotroph tumours {2952,2958,1626}.

Cytology

Although cytology is not used in the routine diagnostic setting, a homogeneous cellular smear consisting of cells with basophilic granular cytoplasm suggests a corticotroph tumour.

Diagnostic molecular pathology

There are no molecular tests required to diagnose corticotroph tumours. A lack of ATRX immunoreactivity is a marker of aggressive and/or metastatic tumours and should be confirmed by molecular genetic analysis. Germline screening for inherited tumours may be considered on the basis of clinicopathological findings.

Essential and desirable diagnostic criteria

Densely granulated corticotroph tumours

Essential: TPIT positivity; diffuse ACTH or PAS reactivity; negativity for PIT1 and SF1; often diffuse keratin; basophilic cytoplasm.

Sparsely granulated corticotroph tumours

Essential: TPIT positivity; variable to absent/scarce ACTH or PAS expression; negativity for PIT1 and SF1; often diffuse keratin; faintly basophilic or amphophilic cytoplasm.

Crooke cell tumours

Essential: TPIT positivity; relocation of ACTH expression and PAS-positive granules to the cell periphery; perinuclear, ring-like keratin.

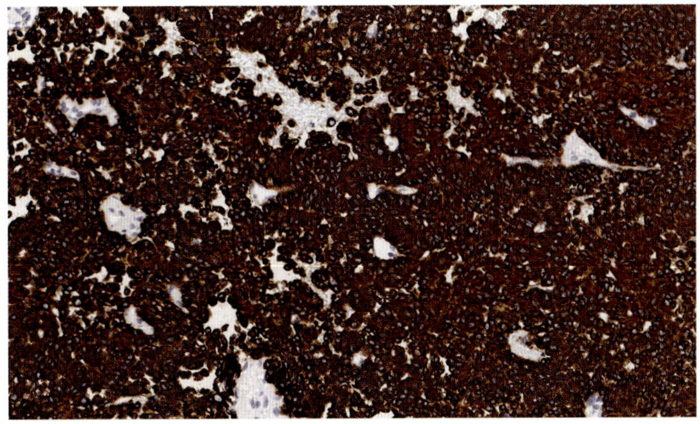

Fig. 2.36 Corticotroph PitNET. CAM5.2 is expressed in densely and sparsely granulated tumours. Both densely and sparsely granulated corticotroph tumours show diffuse and strong cytoplasmic reactivity for CAM5.2. This photomicrograph illustrates CAM5.2 reactivity in a densely granulated corticotroph tumour.

Staging

There is no formal staging system that has been universally applied for pituitary/sellar neoplasms. A CT-era approach based on tumour size and patterns of invasion was proposed in 1973 by Hardy {1786}. Subsequently, a standardized assessment of parasellar tumour extension based on MRI was published by Knosp in 1993 {2354}.

There are no pathology-standardized reporting templates yet endorsed by international pathology organizations. A pathology reporting template for pituitary tumours was introduced in 2011 {3300}, followed by the European Pituitary Pathology Group (EPPG) proposal in 2019 {4707}.

Prognosis and prediction

Persistent untreated Cushing disease is lethal {3573}. Surgery is the treatment of choice and is often curative for microtumours. The surgical cure rate is lower in macrotumours with cavernous sinus invasion. Silent corticotroph tumours may tend to be more aggressive in terms of invasion and recurrence rate {3992, 4991}. However, a recent meta-analysis could not confirm a higher recurrence risk of silent corticotroph tumours compared with other non-functioning PitNETs {1414}.

Crooke cell tumours are often associated with clinically aggressive disease {1533,2414} (a case of invasive and metastatic Crooke cell tumour is demonstrated in *Metastatic PitNET*, p. 79); however, sparsely granulated corticotroph tumours are also associated with some degree of biological aggressivity {1126,3669} that requires further validation.

Like other types of PitNETs, invasive and proliferative corticotroph tumours show an increased risk of disease recurrence/progression {4560,1687} and metastatic spread {2122}. *ATRX*-mutated corticotroph tumours exhibit aggressive behaviour {687}. An absence of Crooke hyaline change of non-tumorous corticotrophs may predict recurrence in patients with functioning corticotroph tumours {66}. SSTR5 immunohistochemistry may help predict responsiveness to pasireotide. Clinically aggressive corticotroph tumours with low or absent MGMT expression have been reported to respond to temozolomide treatment {3908,3907,158,385,4902}.

Gonadotroph PitNET/adenoma

Lopes MBS
Mete O
Nishioka H
Perry A

Definition

Gonadotroph pituitary neuroendocrine tumour (PitNET)/adenoma is a well-differentiated PitNET composed of SF1-lineage adenohypophysial cells with gonadotroph differentiation.

ICD-O coding

8272/3 Gonadotroph PitNET/adenoma

ICD-11 coding

2D12.Y Other specified malignant neoplasms of other endocrine glands or related structures

Related terminology

Acceptable: gonadotroph tumour.

Not recommended: gonadotropin-positive PitNET/adenoma; gonadotropin-producing PitNET/adenoma; gonadotroph cell PitNET/adenoma; gonadotrope PitNET/adenoma; gonadotropinoma.

Subtype(s)

None

Localization

The majority of gonadotroph tumours are intrasellar masses with variable suprasellar and parasellar extension, including the cavernous sinus. Ectopic gonadotroph tumours are extremely uncommon, with only rare reports of cases occurring in the sphenoidal sinus, suprasellar region, third ventricle, and nasopharynx {4086,3629,4475,2332,1458}.

Clinical features

Unlike other PitNETs/adenomas of well-differentiated cell lineage, most gonadotroph tumours are clinically non-functioning (lacking hormone overproduction) and are therefore referred to by some as "silent gonadotroph tumours/adenomas". Generally, these tumours come to medical attention with symptoms related to mass effects, such as visual disturbances, headaches, and hypopituitarism. Hypogonadism, including diminished libido and/or impotence, is present in most male patients {5089}. Among premenopausal women, menstrual disturbances and/or galactorrhoea may be seen, whereas in postmenopausal women clinical manifestations are related to mass effects. Some cases may be diagnosed incidentally through imaging studies performed for other purposes {1288, 1157}. In rare cases, pituitary apoplexy can be the presenting symptom {4062}.

Clinically functioning gonadotroph tumours are rare and diagnosed in patients with elevated levels of FSH/LH or non-suppressed FSH/LH in the presence of elevated gonadal steroids {930,1661}. Functioning tumours are more frequently identified in premenopausal women with a myriad of clinical symptoms, including menstrual irregularities, infertility, galactorrhoea, polycystic ovarian syndrome, and ovarian hyperstimulation syndrome (e.g. abdominal and pelvic pain, bloating, and multiple ovarian cysts) {3305,930,1661}. Functioning tumours in postmenopausal women have been rarely reported, but the clinical presentation is similar to that of clinically non-functioning tumours and related to mass effect {3305}. Likewise, tumours in men may have no symptoms specific to hormonal excess {930}; however, testicular hypertrophy and sexual dysfunction have been reported {4197,1876,877,3305}. Only rare cases have been reported in children with presentation of precocious puberty {3305}.

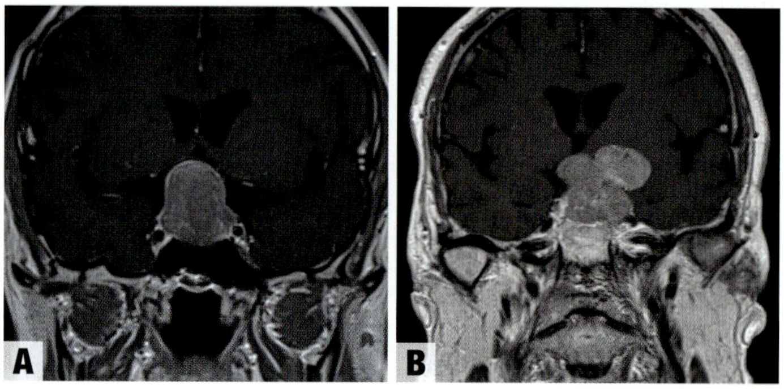

Fig. 2.37 Gonadotroph PitNET/adenoma. T1-weighted coronal MRI. **A** These tumours are often found as larger tumour masses. Typically, they are intrasellar with suprasellar extension. **B** Some are invasive giant tumours.

Biochemical investigations

Preoperative hypersecretion of FSH and LH (defined as a > 2-fold increase above the upper limit of normal) may be observed in men but normally is not seen in premenopausal or postmenopausal women {5089}. Mild hyperprolactinaemia (usually of < 100 ng/mL) is often found, due to pituitary stalk deviation {5089,4659}.

Neuroimaging

Gonadotroph tumours are mostly large masses (mean size: 28 mm) {1881}), often with suprasellar extension and compression of the optic pathways. Radiographic invasiveness (Knosp grade 3 or 4) has been noted in 13.2–56.4% of cases in recent series with updated pathological diagnosis {105,2031,1881}.

Epidemiology

Before the 2017 WHO classification of tumours of endocrine organs, the incidence and prevalence rates of gonadotroph tumours were difficult to estimate, because of the imprecision in distinguishing these tumours from null cell adenomas. Recent pathological series classifying pituitary tumours according to the updated WHO classification have demonstrated that gonadotroph tumours represent about 31–49.5% of surgically removed tumours {3691,2961,3874} and 70–75% of non-functioning pituitary tumours {3269,3379,1157,3874}.

Gonadotroph tumours usually occur in the sixth to eighth decade of life {3379,2961,2031,1881}, with a slight male preponderance {3379,2031,1881}. These tumours are uncommon in paediatric patients (aged ≤ 20 years) {3020,3400,3529,2961,4782}.

Etiology

The etiology for most cases is unknown, although rare case reports have suggested that some may be secondary to longstanding primary hypogonadism {2415,3234}.

Pathogenesis

A small proportion of gonadotroph tumours arise in patients with syndromic diseases, including familial isolated pituitary adenoma (FIPA) {591,4243}. They account for about 20% of surgically resected tumours in the setting of multiple endocrine neoplasia type 1 {4559}, and less commonly in multiple endocrine neoplasia type 4 {109}, SDH-related syndrome {4954}, and *AIP*-associated FIPA {1871}.

Sequencing studies of sporadic gonadotroph tumours showed a lower frequency of somatic mutation rates than in other pituitary tumour types. Somatic mutations involving genes associated with hereditary pituitary tumours (e.g. *MEN1*, *CDKN1B*, *AIP*, and *PRKAR1A*) are rarely observed in sporadic clinically non-functioning pituitary tumours, including gonadotroph tumours {325,4243}.

Genetic events other than recurring somatic mutations, including epigenetic changes, DNA methylation alterations, abnormal microRNAs, and copy-number variations, may play a role in the pathogenesis of most sporadic gonadotroph tumours {3219,3147,418,2359,2360,3208}. Still, sporadic non-functioning tumours including gonadotroph tumours are considered genomically quiet tumours, with rare copy-number gains or losses {418,3208}.

Macroscopic appearance

Gonadotroph tumours are usually large tumours (> 10 mm) with substantial suprasellar or infrasellar extension associated with sellar enlargement or destruction. They are usually soft, tan to dark-brown tumours. Tumours with apoplexy contain areas of necrosis and/or haemorrhage.

Histopathology

Gonadotroph tumours are mostly chromophobic or oncocytic and contain only scant, peripherally situated PAS-positive granules. Unlike normal gonadotrophs, tumour cells are polygonal to elongate with marked cell polarity. Although diffuse and sinusoidal patterns of the tumour cells may be seen, the distinctive trabecular pattern, perivascular pseudorosettes, and even papillary arrangement are consistent and prominent histological features {2385}. Thus, histological neuroendocrine patterns are often seen in gonadotroph tumours.

Immunohistochemistry

Immunohistochemical stains for gonadotropins show variable reactivity for FSH-β, LH-β, or α-subunit. FSH-β alone or combined with LH-β and/or α-subunit is the most common immunohistochemical type {2961,2031}. Tumours positive for only LH-β are rare {2961,2031}.

Immunohistochemistry for the transcription factors SF1, ERα, ERβ, and GATA3 is an additional tool for the characterization of these tumours, particularly in cases in which pituitary hormone immunostaining is faint/uncertain and especially for tumours that lack expression of pituitary hormones. PitNETs that lack expression of gonadotropins but express SF1 represent about 21% of all gonadotroph tumours {3269}. In a large survey of gonadotroph tumours, SF1 and ERα expression was identified in 96% and 82% of these tumours, respectively {2961}. SF1 nuclear labelling is largely strong and diffuse in tumour cells but may be slightly weak or even absent in oncocytic tumour cells {1881}. GATA3 has been reported in the majority (89–98.5%) of gonadotroph tumours {2971,4592,1881}.

Gonadotroph tumours express SSTR2 {3673,819,2031} and SSTR5 {3673} in a variable percentage of the reported cases.

Mitotic count is relatively low in the majority of gonadotroph tumours {2031}. Ki-67 labelling indexes vary in the literature, with 40.2–85.7% of cases reported as having labelling indexes of < 3% {2961,2031}.

Differential diagnosis

Other clinically non-functioning tumours, in particular null cell and hormone-negative corticotroph tumours, should be distinguished from gonadotroph tumours, because they may behave differently. Metastatic carcinomas can mimic gonadotroph tumours, particularly those that lack gonadotropin immunostaining, because some metastatic carcinomas may express ER, GATA3, SF1 {2971}, and INSM1. Because some of the gonadotroph tumours with pseudorosettes mimic gastroenteropancreatic neuroendocrine tumours (GEP-NETs), the possibility of metastatic GEP-NETs must be considered in the differential diagnosis for gonadotroph tumours {3662}. Primary sellar paragangliomas {1787,4165,203} should be distinguished from hormone-negative gonadotroph tumours

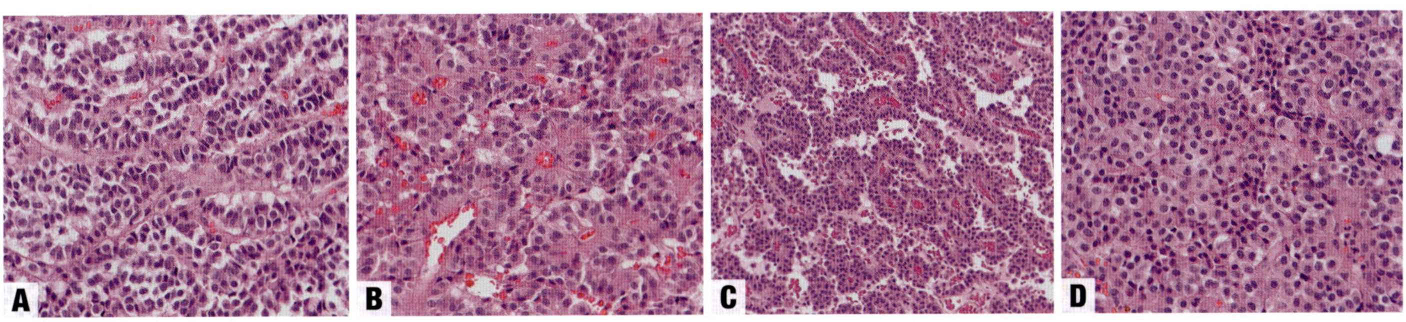

Fig. 2.38 Gonadotroph PitNET/adenoma histopathology. These tumours are composed of chromophobic cells arranged in nests and in diffuse, sinusoidal, and trabecular (**A**) arrangements. Prominent perivascular (**B**) and papillary (**C**) arrangements of elongate cells are also seen. Oncocytic changes characterized by abundant eosinophilic cytoplasm due to mitochondria accumulation may be present (**D**).

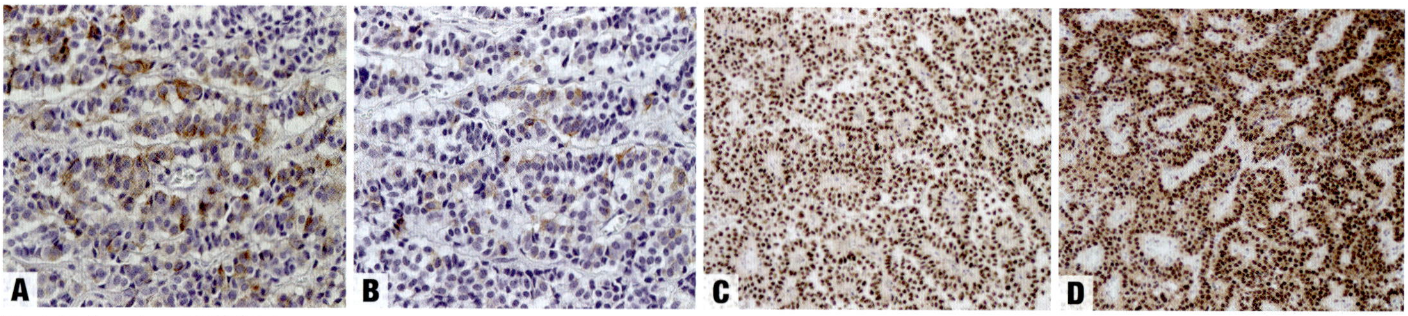

Fig. 2.39 Gonadotroph PitNET/adenoma immunohistochemistry. The tumours may show variable immunopositivity for the gonadotropins FSH-β (**A**), LH-β (**B**), and α-subunit (not shown). Nuclear expression of SF1 (**C**) and GATA3 (**D**) is present in the majority of the tumours.

because of their common positivity for GATA3; expression of SF1 and cytokeratins is helpful in these situations {203}. However, negativity for keratins occurs in about 40% of gonadotroph tumours {2961}. The latter finding along with GATA3 expression should not automatically be taken for a diagnosis of paraganglioma. Positivity for tyrosine hydroxylase and negativity for SF1 can help distinguish paraganglioma. Oncocytic pituicytoma should be ruled out in cases suspicious for a gonadotroph tumour with a more oncocytic appearance; they uniformly stain for thyroid transcription factor 1 (TTF1) and S100 {2565,2973}.

Cytology

Gonadotroph tumours are distinguished by their hypercellularity and homogeneous appearance in cytological preparations. Tumour cells may have enlarged, pleomorphic, or atypical nuclei with variable cytoplasm often embedded in a granular background. Papillary formations are easily recognized on cytological touch or smear preparations.

Diagnostic molecular pathology

There are no specific molecular tests applied to gonadotroph tumours for routine diagnosis. Because a subset of tumours arise in the setting of hereditary syndromes, germline genetic screening has been recommended for all patients aged < 30 years with a macrotumour or any childhood-onset pituitary tumour, regardless of family history {4495,958,4287,591,2855}.

Essential and desirable diagnostic criteria

Essential: a PitNET/adenoma with variable immunoreactivity for gonadotropins (FSH-β, LH-β, α-subunit) and/or SF1; absence of PIT1 and TPIT expression.

Desirable: immunoreactivity for ER and GATA3.

Staging

There is no formal staging system that has been universally applied for pituitary/sellar neoplasms. A CT-era approach based on tumour size and patterns of invasion was proposed in 1973 by Hardy {1786}. Subsequently, a standardized assessment of parasellar tumour extension based on MRI was published by Knosp in 1993 {2354}.

There are no pathology-standardized reporting templates yet endorsed by international pathology organizations. A pathology reporting template for pituitary tumours was introduced in 2011 {3300}, followed by the European Pituitary Pathology Group (EPPG) proposal in 2019 {4707}.

Prognosis and prediction

The majority of gonadotroph tumours have an indolent clinical behaviour. In a recent European Society of Endocrinology survey on aggressive pituitary tumours and pituitary carcinomas, only 4% of aggressive pituitary tumours and 2.5% of pituitary carcinomas were of gonadotroph cell lineage {2914}. No single biomarker has been found to independently predict aggressive behaviour of gonadotroph tumours {1482,2952,3692}.

Surgery is the primary treatment for gonadotroph tumours. Like for other non-functioning tumours, the most significant predictive factor for recurrence is incomplete surgical resection (i.e. postoperative residual tumour), mostly due to cavernous sinus invasion. Tumour invasion is the major risk factor for incomplete removal {536,921,2599}. However, the data associating invasiveness with tumour recurrence/progression are highly conflicting {3439,2735,752,3270,3693,343,921,2599}. Other factors that may be related to recurrence include a young age at diagnosis and large/giant tumours {1173,3704,4823,3439,2735,752,3270,3693,343}.

The Ki-67 (MIB1) proliferation index has been one of the most studied biomarkers in non-functioning tumours, including the gonadotroph types, but its usefulness as a single predictive factor for progression has similarly yielded mixed results {1173,3673,3906,4560,2599,3691}.

Postoperative radiation therapy may be indicated in cases with a large postoperative remnant or regrowth; pharmacotherapy seems to be of limited value in gonadotroph tumours, but it may occasionally be effective {4823,700}. Currently used drugs for the pharmacological treatment of PitNETs/adenomas are somatostatin analogues and DRD2 agonists. SSTR expression and ER expression have been recently studied in gonadotroph tumours as potential predictors of tumour medical responsiveness and tumour clinical behaviour. However, these are exceedingly early data and the results are inconsistent {3379,2031,1832}.

Null cell PitNET/adenoma

Casar-Borota O
Ezzat S
Lopes MBS
Nishioka H
Oyama K
Perry A

Definition

Null cell pituitary neuroendocrine tumour (PitNET)/adenoma is a PitNET that shows no evidence of adenohypophysial differentiation by immunohistochemistry for pituitary hormones and the transcription factors PIT1, SF1, and TPIT.

ICD-O coding

8272/3 Null cell PitNET/adenoma

ICD-11 coding

2D12.Y Other specified malignant neoplasms of other endocrine glands or related structures

Related terminology

Acceptable: pituitary transcription factor and hormone–immunonegative PitNET/adenoma.

Not recommended: immunonegative PitNET/adenoma.

Subtype(s)

None

Localization

Null cell PitNETs are sellar tumours with frequent suprasellar and parasellar growth, sometimes with cavernous and/or sphenoidal sinus extension.

Clinical features

Like patients with other non-functioning PitNETs, patients with null cell tumours usually present with symptoms of mass effect, including visual disturbance, headaches, and various degrees of hypopituitarism. They show no clinical symptoms of hormonal excess apart from occasional mild hyperprolactinaemia due to stalk section effect. A few cases are detected because of a neurological deterioration associated with pituitary apoplexy {105}.

Neuroimaging

Null cell tumours are usually large masses, often with suprasellar extension and compression of the optic chiasm; they are more likely to invade the cavernous sinus than comparable clinically silent gonadotroph tumours {105}.

Epidemiology

There are limited epidemiological data regarding null cell PitNETs as they are currently defined. With the complementary use of antibodies to pituitary transcription factors and anterior pituitary hormones, the proportion of null cell PitNETs has been reduced to < 5% {2961,4175}. One study has shown a reduction to < 1% {3269}. In a recent study, no tumour was classified as a null cell PitNET in a cohort of 171 well-characterized PitNETs {2605}. These data support the previous anticipation that the number of null cell PitNETs/adenomas will diminish with methodological improvements {2416}.

Etiology

Unknown

Pathogenesis

There are no known genetic or epigenetic factors involved in the pathogenesis of transcription factor and hormone–immunonegative PitNETs. The majority of previously diagnosed null cell adenomas probably represent silent, hormone-negative gonadotroph or corticotroph PitNETs that could not be recognized by using immunohistochemistry for pituitary hormones and transcription factors. This has also been suggested by recent molecular genetic studies {3208,955}.

Whether null cell tumours are pathogenetically distinct from their gonadotroph or corticotroph counterparts needs to be determined. Further molecular genetic studies are needed to show whether a proportion of tumours diagnosed as null cell tumours represent true null cell PitNETs originating from pituitary stem cells that show no signs of differentiation towards mature pituitary cell lineages.

Macroscopic appearance

The macroscopic appearance of null cell tumours does not differ from that of other PitNETs. Null cell PitNETs are usually macrotumours. They are mainly solid tumours; however, cystic or haemorrhagic changes can occasionally be identified.

Histopathology

In general, the histopathology of null cell PitNETs does not differ from that of silent gonadotroph or corticotroph tumours. Occasionally, oncocytic change can be seen in the tumour cells. Neuroendocrine markers and synaptophysin, and usually also chromogranin A, are positive. However, immunostains for SF1, TPIT, PIT1, and all adenohypophysial hormones are negative.

Immunohistochemistry

When a tumour fulfils the criteria for null cell PitNET, the use of an expanded set of antibodies to transcription factors involved in pituitary cell differentiation, such as GATA2 {4044}, GATA3 {2971}, ER {4043}, and insulin gene enhancer protein ISL1 {4044}, is recommended. Positivity for GATA3 raises the possibility of paraganglioma. In such cases, the identification of keratin reactivity would support a PitNET, but these tumours are not always positive for keratins; therefore, tyrosine hydroxylase may be helpful for further distinction. Immunopositivity for thyroid transcription factor 1 (TTF1), CDX2 {3998}, or serotonin {688} argues against the diagnosis of PitNET.

Differential diagnosis

Differential diagnosis from rare metastatic neuroendocrine tumours (NETs) is critically important and needs an extensive immunohistochemical panel. Most, but not all, NETs that are metastatic to the pituitary have an appropriate clinical history of a known extracranial primary, unique immunohistochemical features, and transcription factor marks of the tumour's primary site of origin, as well as a generally a higher proliferation index than most PitNETs. In the rare patients with null cell PitNETs, imaging workup such as PET-CT to search for NET in other organs should be considered by the multidisciplinary team {2827}. The important differential with a primary sellar paraganglioma is discussed above (see *Immunohistochemistry*).

Cytology

The cytological features of null cell tumours are identical to those of other PitNETs.

Diagnostic molecular pathology

There are no molecular tests required to diagnose these tumours. Germline screening for inherited tumours should be considered on the basis of clinicopathological findings.

Essential and desirable diagnostic criteria

Essential: a PitNET/adenoma with a lack of immunoreactivity for pituitary-lineage transcription factors and pituitary hormones.

Desirable: additional immunostains to rule out sellar paraganglioma and other neuroendocrine neoplasms (NENs).

Staging

There is no formal staging system that has been universally applied for pituitary/sellar neoplasms. A CT-era approach based on tumour size and patterns of invasion was proposed in 1973 by Hardy {1786}. Subsequently, a standardized assessment of parasellar tumour invasiveness based on MRI was published by Knosp in 1993 {2354}.

There are no pathology-standardized reporting templates yet endorsed by international pathology organizations. A pathology reporting template for pituitary tumours was introduced in 2011 {3300}, followed by the European Pituitary Pathology Group (EPPG) proposal in 2019 {4707}.

Prognosis and prediction

There are data indicating that null cell PitNETs may be more invasive at the time of diagnosis, and associated with a more aggressive clinical course and shorter progression-free survival, than silent gonadotroph tumours {105}. However, data are based on limited case numbers, and no molecular genetic data have been provided to confirm a lack of pituitary cell lineage differentiation.

Plurihormonal PitNET/adenoma

Casar-Borota O
Ezzat S
Perry A

Definition

Plurihormonal pituitary neuroendocrine tumour (PitNET)/adenomas are PitNETs composed of a single population of tumour cells expressing adenohypophysial hormones and/or transcription factors belonging to more than one cell lineage.

ICD-O coding

8272/3 Plurihormonal PitNET/adenoma

ICD-11 coding

2D12.Y Other specified malignant neoplasms of other endocrine glands or related structures

Related terminology

Acceptable: unusual plurihormonal tumour/adenoma.

Subtype(s)

None

Localization

Pituitary gland, with tumour invasion into the parasellar structures in some cases

Clinical features

Plurihormonal PitNETs/adenomas may cause clinical symptoms due to the hypersecretion of any or all hormones expressed in the tumour cells, or they may be clinically non-functioning.

Epidemiology

There are limited data on the epidemiology of plurihormonal PitNETs, because studies in which tumour classification has been based on the complementary use of immunohistochemistry for pituitary hormones and transcription factors are still rare. In a recent study including 1055 PitNETs, only 5 tumours (0.5%) expressed unusual combinations of PIT1, SF1, and various hormones related to the respective cell lineages {2961}. In a case report, a double adenoma composed of a corticotroph component and a plurihormonal component expressing PIT1, SF1, growth hormone, TSH-β, and FSH-β was described {4524}.

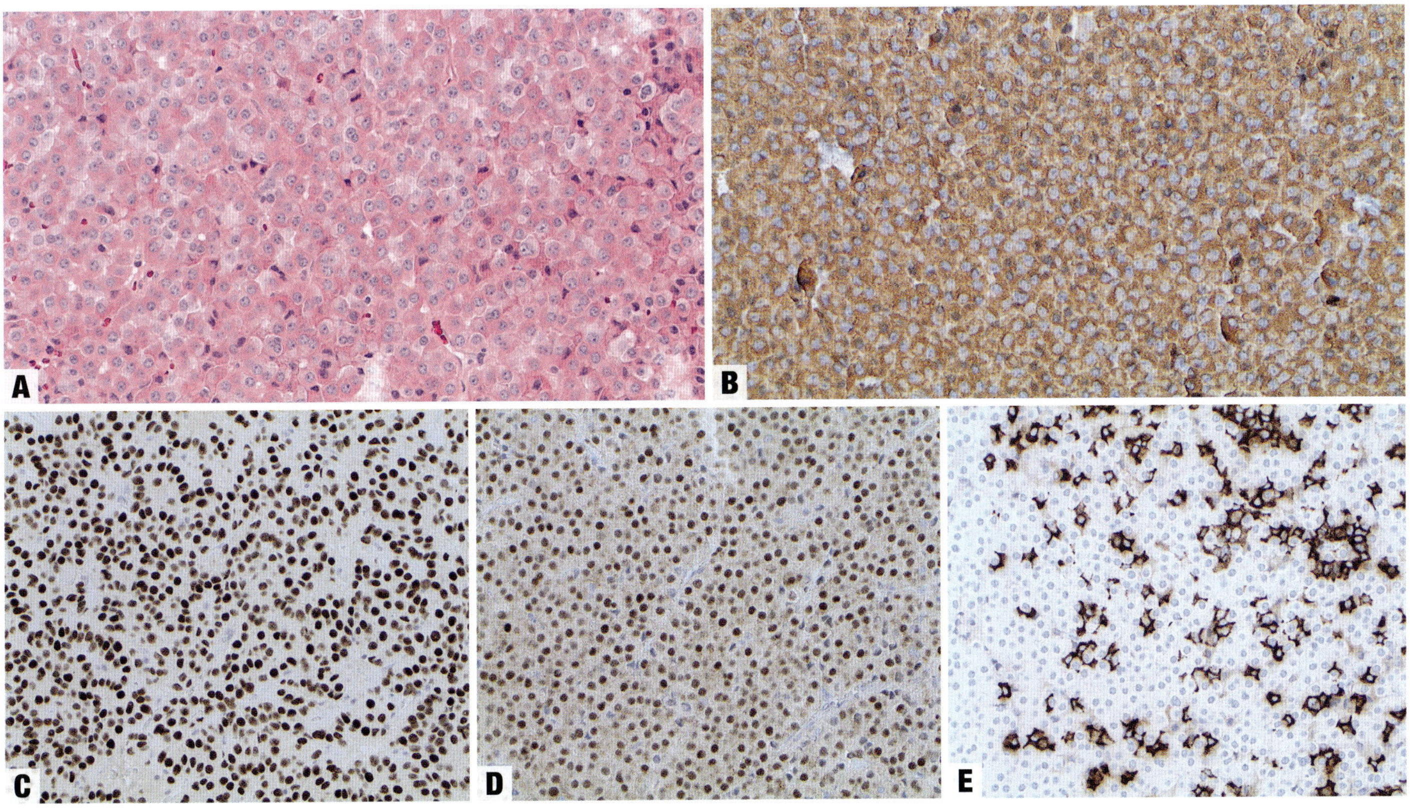

Fig. 2.40 Plurihormonal PitNET/adenoma. **A** A case of plurihormonal PitNET composed mainly of acidophilic tumour cells, in a patient with acromegaly. **B** Extensive expression of growth hormone in a plurihormonal PitNET in a patient with acromegaly. **C,D** Coexpression of PIT1 (**C**) and SF1 (**D**) in tumour cells of a plurihormonal PitNET/adenoma. **E** Positivity for prolactin in a subset of tumour cells in a plurihormonal PitNET in a patient with acromegaly.

Etiology

The etiology of plurihormonal PitNETs/adenomas is unknown.

Pathogenesis

The pathogenesis of plurihormonal PitNETs/adenomas is unknown. An origin from stem cells or progenitor cells with the capacity to differentiate towards multiple cell lineages has been hypothesized {2961}. Gene expression profiles that overlap multiple pituitary cell lineages (SF1/PIT1 and SF1/TPIT) have been recently revealed using whole-genome mRNA transcriptomics analysis {3208}.

Macroscopic appearance

The macroscopic appearance of plurihormonal PitNETs/adenomas does not differ from that of other types of tumours.

Histopathology

The microscopic appearance of plurihormonal PitNET/adenoma is similar to that of its individual cell lineages when found in pure form.

Immunohistochemistry

According to the authors' experience and sparse published literature {4524}, plurihormonal PitNETs/adenomas usually coexpress the transcription factors PIT1 and SF1, along with associated hormones from these two lineages that are present within the tumour. Recently, a plurihormonal tumour expressing all the three transcription factors has been reported in a patient with acromegaly {2605}.

Cytology

The cytology of these tumours is similar to that of other pituitary tumours.

Diagnostic molecular pathology

There are no molecular tests required to diagnose these tumours. Germline screening for inherited tumours should be considered on the basis of clinicopathological findings.

Essential and desirable diagnostic criteria

Essential: immunohistochemical expression of adenohypophysial hormones and transcription factors belonging to at least two different pituitary cell lineages.

Staging

There is no formal staging system that has been universally applied for pituitary/sellar neoplasms. A CT-era approach based on tumour size and patterns of invasion was proposed in 1973 by Hardy {1786}. Subsequently, a standardized assessment of parasellar tumour extension based on MRI was published by Knosp in 1993 {2354}.

There are no pathology-standardized reporting templates yet endorsed by international pathology organizations. A pathology reporting template for pituitary tumours was introduced in 2011 {3300}, followed by the European Pituitary Pathology Group (EPPG) proposal in 2019 {4707}.

Prognosis and prediction

There are no data providing prognostic criteria in plurihormonal PitNETs/adenomas. We anticipate that general prognostic markers combining cell proliferation and tumour invasion {4560} of a PitNET/adenoma may also be applied to this group.

Expression of SSTRs may suggest responsiveness to somatostatin analogues; however, there are no studies describing the effects of somatostatin analogues in patients with plurihormonal tumours.

Multiple synchronous PitNETs/adenomas of distinct lineages

Mete O
Ezzat S
Osamura RY
Perry A

Definition

Multiple synchronous pituitary neuroendocrine tumour (PitNET)/adenomas of distinct lineages are multiple well-differentiated PitNETs consisting of at least two different cell lineages (PIT1, SF1, and TPIT), or a null cell tumour combined with any lineage-specific PitNET.

ICD-O coding

Code as PitNET/adenoma types

ICD-11 coding

2D12.Y Other specified malignant neoplasms of other endocrine glands or related structures

Related terminology

Acceptable: multiple PitNETs of different cell lineages.

Not recommended: double PitNET/adenoma; triple PitNET/adenoma; plurihormonal PitNET/adenoma; mixed somatotroph and lactotroph PitNET/adenoma.

Subtype(s)

None

Localization

These tumours arise within the sella but may show variable extension into parasellar structures {2293,582,3769,2950}.

Clinical features

Although biochemically non-functioning tumours can occur, one or more components of a multiple PitNET of distinct cell lineages can be hormonally functional {2930,3769,2950,890}. Acromegaly (elevated growth hormone / IGF1 levels), Cushing disease (elevated ACTH and cortisol levels), hyperthyroidism (elevated thyroid hormone with inappropriate TSH secretion), and galactorrhoea-amenorrhoea (elevated prolactin levels) have been reported in patients with multiple PitNETs of distinct cell lineages {2384,3939,2293,2789,3769,2950,4524,977}. Non-functioning tumours can manifest with visual field defects or headache {3769}. Multiple PitNETs of distinct cell lineage are often macrotumours

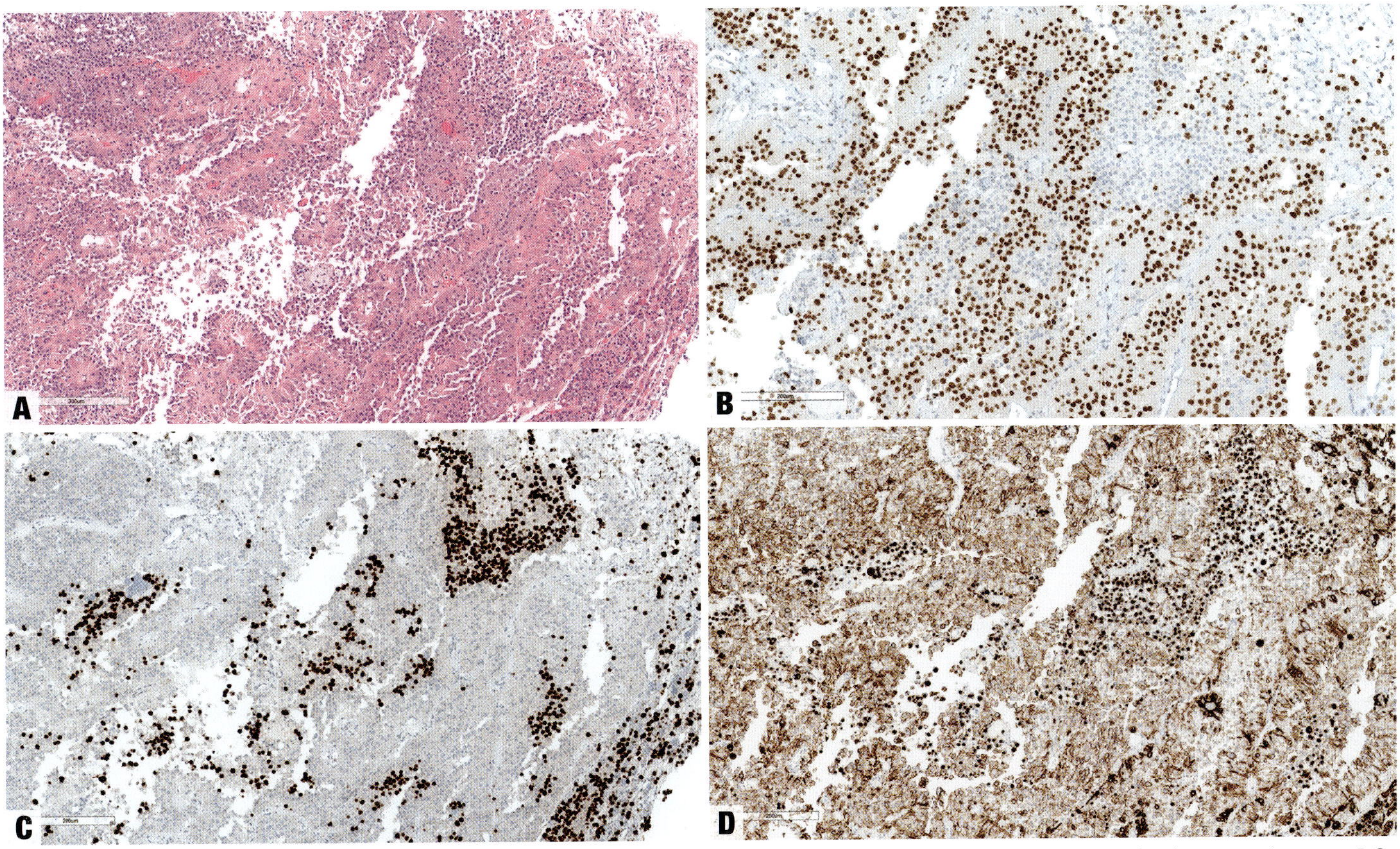

Fig. 2.41 Multiple synchronous PitNETs/adenomas of distinct lineages. Multiple PitNETs consisting of gonadotroph tumour and sparsely granulated somatotroph tumour. **A** On H&E-stained slides, it may be difficult to appreciate the presence of two distinct tumours. **B** SF1 stains the gonadotroph tumour. **C** The sparsely granulated somatotroph tumour component is positive for PIT1. **D** CAM5.2 shows fibrous bodies in the sparsely granulated somatotroph tumour component.

with a mean tumour size of 22.3 mm (range: 9–39 mm), according to a well-characterized clinical series {2950}.

Imaging

Contiguous PitNETs of distinct cell lineages have been reported to occur more frequently than non-contiguous tumours {3769, 2950}. Contiguous multiple PitNETs are often indistinguishable from solitary PitNETs on MRI studies even when examined by expert radiologists {3769}. Occasional multiple PitNETs of distinct cell lineages may be distinguished on preoperative imaging studies or during pituitary surgery if they are clearly separate tumours {2293,3769}.

In patients with Cushing disease due to a small microtumour, an incidental second PitNET may be a decoy lesion that can be mistaken for the source of ACTH and resected, resulting in failure of cure {475}.

Epidemiology

Synchronous multiple PitNETs of distinct cell lineages were reported to account for 1.2% of surgically resected PitNETs in a large series that was assessed using transcription factors in addition to hormone immunohistochemistry {2950}. Non-contiguous double PitNETs were reported to occur in 0.7% of 600 PitNETs surgically resected in a series, wherein half of these were of distinct cell lineages {2293}. In other series, the frequency of double PitNETs of different cell lineages ranged from 0.4% to 1.7% {2384,3686,3939,2789,977}, and autopsy studies have suggested even higher frequencies {2384,582}. Triple PitNETs of distinct cell lineages are rarer {2950}. In one series, a female predominance was reported {3769}; however, there was no significant sex difference in a larger series with a mean age of 55.2 years (range: 36–73 years) at the time of diagnosis {2950}.

Etiology

The etiology is largely unknown, with the exception of reported links to germline susceptibility in some patients with double PitNETs (see *Pathogenesis*) {3939,2293,4559,2950}.

Pathogenesis

The pathogenesis of synchronous multiple PitNETs of distinct cell lineages is largely unknown. Although one may suspect the possibility of an underlying genetic susceptibility, only a few cases showed a link to familial isolated pituitary adenoma (FIPA) {3939,2293} or multiple endocrine neoplasia type 1 {3686, 3939,4559,2950}. The incidence of multiple PitNETs was more frequent in patients with multiple endocrine neoplasia type 1 than in those without it {4559}. Specific genomic studies on sporadic cases of multiple synchronous PitNETs of distinct cell lineages are lacking.

Macroscopic appearance

Multiple PitNETs of distinct cell lineages have been described as white to yellow soft tumours {2293}.

Histopathology

Multiple PitNETs of at least two distinct cell lineages combine a PIT1, SF1, TPIT, or null cell tumour with at least one different PitNET type. Common combinations occur between TPIT- and PIT1-lineage tumours, or between SF1-lineage tumours and either TPIT- or PIT1-lineage tumours {2930,3769,2950, 165}. Immature PIT1-lineage PitNETs and unusual plurihormonal PitNETs {2950,4524} can also be a component of multiple PitNETs of distinct cell lineages. Accurate subtyping of each tumour component is required in the diagnostic workup of these tumours. Specific diagnostic criteria applied to individual PitNETs are identical to those applied to components of multiple PitNETs; however, the diagnosis of multiple PitNETs requires routine application of pituitary transcription factors {2093, 2950,2957,977,213}, because hormone immunohistochemistry alone may result in misclassification or mischaracterization {2957,2605}. These tumours can show variable Ki-67 labelling indexes, ranging from 1% to 5% {2950}.

Cytology

Not reported

Diagnostic molecular pathology

There are no molecular tests required to diagnose multiple PitNETs of distinct cell lineages. Germline screening for genetic susceptibility should be considered on the basis of clinicopathological findings, such as age < 30 years, family history, and other syndrome-associated findings.

Essential and desirable diagnostic criteria

Essential: a PitNET with components of at least two different cell lineages (PIT1, SF1, and TPIT) or a single-lineage tumour combined with a null cell tumour.

Staging

There is no formal staging system that has been universally applied for pituitary/sellar neoplasms. A CT-era approach based on tumour size and patterns of invasion was proposed in 1973 by Hardy {1786}. Subsequently, a standardized assessment of parasellar tumour extension based on MRI was published by Knosp in 1993 {2354}.

There are no pathology-standardized reporting templates yet endorsed by international pathology organizations. A pathology reporting template for pituitary tumours was introduced in 2011 {3300}, followed by the European Pituitary Pathology Group (EPPG) proposal in 2019 {4707}.

Prognosis and prediction

Accurate histological subtyping for each component of multiple PitNETs is of clinical significance {2950}. High-risk (aggressive) histological subtypes of PitNETs and the status of invasive growth were found to predict disease progression in patients with synchronous multifocal PitNETs of different cell lineages {2950}.

Metastatic PitNET

Asa SL
Ezzat S
McCutcheon IE
Perry A
Righi A

Chapter 2

Definition

Metastatic pituitary neuroendocrine tumour (PitNET) is a tumour of adenohypophysial neuroendocrine cells that manifests with metastatic disease to lymph nodes and/or distant sites, or that has discontinuous spread through the CNS.

ICD-O coding

8272/3 PitNET, malignant / pituitary carcinoma, NOS

ICD-11 coding

2D12.Y & XA8J35 & XH7KL6 Other specified malignant neoplasms of other endocrine glands or related structures & Pituitary gland & Pituitary carcinoma, NOS

Related terminology

Acceptable: pituitary carcinoma.

Not recommended: neuroendocrine carcinoma; pituitary neuroendocrine carcinoma.

Subtype(s)

All types and subtypes of PitNET can be metastatic.

Localization

The primary site is usually in the sella turcica but may occasionally be extrasellar, in ectopic locations such as the sphenoidal sinus. Metastatic foci occur in lymph nodes (usually cervical), liver, and bone, and the tumour may spread along the craniospinal axis as the result of dissemination in the subarachnoid space {3525}.

Clinical features

The initial clinical presentation is usually that of a PitNET. Most common is Cushing disease {2411,1446,3876,3564,384,5078,113} and the enhanced tumour growth associated with Nelson syndrome due to a lack of feedback inhibition {3525,2414}; other functioning tumours produce hyperprolactinaemia {3540,4764,3876,551,1689,113}, acromegaly {4286}, or hyperthyroidism due to TSH excess {551,3039}. Hormonally inactive tumours include gonadotroph, null cell, silent corticotroph, silent somatotroph, and poorly differentiated tumours of PIT1 lineage {2457,2767,358,3525,3806,2604,113}. The latency period between the diagnosis of an intrasellar PitNET and the development of metastasis varies widely.

Biochemical investigations

The biochemical features vary with the hormonal activity of the tumour; hypopituitarism may result from tissue destruction.

Neuroimaging

PET imaging using the 68Ga-DOTATATE tracer can identify the extent of disease and SSTR status {282}. The latter can inform on the potential utility of peptide receptor radionuclide therapy (PRRT) {113}.

Epidemiology

Metastatic spread of a PitNET is rare. Most published information is as single case reports; the largest series includes 40 patients {2914}. Metastatic PitNETs accounted for 0.12% of the pituitary tumours in the German Pituitary Tumor Registry {3877} and represented 0.4% and 0.56% of PitNETs in published series from two referral centres of pituitary pathology {113,1687}. Although most patients have been adults, a paediatric case has been reported {1724}.

Etiology

Unknown

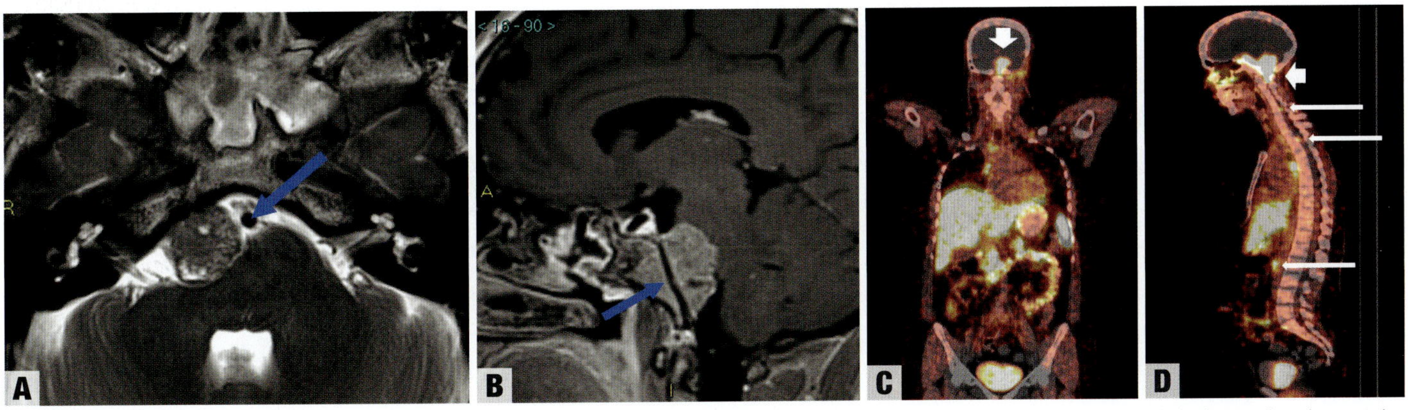

Fig. 2.42 Metastatic PitNET. **A,B** MRI of a multirecurrent corticotroph PitNET in a patient with Cushing disease who developed a metastasis in the pontine cisternae (arrow). **C,D** PET identified extensive 68Ga-DOTATATE reactivity involving the sella, extending into the suprasellar space and inferiorly to the posterior fossa and upper cervical spine (short arrow). Multiple intrathecal deposits in the mid-cervical and upper thoracic spine are also noted, with abnormal radiotracer uptake in the hilar, mediastinal, periportal, and retroperitoneal nodes (long arrows).

Pathogenesis

It is unclear whether metastatic potential is due to genetic or non-genetic (e.g. epigenetic, tissue microenvironment) alterations {1476}. Mutations identified in PitNETs are not implicated in progression to metastatic disease. Mutations in *HRAS* have been identified in metastatic deposits of 3 pituitary carcinomas, but not in their corresponding primary lesions {3485} or in other carcinomas examined {3485,589}. In 1 case, loss of function of *RB1* was implicated in the progression of an ACTH-producing pituitary carcinoma with distant metastases {1892}. Distinct clonal compositions of a primary and metastatic ACTH-producing pituitary carcinoma {5110} suggest the emergence of novel clones. Immunoreactivity for p53 has been reported in pituitary carcinomas {3525,4450} and mutation of *TP53* has been documented in several tumours {2618,4419,2243,3974,687}. Mutations of *ATRX* and *PTEN* have been described in metastatic tumours {687,1709}.

Metastatic PitNETs have been reported in patients with a germline tumour predisposition to neoplasia, including *SDHB* mutation {4582} and Lynch syndrome {384}.

Molecular profiling has shown evidence of multiple alterations in genes implicated in angiogenesis, invasion, and metastasis {5040}.

Macroscopic appearance

The gross appearance of these lesions is similar to that of non-metastasizing PitNETs.

Histopathology

Metastasizing PitNETs are histopathologically similar to their non-metastasizing counterparts. Some have been described as showing hypercellularity, nuclear pleomorphism, mitoses, necrosis, haemorrhage, and invasion, but these are also seen in non-metastatic invasive PitNETs {196}.

Immunohistochemistry

Pituitary immunohistochemical stains and/or electron microscopy are required for the classification of PitNETs, including within metastatic deposits. The Ki-67 labelling index may be high {4449,2914,113}, but this also is not specifically associated with metastatic potential. Metastatic tumours have been reported to exhibit a high microvascular density {4701}, high p53 labelling {4450}, loss of p27 immunoreactivity {2114,2394}, increased TOP2A {4702}, and overexpression of ERBB2 {3301}; however, none of these reliably predict metastatic behaviour.

Cytology

Cytological features are similar to those of non-metastasizing PitNETs.

Diagnostic molecular pathology

At this time, there are no molecular tests required to diagnose metastatic pituitary tumours. Germline screening for inherited somatotroph tumours should be considered on the basis of clinicopathological findings.

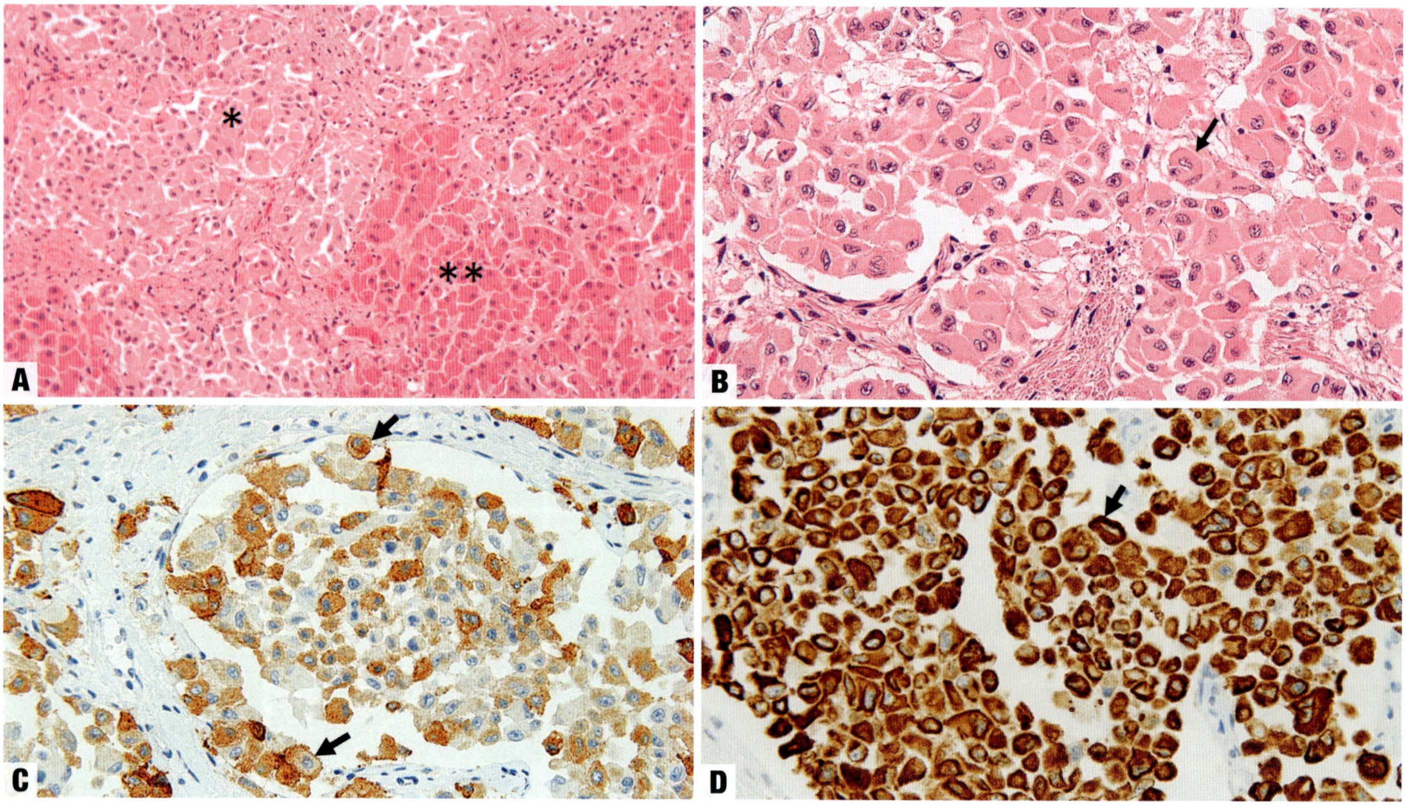

Fig. 2.43 Metastatic PitNET. **A** Crooke cell subtype, liver metastasis. This figure shows the mixture of pleomorphic tumour cells (single asterisk) and admixed hepatocytes (double asterisk). **B** The metastatic tumour cells are mainly large and pleomorphic. Nuclei are atypical. Some cells (arrow) demonstrate the appearance of Crooke cells. **C** Crooke cell subtype. Many tumour cells show positive granular staining for ACTH in the cytoplasm. Some tumour cells (arrow) demonstrate Crooke cell change. **D** Crooke cell subtype. Many tumour cells show strong and ring-like staining for keratin (CAM5.2). Some cells (arrow) exhibit a Crooke cell appearance.

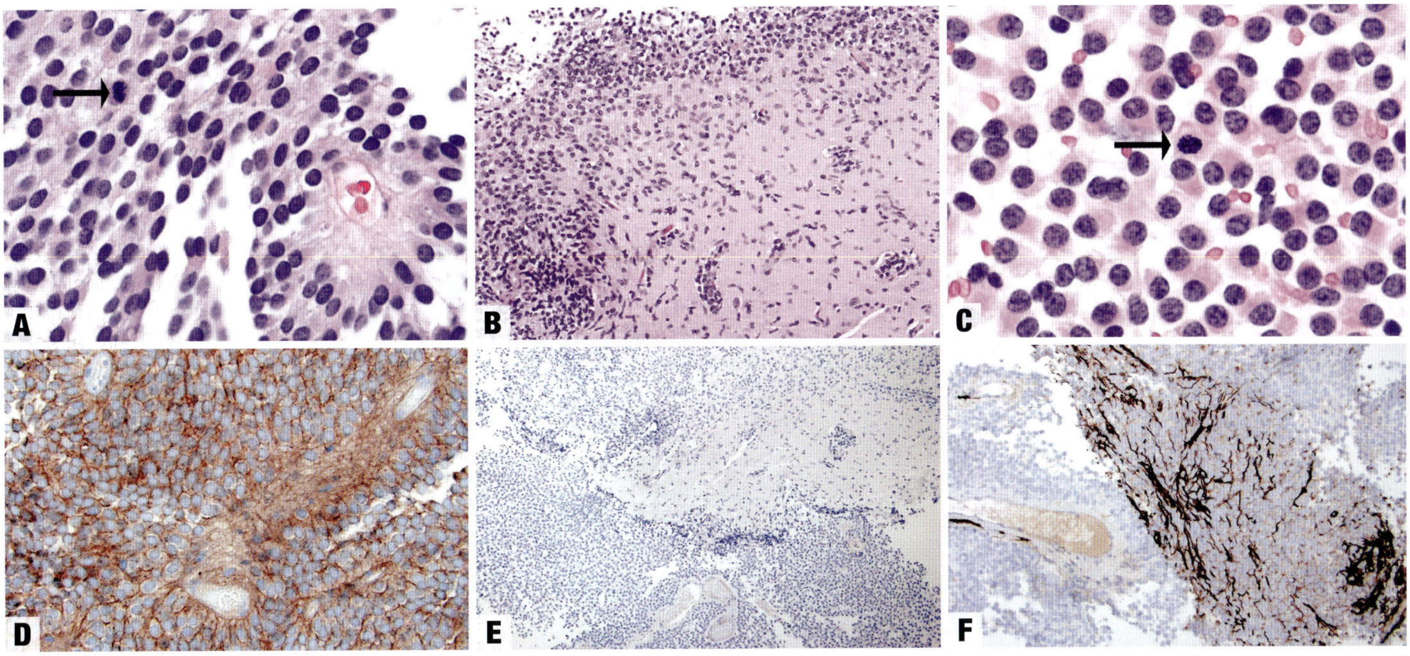

Fig. 2.44 Metastatic PitNET. A PitNET with both extensive cerebrospinal fluid dissemination and focal brain invasion. **A** The tumour cells are relatively homogeneous and there is a pseudorosette around a vascular channel. Note the mitosis (arrow). **B** The tumour invades into surrounding brain parenchyma. **C** A smear preparation shows cellular homogeneity but identifies a mitosis (arrow). **D** Immunohistochemical features of the metastatic PitNET. The tumour shows diffuse synaptophysin positivity. **E** The tumour cells are negative for all pituitary hormones and cytokeratins (shown here). **F** GFAP staining highlights reactive astrocytes in the region of brain invasion. The Ki-67 labelling index of this tumour was very high.

Essential and desirable diagnostic criteria

Essential: diagnostic features of a PitNET with documented metastasis or discontinuous CNS spread.

Staging

There is no formal staging system that has been universally applied for pituitary/sellar neoplasms. A CT-era approach based on tumour size and patterns of invasion was proposed in 1973 by Hardy {1786}. Subsequently, a standardized assessment of parasellar tumour extension based on MRI was published by Knosp in 1993 {2354}.

There are no pathology-standardized reporting templates yet endorsed by international pathology organizations. A pathology reporting template for pituitary tumours was introduced in 2011 {3300}, followed by the European Pituitary Pathology Group (EPPG) proposal in 2019 {4707}.

Prognosis and prediction

The number and variability of published cases is insufficient to draw accurate conclusions concerning appropriate therapy and prognosis. Aggressive surgical resection of metastases has shown survival benefit, whereas radiation therapy has only been palliative {3525}.

Temozolomide has shown some efficacy {1314,1741,2179, 2914,3946}; functioning tumours and those with low expression of MGMT display possibly better responses {2914}. Bevacizumab has also been reported to have efficacy {3846}. The concurrent administration of capecitabine and temozolomide (CAPTEM) has also been used, and subsequent immunotherapy with ipilimumab and nivolumab resulted in a significant reduction of hepatic and intracranial disease burden in a tumour with a somatic mutation burden consistent with alkylator-induced hypermutation that was not seen in the treatment-naïve tumour {2659}. In another study, 2 of 4 corticotroph pituitary carcinomas responded to pembrolizumab after prior exposure to alkylating agents {2800}.

Adamantinomatous craniopharyngioma

Santagata S
Kleinschmidt-DeMasters BK
Komori T
Müller HL
Nishioka H
Yamada S

Definition

Adamantinomatous craniopharyngioma is a mixed solid and cystic squamous epithelial tumour with stellate reticulum and wet keratin (ghost cells), usually localized to the hypothalamic–pituitary axis and characterized by activating *CTNNB1* mutations.

ICD-O coding

9351/1 Adamantinomatous craniopharyngioma

ICD-11 coding

2F7A.Y & XH15X9 Other specified neoplasms of uncertain behaviour of endocrine glands & Craniopharyngioma, adamantinomatous

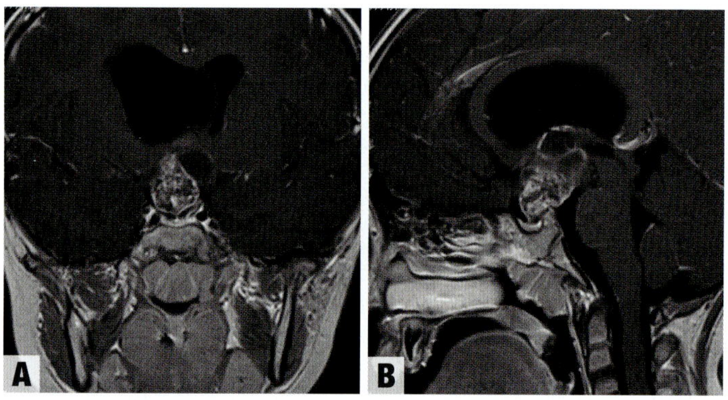

Fig. 2.45 Adamantinomatous craniopharyngioma. **A,B** A 6-year-old girl presented with severe headache and vomiting. MRI disclosed a large cystic and solid mixed suprasellar tumour with unilateral hydrocephalus. She also showed panhypopituitarism.

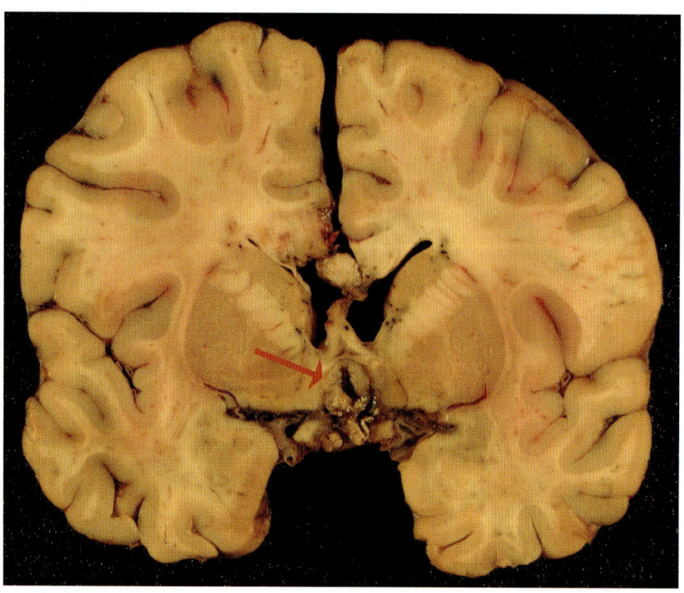

Fig. 2.46 Adamantinomatous craniopharyngioma. A solid and cystic mass with calcification (arrow), first diagnosed 4 years earlier.

Related terminology

None

Subtype(s)

None

Localization

Adamantinomatous craniopharyngioma arises anywhere along the hypophysial canal, but most occur in the sellar and infundibulotuberal region {3131}. The majority (~95%) have a suprasellar component (purely suprasellar, 20–41%; both suprasellar and intrasellar, 53–75%), whereas purely intrasellar craniopharyngiomas are less common (~5%) {2202}. Occasionally, a tumour extends into the anterior (9%), middle (8%), or posterior (12%) fossa. Very rare examples present in the cerebellopontine angle and other ectopic sites {1471}.

Clinical features

Craniopharyngioma rarely presents incidentally (< 2%) {450}. The diagnosis is often made years after the initial manifestation of nonspecific symptoms related to increased intracranial pressure, such as headache {3129,1921}. Primary manifestations include visual impairment (62–84%) {3617} and endocrine deficits (52–87%) affecting growth hormone (75%), LH/FSH (40%), TSH (25%), ACTH (25%), and vasopressin (antidiuretic hormone; 17–27% have central diabetes insipidus at diagnosis) {2202,3131}. Reduced growth rates may be seen in children as young as 12 months, before a diagnosis of craniopharyngioma is made {3129}. Weight gain, predictive of hypothalamic obesity, tends to occur as a later manifestation, shortly before and during the first year after diagnosis {3128}. Almost half of patients develop hypothalamic syndrome from disease- or treatment-related hypothalamic involvement/damage {3128,3129,3130, 1232,453} associated with morbid obesity, cognitive impairment, personality changes, and psychiatric symptoms {3384, 3453}.

Imaging

On MRI and CT, adamantinomatous craniopharyngiomas are intrasellar and parasellar tumours with solid and cystic components {4818}. Imaging features follow a 90% rule: about 90% are predominantly cystic, about 90% have prominent calcifications, and about 90% take up contrast media in the cyst walls {2126, 3131}. Local invasion of hypothalamic, visual tract, and vascular structures, including encasement of the internal carotid arteries, is common (~25%) {5103,3131}. Subarachnoid dissemination or implantation along the spinal cord, the surgical track, or the path of inserted catheters is rare {4003,2395,1922,588}.

Epidemiology

Craniopharyngioma constitutes 1.2–4.6% of all intracranial tumours, accounting for 0.5–2.5 new cases per 1 million person-years {562,3238,5106,3351}. Adamantinomatous craniopharyngioma is the most common non-neuroepithelial intracerebral neoplasm in children (5–11% of intracranial tumours in this age group) {3351,3820}. It accounts for nearly all craniopharyngioma diagnoses in children and about 80% of craniopharyngioma diagnoses in adults {3491,5106,3397}.

There is a bimodal age distribution {3238,5106}, with incidence peaks in children (5–15 years) and adults (45–60 years). Rare neonatal/fetal cases occur {3133,792,2158}. There is no sex predilection {562,5106,3351}.

Etiology

Unknown

Pathogenesis

Craniopharyngiomas are proposed to arise from cellular elements related to the Rathke pouch/hypophysial duct, which is integral to pituitary development {3131}. Expression of oncogenic β-catenin in early embryonic precursors and in SOX2+ stem cell populations of the pituitary drive formation of tumours resembling adamantinomatous craniopharyngioma {1516,142}. SOX2+ progenitors may also underlie formation of papillary craniopharyngioma {1812} and Rathke cleft cyst {535}. Similar stem cell populations for adamantinomatous and papillary craniopharyngiomas {1507} may explain shared patterns of cytokeratin expression {2458,4428,4963,2551}; scattered cells expressing pituitary hormones {4364}, chromogranin A {4994}, and hCG {4368}; and the occasional presence of mixed transitional tumour and cyst phenotypes {3968,1620,1383,3999,2823}. In adamantinomatous craniopharyngioma, SOX2+ stem cells may contribute to the formation of epithelial whorls with nuclear localized β-catenin. The whorls are senescent and function as signalling centres secreting numerous factors including sonic hedgehog, FGF, TGF-β, BMPs, and proinflammatory mediators {578,141,937,1633,938,166,535}. The whorls are analogous to the enamel knot that controls tooth morphogenesis {166,535} and implicate paracrine signalling in tumour formation and signal transduction via primary cilia {937}. Histological and molecular parallels with odontogenic tumours suggest similar cells of origin and similar mechanisms of pathogenesis {402,3474} and explain the occasional presence of teeth in adamantinomatous craniopharyngioma {357}.

Macroscopic appearance

Adamantinomatous craniopharyngiomas are lobulated solid masses with one or several cysts filled with a dark green-brown liquid resembling machine oil.

Histopathology

The well-differentiated tumour epithelium forms cords, lobules, ribbons, nodular whorls, and irregular trabeculae. Peripheral crowding and palisading are prominent. Degenerative features such as fibrosis, calcification, and nodules/whorls of anucleate remnants of ghost-like squamous cells (wet keratin) are common. Loose microcystic areas of stellate reticulum often intermingle between the wet keratin and more densely arranged areas of tumour epithelium. Cysts are often lined by an attenuated, flattened epithelium. Finger-like tumour protrusions extend into surrounding gliotic brain tissue with numerous Rosenthal fibres. A secondary degenerative feature is a xanthogranulomatous reaction to ruptured cyst material, which is characterized by cholesterol clefts, haemosiderin deposits, xanthoma cells, multinucleated giant cells, and lymphoplasmacytic infiltrates. This extensive reaction can constitute a significant, and sometimes near-total, component of the surgically excised material, necessitating a careful search for residual identifiable epithelium and wet keratin. Some xanthogranulomas of the sellar region, however, are associated with a ruptured/haemorrhagic Rathke cleft cyst. Adamantinomatous craniopharyngiomas show a striking resemblance to odontogenic tumours including calcifying odontogenic cyst (50%), ameloblastoma (25%), and mixed calcifying odontogenic cyst and ameloblastoma (15%), and more rarely resemble a few other subtypes {3474}. Malignant progression is exceedingly rare, generally developing after multiple recurrences and radiation therapy, often decades after first diagnosis {3780, 4204,3191,4778}, and resembling squamous cell carcinoma and ameloblastic or odontogenic ghost cell carcinoma {3780,2982}. Primary suprasellar malignant tumour with odontogenic features may represent a morphological pattern of transformed adamantinomatous craniopharyngioma {3780,3271}.

Immunophenotype

Adamantinomatous craniopharyngioma have activating mutations in *CTNNB1*, which encodes β-catenin. The mutation is clonal and present across the tumour epithelium {520,1641, 168}; however, nuclear accumulation of β-catenin is spatially restricted and found in only a small percentage of cells, most pronounced within small epithelial whorls {579,578,938,168}. Nuclear β-catenin is observed even when *CTNNB1* mutations are not detected {1641}. In general practice, immunohistochemistry can replace genetic analysis as an aid in determining the subtype diagnosis of craniopharyngioma {1455}.

Proliferation index

Ki-67 is generally confined to palisading regions and is absent in epithelial whorls. The Ki-67 proliferation index varies widely between cases and provides no prognostic information {3661, 1182,2737,519}.

Grading

Adamantinomatous craniopharyngioma is regarded as CNS WHO grade 1.

Differential diagnosis

The differential diagnosis includes papillary craniopharyngioma, xanthogranuloma, Rathke cleft cyst, epidermoid and dermoid cysts, and pilocytic astrocytoma. The distinction from papillary craniopharyngioma can be made using immunohistochemistry; papillary craniopharyngiomas are positive for BRAF p.V600E using the VE1 antibody, whereas adamantinomatous craniopharyngiomas have β-catenin nuclear staining in the nodular whorls {1455}. Xanthogranuloma of the sellar region is most often a reactive lesion resulting from the leakage, rupture, or haemorrhage of a Rathke cleft cyst, based on strips of columnar or ciliated columnar epithelium in the resected material {3473, 123,1165,2330}, although occasionally it can also be secondary to the leakage of wet keratin from adamantinomatous craniopharyngioma. Epidermoid cysts are distinguished by the presence of a uniloculated cavity lined by keratinizing squamous epithelium and filled with flaky, dry keratin. Dermoid cysts additionally have adnexal structures. Rathke cleft cysts have a cyst

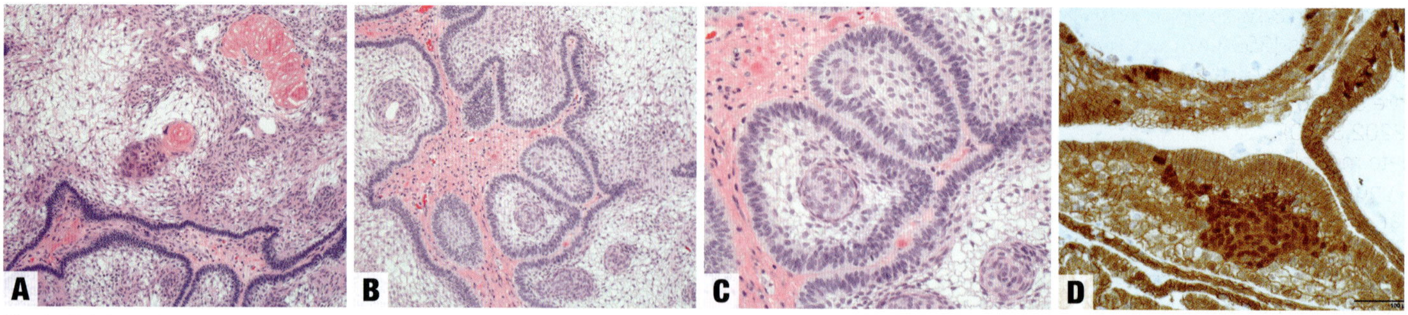

Fig. 2.47 Adamantinomatous craniopharyngioma. **A** Basal palisading of tumour cells along the tumour–brain interface, epithelial whorls, stellate reticulum, and wet keratin. **B** Tumour extending into adjacent brain tissue, which has reactive changes including piloid gliosis and Rosenthal fibres. Epithelial whorling is commonly present in protrusions. **C** High-power view of the interface of adamantinomatous craniopharyngioma and brain tissue; Rosenthal fibres are present in the reactive piloid gliosis. **D** Even though mutations in exon 3 of the *CTNNB1* gene, which encodes β-catenin, are clonal and present across the neoplastic epithelium, β-catenin protein only accumulates in the nucleus in subset of cells, such as those that are scattered individually and present in small clusters.

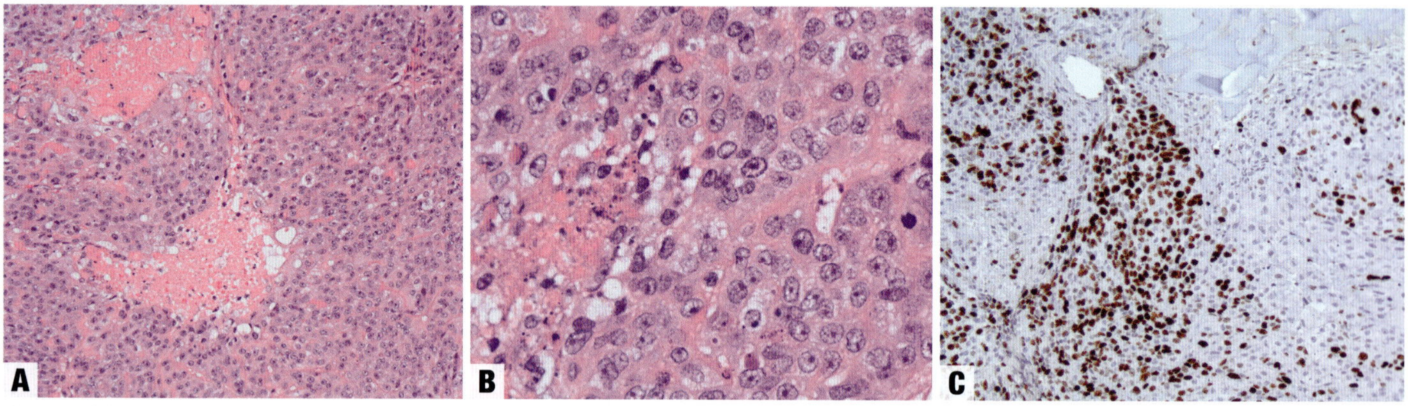

Fig. 2.48 Adamantinomatous craniopharyngioma. **A** Recurrence 19 years after resection and radiation treatment of an adamantinomatous craniopharyngioma that was previously CNS WHO grade 1. Sheets of poorly differentiated cells showing severe cytological atypia, large vesicular nuclei, prominent nucleoli, mitotic activity, and foci of necrosis. **B** High-power view of malignant craniopharyngioma emerging 19 years after resection and radiation treatment of an adamantinomatous craniopharyngioma that was previously CNS WHO grade 1. Sheets of poorly differentiated cells showing severe cytological atypia, large vesicular nuclei, prominent nucleoli, mitotic activity, and necrosis. **C** Characteristic very high tumour cell proliferation in malignant craniopharyngioma, as indicated by the Ki-67 index.

wall lined by simple columnar or cuboidal epithelium, which often is ciliated, with mucinous goblet cells. Myxoid/mucoid cyst contents are common. Rosenthal fibres and dense piloid gliosis adjacent to adamantinomatous craniopharyngioma can mimic pilocytic astrocytoma, but the dense cellularity and biphasic nature characteristic of pilocytic astrocytoma are absent.

Cytology

Although not a specific finding, cyst fluid may contain cholesterol clefts.

Diagnostic molecular pathology

Adamantinomatous craniopharyngiomas are characterized by activating mutations in exon 3 of *CTNNB1*, the gene that encodes the WNT signalling pathway regulator β-catenin {4058,2226,579,520,1933,2815,1641,1776,168}, which lead to the overexpression of β-catenin targets such as *AXIN2* and *LEF1* {1932}. Identification of *CTNNB1* mutations can be variable, ranging from about 60–75% to nearly 100% in some series, depending on the sensitivity of sequencing methods and analytical approaches. *CTNNB1* mutations are clonal driver events {520,167,168}, but nuclear localization of β-catenin is observed in only a fraction of tumour cells, mostly in epithelial whorls. Additional recurrent mutations have not been reported. Germline mutations in *APC* have rarely been identified, but only in combination with *CTNNB1* mutations {1638}. Consistent with the distinct histology and driver mutations of adamantinomatous craniopharyngioma and papillary craniopharyngioma, the tumours also display distinct methylation and transcription profiles {1933}. Although *CTNNB1* and *BRAF* mutations are mutually exclusive, coexistence of the mutations has been (rarely) reported {2531}. Recurrent focal deletions of Xp28 have been described in a subset of samples from male patients, and other recurrent gains have also been described {1641}.

Essential and desirable diagnostic criteria

Essential: a well-differentiated squamous epithelial tumour; stellate reticulum and/or wet keratin foci.

Desirable: nuclear immunoreactivity for β-catenin; mutation in *CTNNB1*; absence of *BRAF* p.V600E mutations.

Staging

Not relevant

Prognosis and prediction

Overall mortality in craniopharyngioma is reported to be three to five times as high as that observed in the general population {3512}. Overall survival (OS) rates reported in paediatric patients range from 83% to 96% at 5 years {3128} and from 65% to 100% at 10 years {3593,4716}; on average, the OS rate at 20 years is 62%. In mixed paediatric and adult patient cohorts, OS rates are 54–96% at 5 years {3512,2202}, 40–93% at 10 years {3512, 2202,3500}, and 66–85% at 20 years {3512,3500}. Increased late mortality without tumour progression results from metabolic syndrome, type 2 diabetes, cerebrovascular and cardiovascular disease, severe infection, and adrenal insufficiency {4716, 3351}. A novel MRI-based grading system of presurgical hypothalamic involvement and surgical hypothalamic lesions shows that posterior hypothalamic involvement/lesions have a major negative impact on hypothalamic function and quality of life {4280,453,1298}.

The optimal treatment for craniopharyngiomas still remains controversial. The debate centres on the need for radical resection for surgical cure, versus limited resection plus adjuvant radiotherapy. Both therapies yield similar rates of disease control and OS {2018}. Therefore, conservative surgical resection is of particular importance in cases with hypothalamic involvement {4280,3127}. In contrast, gross total resection is possible when tumours are small and separate from the hypothalamus and optic pathway. Recent advances in the treatment of craniopharyngioma have focused on minimizing treatment-related toxicity. These advances include endoscopic surgery and precision radiotherapy including stereotactic radiotherapy and proton therapy {3368}. Improved resection, decreased recurrence, and lower complication rates with the application of endoscopic endonasal approaches to paediatric craniopharyngioma are reported in the literature {4217}.

Malignant transformation of craniopharyngioma is rare {3780, 4204,3191,4778}. Tumours with *CTNNB1* T41 mutations or focal deletions of Xp28 may have a worse outcome {1641}. In 1 patient, partial and durable disease control was achieved by MEK inhibition {3459}, consistent with preclinical studies {166}. Distant intraventricular metastasis is extremely rare in childhood craniopharyngioma. A case of an isolated posterior ventricular recurrence of an adamantinomatous craniopharyngioma has been reported {659}.

Papillary craniopharyngioma

Santagata S
Kleinschmidt-DeMasters BK
Komori T
Müller HL
Nishioka H
Yamada S

Definition

Papillary craniopharyngioma is a solid or partially cystic, non-keratinizing squamous epithelial tumour usually localized to the pituitary–hypothalamic axis and characterized by *BRAF* activating mutation.

ICD-O coding

9352/1 Papillary craniopharyngioma

ICD-11 coding

2F7A.Y & XH2BF0 Other specified neoplasms of uncertain behaviour of endocrine glands & Craniopharyngioma, papillary

Related terminology

None

Subtype(s)

None

Localization

Papillary craniopharyngioma arises anywhere along the pituitary–hypothalamic axis, but there is a strong predilection for intrinsic localization within the infundibulum and tuber cinereum of the third ventricle floor. They can expand into the third ventricle cavity and can be located entirely within the ventricle above an intact ventricular floor. Intrasellar involvement is not common {3454,3397,5103,1451,3616}.

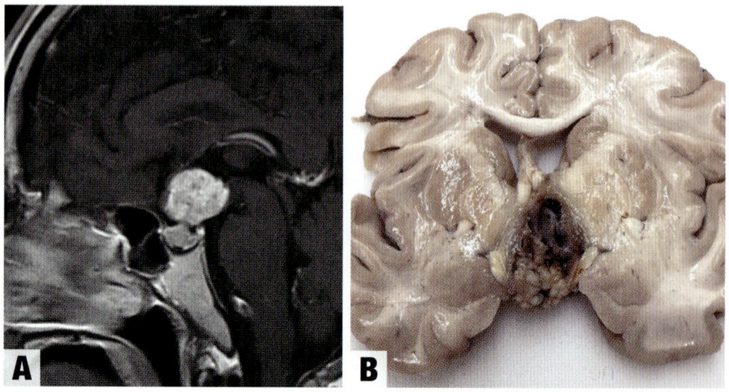

Fig. 2.49 Papillary craniopharyngioma. **A** A solid suprasellar tumour was noted on MRI in this 43-year-old man who presented with visual disturbance and partial hypopituitarism. **B** A fixed coronal section showing a solid and cystic mass involving the infundibulotuberal region and third ventricle in an adult patient without prior surgical intervention. The tumour mass has a cauliflower-like configuration. Calcifications are absent.

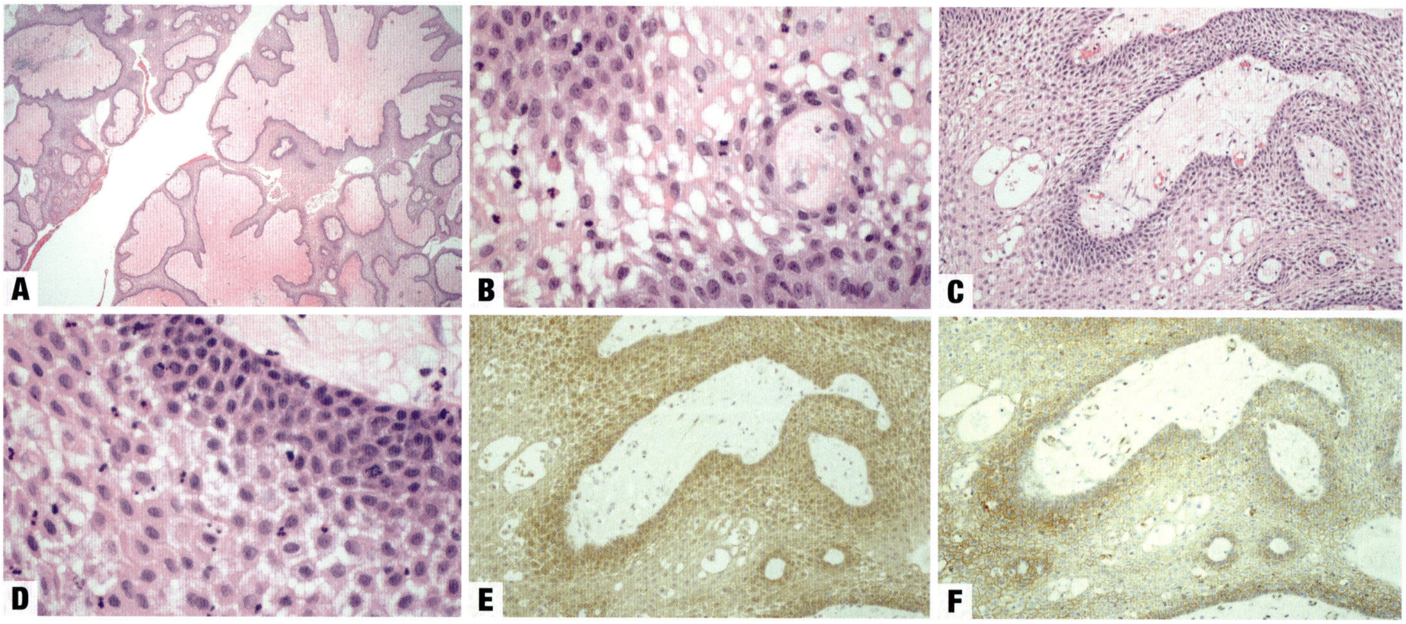

Fig. 2.50 Papillary craniopharyngioma. **A** Low-power view highlights the papillary architecture. **B** Well-differentiated non-keratinizing squamous epithelium with tumour-infiltrating neutrophils, which are common in these tumours. Occasional collagenous whorls and mitoses are found. **C** Well-differentiated non-keratinizing squamous epithelium covering fibrovascular cores that contain a low density of fibroblasts and immune cells including lymphocytes, macrophages, and neutrophils. **D** Well-differentiated non-keratinizing squamous epithelium with intercellular bridges and abundant tumour-infiltrating neutrophils. Occasional mitoses can be found. **E** Essentially all papillary craniopharyngiomas show cytoplasmic (and occasionally nuclear) immunoreactivity for BRAF p.V600E. **F** Whereas adamantinomatous craniopharyngiomas have a subset of cells with nuclear localization of β-catenin, in papillary craniopharyngioma β-catenin localizes to the cytoplasmic membrane.

Clinical features

Primary manifestations include headache (70%) and visual deficits (63%), the latter resulting from compression of the optic chiasm, which often improves or stabilizes postoperatively but rarely worsens after surgery. Nearly all patients have some evidence of hypopituitarism that is either partial (70%) or panhypopituitarism (30%) presenting as hypothyroidism (80%), hypogonadotropic hypogonadism (56%), hypocortisolaemia (50%), and growth hormone deficiency (20%). Hyperprolactinaemia is also seen, due to stalk effect (30%). Diabetes insipidus is a primary manifestation in 25% of patients and often develops anew (70%) after surgery. Hydrocephalus is common (30%). Preoperative hypothalamic disturbances (63%) include weight gain and psychiatric and cognitive disturbances {2476,3453}, as well as alterations in body core temperature and sleep–wake cycle {5193}.

Imaging

Papillary craniopharyngiomas are often solid, but some tumours are mixed solid/cystic or predominantly cystic. They are generally spherical (not lobulated or irregular), and calcification is infrequently seen {3957,2569,2476,1451}. Postcontrast T1-weighted MRI shows homogeneous enhancement, with only a small fraction showing heterogeneous enhancement. The pituitary stalk is often visible and thickened, and the hypothalamus is often below the tumour {5103,3616}. Cystic lesions often have a solid, cauliflower-like nodule. Cysts are hypointense on non-contrast T1-weighted images {3957}.

Spread

Local recurrence occurs in about 25% of patients with involvement of the hypothalamus and other vital neural and vascular structures {3397,3131}. Ectopic recurrence is a rare complication that occurs along the surgical track or at other sites in the CNS via cerebrospinal fluid spread in the subarachnoid space {5034,588}.

Epidemiology

Incidence

Craniopharyngiomas constitute 1.2–4.6% of all intracranial tumours, accounting for 0.5–2.5 new cases per 1 million population per year {562,3238,5106,3351}. Papillary craniopharyngiomas account for about 10% of all craniopharyngioma diagnoses and about 12–33% of those arising in adults {20,1176,3491, 3397,2476,3868}.

Age and sex distribution

Papillary craniopharyngioma is principally a disease of adults (peak incidence: 30–59 years), with tumours arising in paediatric patients only rarely {948,3491,5106,480}. There is no reported sex predilection {948,5106}.

Etiology

Unknown

Pathogenesis

Craniopharyngiomas have been proposed to arise from cellular elements related to the Rathke pouch / craniopharyngeal duct, which is integral to pituitary development {3131}. SOX2+ progenitors may underlie the formation of papillary craniopharyngioma {1812} and Rathke cleft cyst {535}. Rathke cleft cysts with marked squamous metaplasia and craniopharyngiomas with ciliated squamous epithelium overlap histologically, and some authors propose a spectrum of progression from the Rathke cleft cyst, to columnar craniopharyngioma, to the classic papillary craniopharyngioma {4910}. Almost all papillary craniopharyngiomas have *BRAF* p.V600E mutations {520,2531,4035,1933,2815,1641, 1776} leading to the activation of the MAPK/ERK pathway. No other recurrent mutations have been reported. Only a relatively low number of non-synonymous somatic mutations are present in papillary craniopharyngioma, when compared with large cohorts of other tumour types {520}. Consistent with the distinct histology and driver mutations of papillary craniopharyngioma (*BRAF* mutations) and adamantinomatous craniopharyngioma (*CTNNB1* mutations), the tumours also display distinct methylation and transcription profiles {1933}. Papillary craniopharyngiomas show stable genomic copy-number profiles without recurrent chromosomal gains or losses {3741,1641}.

Macroscopic appearance

Although papillary craniopharyngiomas tend to be predominantly solid or mixed solid/cystic, a small fraction can also be mostly cystic, in which case they generally have a cauliflower-like solid nodule. The cyst contents are typically described as viscous and yellow {948}. Calcifications are generally absent. The tumours are generally circumscribed and spherical and are not widely adherent to surrounding brain tissue. The surface can have a papillary pattern.

Histopathology

Papillary craniopharyngiomas have non-keratinizing mature squamous epithelium covering fibrovascular cores or a cyst wall. Stellate reticulum and flaky and wet keratin are absent {20,948}. Calcifications are rare. Crowding is present in the basal cell layer, but pronounced palisading is absent. Epithelial whorls and collagenous whorls are present but are distinct from those of adamantinomatous craniopharyngioma. Mitoses are infrequent. The tumour–brain interface is well demarcated, and invasive protrusions are absent {20}. Tumour-infiltrating neutrophils are common; T cells and macrophages are also present throughout the fibrovascular cores and tumour epithelium. In as many as one third of cases, there are single or small groups of PAS-positive goblet cells within the squamous epithelium, and in a small number of cases there are regions of ciliated epithelium. These histological features overlap with those of Rathke cleft cyst with extensive squamous metaplasia.

Malignant progression of papillary craniopharyngioma has been reported {1496,4778}, but none have been tested for *BRAF* p.V600E mutations.

Immunophenotype

p63 is expressed in all epithelial layers {3069}. Both high-molecular-weight cytokeratins (34βE12 [K903], CK5/6) and low- to intermediate-molecular-weight cytokeratins (CK7, CK17, and CK19) are expressed {4963}. CK7 expression is confined to the superficial epithelial layer {2458}. Some studies indicate that craniopharyngiomas lack CK8 and CK20 expression except in rare cells, in contrast to Rathke cleft cyst; the value for distinguishing these two lesions by cytokeratin expression is unresolved {4963,2551}. Primary cilia are present in the basally oriented tumour cells near the fibrovascular stroma {937}. PDL1 is expressed in multiple layers of tumour cells circumferentially surrounding the fibrovascular stroma {938}. SOX9 is variably expressed, and the expression of SOX2 requires further assessment {1812,4463}.

Nearly all papillary craniopharyngiomas have *BRAF* p.V600E mutations {520}, which can be identified across the tumour epithelium using mutation-specific antibodies, thereby distinguishing papillary craniopharyngioma from adamantinomatous craniopharyngioma and Rathke cleft cyst {2132,4035,2288}; the latter displays antibody cross-reactivity in motile cilia {2132}. In papillary craniopharyngioma, β-catenin is confined to the cytoplasmic membrane {520}. In general practice, immunohistochemistry can replace genetic analysis as an aid to determining the subtype diagnosis of craniopharyngioma {1455}.

Grading
Papillary craniopharyngioma is regarded as CNS WHO grade 1.

Proliferation index
Ki-67 is generally confined to the basal layers {519,1812}. The proliferation index varies widely between cases and provides no prognostic information {1182,2737}.

Differential diagnosis
The differential diagnosis of papillary craniopharyngioma includes adamantinomatous craniopharyngioma, xanthogranuloma, Rathke cleft cyst, epidermoid and dermoid cysts, and pilocytic astrocytoma. When accompanied by extensive squamous metaplasia, Rathke cleft cyst can be difficult to discriminate from papillary craniopharyngioma, because the latter can also contain ciliated columnar cells and goblet cells. Importantly, Rathke cleft cyst lacks *BRAF* p.V600E mutations {2132, 4035}.

Cytology
Not clinically relevant

Diagnostic molecular pathology
Demonstration of *BRAF* mutation confirms the diagnosis, whereas *CTNNB1* mutation suggests adamantinomatous craniopharyngioma {1776}. Although *BRAF* and *CTNNB1* mutations are mutually exclusive, rare examples of the coexistence of these mutations have been reported in adamantinomatous craniopharyngioma {2531}.

Essential and desirable diagnostic criteria
Essential: a well-differentiated non-keratinizing squamous epithelial tumour; fibrovascular cores.

Desirable: demonstration of *BRAF* p.V600E mutations by immunohistochemistry and/or molecular testing; absence of nuclear β-catenin immunoreactivity; absence of *CTNNB1* mutation.

Staging
Not relevant

Prognosis and prediction
Papillary craniopharyngiomas are less adherent to hypothalamic structures than are adamantinomatous craniopharyngiomas, which could, in theory, favour better and safer gross total removal. In contrast, there appear to be no significant differences between papillary and adamantinomatous craniopharyngioma with respect to resectability, efficacy of radiation therapy, and overall survival {948}. Similarly, a systematic review and meta-analysis of adult patients with craniopharyngioma (34.3% of whom had papillary craniopharyngiomas) showed no statistically significant difference in rates of recurrence between the two types of tumours whether treated with gross total resection or with incomplete resection plus radiotherapy after surgery {981}. Indeed, the current standard-of-care treatments for both types of craniopharyngioma are similar, but the vast majority of papillary craniopharyngiomas harbour targetable *BRAF* p.V600E mutations, offering promising new perspectives for the treatment of this tumour {94}.

Pituitary blastoma

Mete O
de Kock L
Foulkes WD
Jarzembowski JA
Schultz KAP

Definition

Pituitary blastoma is an embryonal sellar neoplasm composed of primitive blastemal cells, neuroendocrine cells, and Rathke pouch epithelium.

ICD-O coding

8273/3 Pituitary blastoma

ICD-11 coding

2D12.Y & XH5QV8 Other specified malignant neoplasms of other endocrine glands or related structures & Pituitary blastoma

Related terminology

Not recommended: pituitary embryoma.

Subtype(s)

None

Localization

Pituitary blastoma originates within the sella and frequently extends into the suprasellar region and invades the cavernous sinus {3989}.

Clinical features

Cushing disease is one of the most common presenting symptoms {3989,1020}. Other hormones may also be overexpressed {814}. Ophthalmoplegia frequently occurs due to tumour growth into the optic chiasm {3989}.

Epidemiology

Pituitary blastoma is extremely rare, with < 20 well-characterized cases. It usually occurs in children aged < 2 years (median age: 9 months), with a slight female predominance {3989,1020}. Recent evidence suggests that pituitary blastoma may also occur in young adults {814,836}. Patients may present with or subsequently develop other *DICER1*-related tumours {1020}.

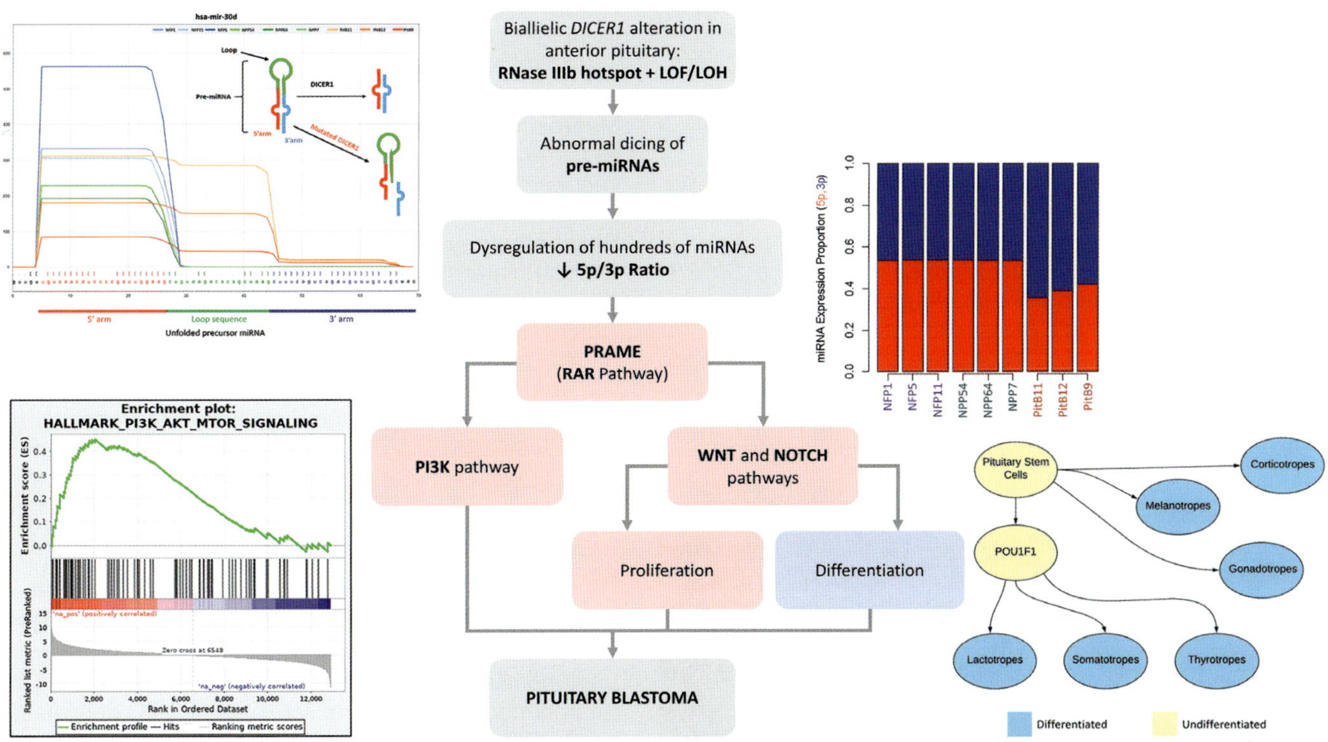

Fig. 2.51 Pituitary blastoma pathogenesis. From *DICER1* mutation to tumorigenesis. Each tumour starts with presumptively biallelic mutations in *DICER1* (RNase IIIb hotspot mutation coupled with a loss-of-function variant [LOF] or loss of heterozygosity [LOH]). Because the RNase IIIa domain of *DICER1* remains functional, the processing of microRNA precursors (pre-miRNAs) will generate a skewed distribution of 5p/3p mature microRNA; as shown in the graphic, this improper dicing of precursors results in aberrant 5p products and a skewed distribution of microRNAs favouring 3p over 5p microRNAs. This in turn leads to the dysregulation of hundreds of 5p and 3p microRNAs, with the concomitant dysregulation of many target mRNAs. In the case of pituitary blastoma (PitB), this includes the upregulation of PRAME (fold-change: > 500). Gene-set analyses showed that the retinoic acid receptor (RAR) pathway and the WNT, NOTCH, and PI3K pathways are activated in pituitary blastoma tumours, as compared with normal postnatal pituitary (NPP) samples. The analysis revealed that, like normal fetal pituitary (NFP), PitB samples have a high level of undifferentiated cells as compared with NPP samples. PitB tumours have the lowest level of differentiated cells, as compared with NPP and NFP samples. Pink represents upregulated processes and blue represents a downregulated process.

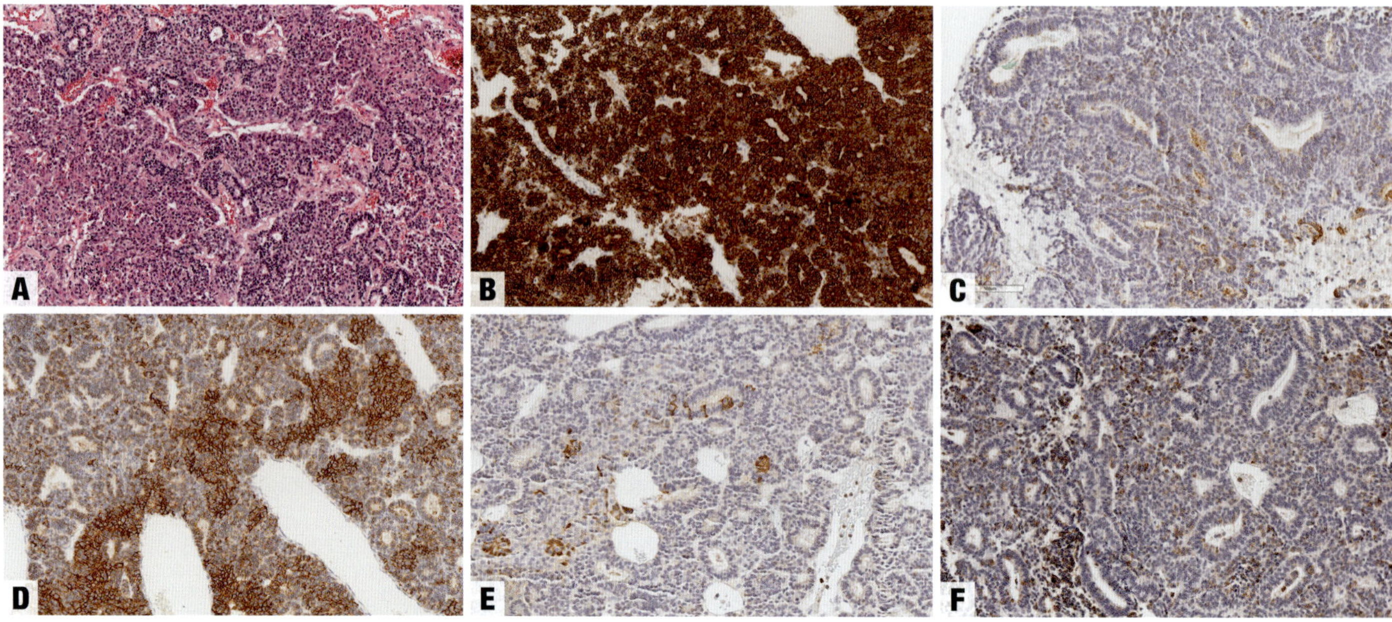

Fig. 2.52 Pituitary blastoma. **A** The cellular components of pituitary blastomas include large adenohypophysial neuroendocrine cells arranged in lobules or diffuse sheets, cuboidal primitive Rathke pouch epithelium with rosette or gland/follicle formation, and scattered undifferentiated blastemal cells. **B** CAM5.2 (low-molecular-weight cytokeratin) immunohistochemistry stains almost all cellular components in pituitary blastomas. **C** EMA shows variable staining in cellular components, with stronger staining in areas with rosette- or follicle-forming cuboidal or columnar primitive Rathke pouch epithelium. **D** Strong membranous CD56 expression distinguishes areas of neuroendocrine cells, whereas other cellular elements show reduced staining intensity for CD56. **E** S100 stains scattered folliculostellate cells in a pituitary blastoma. **F** The adenohypophysial neuroendocrine tumour cells are arranged in diffuse sheets or lobules and are variably positive for ACTH. Unlike the cells arranged in sheets, rosette- or follicle-forming cuboidal or columnar primitive Rathke pouch epithelium and blastemal undifferentiated cells tend to be negative for ACTH.

Etiology

Pituitary blastoma is linked to germline and somatic *DICER1* variants {1020}.

Pathogenesis

Pituitary blastoma appears to arise due to genetic alteration of *DICER1*, which encodes an enzyme involved in microRNA processing; mature microRNAs in turn regulate the translation of mRNAs. Virtually all tumours harbour at least one *DICER1* alteration, typically a germline loss-of-function pathogenic variant coupled with a somatic RNase IIIb hotspot missense mutation {3885,1020}. In a minority of cases, the second somatic alteration may be the loss of the wildtype allele {1020}. Defective *DICER1* leads to a reduced 5p:3p microRNA ratio with altered target RNAs and *PRAME* gene upregulation in the retinoic acid receptor signalling pathway, as well as activation of PI3K, WNT, and NOTCH pathways {3151}.

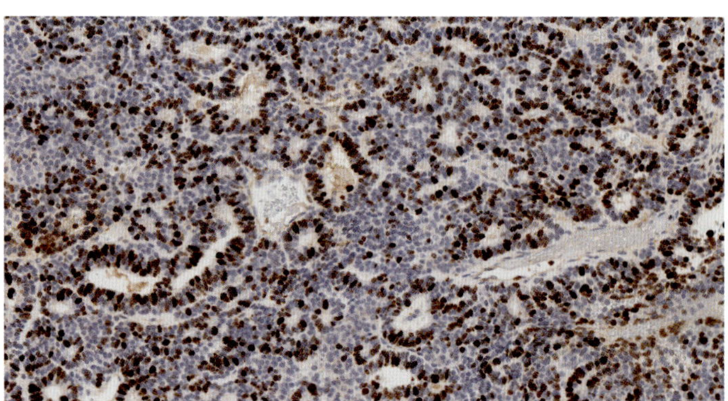

Fig. 2.53 Pituitary blastoma. Proliferative heterogeneity of the various cellular components. The follicle-forming cuboidal or columnar primitive Rathke pouch epithelium shows a higher Ki-67 proliferation index than other cellular elements.

Macroscopic appearance

Gross examination details are largely unknown. Focal cystic or haemorrhagic changes and partial necrosis can be seen {3993}.

Histopathology

Pituitary blastomas are composed of three cellular components: (1) large adenohypophysial neuroendocrine cells arranged in lobules or diffuse sheets, (2) cuboidal or columnar primitive Rathke pouch epithelium with rosette or gland/follicle formation, and (3) small undifferentiated blastemal cells {3993,3989, 1020}. Ultrastructural features resemble fetal pituitary gland of 10–12 weeks but are distinguished by a marked complex cellular proliferation of mature TPIT-lineage corticotroph cells (some with Crooke hyaline change) and PIT1-lineage somatotrophs in the background of adenohypophysial cells with small secretory granules that simulate null cells, and other elements including undifferentiated Rathke pouch epithelial cells and folliculostellate cells {3993,3989}.

Immunohistochemistry

Neuroendocrine cells variably express POMC derivates, including ACTH, β-endorphin, MSH, and (to a lesser extent) growth hormone {3993}. Rare LH-β {3993} and/or FSH-β {3993, 3885} staining has also been reported. Unlike neuroendocrine cells, blastemal and Rathke pouch cells rarely show pituitary transcription factor expression {3989}. EMA and keratins are expressed in various components, with stronger staining in the Rathke pouch epithelium {3993}. Galectin-3 variably stains cellular components {3993}. Unlike postnatal normal pituitaries, these tumours often express biomarkers of fetal pituitary including PRAME and EZH2 {3151}. Proliferative heterogeneity varies among cases and tumour components {3993,3989}. An increased Ki-67 labelling index (as high as 60%) along with p53 expression is more frequent in the Rathke pouch epithelium {3993,3989,1020}. Necrosis can occur {3989}.

Differential diagnosis

The differential diagnosis of these tumours includes sellar teratoma and other germ cell tumours or pituitary neuroendocrine tumours (PitNETs) with synchronous Rathke cleft cyst {3873,1010}.

Cytology

The details of intraoperative touch and/or squash preparations of these tumours are unknown.

Diagnostic molecular pathology

DICER1 variants may be considered a diagnostic molecular marker of pituitary blastoma. Germline and tumour sequencing should be performed.

Essential and desirable diagnostic criteria

Essential: Rathke pouch epithelial glands; primitive blastomatous cells; secretory and folliculostellate adenohypophysial cells; *DICER1* alterations.

Desirable: diagnosis in children aged < 24 months (although possible in young adults); Cushing disease; personal or family history of *DICER1* syndrome or related tumours.

Staging

There is no formal staging system that has been universally applied for pituitary/sellar neoplasms. A CT-era approach based on tumour size and patterns of invasion was proposed in 1973 by Hardy {1786}. Subsequently, a standardized assessment of parasellar tumour invasiveness based on MRI was published by Knosp in 1993 {2354}.

There are no pathology-standardized reporting templates yet endorsed by international pathology organizations. A pathology reporting template for pituitary tumours was introduced in 2011 {3300}, followed by the European Pituitary Pathology Group (EPPG) proposal in 2019 {4707}.

Prognosis and prediction

The prognostic factors are not yet fully understood; however, the extent of tumour excision is a significant factor in survival {2676}. In the largest series of 17 patients, 1 out of 8 deaths were related to tumour progression {2676}. Evidence suggests the most deaths are linked to early or late treatment-related complications {1020,2676}.

Pituicytomas

Mete O
Asa SL
Kleinschmidt-DeMasters BK
Perry A
Shibuya M

Definition

Pituicytomas are a distinct group of related low-grade neoplasms composed of pituicytes of the posterior pituitary and infundibulum.

ICD-O coding

9432/1 Pituicytoma
9582/0 Granular cell tumour of the sellar region / granular cell pituicytoma
8290/0 Spindle cell oncocytoma / oncocytic pituicytoma
9391/1 Ependymal pituicytoma

ICD-11 coding

2F7A.Y & XH59V4 Other specified neoplasms of uncertain behaviour of endocrine glands & Pituicytoma
2F7A.Y & XH2XW8 Other specified neoplasms of uncertain behaviour of endocrine glands & Granular cell tumour of the sellar region
2F7A.Y & XH26P7 Other specified neoplasms of uncertain behaviour of endocrine glands & Spindle cell oncocytoma
2F7A.Y & XH1Q28 Other specified neoplasms of uncertain behaviour of endocrine glands & Sellar ependymoma

Related terminology

Pituicytoma

Not recommended: pilocytic astrocytoma of the posterior pituitary; posterior pituitary astrocytoma; infundibuloma.

Granular cell tumour of the sellar region / granular cell pituicytoma

Acceptable: pituicytoma with granular cell features.
Not recommended: Abrikossoff tumour; choristoma; granular cell myoblastoma; granular cell neuroma; granular cell schwannoma.

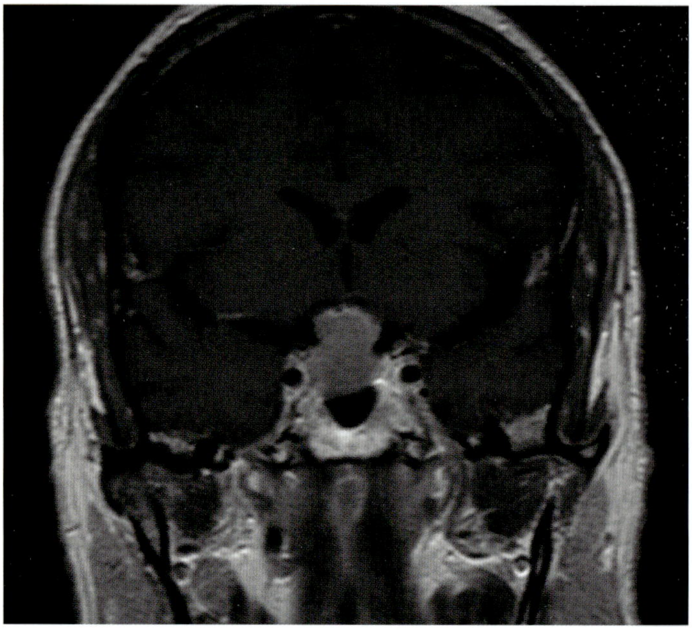

Fig. 2.54 Pituicytoma. This 55-year-old man presented with symptoms of a non-functioning sellar tumour, and his preoperative neuroimaging studies were thought to indicate non-functioning PitNET/adenoma on the basis of the presence of a homogeneous, well-demarcated sellar/suprasellar mass, as seen here; biopsy, however, proved this to be a pituicytoma.

Spindle cell oncocytoma / oncocytic pituicytoma

Acceptable: pituicytoma with oncocytic features.
Not recommended: spindle cell oncocytoma of the anterior pituitary.

Ependymal pituicytoma

Acceptable: pituicytoma with ependymal features.
Not recommended: pituitary ependymoma; sellar ependymoma.

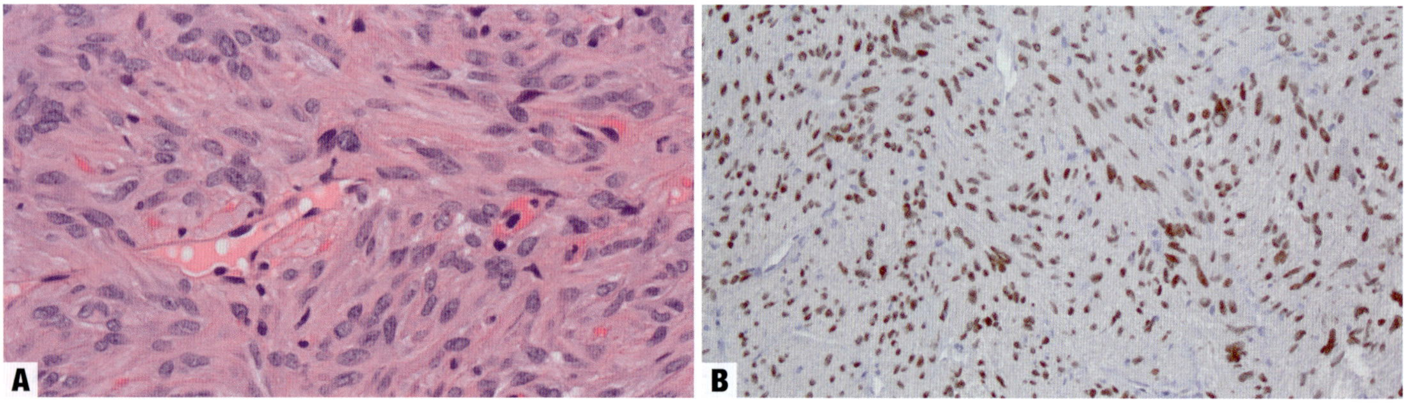

Fig. 2.55 Pituicytoma. **A** The tumour cells are cytologically bland, with oval nuclei, minimal hyperchromatism, and eosinophilic cytoplasm. **B** Diffuse nuclear immunoreactivity for thyroid transcription factor 1 (TTF1) is typical of pituicytoma and confidently distinguishes it from schwannoma, meningioma, or pituitary adenoma, all of which are immunonegative.

Chapter 2

Subtype(s)

Granular cell tumour of the sellar region / granular cell pituicytoma; spindle cell oncocytoma / oncocytic pituicytoma; ependymal pituicytoma

Localization

These tumours arise along the length of the posterior pituitary, forming suprasellar or sellar/suprasellar masses {1806}. They may extend into the cavernous sinus and invade the sellar floor {4114,1806} and have been reported to erode the clinoid process {3954}.

Clinical features

Tumour presentations are clinically indistinguishable from nonfunctioning pituitary neuroendocrine tumours (PitNETs)/adenomas and include headaches, visual field defects, and hypopituitarism {4801,4114}. Diabetes insipidus is uncommon {935}. The tumours have been reported in association with synchronous functioning corticotroph and somatotroph tumours {600,3857, 2027}; a small number have presented with hypercortisolism or acromegaly without demonstration of a synchronous PitNET/ adenoma {2027}. Massive intraoperative bleeding or spontaneous haemorrhage can occur, possibly owing to their hypervascularity {2331}.

Neuroimaging

No specific features have been identified to distinguish these lesions from other clinically non-functioning pituitary tumours. They are isointense on T1-weighted MRI and show either homogeneous or heterogeneous enhancement. T2-weighted MRI reveals various intensities {935,4801,4114}.

Epidemiology

These tumours are rare; there are no epidemiological data available currently. A recent meta-analysis of literature published in English or Spanish identified about 270 examples {1698}. The ependymal type is the rarest, with only 14 cases reported {3995,4635,2472,3872,5084,4801,2574}.

The majority of these tumours occur in adults in their fifth or sixth decade of life {1698,4801}, with a higher mean age (61.6 years) in patients with oncocytic tumours {3805}. Sex distribution varies in the literature; a slight male predominance is reported for pituicytomas and ependymal types {935, 4801,3911}, whereas a slight female predominance has been reported for oncocytic tumours {935} and granular cell tumours {935,5151}.

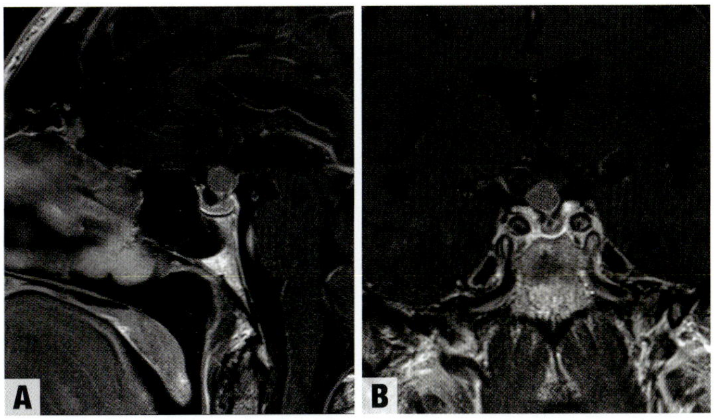

Fig. 2.56 Granular cell tumour of the sellar region / granular cell pituicytoma. Sagittal (**A**) and coronal (**B**) postcontrast images demonstrating homogeneous mild enhancement within the mass and a relatively normal calibre of the more caudal stalk.

Etiology

The etiology of these neoplasms is unknown. No germline susceptibility has been identified.

Pathogenesis

Ubiquitous nuclear thyroid transcription factor 1 (TTF1) expression indicates a common derivation of pituicytoma, granular cell tumour, and spindle cell oncocytoma from the pituitary infundibulum / forebrain ganglionic eminence (ventral neuroectoderm) rather than from the endocrine cells of the anterior pituitary or from folliculostellate cells {2565,4635,3872,5084}. Similarities between these tumours and subtypes of normal light, dark, granular, oncocytic, and ependymal pituicytes are in keeping with an origin from the posterior pituitary {4384,3990,2565, 2973}.

Genetic profile

Molecular genetic studies have been restricted to the most common tumours of this group, i.e. pituicytomas, granular cell tumours, and spindle cell oncocytomas. Methylation-based classification studies show close clustering, suggesting that these tumours may be a single spectrum of tumour types with

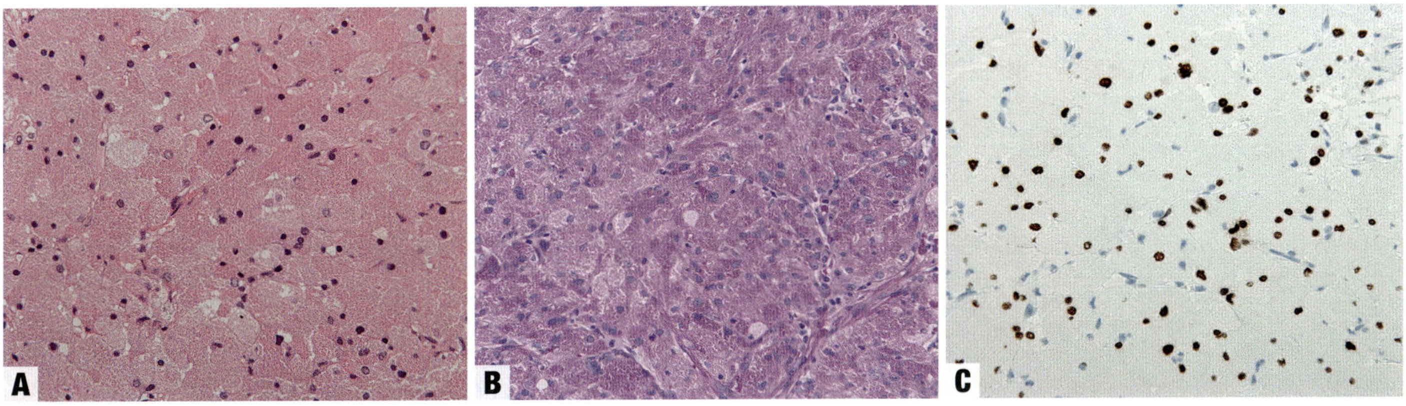

Fig. 2.57 Granular cell tumour of the sellar region / granular cell pituicytoma. **A** These tumours are characterized by eosinophilic polygonal cells with abundant granular eosinophilic cytoplasm. **B** The cells show marked PAS positivity. **C** The cells show nuclear thyroid transcription factor 1 (TTF1) immunoexpression.

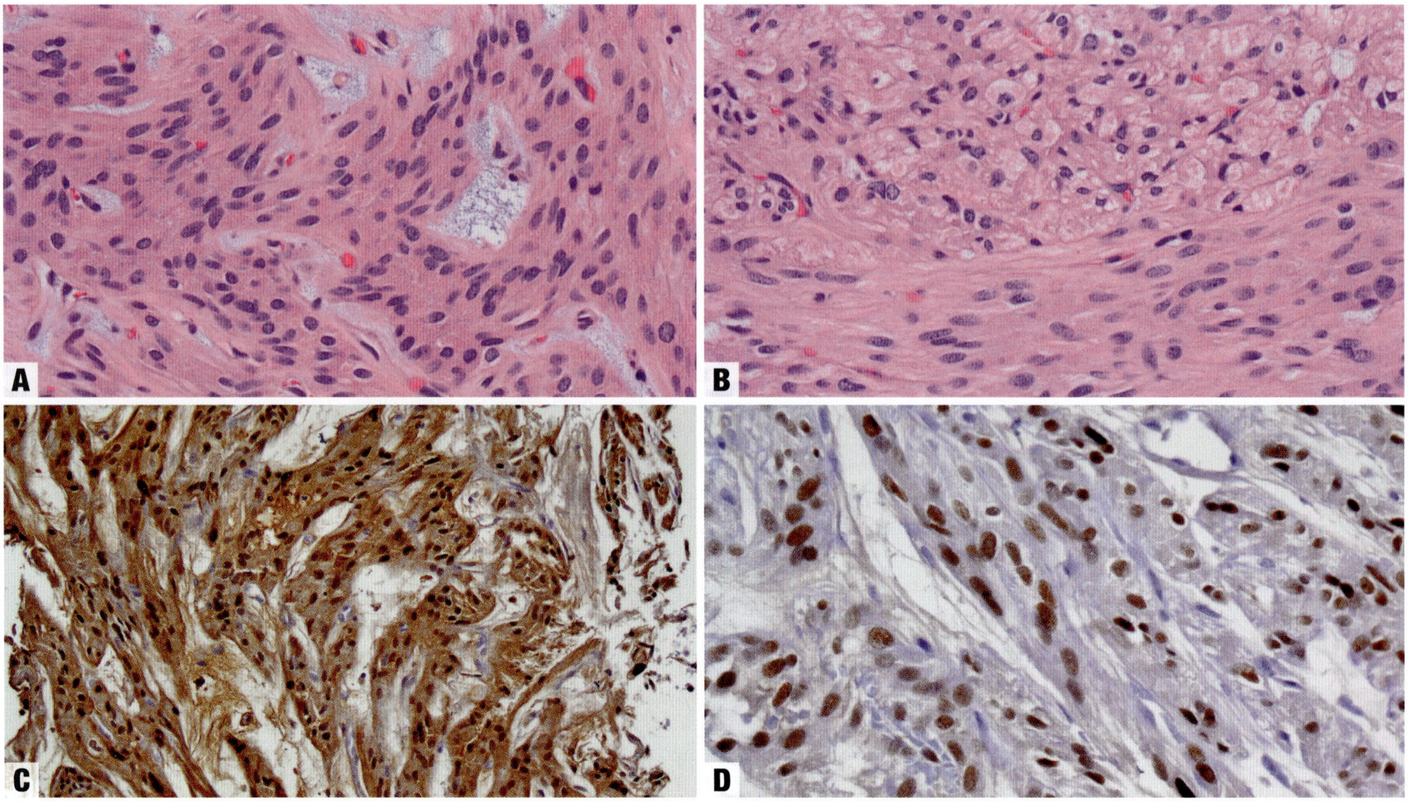

Fig. 2.58 Spindle cell oncocytoma / oncocytic pituicytoma. **A** Tumour cells generally show more oval nuclei than those seen in schwannoma, which usually contains tapering nuclei with pointed ends. Note the absence of nuclear pseudoinclusions, which are seen in some meningioma cells. Note also the uniformity of nuclear features and absence of mitotic activity. **B** Intersecting fascicles of tumour cells show the plump eosinophilic cytoplasm typical of this tumour; increased cytoplasmic volume is due to increased mitochondrial content. **C** These sellar/suprasellar tumours are composed of small groups of cytologically bland spindle cells that usually show strong diffuse cytoplasmic immunoreactivity for S100. **D** These tumours show diffuse nuclear immunoreactivity for thyroid transcription factor 1 (TTF1), but so do pituicytomas, granular cell tumours of the posterior pituitary, and even normal posterior pituitary gland, so this immunostain does not distinguish between these lesions.

a shared histogenesis, yet with distinctive morphologies {641, 4004}. The *IDH1* p.R132H mutation and *KIAA1549::BRAF* oncogene fusion are absent {2973}. A limited number of case series identified various somatic alterations, with some evidence supporting the MAPK pathway activation in pituicytomas and spindle cell oncocytomas {3014,4697}. Whole-exome sequencing identified several mutations, including in *HRAS*, *SND1*, and *FAT1*, in 4 spindle cell oncocytomas from 3 patients {3014}. The *HRAS*-mutant tumour also had a *MEN1* frameshift mutation {3014}. Similarly, constitutive MAPK activation was found in 10 of 11 pituicytomas and included *HRAS* somatic mutations as well as pathogenic *BRAF* p.V600E, *NF1*, and *TSC1* sequence variants {4697,324}. A spindle cell oncocytoma with *BRAF* p.V600E mutations has been shown to respond to targeted inhibition of the MAPK/ERK signalling pathway {4218}. The whole microRNA signature of spindle cell oncocytomas shows global downregulation of microRNA expression, with a differential profile between primary and recurrent tumours versus the normal pituitary gland {2437}. A recent study showed chromosome 1 alterations in spindle cell oncocytomas, including 1p deletion (in 4 of 5 cases) and 1p gain (in 1 of 5 cases) {324}. A more detailed analysis of a large number of tumours (47 cases) detected two epigenomic DNA methylation subgroups with only subtle overall methylation differences. The first subgroup, composed mainly of granular cell tumours and some spindle cell oncocytomas, lacked identifiable genetic alterations. Pituicytomas and a subset of spindle cell oncocytomas formed the largest cluster, with a high number of pathogenic mutations in genes of the MAPK/PI3K pathways (*FGFR1*, *HRAS*, *BRAF*, *NF1*, *CBL*, *MAP2K2*, *PTEN*); rare tumours had accompanying *TERT* promoter mutation. Pituicytomas and a subset of spindle cell oncocytomas were further segregated by the presence of copy-number alterations into a favourable group (no copy-number changes) and a less favourable group (copy-number imbalances present) that had a significantly reduced progression-free survival {4004}.

Macroscopic appearance

These tumours cannot be distinguished on the basis of gross features. Texture reportedly ranges from similar to normal brain, to firm and vascular, with a grey to tan colour {3995,3122}. They can occasionally be associated with haemorrhage {478,1698}.

Histopathology

Pituicytoma

Pituicytomas are composed of elongate bipolar spindle cells often arranged in solid sheets and short fascicles that can have a storiform pattern {522,2331,2973,2972}. Tumour cells tend to show distinct cell borders. These tumours lack eosinophilic granular bodies, Rosenthal fibres, and hyalinized blood vessels {2331}. Inflammatory infiltrates can sometimes be present {2565,2331}. Some pituicytomas may display regions with ependymal and oncocytic changes {3872,5084}, again raising the possibility of morphological continuity among pituicyte-related tumours of the posterior lobe {2973,3872,4114}.

Pituicytomas typically show low mitotic activity, but rare examples with atypical features characterized by increased cellularity, pleomorphism, and mitotic activity have been reported {1739,4697}. Their ultrastructural characteristics resemble light and dark pituicytes (two of the five ultrastructural classes of non-tumorous pituicytes) {4384} that are enriched in intermediate filaments {2973}.

Granular cell tumour of the sellar region / granular cell pituicytoma

Granular cell tumours consist of densely packed polygonal cells with granular eosinophilic cytoplasm due to lysosomal accumulation. The architecture is typically nodular; sheets and/or spindled/fascicular patterns can also be seen. PAS staining of cytoplasmic granules is resistant to diastase digestion {2331}. The tumour cell nuclei are small, with inconspicuous nucleoli and evenly distributed chromatin. Perivascular lymphocytic aggregates are common. Mitotic activity is usually inconspicuous. Ultrastructural analysis highlights the abundant cytoplasmic lysosomal population of the tumour cells that confers the granular aspect of the cytoplasm seen with light microscopy. Neurosecretory granules are absent.

Spindle cell oncocytoma / oncocytic pituicytoma

Spindle cell oncocytomas are typically composed of interlacing fascicles and poorly defined lobules of spindle to epithelioid cells with eosinophilic, variably granular cytoplasm. Oncocytic change can be focal to widespread. Whorls, myxoid change, clear cells, osteoclast-like giant cells, and follicle-like structures can also be features of this tumour {4635,3845,5084}. Mild to moderate nuclear atypia and (less commonly) marked pleomorphism can be observed. Focal infiltrates of mature lymphocytes are common. Hallmark ultrastructural features include an increased number of (often abnormal) mitochondria, intermediate filaments, and cell–cell junctions including well-formed desmosomes and intermediate-type junctions {3805,1684}. Follicular structures {887} and intracytoplasmic lumina with microvillous projections have been reported {4635,3122}.

Ependymal pituicytoma

Ependymal pituicytomas (previously known as sellar ependymomas) are described as tumours resembling either pituicytomas or spindle cell oncocytomas composed of spindled to plump epithelioid and oncocytic cells arranged in sheets and small fascicles {3995,4635,2472,3872,5084}. Remarkably, the tumours show variable ependymal histological features, including perivascular pseudorosettes and true rosettes. Mitoses are rare and no necrosis is evident. Rosenthal fibres and eosinophilic granular bodies have not been reported in these tumours. Despite the presence of ependymal features, these tumours appear not to be biologically related to ependymal tumours arising in the supratentorium, posterior fossa, and spinal cord {1228}. Ultrastructural analyses reveal tumour cells with ependymal-like features, including intracellular and intercellular microlumina containing microvilli and occasional cilia and desmosomal junctions, in addition to moderate numbers of intermediate filaments, rare microtubules, occasional lysosomes, and mitochondria {3125,3995,4635,5084}. However, all these features have also been described in non-tumorous pituicytes with ependymal features {3990,4384}.

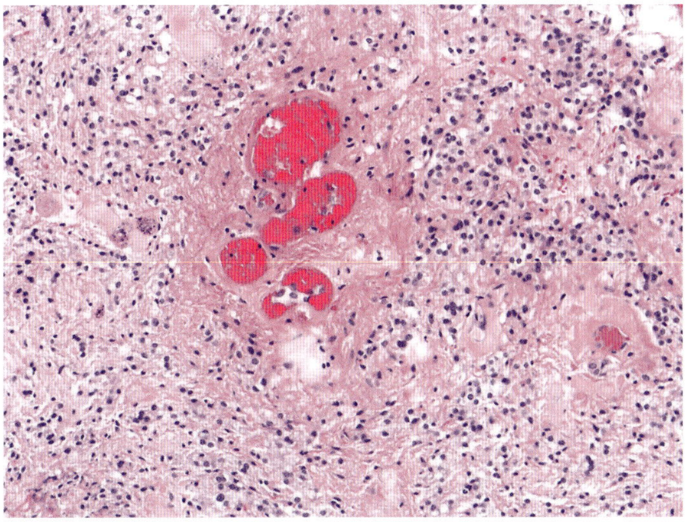

Fig. 2.59 Ependymal pituicytoma. This pituicytic tumour shows perivascular pseudorosettes similar to those seen in ependymomas of the CNS.

Immunohistochemistry

These tumours invariably express TTF1 {2565,2973,4635,3872,5084} and are negative for cytokeratins, pituitary hormones and transcription factors, chromogranin A, synaptophysin, and neurofilaments, as well as CD34 and markers of skeletal and smooth muscle differentiation {2331,2973}. They show reactivity for S100 and vimentin; they may express GFAP, EMA, CD56, annexin, galectin-3, CD68, BCL2, CD44, nestin, and αB-crystallin {95,2331,2973,1221,2828,1700,1564,3125,3995,4635,3872,2574}. Granular cell tumours are also positive for CD68, α1-antitrypsin, α1-antichymotrypsin, and cathepsin B, whereas spindle cell oncocytomas are strongly immunoreactive for antimitochondrial antigen {3801,5198}. Studies documented phosphorylated ERK, AKT, and S6 expression {95,3014}. SSTRs and DRD2s have been found {4239,2639}.

Although these tumours typically show low a Ki-67 labelling index (often < 3%) {1739,4697}, rare examples with an elevated Ki-67 labelling index (> 5%) have been reported {1739,4697,1564,1806}.

Differential diagnosis

Pituicytomas may be distinguished from normal posterior pituitary by the identification of Herring bodies and the presence of axons, the latter identified by the expression of NFP. Unlike schwannomas, reticulin histochemistry shows no pericellular staining {2331}.

Cytology

In cytological preparations, pituicytomas can display fibrillary to fine and wispy cytoplasm with occasional spindled cell morphology, sharing glial and meningioma-like features {4696}. Granular cell tumour cytological preparations are characterized by a uniform appearance of the polygonal cells, with round to ovoid nuclei and abundant eosinophilic granular cytoplasm dispersed in a granular background {3583}.

Diagnostic molecular pathology

No specific molecular test results are used in the diagnosis.

Essential and desirable diagnostic criteria

Essential: a spindle cell or epithelioid sellar neoplasm with diffuse S100 and nuclear TTF1 positivity and lacking reactivity for adenohypophysial neuroendocrine markers, transcription factors, and hormones.

Desirable: GFAP immunoexpression; for the granular cell subtype: PAS positivity (diastase resistance) and CD68 or α1-antitrypsin positivity; for the oncocytic subtype: antimitochondrial antibody positivity; for the ependymal subtype: EMA positivity with a dot-like, cellular apical, and/or luminal pattern.

Staging

Not relevant

Prognosis and prediction

Pituicytoma, granular cell tumour, and spindle cell oncocytoma are usually indolent, slow-growing tumours, curable by gross total surgical excision. However, there seems to be a higher frequency of recurrence in spindle cell oncocytomas, and most likely secondary to low rates of tumour gross total resection due to their rich vascularity and extensive adhesion to adjacent structures {2347,478,2331,2828,1564,732,1806}. As noted above, the presence of copy-number imbalances in pituicytomas and spindle cell tumours has been significantly associated with reduced progression-free survival {4004}. The prognosis of the rare sellar ependymoma is unknown; only 1 case with established follow-up has been described, with a lack of tumour progression and residual tumour control after radiation therapy within a 10-year follow-up after initial surgery {2574}. Malignant transformation and distant metastases have not been reported in any of these tumours.

Gangliocytoma and mixed gangliocytoma–PitNET/adenoma

Roncaroli FR
Wesseling P
Yamada S

Chapter 2

Definition

Gangliocytoma and mixed gangliocytoma–pituitary neuroendocrine tumour (PitNET)/adenoma is a tumour composed of mature ganglion cells resembling hypothalamic neurons, in some instances admixed with neoplastic pituitary neuroendocrine cells.

ICD-O coding

9492/0 Gangliocytoma
9492/0 Mixed gangliocytoma–PitNET/adenoma
9505/1 Ganglioglioma

ICD-11 coding

2A00.21 & XH6KA6 Mixed neuronal-glial tumours & Gangliocytoma

Related terminology

Not recommended: pituitary tumour/adenoma–neuronal choristoma; PitNET/adenoma with gangliocytic component.

Subtype(s)

Mixed gangliocytoma–PitNET/adenoma; ganglioglioma

Localization

These lesions usually arise within the sella turcica, although suprasellar and cavernous sinus extension is frequent, and bone invasion has been reported. One ectopic case involved the sphenoid and was associated with empty sella {2050}.

Clinical features

Headache and visual impairment are common at onset. Acromegaly and hyperprolactinaemia are the most frequent hormonal dysfunctions, followed by Cushing disease {926,5013, 202,3895}. The duration of signs and symptoms ranges from weeks to several years. Clinically non-functioning examples are exceedingly rare {926}.

Imaging

Mixed and pure forms are heterogeneously enhancing solid or solid/cystic masses. CT may reveal calcification {5013}.

Epidemiology

Pure and mixed gangliocytomas represent < 0.5% of sellar tumours {926,5013}, with about 15% being pure forms. The incidence of gangliocytomas associated with prolactinoma is probably underestimated, because they may respond to medical treatment and therefore are not operated. Literature reviews reported a wide range of age at presentation (average: 44 years); > 75% of patients are female {3642,926,5013}.

Etiology

Unknown

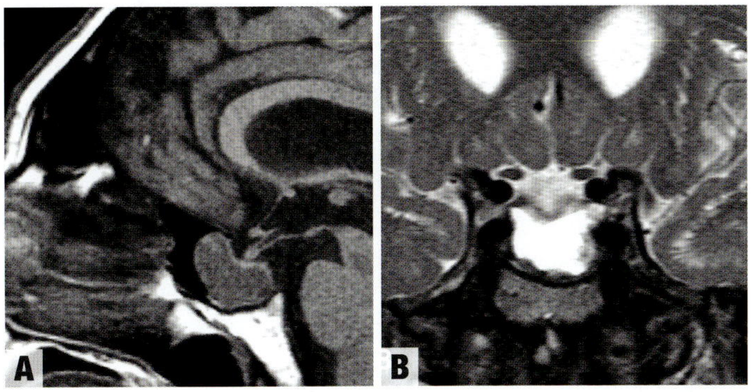

Fig. 2.60 Mixed gangliocytoma–adenoma/PitNET. **A** This postcontrast sagittal T1-weighted image shows a sellar tumour extending downward into the sphenoidal sinus. **B** The lesion has a cystic component, evidenced in this coronal T2-weighted sequence.

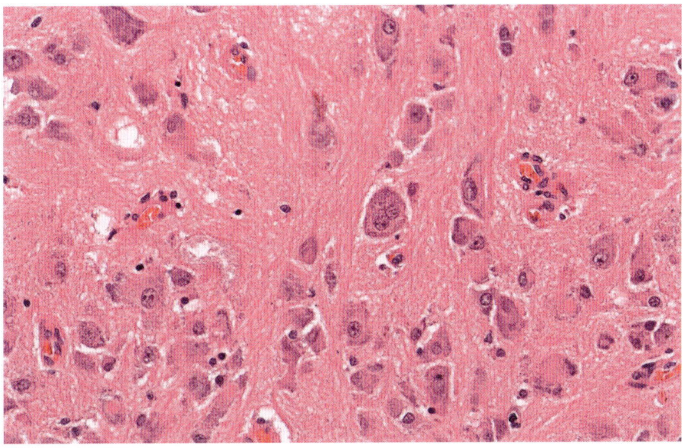

Fig. 2.61 Gangliocytoma. The tumour was associated with acromegaly, without a PitNET.

Pathogenesis

Transdifferentiation of neoplastic endocrine cells into ganglion cells is the most current hypothesis, based on the expression of pituitary transcription factors in ganglion cells {2386,2127,3229, 3895}. Cells with intermediate features between neurons and adenohypophysial cells, as well as NeuN and neurofilament expression in neuroendocrine cells, corroborate this hypothesis {1947}. A common pituitary stem/progenitor cell {2386} and neoplastic transformation of adenohypophysial cells induced by hypothalamic hormones are also postulated {926}. Cases in patients with multiple endocrine neoplasia type 1 may represent multiple primary tumours (i.e. collision tumours) {4067}.

Macroscopic appearance

Pure and mixed forms are described as well-demarcated grey tumours with a soft or heterogeneous texture {1861,5013}.

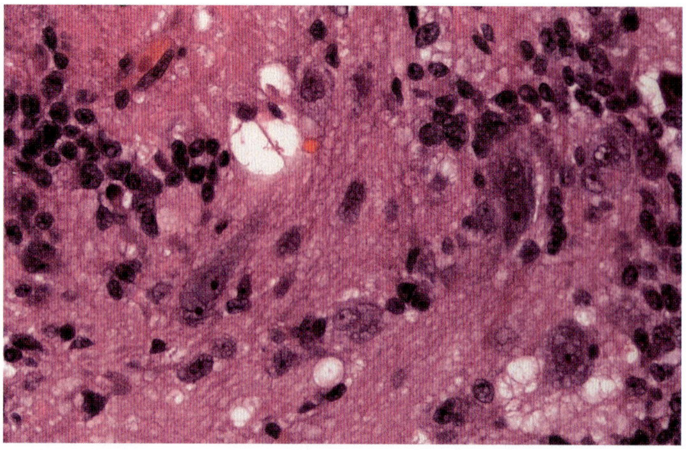

Fig. 2.62 Mixed gangliocytoma–PitNET/adenoma. Ganglion cells in a fibrillary matrix resembling neuropil are admixed with groups of uniform epithelial cells.

Histopathology

Gangliocytoma

These tumours are composed of large mature ganglion cells in abundant neuropil. The ganglion cells often show dysplastic features with binucleation and multinucleation {3625}. They express synaptophysin, NeuN, NSE, NFPs, and MAP2 {210,199}. They have been reported in patients with acromegaly, where they produce GHRH {218}, and in patients with Cushing disease, where they produce CRH {206} or vasopressin {202}. Thyroid transcription factor 1 (TTF1) expression is reported {202}.

Mixed gangliocytoma–PitNET/adenoma

These tumours can be stratified on the basis of hormonal profile and immunoprofile. Dispersed single cells or clusters of ganglion cells are admixed with neoplastic adenohypophysial neuroendocrine cells. The proportion of ganglion cells and the fibrillary matrix vary among cases and within tumours. Intermediate features between epithelial and neuronal cells are documented {2730}.

Immunohistochemically, ganglion cells express synaptophysin, NeuN, NSE, NFPs, and MAP2, as well as one or more pituitary hormones, GHRH, GnRH, CRH, and vasopressin; expression of the pituitary transcription factors PIT1, TPIT, and SF1 has also occasionally been described. VIP {2633}, somatostatin, and glucagon {206} can be observed. Gangliocytomas secreting GHRH only {218,2050,949}, ACTH, CRH {1133}, and TSH/TRH {3895} are exceedingly rare. The neuropil is positive for synaptophysin, neurofilaments, and MAP2. The ganglion cells are negative for GFAP and cytokeratins {2730}.

About 50% of mixed forms contain a growth hormone–producing tumour, most commonly a sparsely granulated somatotroph tumour with its characteristic fibrous bodies. Lactotroph and corticotroph cells are less frequent. FSH-β, LH-β, and α-subunit are exceptional. A case with distinct corticotroph and

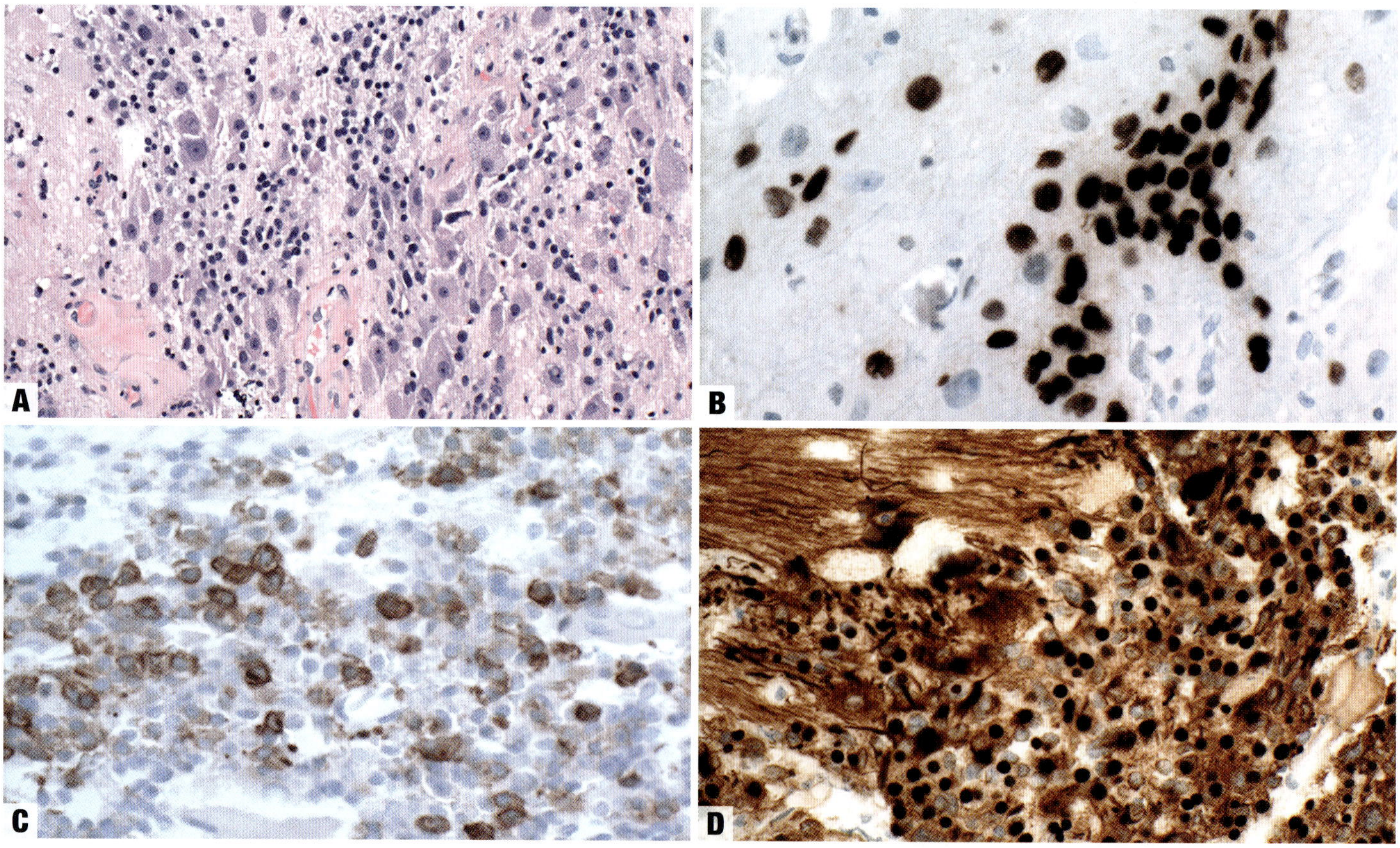

Fig. 2.63 Mixed gangliocytoma–PitNET/adenoma: gangliocytoma with sparsely granulated somatotroph tumour. **A** Ganglion cells resembling those of the hypothalamic magnocellular nuclei are dispersed within a rich neuropil and admixed with small round epithelial cells of a somatotroph tumour. **B** PIT1 immunohistochemistry yields strong nuclear staining in the somatotroph component. **C** Growth hormone immunohistochemistry shows variable positivity in the somatotrophs. **D** CAM5.2 immunohistochemistry decorates fibrous bodies in the somatotroph component, confirming that this is a sparsely granulated somatotroph tumour.

lactotroph tumours has been reported in a patient with multiple endocrine neoplasia type 1 {4067}. The pattern of cytokeratins reflects that of conventional adenohypophysial tumours. SSTR2 can be expressed in neuroendocrine cells. Its therapeutic significance is unclear; SSTR5 is reportedly absent {926,3895}. The Ki-67 labelling index is typically < 5%.

Ganglioglioma

Occasional tumours, defined as gangliogliomas, either alone or mixed with PitNET/adenoma, contain a glial component {2155, 1936,3228,3352}.

Cytology

A report of 2 mixed gangliocytoma–adenoma/PitNETs describes variable proportions of ganglion cells, neuroendocrine cells, and fibrillary background {4356}.

Diagnostic molecular pathology

The molecular profile has not been investigated.

Essential and desirable diagnostic criteria

Essential: intrasellar/suprasellar location; dispersed or clustered ganglion cells and neoplastic or hyperplasic neuroendocrine cells (in mixed gangliocytoma–PitNET/adenoma); dispersed or clustered ganglion cells without an epithelial component (in pure gangliocytoma).

Desirable: fibrillary matrix resembling neuropil; expression of one or more pituitary hormones and transcription factors in the neuroendocrine component; expression of epithelial and neuroendocrine markers in neuroendocrine cells; expression of pituitary transcription factors in ganglion cells (not a consistent finding); expression of hypothalamic releasing hormones in ganglion cells.

Staging

Not relevant

Prognosis and prediction

Complete surgical resection can be curative with postoperative biochemical normalization; recurrence is rare even after incomplete resection {3642,5041}. Response to medical treatment depends on the subtype of the neuroendocrine component {926}. Resistance to medical therapy is reported {949, 5041}. Brain metastasis from the neuroendocrine component of a mixed gangliocytoma with a lactotroph component has been documented {3991}.

Sellar neurocytoma

Sievers P
Ezzat S
Park SH
Wesseling P

Definition
Sellar neurocytoma is a tumour composed of uniform round cells with neuronal differentiation and immunohistochemical resemblance to hypothalamic neurons.

ICD-O coding
9506/1 Sellar neurocytoma

ICD-11 coding
2F9A & XA8J35 Neoplasms of unknown behaviour of endocrine glands & Pituitary gland

Related terminology
Acceptable: neurocytoma of the sellar region; hypothalamic neurocytoma.

Subtype(s)
None

Localization
Sellar neurocytomas are located in the sellar or hypothalamic region. Ectopic neurocytomas with immunohistochemical resemblance to hypothalamic neurons have been reported {1695}.

Clinical features
Patients often present with visual disturbances and hypothalamic–pituitary dysfunction {3505,4786,202,4403}. Like other lesions within the sellar region, they can interfere with stalk delivery of dopamine. The resulting prolactin excess contributes to galactorrhoea, menstrual irregularities, and infertility. However, unlike other sellar lesions, they can also present with neurological features including nausea, vomiting, and speech difficulties {202}. Neurocytomas can also be an important source of hormone excess. In particular, vasopressin overproduction contributes to water retention with significant hyponatraemia {202}. The resulting syndrome of inappropriate antidiuresis (SIAD) can be enigmatic until histopathological examination confirms the diagnosis. Acromegaly has been reported in a single case {170}.

Imaging
Neurocytoma represents one of the differential diagnoses of large sellar or suprasellar masses. They are typically detected as partially calcified lesions on CT. On MRI they show mixed cystic changes with heterogeneous enhancement after gadolinium administration. The solid portion is frequently isointense to hypointense on T1-weighted images and predominantly hyperintense on T2-weighted images {4786,3212}. Suprasellar extension and/or invasion of the parasellar sinuses have been reported {4786,202}.

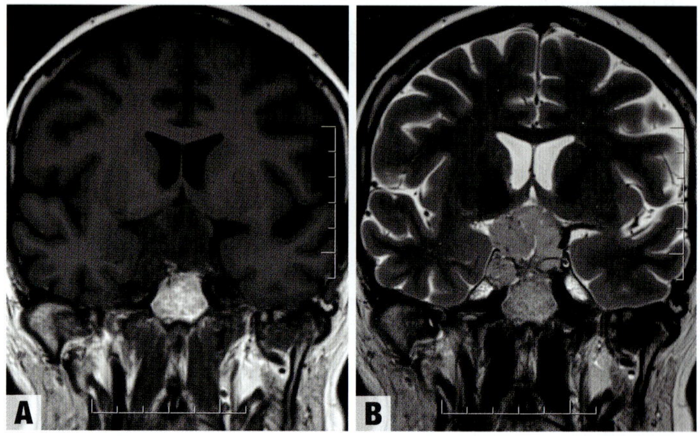

Fig. 2.64 Neurocytoma. MRI of a neurocytoma in the sellar region. The large mass is heterogeneous on T1-weighted (**A**) and T2-weighted (**B**) MRI. The predominant component is in the suprasellar space, with extension into the right cavernous sinus and circumferential involvement of the carotid. Note that the sella itself is only minimally enlarged.

Epidemiology
Sellar neurocytomas are rare tumours typically diagnosed in adults with a median age of approximately 45 years, although age at presentation varies widely {4786,4403,4509}. According to the population-based data reported by the Central Brain Tumor Registry of the United States (CBTRUS), it is estimated that extraventricular neurocytomas in all localizations occur with an incidence rate of approximately 0.01 cases per 100 000 person-years {4508}. A female predominance has been noted for sellar neurocytomas {4786,202,4403}.

Etiology
The etiology of sellar neurocytoma is unknown. No risk factors or inherited genetic susceptibility have been reported to date.

Pathogenesis
The cellular origin of neurocytoma of the sellar region is unknown. The fact that central and extraventricular neurocytomas form a distinct molecular group suggests that these tumours may arise from a specific precursor cell population {4137}. However, it is not clear whether these findings can be extrapolated to neurocytomas of the sellar region. Evidence for coexpression of thyroid transcription factor 1 (TTF1) and vasopressin in at least a proportion of tumours {202} may indicate that these neoplasms originate from neurons of the paraventricular or supraoptic nuclei of the hypothalamus {2559,3162}.

Genetic profile
Genetic data specifically addressing sellar neurocytomas have not been reported. It is unclear whether these tumours can be regarded as part of the spectrum of other (extraventricular) neurocytomas, which have been reported to share a unique DNA methylation profile {641,4137}, or as a separate type of tumour.

Macroscopic appearance

Neurocytoma of the sellar region usually appears as a large, mostly round mass, often with focal calcifications.

Histopathology

Sellar neurocytomas are histologically characterized by uniform neoplastic cells with small round nuclei, often with finely speckled chromatin and clear cytoplasm embedded in a finely fibrillar neuropil matrix {521,3505,4786,202}. Tumour cells can be arranged in sheets, cell clusters with neuropil islands, or neurocytic rosettes {4814,4786,202}. A subset of tumours contain ganglion cells. Microcalcifications may be present. Microvascular proliferation and necrosis are not commonly observed in sellar neurocytomas. Mitotic activity is typically very low. Electron microscopy confirms neuronal differentiation {2238, 2792}.

Grading

The majority of sellar neurocytomas present histologically as well-differentiated low-grade tumours and correspond to CNS WHO grade 2. However, a subset of tumours may show increased mitotic and proliferative activity, which has been reported to be associated with a more aggressive clinical behaviour.

Immunohistochemistry

Sellar neurocytomas are characterized by diffuse cytoplasmic positivity for synaptophysin present in the tumour cells and neuropil islands {4786,202,4403}. NeuN, chromogranin A, and neurofilament labelling confirms neuronal differentiation but might be very focal {4786,202}. GFAP staining is typically absent in the tumour cells {4786,3212}. Cytokeratin, pituitary transcription factors, and hormone stains are negative {3505,4786,202}. Expression of TTF1 and vasopressin has been reported in a subset of cases {202,2792}. The Ki-67 proliferation index is usually low (1–3%), but it can be elevated in a subset of cases.

Differential diagnosis

The differential diagnosis usually includes pituitary neuroendocrine tumour (PitNET)/adenoma, sellar paraganglioma, gangliocytoma, neuroblastoma, and pituicytoma. The diffuse cytoplasmic immunoreactivity for synaptophysin and neurofilament, as well as nuclear NeuN and TTF1, and vasopressin in a subset of cases, in the absence of reactivity for cytokeratins, pituitary transcription factors, and hormones, usually allows the recognition of a sellar neurocytoma. Glial tumours can typically be distinguished by their GFAP immunoreactivity and/or the presence of characteristic molecular markers.

Cytology

Not clinically relevant

Diagnostic molecular pathology

Genome-wide DNA methylation profiling has provided evidence for a specific epigenetic signature of both central and extraventricular neurocytoma {4137,641}. However, it is not clear whether these findings can be extrapolated to neurocytomas of the sellar region.

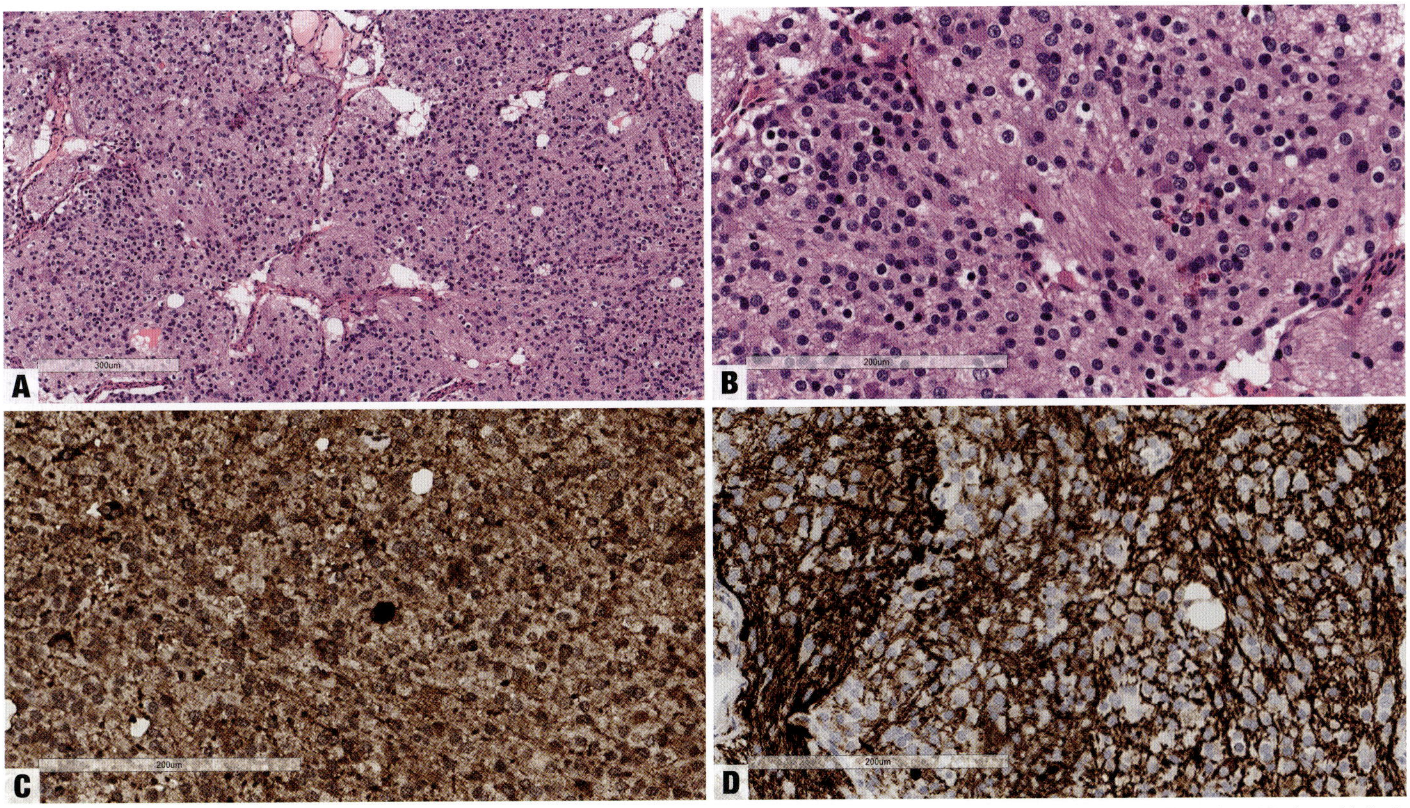

Fig. 2.65 Neurocytoma. **A** The tumour is composed of lobules of uniform neoplastic cells in a rich fibrillar neuropil. **B** The tumour cells have small round nuclei, often with finely speckled chromatin and clear cytoplasm that merges with the fibrillary matrix. **C** Chromogranin A is diffusely positive and highlights axonal terminals that resemble the Herring bodies of the normal posterior pituitary. **D** The tumour cells are strongly positive for neurofilament.

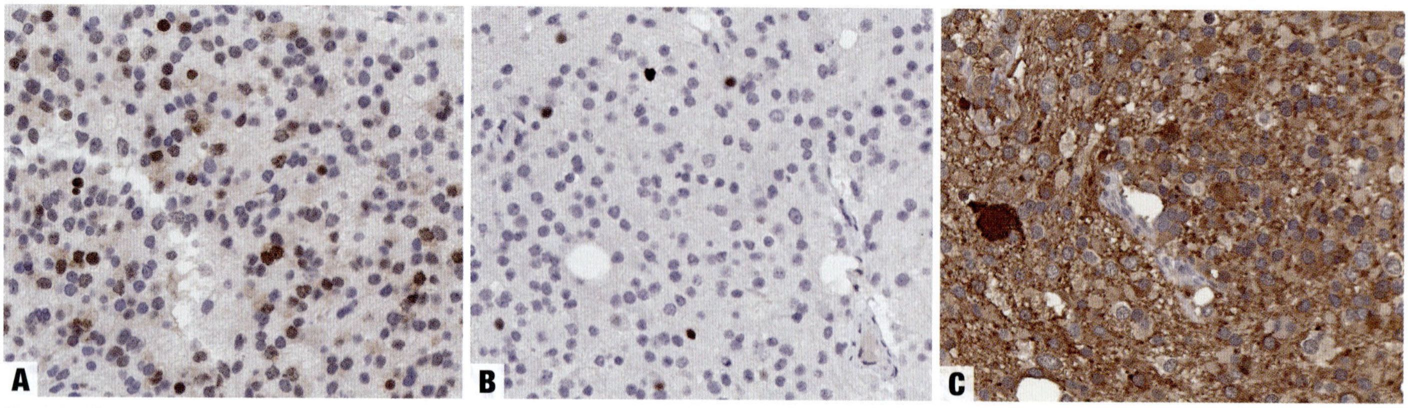

Fig. 2.66 Neurocytoma. **A** Tumour cell nuclei stain for NeuN, confirming neuronal differentiation. **B** Thyroid transcription factor 1 (TTF1) reactivity is variable and is a feature of tumours of the basal hypothalamus. **C** Vasopressin reactivity is very strong, especially in axon terminals resembling Herring bodies.

Essential and desirable diagnostic criteria

Essential: sellar or parasellar neoplasms composed of monomorphic round cells showing neuronal differentiation.

Desirable: focal NeuN expression; neurofilament expression; TTF1 expression; vasopressin expression.

Staging

Not clinically relevant

Prognosis and prediction

The clinical course of sellar neurocytomas is usually favourable, with the extent of resection and the absence of atypical morphological features being the most important prognostic factors {2187,4786,202,4403}. However, growth of the tumour and dissemination is observed in a subset of cases, and long-term follow-up is recommended {2238,4786}. SSTR ligand therapy has been suggested as a potential therapeutic approach for residual tumours {5131}.

Meningiomas

Sahm F
Perry A
Roncaroli FR

Definition

Meningiomas are a family of neoplasms that are most likely derived from the meningothelial cells of the arachnoid (CNS WHO grades 1, 2, or 3).

ICD-O coding

9530/0 Meningioma, NOS
9531/0 Meningothelial meningioma

ICD-11 coding

2A01.0Z Meningiomas, unspecified

Related terminology

Acceptable: tuberculum sellae meningioma; diaphragma sellae meningioma; suprasellar meningioma.

Subtype(s)

Meningothelial meningioma is the most common subtype; for other subtypes, see the *Central nervous system tumours* volume {4865}.

Localization

Most tumours in the sellar region are suprasellar; they can originate in the planum sphenoidale, tuberculum sellae, and diaphragma sellae {104}. Intrasellar meningiomas are derived from the inferior leaf of the diaphragma sellae {2315}.

Other endocrine organs are uncommon sites of meningioma development, with single case reports of incidental meningioma in the adrenal gland {904,3675} or metastatic meningioma in the thyroid gland {1805}.

Clinical features

Visual deficits and headache are the most common signs and symptoms at presentation {3656,334,1325,2696}. Endocrine abnormality is uncommon {2315,3965,2696}. Cranial nerve palsies may be seen in cases with cavernous sinus invasion {334}. Sellar meningioma can become symptomatic during pregnancy {5191}. Coexistence of meningioma and pituitary neuroendocrine tumour (PitNET)/adenoma has been reported {3785}.

Imaging

On imaging, the tumours are typically well-circumscribed, homogeneously isodense or hyperdense masses, with diffuse enhancement on CT. The tumours are isointense to grey matter on T1-weighted MRI, but variable on T2-weighted images, with most being T2-hyperintense {640}. Contrast enhancement is strong and uniform, allowing most meningiomas to be distinguished from PitNETs/adenomas {4432,640}. Involvement of the dura mater can occur in about 30% of cases {2466}. Invasion of the sellar floor is uncommon.

Epidemiology

Meningiomas account for about 5% of all sellar neoplasms {3877,1341} and are the second most common suprasellar neoplasm in adults {2315,1341}. The peak incidence is in the fifth or sixth decade of life, and there is a female predominance {3656, 334,3965,2466,3369}.

Etiology

Ionizing radiation is an established risk factor for meningioma {498,497}. However, after radiation to the skull, meningiomas typically arise at the convexity, not in the sellar region {3888,45}.

The expression of hormone receptors in meningioma {681, 682}, the higher incidence of meningioma in women than in men, and the increased risk after hormone treatment {875,4875} suggest an as yet mechanistically unproven role of hormones. Meningiomas developing after progestin therapy typically arise at the skull base and harbour *PIK3CA* mutations according to one study {1161}. Neurofibromatosis type 2 is the most common among tumour syndromes associated with meningiomas.

Pathogenesis

Meningiomas are believed to originate from arachnoid cells. Whereas the molecular genetics of intracranial meningiomas is well studied, little is known about those arising in the sellar region.

Macroscopic appearance

Meningiomas are typically solid and firm lesions with a whorled or lobulated appearance; psammomatous subtypes may have a gritty texture. Invasion of the dura and cavernous sinus is common.

Histopathology

Meningiomas have several histopathological appearances, varying in grade and biological behaviour. The most common subtypes are meningothelial, fibrous (fibroblastic), and transitional

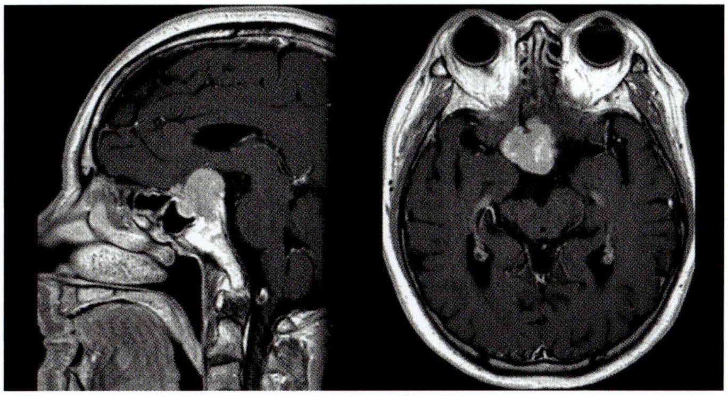

Fig. 2.67 Sellar meningioma. A 76-year-old man with visual disturbance. Gadolinium-enhanced T1-weighted MRI shows a well-demarcated suprasellar tumour.

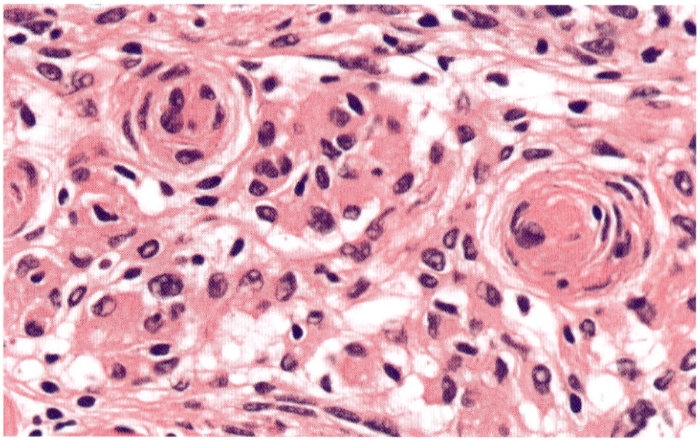

Fig. 2.68 Sellar meningioma, meningothelial. Frequent whorling pattern of uniform spindle cells.

(mixed). The exact characteristics of the subtypes are discussed in the *Central nervous system tumours* volume {4865}.

Grading

The WHO grading system for meningiomas designates the tumours as benign (grade 1), atypical (grade 2), or anaplastic (grade 3) according to specific histopathological criteria. Recognized histological subtypes with a greater likelihood of recurrence and/or aggressive behaviour include chordoid and clear cell meningiomas (grade 2). Mitotic activity and the Ki-67 proliferation index increase with tumour grade.

Atypical meningiomas are characterized by increased mitotic activity (≥ 2.5 mitoses/mm^2 or ≥ 4 mitoses/10 HPF of 0.16 mm^2, as originally described) {3532}, brain invasion, or any three of the following features: increased cellularity, loss of pattern or sheet-like growth, small cells with a high N:C ratio, prominent nucleoli, and foci of spontaneous necrosis.

Anaplastic meningiomas can be histologically similar to but are biologically distinct from meningeal sarcomas. Anaplasia is diagnosed in the presence of morphology resembling carcinoma, high-grade sarcoma, or melanoma; increased mitotic activity (≥ 12.5 mitoses/mm^2 or ≥ 20 mitoses/10 HPF of 0.16 mm^2, as originally described) {3532}; *TERT* promoter mutation; or homozygous deletion of *CDKN2A* and/or *CDKN2B*.

Immunohistochemistry

Meningiomas are typically immunoreactive for vimentin and EMA, but the latter can be weak, especially in the fibroblastic subtype. S100 reactivity is variable. PR is expressed in most benign meningiomas, whereas ER is less common. SSTR2A is strongly expressed in most meningiomas, including atypical and anaplastic tumours {2941}. STAT6 (nuclear) and thyroid transcription factor 1 (TTF1) are not expressed.

Ultrastructure

Features include complex interdigitating cellular processes, abundant intermediate filaments, and desmosomal junctions.

Differential diagnosis

The entities include TTF1-expressing tumours of the posterior lobe, schwannoma, and solitary fibrous tumour of the sella.

Cytology

Fibrous meningiomas can be difficult to smear; cellularity can be low on touch imprints. Compact fascicles of spindle cells, a whorling pattern, calcification, and nuclear pseudoinclusions are features of meningioma on squash preparation {3178}. Distinction from pituicytoma and spindle cell oncocytoma is challenging.

Diagnostic molecular pathology

Meningothelial meningiomas, the most common subtype in the sellar region, typically carry *AKT1* p.E17K mutations (often combined with *TRAF7* mutations) or, alternatively, isolated *PIK3CA* or *SMO* mutations {872,6}. They rarely show any copy-number alterations {872}.

Essential and desirable diagnostic criteria

Essential: classic histopathological features matching at least one of the meningioma subtypes; suggestive histopathological features combined with biallelic inactivation of *NF2* or other classic drivers of conventional meningioma (*TRAF7, AKT1, KLF4, SMO, PIK3CA*), clear cell meningioma (*SMARCE1*), or rhabdoid meningioma (*BAP1*); suggestive histopathological features combined with one of the defined DNA methylation classes of meningioma.

Desirable: dural or meningeal localization; EMA immunoreactivity; strong and diffuse SSTR2A immunoreactivity; classic copy-number alterations of *NF2*-mutant meningioma, such as monosomy 22/22q in lower-grade meningiomas, with additional losses of 1p, 6, 10q, 14q, and/or 18 in higher-grade meningiomas.

Staging

Not applicable

Prognosis and prediction

Prognosis depends on invasion of parasellar structures, tumour histopathology (see subtypes), and tumour grade. Outcomes are favourable in patients aged < 50 years and patients with clinical presentation for < 1 year {1315}. Recurrence is associated with incomplete surgical resection {1315,334,2466}. Perioperative mortality rates are low {334}, but postoperative persistence of disease and hypopituitarism are not uncommon {3965}.

Chordoma

Varlet P
Perry A
Roncaroli FR

Chapter 2

Definition
Chordoma is a primary malignant bone neoplasm showing notochordal differentiation.

ICD-O coding
9370/3 Conventional chordoma
9371/3 Chondroid chordoma
9370/3 Poorly differentiated chordoma
9372/3 Dedifferentiated chordoma

ICD-11 coding
2B5K & XH9GH0 Unspecified malignant soft tissue tumours or sarcomas of bone or articular cartilage of other or unspecified sites & Chordoma, NOS
2B5K & XH17D8 Unspecified malignant soft tissue tumours or sarcomas of bone or articular cartilage of other or unspecified sites & Chondroid chordoma
2B5Z & XH7303 Malignant mesenchymal neoplasm of unspecified type & Dedifferentiated chordoma

Related terminology
None

Subtype(s)
Conventional chordoma; chondroid chordoma; poorly differentiated chordoma; dedifferentiated chordoma

Localization
Skull base chordomas typically arise from the clivus. Parasellar or suprasellar extension is common. Entirely intrasellar lesions are rare {50}. Coexistence of chordoma and pituitary neuroendocrine tumour (PitNET)/adenoma is exceptional {3440}.

Clinical features
Patients with intrasellar chordomas present with cranial nerve deficit (88.1%), visual disturbances, and endocrine abnormalities (52.8%) including hyperprolactinaemia and/or hypopituitarism {4940,50}. Headache alone is rare {50}.

Imaging
Chordomas are bone destructive midline lesions. On MRI, they are usually hypointense on T1 sequences (lower intensity than the clival fat), are hyperintense on T2 sequences, and show variable contrast enhancement.

Epidemiology
The prevalence is 0.088 cases per 1 million individuals, representing 0.5% of primary CNS tumours {992}. Chordomas account for 0.5% of sellar lesions {3877,16}. The skull base is the primary site in approximately 38% of cases {4049,992}. Both children and adults are affected. Adults with intrasellar chordoma (mean age: 55.5 years) are older than patients with non-intrasellar skull base chordoma (mean age: 43.3 years). There is a slight female predominance (M:F ratio: 1:1.16) {50}.

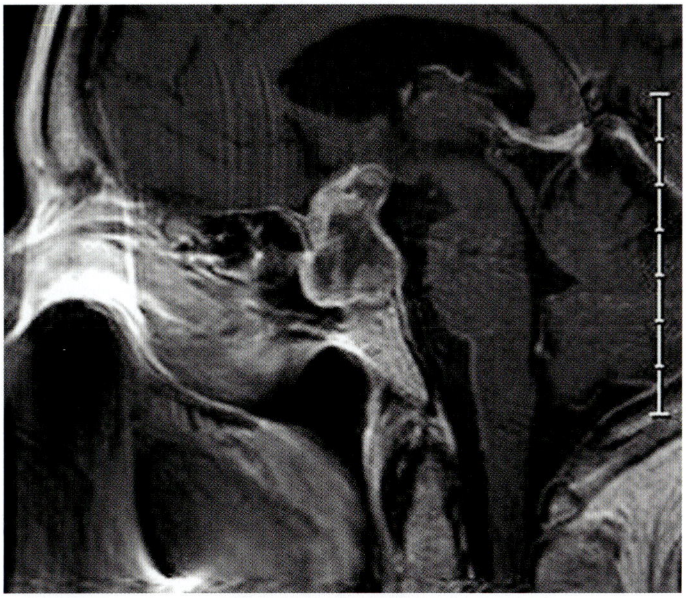

Fig. 2.69 Chordoma. Midsagittal postcontrast MRI showing a clival chordoma that invaded upward into the sella and suprasellar space.

Etiology
The majority of chordomas are sporadic. Germline *TBXT* gene duplication has been reported in a subset of familial cases {2252}. An association with tuberous sclerosis is documented {968}.

Pathogenesis
Chordomas probably derive from notochordal remnants that persist after development in a subset of individuals. The molecular mechanism underlying the transformation of notochordal rests is poorly understood. *TBXT* gene duplication (27% of cases) and *PIK3CA* signalling mutations (16%) have been described {2252,4423,264}. A novel *LYST* inactivating mutation (10%) has also been reported {4423,264}. Alterations of *PBRM1/SETD2*, members of the SWI/SNF complex, represent the most common events (in 16%) in skull base chordomas, along with homozygous *CDKN2A* deletion {264}. Loss of SMARCB1 (INI1) expression resulting from homozygous *SMARCB1* gene deletion occurs in poorly differentiated chordomas {1810}.

Macroscopic appearance
Chordomas appear as lobulated solid tumours with a gelatinous appearance, typically invading the bone and extending into the surrounding tissue.

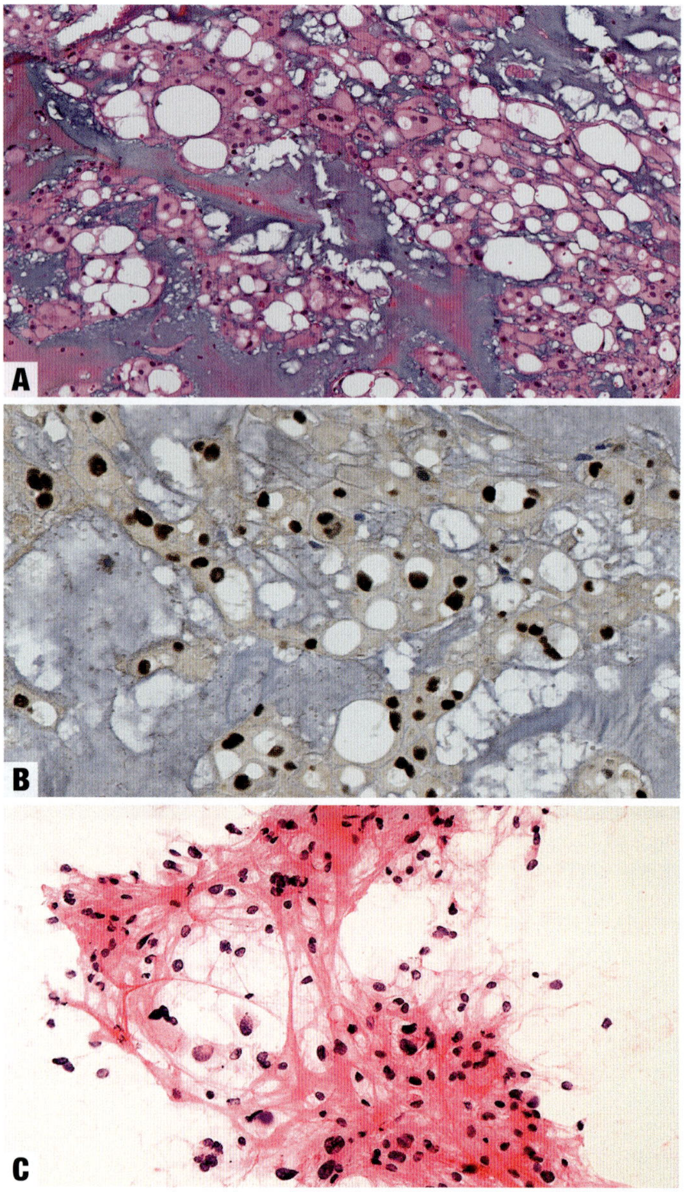

Fig. 2.70 Chordoma. **A** Conventional chordoma. Chords of tumour cells in a myxoid stroma. Note that occasional cells display a bubbly cytoplasm (physaliphorous cells). **B** Conventional chordoma. Chordomas typically show nuclear immunoreactivity for brachyury. **C** Chordoma of the clivus. Neoplastic cells, including clusters of physaliphorous cells, in a fibrillary matrix in this squash preparation.

Histopathology

Conventional chordoma shows a lobular architecture with lobules delimited by fibrous septa. Tumour cells form cords or ribbons within a myxoid matrix. Cells are large with clear to eosinophilic cytoplasm. They are defined as physaliphorous cells when the cytoplasm is vacuolated or bubbly. Anisokaryosis and nuclear inclusions may be observed. Prominent nucleoli, mitoses, and apoptotic bodies are seldom seen.

Subtypes

Chondroid chordoma represents a subtype composed predominantly of hyaline cartilage–like extracellular matrix.

Dedifferentiated chordomas are biphasic tumours composed of conventional chordoma juxtaposed to high-grade sarcoma. Brachyury and cytokeratin expression is preserved in the conventional component, whereas the sarcomatous areas can lose these proteins {235,1991}.

Poorly differentiated chordoma consists of epithelioid or rhabdoid cells and lacks myxoid areas and physaliphorous cells. Immunostaining for brachyury is retained. SMARCB1 (INI1) expression is lost {1810,4116}.

Immunohistochemistry

Brachyury expression is the diagnostic hallmark {4747,4505,2995}.

Differential diagnosis

The differential diagnosis includes benign {4627} and atypical {684} notochordal cell tumours. Chondroid chordoma should be distinguished from low-grade chondrosarcoma.

Cytology

Squash or imprint preparations show clustered or dispersed uniform cells with weakly eosinophilic or clear vacuolated cytoplasm (physaliphorous cells) in a myxoid and/or fibrillary matrix.

Diagnostic molecular pathology

No diagnostic molecular markers have been reported for conventional chordoma. Homozygous *SMARCB1* deletions support the diagnosis of poorly differentiated chordoma.

Essential and desirable diagnostic criteria

Conventional chordoma and chondroid chordoma

Essential: epithelioid and physaliphorous cells in a myxoid to chondroid matrix; brachyury expression.

Dedifferentiated chordoma

Essential: an additional sarcomatous component.

Poorly differentiated chordoma

Essential: aggregates of atypical epithelioid to rhabdoid cells; loss of SMARCB1 (INI1) expression; retained brachyury.

Staging

Chordoma staging follows bone sarcoma protocols.

Prognosis and prediction

Chordomas are slow-growing but locally aggressive tumours. Incomplete resection represents the main prognostic factor. Adult patients with intrasellar chordoma have a worse prognosis than patients with skull base chordoma {50}, possibly due to incomplete removal and postoperative endocrine sequelae.

Dedifferentiated and poorly differentiated chordomas are highly aggressive neoplasms {1810,359,4116,5162}.

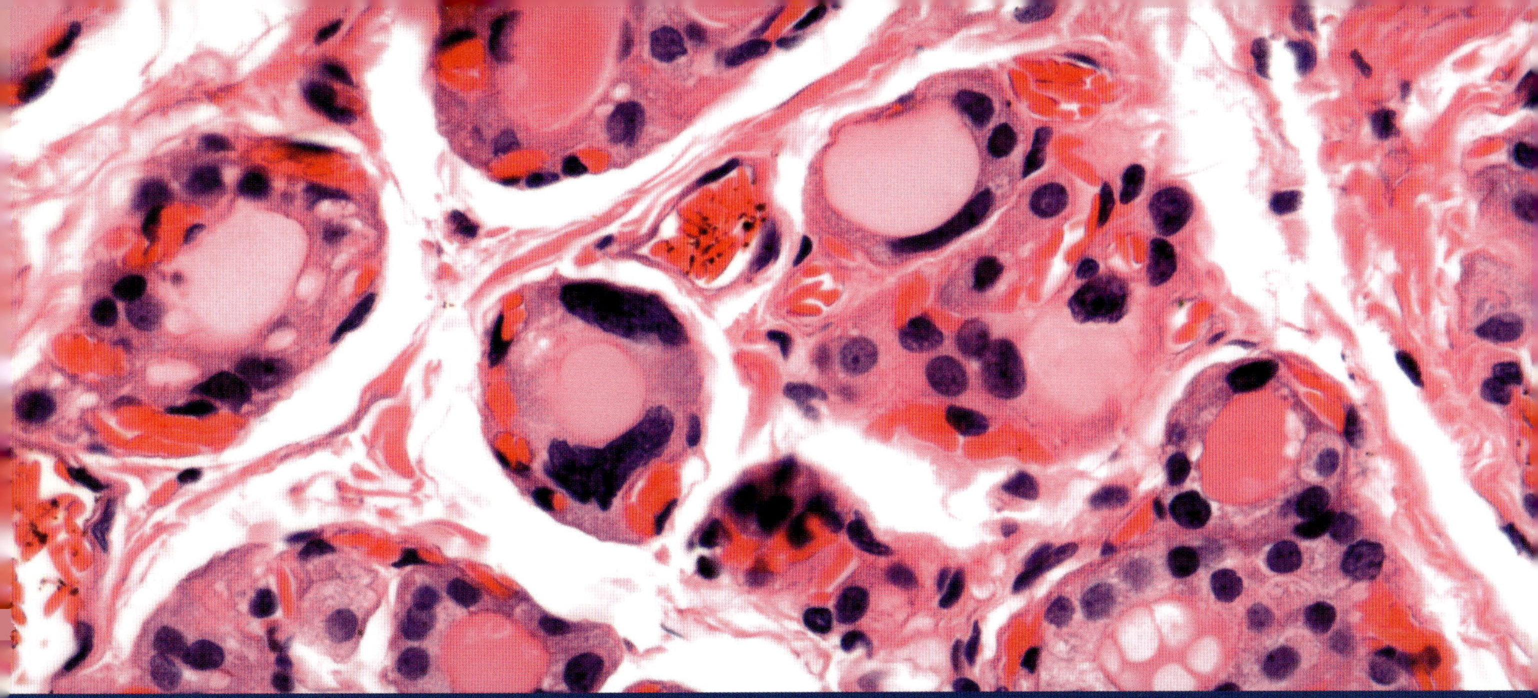

3

Thyroid tumours

Edited by: Asa SL, Baloch ZW, Erickson LA, Ghossein RA, Gill AJ, Lax SF, Mete O, Papotti M, Sobrinho-Simoes M, Tallini G, Thompson LDR

Thyroid tumours: Introduction

Asa SL
Durante C
Tuttle RM

Tumours of the thyroid gland are the most common endocrine neoplasms. The vast majority are derived from follicular epithelial cells that form the greater part of the gland. A much smaller number arise from calcitonin-secreting C cells, a component of the dispersed neuroendocrine system. Rarely, thyroid tumours are composed of both C cells and follicular cells. Tumours of parathyroid, thymus, and salivary glands can present as primary thyroid neoplasms because of their proximity to, and occasional location within, the gland. As in any organ, there can be primary tumours of stromal elements, and because the thyroid is a midline organ, germ cell tumours may arise.

Tumours of thyroid follicular cell derivation

Tumours of thyroid follicular cell derivation include benign adenomas, low-risk neoplasms, and malignancies that span the spectrum from minute, incidental findings to aggressive, rapidly lethal tumours (see Table 3.01).

Benign

Benign neoplasms are classified as adenomas. The majority have simple microfollicular or macrofollicular architecture and exhibit a RAS-like molecular profile {622}. Some adenomas are composed of oncocytic cells (previously called Hürthle cells, although this is actually a misnomer and the term "Hürthle" is now discouraged {212}). A distinct form of adenoma has an intrafollicular papillary architecture sometimes reflecting a hyperfunctional status due to mutations that activate the cAMP pathway {3824}. A common abnormality of the thyroid is the presence of multifocal benign nodules that span a hyperplasia–neoplasia sequence; morphological criteria cannot always distinguish hyperplastic lesions from neoplastic lesions in nodular disease of follicular cells in this disorder that has, by consensus, been designated by pathologists as thyroid follicular nodular disease. These lesions may give rise to clinically detectable thyroid enlargement, known as multinodular goitre, but they are

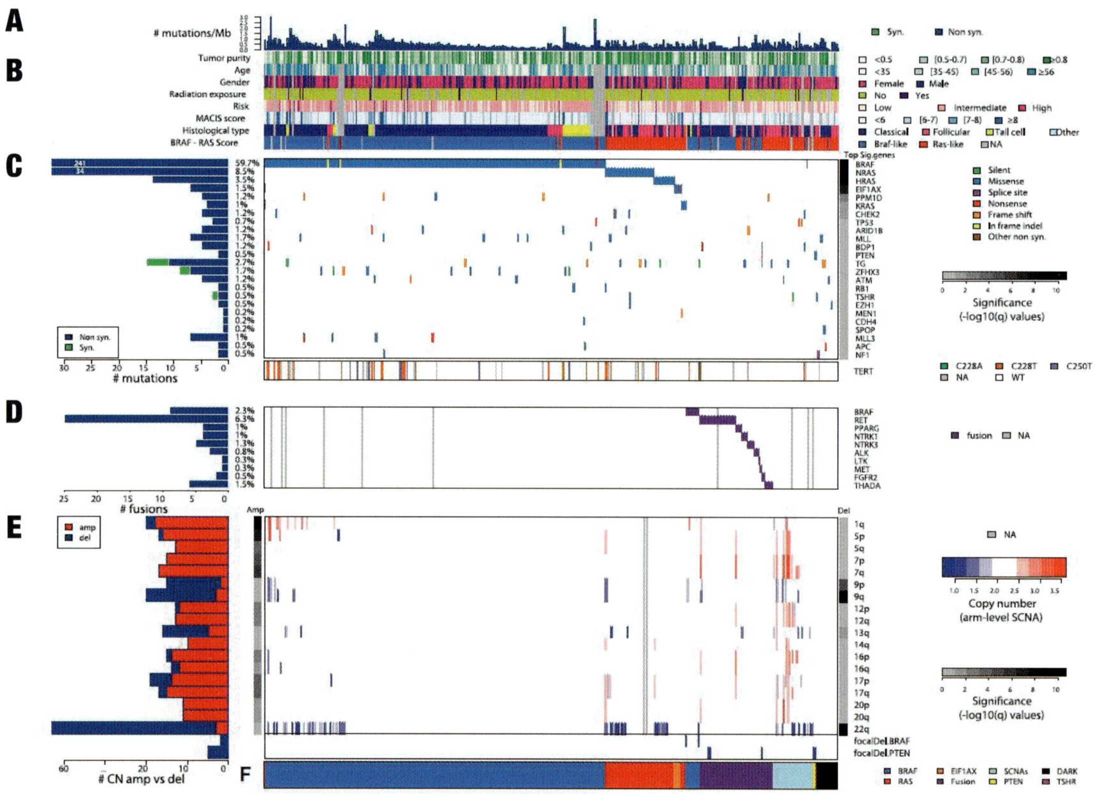

Fig. 3.01 Landscape of genomic alterations in 402 papillary thyroid carcinomas. **A** Mutation density (mutations/Mb) across the cohort. **B** Tumour purity, patient age, patient sex, history of radiation exposure, risk of recurrence, MACIS score (distant metastasis, patient age, completeness of resection, local invasion, and tumour size), histological type, and BRAF p.V600E–RAS score (BRS). **C** Number and frequency of recurrent mutations in genes (left) ranked by MutSig significance (right), gene-sample matrix of mutations (middle) with *TERT* promoter mutations (bottom). **D** Number and frequency of fusion events (left), gene-sample matrix of fusions across the cohort (middle). **E** Number and frequency of somatic copy-number alterations (left), chromosome-sample matrix of somatic copy-number alterations across the cohort (middle) with focal deletions in *BRAF* and *PTEN* (bottom), GISTIC2 significance (right). **F** Driving variant types across the cohort. Samples were sorted by driving variant type with dark matter on the left.

Table 3.01 Prognostic risk-based classification of follicular cell–derived carcinomas of the thyroid gland

Grade (mitoses, tumour necrosis)	Histological differentiation (architecture: papillae, follicles, solid/trabecular/insular patterns)	Histotype	Outcome
Low	Present, well differentiated	Papillary carcinoma	Favourable
		Follicular carcinoma	Favourable
		Oncocytic carcinoma	Favourable
High	Present, well differentiated	High-grade differentiated thyroid carcinoma: papillary, follicular, oncocytic	Intermediate
	Present, poorly differentiated	Poorly differentiated thyroid carcinoma	Intermediate
	Absent	Anaplastic thyroid carcinoma	Poor

Note: Tumours with mixed histological features should be typed according to the component of highest grade and least differentiation.

also present in glands that do not qualify for this designation because the gland is not enlarged.

Low-risk

A category of low-risk neoplasms has been created to bridge the gap between benign and malignant. They include neoplasms that have been reported to give rise to metastases but have an extremely low incidence of spread. The designation "tumour", rather than "carcinoma", is intended to reduce the risk of overtreatment. These include tumours that have cytological features of malignancy but no evidence of invasive growth (non-invasive follicular thyroid neoplasm) {3255}, tumours with uncertain invasiveness (uncertain malignant potential) {4883,1925}, and tumours with striking nuclear features of papillary carcinoma and hyaline cytoplasm (hyalinizing trabecular tumour) {668}.

Malignant

Malignancies of thyroid follicular cells have been characterized at the molecular level, and it is clear that the majority of well-differentiated thyroid carcinomas fall into one of two categories. Tumours with a predominant expansile but not infiltrative growth pattern, often (but not always) clear encapsulation, and follicular architecture are classified as RAS-like tumours because of the high prevalence of RAS mutations and a common mRNA and protein expression profile {622}. They may have no nuclear atypia (follicular carcinoma), or they may have mild to moderate nuclear convolution and clearing of nucleoplasm (encapsulated follicular variant of papillary thyroid carcinoma); the degree of nuclear atypia is a highly subjective feature accounting for geographical and interobserver variability in the distinction of these two entities, and they may be

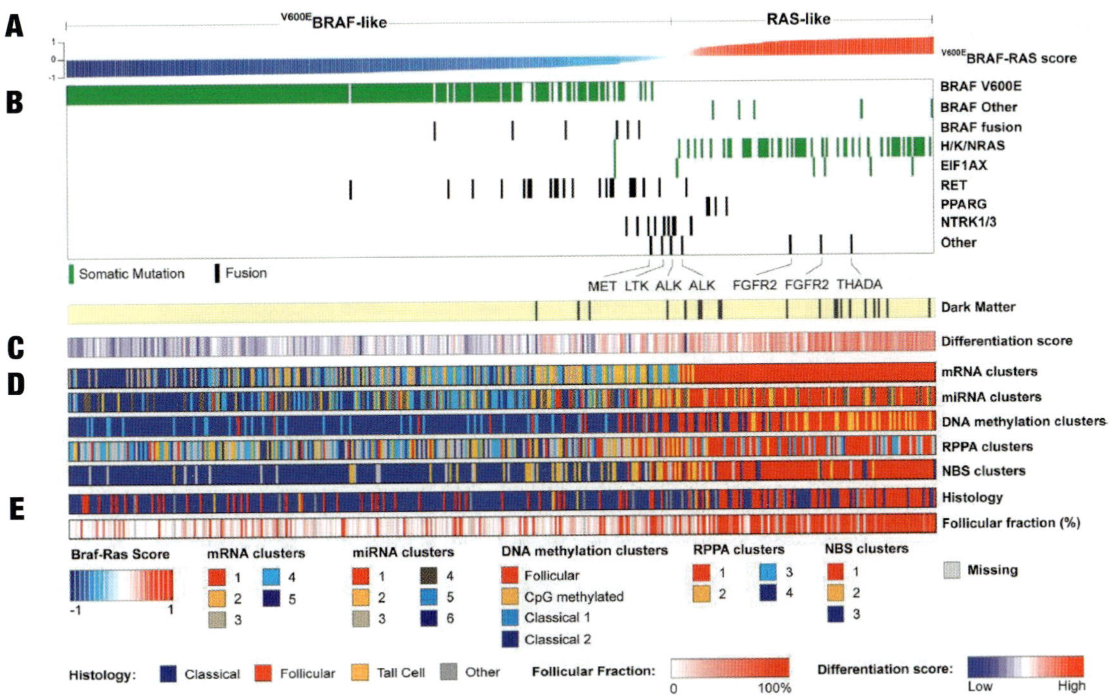

Fig. 3.02 The BRAF p.V600E–RAS score (BRS) with the list of RAS-like and *BRAF* p.V600E–like molecular alterations. **A** Thyroid samples (*N* = 391) were ranked by BRS, with BRAF p.V600E–like and RAS-like samples having negative (−1 to 0) and positive (0 to 1) scores, respectively. The BRS is strongly associated with driver mutation status (**B**), thyroid differentiation score (**C**), single data-type clusters (**D**), and histology and follicular fraction (**E**). The RAS-like samples (normalized score > 0, in red on the top bar) consistently emerged as a distinct subgroup characterized by a higher thyroid differentiation score.

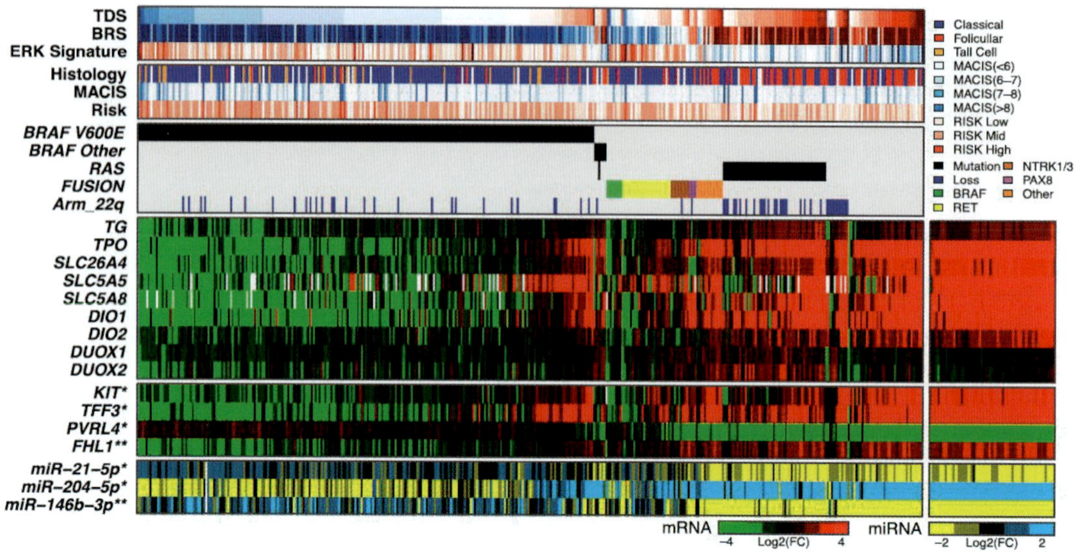

Fig. 3.03 Role of thyroid differentiation in papillary thyroid carcinomas. Thyroid differentiation score (TDS) across the cohort, with tumours sorted by driver mutation and TDS. Below the TDS are the BRAF p.V600E–RAS score (BRS), ERK signature, histological type, MACIS score (distant metastasis, patient age, completeness of resection, local invasion, and tumour size), risk of recurrence, driver mutations, and gene expression data for nine thyroid genes used to derive the TDS (*TG*, *TPO*, *SLC26A4* [encoding pendrin], *SLC5A5* [encoding the sodium/iodide symporter], *SLC5A8* [apical iodide transporter], *DIO1*, *DIO2*, *DUOX1*, and *DUOX2*), four selected mRNAs correlated to the TDS, and three selected microRNAs correlated to the TDS. Featured mRNA (except for 16 thyroid genes) and microRNA genes were selected on the basis of the Spearman correlation to the TDS in the BRAF p.V600E cohort (single asterisk) and the full cohort (double asterisk).

merged in the next edition of the WHO classification of endocrine and neuroendocrine tumours. These are the most differentiated carcinomas according to their morphology and iodide metabolism / functional thyroid differentiation expression profiles. Tumours with architectural abnormalities including papillary and/or infiltrative growth have a high frequency of *BRAF* p.V600E mutations (or *RET* or NTRK gene fusions) and are designated as *BRAF* p.V600E–like tumours {622,4591}. These *BRAF* p.V600E–like carcinomas usually have florid nuclear atypia, the hallmark of papillary carcinoma, and they frequently contain psammoma bodies. Although still histologically differentiated, the family of papillary thyroid carcinomas are less differentiated at the molecular level than follicular carcinoma or encapsulated follicular variant of papillary thyroid carcinoma, being associated with impairment of iodide-metabolizing machinery and reduced radioactive iodine avidity {622}. Both RAS-like and *BRAF* p.V600E–like carcinomas can have high-grade features, i.e. tumour necrosis and/or mitotic activity, which correlate with additional molecular events conferring more aggressive behaviour. Thus, progression, associated

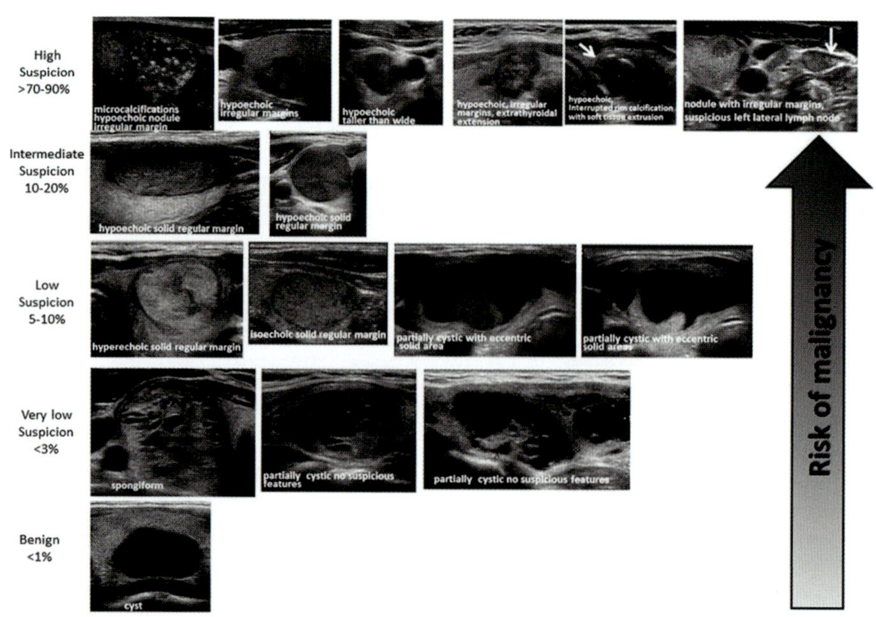

Fig. 3.04 American Thyroid Association (ATA) nodule sonographic patterns and risk of malignancy.

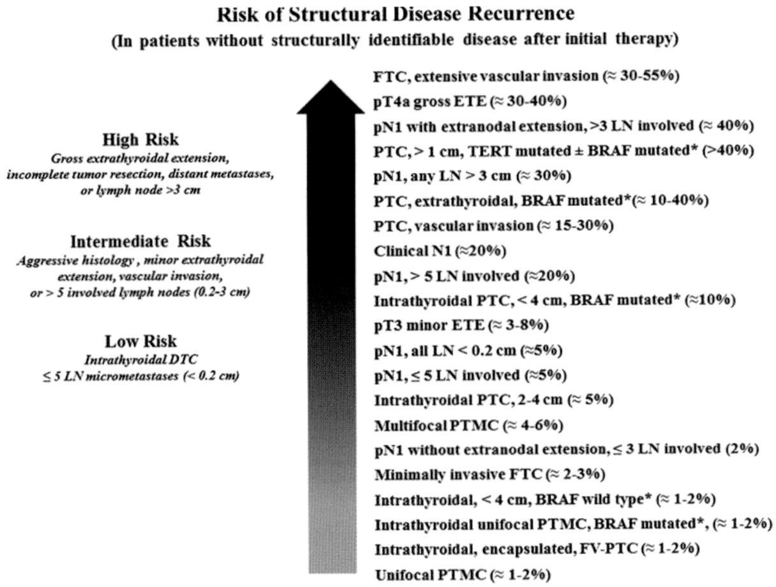

Fig. 3.05 Risk of structural disease recurrence in patients without structurally identifiable disease after initial therapy. The risks of structural disease recurrence associated with selected clinicopathological features are shown as a continuum of risk with percentages (ranges, approximate values) presented to reflect our best estimates based on the published literature reviewed in the text. On the left, the 3-tiered risk system proposed as the Modified Initial Risk-Stratification System is also presented to demonstrate how the continuum of risk estimates informed our modifications of the 2009 American Thyroid Association (ATA) Initial Risk System (see Recommendation 48). Although analysis of *BRAF* and/or *TERT* status (asterisks) is not routinely recommended for initial risk stratification, we have included these findings to assist clinicians in proper risk stratification in cases where this information is available. ETE, extrathyroidal extension; FTC, follicular thyroid carcinoma; FV, follicular variant; LN, lymph node; PTMC, papillary thyroid microcarcinoma; PTC, papillary thyroid carcinoma.

with secondary genetic events (typically mutations of *TP53*, *PIK3CA*, *PTEN*, or *TERT* promoter), gives rise to high-grade follicular cell–derived carcinomas that may be RAS-like, such as most poorly differentiated (insular) thyroid carcinomas, or *BRAF* p.V600E–like, such as the high-grade papillary carcinomas. Therefore, a prognostically relevant classification of thyroid carcinoma of follicular cells must take into account differentiation and grade (mitotic activity and/or necrosis). All malignancies of follicular thyroid cells can have histological subtypes, but the most challenging are those with oncocytic cytology {212}. Oncocytic neoplasms can have genetic alterations characteristic of their corresponding non-oncocytic neoplasms (e.g. oncocytic papillary carcinomas may have *BRAF* p.V600E mutations) but in addition, mutations of mitochondrial genes that typically encode oxidative phosphorylation complex I subunits and genome haploidization with uniparental disomy are their defining molecular features {1515,1637}. In this chapter, there is a separate discussion of oncocytic follicular carcinomas.

The most aggressive follicular-derived carcinoma is anaplastic thyroid carcinoma, a rapidly lethal malignancy. These tumours are by definition undifferentiated and therefore represent a diagnosis of exclusion. In most cases, the presence of a differentiated precursor lesion and mutations that are characteristic of thyroid carcinoma, such as RAS or *BRAF* p.V600E, combined with secondary genetic events (usually *TP53* and/or *TERT* promoter mutation) provide evidence for the diagnosis {4970}. Primary squamous cell carcinoma of the thyroid, listed separately in the previous edition of the WHO classification of tumours of endocrine organs, is now considered a subtype of anaplastic thyroid carcinoma. Previous reports of thyroid angiosarcoma and other high-grade mesenchymal tumours may represent misdiagnosed anaplastic thyroid carcinoma. However, there is also good evidence of primary thyroid angiosarcomas that appear to be geographically clustered {3419}.

Tumours of thyroid C-cell derivation

Tumours of thyroid C-cell derivation are known as medullary thyroid carcinoma. This neuroendocrine neoplasm (NEN) is not known to have a benign counterpart. *RET* and RAS mutations are the predominant drivers of medullary thyroid carcinoma, being detected in as many as 80–90% of cases {4985}. *RET* mutation is inherited in the germline of patients with multiple endocrine neoplasia types 2A and 2B. C-cell hyperplasia is a precursor lesion in patients with familial predisposition {857,2705}.

Cribriform-morular thyroid carcinoma

Cribriform-morular thyroid carcinoma is an unusual thyroid tumour that may be either sporadic or a harbinger of familial adenomatous polyposis syndrome. Originally called a subtype of papillary thyroid carcinoma because of its papillary architecture, it was recently recognized as a distinct thyroid tumour because of its characteristic genetic features of WNT signalling alterations {615}. A recent study has shown a lack of thyroid follicular differentiation in these tumours, and they remain of uncertain histogenesis {507}.

Thyroblastoma

Thyroblastoma is an extremely rare embryonal high-grade thyroid neoplasm composed of primitive follicular cells, small cells, and mesenchymal stroma. As in other organs where blastomas arise, this malignancy is due to mutations in the *DICER1* gene, which encodes an enzyme involved in microRNA processing {32}. Thyroblastoma was commonly previously classified as malignant (grade 3) teratoma of the thyroid gland.

Parathyroid tumours

Parathyroid tumours are occasionally intrathyroidal. These tumours are discussed separately in Chapter 4: *Parathyroid tumours*.

Salivary gland tumours

Salivary gland tumours can arise in or around the thyroid. They include mucoepidermoid carcinoma and secretory carcinoma (previously known as mammary analogue secretory carcinoma). A recent report adds to this list a perithyroidal acinic cell carcinoma {2140}. The previous category "mucinous carcinoma" is now regarded as a subtype of mucoepidermoid carcinoma. In contrast, the tumour known as sclerosing mucoepidermoid carcinoma with eosinophilia, although previously thought to be related to salivary gland–type mucoepidermoid carcinoma, is now recognized to be of uncertain histogenesis.

Thymic tumours

Thymic tumours that arise in or near the thyroid include thymoma, thymic carcinoma, and spindle epithelial tumour with thymus-like elements.

Other thyroid lesions

Other thyroid lesions include haematolymphoid, stromal, and mesenchymal tumours, as well as germ cell tumours that can arise in the thyroid. They are discussed in separate chapters. The thyroid is also a common site for metastatic malignancy, and this, too, is discussed in a chapter on metastatic disease.

Cytopathology

FNA plays an essential role in the management of patients with thyroid nodules {1817,1380}. Which nodule to aspirate depends on the size and sonographic features of the nodule {1817,1380}. Most malignant thyroid tumours can be diagnosed on cytology FNA material. Reporting follows established diagnostic criteria associated with different risks of malignancy to include benign, indeterminate, and malignant categories {2362,858}.

Ancillary markers

The application of ancillary immunohistochemical biomarkers is important to confirm the thyroid cell of origin (follicular vs C-cell derivation) and in the distinction between primary and metastatic tumours {284}. Immunohistochemistry using mutation-specific antibodies is becoming widely used in clinical practice to provide additional information on the pathogenesis and molecular classification of thyroid tumours. Molecular testing of FNA material is a useful adjunct for malignancy risk assessment in cases with indeterminate cytology {1817}.

Thyroglossal duct cyst

Thompson LDR
Hyrcza MD
Prasad ML
Richardson MS
Wenig BM

Definition

A thyroglossal duct cyst (TGDC) is the persistence and cystic dilatation of the thyroglossal duct in the anterior neck, commonly midline.

ICD-O coding

None

ICD-11 coding

DA05.Y Other specified cysts of oral or facial-neck region

Related terminology

None

Subtype(s)

None

Localization

The majority (> 95%) of TGDCs occur in the midline neck, at or just below the level of the hyoid bone (75% are infrahyoid), with 2–4% just at the tongue base {3926,3602,4473}. Rarely, TGDC may be seen within the thyroid gland (pyramidal lobe, isthmus) {3291}. The lateral (non-midline) neck cases are usually displaced by recurrent infections or prior surgery {4473}.

Clinical features

Patients generally present with a mobile, midline, infrahyoid, painless neck mass that moves upward with swallowing {1902, 3724,5003,4473}. An associated skin fistula (~10% of patients) is twice as common in paediatric patients as it is in adult patients {1902,5003,4473}. A malignancy may be identified in about 3% {1361,1877,1145,835,4473}.

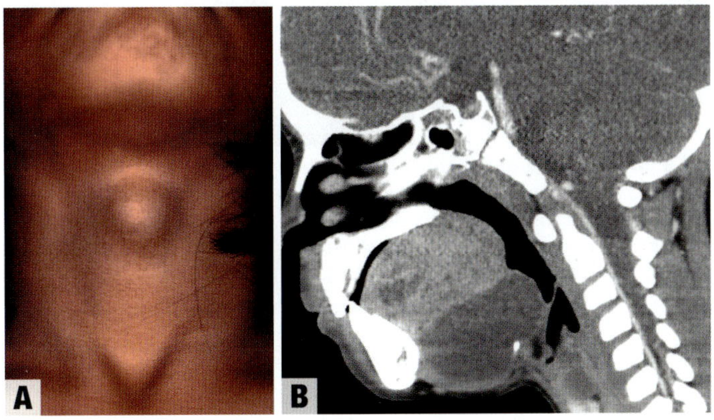

Fig. 3.06 Thyroglossal duct cyst. **A** A midline subcutaneous mass is identified at the level of the hyoid bone in this young man. **B** Sagittal CT of a cystic mass just below the tongue and above the hyoid bone.

Imaging

By imaging, a midline round or elongated cystic lesion, sometimes with irregular walls, septa, and solid components, may expand into or destroy the hyoid bone {5003,842,3378,3570, 3461}. The amount of thyroid follicular tissue is usually insufficient to be detected on radioisotope studies. Nodular soft tissue excrescences may suggest carcinoma.

Epidemiology

About 2.23 individuals per 100 000 general population have TGDCs, representing 60–70% of patients with congenital neck cysts {4473}. Furthermore, in adult patients undergoing neck ultrasound, 0.9% were noted to have a TGDC {2296}, and 7% of adult laryngectomy specimens demonstrate thyroglossal duct remnants {1226}. There is a wide age range (0.8–87.0 years), with a median age of 32 years {4473,4599}, but with bimodal peaks in the first and fifth decades of life {3724,3602,4473}.

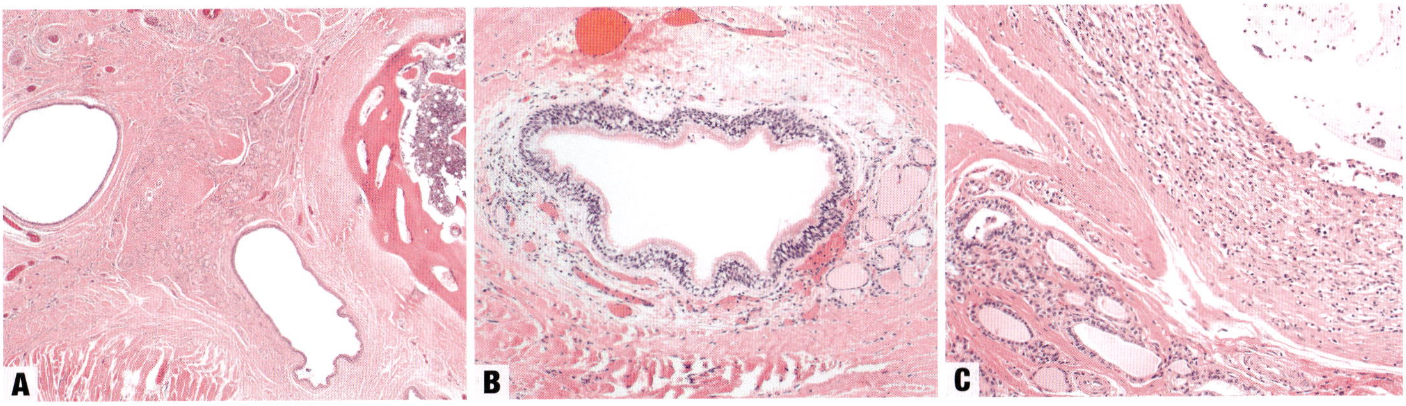

Fig. 3.07 Neck thyroglossal duct cyst. **A** Immediately adjacent to the hyoid bone, within the soft tissue are follicles of thyroid epithelium adjacent to a respiratory epithelium–lined cyst. **B** Thyroid follicles are usually identified in the soft tissues immediately adjacent to the cyst. This cyst shows a respiratory epithelium. **C** Cysts commonly rupture or become inflamed, here seen with a metaplastic squamous lining. Note the thyroid follicles in the cyst wall.

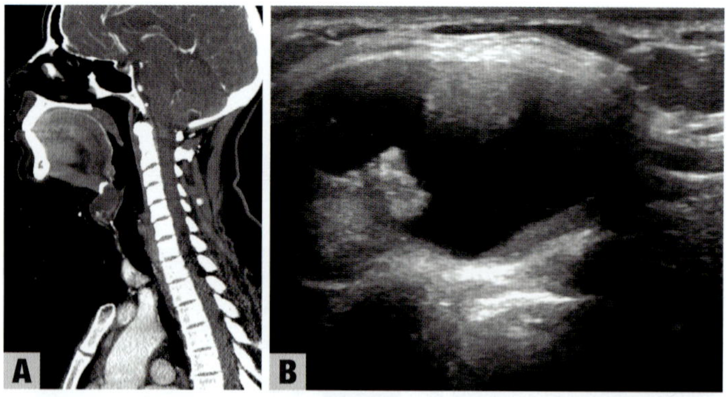

Fig. 3.08 Papillary carcinoma arising in a neck thyroglossal duct cyst. **A** This sagittal CT shows a cystic lesion immediately adjacent to the hyoid bone. Nodular soft tissue excrescences within the cyst suggested carcinoma, which was confirmed histologically. **B** An ultrasound image of a midline neck cyst with an irregular contour and a nodular, soft tissue excrescence projecting into the lumen. This finding is worrisome for carcinoma, which was identified histologically.

There is an equal sex distribution overall, although there is a slight male prevalence in the paediatric population and a slight female prevalence in the adult population {3724,4599,1526, 4834,4473}. In patients with carcinoma there is a female predominance (M:F ratio: 1:2.3), with a mean age at presentation of 40 years {1145,1407,835,845,4484,3696}, although children can be affected {3382,4484,4483}.

Etiology

Unknown

Pathogenesis

The thyroglossal duct is an embryonic developmental structure whose remnant remains anywhere along the thyroid anlage migration pathway from the tongue foramen caecum to a final pretracheal position. Normal involution between 7 and 10 weeks of gestation may anomalously persist, with dilatation resulting in a TGDC {98,3074,842,4834,4473}.

Macroscopic appearance

A smooth-walled cystic structure includes clear, mucinous fluid, which can become purulent when secondarily infected. The size ranges from 2 to 85 mm (median: 25 mm); cysts are smaller in children than in adults {4473,2665}.

Histopathology

There is an epithelial-lined cyst adjacent to the hyoid bone, containing respiratory or squamous epithelium alone, or a mixture of both (50% of cases show both), with squamous epithelium alone being more common in inflamed cases {4473}. Some cases lack an epithelial lining. Cysts rupture frequently (65%), inciting fibrosis, with histiocytes, cholesterol clefts, and foreign body giant cell reaction. Thyroid follicular epithelium, commonly localized in the cyst wall as several millimetres of tissue, is identified in about 70% {4473,748}. Mucoserous salivary gland tissue (15%) and cartilage (< 1%) may also be identified.

Malignant neoplasms are identified in about 3% of TGDCs {4484,4473,3067,4483,4834,1361}, with papillary thyroid carcinoma accounting for > 95% of malignancies {1361,1145,1802, 1407,835,4834,4473,4484,4483,3696} and with other carcinoma types rarely detected {1756,2017}. Soft tissue involvement is common (60%). Some patients may show concurrent malignancy in thyroidectomies performed as part of management {1802,1407,845,4834,4473,4484,4930}. C cell–derived tumours are not identified, because of an origin from the ultimobranchial apparatus, which is not seen in lingual-based foramen caecum lesions {4473,4273}.

Differential diagnosis

The entities include epidermal inclusion cyst, dermoid cyst, branchial cleft cyst, bronchogenic cyst, cervical thymic cyst, and metastatic papillary thyroid carcinoma, which can usually be separated on the basis of the anatomical site of involvement, imaging findings, and pertinent histological features.

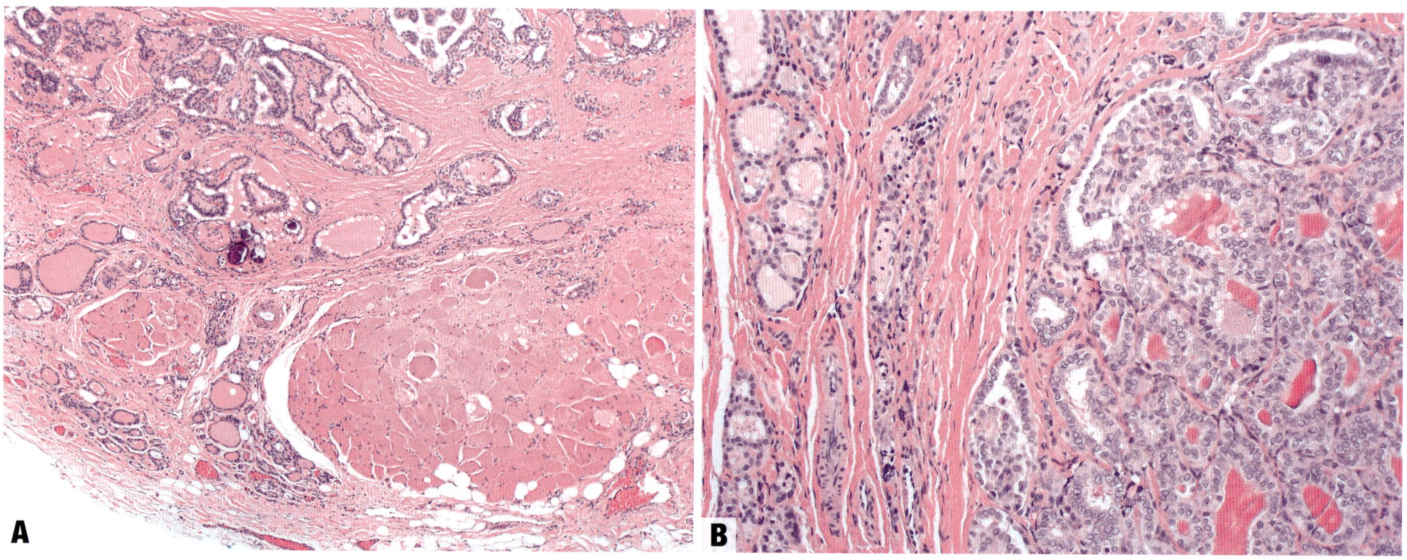

Fig. 3.09 Papillary carcinoma arising in a neck thyroglossal duct cyst. **A** The characteristic histological features of conventional papillary thyroid carcinoma are noted, including psammoma bodies. Note the uninvolved thyroid gland follicles within the skeletal muscle. **B** The histological features of papillary thyroid carcinoma are easily identified at high magnification. Note the adjacent uninvolved thyroid follicles (left).

Cytology

Smears from TGDCs are often nondiagnostic, with a low cellularity and more inflammatory cells than epithelial cells {4076, 1902,2564,4834,4473}. The epithelial cells are usually squamous or respiratory, seldom containing thyroid follicular cells. Smears obtained from firm, fixed lesions may show nuclear features of papillary thyroid carcinoma when malignancy is concurrently present {4834,4473,4484}.

Diagnostic molecular pathology

Not clinically relevant

Essential and desirable diagnostic criteria

Essential: perihyoidal location.

Desirable: a midline lesion; a respiratory- or squamous-lined cyst with associated thyroid follicular epithelium.

Staging

Not applicable

Prognosis and prediction

Recurrence is higher in patients with infected cysts and in cases not managed by the Sistrunk procedure, with perihyoidal thyroglossal duct remnants resulting in persistent clinical disease {1506,978,1484,3523}. Infection, rupture, haemorrhage, and fistula formation are recognized complications {1902,4153,4599, 1526,3646,978}. When carcinoma is identified, the outcome is excellent, although staging is not presently required for extrathyroidal sites {1802,4473,261}.

Other congenital thyroid abnormalities

Baloch ZW

Definition

Defects in thyroid organogenesis can lead to a variety of congenital thyroid abnormalities, including agenesis (athyreosis), hemiagenesis, ectopic thyroid, and hypoplasia, collectively termed thyroid dysgenesis (TD). Dyshormonogenetic goitre (DG) is due to inborn defects in any of the proteins indispensable for thyroid hormone synthesis.

ICD-O coding

None

ICD-11 coding

5A0Y Other specified disorders of the thyroid gland or thyroid hormones system

Related terminology

Acceptable: congenital hypothyroidism; athyreosis; agenesis; aplasia; thyroid ectopy; aberrant thyroid; thyroid hemiaplasia; thyroid dyshormonogenesis.

Subtype(s)

Agenesis (athyreosis); hypoplasia; hemiagenesis; ectopic thyroid

Localization

Ectopic thyroid tissue is found in the base of tongue (lingual thyroid), adjacent to the hyoid bone, in the midline infrahyoid, and (very rarely) in the lateral neck. Lingual thyroid is the most common site of ectopic thyroid tissue (90% of cases). Other ectopic sites include adjacent to the mandible, trachea, oesophagus or para-oesophageal region, and inferior to the aortic arch, as well as unexpected locations such as the heart, duodenum, and gallbladder {76,313,759,4455,4363,15}. Exceptionally, islands of ectopic thyroid tissue (usually comprising few follicles) may be seen in the central lymph nodes (also known as thyroid inclusions) {1570,4546,2607,2020}. Because of the thyroid gland's close proximity to other branchial apparatus derivatives, adipose tissue, salivary gland remnants, or skeletal muscle may be identified within the thyroid gland parenchyma {3822,3821,676}. DG affects both thyroid lobes {3081,599,3672}.

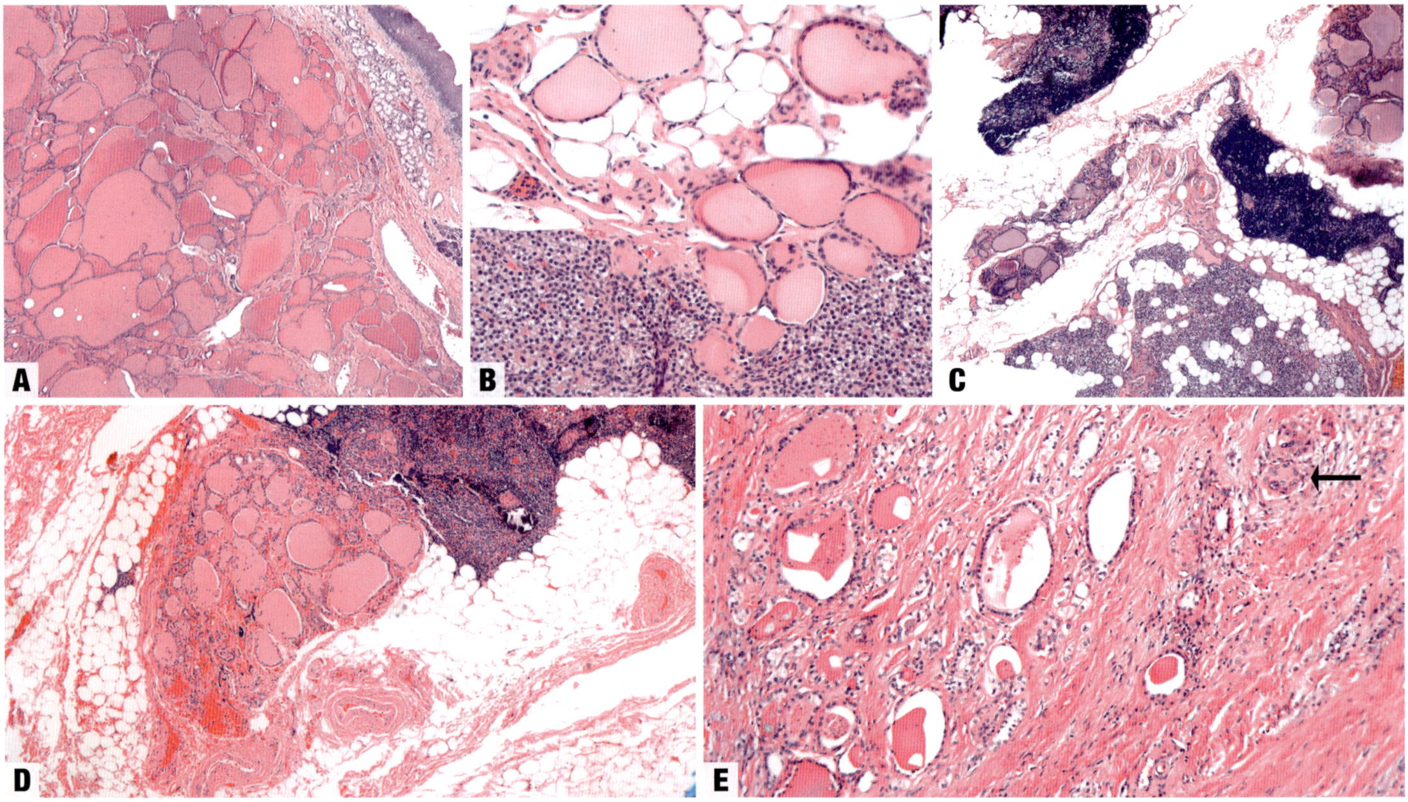

Fig. 3.10 Ectopic thyroid. **A** Lingual thyroid demonstrates an intact squamous epithelium with subepithelial minor mucoserous glands in addition to the follicles of unremarkable thyroid gland parenchyma. **B** Islands and follicles of normal-appearing thyroid gland tissue are noted in the adipose tissue and within the parathyroid gland parenchyma. **C** Normal-appearing thyroid and parathyroid tissue are noted in the adipose tissue of the mediastinum, along with thymic tissue. **D** Ectopic thyroid tissue in the thymus. **E** Laryngectomy specimen showing ectopic thyroid tissue in soft tissue and muscle, infiltrated by squamous cell carcinoma (arrow).

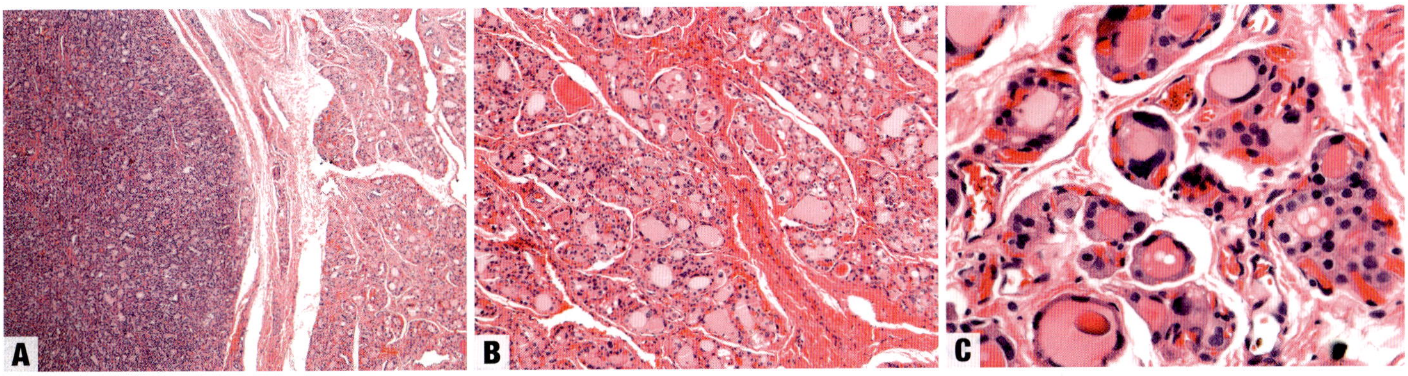

Fig. 3.11 Dyshormonogenetic goitre. **A** The thyroid is composed of nodules (usually hypercellular) separated by internodular fibrous tissue. **B** Random nuclear atypia, concentrated in the internodular regions, is one characteristic feature of this disease. **C** The nuclear atypia consists of irregularly shaped enlarged and hyperchromatic nuclei.

Clinical features

Most cases of ectopic thyroid are asymptomatic; however, cases associated with compressive symptoms (dysphagia, dyspnoea, airway obstruction) occur during puberty and pregnancy. In 75% of cases of lingual thyroid, it is the only source of thyroid hormone production. Thyroid malignancies of follicular cell derivation (papillary and follicular carcinomas) have been reported in ectopic locations {76,313,759,4455,4363,15,1217}. DG is one of the commonest causes of hypothyroidism in children and adolescents, along with chronic lymphocytic thyroiditis and iodine deficiency {3534,4658}.

Epidemiology

TD is responsible for > 80% of cases of congenital hypothyroidism; the overall incidence of congenital hypothyroidism is 1 in 3500 live births {3536}. TD is common in people who are genetically female and shows a higher prevalence in White and Hispanic people {1053,3381,2393,3534}. DG is the second most common cause of congenital hypothyroidism and afflicts 1 in 30 000–50 000 live births {514}.

Etiology

TD is predominantly sporadic, with about 2% of cases being familial. It has been shown that some cases of TD are due to the defective function of genes regulating various aspects of thyroid development, including *NKX2-1* (encoding thyroid transcription factor 1 [TTF1]), *FOXE1*, *PAX8*, *HHEX*, and *TSHR* {1053,3381, 2393,3534}. DG can be caused by the following: defects in iodide uptake by the follicular cells due to mutations in the gene encoding the sodium/iodide symporter (*SLC5A5* [*NIS*]); organification defects due to mutation in *TPO*, *DUOX2*, *DUOXA2*, and *SLC26A4* (encoding pendrin); defects in thyroglobulin synthesis, storage, or release; and defective IYD1 (DEHAL1) causing failure of iodide recycling {3534,4658,4293}.

Pathogenesis

Agenesis (athyreosis): Total absence of thyroid follicular tissue in normal or ectopic location, due to the failed formation of the median anlage or alterations causing defects in its growth and proliferation {2393,1053,3381}.

Hypoplasia: Reduced thyroid gland volume (~5% of total cases of TD) {2393,1053,3381}.

Hemiagenesis: Failed development of one of the lateral lobes of the thyroid gland {2393,1053,3381}.

Ectopic thyroid: Descent of the entire thyroid primordium, or a portion of it, is halted, leading to thyroid development in an abnormal position (between the foramen caecum and mediastinum).

Macroscopic appearance

Lingual thyroid tissue usually appears as a circumscribed mass covered by mucosa. Carcinomas in this location will show the gross characteristics of their counterparts in the normal location {1217,4354,313}. The thyroid gland in DG is asymmetrically enlarged and shows multiple nodules and degenerative changes such as cystic change, haemorrhage, and fibrosis {1556,599,3672}.

Histopathology

Ectopic thyroid tissue shows normal follicular architecture intermixed with surrounding structures (skeletal muscle, adipose) native to the location. Carcinomas arising in ectopic tissue maintain their histopathological features {1217,4354,313}.

Thyroid inclusions in the lymph nodes can be diagnostically challenging {1570,4546,2607,2020}. Strict criteria must be applied when diagnosing benign thyroid follicular tissue in a lymph node: identified in lymph nodes medial to the jugular vein; identified within the capsule; and composed of normal-appearing thyroid without atypical nuclei, psammoma bodies, or papillary formation. Even though normal thyroid gland tissue may be present in lateral neck soft tissues, thyroid tissue in a lymph node lateral to the jugular vein, no matter the appearance, most likely represents metastatic papillary thyroid carcinoma {1570,4546,2607,2420,2979}. Thyroid nodules in DG are hypercellular and can show papillary, trabecular/solid, microfollicular, and microcystic architecture. The colloid is usually pale-staining. The follicular cells can show cytoplasmic clearing. Random nuclear atypia is often observed in the form of irregularly shaped enlarged and hyperchromatic nuclei, most commonly identified between nodules. The extreme hypercellularity and the random nuclear atypia can lead to a misdiagnosis of carcinoma. Nevertheless, differentiated thyroid carcinoma (usually papillary carcinoma) can arise in the background of DG {4698,1556,599,3672}.

Cytology

FNAB (usually ultrasound-guided) can help identify normal thyroid tissue and diagnose malignancy {624,5186,4776,4267}.

The aspirates from nodules in DG are usually hypercellular and show a microfollicular growth pattern with focal cytological atypia {1101,2199}.

Diagnostic molecular pathology

Molecular testing on specimens from ectopic locations can help differentiate between reactive and neoplastic thyroid conditions.

Essential and desirable diagnostic criteria

Ectopic thyroid

Essential: normal thyroid follicular architecture intermixed with surrounding structures native to the location; if lymph node, must be medial to jugular vein.

Dyshormonogenetic goitre

Essential: multinodular gland showing hypercellular nodules with a microfollicular growth pattern and random nuclear atypia.

Staging

Not applicable (carcinomas in ectopic sites are not staged)

Prognosis and prediction

Ectopic thyroid has no significant functional impact, unless it is the sole tissue responsible for hormone production. Carcinomas arising in ectopic thyroid tissue carry a prognosis similar to that of their counterparts arising in the normal location.

Thyroid follicular nodular disease

Barletta JA
Erickson LA
Kakudo K
Kondo T
LiVolsi V
Mete O
Tallini G

Definition

Thyroid follicular nodular disease is a multifocal non-inflammatory benign proliferation of thyroid follicular cells that results in multiple clonal and non-clonal nodules with highly variable architecture. Multinodular goitre (MNG) is a clinical term referring to an enlarged thyroid gland with multiple nodules caused by follicular nodular disease (FND).

ICD-O coding

None

ICD-11 coding

5A01.2 Non-toxic multinodular goitre

Related terminology

Acceptable: nodular follicular disease; follicular nodular disease; adenomatous nodules; nodular hyperplasia; adenomatous hyperplasia; multinodular thyroid hyperplasia; multinodular goitre (clinical).

Not recommended: goitre; adenomatoid hyperplasia; diffuse goitre; colloid nodule/goitre.

Subtype(s)

None

Localization

MNG can cause bilateral or unilateral enlargement of the thyroid gland. In some cases, enlarging thyroid nodules may extend into the superior mediastinum, known as retrosternal goitre {3220}. Nodular hyperplasia has also been reported in thyroid tissue in ectopic locations, including in association with thyroglossal duct cysts, lingual thyroid tissue, and struma ovarii {2413,1852, 2353,4520,3359}.

Clinical features

MNG has variable signs and symptoms, ranging from being asymptomatic to producing compressive symptoms (upper airway compression, respiratory insufficiency, dysphagia, odynophagia, hoarseness). Retrosternal goitre can lead to stridor and superior vena cava syndrome. Rapid growth in a thyroid nodule can be due to the following: haemorrhage, infection, and malignancy (anaplastic carcinoma, lymphoma) {2353,262,4922,1115}.

The evaluation of thyroid nodules involves clinical history, physical examination, associated malignancy risk assessment, thyroid function tests, ultrasound evaluation, and (if needed) FNAB {3499,4922,2935,3176}. Ultrasound evaluation of MNG has proved helpful in selecting thyroid nodules for FNA on the basis of specific features such as echogenicity, shape, microcalcifications (echogenic foci), and extrathyroidal extension {1818,4263}. Various radiological societies have devised ultrasound risk-assessment schemes to help triage thyroid nodules for FNAB {1910,5143,5031}. Most hyperplastic nodules on ultrasound will show mixed cystic and solid features or a spongiform appearance {1818}.

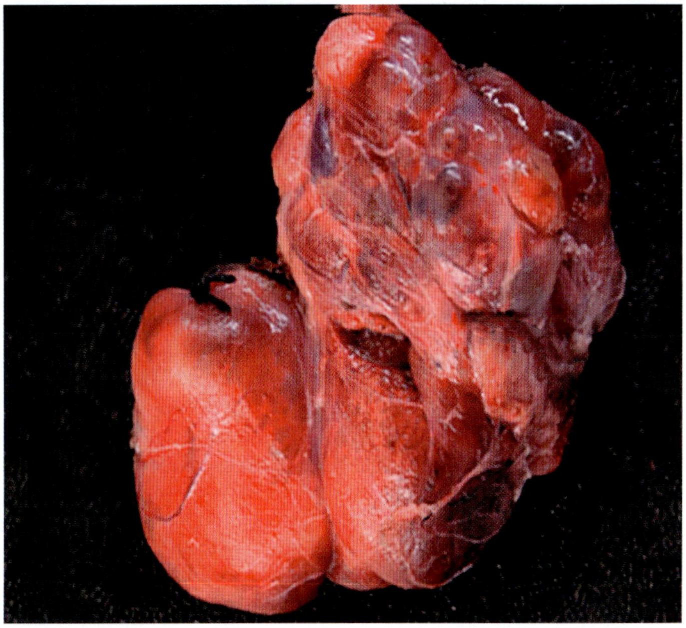

Fig. 3.12 Multinodular goitre. Gross picture of multinodular goitre. One side of the gland is often more affected than the other.

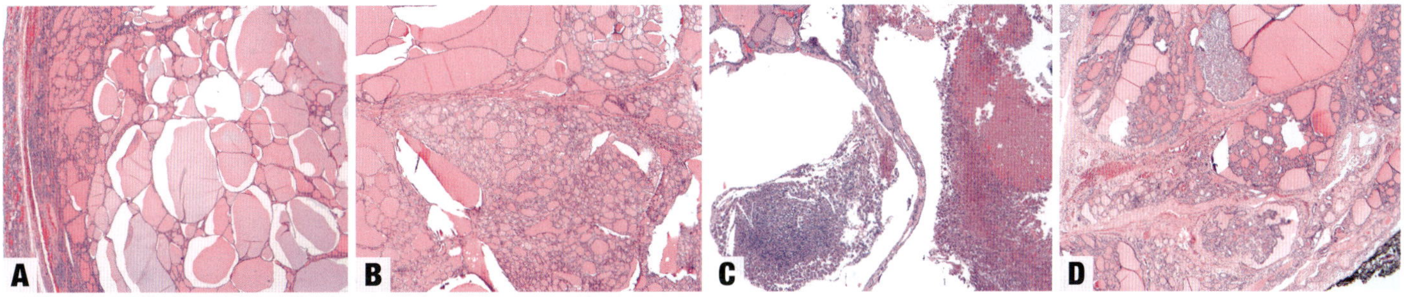

Fig. 3.13 Hyperplastic nodule. **A** Hyperplastic nodule with dilated macrofollicles. **B** Hyperplastic nodule with mixed macrofollicular and microfollicular architecture. **C** Hyperplastic nodule with degenerative changes. **D** Hyperplastic nodule with areas of papillary architecture.

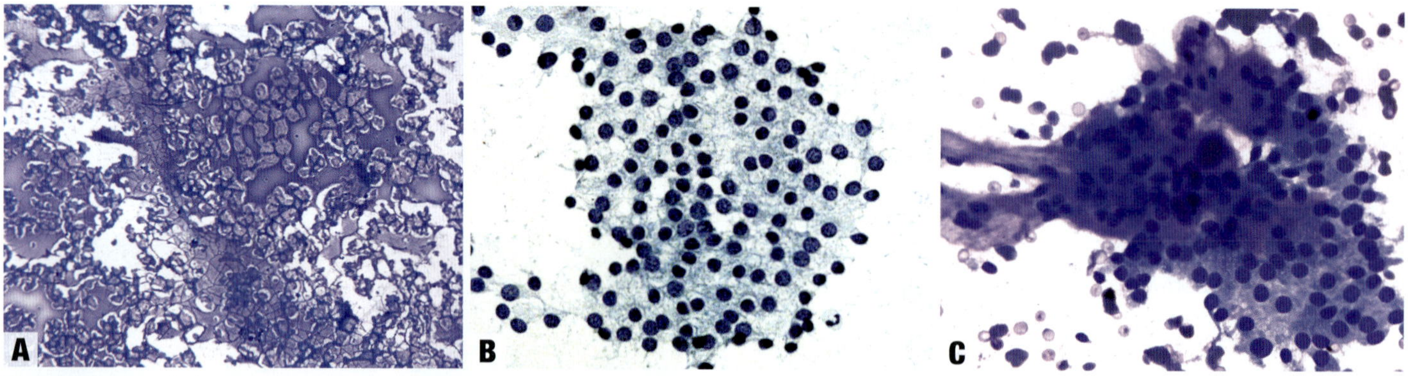

Fig. 3.14 Cytology of a hyperplastic nodule of multinodular goitre. **A** This nodule has abundant colloid showing the chicken-wire artefact (Giemsa stain). **B** A monolayer sheet of cells lacking nuclear atypia (Pap). **C** The cells are arranged in a cohesive tissue fragment (Giemsa stain).

Most patients with MNG are euthyroid; TSH screening is essential to exclude the possibility of toxic MNG. Radionuclide scanning is usually not performed in patients with MNG; however, it can be helpful in identifying hypofunctioning nodules for FNA in patients with subclinical hyperthyroidism or toxic MNG {3176}.

The majority of asymptomatic cases of MNG classified as benign by ultrasound and FNA can be managed clinically; however, surgery may be indicated for cases causing symptoms {1818,4263}.

Epidemiology

MNG has a female predilection (M:F ratio: 1:6–15). The incidence increases with age and is highest in individuals aged > 65 years {1852,2353,4520,3359}. MNG is commonly encountered throughout the world; however, it is more prevalent in iodine-deficient regions (endemic MNG) than in non–iodine-deficient regions (sporadic MNG).

Etiology

Iodine deficiency is a well-known etiological factor for MNG, especially the endemic type. However, it is understood that iodine deficiency is not the sole etiological factor for the development of MNG {1096,1095,2635}. It is probably a multifactorial process that involves an inherent predisposition (susceptibility to developing thyroid nodules, familial euthyroid goitre) and environmental factors {5145}. Thus, risk factors for MNG include age; sex; smoking; iatrogenic and dietary goitrogens; dietary deficiency in selenium, iron, and vitamin A; iodine excess; estrogen; and genetic predisposition {2560,2647,592,5071,4900,961,3153}. Inborn errors of thyroid metabolism consist of a spectrum of inherited biochemical abnormalities that can affect any step in the pathway of thyroid hormone synthesis, secretion, or action. These can lead to hypothyroidism and MNG, known as dyshormonogenetic goitre {599,1556,4470}.

Pathogenesis

Follicular nodules in MNG are caused by the proliferation of multiple cells in response to growth factors and cytokines. However, clonal nodules do occur in the background of MNG and represent true neoplasms {1094,1796,2135,2436,164}. It has been shown that the genes that play an important role in the thyroid hormone pathway (*TG*, *TPO*, *SLC5A5* [*NIS*], *DUOX2*, *AFAP1L2* [*XB130*], and *TSHR*) are the most likely candidates in the pathogenesis of MNG {1685,2884,1904,1657,920,824}. Other loci involved in the pathogenesis of MNG are the multinodular goitre 1 (MNG) locus on chromosome 14 and loci on chromosomes Xp22 (MNG2), 2q, 3p, 3q (MNG3), 7q, and 8p. Molecular analyses of multigenerational families with MNG inherited in an autosomal dominant inheritance pattern have identified genetic variants (*RGS12*, *GRPEL1*, *CLIC6*, and *WFS1*) in familial goitre {920,487,1565,3216,353}. Additional studies have also identified somatic alterations in *SPOP*, *ZNF148*, and *EZH1* in about 25% of nodules of MNG {5056}.

Functioning or toxic MNG often consists of multiple clonal proliferations due to *TSHR* and *GNAS* {2678,3931}, *PRKAR1A* (typically in the setting of Carney complex), and *EZH1* mutations {595} (see *Follicular thyroid adenoma with papillary architecture*, p. 126). Familial and early-onset FND can also be associated with *DICER1* syndrome {2269}.

Macroscopic appearance

MNG glands can be slightly to massively enlarged, with reported weights ranging from 50 g to > 2000 g. The external surface can be vaguely to prominently nodular. Some nodules may be barely attached to the gland or totally separate from the gland in the surrounding soft tissue (known as parasitic nodules). The cut surface displays nodules with a range of sizes and shapes that show variable degrees of encapsulation, cystic change, fibrosis, calcification, and haemorrhage.

Histopathology

The characteristic histopathological finding in MNG is thyroid FND. The nodules usually show an admixture of large and small follicles, often with papillary formations. A dominant follicular or papillary growth pattern can also be present (see also the sections on follicular adenoma). The epithelium lining the follicles and papillae can range from tall columnar to low cuboidal. Nuclear features of papillary thyroid carcinoma are absent. Large follicles lined by flattened epithelium and distended with colloid often merge to form large cystic spaces filled with thin colloid, known as colloid nodules. Encapsulated cellular nodules with either a follicular or papillary growth pattern morphologically appear similar to follicular adenoma and have therefore been termed adenomatous nodules or adenomatoid nodules. It is common to encounter foci of nodular hyperplasia intermixed with foci of haemorrhage (either due to degenerative changes or related to preoperative FNA), haemosiderin-laden macrophages, fibrosis, calcifications, and even ossification.

Cytology

Smears show usually abundant thin colloid and a variable cellularity consisting of follicular monolayer sheets and larger tissue fragments consisting of macrofollicles, sometimes containing colloid, separated by thin fibrovascular strands. Intact follicles and a variable number of stripped follicular nuclei can be seen. Cystic degeneration adds macrophages, haemosiderophages, and other inflammatory cells, and these may be the prominent feature with scant follicular epithelium in cyst aspirates. Follicular nuclei in the sheets are evenly spaced and round, with fine, even chromatin and small nucleoli in some cells, although enlarged round nuclei can be scattered through the sheets. Colloid follicular nodules show abundant thin colloid with scant follicular epithelium. Hyperplastic follicular nodules are usually highly cellular with follicular and sometimes papillary tissue fragments, and exuded colloid fire flares ring the epithelium. However, the cells exhibit bland nuclei. FNAB is an accurate diagnostic test for distinguishing benign follicular and colloid nodules from thyroid carcinomas {3499,4922,2935,3176}.

Diagnostic molecular pathology

Molecular analysis of FNA specimens of thyroid nodules has proved to be useful in differentiating between hyperplastic nodules and neoplasms {3249,3266}.

Essential and desirable diagnostic criteria

Essential: follicular cell proliferations lacking invasive growth and nuclear features of papillary thyroid carcinoma.

Desirable: an admixture of follicular and papillary growth patterns along with varying degrees of degenerative and reparative changes.

Staging

Not applicable

Prognosis and prediction

Benign follicular nodules do not metastasize and do not recur when completely excised. A recurrence rate of 30% has been reported in patients undergoing subtotal thyroidectomy {883,4441,5076}.

Follicular thyroid adenoma

Barletta JA
Erickson LA
Kakudo K
Kondo T
LiVolsi V
Rossi ED
Tallini G

Definition

Follicular adenoma (FA) is a benign, encapsulated, follicular cell–derived neoplasm without invasion or the nuclear features of papillary thyroid carcinoma (PTC).

ICD-O coding

8330/0 Follicular thyroid adenoma

ICD-11 coding

2F37.Y & XH0LM0 Other specified benign neoplasm of endocrine glands & Follicular adenoma

Related terminology

None

Subtype(s)

None

Localization

FAs can occur anywhere in the thyroid gland. They have also been reported in ectopic locations, including in association with thyroglossal duct cysts, lingual thyroid tissue, and struma ovarii {1106,860,3766,1100}.

Clinical features

The mean age at diagnosis of FA is 45–55 years {2753,2677, 1870}. Although FAs commonly occur in adults, they can also occur in children {4781}. FAs usually present as painless, palpable thyroid masses that are detected on routine physical examination or are incidentally discovered on imaging studies. A small subset of large FAs are associated with compressive symptoms such as dysphagia or dyspnoea {2878}. On ultrasound, FAs are typically solitary, well-demarcated, solid, homogeneous, ovoid, isoechoic or hypoechoic nodules. Most cases also show a prominent halo. Although there are some sonographic features that are more common in follicular thyroid carcinoma (FTC) than FA (irregular margins, interrupted capsular calcification), FA and FTC are usually indistinguishable on ultrasound because of their overlapping features {4066,2452,1870}. Most patients with FA are euthyroid {1870}. On radionuclide scan, FAs generally show less radioiodine uptake than the adjacent thyroid parenchyma (i.e. they are hypofunctioning, cold nodules). Rare FAs are hyperfunctioning and hot on radionuclide scan, showing increased uptake compared with the adjacent gland (see *Follicular thyroid adenoma with papillary architecture*, p. 126).

Epidemiology

The incidence of FA is difficult to assess because there is histological overlap between FA and hyperplastic/adenomatous thyroid nodules, and because most population-based studies report the incidence of malignant tumours only {2838,287}. However, from data from autopsy series, the incidence of FA in adults is estimated to be approximately 5% {435,436,2373, 4146}. FA shows a female predominance {1870}.

Etiology

Radiation exposure during childhood is a known risk factor for FA. A relative risk ratio as high as 15 has been reported, with increased risk associated with a younger age at the time of radiation exposure and with a similar risk generally reported for male and female patients {4132,1737,3803,2032}. FAs typically develop 10–15 years after radiation exposure, but the risk persists for > 50 years {4132,2032,17}. Iodine deficiency has also been associated with the development of FA {5189}.

Most FAs are sporadic; however, they can occur as part of a tumour syndrome, such as *PTEN* hamartoma tumour syndrome (which includes Cowden syndrome), *DICER1* syndrome, and Carney complex {614,1703}. Thyroidectomy specimens from patients with Cowden syndrome are characterized by multiple adenomatous nodules, FA (often multiple), and C-cell hyperplasia, with or without follicular or papillary thyroid carcinoma {1781,317}. *DICER1* syndrome is an autosomal dominant disorder caused by heterozygous inactivating germline *DICER1* gene mutations {4031}. It is associated with nodular hyperplasia and an increased risk (as high as 16-fold) of thyroid cancer; however, FA can also occur in patients with *DICER1* syndrome

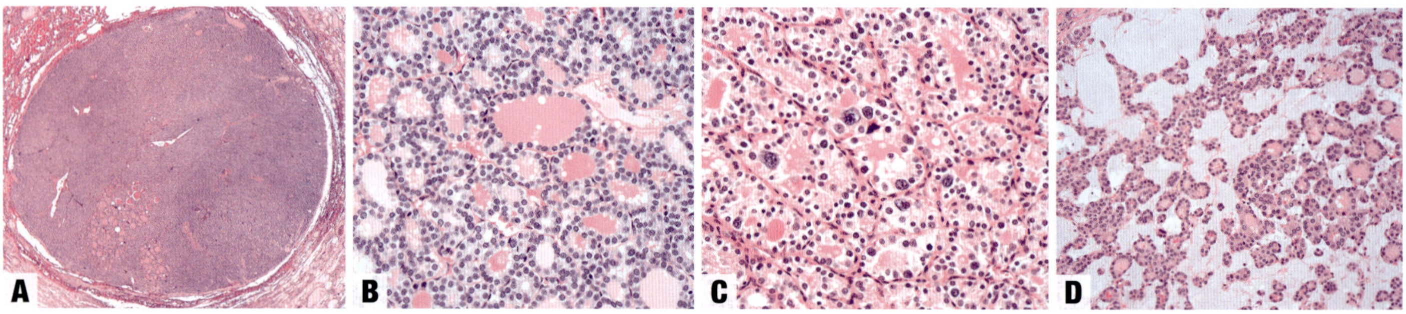

Fig. 3.15 Follicular adenoma. **A** Low-power photomicrograph. **B** Microfollicular architecture composed of cells with round nuclei with variably coarse chromatin. **C** Scattered cells demonstrating endocrine atypia. **D** Myxoid stroma.

{2269,2590,1021,614}. About a quarter of patients with Carney complex, an autosomal dominant disorder usually caused by germline mutations in *PRKAR1A*, have thyroid tumours, including FAs (which are often multiple) {407,670}. The finding of a FA in a background of multiple adenomatous nodules and nodular hyperplasia with or without an associated thyroid carcinoma raises the possibility of an underlying hereditary syndrome, especially if the FAs are multiple or occur in childhood. PTEN immunohistochemistry can be used to evaluate for Cowden syndrome; loss of staining in all or a subset of adenomatous nodules is suggestive of Cowden syndrome {317}, although clinical evaluation is required to confirm the diagnosis.

Pathogenesis

FAs are clonal neoplasms {1883,3174,852}. The most common somatic mutations in FA are RAS point mutations. RAS mutations have been reported in approximately a quarter of FAs {1280,1454,4675,3257}. *NRAS* mutations are most common, with less frequent *HRAS* mutations and *KRAS* mutations {1280, 1454}. Most *NRAS* and *HRAS* mutations involve codon 61, whereas most *KRAS* mutations involve codon 12/13 {1280, 1454}. *PAX8::PPARG* rearrangements occur in about 5–10% of FAs {3257,2852,3256}. RAS mutations and *PAX8::PPARG* rearrangements are generally mutually exclusive. *EIF1AX* mutations are identified in about 5% of FAs {2210}. The most common mutation hotspot is the A113_splice, followed by a cluster of mutations in exon 2. In FA, *EIF1AX* mutations generally do not co-occur with RAS mutations as has been reported for some thyroid malignancies {2210}. *DICER1* RNase IIIb–domain mutations resulting in impaired microRNA processing have been reported in FA, demonstrating that somatic *DICER1* mutations are not confined to thyroid malignancies {3588}. *THADA::IGF2BP3* fusions, associated with aberrant insulin growth factor receptor signalling, can be encountered in a small subset of FAs {3088}. Hyperfunctioning FAs are characterized by *TSHR* and *GNAS* mutations (for additional information see *Follicular thyroid adenoma with papillary architecture*, p. 126). Mutations in genes of the PI3K/PTEN/AKT pathway are absent or rare in FA {4810}. FAs also lack *TERT* promoter mutations, although they have been reported (rarely) in FA with atypical features {942}.

Macroscopic appearance

FAs are usually solitary, round to oval encapsulated nodules, with a mean size of 20–30 mm {5027,2677,1870}; however, tumours measuring > 40 mm occur {1107}. It is important to adequately examine the tumour capsule in large FAs to exclude invasion. Of note, size cannot be used to differentiate between FA and FTC {2753,4597,5027,2677}. The cut surface is usually homogeneous and can be greyish-white, tan, or brown. Tumours that are greyish-white are more cellular, whereas tan to brown tumours have more colloid. Haemorrhage secondary to FNA may be present.

Histopathology

FAs are encapsulated, follicular-patterned tumours that lack capsular or vascular invasion. The capsule of FA ranges from thin to thick, although it is generally thinner than that seen with FTC {5005,4202}. FAs can have a microfollicular, normofollicular, or macrofollicular growth pattern. Solid or trabecular growth can also occur, usually in combination with follicular-patterned growth. The tumour cells are generally cuboidal or polygonal and they have a moderate amount of eosinophilic cytoplasm, round nuclei with smooth nuclear contours, and variably coarse chromatin. Scattered cells with marked nuclear enlargement and hyperchromasia (endocrine atypia) may be present. However, nuclear features of PTC are absent. Mitoses are usually rare (< 3 mitoses/2 mm^2), and coagulative tumour necrosis is absent. Although the stroma of FA is often scant, it can be oedematous, myxoid, or hyalinized. Calcification and osseous metaplasia may be present in tumours with extensive hyalinization. Infrequently, FAs have areas of lipomatous metaplasia. Fibrosis and/or haemorrhage secondary to prior FNA may be present.

The histological distinction between FA and hyperplastic nodule is straightforward when the FA is solitary and has a well-defined capsule and an architecture that differs from the surrounding parenchyma. However, FA occurring in a background

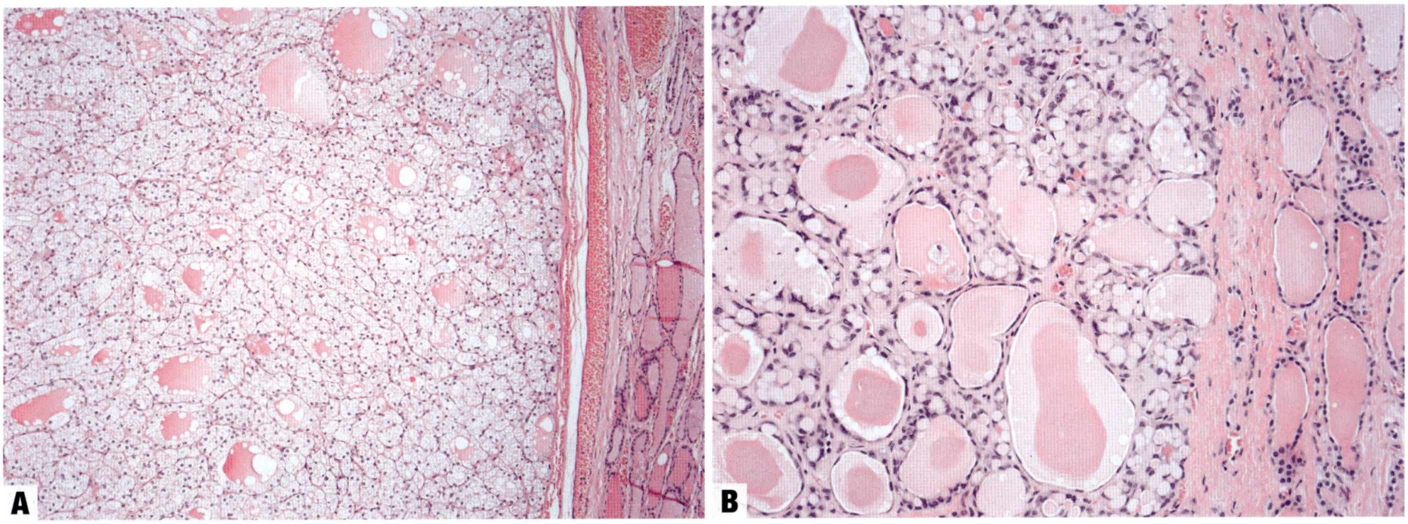

Fig. 3.16 Follicular adenoma. **A** Clear cell pattern. Rare follicular adenomas are composed of cells with clear cytoplasm. **B** Signet-ring cell pattern. This tumour is composed of cells with a signet-ring cell morphology.

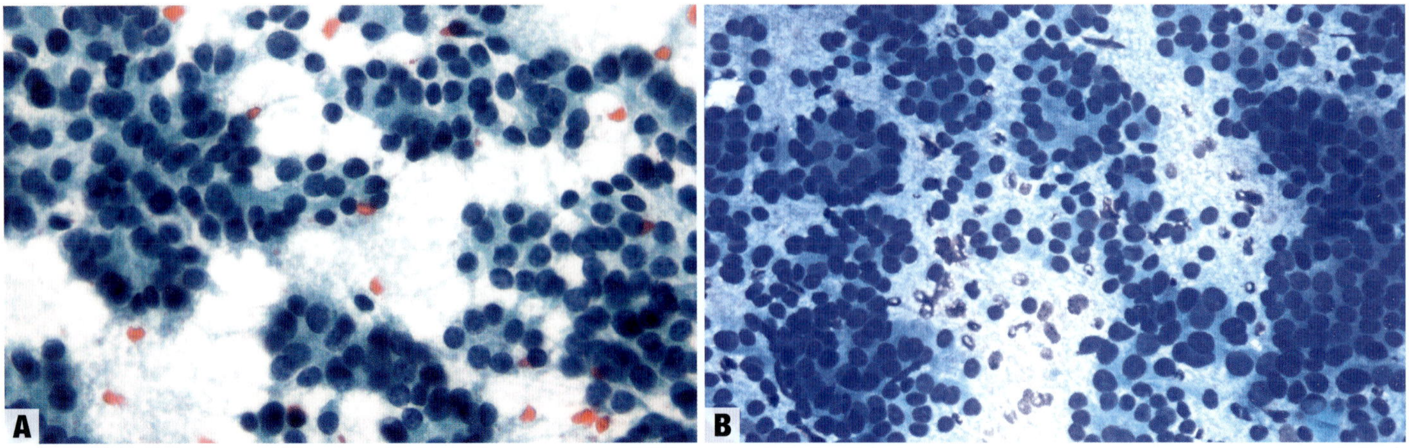

Fig. 3.17 Follicular adenoma. **A** This FNA specimen from a follicular adenoma was diagnosed as suspicious for a follicular neoplasm. Note the microfollicular architecture and round nuclei. Follicular adenomas and follicular thyroid carcinomas cannot be distinguished in FNA specimens because the distinction is based on assessment of invasion (Pap). **B** FNA specimen of a follicular adenoma diagnosed as suspicious for a follicular neoplasm because of the presence of a monotonous population of follicular cells arranged in microfollicles (Giemsa stain).

of FND, clinically known as multinodular goitre, can be difficult to distinguish from hyperplastic nodules with adenomatous change, and it should be acknowledged that without mutation status the distinction may be arbitrary.

Because distinction between follicular thyroid carcinoma and FA rests on the histological evaluation of the capsule, the capsule should be sampled as extensively as resources permit. Moreover, serial/deeper sections should be considered to resolve foci of questionable capsular or vascular invasion. If deeper levels do not allow for the definitive classification of a tumour as FA or follicular thyroid carcinoma, a diagnosis of follicular tumour of uncertain malignant potential can be rendered (see *Thyroid tumours of uncertain malignant potential*, p. 135). However, this category should be used sparingly.

Immunophenotype

FAs are positive for CAM5.2, EMA, CK7, and the transcription factors PAX8 and thyroid transcription factor 1 (TTF1), whereas they are negative for CK20 and calcitonin {4895,370,2546}. The cytoplasm and associated colloid of FA are positive for thyroglobulin {370}. FAs are usually negative for galectin-3, HBME1, and CITED1 {4039,3163}. Consistent with the low mitotic rate of FA, the Ki-67 proliferation index is low (usually < 5%) {1269}. There are no immunohistochemical stains that reliably distinguish FTC from FA (although stains that highlight endothelial cells can be used to evaluate vascular invasion).

Histological patterns

Specific patterns of FA are rare. Hyperfunctioning (so-called toxic or hot) adenomas are discussed separately (see *Follicular thyroid adenoma with papillary architecture*, p. 126). Some FAs that are not hyperfunctioning demonstrate papillary hyperplasia (FA with papillary hyperplasia). FAs with papillary hyperplasia are often cystic and have papillae that are usually non-branching. Collections of follicles may be present within the papillary structures. The papillae are lined by cells that range from cuboidal to columnar. Unlike in hyperfunctioning FA, the cytoplasm is not vacuolated and the associated colloid is not bubbly and lacks peripheral scalloping. It is important that FAs with papillary hyperplasia are not mistaken for PTC. FAs with papillary hyperplasia have round nuclei without pallor, grooves, or pseudoinclusions, i.e. they lack the nuclear features of PTC. Additionally, psammomatous calcifications are absent.

Clear cell FAs have a predominance of clear cells. Clear cell change, which can occur in a range of benign and malignant thyroid tumours {251,647,4023,2142,2147}, occurs secondary to an accumulation of glycogen, lipids, thyroglobulin, or vesicles of apparent mitochondrial derivation {4023,647}. Because clear cell FA is a rare tumour, other tumours with clear cytoplasm should be excluded, including metastatic clear cell renal cell carcinoma, medullary thyroid carcinoma, and parathyroid tumours. It should be noted that thyroglobulin staining can be focal or weak in thyroid tumours with clear cytoplasm {1778}; hence, the combined use of TTF1 and PAX8 may be more helpful diagnostically.

The signet-ring cell pattern of FA has cells with cytoplasmic vacuoles with eccentrically displaced nuclei {647,4024}. The cytoplasmic vacuoles, which have been shown to be similar to follicular lumina, have accumulation of thyroglobulin {4024}. The nuclei are generally uniform and bland. The signet-ring cell pattern of FA should be distinguished from a metastatic adenocarcinoma with signet-ring cell morphology, which can rarely present as a thyroid nodule {4860}.

Mature adipose tissue can be seen in a range of neoplastic and non-neoplastic conditions of the thyroid {1612}. Lipoadenoma (also called adenolipoma or thyrolipoma) may have areas of yellow on cut surface. Histologically, the tumour has variable proportions of mature adipose cells dispersed throughout {4025,1906}. Lipoadenomas have been reported in patients with Cowden syndrome {607,1781} and after exposure to radiation {1612}.

FA with bizarre nuclei is characterized by markedly enlarged and hyperchromatic tumour cells arranged singly or in clusters throughout the tumour. These bizarre nuclei can be considered as endocrine atypia and are not a marker of malignancy. Mitotic activity and tumour necrosis are absent in these tumours.

In the rare spindle cell pattern of FA, the tumour demonstrates extensive spindle cell metaplasia {4689,58}. The spindle cells are bland and have nuclei that range from elongated to more plump with chromatin that may be finely granular or coarse, and with variably distinct nucleoli. Because of the rarity of this tumour, it is essential to rule out the spindle cell subtype of medullary thyroid carcinoma and anaplastic thyroid carcinoma, which rarely may be encapsulated {1116}. To render a diagnosis of the spindle cell pattern of FA, the tumour must have a low mitotic count (< 3 mitoses/2 mm^2) and must lack tumour necrosis. The tumour should be positive for TTF1 and thyroglobulin, negative for calcitonin, and have a Ki-67 proliferation index < 5%.

Black FA can be seen in patients treated with minocycline, as similarly reported in patients with black thyroid {2396}. On cut section the tumour is black. Histologically, brown to black pigment is seen within the colloid and cytoplasm of the follicular cells. Dense osmophilic material present within the lysosomes of the follicular cells can be seen by electron microscopy.

Cytology

Smears are usually highly cellular and show a monotonous population of follicular cells, arranged singly, in cohesive sheets, and as microfollicles, in a bloody background with limited thin colloid. Some cases may show prominent nuclear overlapping and crowding. Nuclei are round with even chromatin, although some larger nuclei, a degree of nuclear pleomorphism, and more prominent single nucleoli may be seen in some cases. FA and FTC cannot be distinguished on FNAB, because the diagnosis of carcinoma is based on the demonstration of capsular and/or vascular invasion. Because nuclear features of non-invasive follicular thyroid neoplasm with papillary-like nuclear features and encapsulated follicular variant of PTC may be subtle, it can be difficult to distinguish these tumours from FA on FNAB, and many will be reported as follicular neoplasm / suspicious for follicular neoplasm.

Diagnostic molecular pathology

Not relevant

Essential and desirable diagnostic criteria

Essential: a non-invasive, encapsulated, follicular-patterned tumour; absence of nuclear features of PTC; architecture and cytomorphology of FA should be distinct from the background thyroid parenchyma.

Staging

Not relevant

Prognosis and prediction

FAs are benign tumours that do not metastasize and do not recur if completely excised.

Follicular thyroid adenoma with papillary architecture

Barletta JA
Asa SL
Erickson LA
Kakudo K
Kondo T
LiVolsi V
Rossi ED
Tallini G

Definition

Follicular thyroid adenoma with papillary architecture is a benign, non-invasive, encapsulated follicular cell–derived neoplasm that is characterized by an intrafollicular papillary architecture, lacks nuclear features of papillary thyroid carcinoma (PTC), and is often associated with autonomous hyperfunction.

ICD-O coding

8330/0 Follicular thyroid adenoma with papillary architecture

ICD-11 coding

2F37.Y & XH0LM0 Other specified benign neoplasm of endocrine glands & Follicular adenoma

Related terminology

Acceptable: hyperfunctioning thyroid adenoma; toxic thyroid adenoma.

Not recommended: papillary thyroid adenoma; papillary hyperplastic thyroid nodule.

Subtype(s)

None

Localization

These neoplasms can occur anywhere in the thyroid gland. They may also arise in ectopic thyroid tissue, including satellite thyroid tissue (i.e. parasitic thyroid nodules) in the perithyroidal soft tissues.

Clinical features

Solitary autonomous hyperfunctioning follicular adenomas with papillary architecture occur predominantly in women and were initially described in young women at the age of menarche {4699}. Most patients have subclinical hyperthyroidism and present with a thyroid mass; however, 15–60% of patients present with symptoms of hyperthyroidism, including cardiac signs and symptoms, nervousness, muscle weakness, heat intolerance, and weight loss {445,1942,4147,3045}. The rate of overt hyperthyroidism increases with the size of the adenoma

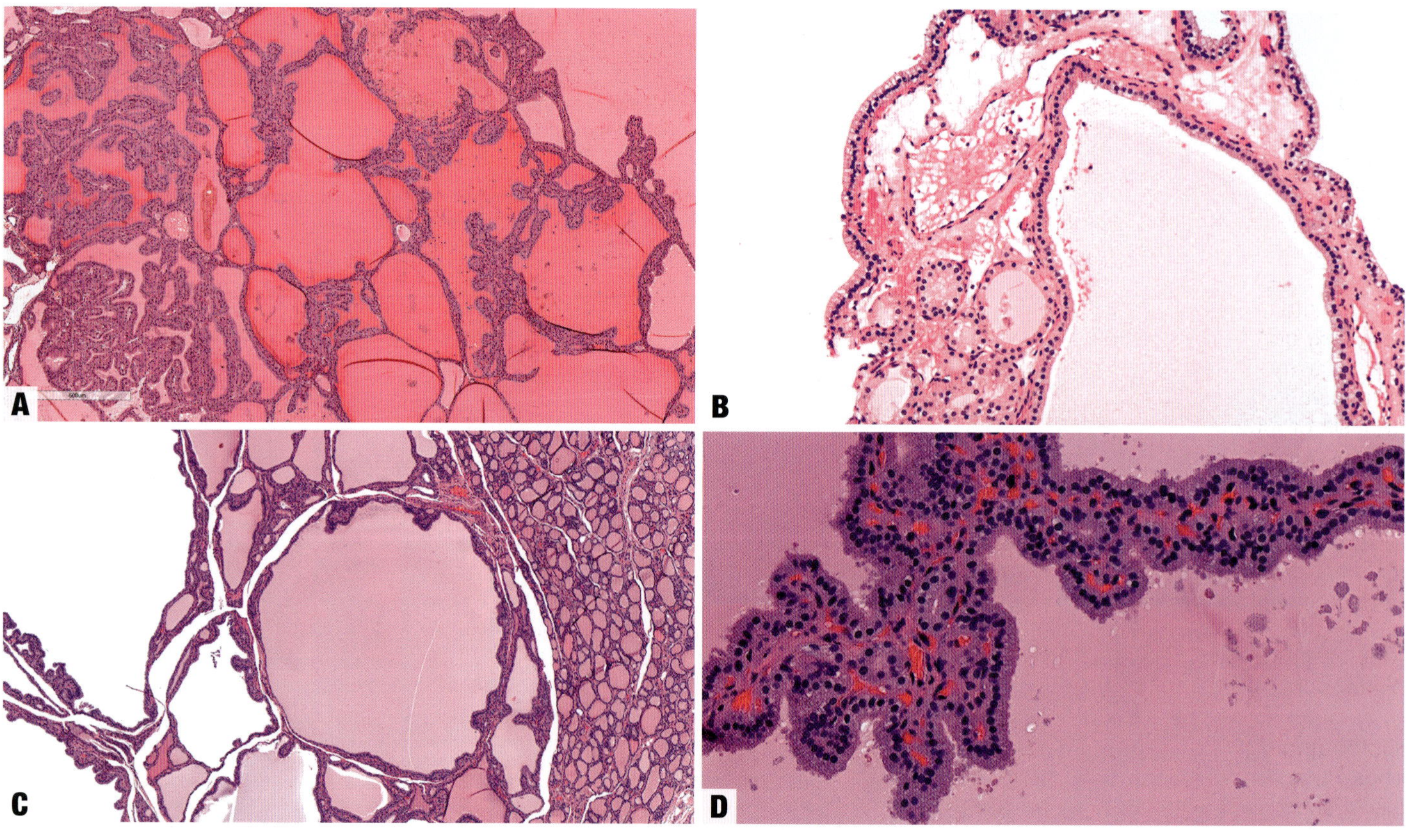

Fig. 3.18 Follicular adenoma with papillary architecture. **A** Low-power view showing large colloid-filled follicles and complex papillary infoldings of the lining epithelium. **B** At high magnification the cells are often columnar. The nuclei are basally located and are small, round, and dark. Nuclear features of papillary thyroid carcinoma are always absent. The oedematous fibrovascular cores show embedded follicles. **C** This example is from a patient with McCune–Albright syndrome. **D** Cytological features. The papillae are lined by follicular epithelial cells that have uniform round basophilic nuclei.

{445,1942,4147,3045} and with iodine deficiency {2756,2544, 658}. Thyroid hormone levels are variably elevated and, therefore, TSH levels are variably suppressed {1942,3045}. On ultrasound they can be solid and isoechoic to hypoechoic with increased vascularity {861}. These neoplasms usually demonstrate increased radioiodide uptake compared with the adjacent gland (they are "hot").

Epidemiology

These neoplasms have been reported to account for approximately 3% of thyroid nodules {3045}. However, it should be acknowledged that the incidence of these tumours is difficult to assess because they are associated with a variable rate of clinical hyperthyroidism that is impacted by the rate of iodine deficiency {658}. Additionally, cases of hyperthyroidism attributed to "toxic nodular hyperplasia" actually represent a clonal hyperfunctioning follicular adenoma arising in multinodular goitre {4519}.

Etiology

The etiology of these lesions is usually unknown. A few have arisen in the setting of thyroid FND (multinodular goitre) {4519} and some occur in patients with McCune–Albright syndrome, Carney complex, and *DICER1* syndrome {1378,4825,670}.

Pathogenesis

These neoplasms are caused by genetic alterations that stimulate thyroid hormone synthesis and secretion as well as follicular cell proliferation. Activating *TSHR* mutations are detected in as many as 70%, whereas *GNAS* mutations are found in a small subset {3448,4566,1655}. These mutations result in the activation of adenylyl cyclase, which leads to increased intracellular cAMP, which, in turn, produces unrestrained stimulation of thyroid follicular cell function and proliferation {3592}. Additionally, almost 30% of these tumours harbour an *EZH1* mutation in combination with a *TSHR* or a *GNAS* mutation {595}. *EZH1* mutations have been shown to result in increased histone H3 trimethylation and increased proliferation of thyroid cells. In patients with McCune–Albright syndrome, germline mosaicism for activating mutations in *GNAS* are implicated {1378,2759}. In Carney complex, germline inactivating mutations in *PRKAR1A* result in constitutive activation of the cAMP/PKA pathway through loss of regulation of the catalytic subunits of PKA {2174}. The pathogenesis of tumours lacking *TSHR*, *GNAS*, or *PRKAR1A* mutations is not established.

Macroscopic appearance

These neoplasms are usually well-delineated thyroid nodules that may have a distinct capsule. The cut surface is usually beefy-red with colloid translucence. There may be foci of haemorrhage and cystic degeneration, especially if the lesion has been biopsied before resection. In McCune–Albright syndrome, the tumours may be multiple.

Histopathology

These tumours have a characteristic morphology. They are usually cystic and show a mixture of follicular and papillary architecture that is neither random nor complex. Instead, the overarching theme is one of large follicles with complex papillary infoldings of the lining epithelium, with broad papillae showing an organized centripetal orientation and oedematous cores with embedded follicles. The formation of Sanderson polsters (subfollicles within follicles) is common. The colloid may appear bubbly and often has peripheral scalloping, consistent with the rapid resorption of colloid for active hormone synthesis. The follicular epithelial cells lining the papillae are crowded. If there is haemorrhage, the epithelial cells usually show a striking accumulation of haemosiderin, reflecting active uptake of colloid. The cells are often columnar and have variably vacuolated cytoplasm; oncocytic metaplasia has been reported in a few cases. The nuclei, which are often basally located, are round and uniform in size and shape. They lack clearing and peripheral margination of chromatin. Intranuclear grooves and pseudoinclusions are not seen. There may be focal nuclear atypia around sites of degeneration, but this is considered to be reactive and should not alter the diagnosis. Psammoma bodies are not seen in these tumours. The presence of nuclear enlargement, clearing, contour irregularities, grooves, pseudoinclusions, or psammoma bodies should prompt a diagnosis of PTC {4699,2115, 618,3636,2709}. These neoplasms generally lack immunoreactivity for HBME1, galectin-3, and BRAF p.V600E (VE1); CK19 can be focally positive, especially in cases that have undergone preoperative biopsy {3905,3,1261,309}.

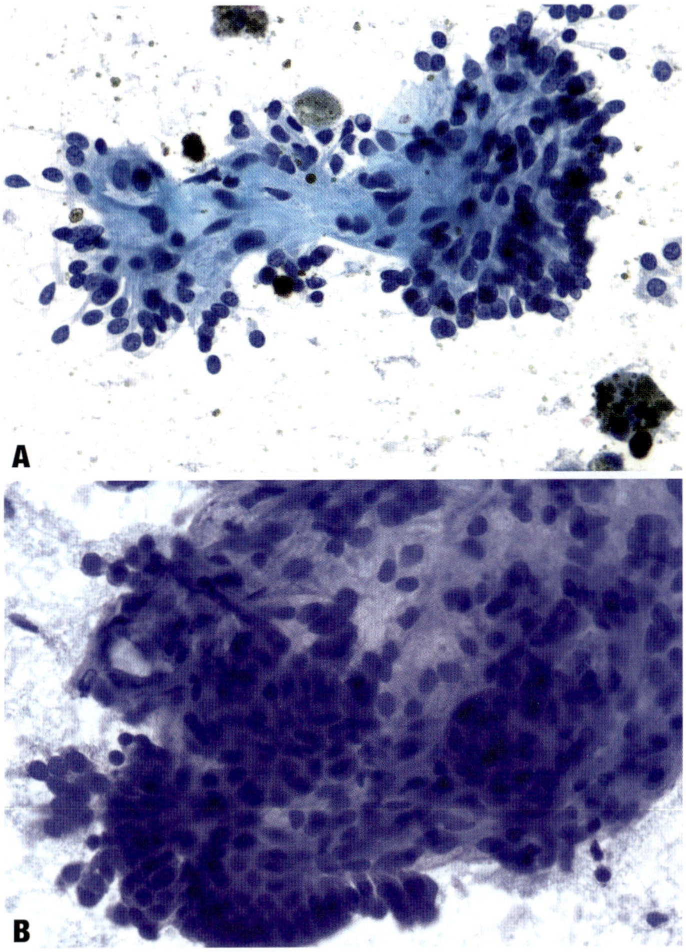

Fig. 3.19 Follicular adenoma with papillary architecture. **A** Pap-stained FNA specimen showing a monotonous population of follicular cells arranged in non-branching papillary groups in a background of thin colloid and macrophages. **B** Giemsa-stained FNA showing a monotonous population of follicular cells arranged in non-branching papillary groups.

Cytology

FNA specimens are usually cellular and show a monotonous population of follicular cells, some with oncocytic change, arranged in non-branching papillary groups in a background of thin colloid and macrophages. The cells usually have readily identifiable prominent nucleoli, especially those with oncocytic change. Rare cases of this neoplasm on FNA can show intranuclear grooves and nuclear chromatin clearing. Because of the papillary architecture and atypical nuclear features, some cases are mistaken for PTC {2272,2115,3636}.

Diagnostic molecular pathology

TSHR, *DICER1*, and *GNAS* mutations can be detected in FNA specimens of these neoplasms diagnosed as atypical or suspicious for PTC. This molecular profile usually triggers investigations to confirm the possibility of a hyperfunctioning nodule {3253,837,2521}.

Essential and desirable diagnostic criteria

Essential: an encapsulated thyroid neoplasm; follicular epithelial cells with an organized intrafollicular papillary architecture, with subfollicle formation; broad papillae with oedematous cores; no nuclear atypia of PTC; no capsular invasion; no psammoma bodies.

Staging

Not applicable

Prognosis and prediction

Like conventional follicular adenomas, these are benign tumours that do not recur once resected.

Oncocytic adenoma of the thyroid gland

Barletta JA
Asa SL
Erickson LA
Ghossein RA
Kakudo K
Kondo T
LiVolsi V
Mete O
Morreau H
Rossi ED
Sadow PM
Tallini G

Definition

Oncocytic adenoma (OA) is a benign, non-invasive, encapsulated, follicular cell–derived neoplasm composed of > 75% oncocytic cells.

ICD-O coding

8290/0 Oncocytic adenoma of the thyroid gland

ICD-11 coding

2F37.Y & XH5SM2 Other specified benign neoplasm of endocrine glands & Follicular adenoma, oxyphilic cell

Related terminology

Not recommended: Hürthle cell adenoma; oxyphilic adenoma; follicular adenoma, oncocytic variant; follicular adenoma, Hürthle cell type.

Subtype(s)

None

Localization

OA can occur anywhere in the thyroid. It has also been reported in ectopic locations, such as in association with thyroglossal duct cysts and arising from thyroid tissue within the mediastinum {4533,1026}.

Clinical features

The median age at diagnosis of OA is 50–55 years {967,1224, 3942,4917,1123}. They are uncommon in children {4237}. OAs usually present as painless, palpable thyroid masses or are incidentally detected on physical examination or imaging studies, although a small subset of large OAs are associated with compressive symptoms. On ultrasound, OAs are typically solitary, well-demarcated, solid, ovoid nodules with smooth borders, variable echogenicity (they may be either isoechoic to hypoechoic, or hyperechoic), and no associated calcifications. The sonographic features of OA and oncocytic carcinoma (OCA) show considerable overlap, so benign and malignant tumours usually cannot be differentiated on ultrasound {3942}. Most patients with OA are biochemically euthyroid. On radionuclide scan, OAs show less radioiodide avidity than the adjacent thyroid parenchyma (they are “cold” nodules). OAs show significantly higher focal FDG uptake than non-oncocytic follicular adenomas and can be mistaken for primary or secondary malignant thyroid tumours {5118,3465}.

Epidemiology

The incidence of OA is difficult to assess, because many studies combine OA with follicular adenoma and there is histological overlap between OA and oncocytic adenomatous nodules. However, OAs have been reported to account for about 10–15% of thyroid nodules with a preceding indeterminate FNA diagnosis {3623,90}. OAs are more frequently diagnosed in women than in men {967,1224,4917}.

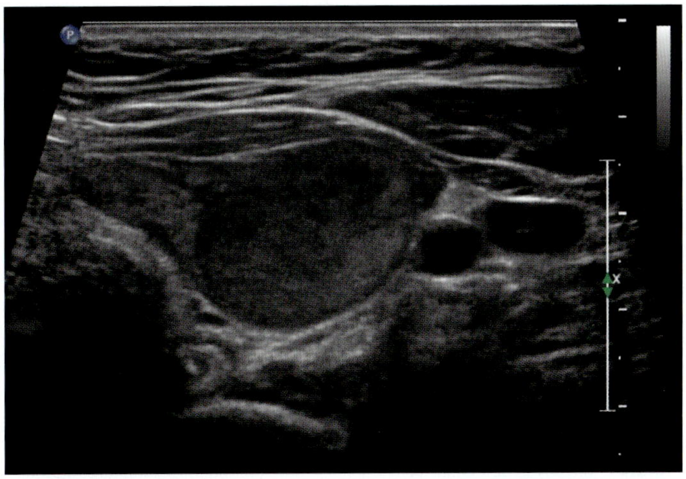

Fig. 3.20 Oncocytic adenoma. An ultrasound image of an oncocytic adenoma showing a well-demarcated, solid, ovoid nodule with smooth borders, variable echogenicity (isoechoic to hypoechoic and hyperechoic), and no associated calcifications.

Etiology

There are no known exogenous risk factors for OA. Rarely, OA can be seen in the context of tumour syndromes, including Cowden syndrome (most frequently associated with a germline *PTEN* mutation) and Carney complex (most frequently associated with a germline *PRKAR1A* mutation). Although most benign neoplasms that occur in these syndromes represent follicular adenomas, OA can be rarely seen {1781,4298}.

Pathogenesis

The genomics of OA is distinct from that of follicular adenoma. OAs are characterized by alterations in the mitochondrial genome; specifically, disruptive mutations in mitochondrial DNA complex I subunit genes {472,1515,1637,1490}. These mitochondrial DNA mutations affect the majority of copies of the mitochondrial genome (near-homoplasmy) and lead to global mitochondrial respiratory dysfunction. OAs also harbour mutations in *NDUFA13* (*GRIM19*), a nuclear gene that contributes to a component of the complex I subunit {2896}. The mitochondrial respiratory dysfunction of OA is thought to underlie the mitochondrial accumulation that characterizes these tumours. Copy-number alterations have been reported in OA; however, the rate has been reported to be lower than in OCA (38% for OA vs 81% for OCA) {1123}. In OCA, near-genome-wide haploidization as a consequence of widespread whole-chromosome loss is often found, with subsequent genome endoreduplication. Allelic state analysis in a small series showed that only a small proportion of OAs showed similar features, and to a far lesser extent. Furthermore, a larger fraction of OAs seem to

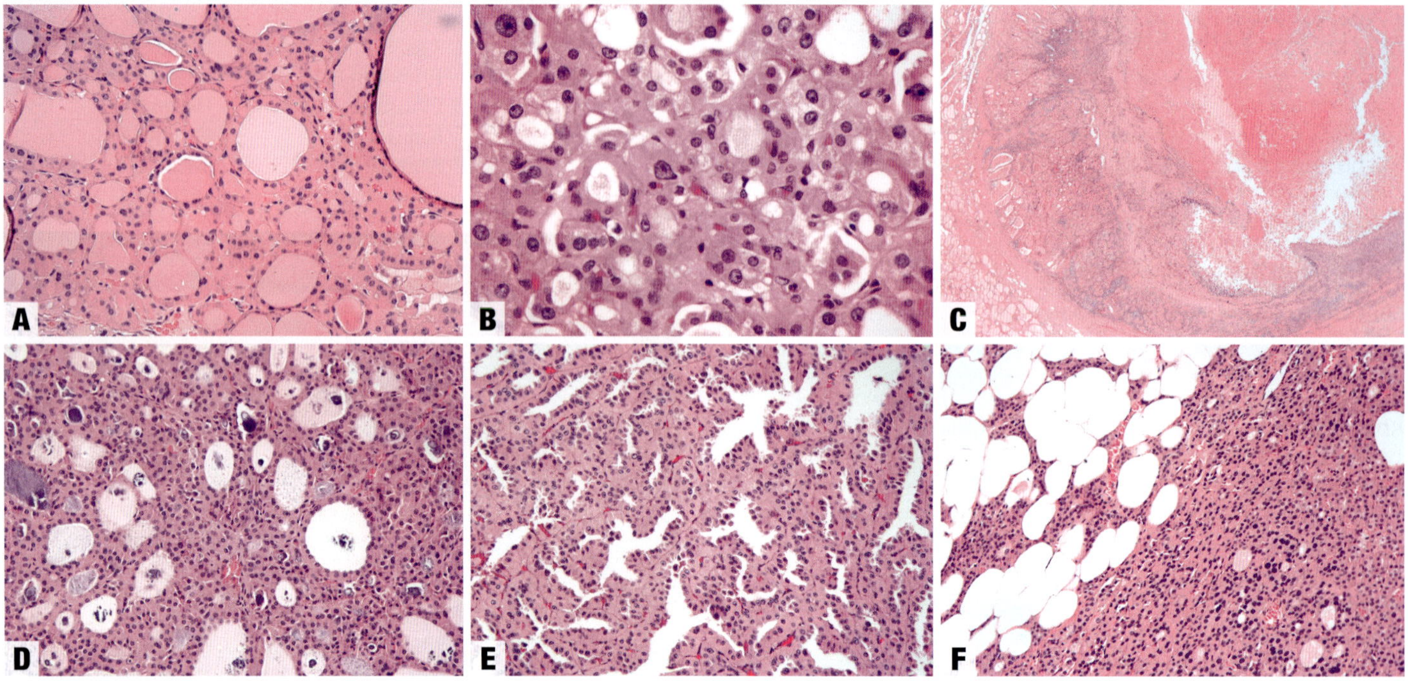

Fig. 3.21 Oncocytic adenoma. **A** The tumour has a follicular architecture, and the cells lining the follicles have bland round uniform nuclei with evenly distributed chromatin; they lack nuclear irregularity including overlap, moulding, grooves, and clearing of nucleoplasm. **B** Tumour cells with abundant eosinophilic cytoplasm and nuclei with prominent nucleoli. Focal nuclear atypia is frequently seen in oncocytic tumours. **C** A low-power photomicrograph of an oncocytic adenoma showing extensive infarction secondary to FNA. **D** An oncocytic adenoma with calcifications. Note that the calcifications are within follicles and are associated with colloid. **E** A minor subset of oncocytic adenomas has areas of papillary architecture. However, in contrast to the oncocytic subtype of papillary thyroid carcinoma, this tumour lacks the nuclear features of papillary thyroid carcinoma. **F** Lipomatous metaplasia.

show whole-chromosome gains as if being the reciprocal mirror of OCA {923}. Interestingly, in oncocytic cell hyperplasia no such abnormalities are seen {3258}. A subset of OAs have RAS and *EIF1AX* mutations (together present in about 10% of tumours). The rate of these mutations is similar to that seen in OCAs, although in contrast to OCAs, in OAs these mutations occur in tumours without copy-number alterations {1123}. *TERT* promoter mutations and *TP53* mutations, found in a subset of OCAs, are very rare in OA {3987,1123}. Additionally, OAs lack the fusions found in follicular adenomas, such as *PAX8*::*PPARG* rearrangements and *THADA*::*IGF2BP3* fusions.

Macroscopic appearance

OAs are usually solitary, round or oval encapsulated nodules, with a mean size of 20–30 mm {1224,3942,4917}. Larger oncocytic nodules have a higher rate of malignancy than smaller nodules {967,1123}. For example, oncocytic tumours measuring > 40 mm have been reported to have double the malignancy rate of those < 40 mm {967}. However, OAs can be well over 40 mm, and therefore size cannot be used to differentiate between OA and OCA {3942}. The cut surface of OA is usually homogeneous and is tan to mahogany brown. Oncocytic neoplasms are prone to haemorrhage and infarction secondary to FNA, and these secondary changes may be grossly apparent.

Histopathology

OAs are encapsulated, follicular-patterned tumours that lack capsular or vascular invasion. The capsule of OA ranges from thin to thick, although it is generally thinner than that of OCA. OA can have a microfollicular, normofollicular, or macrofollicular growth pattern. It can also have solid or trabecular growth, although these growth patterns are more frequent in OCA. OAs comprise > 75% oncocytic cells. Oncocytic cells are characterized by abundant granular eosinophilic cytoplasm, sharp cytoplasmic borders, and round to oval nuclei with an even chromatin pattern and prominent nucleoli. In contrast to other tumours that may have granular eosinophilic cytoplasm (e.g. oncocytic, tall cell, and Warthin-like subtypes of papillary thyroid carcinoma [PTC]), there is a complete loss of cell polarity in OA {4580}. Moreover, at an ultrastructural level, although these PTC subtypes may be rich in mitochondria, the accumulation of mitochondria is less than that seen in OA. The nuclei of OA cells are usually round; however, nuclear contour irregularities and even nuclear grooves (raising the diagnostic consideration of PTC) may be present. However, unlike PTC, which has small, peripherally located nucleoli, OA characteristically has larger, centrally placed nucleoli. OAs often show focal nuclear atypia, with scattered cells with large hyperchromatic nuclei, consistent with endocrine atypia. Mitoses are usually rare (< 3 mitoses/2 mm^2). OAs are prone to infarction induced by prior FNA; however, coagulative tumour necrosis is absent. Necrosis secondary to FNA is usually associated with fibrosis, haemorrhage, granulation tissue formation, and haemosiderin-laden macrophages. FNA can also result in capsular disruption that must be differentiated from true capsular invasion, and it can induce vascular changes that can mimic vascular invasion {290}. Some OAs have calcifications within follicles that are often associated with colloid and should not be confused for psammomatous calcifications found in PTC. The stroma of OA is often scant, but it can be oedematous, myxoid, or hyalinized.

In some cases of OA with extensive hyalinization, the stroma may be calcified and even ossified showing cancellous bone. A lymphocytic infiltrate may be present in OA (usually denser at the periphery) that occurs in a background of Hashimoto thyroiditis. Lipomatous metaplasia can occur in OA.

The histological distinction between OA and an oncocytic hyperplastic nodule is straightforward when the tumour is solitary and has a well-defined capsule; however, the distinction is less clear when there is a background of hyperplastic nodules with adenomatous and oncocytic change. In some cases, histological distinction between a clonal OA and a hyperplastic nodule with oncocytic change is not possible.

The distinction between OA and OCA is based on the histological evaluation of the tumour capsule. Therefore, the capsule should be thoroughly sampled. Serial/deeper sections should be considered to resolve foci of questionable capsular or vascular invasion. If deeper levels do not allow for the definitive classification of a tumour as OA or OCA, a diagnosis of oncocytic tumour of uncertain malignant potential can be rendered (see *Thyroid tumours of uncertain malignant potential*, p. 135). However, this category should be used sparingly.

A subset of OAs have a papillary architecture that may be focal or extensive. In contrast to PTCs, these tumours lack nuclear clearing, peripheral margination of chromatin, and pseudoinclusions (although nuclear contour irregularities may be present). Additionally, psammomatous calcifications are absent. For oncocytic tumours with a papillary architecture, malignancy is based on the same criteria as are used for conventional oncocytic neoplasms.

Non-invasive, encapsulated, follicular cell–derived neoplasms composed of < 75% oncocytic cells are considered follicular adenomas with oncocytic features {4392,1492}.

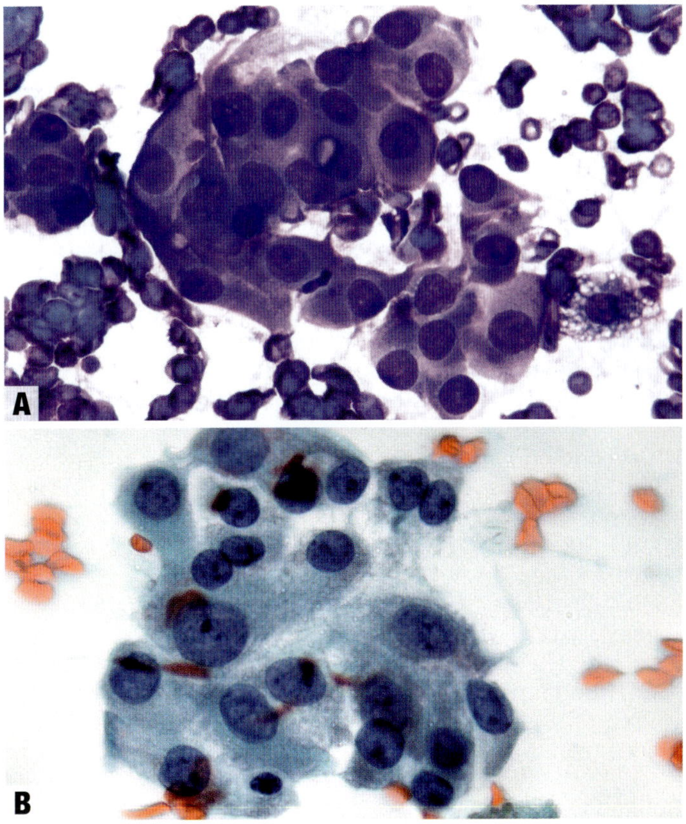

Fig. 3.22 Oncocytic adenoma. A Giemsa-stained FNA specimen (**A**) and a Pap-stained FNA specimen (**B**) showing a cluster of cells exhibiting abundant coarsely granular cytoplasm and uniform central round nuclei with prominent single nucleoli. Intracytoplasmic lumina can be seen.

Immunophenotype

OAs have an immunohistochemical profile similar to that of other differentiated thyroid tumours. They are positive for PAX8 and thyroid transcription factor 1 (TTF1) and negative for calcitonin {4895,370,2546}. The cytoplasm and associated colloid of OA is positive for thyroglobulin {370}. There are no immunohistochemical stains that reliably distinguish OA from OCA.

Cytology

Smears are moderately cellular and show oncocytic cells as sheets, as tissue fragments of nested oncocytic cells separated by transgressing vessels, and as single cells. The oncocytic cells constitute more than 90% of epithelial cells, in distinction to the common finding of focal metaplastic, oncocytic change frequently associated with cystic degeneration in follicular nodules. Thin colloid is usually absent, chronic inflammatory cells are scant, and intracytoplasmic lumina can be seen. The cells have abundant coarsely granular cytoplasm and uniform central round nuclei with prominent single nucleoli {1224}. Although cytopathological features favouring OCA over OA (and other benign conditions with oncocytic metaplasia) have been reported, including small cell dysplasia, large cell dysplasia, nuclear crowding, and prominent cellular dyscohesion {4946}, ultimately OA and OCA have overlapping features and cannot be definitively distinguished on FNAB, because the distinction is based on capsular and vascular invasion, similar to the problematic distinction between follicular adenoma and follicular carcinoma. Diagnostic pitfalls for OA include oncocytic, Warthin-like, and tall cell subtypes of PTC, which also have cells with abundant granular cytoplasm and a variable number of nuclear pseudoinclusions and grooves {37}, as well as the oncocytic subtype of medullary thyroid carcinoma {3927} and autonomously functioning follicular adenomas {2521}.

Diagnostic molecular pathology

Oncocytic neoplasms (adenoma and carcinoma) have a low prevalence of mutations in genes that are commonly altered in non-oncocytic thyroid tumours {1637,1490}. Therefore, a negative result obtained from molecular analysis performed on preoperative cytology samples should not influence the decision for thyroid surgery, especially when limited molecular panels {375} are employed.

Essential and desirable diagnostic criteria

Essential: a non-invasive, encapsulated tumour; > 75% oncocytic cells.

Staging

Not relevant

Prognosis and prediction

OAs are benign tumours that do not recur if completely excised.

Non-invasive follicular thyroid neoplasm with papillary-like nuclear features

Ghossein RA
Bongiovanni M
Jung CK
Kakudo K
Katoh R
Sadow PM

Definition

Non-invasive follicular thyroid neoplasm with papillary-like nuclear features (NIFTP) is a non-invasive, encapsulated/well-demarcated follicular cell–derived tumour with a follicular growth pattern and nuclei resembling those of papillary thyroid carcinoma (PTC), with an extremely low malignant potential.

ICD-O coding

8349/1 Non-invasive follicular thyroid neoplasm with papillary-like nuclear features
8349/1 Subcentimetre non-invasive follicular thyroid neoplasm with papillary-like nuclear features
8349/1 Oncocytic non-invasive follicular thyroid neoplasm with papillary-like nuclear features

ICD-11 coding

2F9A & XA8RK3 Neoplasms of unknown behaviour of endocrine glands & Thyroid gland

Related terminology

Not recommended: non-invasive follicular variant of papillary thyroid carcinoma.

Subtype(s)

Subcentimetre NIFTP (< 10 mm); oncocytic NIFTP (≥ 75% oncocytic cells)

Localization

Thyroid lobe or isthmus

Clinical features

Patients usually present with an asymptomatic nodule detected during routine physical examination or by imaging. By ultrasonography, NIFTP typically appears as a solid, mildly hypoechoic or isoechoic mass, round to ovoid in shape, with smooth borders and lacking calcifications {2473}.

Epidemiology

The incidence of NIFTP varies between different regions of the world. Tumours currently classified as NIFTP were formerly classified as non-invasive encapsulated follicular variant of PTC (FVPTC). Among retrospectively reviewed PTCs, the prevalence of cases reclassified as NIFTP or previously labelled as non-invasive encapsulated FVPTC is much lower in Asia (0.5–5%) than in countries with populations largely of European descent (15–20%), especially North America {3814,4471,2582,585}. There are also significant variations between different institutions within the same geographical location {3388}. Most of these discrepancies are related to different thresholds used to diagnose the nuclear features of papillary carcinoma and NIFTP {3814,4395,585,3388}. There is a female preponderance (M:F ratio: ~1:5) {3255,3818,3388}. NIFTP can occur at any age, including in childhood {4780,3388}. In most series, the mean and median age at diagnosis fall within the fifth decade of life {3255,3818,3737,3388}.

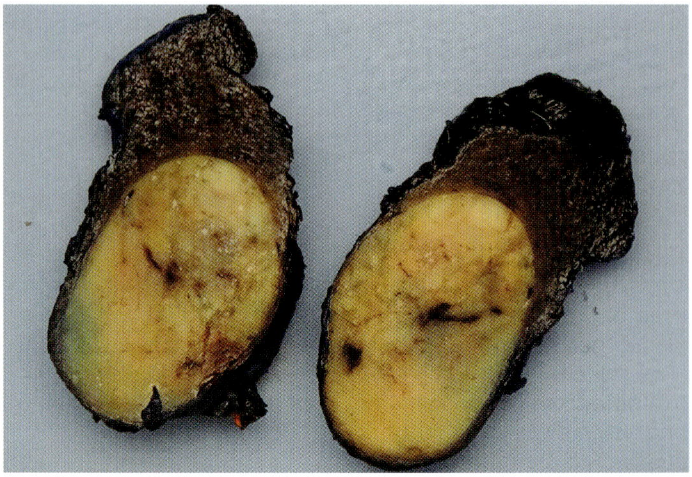

Fig. 3.23 Non-invasive follicular thyroid neoplasm with papillary-like nuclear features. Grossly, the tumour is well demarcated, with smooth borders, a homogeneous yellow-tan cut surface, and focal areas of haemorrhage.

Etiology

There are no known etiological factors in NIFTP.

Pathogenesis

RAS-like molecular alterations promote the development of NIFTP {622}. RAS mutations are the main drivers of NIFTP, occurring in 52% of cases, with most located in *NRAS* {3255,5155,517,4976}. Rearrangements of *PPARG* and *THADA*, as well as *EIF1AX* mutations, have also been reported but at a lower frequency (6–17%) {3255,5155,517,4976}. *BRAF* p.V600E is now considered an exclusion criterion for NIFTP {4982}; however, *BRAF* mutations other than p.V600E, such as p.K601E, have been detected in 4% of these tumours {3255,517,4976}. In rare instances, RAS mutations have been found to coexist with *TP53* and *PTEN* mutations {517}.

Macroscopic appearance

NIFTP is a well-delineated or encapsulated solid nodule that usually looks white/tan to brown on cross-section {2137}. When present, the capsule is usually thin. If necrosis and haemorrhage are found, they are almost always due to a previous FNA procedure. There is a wide variation in the reported size, with tumours ranging from < 10 mm to 100 mm, with an average of approximately 30 mm {4052,3388}. Because most NIFTP studies have excluded subcentimetre tumours, most publications do not reflect the accurate average dimension of this tumour type. In the rare series that include subcentimetre NIFTP, the median size is 17 mm {3388}.

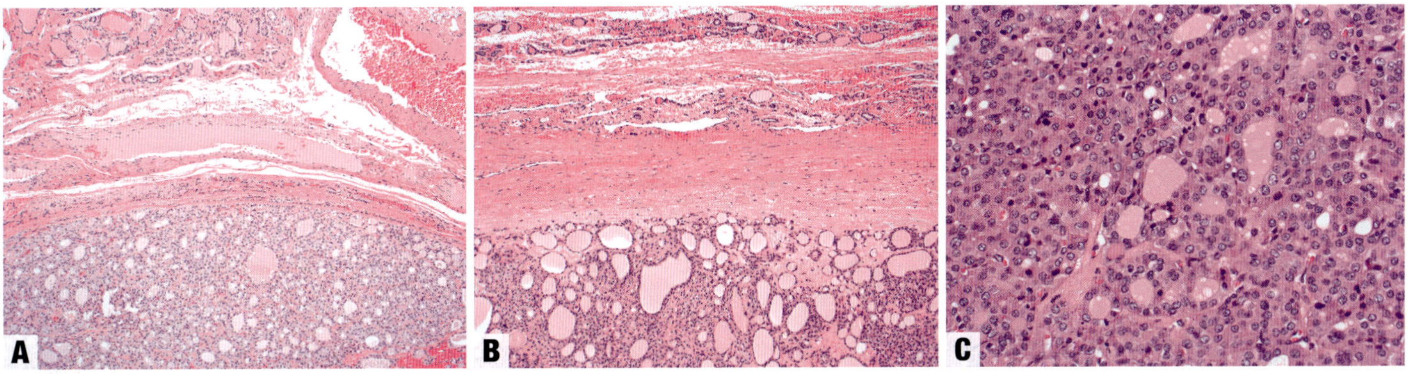

Fig. 3.24 Non-invasive follicular thyroid neoplasm with papillary-like nuclear features. The capsule can be thin (**A**) or thick (**B**), and the neoplasm shows a predominantly follicular growth pattern. **C** This tumour has a diffuse distribution of papillary carcinoma–like nuclei, and the neoplastic cell cytoplasm is oncocytic (oncocytic non-invasive follicular thyroid neoplasm with papillary-like nuclear features).

Histopathology

In order to qualify as NIFTP, a tumour must be totally encapsulated or completely demarcated from the surrounding non-neoplastic parenchyma. Because NIFTP is by definition non-invasive, the entire periphery of the lesion should be submitted for microscopic examination to rule out infiltration, capsular invasion, and vascular invasion. A third requisite is the presence of nuclear atypia. The nuclear atypia is usually not very pronounced and often multifocal, and therefore difficult to assess. A scoring system composed of a set of three nuclear features can assist in that endeavour. These categories are size and shape (nuclear enlargement/elongation/overlapping/crowding), nuclear membrane irregularities (including grooves and pseudoinclusions), and chromatin characteristics (clearing) {3255,4052}. For each category of nuclear features, a tumour is assigned a score of 0 or 1, such that a neoplasm's total score can range from 0 to 3 {3255,4052,4487}. A score of 2–3 is necessary for the diagnosis of NIFTP {3255}. Although the presence of diffuse well-developed PTC nuclear features does not preclude a diagnosis of NIFTP, these lesions need to be entirely examined histologically. This is essential because diffuse overt nuclear PTC features increase the probability of the lesion being classic PTC with a predominantly follicular pattern {1990,4052}. The presence of a predominantly follicular growth pattern is the fourth mandatory element. The follicles can vary in size (microfollicular, normofollicular, and macrofollicular) and colloid content. A minor solid growth pattern (< 30% of the tumour) is allowed. Although abortive (short, rudimentary) papillary formations or hyperplastic Sanderson polster foci can be seen {3255,4052}, true papillae (with a fibrovascular core and lined by cells with score 2–3 nuclei) should be very rare or absent altogether (< 1% of the lesion). There is a debate regarding the proportion of true papillae allowed. Because three studies have reported a small rate of metastasis in cases with < 1% papillae {829,2295,3429}, several authors have proposed that a complete absence of true papillae is a requirement for the diagnosis of NIFTP {3252}. Subsequent series assessing the proportion of papillae in 235 encapsulated tumours with PTC nuclei found no metastasis in all non-invasive tumours with < 10% papillae, including 120 tumours fulfilling the original NIFTP criteria (< 1% true papillae) {4982}. Because the vast majority of studies using < 1% papillae as a cut-off point did not report adverse oncological events {3255,4471,3818,4984,4969,4980,4982,1403}, the original threshold permitting < 1% true papillae remains valid {4982}. In addition to a papillary architecture, any of the following findings are exclusion criteria for NIFTP: psammoma bodies, a mitotic count of ≥ 3 mitoses/2 mm^2, tumour necrosis, and cytological and architectural features characteristic of other PTC subtypes {3255,4052}. For example, the presence of even a small number of tall or columnar cells is sufficient to exclude a lesion from the NIFTP category {4052}. The presence of a *BRAF* p.V600E mutation (which is usually associated with other exclusion criteria such as papillae, psammoma bodies, or tall cells when complete histological examination of the entire tumour is performed) is now also considered an exclusion

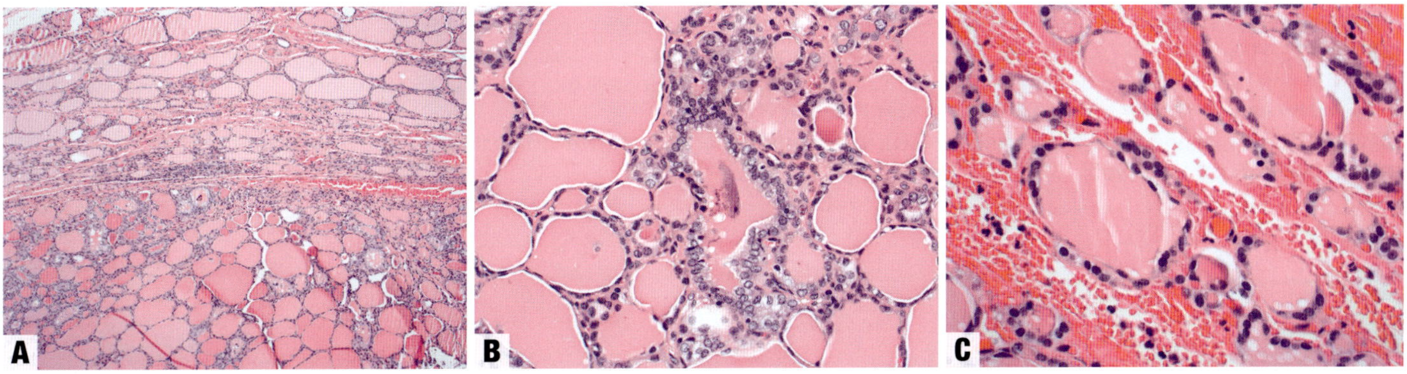

Fig. 3.25 Non-invasive follicular thyroid neoplasm with papillary-like nuclear features. **A** The tumour lacks a capsule but is well demarcated from adjacent non-neoplastic thyroid. The neoplasm shows a predominantly follicular growth pattern. **B** This tumour shows follicles with papillary carcinoma–like nuclei intermixed with follicles lined by normal-appearing follicular cells. **C** Normal follicles lined by cells with small round normochromatic nuclei are adjacent to a non-invasive follicular thyroid neoplasm with papillary-like nuclear features and are used as a reference.

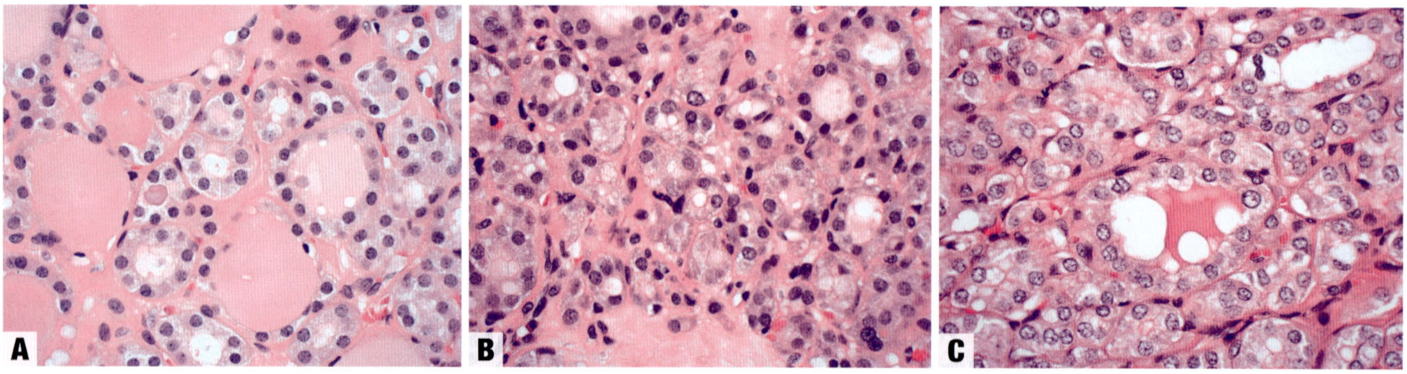

Fig. 3.26 Non-invasive follicular thyroid neoplasm with papillary-like nuclear features (NIFTP). **A** Nuclear score of 1. The cells in this field are enlarged as compared with normal thyroid but lack significant nuclear irregularity and chromatin clearing. These features are insufficient for a diagnosis of NIFTP. **B** Nuclear score of 2. The cells of this NIFTP have enlarged nuclei (as compared with normal thyroid) and irregular nuclear membranes but no substantial chromatin clearing. These features meet the criteria for NIFTP. **C** Nuclear score of 3. The cells in this example have enlarged nuclei (as compared with normal thyroid), irregular nuclear membranes, and chromatin clearing. These features meet the criteria for NIFTP.

criterion for NIFTP {4052,3252,4982}. NIFTP can have cells with oncocytic cytoplasm (oncocytic NIFTP) {4980} and measure < 10 mm (subcentimetre NIFTP) {4471,4969,4393}. Although NIFTP can be very small, the diagnosis is almost unattainable in tumours measuring < 2 mm and difficult in those < 5 mm if a capsule is not present.

Differential diagnosis

NIFTP is differentiated from invasive FVPTC by its lack of invasion, from classic follicular predominant PTC by its very scant papillary component (< 1% papillae), and from other PTCs by the absence of the cytoarchitectural features of these subtypes (e.g. tall cells). Those rare non-invasive follicular-patterned tumours with PTC nuclei that are excluded from NIFTP because of a mitotic count of ≥ 3 mitoses/2 mm^2 are best reported as mitotically active encapsulated PTC with a predominant follicular growth pattern, and if the mitotic count is ≥ 5 mitoses/2 mm^2 or if there is tumour necrosis they should be reported as non-invasive encapsulated FVPTC with high-grade features {4968}. Follicular adenomas are separated from NIFTP by the lack of PTC nuclear alterations (PTC nuclear score: 0–1).

Cytology

Smears are composed predominantly of microfollicles consisting of crowded cells with enlarged, pale, irregular nuclei with grooves {439,3827}. Nuclear pseudoinclusions are rarely observed, and papillae and psammoma bodies are absent {439,3827}. Histologically proven NIFTP cases are diagnosed predominantly as atypia of undetermined significance (30%), followed by suspicious for malignancy (24%) and follicular neoplasm (21%). A malignant diagnosis, usually PTC, is rendered in a minority (8%) of cases {465}.

Diagnostic molecular pathology

BRAF p.V600E mutation detected by immunostaining or genotyping excludes the diagnosis.

Essential and desirable diagnostic criteria

Essential:

- Encapsulation or clear demarcation
- Follicular growth pattern with all of the following: < 1% true papillae, no psammoma bodies, and < 30% solid/trabecular/insular growth pattern
- Nuclear features of papillary carcinoma (nuclear score of 2–3)
- No vascular or capsular invasion
- No tumour necrosis
- Low mitotic count (< 3 mitoses/2 mm^2)
- Lack of cytoarchitectural features of papillary carcinoma subtypes other than the follicular subtype (tall cell features, solid, etc.)

Desirable: immunohistochemistry or molecular testing for *BRAF* and *NRAS* mutation (in selected cases).

Staging

Staging is not performed for NIFTP {1551}.

Prognosis and prediction

NIFTPs, including the oncocytic and subcentimetre forms, are extremely indolent neoplasms provided they are completely resected. A compilation of studies including > 1500 NIFTP cases reveals a rate of adverse oncological events < 1% and no reported mortality {1895,4969,4980,3817}. Inadequate resection can lead to tumour recurrence {4717}. Lobectomy without radioactive iodine therapy is the treatment of choice.

Thyroid tumours of uncertain malignant potential

Tallini G
Bongiovanni M
Jung CK
Katoh R
LiVolsi V

Chapter 3

Definition

Thyroid tumours of uncertain malignant potential (UMP tumours) are well-differentiated thyroid tumours with follicular architecture that are encapsulated or unencapsulated but well circumscribed, in which invasion remains questionable after thorough sampling and exhaustive examination.

ICD-O coding

8335/1 Follicular tumour of uncertain malignant potential

8348/1 Well-differentiated tumour of uncertain malignant potential

ICD-11 coding

2F9A & XA8RK3 Neoplasms of unknown behaviour of endocrine glands & Thyroid gland

Related terminology

Not recommended: atypical adenoma.

Subtype(s)

Follicular tumour of uncertain malignant potential (FT-UMP); well-differentiated tumour of uncertain malignant potential (WDT-UMP)

Localization

UMP tumours occur in the thyroid gland, although they may arise at any site where thyroid parenchyma may be present {331,3645}.

Clinical features

Like patients with follicular adenoma or non-invasive follicular thyroid neoplasm with papillary-like nuclear features, patients with an UMP tumour usually present with single, oval, solid, slightly hypoechoic or isoechoic nodules with a hypoechoic halo by ultrasound that are typically cold by scintigraphy {331}.

Epidemiology

The prevalence is 0.5–3% of all thyroidectomies in institutions where UMP terminology is used in routine diagnostic practice {1925,331}. The mean age at diagnosis is 50–55 years, but the age range is wide {1925,331}. Female patients predominate (M:F ratio: 1:2–3) {1925,331}. The proportions of cases diagnosed as FT-UMP and WDT-UMP are similar {1925,1164}.

Etiology

None

Pathogenesis

RAS-like molecular alterations promote the development of UMP tumours {622}. *EIF1AX* and *TSHR* mutations, as well as *PAX8::PPARG* rearrangement, have been reported in a minority of cases {1925,1164,5132}.

Table 3.02 Terminology for well-differentiated encapsulated follicular-patterned tumours, taking into account alterations of nuclear morphology and tumour invasion

PTC-type nuclear alterations	Invasion[a]		
	Present	**Questionable**	**Absent**
Present	IEFVPTC	WDT-UMP	NIFTP
Questionable	WDC-NOS	WDT-UMP	NIFTP
Absent	FTC	FT-UMP	FA

FA, follicular adenoma; FTC, follicular thyroid carcinoma; FT-UMP, follicular tumour of uncertain malignant potential; IEFVPTC, invasive encapsulated follicular variant of papillary thyroid carcinoma; NIFTP, non-invasive follicular neoplasm with papillary-like nuclear features; PTC, papillary thyroid carcinoma; WDC-NOS, well-differentiated carcinoma not otherwise specified; WDT-UMP, well-differentiated tumour of uncertain malignant potential.

[a]Invasion into vessels or through the tumour capsule (or into the thyroid parenchyma for well-circumscribed unencapsulated tumours).

Macroscopic appearance

The size is variable, with a mean of 20–30 mm and a few cases reaching ≥ 50 mm {1925,331,1164,942}. FT-UMPs tend to be larger than WDT-UMPs {3472,1164}.

Histopathology

General features are the same as those of other encapsulated well-differentiated follicular-patterned neoplasms such as follicular adenoma, follicular carcinoma, or encapsulated follicular variant papillary carcinoma. When the nodule is large its interface with the surrounding tissues should be examined particularly carefully. There are two histological subtypes of thyroid UMP tumours: FT-UMP, in which tumour cells have regular, round nuclei that lack the nuclear features of papillary thyroid carcinoma (nuclear score: 0–1 {3255}); and WDT-UMP, in which tumour cell nuclei have papillary thyroid carcinoma–type nuclear alterations (nuclear score: 2–3 {3255}). For the latter, if invasion has been thoroughly excluded, the term "non-invasive follicular thyroid neoplasm with papillary-like nuclear features" should now be used (see *Non-invasive follicular thyroid neoplasm with papillary-like nuclear features*, p. 132, and Table 3.02). Some tumours are oncocytic {1925,1164,942}, others may display unusual features such as clear cells {2142} or a glomeruloid architecture {586}. If there is high mitotic activity or tumour necrosis, the tumour should be diagnosed as high-grade encapsulated follicular cell–derived carcinoma with questionable vascular invasion. The term "UMP" should not be used for cases in which the question of invasion remains unresolved because of incomplete resection of a thyroid tumour or inadequate sampling. Pseudoinvasive artefacts such as those induced by FNA or surgical manipulation must be distinguished from true invasion {3815}.

The tumour capsule is usually well defined and thicker in FT-UMP, and it tends to be thinner and sometimes incomplete or

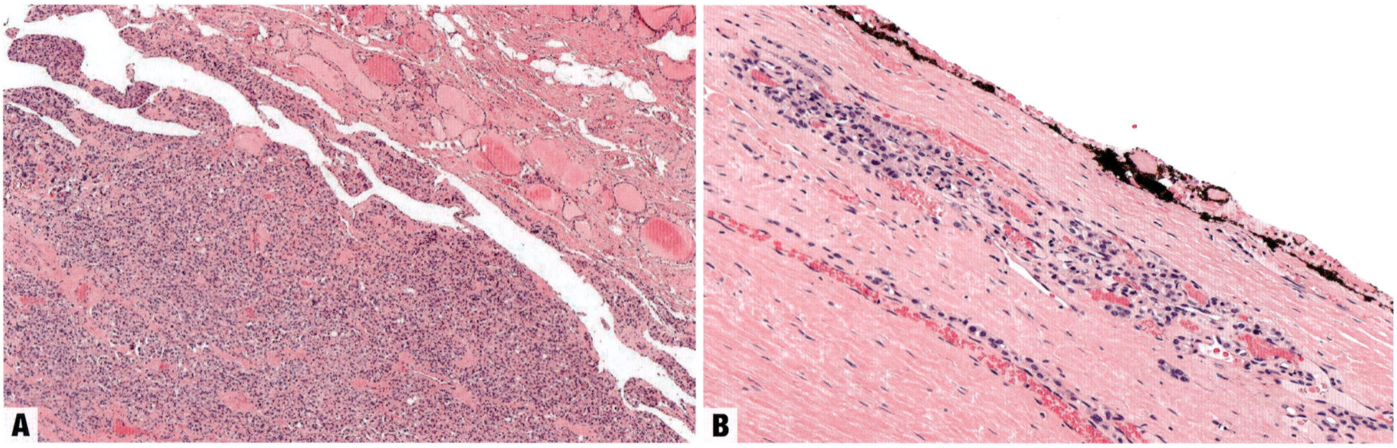

Fig. 3.27 Questionable vascular invasion in a follicular tumour of uncertain malignant potential. **A** Sharply outlined collections of tumour cells covered by endothelium protrude and float into vascular spaces at the parenchymal interface of a well-circumscribed nodule that has a thin, poorly defined capsule. It is difficult to be sure whether intravascular tumour nests belong to the inside of the nodule and are therefore not to be regarded as evidence of vascular invasion, or whether the tumour nests are within the capsule and are therefore diagnostic of vascular invasion. The tumour cells lack the nuclear alterations of papillary carcinoma. **B** Irregular outgrowths of tumour cells undermining the endothelium of small blood vessel cells within a thick fibrous capsule: the close intertwining of vascular spaces and tumour cells raises concern for early vascular invasion. The tumour cells lack the nuclear alterations of papillary carcinoma.

absent in WDT-UMP {1925}. Invasion is questionable when there are broad protrusions of neoplastic cells deep into the capsule casting doubt as to the completeness of its penetration, such as tumour mushrooms abutting the outer surface of the capsule. In some well-circumscribed nodules, particularly in those where the capsule is thin or incomplete, irregularities of the contour of the nodule with outpouching of tumour cells may be inconsistently regarded as a sign of invasion.

The possibility of vascular invasion is more worrisome than that of capsular invasion, because of the higher associated risk of tumour dissemination. Cases with doubtful (or certain) capsular invasion upon close scrutiny may represent doubtful (or certain) vascular invasion. Intertwining of vascular spaces and tumour cells raises concern for early vascular invasion. Tumour cell nests may undermine vascular endothelium in the tumour capsule, and the variable protrusion of the nests within vessels can be variably interpreted as evidence for vascular invasion. Vascular invasion is questionable in the case of intraluminal tumour cell nests with a regular contour that have neither endothelial lining nor definite evidence of associated thrombus. In well-circumscribed nodules (particularly in those with an incomplete or thin fibrous capsule), it can be impossible to define whether intravascular tumour nests belong to the inside of the tumour and are therefore not to be regarded as evidence of vascular invasion, or whether the tumour nests are within the tumour capsule and are therefore diagnostic of vascular invasion.

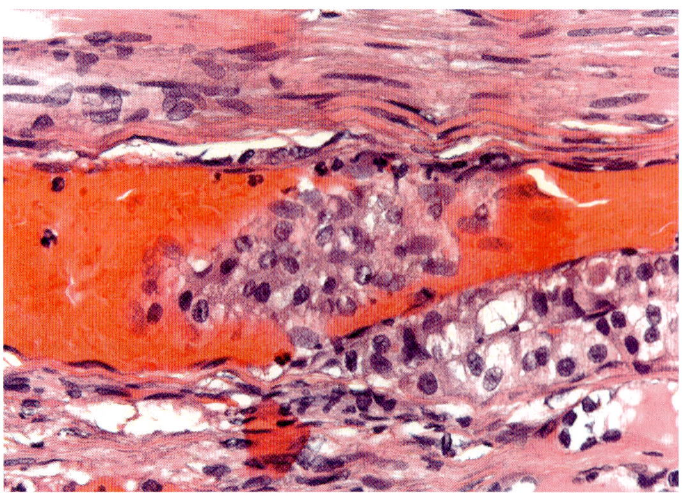

Fig. 3.28 Questionable vascular invasion in a well-differentiated tumour of uncertain malignant potential. An intraluminal tumour cell nest, showing neither an endothelial lining nor definite evidence of an associated thrombus, loosely attached to the wall of a vessel within the tumour capsule. The neoplastic cells show some of the nuclear alterations of papillary carcinoma: chromatin clearing and occasional nuclear grooves.

Cytology

FT-UMP has the same cytological features as follicular adenoma or carcinoma, whereas WDT-UMP exhibits enlarged, clear nuclei and few nuclear grooves, but no pseudoinclusions. Most cases belong to the follicular neoplasm and atypia of undetermined significance categories (IV and III of the Bethesda system) {1925,3264,331}.

Diagnostic molecular pathology

HRAS, *KRAS*, or *NRAS* mutations are identified in as many as 30–40% of cases, *NRAS* p.Q61R being the most common. If *BRAF* p.V600E mutation is present, the diagnosis of NIFTP is excluded. If *TP53* or *TERT* promoter mutations are detected, the tumour should be meticulously examined to rule out carcinoma {3472,1164,2009,942,5132}.

Essential and desirable diagnostic criteria

Essential: questionable invasion; the feature of concern (i.e. invasion of vessels and/or of the tumour capsule) must be specified; no high-grade morphology.

Desirable: molecular investigation for *HRAS*, *KRAS*, or *NRAS* mutations; *BRAF* p.V600E, *TP53*, or *TERT* promoter mutations in selected cases.

Staging

Not applicable

Prognosis and prediction

Most series have not reported nodal or distant metastases, tumour recurrence, or tumour-related deaths {3546,4202, 2702,331,1164}. The risk of recurrence or metastases is extremely low for encapsulated follicular-patterned tumours where invasion of the tumour capsule is the only concern {4650,4479,2686,4874,3546,4202,2161,1493}. In retrospective studies of cases that metastasized after an initial benign diagnosis, some have been reclassified as UMP tumours. In one series of 2978 cases originally diagnosed as benign thyroid nodule/tumour, 5 were found to later develop distant metastases: among these, 2 would qualify as FT-UMP (1 with questionable vascular invasion and 1 with questionable invasion of the thyroid parenchyma) {2161}. In another series of 10 992 consecutive patients with differentiated thyroid cancer, slide review in 26 of the 39 cases with distant metastases after an initial benign diagnosis reclassified 10 cases as FT-UMP and 5 cases as WDT-UMP {3645}.

Hyalinizing trabecular tumour

Volante M
Asa SL
Bongiovanni M
Erickson LA
Tallini G

Definition

Hyalinizing trabecular tumour (HTT) is a follicular cell–derived neoplasm composed of large trabeculae of elongated/polygonal cells with hyaline cytoplasm admixed with intratrabecular hyaline material and with nuclear features characterized by prominent grooves, vacuoles, and membrane irregularities.

ICD-O coding

8336/1 Hyalinizing trabecular tumour

ICD-11 coding

2F9A & XH1Y66 Neoplasms of unknown behaviour of endocrine glands & Hyalinizing trabecular tumour

Related terminology

Acceptable: hyalinizing trabecular neoplasm; hyalinizing trabecular adenoma.

Not recommended: paraganglioma-like adenoma of thyroid.

Subtype(s)

None

Localization

HTT occurs anywhere in the thyroid, with a slight predilection for the right lobe {668}. No ectopic locations are described.

Clinical features

HTT is found incidentally by ultrasonography in asymptomatic patients or during clinical examination. It may be solitary or associated with other thyroid pathologies. At ultrasonography HTT is hypoechoic and solid, with peripheral or poor vascularity {2086}. Microcalcifications are usually absent. HTT cannot be reliably diagnosed by ultrasound alone, and a clinical suspicion of malignancy is rendered in a variable percentage of cases {2580,834}. HTT is cold on a radioactive scan {668} and may be positive with 99mTc sestamibi (MIBI) {349}.

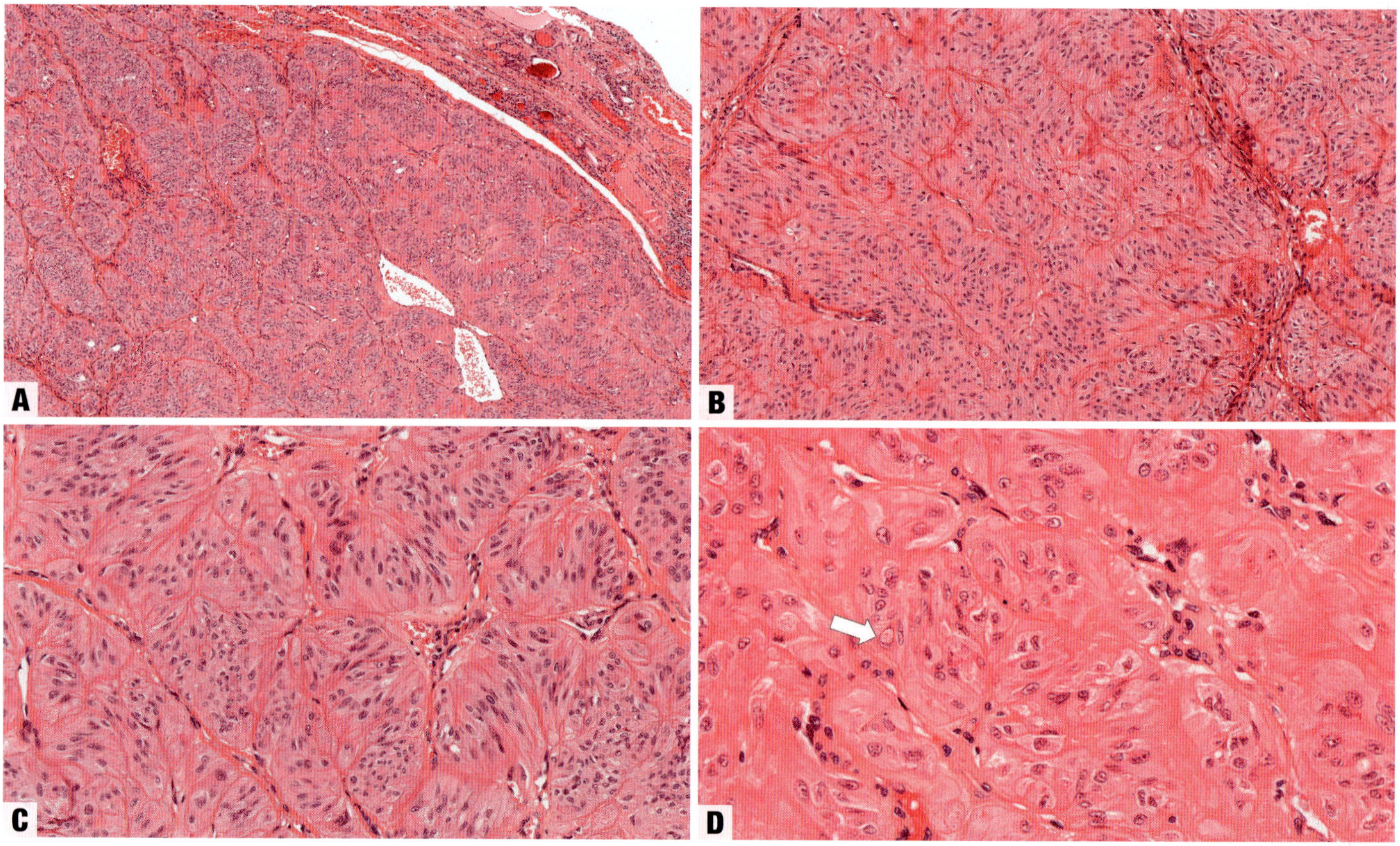

Fig. 3.29 Hyalinizing trabecular tumour with metachronous lymph node metastases. **A** A circumscribed but unencapsulated neoplasm composed of nests and cords of elongated cells with hyaline cytoplasm and prominent eosinophilic hyaline amorphous material in the stroma. **B** Large polygonal or elongated tumour cells have abundant eosinophilic cytoplasm. **C** The tumour cells have abundant hyaline cytoplasm and bizarre convoluted nuclei. **D** The tumour cell nuclei are convoluted with prominent membrane irregularities that form grooves and pseudoinclusions (arrow).

Epidemiology

HTT represents < 1% of thyroid neoplasms. It has a strong female predominance (> 80% of cases) and a mean age of 50 years (range: 21–79 years) {668}.

Etiology

The etiology and risk factors are unknown; previous radiation exposure has been reported {668}.

Pathogenesis

HTT is characterized by the presence of GLIS rearrangements (*PAX8::GLIS1* and *PAX8::GLIS3*, the latter being the most frequent) detected in virtually all cases analysed and not in other thyroid tumours, when stringent diagnostic criteria are applied {3260,2842}. The *GLIS1* and *GLIS3*-encoded proteins are activators of transcription belonging to the Krüppel-like zinc finger family {3566}. The oncogenic activity of the *PAX8::GLIS3* fusion gene implies a significant activation of the sonic hedgehog pathway {332}. Neither RAS nor *BRAF* mutations have been detected in HTT {3919}. The relationship between HTT and papillary thyroid carcinoma was originally suggested by the detection of *RET::CCDC6* rearrangements {805,3425,3919}, although these findings were not confirmed by others {4107,2842}.

Macroscopic appearance

HTT is a well-circumscribed, solid neoplasm with a round or oval shape, a firm to soft consistency, a lobulated appearance, and a white to yellow colour. The size ranges from 5 to 75 mm; about half of all reported cases measure < 30 mm {668}.

Histopathology

The morphological characteristics of HTT include architectural and cytological features {671}. The lesion is usually well circumscribed or encapsulated. Tumour cells are arranged in wide trabeculae or small nests delimited by stromal bundles. Within the trabeculae, a variably abundant eosinophilic hyaline amorphous material (resembling amyloid but Congo red–negative) is present, sometimes enveloping tumour cells. This material is diastase-resistant, PAS-positive, and made of basal membrane material. The amount of intertrabecular stroma is variable, but, even when conspicuous, it is not diagnostic of HTT in the absence of intratrabecular hyalinization. Tumour cells are large or medium-sized and polygonal or elongated, oriented perpendicular to the trabeculae. The cytoplasm is variably eosinophilic (occasionally clear) with hyaline material that contains finely granular deposits and with focal perinuclear yellowish cytoplasmic bodies of lysosomal origin {3843}. These bodies may be present in thyroid lesions other than HTT but at a much lower frequency {3844}. The nuclei are large, elongated, and convoluted, with prominent grooves, vacuoles, and membrane irregularities, but they are not usually as clear as in papillary carcinoma. Mitoses are rare. Intratrabecular and stromal calcifications are frequent {668,1891}. Rare tumours with HTT features have been described showing capsular, vascular, or thyroid parenchymal invasion and these demonstrate a (small) recurrence/metastasis risk {3065,2912, 1651,668,3924}.

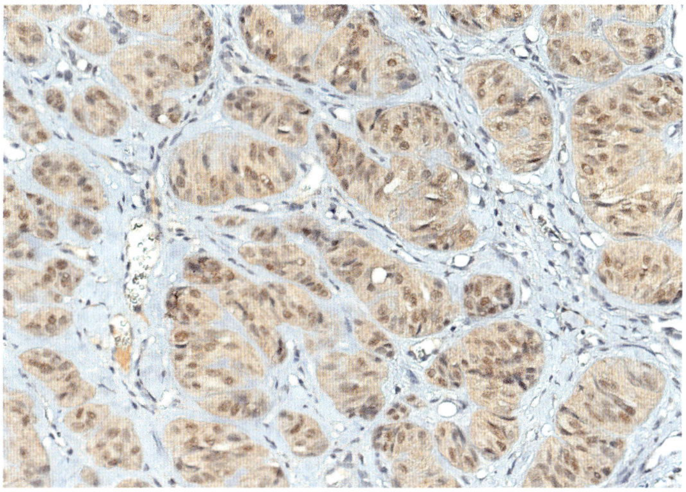

Fig. 3.30 Hyalinizing trabecular tumour. Cytoplasmic and nuclear expression of GLIS3 in the presence of a *PAX8::GLIS3* rearrangement.

Immunophenotype

Thyroglobulin and thyroid transcription factor 1 (TTF1) are invariably positive. Malignancy-related markers of follicular cells (e.g. galectin-3) are variably expressed {1478}. The hyaline material is positive for collagen IV {668,2634}. Anomalous Ki-67 cell membrane reactivity is unique in HTT {1894} but occurs only when the monoclonal antibody MIB1 is used, and only at room temperature {2608,4376}. MIB1 membranous staining is also a

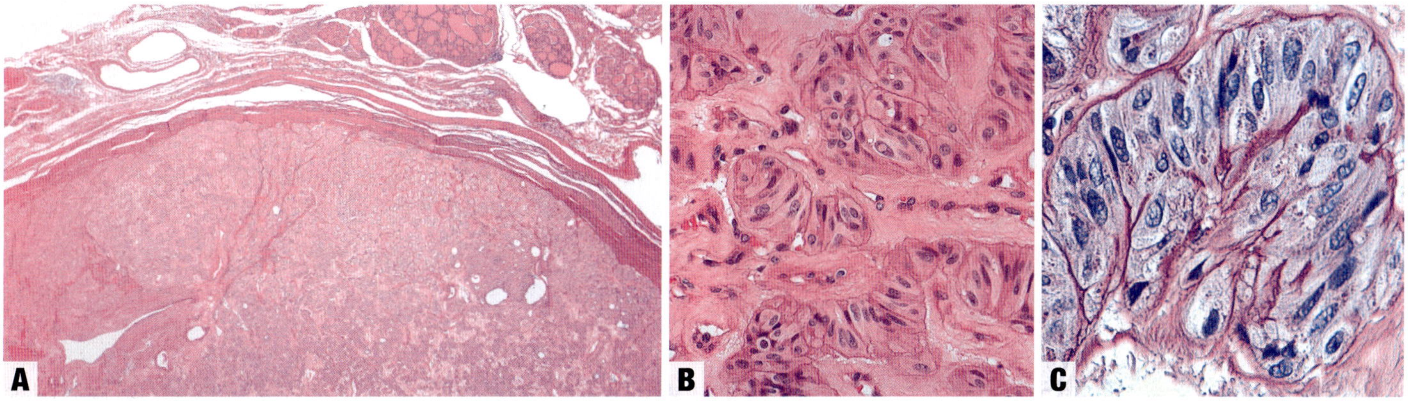

Fig. 3.31 Hyalinizing trabecular tumour. **A** A well-circumscribed nodule with a thin capsule. **B** Typical trabecular growth, marked cytoplasmic hyalinization, and irregular nuclei with irregular contours and pseudoinclusions. **C** PASD-positive intratrabecular material, with cells oriented perpendicularly to the trabeculae.

Table 3.03 Differential diagnosis of hyalinizing trabecular tumour (HTT)

Key features	HTT	Follicular adenoma with trabecular growth	Papillary carcinoma with trabecular growth	Poorly differentiated carcinoma with trabecular growth	Medullary thyroid carcinoma	Paraganglioma
Trabecular growth	Present	Present	Present	Present	Present	Present
Tumour borders	Well defined (encapsulation)	Encapsulated	Well defined or infiltrative	Infiltrative	Well defined or infiltrative	Well defined (encapsulation)
Capsular/vascular invasion	Absent (present in extremely rare malignant cases)	Absent	Variable	Present	Variable	Usually absent
Intertrabecular hyalinization	Present, variable extent	May be present	May be present	May be present	May be present, but to be distinguished from amyloid material (Congo red+) in medullary thyroid carcinoma	Usually absent
Intratrabecular stromal hyalinization	Present, variable extent	Absent	Absent	Absent	Absent	Absent
Nuclear features	Diffuse membrane irregularities, grooves, intranuclear pseudoinclusions, no peripheral margination of chromatin (clearing)	Usually dark and small; may show nuclear enlargement and grooves	RAS-like carcinomas have enlarged nuclei, irregular nuclear membranes with convolutions, grooves; BRAF-like carcinomas have florid irregularity, clearing, intranuclear pseudoinclusions	Usually dark and small; irregular nuclear membranes with convolutions in some cases	Finely granular chromatin; may show membrane irregularities and intranuclear pseudoinclusions	Hyperchromatic nuclei with small nucleoli; may show membrane irregularities
MIB1 staining (in appropriate conditions; see text)	Membranous (+ nuclear in proliferative cells)	Only nuclear	Only nuclear	Only nuclear	Only nuclear	Only nuclear
Follicular cell markers (thyroglobulin, TTF1, PAX8)	Positive	Positive	Positive	Positive (focal dot-like thyroglobulin pattern)	Negative (may be focal TTF1)	Negative
GLIS fusion	Present	Absent	Absent	Absent	Absent	Absent

TTF1, thyroid transcription factor 1.

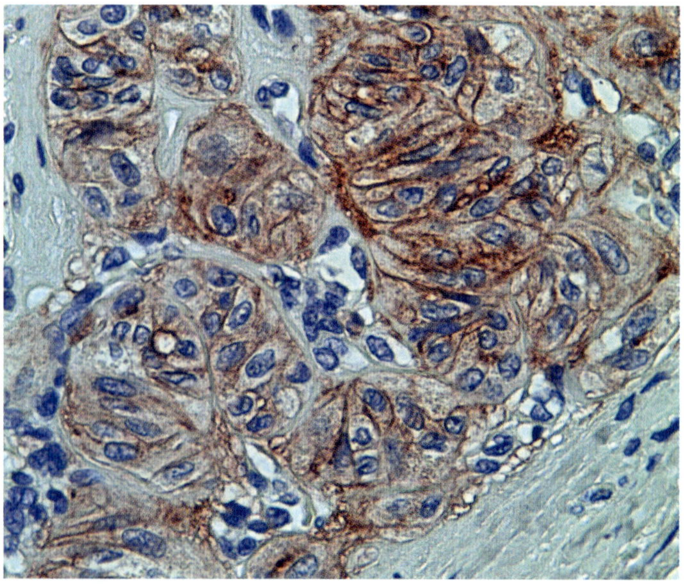

Fig. 3.32 Hyalinizing trabecular tumour. Membranous Ki-67 staining using the MIB1 clone in a histological sample. Immunoperoxidase with DAB staining.

useful diagnostic tool in cytological samples {690,278}. Expression of GLIS3 is associated with the presence of a *PAX8::GLIS3* fusion.

Differential diagnosis

The most relevant differential diagnoses include follicular cell–derived neoplasms with trabecular growth (follicular adenoma, papillary and poorly differentiated carcinomas), medullary thyroid carcinoma, and paraganglioma {4733,3831}. Key differential diagnostic features are summarized in Table 3.03.

Cytology

These cytological features are not specific {3883}. HTT features include loosely cohesive groups of tumour cells with abundant cytoplasm and a trabecular or syncytial pattern radiating outwards from a hyaline core and amyloid-like material in the background {278,691,1075}. Papillary structures with fibrovascular stalks are absent. It is frequently classified as papillary carcinoma (category VI in the Bethesda system) or less frequently as follicular neoplasm or suspicious for malignancy (category IV–V in the Bethesda system) {3883}.

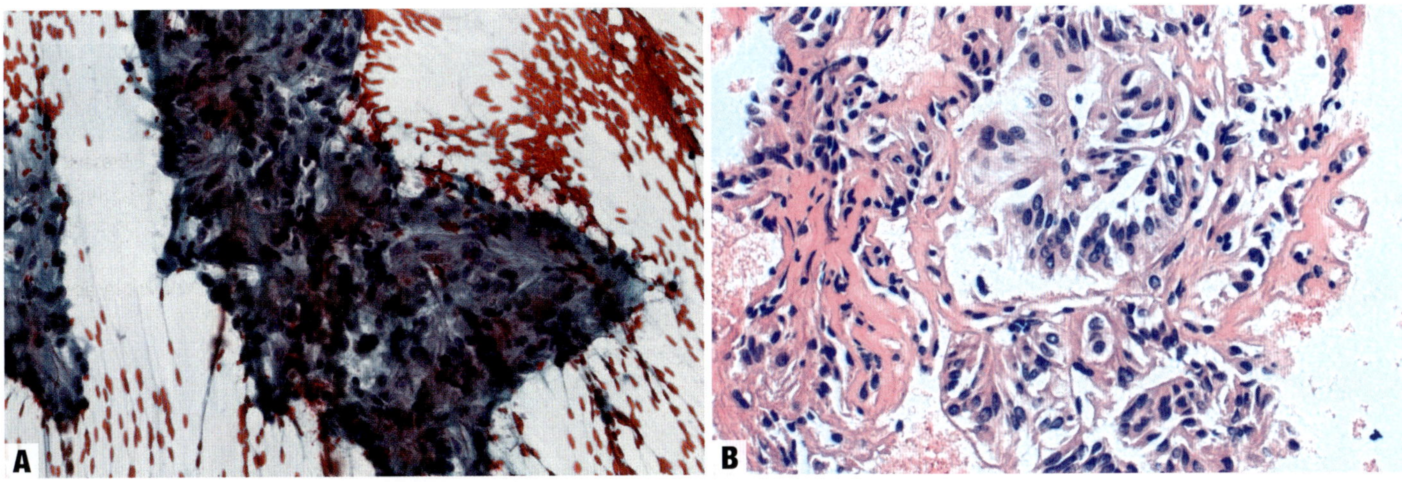

Fig. 3.33 Cytological features of hyalinizing trabecular tumour. Sheets of cells with a trabecular arrangement. **A** Pap. **B** Cell-block preparation.

Diagnostic molecular pathology

The detection of the GLIS fusions (or GLIS protein expression) may be of clinical relevance in the preoperative setting, in the presence of a suggestive cytology, to tailor the most adequate surgical therapy {3259}. To date, GLIS fusions have not been investigated in metastatic tumours, so it is unclear whether their identification can be used to exclude metastatic risk.

Essential and desirable diagnostic criteria

Essential: follicular cell differentiation; pure trabecular architecture with intratrabecular hyalinization and nuclear features characterized by prominent grooves, vacuoles, and membrane irregularities.

Desirable: membranous Ki-67 staining (MIB1 clone); detection of GLIS rearrangements in selected cases.

Staging

Not relevant

Prognosis and prediction

The overwhelming majority of HTTs are clinically benign even after a long follow-up, and complete excision is generally curative {668}. The rare cases with lymph node or distant metastases usually show invasive growth or vascular invasion {668, 3065,1651,2912,3924}.

Follicular thyroid carcinoma

Barletta JA
Asa SL
Fadda G
Juhlin CC
Jung CK
Kakudo K
Kondo T
LiVolsi V

Definition

Follicular thyroid carcinoma (FTC) is a malignant well-differentiated follicular cell–derived neoplasm that has invasive growth and lacks nuclear features of papillary thyroid carcinoma (PTC) and high-grade features.

ICD-O coding

8330/3 Follicular thyroid carcinoma
8335/3 Minimally invasive follicular thyroid carcinoma (capsular invasion only)
8339/3 Encapsulated angioinvasive follicular thyroid carcinoma
8330/3 Widely invasive follicular thyroid carcinoma

ICD-11 coding

2D10.0 Follicular carcinoma of thyroid gland

Related terminology

Acceptable: follicular carcinoma.

Subtype(s)

Minimally invasive follicular thyroid carcinoma (capsular invasion only); encapsulated angioinvasive follicular thyroid carcinoma; widely invasive follicular thyroid carcinoma

Localization

FTC can occur anywhere in the thyroid, in ectopic locations and in association with struma ovarii {1106,3766,4833}.

Clinical features

FTC occurs predominantly in adults (mean age at diagnosis: 45–50 years at diagnosis) and is rare in children {1987,3317, 4319,3577,2614,3515}. Most patients present with a painless thyroid mass that is detected on self-examination, routine physical examination, or incidentally on imaging. As many as 25–35% of FTCs are > 40 mm {223,3515}; however, only a subset of these tumours produce dysphagia, hoarseness, or stridor. Regional lymph node enlargement at presentation essentially does not occur with FTC. Approximately 5–10% of patients with FTC have distant metastases at diagnosis {4319,3515}. In some of these patients, the metastases may be the presenting symptom, especially in patients with bone metastases at diagnosis. Very rare examples of FTC are associated with hyperthyroidism {1780,2687}. On ultrasound, the majority of FTCs are indistinguishable from follicular adenoma (FA). Most FTCs are solitary, well-defined, solid, homogeneous, ovoid, isoechoic or hypoechoic nodules, with or without lobulated margins {4920, 698}.

Epidemiology

While an increase in PTC has driven a global rise in thyroid cancer over the past four decades, the absolute incidence of FTC has been relatively stable {897,4678,3515}. The incidence of FTC in the USA in 1980–2009 was 0.88 cases per 100 000 person-years, with the rate in women about 2.2 times as high as that seen in men {223}. FTC currently accounts for approximately 5–15% of thyroid carcinomas, although this percentage varies geographically, in part because of a variable rise in PTC across countries {4678,3401,3577,657,2656,1160}.

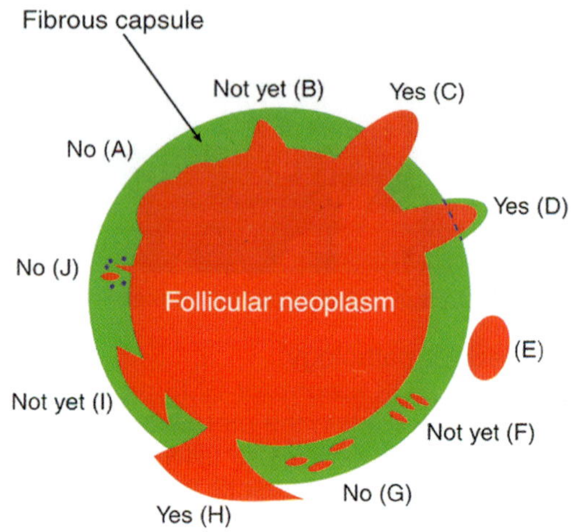

Fig. 3.34 Schematic drawing for the interpretation of the presence or absence of capsular invasion. The diagram depicts a follicular neoplasm (red) surrounded by a fibrous capsule (green). **A** Bosselation on the inner aspect of the capsule does not represent capsular invasion. **B** Sharp tumour bud invades into but not through the capsule, suggesting invasion and requiring deeper sections to exclude. **C** Tumour totally transgresses the capsule invading beyond the outer contour of the capsule, qualifying as capsular invasion. **D** Tumour clothed by thin (probably new) fibrous capsule but already extending beyond an imaginary (dotted) line drawn through the outer contour of the capsule, qualifying as capsular invasion. **E** A satellite tumour nodule with similar cytoarchitecture to that of the main tumour lying outside the capsule, qualifying as capsular invasion. If there is a background of adenomatous nodules, level sections should be considered to confirm that the focus is contiguous with the main mass. **F** Follicles aligned perpendicularly to the capsule, suggesting invasion and requiring deeper sections to exclude. **G** Follicles aligned parallel to the capsule do not represent capsular invasion. **H** Mushroom-shaped tumour with total transgression of the capsule qualifies as capsular invasion. **I** Mushroom-shaped tumour within but not through the capsule suggests invasion, requiring deeper sections to exclude. **J** Neoplastic follicles in the fibrous capsule with a degenerated appearance accompanied by lymphocytes and siderophages do not represent capsular invasion but rather capsular rupture related to prior FNA.

Etiology

Iodine deficiency is considered a risk factor, based on studies demonstrating a higher incidence of FTC and an increased FTC:PTC ratio in iodine-deficient areas compared with iodine-sufficient areas and series demonstrating a decrease in FTC incidence with iodine supplementation {1777,2670,5189}. FTC incidence has also been reported to be increased after exposure to ionizing radiation {2184}, although it is possible that some, or even most, of these FTCs may actually represent the follicular variant of PTC.

Although the majority of follicular cell–derived thyroid carcinomas are sporadic, almost 10% are hereditary {3101}. FTC can occur in the setting of syndromes predominantly defined by extrathyroidal manifestations, including *PTEN* hamartoma tumour syndrome (which includes Cowden syndrome), *DICER1* syndrome, Werner syndrome, and Carney complex {1703,614}. Cowden syndrome is an autosomal dominant disorder most frequently caused by germline mutations in the tumour suppressor gene *PTEN*. In addition to the numerous adenomatous nodules and FA that are often seen in thyroids from patients with Cowden syndrome {2545,317}, approximately 25% of patients with Cowden syndrome have FTC that may present in childhood (for additional features of Cowden syndrome, see the section on Cowden syndrome) {3224,2590,614}. *DICER1* syndrome is an autosomal dominant disorder with reduced penetrance caused by heterozygous inactivating germline *DICER1* mutations {4031}. People with *DICER1* syndrome have a 16-fold increased risk of thyroid cancer, with FTC accounting for a significant subset of these cancers, some of which present in childhood {1021,2269, 2590}. FTC can also occur in people with Werner syndrome, an autosomal recessive disease characterized by premature aging and cancer predisposition caused by biallelic *WRN* mutations {3365}. Thyroid neoplasms occur in approximately 15% of patients with Werner syndrome {2543}. In Japanese patients with Werner syndrome, FTC has been reported to account for 48% of thyroid malignancies {2049}. About a quarter of patients with Carney complex, an autosomal dominant disorder most often caused by germline mutations in *PRKAR1A*, have thyroid tumours (including FA, follicular adenomatosis, and toxic adenomas) and 2.5% have thyroid carcinomas {407}. In a cohort of patients with Carney complex who underwent thyroid surgery, it was reported that approximately a quarter had FTC {670}. A family history of thyroid carcinoma is identified in 3.7% of patients diagnosed with FTC in the USA {1987}.

Pathogenesis

The most common somatic mutations in FTC are RAS point mutations, which are reported in as many as half of all FTCs, with an overall rate of approximately 30% in published studies {3314}. *NRAS* mutations are most common, followed by *HRAS* and *KRAS* mutations {3052,2102}. Most *NRAS* and *HRAS* mutations involve codon 61, whereas most *KRAS* mutations involve codon 12/13 {2102}. *PAX8::PPARG* rearrangements occur in 10–40% of FTCs {474}, with the frequency showing more geographical variability than is seen with RAS mutations {3052}. RAS mutations and *PAX8::PPARG* rearrangements are generally mutually exclusive. Compared to RAS-mutant FTCs, FTCs with *PAX8::PPARG* rearrangements have been reported to occur in younger patients and to be smaller in size but with more overt invasion {1435,3257}. Rare *CREB3L2::PPARG* gene fusions have also been reported in FTC {2757}. *EIF1AX* mutations are identified in about 5% of FTCs and may co-occur with RAS mutations {2210,1164}.

FTCs also harbour mutations and copy-number gains in genes involved in the PI3K/PTEN/AKT pathway. *PIK3CA* mutations and copy-number gain are found in approximately 8% and 30% of FTCs, respectively {1956,4810}. Inactivating *PTEN* mutations are identified in approximately 10% of FTCs {1956, 4810}. Alterations in the PI3K/PTEN/AKT pathway are more frequent in FTC than in FA {4810}.

A small subset of FTCs harbour somatic *DICER1* or somatic *NF1* mutations {3235}. FTCs with *DICER1* mutations may have a macrofollicular architecture {468,2152}. *TERT* promoter mutations are found in approximately 15% of FTCs (often in combination with a RAS mutation), with NC_000005.9:g.1295228G>A (228C>T) as the predominant form of this mutation {2695,2297, 1164}. *TERT* promoter mutations are enriched in FTC with distant metastases (found in approximately half) {940,942}. FTC can also rarely have activating *TSHR* mutations {3070}. In contrast to oncocytic carcinoma, conventional FTC generally lacks *TP53* mutations {3261}.

Macroscopic appearance

The vast majority of FTCs are grossly encapsulated, representing either minimally invasive FTC or encapsulated angioinvasive FTC {998,3354,4319}. Most FTCs are > 20 mm {223}; however, tumour size cannot be used to differentiate FTC from FA. FTCs are usually solid and tan/grey on cut surface. The capsule of minimally invasive FTC and encapsulated angioinvasive FTC can vary in thickness, although it is generally thicker in FTC than in FA {5005,4202}. Gross evidence of invasion in encapsulated FTC is rare. A diagnosis of widely invasive FTC is based

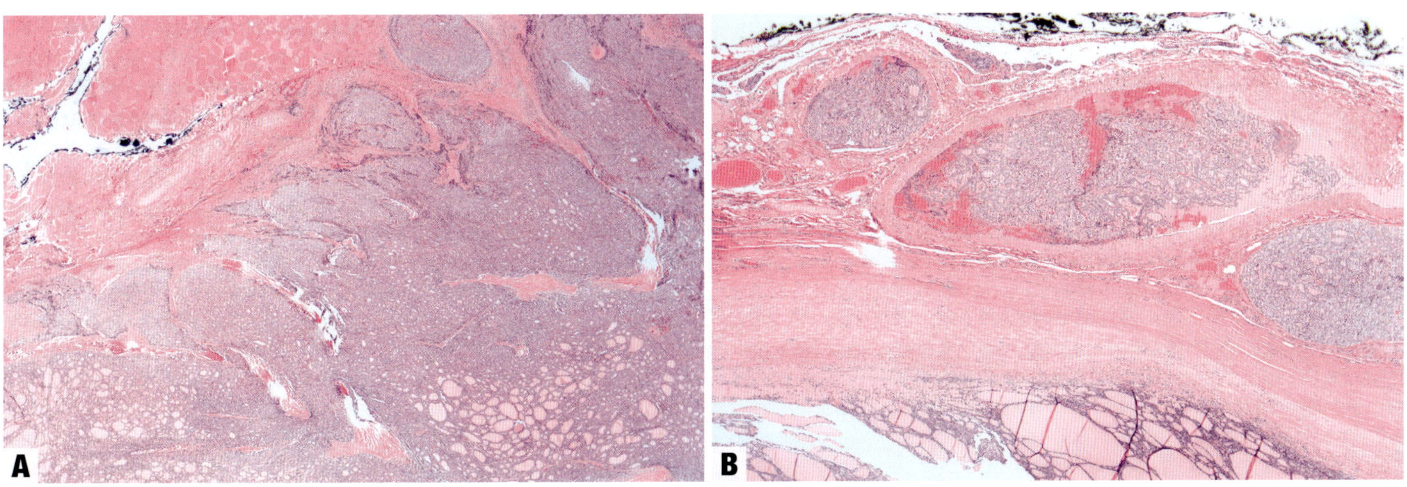

Fig. 3.35 Follicular thyroid carcinoma, widely invasive. **A** Low-power photomicrograph showing tumour involving the thyroid in a multinodular pattern. **B** Vascular invasion is frequently present. Frequently, large vessels are involved.

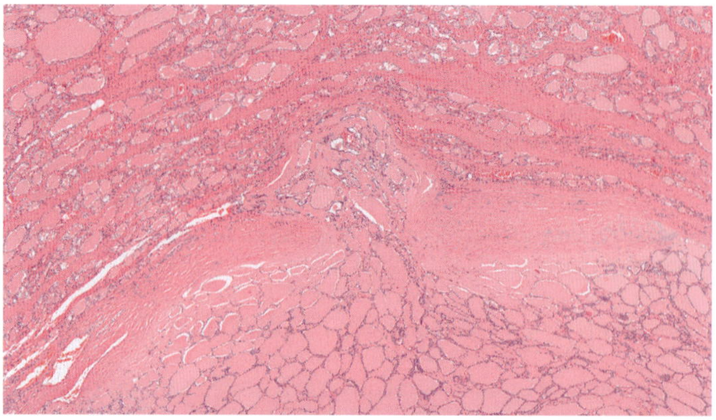

Fig. 3.36 Follicular thyroid carcinoma, minimally invasive. Mushrooming capsular invasion with a predominantly macrofollicular architecture. This tumour was found to harbour a somatic *DICER1* mutation.

on tumour grossly invading through the thyroid parenchyma, often in a multinodular pattern. Widely invasive FTC can grossly invade extrathyroidal tissue. In some of these cases, some of the tumour nodules represent large tumour thrombi within vessels. Widely invasive tumours tend to be larger than minimally invasive FTCs {1015,3577}. It should be noted that widely invasive FTCs are very rare tumours. Many tumours previously diagnosed as such probably represent poorly differentiated thyroid carcinoma (PDTC).

Histopathology

The diagnosis of FTC requires capsular and/or vascular invasion. FTC is divided into three subtypes: (1) minimally invasive (capsular invasion only), (2) encapsulated angioinvasive (venous invasion present with or without capsular penetration), and (3) widely invasive. Although the distinction between FTC and FA is seemingly straightforward, it is recognized that there is debate over what constitutes capsular invasion {4479,292} and vascular invasion {2955}, and there are issues with interobserver reproducibility {5182}.

Minimally invasive FTC: To render this diagnosis, most authors require full-thickness capsular penetration. Tumour that has invaded through the capsule often shows mushroom-shaped growth. The leading edge of the tumour may induce fibrosis, which can complicate assessment of invasion; however, the fibrosis at the leading/invasive edge of the tumour is beyond the contour of the tumour capsule. For cases with foci of invasion into but not through the capsule, serial/deeper sections should be considered, because full-thickness invasion may be identified on deeper sections. In a subset of cases, tumour is present outside the capsule but the focus of capsular invasion connecting the focus to the main mass is not present on the section examined. To be considered evidence of invasion, the focus being considered must have the same cytomorphology as that seen in the main mass. Also, the background thyroid should be considered. If there is a background of multiple adenomatous nodules, caution is advised and serial/deeper sections should be considered to confirm that the focus is contiguous with the main mass. Capsule rupture due to surgical manipulation or tissue grossing, capsular disruption secondary to prior biopsy, and curling of tumour beyond the capsule at tissue edges should not be equated with invasion. Capsular disruption secondary to FNA can often be recognized by the presence of haemosiderin-laden macrophages, inflammatory cells, and fresh haemorrhage.

Encapsulated angioinvasive FTC: Most authors define vascular invasion as the invasion of vessels within the tumour capsule or beyond, with intravascular tumour attached to the vessel wall, or admixed with fibrin or covered by endothelium. In some cases with vascular invasion, the tumour is seen directly invading into the capsule and into a vessel within the capsule as a polypoid protrusion within the lumen. Foci of tumour that only push up against vessels should not be considered foci of vascular invasion because this can frequently be seen at the tumour capsule interface or in the context of tumour buds within the capsule that are located next to vessels. Additionally, foci resembling vascular invasion that are located within the tumour or tumour floating within a vessel lumen (without associated endothelium) are not diagnostic of vascular invasion. There are also vascular alterations, including pseudoangiosarcomatous changes (Masson lesion) and endothelial proliferations, that may be associated with the needle tract from the prior FNA and can mimic vascular invasion {290}. The presence and extent of vascular invasion is prognostically relevant {998,2059,4986}. Tumours with limited invasion of vessels (< 4 foci) have a better prognosis than do those with extensive vascular invasion (≥ 4 foci of invasion). Therefore, foci of vascular invasion should be counted (with foci in adjacent vessels counted separately). ERG or CD31 immunohistochemistry may be considered, to highlight vascular endothelial cells {2668,284}. Vascular invasion represents venous invasion, regardless of the vessel size; moreover, consistent with the fact that FTC rarely spreads to lymph nodes, lymphatic invasion is essentially not seen with FTC {2668}. In one study, vascular invasion was diagnosed only when the intravascular tumour was associated with fibrin or invaded the vessel wall {2955}. These stringent criteria resulted in a higher risk of distant metastasis and a diminished impact of the extent of vascular invasion in prognosis, highlighting the importance of fibrin-associated tumour thrombi {2955}. In that study, the number of foci of vascular invasion did not impact the outcome {2955}. In cases with questionable capsular or vascular invasion, a diagnosis of follicular tumour of uncertain malignant potential can be rendered. However, this category should be used sparingly.

Widely invasive FTC: The capsule of widely invasive FTC may be entirely obliterated or only focally intact. Widely invasive FTCs show extensive invasion of the thyroid and often of extrathyroidal soft tissues. Vascular invasion is often prominent, but alone it does not categorize an FTC as widely invasive.

The cytoarchitectural features of FTC are similar to those of FA. The tumour can have a microfollicular, normofollicular, or macrofollicular growth pattern. Solid or trabecular growth can occur (alone or in combination with follicular-patterned growth); however, it is important that in tumours showing these growth patterns, a diagnosis of PDTC should be excluded (see *High-grade follicular cell–derived non-anaplastic thyroid carcinoma*, p. 165). For all cases, the tumour should be examined for mitoses. The mitotic count should be < 3 mitoses/2 mm^2 in areas of solid or trabecular growth and < 5 mitoses/2 mm^2 if the tumour has an entirely follicular architecture (see *High-grade follicular cell–derived non-anaplastic thyroid carcinoma*, p. 165). Tumour necrosis should not be seen in FTC, but infarct-like necrosis (often secondary to preoperative FNAB) is permissible. FTC also lacks the nuclear features of PTC. Instead, the nuclei are round and have coarse chromatin. All potential FTCs should be examined for nuclear features of PTC to exclude a diagnosis of the encapsulated follicular variant of PTC. The stroma of FTC can vary from scant to hyalinized or myxoid. Occasionally, lipomatous metaplasia is present within the tumour. Extensive intratumoural fibrosis (often with associated calcification), a finding that has been associated with FTC with distant metastases at diagnosis, can variably obscure evidence of invasion {940}. Although it is difficult to identify vascular invasion in such lesions, it seems logical that venous involvement was present at some time during the evolution of the tumour.

Histological patterns

Other histological patterns of FTC are extremely rare. Clear cell FTC, the most frequent non-conventional pattern of FTC, is defined as having > 50% clear cells. Clear cell change can occur in a range of benign and malignant thyroid tumours {251, 647,4023,2142,2147} and occurs secondary to an accumulation of glycogen, lipids, thyroglobulin, or vesicles of apparent mitochondrial derivation {4023,647}. A diagnosis of malignancy is rendered according to the criteria used for conventional FTC. Clear cell FTC can have areas of solid architecture {647}; in such cases, progression to PDTC should be excluded. Because clear cell FTC is a rare tumour, other tumours with clear cytoplasm should be excluded, including metastatic clear cell renal cell carcinoma, medullary thyroid carcinoma, and parathyroid tumours. Thyroglobulin staining can be focal or weak in clear cell FTC {1778}; therefore, the combined use of thyroid transcription factor 1 (TTF1) and PAX8 may be more helpful diagnostically. The prognostic significance of clear cell change has not been established, because of the rarity of the tumour. Like patients with conventional FTC, some reported patients have no further evidence of disease after resection, whereas others die of disease progression {251,4023}. Clear cell FTCs have molecular alterations similar to those seen in conventional FTC, with RAS mutations and *PAX8::PPARG* rearrangements reported {251}. Malignant oncocytic tumours are discussed separately in the section on oncocytic carcinoma (see *Oncocytic carcinoma of the thyroid gland*, p. 161).

The signet-ring cell pattern of FTC is characterized by cells with cytoplasmic vacuoles with eccentrically displaced nuclei {4024,647,3800,2008}. The cytoplasmic vacuoles are similar to follicular lumina and have an accumulation of thyroglobulin {4024}. The nuclei are generally uniform and bland. These tumours must be distinguished from metastatic adenocarcinomas with signet-ring cell morphology. Other extremely rare lesions are FTC with a glomeruloid pattern, characterized by follicles with round to oval epithelial tufts growing within them, mimicking a renal glomerulus {610}; and spindle cell FTC {1601}, characterized by cells arranged in intersecting fascicles. Differentiating spindle cell FTC from anaplastic thyroid carcinoma is essential. To render a diagnosis of spindle cell FTC, pleomorphism, marked mitotic activity, and tumour necrosis must be absent.

Immunohistochemistry

FTC is positive for CAM5.2, EMA, and CK7 and negative for CK20 {4895,370}. These tumours also have strong nuclear staining for the transcription factors PAX8 and TTF1 {370,2546}. The cytoplasm and associated colloid of FTC is positive for thyroglobulin {370}. There are no immunohistochemical stains that reliably distinguish FTC from FA. Ki-67 immunohistochemistry may be helpful when considering a differential diagnosis of PDTC. Consistent with the low mitotic count of FTC, the Ki-67 proliferation index is < 5% in the majority of FTCs, whereas most PDTCs have a higher Ki-67 proliferation index {228}.

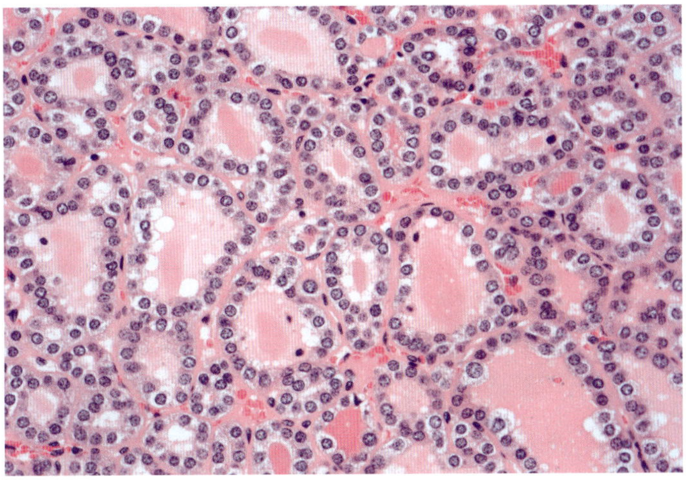

Fig. 3.37 Follicular thyroid carcinoma. The tumours have a follicular architecture and are composed of cells with round normochromatic nuclei.

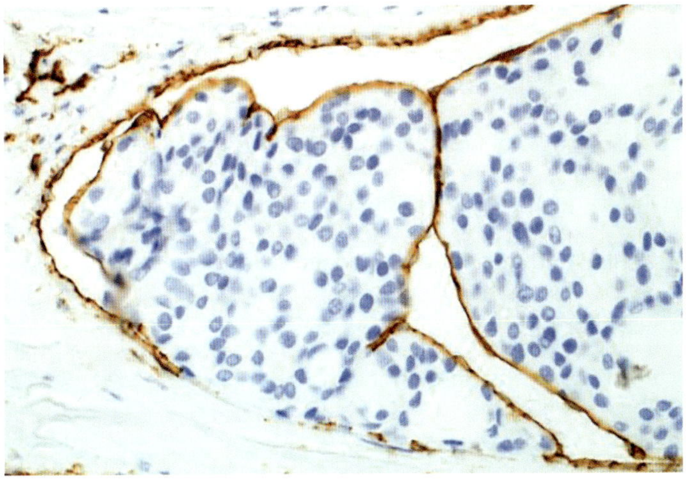

Fig. 3.38 Follicular thyroid carcinoma, encapsulated angioinvasive. CD31 immunohistochemistry highlights endothelial cells in this focus of vascular invasion.

Cytology

Benign and malignant follicular-patterned lesions cannot be distinguished using thyroid FNA. The cytological diagnosis of follicular neoplasm or suspicious for follicular neoplasm reflects the limitations of thyroid cytology, because the diagnosis of FTC is based on the demonstration of capsular and/or vascular invasion.

Diagnostic molecular pathology

In preoperative fine-needle biopsies, the presence of RAS mutations and *PAX8::PPARG* rearrangements raise the possibility of FTC {1368}. However, these genetic events are not

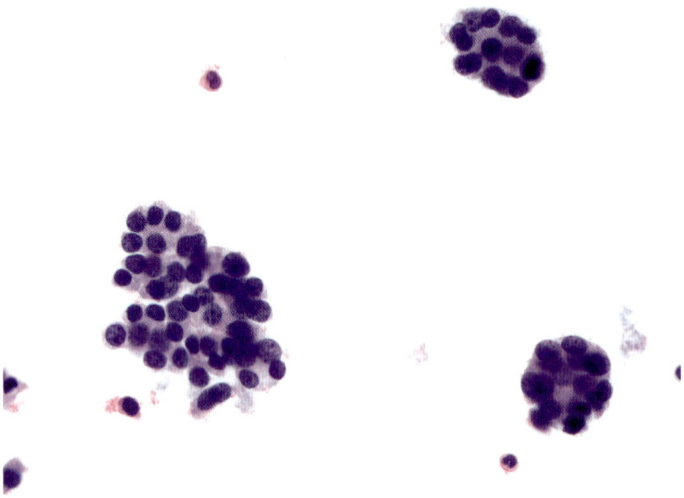

Fig. 3.39 Follicular neoplasm. FNA specimen diagnosed as suspicious for a follicular neoplasm. Note the microfollicular architecture, round nuclei, and coarse chromatin. The cytological findings are not diagnostic of malignancy, because malignancy is based on the assessment of invasion in the resection specimen. The resection specimen was a minimally invasive follicular thyroid carcinoma.

specific, being encountered in FA and encapsulated follicular variant of PTC. There is currently no role for molecular pathology in the diagnosis of FTC in the postoperative setting.

Essential and desirable diagnostic criteria

Essential: follicular cell–derived tumours lacking nuclear features of PTC and lacking high-grade features; capsular and/or vascular invasion; widely invasive FTCs have grossly apparent invasion through the thyroid parenchyma and (typically) harbour extensive vascular invasion.

Staging

FTC is staged according to the Union for International Cancer Control (UICC) and American Joint Committee on Cancer (AJCC) staging systems, incorporating age at diagnosis.

Prognosis and prediction

Extent of invasion significantly impacts survival for patients with FTC. Disease-free survival rates of 97%, 81%, and 45% at 40 months have been reported for minimally invasive, encapsulated angioinvasive, and widely invasive FTC, respectively {3354}. For the rare minimally invasive FTC that results in death, distant metastases are usually present at the time of initial diagnosis {4986,3354}. For encapsulated angioinvasive FTC, the extent of vascular invasion has been shown to be prognostically significant, with an odds ratio of 13.7 reported for extensive vascular invasion in a multivariate analysis of 10-year cause-specific survival {2059}. For M0 patients with minimally invasive or encapsulated angioinvasive FTC, an age of ≥ 55 years and a tumour size of > 40 mm have been shown to be prognostic for decreased disease-free survival in multivariate analyses {5008,3577,2059}. The presence of distant metastases is the most important prognostic feature for FTC. The most common sites of distant metastases are lung and bone {4320}, with bone metastases more common in patients with metastatic disease at the time of initial diagnosis, and lung metastases more common in patients who are M0 at initial diagnosis {940}. The prognosis appears to be similar for patients who present with or subsequently develop distant metastases {940}. *TERT* promoter mutations have been shown to be associated with more aggressive clinical behaviour in FTC, including a more advanced stage at presentation, distant metastases, and increased disease-specific mortality {2934,4215,2297}. Increased mutation burden has also been associated with a worse prognosis in FTC {3235}.

Invasive encapsulated follicular variant of papillary thyroid carcinoma

Barletta JA
Asa SL
Fadda G
Juhlin CC
Jung CK
Kakudo K
Kondo T
LiVolsi V

Definition

Invasive encapsulated follicular variant of papillary thyroid carcinoma (IEFVPTC) is a malignant well-differentiated follicular cell–derived neoplasm that is encapsulated and has an exclusive or almost exclusive follicular architecture, nuclear features of papillary thyroid carcinoma (PTC), and invasive growth.

ICD-O coding

8340/3 Invasive encapsulated follicular variant of papillary thyroid carcinoma
8340/3 Minimally invasive encapsulated follicular variant of papillary carcinoma (capsular invasion only)
8340/3 Encapsulated angioinvasive follicular variant of papillary carcinoma
8340/3 Widely invasive follicular variant of papillary carcinoma

ICD-11 coding

2D10.1 & XH0Q59 Papillary carcinoma of thyroid gland & Papillary carcinoma, encapsulated, of thyroid

Related terminology

Acceptable: invasive encapsulated follicular subtype of papillary thyroid carcinoma.

Subtype(s)

Minimally invasive encapsulated follicular variant of papillary thyroid carcinoma (capsular invasion only); encapsulated angioinvasive follicular variant of papillary thyroid carcinoma; widely invasive follicular variant of papillary thyroid carcinoma

Localization

IEFVPTC can occur anywhere in the thyroid and in ectopic locations, including in association with thyroglossal duct cysts and struma ovarii {4005,3766,4834,4833}.

Clinical features

IEFVPTC occurs predominantly in adults, with a median age of 40–50 years at diagnosis and an M:F ratio of < 1:3 {2686, 4717,2295}. Approximately 15% of PTCs in children represent IEFVPTC {3317,2614,279,3928}. Most patients present with a painless thyroid mass. Regional lymph node enlargement at presentation, a finding often observed with classic PTC or infiltrative follicular variant of papillary thyroid carcinoma (FVPTC), is not seen with IEFVPTC {2686,4717}. Distant metastases are present at diagnosis in as many as approximately 5% of patients {3758}. The ultrasound characteristics of IEFVPTC overlap with those of non-invasive follicular thyroid neoplasm with papillary-like nuclear features (NIFTP): both tumours are typically solitary and round to ovoid, with smooth margins, variable echogenicity, and no calcifications {1747,5022}. The invasive nature of a subset of IEFVPTC may be apparent on ultrasound {5023}.

Epidemiology

The incidence of IEFVPTC is difficult to establish, because most population-based studies rely on data that predate the introduction of the name NIFTP or do not differentiate IEFVPTC from infiltrative FVPTC. In the USA, FVPTC overall has been reported to account for approximately a quarter of PTCs according to SEER data, with the incidence dropping after the introduction of the NIFTP terminology {3515}. In a study evaluating tumours diagnosed in Japan, the Republic of Korea, China (including Taiwan, China), Thailand, and Viet Nam, IEFVPTC was reported to account for 1% of PTCs {585}.

Etiology

Although the vast majority of cases of IEFVPTC are sporadic, FVPTC has been reported in association with tumour syndromes including *PTEN* hamartoma tumour syndrome, *DICER1* syndrome, and Carney complex {1430,2545,3224,1021,670}. The finding of IEFVPTC in a background of multiple adenomatous

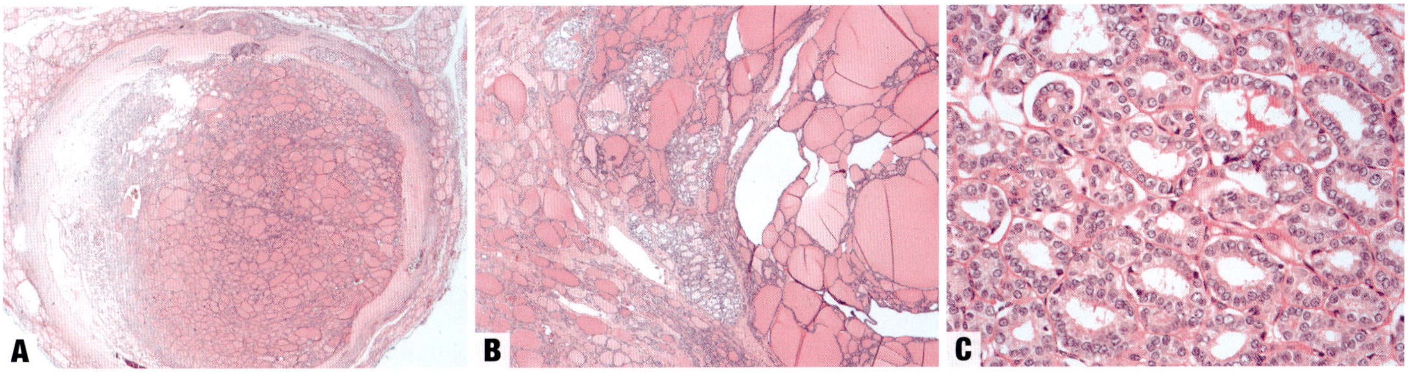

Fig. 3.40 Invasive encapsulated follicular variant of papillary thyroid carcinoma. **A** Low-power photomicrograph showing capsular invasion. **B** The tumour demonstrates foci with more well-developed nuclear features of papillary thyroid carcinoma. This phenomenon, known as the sprinkling sign, can be appreciated at low magnification. **C** The tumour is characterized by a follicular architecture and nuclei that demonstrate enlargement, clearing, contour irregularities, and grooves.

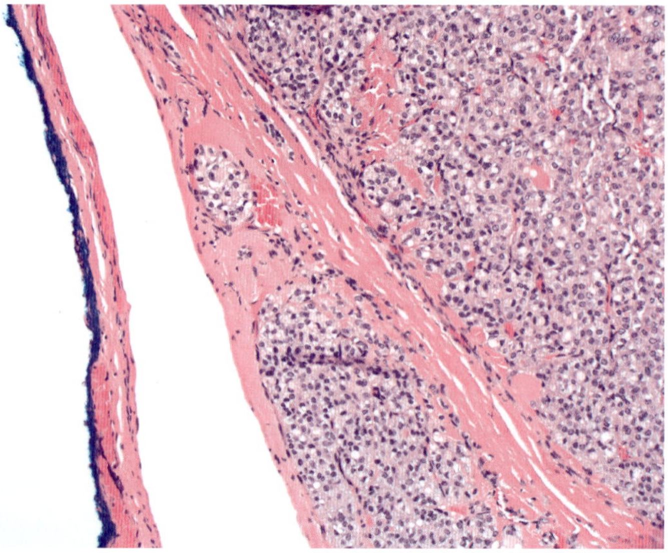

Fig. 3.41 Invasive encapsulated follicular variant of papillary thyroid carcinoma, angioinvasive. Vascular invasion.

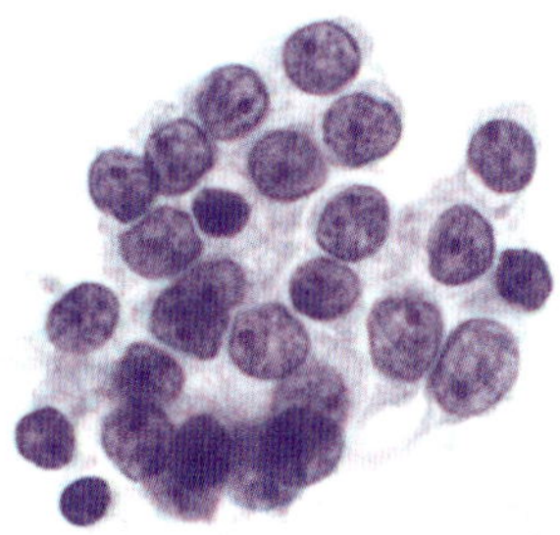

Fig. 3.42 Follicular neoplasm. FNA specimen diagnosed as suspicious for follicular neoplasm. Note the microfollicular architecture. Additionally, there is nuclear pallor and there are mild contour irregularities. The cytological findings are not diagnostic of malignancy, because malignancy is based on the assessment of invasion in the resection specimen. The resection specimen was an encapsulated follicular-variant papillary thyroid carcinoma with invasion.

nodules, adenomas, and nodular hyperplasia raises the possibility of an underlying hereditary syndrome, especially if the tumour occurs in childhood.

Pathogenesis

IEFVPTC has a molecular profile similar to that of follicular adenoma and follicular thyroid carcinoma (FTC). RAS point mutations, the most frequent somatic alteration detected in encapsulated FVPTC (EFVPTC), are present in as many as two thirds of cases {3756,2298}. Additionally, *PAX8::PPARG* rearrangements, although less frequent than RAS mutations, are also characteristic of EFVPTC {703,178}. In contrast to classic PTC and infiltrative FVPTC, *BRAF* p.V600E mutations are infrequent in strictly defined IEFVPTC {3756,2298,4982}. A small subset of IEFVPTC cases have a *BRAF* p.K601E mutation {2298}, an *EIF1AX* mutation {2210}, a *TSHR* mutation {3261}, or a *THADA::IGF2BP3* fusion {3088}. *TERT* promoter mutations are uncommon in IEFVPTC, occurring in < 5% of tumours {3622}.

Macroscopic appearance

Although IEFVPTC can be large (> 40 mm), the mean size of EFVPTC is 20–30 mm and most are < 40 mm {2686,4717, 5023,2295}. IEFVPTC tends to be larger than infiltrative FVPTC {5023,1747,2295}. The capsule of IEFVPTC can vary in thickness, although it has been reported to be thicker than that of NIFTP {5005,4202,4717,1434}. Gross evidence of invasion in IEFVPTC is rare. A diagnosis of widely invasive FVPTC is based on tumour grossly invading through the thyroid parenchyma.

Histopathology

A diagnosis of IEFVPTC requires capsular and/or vascular invasion. IEFVPTC is subclassified into three groups: (1) minimally invasive (capsular invasion only), (2) encapsulated angioinvasive (venous invasion present with or without capsular penetration), and (3) widely invasive. It is recognized that there are issues with interobserver reproducibility for IEFVPTC that reflect different definitions of capsular and vascular invasion, as well as different thresholds for assessment of nuclear features of PTC {4479,292,1238,2955,2162,5182,268}.

To render a diagnosis of minimally invasive IEFVPTC, most authors require full-thickness capsular penetration. For cases with foci of invasion into but not through the capsule, serial/deeper sections should be considered to evaluate for complete capsular transgression in deeper levels. In a subset of cases, tumour is present discontinuously on the outside of the tumour capsule. For such foci to be considered evidence of invasion, they must have the same cytomorphology as that seen in the main mass.

Most authors define vascular invasion as the invasion of vessels within the tumour capsule or beyond, with intravascular tumour attached to the vessel wall, or admixed with fibrin or covered by endothelium. Foci of tumour that only push up against a vessel should not be considered vascular invasion. Additionally, foci resembling vascular invasion that are located within the tumour or tumour floating within a vessel lumen (without associated endothelium) are not diagnostic of vascular invasion. Because the extent of vascular (i.e. venous) invasion is likely to be prognostically significant, as has been demonstrated for FTC {998, 2059,4986}, foci of vascular invasion should be counted (with foci in adjacent vessels counted separately). ERG or CD31 immunohistochemistry may be considered, to highlight vascular endothelial cells to aid in the evaluation of vascular invasion {2668,284}.

IEFVPTC and FTC are both encapsulated tumours with a follicular architecture and invasive growth; therefore, the distinction between entities is based on the presence of nuclear features of PTC in IEFVPTC. Compared with the adjacent non-neoplastic follicular cells, the nuclei of FVPTC are enlarged, elongated, crowded, and overlapping. Additionally, IEFVPTC has nuclear contour irregularities and longitudinal grooves; variable degrees of nuclear clearing with margination of chromatin to the nuclear membrane; and small, peripherally located nucleoli. The nuclear features of IEFVPTC tend to be more subtle than those seen with infiltrative FVPTC {2686}. Nuclear pseudoinclusions are uncommon in IEFVPTC. PTC nuclear features are often variable throughout the tumour. In general, nuclear features tend to be more pronounced at the periphery of the nodule or in the areas of invasive growth. In some cases, IEFVPTC has scattered foci of follicular cells with well-developed nuclear features of PTC distributed throughout a tumour with subtle to essentially absent nuclear atypia – a phenomenon described as the sprinkling sign of FVPTC {4668}. Bone metastases of IEFVPTC may lack nuclear features of PTC {289}.

IEFVPTC has microfollicular, normofollicular, or macrofollicular growth. Solid or trabecular growth can occur (alone or in combination with follicular-patterned growth); however, it is important that in tumours showing these growth patterns, a diagnosis of poorly differentiated thyroid carcinoma is excluded. In areas of solid or trabecular growth, nuclear features of PTC should be maintained and the mitotic count should be < 3 mitoses/2 mm^2. Tumour necrosis should not be seen in IEFVPTC. Some cases of IEFVPTC have deeply eosinophilic colloid. True papillae (i.e. with fibrovascular cores and lined by PTC nuclei) can be found occasionally but should be limited to < 1% of the tumour. Extensive intratumoural fibrosis, a finding that has been associated with distant metastases at diagnosis, can variably obscure evidence of invasion {4986}.

Immunohistochemistry

IEFVPTC is positive for CAM5.2, EMA, CK7, PAX8, thyroid transcription factor 1 (TTF1), and thyroglobulin. Ki-67 immunohistochemistry may be helpful when evaluating for progression to poorly differentiated thyroid carcinoma, because the Ki-67 index is < 5% in the majority of IEFVPTC cases but > 5% in most poorly differentiated thyroid carcinomas {228,3918}.

Differential diagnosis

NIFTP is differentiated from IEFVPTC by the absence of capsular and vascular invasion. Therefore, tumours fulfilling all the criteria for NIFTP except capsular/vascular invasion are labelled as IEFVPTC. The latter is separated from FTC by the presence of PTC nuclear features.

Cytology

On FNA, IEFVPTC is characterized by a microfollicular architecture along with variably prominent nuclear features of PTC that include nuclear enlargement, crowding, contour irregularities, longitudinal grooves, and chromatin clearing {5155,2295}. Because nuclear features of IEFVPTC are variably present throughout the tumour, the nuclear atypia of IEFVPTC may not always be apparent on FNA. Thus, there is overlap in the cytology of IEFVPTC and tumours such as follicular adenoma and FTC. In contrast to classic PTC, IEFVPTC lacks papillae and psammomatous calcifications. Additionally, the nuclear features of IEFVPTC are generally more subtle than those of classic PTC (and infiltrative FVPTC), with pseudoinclusions rare to absent. IEFVPTC cannot be distinguished from NIFTP on cytology because the distinction is based on the demonstration of invasion {2426,5155,858}.

Diagnostic molecular pathology

In preoperative fine-needle biopsies, the presence of RAS and *BRAF* p.K601E mutations as well as *PAX8::PPARG* rearrangements raises the possibility of IEFVPTC {178,703,2298}. However, these genetic alterations are not specific, being encountered in follicular adenoma, FTC, and NIFTP {3255}. There is currently no role for molecular pathology in the diagnosis of IEFVPTC in the postoperative setting.

Essential and desirable diagnostic criteria

Minimally invasive and angioinvasive EFVPTC

Essential: encapsulated tumours with an exclusive or almost exclusive follicular architecture, nuclear features of PTC, and capsular and/or vascular invasion.

Widely invasive FVPTC

Essential: grossly apparent invasive growth; histologically characterized by an exclusive or almost exclusive follicular architecture, nuclear features of PTC, and (typically) extensive vascular invasion.

Staging

IEFVPTCs are staged according to the Union for International Cancer Control (UICC) and American Joint Committee on Cancer (AJCC) staging systems, incorporating age at diagnosis.

Prognosis and prediction

Like FTC, IEFVPTC spreads to distant sites, often bypassing lymph nodes {1493}. Most patients with IEFVPTC that pursues an adverse clinical course present with distant metastases {1493}. Minimally invasive EFVPTC is an extremely indolent tumour if distant metastasis is absent at presentation {4986}. Widely invasive FVPTC and EFVPTC with extensive vascular invasion are at higher risk of distant metastasis and pursuing an aggressive clinical course than are minimally invasive EFVPTCs or encapsulated tumours with only focal vascular invasion (< 4 foci).

Papillary thyroid carcinoma

Baloch ZW
Barletta JA
Bongiovanni M
Fadda G
Jung CK
Kakudo K
Kondo T
LiVolsi V
Mete O
Piana S
Sadow PM

Definition

Papillary thyroid carcinoma (PTC) is a malignant tumour of follicular cell derivation characterized by distinct nuclear features. PTC diagnosis requires either papillary or solid/trabecular architecture, or invasive growth in follicular-patterned tumours.

ICD-O coding

8260/3 Papillary thyroid carcinoma
8340/3 Infiltrative follicular variant of papillary thyroid carcinoma
8342/3 Oncocytic papillary thyroid carcinoma
8260/3 Classic papillary thyroid carcinoma
8343/3 Encapsulated classic papillary thyroid carcinoma
8350/3 Diffuse sclerosing papillary thyroid carcinoma
8260/3 Solid/trabecular papillary thyroid carcinoma
8260/3 Warthin-like papillary thyroid carcinoma
8260/3 Clear cell papillary thyroid carcinoma
8260/3 Spindle cell papillary thyroid carcinoma
8260/3 Papillary thyroid carcinoma with fibromatosis/fasciitis-like/desmoid-type stroma
8344/3 Tall cell papillary thyroid carcinoma
8260/3 Hobnail papillary thyroid carcinoma
8344/3 Columnar cell papillary thyroid carcinoma

ICD-11 coding

2D10.1 Papillary carcinoma of thyroid gland
2D10.1 & XH0426 Papillary carcinoma of thyroid gland & Papillary carcinoma, diffuse sclerosing
2D10.1 & XH85E5 Papillary carcinoma of thyroid gland & Papillary carcinoma, tall cell
2D10.1 & XH0Q59 Papillary carcinoma of thyroid gland & Papillary carcinoma, encapsulated, of thyroid
2D10.1 & XH5YT2 Papillary carcinoma of thyroid gland & Papillary carcinoma, oxyphilic

Related terminology

Acceptable: papillary thyroid adenocarcinoma; infiltrative follicular subtype of papillary thyroid carcinoma (for infiltrative follicular variant of papillary thyroid carcinoma).

Subtype(s)

Infiltrative follicular variant of PTC; oncocytic PTC; classic PTC; encapsulated classic PTC; diffuse sclerosing PTC; solid/trabecular PTC; Warthin-like PTC; clear cell PTC; spindle cell PTC; PTC with fibromatosis/fasciitis-like/desmoid-type stroma; tall cell PTC; hobnail PTC; columnar cell PTC

Localization

PTC can arise anywhere in the thyroid gland in its orthotropic and ectopic locations {2685}. It can also occur in thyroglossal duct cyst and teratomas including struma ovarii {4834,4833, 4484,322}.

Clinical features

PTC usually presents as a painless thyroid nodule with or without associated cervical lymphadenopathy. Dysphagia and stridor due to local compression on the trachea and oesophagus, as well as voice complaints, can be encountered in as many as 20% of patients. Rare cases of PTC will initially present as distant metastasis (usually lung or bone) {1817,3150}. PTC in paediatric patients shows high rates of bilateral and multifocal disease, regional lymph node metastasis, and an increased risk of pulmonary metastasis {347,1420}.

In most cases of PTC, thyroid function tests are within normal limits. Extremely rare cases of PTC can be associated with hyperthyroidism (autonomously functioning tumour or arising in a background of toxic nodular goitre) {1817,3150}. On radionuclide scanning, PTCs are typically hypofunctioning (cold) as compared with the surrounding thyroid parenchyma {4332, 1817,2575}.

A typical case of PTC will appear on thyroid ultrasound as a solid and hypoechoic nodule with microcalcifications / echogenic foci and poorly defined margins. Cystic elements can occur within a solid nodule. Doppler ultrasound may show disorganized and increased vascularity. Ultrasound examination can also confirm cervical lymph node involvement by PTC. Additional imaging modalities employed in the detection and staging of PTC include CT, MRI, and FDG PET-CT. These help

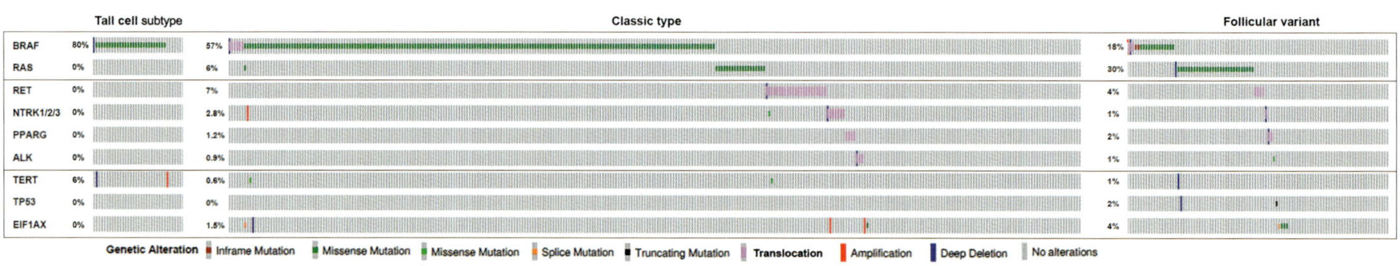

Fig. 3.43 Papillary thyroid carcinoma. Main genetic alterations. Frequency of genetic alterations in 324 classic papillary thyroid carcinomas, 99 follicular-variant papillary thyroid carcinomas, and 31 cases of the tall cell subtype genotyped by The Cancer Genome Atlas (TCGA) Research Network {622} and obtained through cBioPortal {1494;717}.

to identify the extent of extrathyroidal invasion, lymphadenopathy and metastatic foci not visualized by ultrasound (mediastinum, posterior to trachea, skull base), and distant metastasis especially from non–radioiodine-avid tumours {4332,1817,3035, 697,4543,2575}.

Epidemiology

PTC is the most common endocrine malignancy in both the adult population and the paediatric population. In adults, it accounts for 80–85% of all thyroid malignancies, and in children it accounts for 90% {2324}.

The incidence of PTC has been increasing worldwide in recent decades across all age groups and in both sexes; the reported rates are related to screening and diagnostic practices {1002,3829,3025,1032}. According to recent data, in the USA, the incidence rates of PTC have almost quadrupled between 1975 and 2016, with an average annual increase of 3.30%, compared with a decrease of 0.02% for follicular thyroid carcinoma and a decrease of 0.41% for anaplastic thyroid carcinoma {2323}. The extreme example of increased incidence rates of PTC comes from the Republic of Korea, where there was a 15-fold increase between 1993 and 2011 {3319,4897}. Similar but more subtle trends have been reported from Italy, France, and Australia. Approximately half of all diagnosed PTC cases measure ≤ 10 mm, and despite the increasing incidence of PTC, the mortality rate remains stable. However, some authors have also reported an increase in the number of large PTCs; this remains to be validated as a true increase in incidence {4897, 828,2101,3025}.

Etiology

PTC commonly occurs as a sporadic tumour. However, familial forms are being increasingly recognized {1703,1049,847,636}. Exposure to radiation during childhood is the most extensively studied and well-documented environmental factor in the development of PTC {4002,42,3214}. The factors that increase the risk of developing PTC after radiation include female sex, radiation therapy for childhood cancer, and a family history of thyroid cancer.

High levels of dietary iodine have also been implicated in the development of PTC, because of the increasing rates in the dietary iodine–sufficient regions of the world {2573,2571}. Other risk factors studied in the development of PTC include exposure to specific chemical compounds found in volcanic regions, polybrominated diphenyl ethers, obesity, hormonal reproductive factors, and hereditary syndromes {2810,4897,1703,3214, 1049,847,636}.

As mentioned, most PTCs (> 90%) are sporadic and approximately 5–10% are familial. Familial PTCs have been divided into two groups: syndromic with a preponderance of non-thyroidal tumours such as familial adenomatous polyposis, designated as syndromic familial non-medullary thyroid carcinoma; and those with PTC as the main tumour, designated as non-syndromic familial non-medullary thyroid carcinoma {3488,1703,1049, 614,636} (see Chapter 13: *Genetic tumour syndromes associated with endocrine lesions and tumours*).

Pathogenesis

The majority of molecular alterations seen in PTC are somatic mutations that probably occur in the early stage of pathogenesis.

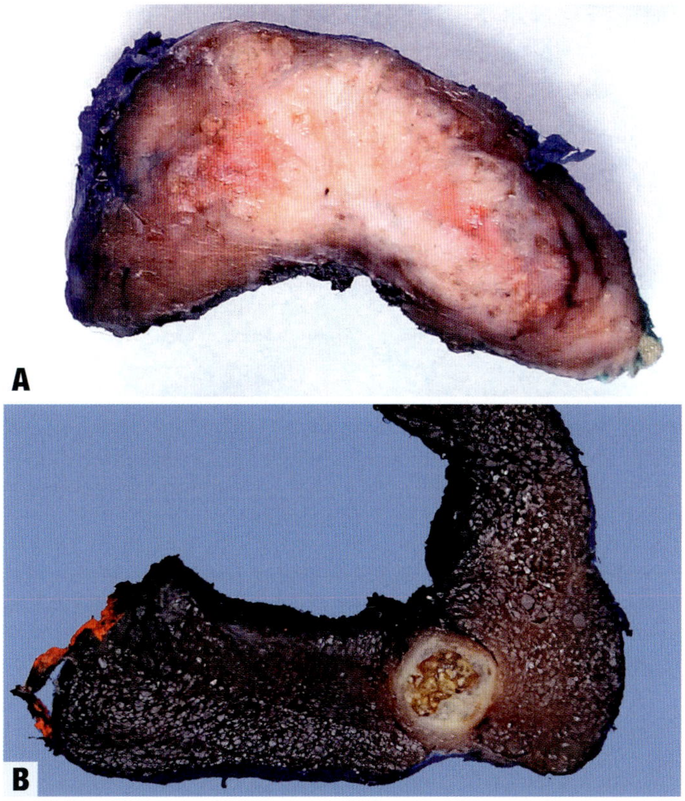

Fig. 3.44 Papillary thyroid carcinoma. **A** Gross photograph of a tumour with sclerosis and infiltrative margins. **B** This papillary carcinoma is encapsulated, and partly solid and cystic. There is granularity in the cystic component, suggestive of papillary formations.

Interestingly, PTCs show a low somatic tumour mutation burden (~0.41 non-silent mutations/Mb), the lowest among all cancer types {622,928,3611,2777,3795}.

The most frequent driver events are either point mutations or gene rearrangements, mostly involving the MAPK pathway. The most common molecular alterations in PTC involve somatic mutations in *BRAF* and in RAS genes (mainly *NRAS*) and *RET* fusions. *BRAF* p.V600E mutations are common in classic PTC and in subtypes showing a papillary architecture; this is in contrast to RAS mutations and the rare *BRAF* p.K601E in follicular-patterned tumours {23,1593,622} (see *Invasive encapsulated follicular variant of papillary thyroid carcinoma*, p. 147).

BRAF p.V600E mutations are the most common (98–99%) of all *BRAF* mutations in PTC. The prevalence of *BRAF* mutations varies with different histological subtypes of PTC and is highest in tall cell PTC (TCPTC) {622,4201,3569,3681}.

The infiltrative follicular variant of PTC shows *BRAF* p.V600E mutations, and some cases may show *RET* translocations and NTRK and *ALK* fusions {3756,1964,4214,337}.

BRAF mutations have been reported in oncocytic PTC (OPTC). Somatic and germline mutations of *NDUFA13* (*GRIM19*) and *RET* rearrangements have also been reported in limited case series {4561,2521,1286,4934,2896}.

BRAF p.V600E mutations have been found in some cases of Warthin-like PTC (WLPTC) {5063,1762}.

Molecular studies have shown that radiation-associated solid/trabecular PTC (SPTC) commonly harbour *NCOA4*::*RET* rearrangements, as compared with non–radiation-associated cases demonstrating *CCDC6::RET* and *ETV6::NTRK3* fusions. *BRAF* p.V600E mutations are rare in SPTC {3254,4562,820, 3605}.

Molecular analyses have shown that the spindle cells in PTC with fibromatosis/fasciitis-like stroma show *CTNNB1* (β-catenin) mutations, and the epithelial component frequently harbours *BRAF* p.V600E mutations {4923,5171,4344}.

BRAF p.V600E mutations are common in TCPTC (~80% of cases), and some cases have shown *TERT* promoter mutations. Loss of heterozygosity at chromosome 1 (D1S243) and the *TP53* mutation have been reported in TCPTC, although not consistently {3811,4879,4809,3860,1952}.

Mutations involving *TERT* promoter genes occur in approximately 10% of PTCs {622}. The two most common *TERT* promoter mutations in PTC are NC_000005.9:g.1295228G>A (*TERT* promoter p.C228T) and NC_000005.9:g.1295250G>A (*TERT* promoter p.C250T); these are considered as secondary pathogenic mutations in PTC {2583,3509,768,2682,5156}.

Less common molecular alterations in PTC include mutations in *HRAS*, *KRAS*, *PPM1D*, *CHEK2*, and *MAP2K1* (*MEK1*), and fusions in *BRAF*, *PPARG*, *THADA*, *LTK*, *MET*, and *FGFR2*. NTRK fusions (*NTRK1* and *NTRK3*) can be detected in 3–5% of PTCs {3088,3403,3605,479,3250,4993,3492}.

Fusions involving *RET* occur in PTC {3386,3794,4993}. The prevalence of *RET* rearrangement in papillary carcinoma varies significantly among various geographical regions. In sporadic tumours, *CCDC6::RET* is the most common form of *RET* rearrangement (60–70%), followed by *NCOA4::RET* (20–30%). A strong association between radiation-induced papillary carcinoma and expression of *RET* rearrangement has been found. In PTC occurring among children affected by the Chernobyl nuclear accident, *NCOA4::RET* was found to be the most common form of rearrangement, followed by *CCDC6::RET* {2594, 3250,3037}. The other molecular targets involved in the pathogenesis of radiation-associated PTC involve primary chromosomal rearrangements causing gene fusions in NTRK and other oncogenes {2785,1202,3100,4348}.

Alterations in copy number, gene expression, and microRNA expression have been reported in PTC {4800,815}.

Although the pathogenesis of syndromic familial non-medullary thyroid carcinoma is well known (e.g. germline mutation in *APC* for familial adenomatous polyposis), the genetic basis of non-syndromic familial non-medullary thyroid carcinoma remains poorly understood {636,1049,3488,614} (see *Non-syndromic familial follicular cell–derived thyroid tumours*, p. 488).

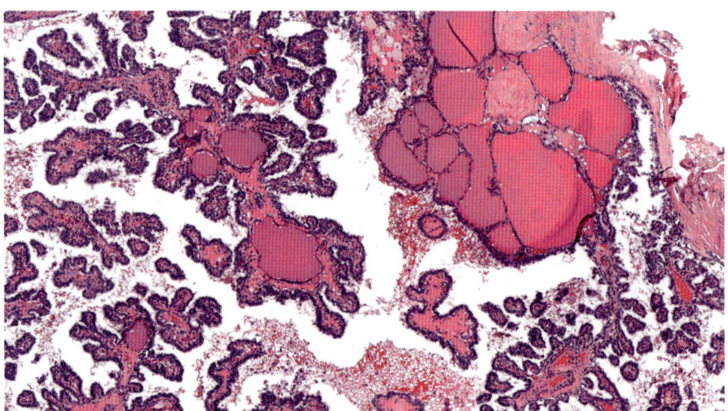

Fig. 3.45 Papillary thyroid carcinoma, classic. The tumour is composed of papillae and follicles.

Macroscopic appearance

The gross appearance of PTC can be quite variable. Most variations in the gross appearance of PTC are related to subtypes and are discussed in their descriptions. Typically, PTC measures more than 10–15 mm, often averaging 20–30 mm, although large tumours can also occur. The tumour nodule is usually firm and white in colour, with an infiltrative appearance. Focal intratumoural calcification is a common feature; however, in some cases it may be extensive or (rarely) associated with ossification. Because of extensive sclerosis, some PTCs may grossly resemble a scar. Cystic formation of varying degrees is not uncommon in PTC; rarely, some lesions may be entirely cystic. Necrosis (in the absence of a prior needle biopsy) is not a feature of PTC and suggests transformation to high-grade follicular cell–derived carcinoma or undifferentiated carcinoma {648,2706,1987}.

Histopathology

The hallmark features of classic (conventional) PTC are the papillae and the nuclear features. The neoplastic papillae contain a central thin core of fibrovascular (occasionally just fibrous) tissue lined by one or (occasionally) several layers of tumour cells with crowded oval nuclei. The papillae may be long, straight, or arborizing; arranged in a parallel regimented fashion, short and stubby; or tightly packed, imparting a solid appearance to the tumour on low magnification. The cores of the papillae are usually composed of loose connective tissue and thin-walled vessels of various sizes. It is rare to encounter cases of PTC showing exclusively papillary formations. Most PTCs will show interspersed neoplastic follicles containing thick colloid and lined by cells with nuclear features similar to those of the cells lining the papillae {4699,648,4700,2511,2706}.

The tumour cells of PTC show a distinct set of nuclear features that can be categorized as changes in size and shape, irregularities of the membrane, and chromatin characteristics {3421}. The nuclei are larger and more elongated or oval in shape than normal follicular cell nuclei and often show overlapping. The nuclear envelope shows marked remodelling, which is evident from irregular contours, nuclear pseudoinclusions, and/or prominent intranuclear grooves {4699,4700,648,2706}. The characteristic nuclear pseudoinclusions seen in PTC are due to deep cytoplasmic invaginations into the nucleus, often eccentrically placed, lightly acidophilic, and round in shape, with sharp outlines due to the peripheral condensation of chromatin. Intranuclear grooves are another characteristic feature of PTC. However, these can occur in other non-neoplastic lesions and neoplasms of the thyroid {1074,85,288}. The other characteristic feature of PTC nuclei is an empty appearance of the nucleoplasm. This feature has been variously described as optically clear, empty, or ground glass {1773}.

The cytoplasm of the tumour cells is generally slightly eosinophilic. Mitotic figures are usually rare or absent {2587} (excluding foci of reactive changes due to preoperative FNAB). A focal solid growth pattern can be seen in classic PTC and does not indicate a different subtype or high-grade transformation {85, 294,613}.

Psammoma bodies, round calcific concretions that exhibit concentric lamination, are found in 40–50% of cases of PTC

{2123,2339}. They are commonly seen in the PTC subtypes with papillary growth patterns {2123,2511}. True psammoma bodies are seen within the main tumour mass, in associated tumour stroma, and within lymphatic channels {2123,3597}. Psammoma body–like calcifications of the colloid (pseudopsammoma bodies) can be encountered in benign conditions such as chronic lymphocytic thyroiditis, toxic goitre {3458,1178, 1229}, and non-papillary follicular-patterned and oncocytic follicular tumours and they should not be considered diagnostic of PTC {1993,85,1764}.

Focal or extensive squamous differentiation can be encountered in PTC (in ~15–45% of cases) {3441,648}. Desmoplasia, in either the central or the peripheral zone of the tumour, is seen in PTC; encapsulated tumours will show dense sclerosis in the areas of capsular invasion {648}. Scattered lymphocytes are common (rarely, there is extensive infiltrate) at the invasive edges of the tumour {648,2706,4708,4585}. Cyst formation of varying proportions may occur in PTC. Most cases of cystic PTC will show readily identifiable papillary formations lined by tumour cells. However, in other instances the papillae can be few in number and lined by attenuated, flattened, benign-appearing epithelium {648,5020,2706}.

PTC invades the thyroid gland lymphatics, which accounts for its high incidence of regional node metastases {648,2706}. PTC can also present as multifocal tumours within the same gland {3581,3389}. Multifocality of PTC can be due to intrathyroidal lymphatic spread from one tumour source or multifocal primary tumours {2443,1530,2749,3149}.

Vascular (blood vessel) invasion is rare in PTC and can be identified in up to 7% of cases {2796,1466,1324,4986}. It is more often seen in encapsulated PTC or TCPTC {2796,1466, 1324,1550,4986,4749}. Regional lymph node metastases are extremely common (≥ 80%) at the initial presentation of usual papillary carcinomas {3150,2988,4200,4619}. Histological grading is of no use in papillary carcinoma because > 95% of these lesions are low-grade {1676}. See also *High-grade follicular cell–derived non-anaplastic thyroid carcinoma* (p. 165).

PTC measuring ≤ 10 mm has been termed PTC-microcarcinoma (also termed occult sclerosing carcinoma, occult papillary carcinoma, or incidental PTC). Although not endorsed, this same terminology has been applied by some authors to tumours measuring up to 15 mm {4318,291,3898,1827,3444, 1931}. These lesions are common and are often encountered during autopsy or in thyroidectomies for benign thyroid disease, completion thyroidectomy, and thyroid removal during surgery for carcinoma of a neighbouring organ (laryngeal carcinoma). The incidence of PTC-microcarcinoma has been reported to be as high as 36% in meticulously sectioned thyroid specimens. Because of their small size, these lesions can be missed on gross examination. By histology, a typical case of microcarcinoma will show an infiltrative scar-like pattern with neoplastic elements either at the periphery or embedded within. Some cases are completely encapsulated by a thick fibrous capsule, which may be focally calcified. Histologically, the tumours may be totally follicular-patterned or demonstrate papillary areas as well; they can also occur as other histological subtypes of PTC {1552,3483,959}. Overall, the prognosis of PTC-microcarcinoma is excellent. However, lymph node metastasis and distant metastasis have been reported, almost always at presentation {3816,97,1246,1552,1497}. Aggressive clinical behaviour in PTC-microcarcinoma is associated with specific PTC-subtype histology, vascular invasion, location within the thyroid gland (peripheral vs central), molecular profile, and family history of PTC {4321,5099,4096,2562,1931,1690}. In 2003, during a meeting held in Porto, Portugal, some authors proposed renaming papillary microcarcinomas as papillary microtumours if they lack aggressive clinicopathological features {3816}. More recently, Aliyev et al. defined papillary microtumour on the basis of the following exclusion criteria: (1) patient aged < 19 years, (2) multiple tumour foci measuring in aggregate > 10 mm when all foci diameters are added, and (3) aggressive histological features (extrathyroidal extension, angioinvasion, tall and/or hobnail cells) {97}. This approach, named the updated Porto proposal, has been shown in one study to identify those papillary microcarcinomas with extremely low malignant potential {97}.

It is recommended that papillary microcarcinoma should not be considered a distinct subtype, because size alone is not a sufficient criterion to consider it a subtype. For this reason, the current classification requires the subtyping of papillary microcarcinomas (e.g. classic microcarcinoma).

Immunohistochemistry

By immunohistochemistry, PTC cells express thyroid transcription factor 1 (TTF1), PAX8, thyroglobulin, and cytokeratins

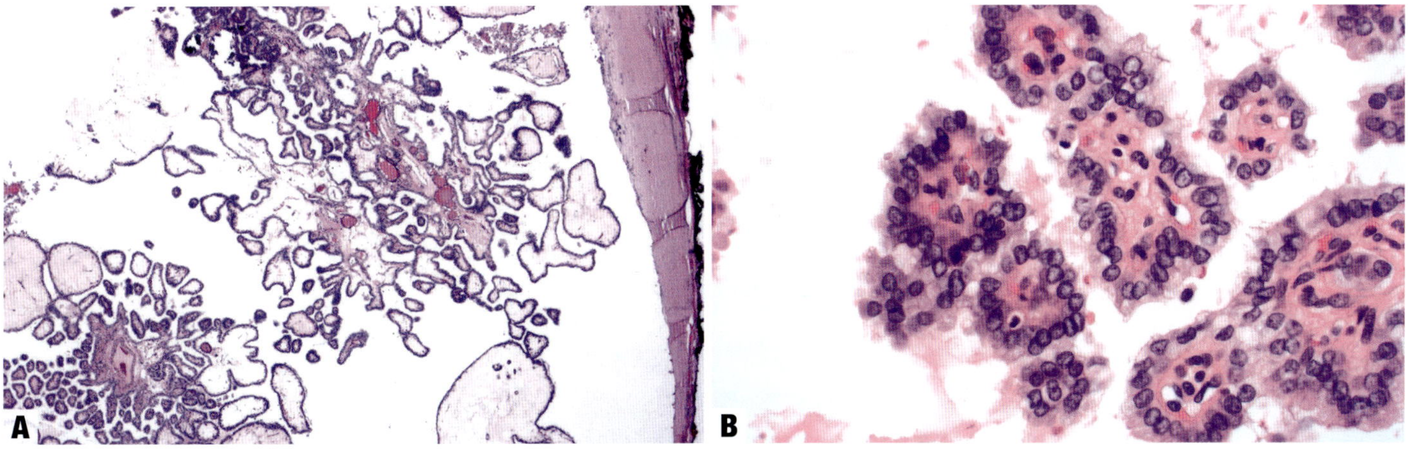

Fig. 3.46 Papillary thyroid carcinoma, encapsulated subtype. **A** Low-magnification view showing an encapsulated tumour with partial cystic change and papillary architecture. **B** The papillae are lined by tumour cells with enlarged, irregular, overlapping nuclei with chromatin clearing and grooves.

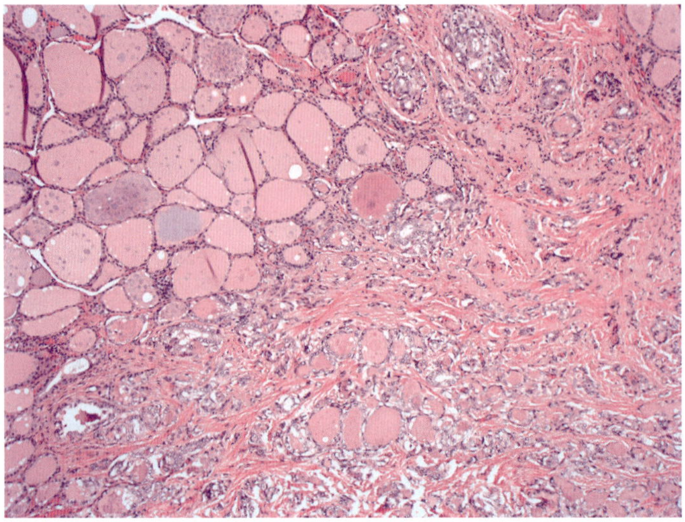

Fig. 3.47 Papillary thyroid carcinoma, infiltrative follicular variant. The tumour is exclusively composed of follicles infiltrating the normal thyroid. Intratumoural fibrosis can be seen.

(pancytokeratin, AE1/AE3, CK7, and CAM5.2) {284}. They are negative for CK20, calcitonin, and neuroendocrine markers {284}. Mucicarmine positivity of varying proportions can be encountered in PTC {746,1329,5019,613}. Immunostains for HBME1, galectin-3, CK19, and CD56 have been shown to help differentiate between PTC and benign lesions with either papillary architecture and/or atypical nuclei {3680,3813,4072, 1028,1691,729}. However, none of these markers is specific and may be seen in benign lesions {3832,4053,1691}, as well as in low-risk follicular-patterned tumours including non-invasive follicular thyroid neoplasm with papillary-like nuclear features {1691}. Immunostaining for BRAF p.V600E using the VE1 clone is highly sensitive and specific for the detection of the mutation in PTC {560}. To be considered positive, the staining should be cytoplasmic and diffuse throughout the tumour (≥ 90% staining) {560,3445,4156}. Other potential biomarker immunostains employed in the diagnosis of PTC include mutation-specific antibodies to RAS, and antibodies to RET, ALK, and pan-TRK, which are overexpressed in tumours with oncogenic fusions {181,3303,3914}.

Histological subtypes of PTC

Encapsulated PTC

Encapsulated PTC is defined as classic PTC enveloped by a thick fibrous capsule, which may be intact or infiltrated by tumour with or without extension into the surrounding thyroid parenchyma {1550,4972,4973,268}. It accounts for approximately 10% of all cases. The differential diagnosis includes follicular adenoma with papillary architecture and papillary hyperplastic nodule {1550,4972,4973}.

Infiltrative follicular variant of PTC

After classic PTC, the follicular variant of PTC (FVPTC) is the second most common histological subtype of PTC {742,1550, 797,4395,3986}. It exclusively or almost exclusively shows a follicular growth pattern {742,3986,2708}. Two major forms are known: infiltrative FVPTC and invasive encapsulated FVPTC {3756,4972,1550}. The majority of follicular PTCs are encapsulated FVPTCs, which are RAS-like tumours; these are described in *Invasive encapsulated follicular variant of papillary thyroid carcinoma* (p. 147). Infiltrative FVPTC is quite rare and clinically behaves like classic PTC {3756,4972,2295}. Despite the almost exclusive follicular-patterned growth in the primary site, features that suggest that a tumour is a papillary carcinoma include clear nuclei, psammoma bodies, and sclerosis in the foci of infiltration. In addition, some of these tumours are accompanied by multicentric tumour foci of classic PTC within the same gland and cervical lymph node metastasis, with some showing papillary architecture (classic PTC features) {3756,1550,4972,3406}.

Oncocytic PTC

Oncocytic changes can occur in PTCs with a follicular growth pattern as well as in those with a solid pattern. The term "OPTC" (or "pure OPTC") is reserved for those very rare neoplasms composed of well-developed papillae (and rare follicles) all lined by oncocytic cells with nuclear features of PTC {398,678, 1128,212}. The nuclei can be similar to those of papillary carcinoma, although in a few studied cases, large nucleoli reminiscent of those seen in oncocytes were seen. OPTC should be distinguished from TCPTC. In contrast to OPTC cells, TCPTC cells have a height that is at least three times their width and a polarized nucleus (in a basal or apical position).

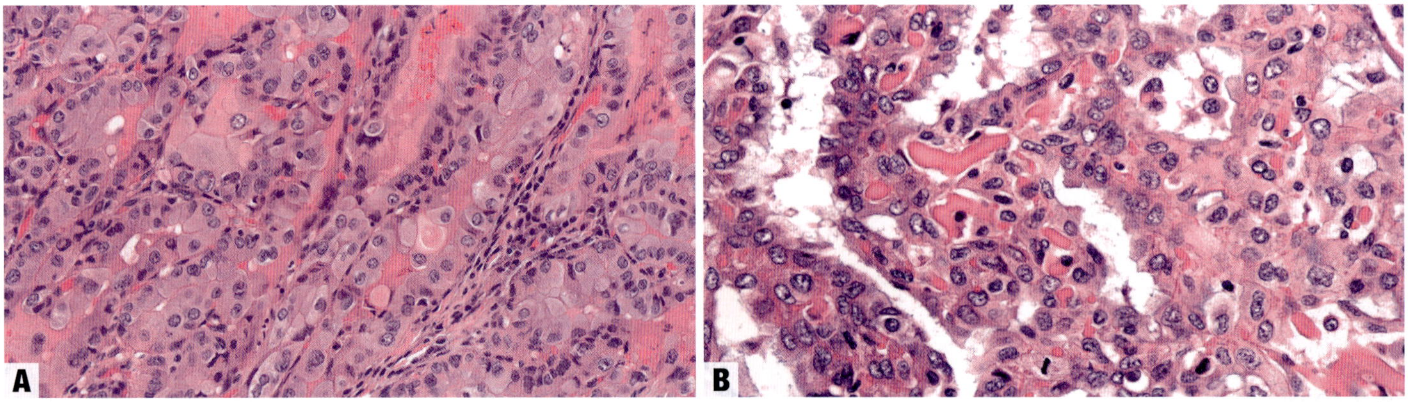

Fig. 3.48 Papillary thyroid carcinoma, oncocytic subtype. **A** The tumour is composed of papillae and follicles lined by follicular epithelial cells that have abundant granular eosinophilic cytoplasm and the characteristic nuclear atypia of papillary carcinoma. **B** High-magnification view showing papillae lined by tumour cells with oncocytic cytoplasm and papillary thyroid carcinoma nuclei that lack polarization.

Warthin-like PTC

WLPTC can present as a well-circumscribed or infiltrative tumour and shares morphological similarities with Warthin tumour of the salivary gland. It is composed of papillae lined by oncocytic cells, with the papillary cores rich in lymphocytes and plasma cells. It almost always occurs in a background of well-developed to severe chronic lymphocytic thyroiditis (Hashimoto thyroiditis) {163,297,1278,2447}. The neoplastic cells resemble the metaplastic follicular cells in the thyroiditis so the neoplasm is sometimes overlooked at low magnification. Transition to TCPTC can occur in WLPTC and it is usually found at the invasive edge of the tumour.

Clear cell PTC

Clear cell changes occur in both benign and malignant thyroid lesions and are usually associated with other usual features, such as oncocytic changes {647,4023,220,866}. Histologically, clear cells can grow in papillae or solid sheets and often show typical PTC nuclei {4669,647,866,3819}.

Metastatic clear cell renal cell carcinoma, intrathyroidal parathyroid tumours, and clear cell medullary thyroid carcinoma are the main differential diagnoses; immunostains for thyroid transcription factor 1 (TTF1), chromogranin, calcitonin, PTH, or renal cell carcinoma markers may be required {866}.

Diffuse sclerosing PTC (DSPTC)

DSPTC is a rare subtype of PTC, representing only about 3% of all PTCs {3560,4748,879}. It is characterized by diffuse involvement of a single lobe or the entire thyroid gland with extensive lymphatic permeation, dense sclerosis, numerous psammoma bodies, and associated chronic lymphocytic thyroiditis. Tumour appears as solid nests and papillary formations with squamous metaplasia. Some cases may show a large focus of classic PTC. The lymphatics are extensively involved by psammoma bodies with or without accompanying viable tumour cells {3560, 1907}. This tumour is common in children and young adults, and it represented 10% of PTCs seen in children exposed to radioactive iodine after the Chernobyl accident {5105,1437}. Compared with other PTCs, there is a higher incidence of potentially actionable gene rearrangements, usually involving *RET*, *NTRK3*, *NTRK1*, *ALK*, or *BRAF*, and a relatively lower incidence of the *BRAF* p.V600E mutations, which are found in about 20% of cases {841,4016}.

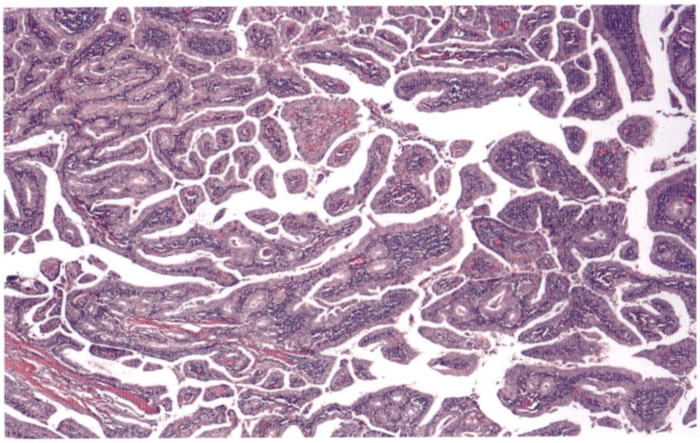

Fig. 3.49 Papillary thyroid carcinoma, Warthin-like subtype. Medium-power view showing papillary structures lined by oncocytic tumour cells and a lymphocytic plasmacytic infiltrate in the core of the papillae.

Solid/trabecular PTC

SPTC represents 1–3% of all adult PTCs. It is common in children and was reported in > 30% of children after the Chernobyl accident {3254,3326,3197,3325,4753}. A diagnosis of SPTC requires the presence of a solid, trabecular, or nested growth pattern in > 50% of the tumour mass {294}. The stroma separating the tumour sheets and nests usually shows thin and delicate fibrovascular bands; however, some cases may show foci of dense sclerosis. A few well-formed neoplastic papillae and abortive follicular groups can occur. The tumour cells show mostly rounded nuclei with other features of PTC {4751,3325, 4753}. Because of its growth pattern, SPTC should not be mistaken for aggressive high-grade follicular cell–derived thyroid carcinoma. In contrast to the latter, SPTC lacks tumour necrosis and a high mitotic rate (see also *High-grade follicular cell–derived non-anaplastic thyroid carcinoma*, p. 165).

PTC with fibromatosis/fasciitis-like/desmoid-type stroma

The hallmark diagnostic feature of this very rare (< 1% of all adult PTCs) subtype of PTC is characterized by abundant cellular stroma resembling nodular fasciitis, desmoid fibromatosis, or other myofibroblastic processes {2511,1588,3701,4375, 4344}. The epithelial tumour cells embedded within the stroma usually form cords, tubules, and compressed papillae, and

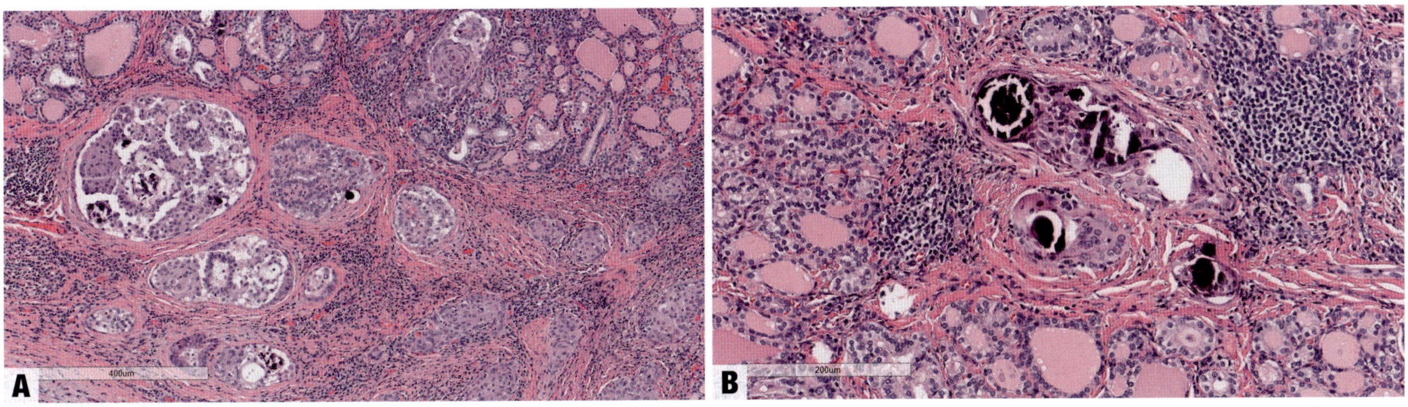

Fig. 3.50 Papillary thyroid carcinoma, diffuse sclerosing subtype. **A** The tumour infiltrates throughout the gland in small nests with prominent calcifications and focal squamous metaplasia. **B** The infiltrating tumour nests are associated with numerous psammoma bodies.

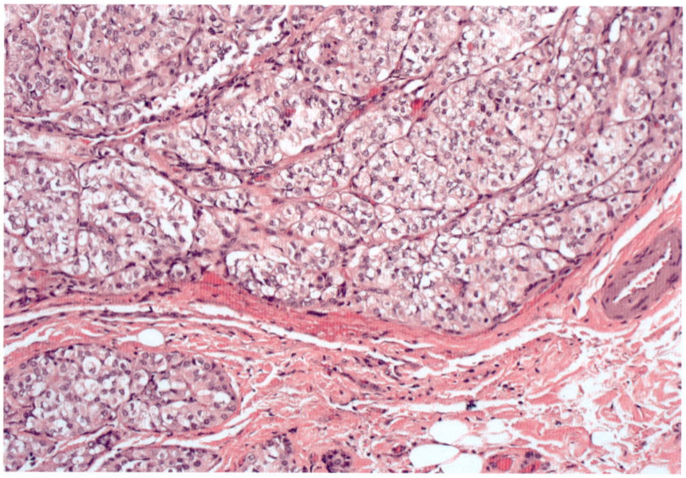

Fig. 3.51 Papillary thyroid carcinoma, solid subtype. The tumour is composed of solid nests separated by thin fibrovascular bands.

show nuclear features of PTC. Varying degrees of squamous metaplasia can occur in these tumours. The stroma can be cellular, show myxoid change, or be densely collagenous, like the stroma seen in scar/keloid and desmoid tumours {3701}. The stromal cells do not demonstrate nuclear atypia. PTC with fibromatosis/fasciitis-like stroma should be distinguished from spindle cell anaplastic carcinoma arising in PTC and the paucicellular subtype of anaplastic carcinoma. Immunohistochemical analysis should help in arriving at the correct diagnosis. The stromal cells in PTC with fibromatosis/fasciitis-like stroma are negative for cytokeratins and show expression of desmin, SMA, β-catenin (nuclear accumulation), and cytoplasmic SOX11 {3701,4377,4923,4344}. The epithelial cells express TTF1, PAX8, and thyroglobulin {3701,4375}.

Spindle cell PTC

Thyroid spindle cell lesions are rare {3416}, and spindle cell metaplasia in PTC is even rarer. Spindle cell areas may be focal or diffuse in PTC, but this subtype is characterized by a predominance (> 50%) of spindle cells with nuclear features of PTC. Their presence does not modify the prognosis of the tumour, but a case of spindle cell transformation carrying a poor prognosis has been reported {518}; however, data are generally lacking. Spindle cell areas are made up of cytologically bland, elongated cells arranged in bundles, with less-pronounced nuclear clearing or pseudoinclusions than in classic PTC {613}. Spindle cells do not show increased mitotic activity or necrosis. They are immunoreactive for pancytokeratin and markers of thyroid lineage (thyroglobulin, TTF1, and PAX8) {2885,2773,613}, but negative for calcitonin/chromogranin, confirming their follicular origin. These cells are not associated with post-FNA reactive change. The main differential diagnoses include PTC with fibromatosis stroma, anaplastic carcinoma, medullary carcinoma, and spindle epithelial tumour with thymus-like elements.

Tall cell PTC

By definition, TCPTC is composed of cells whose height is at least three times their width and that show abundant eosinophilic cytoplasm with a prominent cell membrane {4916}. The typical nuclear features of PTC, especially intranuclear pseudoinclusions, are easily found. Tall cells should represent ≥ 30% of the PTC cells to make the diagnosis of TCPTC {1869,294, 3197,4588}.

TCPTC shows an exuberant and tightly knitted growth pattern of elongated follicles, giving rise to a tram-track appearance. The differential diagnosis of TCPTC includes thyroid tumours with papillary architecture and oncocytic features, such as WLPTC, OPTC, and rare cases of oncocytic carcinoma with papillary architecture. Like other differentiated follicular-derived carcinomas, these tumours express TTF1, PAX8, and thyroglobulin. A high Ki-67 labelling index (≥ 5%) has been reported in TCPTC {2060}.

Hobnail PTC (HNPTC)

HNPTC is an aggressive subtype of PTC, which derives its name from the peculiar feature of its tumour cells having enlarged nuclei that bulge from the apical surface (hobnail appearance). This subtype is defined by the presence of > 30% hobnails and accounts for < 1% of PTCs {229,227,126,294,3197,2058,3313}. There is a female predominance and a mean age of > 55 years at diagnosis. These tumours usually have a complex papillary or micropapillary architecture, although areas of follicular architecture may be present. Nuclear features of PTC are present; however, there is often more pleomorphism than is typically seen in classic PTC. High-grade features are often present (i.e. frequent mitoses and/or tumour necrosis), and thus many HNPTCs qualify as high-grade follicular cell–derived carcinomas {4915}.

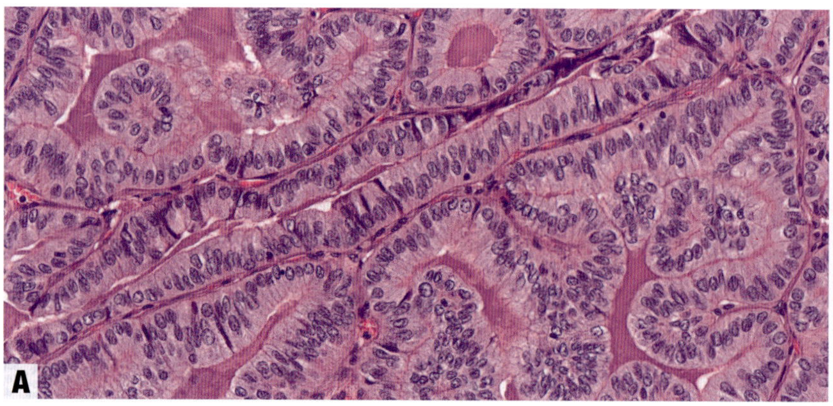

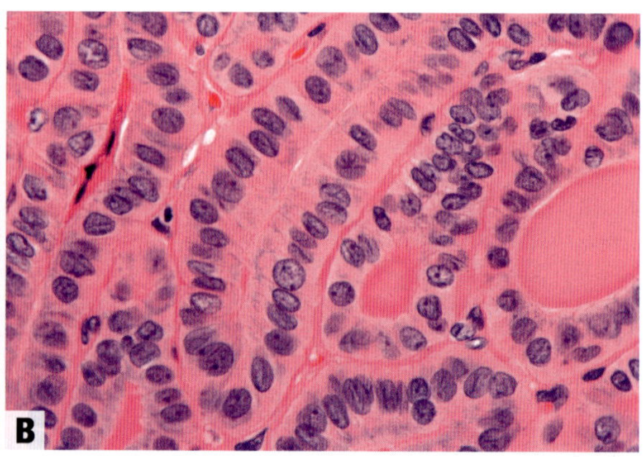

Fig. 3.52 Papillary thyroid carcinoma, tall cell subtype. **A** The tumour is composed of complex papillary and elongated trabecular formations that have a tram-track appearance. They are lined by crowded cells that have a height-to-width ratio of ≥ 3:1. **B** Tumour cells with an eosinophilic cytoplasm and a height three times their width.

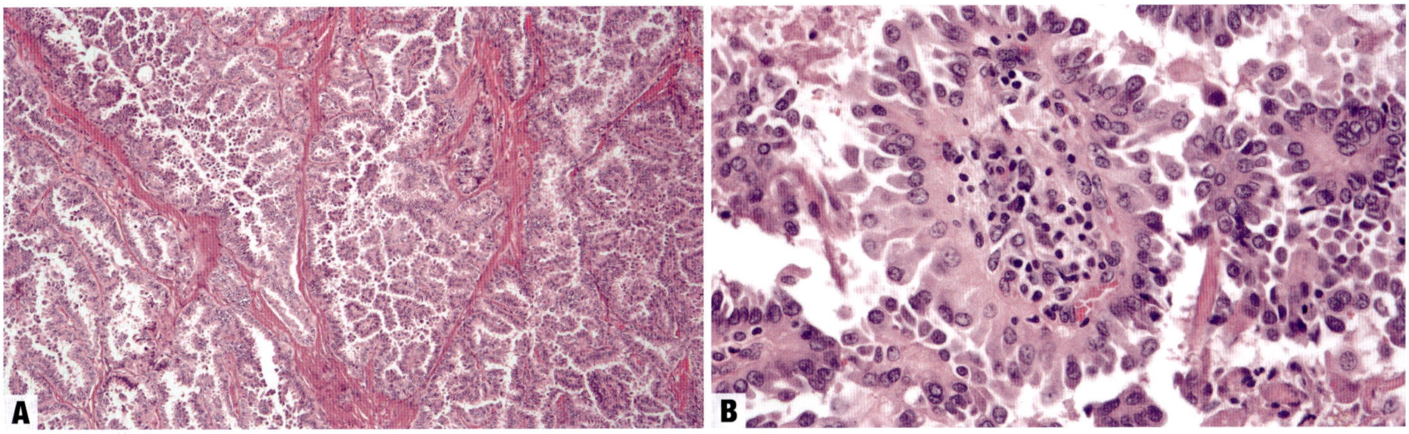

Fig. 3.53 Papillary thyroid carcinoma, hobnail subtype. **A** These tumours usually have a complex papillary or micropapillary architecture. **B** This subtype of papillary thyroid carcinoma contains tumour cells with enlarged nuclei that bulge from the apical surface (hobnail appearance).

Vascular invasion and gross extrathyroidal extension are frequently present, and there is a high rate of lymph node and distant metastases detected either at the time of initial presentation or with disease progression.

These tumours are extremely rare in pure form and should be generously sampled and carefully examined, because they are usually intermixed with areas showing progression to high-grade differentiated, poorly differentiated, and anaplastic thyroid carcinoma {2752,122,616}.

HNPTC generally has an immunohistochemical profile similar to that of classic PTC; however, the Ki-67 proliferation index is often > 5% and a subset of tumours overexpress p53 {229}. Molecular analysis has shown that most tumours harbour *BRAF* p.V600E mutations {3087,4434,4829,2592,2752}, although *RET* rearrangements have been reported {2752}. Additionally, *TP53* mutations, *TERT* promoter mutations, and *PIK3CA* mutations are common {3087,4434,4829}. Additional genes with alterations reported include *CTNNB1*, *EGFR*, *AKT1*, *ATM*, *ARID2*, and *NOTCH1* {3087,4914}.

Columnar cell PTC (CCPTC)

CCPTC is a rare PTC subtype, composed of columnar cells with pale eosinophilic to clear cytoplasm, and prominent nuclear pseudostratification. Subnuclear vacuoles may be present that impart an appearance reminiscent of secretory endometrium. Nuclear clearing and grooves are evident in some tumours but subtle in others. Pseudoinclusions are generally absent. The tumour is hypercellular, with areas of crowded elongated follicles admixed with thin papillae. Morphologically, these tumours can be distinguished from TCPTC by their typical cellular features. Because of the unusual morphology of CCPTC, metastases from other sites may be considered (e.g. endometrial or colorectal primaries). Like other PTCs, these tumours are positive for PAX8, TTF1, and thyroglobulin. Additionally, as many as 55% have been shown to be positive for CDX2 {1254,4327}. The prognosis of this subtype depends on its encapsulation and infiltrative status {4853}. Infiltrative CCPTCs are usually large (often > 40 mm), invasive tumours with frequent gross extrathyroidal extension {4203,1297,779,1254,2090}. These tumours often have high-grade features (necrosis and increased mitotic count) and many can be classified as high-grade follicular cell–derived thyroid carcinoma {2090}. Distant metastases are frequently present at the time of initial diagnosis or develop with disease progression.

Cytology

Smears are usually moderate to highly cellular and demonstrate complex papillary structures with fibrovascular cores, rounded papillary fragments without cores, crowded monolayered sheets showing nuclear overlapping and often moulding, and 3D groups with cellular swirls in a background of watery or ropy (chewing-gum like) colloid. The background may also contain calcific debris,

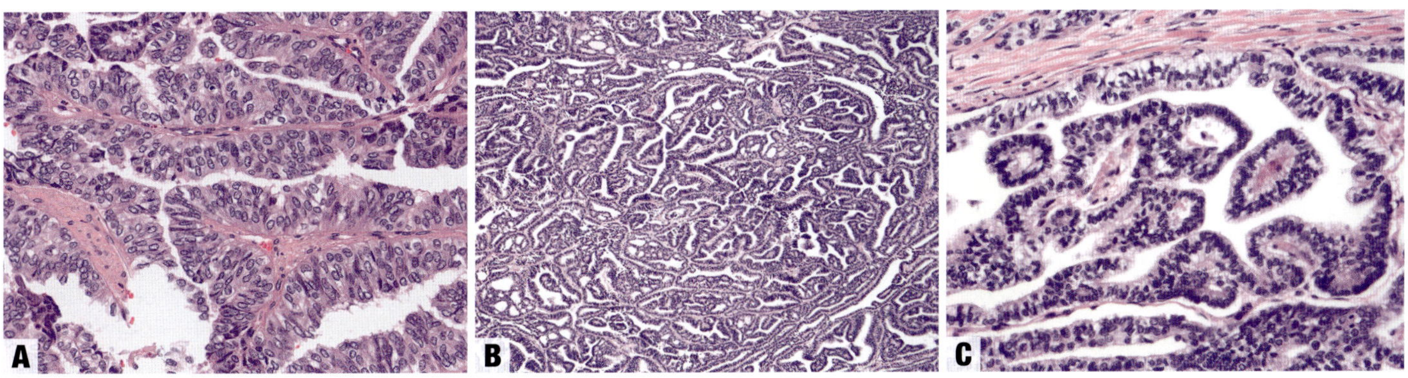

Fig. 3.54 Papillary thyroid carcinoma, columnar cell subtype. **A** The tumour is composed of complex papillae lined by crowded elongated pseudostratified epithelial cells. **B** The tumour is hypercellular with areas of crowded elongated follicles admixed with thin papillae. **C** Subnuclear vacuoles may be present that impart an appearance reminiscent of secretory endometrium.

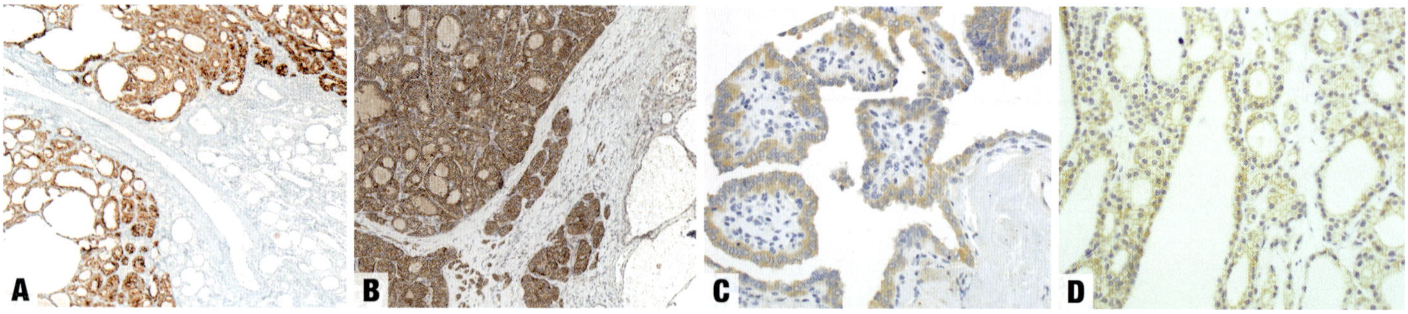

Fig. 3.55 Papillary thyroid carcinoma. **A** This photomicrograph shows a papillary thyroid carcinoma harbouring *ALK* fusion, highlighted by immunohistochemistry using the 5A4 antibody, which is optimized to detect *ALK* fusions. **B** This photomicrograph shows an NTRK fusion–harbouring papillary thyroid carcinoma that is positive for pan-TRK antibody. **C** Papillae and follicles lined by cells that have the characteristic nuclear features of papillary thyroid carcinoma and are strongly immunopositive for BRAF p.V600E. **D** Encapsulated follicular variant of papillary thyroid carcinoma. The tumour is composed of follicles lined by cells with enlarged, clear, irregular, overlapping nuclei. An immunostain directed against the NRAS p.Q61R–mutated protein shows cytoplasmic and membranous staining in the tumour.

macrophages, multinucleated giant cells, and stromal fragments. The individual tumour cells are enlarged and elongated or oval, with well-defined cytoplasm. The diagnostic feature of PTC is the typical nuclei, which are elongated, with thickened membranes and often a pleomorphic shape; pale, powdery, even chromatin (Pap); grooves (often delicate and more easily seen on Pap); and pseudoinclusions. The one or more nucleoli are small and eccentrically placed {2314,1421,990,4366}.

Cytopathological features of PTC subtypes

FNAB diagnosis of FVPTC can be challenging in some cases, because of the paucity of the nuclear features of PTC. FVPTC shows enlarged follicular cells arranged in monolayer sheets and microfollicles in a background of thin and thick colloid {2080,990,1746,4535}. Thin colloid can be abundant in cases containing an appreciable number of enlarged, dilated follicles {5107,2720}. The intranuclear grooves in FVPTC are delicate and do not traverse the entire length of the nucleus {2720,285}, and intranuclear pseudoinclusions can be scarce, especially in liquid-based cytology {285,2720,5149}. Diffuse sclerosing PTC shows ball-like tissue fragments of tumour cells with or without flat sheets and papillary fragments, consisting of cells with well-demarcated squamoid dense cytoplasm and nuclear features of PTC, although inclusions and grooves may be scant. A hobnail outer margin to the tissue fragments, squamous metaplasia, and unilocular vacuoles in the cytoplasm are frequent. Psammoma bodies along with specks of coarse calcifications and calcific debris are numerous. A brisk lymphocytic infiltrate is always seen closely associated with tumour cell fragments and in the background {4378,3833,2572,1299}. The diagnosis of WLPTC can be difficult in FNAB preparations because of the presence of a heavy lymphoplasmacytic infiltrate into the fibrovascular stalks and oncocytic cells of papillary tissue fragments and in the background chronic lymphocytic thyroiditis. Oncocytic tumour cells with nuclear features of PTC are present {4672,3391,4952}. TCPTC smears show elongated cells with distinct cytoplasmic borders, granular cytoplasm, and elongated variably sized nuclei with readily identified PTC features including relatively frequent pseudoinclusions and more prominent central nucleoli {4219,4625,1686,4408}. Intranuclear inclusions can be multiple and variably sized within the same nucleus, giving rise to a soap-bubble appearance {4219}. HNPTC smears tend to be highly cellular, with a bloody background and scant colloid with micropapillary tissue fragments consisting of elongated cells with polarized eccentric nuclei and tapering cytoplasm attached to the tissue fragment, leading to a teardrop or comet-like appearance {231,2592,3828}. Similar single cells are present. Multiple intranuclear inclusions may also result in a soap bubble–like nuclear appearance similar to that seen in TCPTC. CCPTC can have cytopathological features that overlap with those of classic PTC, showing marked cellularity, with papillary tissue fragments covered by elongated cells with pseudostratified oval nuclei, which are more hyperchromatic and show infrequent to absent nuclear pseudoinclusions and grooves {467}. Necrosis and mucin are not seen in the background.

The cytopathological features of other rare subtypes of PTC have been described in the literature {1144,4628,3327,1299}.

Diagnostic molecular pathology

Currently, molecular genetics is not required for the histopathological diagnosis of PTC but is increasingly being relied upon for clinical decision-making, particularly for surgical planning in cases with indeterminate cytology as well as for additional decision-making surrounding treatment goals (inoperable tumour with possibilities for neoadjuvant treatment) {3265,2703,1884}. Currently, platforms for preoperative and postoperative molecular testing are either commercially available or developed in laboratories in academic medical centres. Preoperative testing determines the need for surgery. Postoperative molecular testing typically is for the purposes of subclassification and/or the documentation of targetable/actionable mutations {375,4912, 3251}. Germline screening for genetic susceptibility is considered on the basis of clinicopathological findings.

Essential and desirable diagnostic criteria

Essential: a carcinoma of follicular cell derivation characterized by a set of distinct nuclear features, with either papillary or solid growth or invasive features.

Staging

PTC is staged according to the Union for International Cancer Control (UICC) and American Joint Committee on Cancer (AJCC) staging systems, incorporating age at diagnosis.

Prognosis and prediction

PTC is typically associated with long-term survival; survival rates are 96% at 5 years, 93% at 10 years, and > 90% at 20 years.

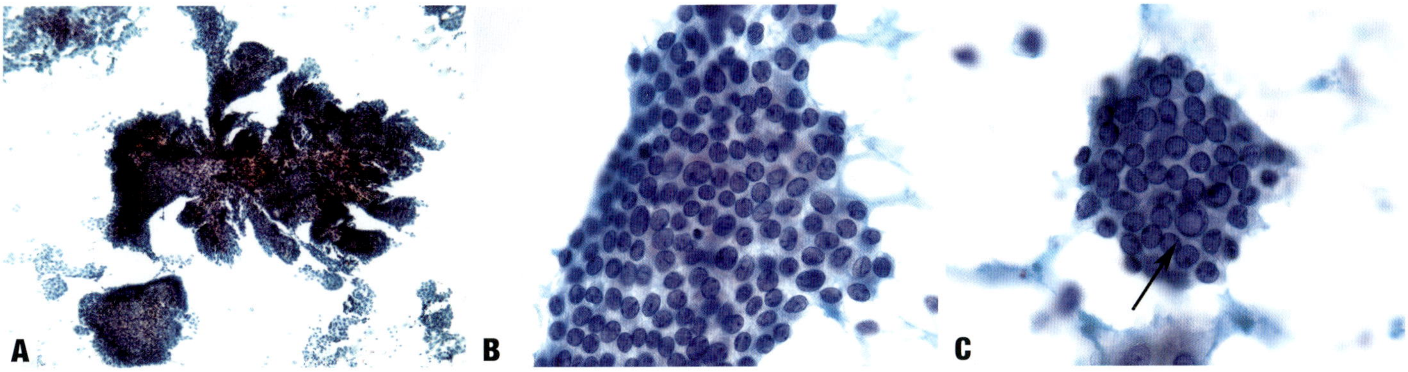

Fig. 3.56 Papillary thyroid carcinoma, classic, FNA. **A** Low-magnification view showing complex papillary architecture. **B** Typical nuclear features. **C** Typical nuclear features with an intranuclear inclusion (arrow).

Overall, mortality rates for PTC are 1–6.5%, and reported overall recurrence rates are 15–35%, with tumour recurrence occurring either in the tumour bed or cervical neck lymph nodes, or rarely at distant sites {4975,4796,3001,865}.

The prognosis in PTC is influenced by the clinical extent of the disease; the 10-year survival rate is > 99% for stage I disease and drops to < 50% for stage IV disease. Poor prognostic factors in PTC include older age at diagnosis, male sex, large tumour size, and gross extrathyroidal growth. Pathological variables associated with a more guarded prognosis include vascular invasion (specifically venous invasion) {2955,3105,4796,4975,3001,4236,2289}.

Although some studies found that non-syndromic familial non-medullary thyroid carcinoma-PTCs have a similar behaviour to sporadic PTCs {3767}, other publications reported a higher risk of multifocality, extrathyroidal invasion, lateral lymph node involvement, and recurrence in the familial cases {2901,2591} (see also *Syndromic familial follicular cell–derived thyroid tumours*, p. 482, and *Non-syndromic familial follicular cell–derived thyroid tumours*, p. 488).

Complete excision of a PTC that is confined to the thyroid gland, including central and cervical lymph nodes, is an important determinant of outcome. Incomplete surgical resection and a tumour with gross extrathyroidal extension and extranodal extension of lymph node metastases is associated with increased recurrence. Various professional societies have devised dynamic risk-stratification schemes, which take into account clinical, histopathological, and follow-up data, to care for patients with PTC {1819,1817,2935,1380,2065,2300}.

Early studies suggested that *BRAF* p.V600E mutations are associated with an aggressive clinical course; however, this was predictive only in univariate and not multivariate analysis, and the association may fall away when adjusted for aggressive clinicopathological factors {642,1076,4965}. Therefore, the *BRAF* p.V600E mutation status of a tumour will most probably not alter clinical management; for example, *BRAF*-mutant and *BRAF*-wildtype subcentimetre papillary thyroid carcinomas are treated similarly. Some studies have also identified *TERT* promoter mutation alone as an independent prognostic variable that may play a role in distant metastasis. PTCs with coexistent *BRAF* p.V600E and *TERT* promoter mutations were shown to have worse disease-specific survival than those with either mutation alone {2690,3436,962,4201}. Although these molecular markers are not currently recommended for the postoperative prognostication and management of PTC {1817}, they can provide valuable targets for those PTCs that are refractory to conventional treatment protocols.

Children with PTC have larger primary tumours, more regional nodal metastasis, and a higher rate of distant disease at presentation than adults with PTC {1828}. In a comparative study of 190 children and 4242 adults with PTC, 75% of the children presented with regional nodal metastasis, 17% with extrathyroidal

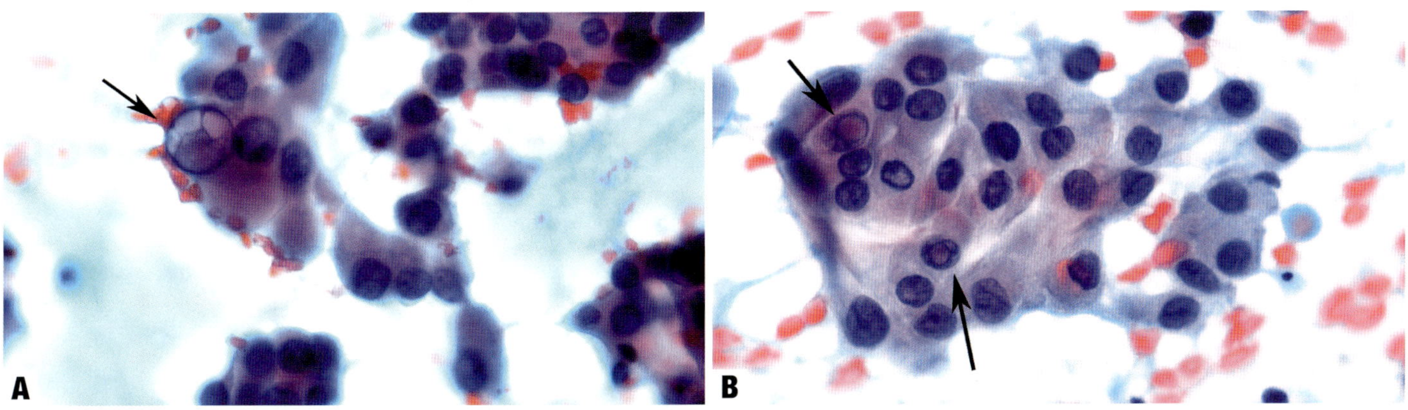

Fig. 3.57 Papillary thyroid carcinoma. **A** Oncocytic subtype. FNA specimen (Pap-stained alcohol-fixed smear preparation). Smear showing elongated tumour cells with dense cytoplasm and nuclei with soap-bubble intranuclear inclusions (arrow). **B** Tall cell FNA (Pap-stained alcohol-fixed smear preparation). Smear showing a tissue fragment of elongated tumour cells with dense cytoplasm and multiple intranuclear inclusions (arrows).

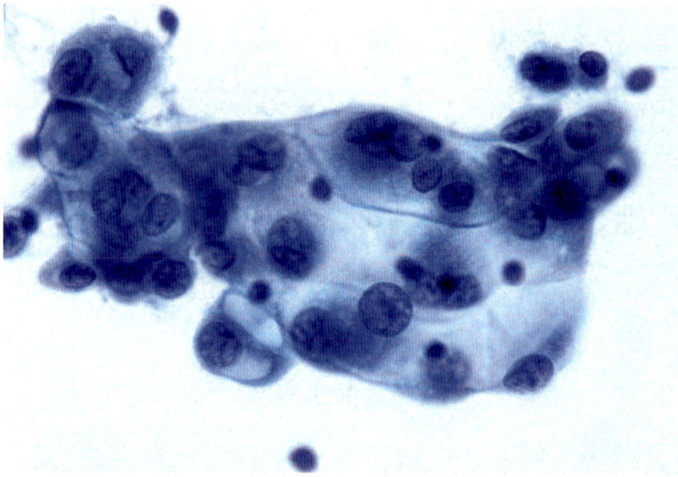

Fig. 3.58 Papillary thyroid carcinoma, diffuse sclerosing subtype. Smear showing tumour cells with foamy cytoplasm arranged in a cohesive group (liquid-based cytology).

extension, and 5% with distant disease, whereas in the adults, regional nodal disease, extrathyroidal extension, and distant metastases were found in 40%, 9%, and 2%, respectively {1828}. Despite presenting with more extensive disease than adults, children with PTC have similar recurrence rates and a much lower mortality {1828}. The difference in mortality is particularly striking in patients with distant metastasis at presentation, where the 20-year disease-specific mortality rate is 63% in adults and 0% in children {1828}.

Encapsulated PTC carries an excellent prognosis, with survival rates nearing 100% {649,646,1818}.

The prognosis for diffuse FVPTC appears to be poor {3047, 2066,1714,2643,294}.

OPTC can metastasize to lymph nodes, but too few cases diagnosed according to the above criteria have been systematically studied to understand their prognosis and clinical outcomes {73,136,4855}.

WLPTC has an excellent long-term prognosis, similar to that of low-risk PTC {297,1278}.

The clear cell subtype has a prognosis similar to that of PTC without cell clearing.

DSPTC is often associated with extrathyroidal extension, extensive cervical lymph node involvement, and distant metastasis {2809,4748,4222,4251,879,4264,841}. Although DSPTC has a lower disease-free survival than classic PTC, its mortality rate is similar to that of classic PTC {4251}. Molecular analyses of DSPTC have revealed a high rate of potentially actionable rearrangements in *RET*, *NTRK3*, *NTRK1*, *ALK*, and *BRAF* {841, 4016}. *BRAF* p.V600E mutations are reported in 20% of cases {3164,4106,839,3111,451,879,841,4016}.

Higher rates of less favourable clinicopathological features have been reported in SPTC. In adults, the prognosis of SPTC appears to be less favourable than that of classic PTC {3254, 3326,3197,4751,3325,4753}.

Typically, TCPTCs occur at an older age than classic PTCs; are large and often associated with extrathyroidal extension; and show mitotic activity, vascular invasion, and locoregional and distant metastasis more often than classic PTCs {1553, 4809,4979,3859,4711,2701}. TCPTCs can follow an aggressive clinical course, with a lower 5-year disease-specific survival rate than classic PTC, and they probably represent a significant proportion of radioiodine-refractory thyroid carcinomas. This aggressive clinical course in TCPTC is probably related to its association with poor prognostic variables: old age, large tumour size, extrathyroidal extension, and high mitotic rate {4588}. Local tumour recurrences and distant metastasis (even to unusual sites) are not uncommon in TCPTC. Even though a diagnosis of TCPTC should be reserved for tumours with TCPTC features constituting ≥ 30% of the tumour, tumours with a smaller TCPTC component (especially > 10% but < 30%) can pursue an aggressive clinical course {1555,3345,4809,4979, 2701,3859,4711,463,4588}. Therefore, it is recommended to document focal tall cell change (< 30% of the tumour) in PTC. Dedifferentiation of TCPTC to the spindle squamous subtype of anaplastic thyroid carcinoma has been described {541,1636}.

HNPTC is an aggressive PTC subtype, with most patients demonstrating rapid disease progression and many dying of the disease within 5 years. It is important to note that hobnail cells can be seen in classic PTC with an indolent course, sometimes in > 30% of the tumour {4914}. In contrast to HNPTC, these hobnail-like PTCs occur in younger patients, have a low mitotic rate, and lack gross extrathyroidal extension and secondary pathogenic mutations {4914,613}. A diagnosis of HNPTC without the presence of aggressive clinicopathological features (e.g. a high mitotic count) should therefore be rendered with caution {4914}.

Most patients with CCPTC demonstrate rapid disease progression, and many die of the disease within 5 years {4203, 1297,1372,779,2090}. The encapsulated/circumscribed form of CCPTC has limited invasion. In contrast to infiltrative CCPTC, these circumscribed tumours have been shown to have an indolent clinical course {1372,4853,779,826} and may also lack secondary molecular alterations associated with aggressive clinical behaviour {2090}.

Oncocytic carcinoma of the thyroid gland

LiVolsi V
Baloch ZW
Barletta JA
Erickson LA
Kakudo K
Kondo T
Mete O
Morreau H
Rossi ED
Sadow PM

Definition

Oncocytic carcinoma (OCA) is an invasive malignant follicular cell neoplasm composed of oncocytic cells (≥ 75%) in which the nuclear features of papillary thyroid carcinoma (PTC) and high-grade features are absent.

ICD-O coding

8290/3 Oncocytic carcinoma of the thyroid gland
8290/3 Minimally invasive oncocytic carcinoma of the thyroid gland (capsular invasion only)
8290/3 Encapsulated angioinvasive oncocytic carcinoma of the thyroid gland
8290/3 Widely invasive oncocytic carcinoma of the thyroid gland

ICD-11 coding

2D10.Y & XH09D6 Other specified malignant neoplasms of thyroid gland & Oxyphilic adenocarcinoma

Related terminology

Not recommended: Hürthle cell carcinoma; oxyphilic carcinoma; follicular carcinoma, oncocytic variant; follicular carcinoma, Hürthle cell type.

Subtype(s)

Minimally invasive oncocytic carcinoma of the thyroid gland (capsular invasion only); encapsulated angioinvasive oncocytic carcinoma of the thyroid gland; widely invasive oncocytic carcinoma of the thyroid gland

Localization

OCA can arise anywhere in the thyroid, including in ectopic locations such as lingual thyroid and the mediastinum {3302, 2954,4448,2083,1333}.

Clinical features

OCA usually presents as a slowly enlarging, painless solitary thyroid nodule. Patients with widely invasive tumours report a palpable neck mass with compressive symptoms, whereas minimally invasive tumours are usually either identified as a palpable thyroid nodule or found incidentally on radiological screening {5021,4612,4125}. Distant metastasis at the time of presentation is seen in 15–27% of cases, and in as many as 40% of cases with extensive vascular invasion {2453}. Thyroid function tests are usually within normal ranges in most patients with OCA {2453,1817}.

Thyroid ultrasound cannot differentiate between oncocytic adenoma and OCA. Most OCAs show a variety of ultrasound appearances, ranging from hypoechoic to hyperechoic nodules with a peripheral halo due to the tumour capsule and compressed peripheral vessels {2453}. Tumours with invasion beyond the tumour capsule will show irregular margins, and extrathyroidal extension can be seen on ultrasound. On radionuclide scan most OCAs are hypofunctioning; however, rare hyperfunctioning cases have been reported {2687}. Most OCAs are FDG-avid tumours {4544,699}.

Epidemiology

OCA is an uncommon thyroid malignancy, accounting for 3.6% of thyroid carcinomas in the USA {1987}. OCA is rare in children and occurs across a wide age range in adults (mean age: 58 years) {1615,2453}. OCA is more common in women (M:F ratio: 1:2.2) {1615,5138}.

Etiology

There are no known etiological factors for OCA. Some of these tumours occur in individuals with genetically defined tumour syndromes such as *PTEN* hamartoma tumour syndrome (e.g.

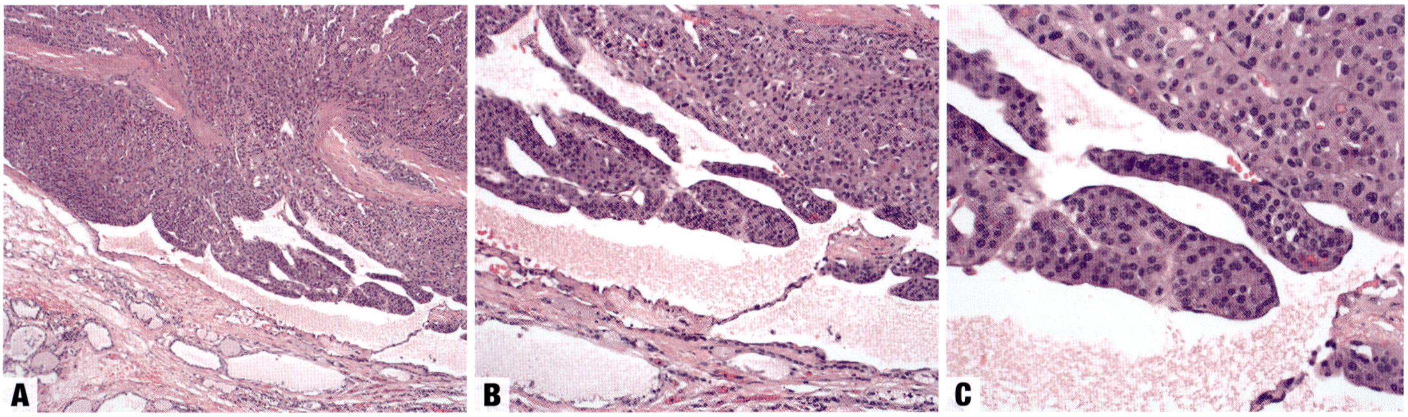

Fig. 3.59 Oncocytic carcinoma, encapsulated with angioinvasion. **A** Encapsulated tumour with a lesional bud penetrating the capsule and hanging in the lumen of an intracapsular vessel. **B** Several tumour plugs are hanging in the lumen of an intracapsular vessel and covered by endothelial cells. **C** Intravascular tumour plugs of oncocytic cells with vesicular nuclei and central nucleoli covered by endothelial cells.

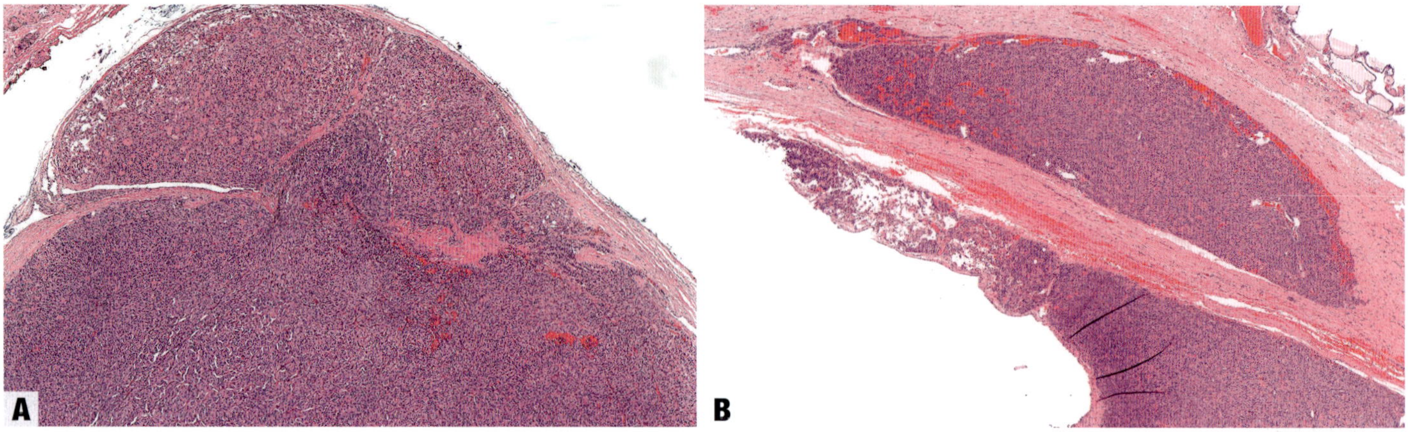

Fig. 3.60 Oncocytic carcinoma. **A** Mushroom invasion of the full thickness of the tumour capsule. **B** Venous invasion in the tumour capsule. At the lower left, partial cystic change was noted in the tumour.

Cowden syndrome) and Carney complex (*PRKAR1A* mutation) {2897,2901,1703,3870,4361,4835}.

Pathogenesis

Accumulation of abnormal mitochondria in follicular cells is a defining feature of oncocytic neoplasia of the thyroid. Complete mitochondrial DNA sequencing of 45 benign and malignant oncocytic tumours identified mitochondrial DNA mutations clustering within complex I of the electron transport chain in a majority of cases {1515}. These mutations were homoplasmic or highly heteroplasmic (> 70%), above the threshold for a biochemically damaging effect on mitochondria, and they are responsible for the oncocytic phenotype {472,1515}. A recent OCA study confirmed the findings and identified mitochondrial DNA mutations in 24 (60%) of 40 primary and metastatic tumours {1637}. The high prevalence of deleterious complex I mitochondrial DNA mutations in OCA suggests that dysfunctional complex I may be advantageous for tumour growth {1637}.

In OCA, chromosome losses are widespread, leading to near-haploidy, and they are observed more frequently than chromosomal gains {2903,924}. Specifically, monosomies of chromosomes 8, 22, and 2, as well as gains of chromosomes 7, 12, and 17, are most common {2903}. Tumours with a greater number of chromosome losses exhibited poorer outcomes by retrospective analysis {1266}. Minimally invasive OCAs and those with limited vascular invasion are frequently diploid, whereas widely invasive OCAs and those with extensive vascular invasion are polysomic and almost always exhibit amplification of chromosome 7 {1490}. A subset of near-haploid OCAs undergo whole-genome duplication, resulting in uniparental disomy of much of the genome {1490}. A comparison of related primary and metastatic tumours revealed that chromosomal content is stable, suggesting it does not play a role in metastatic progression {1637}.

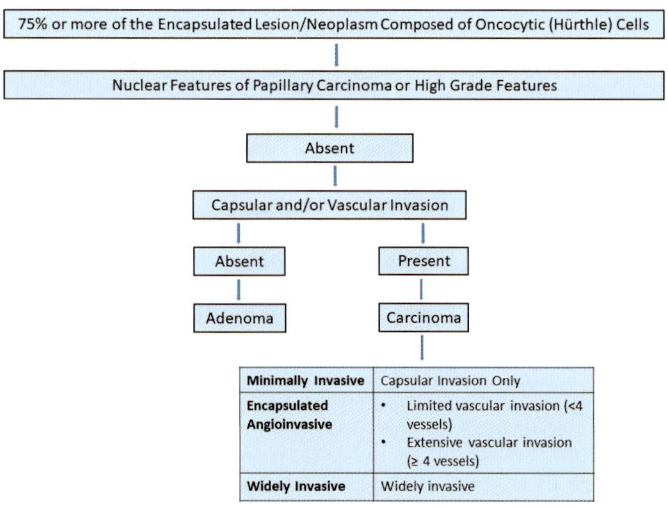

Fig. 3.61 Oncocytic neoplasm diagnostic paradigm.

Macroscopic appearance

OCAs are usually solitary round to oval nodules, usually encapsulated, with an average size of 30–40 mm {1697,3929}. The capsule of an OCA is thicker than that of an oncocytic adenoma and is often partly calcified. The tumour itself ranges from tan to mahogany in colour and is usually solid. The larger the neoplasm, the greater the risk of malignancy, with an estimated two thirds of lesions > 35 mm showing invasive growth. Some OCAs that have been biopsied (either FNAB or core biopsy) undergo partial or complete infarction that can be noted grossly.

OCAs can show gross capsular invasion and (rarely) vascular invasion in the extrathyroidal soft tissues.

Histopathology

OCAs are usually thickly encapsulated neoplasms that demonstrate capsular and/or vascular invasion. By convention, ≥ 75% of the tumour cells should display oncocytic cytology {4392, 1492}. Although some tumours show a follicular (often microfollicular) pattern, most have solid or solid/trabecular growth. The lesional capsule may have multiple foci of dystrophic calcifications. The intraluminal non-lamellated calcifications seen in oncocytic adenomas or oncocytic hyperplastic nodules are seen less often in OCA, because most of these lack a follicular growth pattern {1128,619,2954,2083,2898}.

Like follicular thyroid carcinoma, OCA is classified as minimally invasive, encapsulated with vascular invasion, and widely invasive. The term "minimally invasive" is restricted to tumours showing only tumour capsule invasion, whereas the encapsulated tumours showing vascular invasion are further subdivided into tumours with limited (< 4 vessels) or extensive (≥ 4 vessels) vascular invasion. The criteria for capsular and vascular invasion are similar to those used in follicular carcinoma {2954, 2898,619,1128,2083}.

Infarcted areas encountered in OCAs that have been biopsied are often associated with haemosiderin and macrophages, distinguishing them from true tumour necrosis that portends a poorly differentiated carcinoma or high-grade differentiated thyroid carcinoma. Some of the post-FNA changes can mimic capsular invasion, but linear geography and associated inflammatory changes can assist in differentiating these phenomena from true capsular invasion {2710,293}.

Tumour cells have abundant eosinophilic granular cytoplasm with round nuclei and prominent central nucleoli. Areas of random nuclear atypia, including multinucleated giant cells, may be seen. Electron microscopy shows numerous abnormal mitochondria {2083,2954,2453,4913,1664,4973,915,4972}.

The stroma of OCA is often sparse, with rare (usually very large) tumours showing significant fibrous stroma. Because the neoplasms are usually stroma-poor, a pseudopapillary architecture as an artefact of tissue processing can be mistaken for PTC. Nuclear cytology is helpful in distinguishing these entities.

OCAs have a different biological potential to non-OCA follicular carcinomas. Although the latter spread exclusively through the venous system, OCAs can metastasize to lymph nodes as well as haematogenously. However, it is important to note that some examples of locoregional node metastasis represent tumour plugs in veins in the soft tissues of the neck, and not lymph nodes replaced by tumour {434}.

Distant metastases of OCA target lungs, bones, and liver. Some hepatic metastases are solitary and may be misdiagnosed as primary hepatocellular carcinoma {5175,4055,3920}.

Small series of OCA with certain histological features have been reported to have a more guarded prognosis than usual OCA. The microscopic features of concern include tumour necrosis, numerous mitoses (≥ 1.5/mm^2), abnormal mitoses, and foci of small cell change (cytoplasmic loss) {266}. Tumours with these features are likely to be radioiodine resistant {1640} and in metastatic sites may fail to express thyroid transcription factor 1 (TTF1) and thyroglobulin, causing diagnostic confusion. OCAs with necrosis and mitotic activity are best classified as high-grade differentiated thyroid carcinoma, oncocytic type (see *High-grade follicular cell–derived non-anaplastic thyroid carcinoma*, p. 165).

No immunostains can distinguish OCA from oncocytic adenoma. All oncocytic follicular tumours show an immunoprofile similar to that of other follicular-derived neoplasms, with positivity for thyroglobulin, CK7, PAX8, and TTF1. Calcitonin staining is negative. In some cases, thyroglobulin will show punctate staining confined to the perinuclear area {284}.

Cytology

Smears are usually cellular and show > 75% oncocytic follicular cells, but the features of oncocytic adenomas and OCA are the same, and distinguishing between oncocytic follicular adenoma and carcinoma is not possible on FNAB alone {3726,2083,5054, 3786,3623,5018}. Smears show a monotonous population of oncocytic follicular cells with characteristic voluminous granular cytoplasm, sharp cytoplasmic borders, usually centrally located nuclei with an even chromatin pattern, and prominent round single nucleoli. Thin fibrovascular strands (transgressing vessels) can be seen in the tissue fragments, separating the oncocytic cells. Intracytoplasmic lumina can be seen {5037,991,1224}. Prominent or large irregular nucleoli and multinucleation are not diagnostic of carcinoma {4946,3729}, and prominent nuclear grooves can be seen in oncocytic follicular cells leading to a mistaken diagnosis of subtypes of PTC that can have oncocytic cytoplasm. In some cases, the nucleus of the oncocytic follicular cells can be located eccentrically, mimicking medullary thyroid carcinoma {2083,1224}.

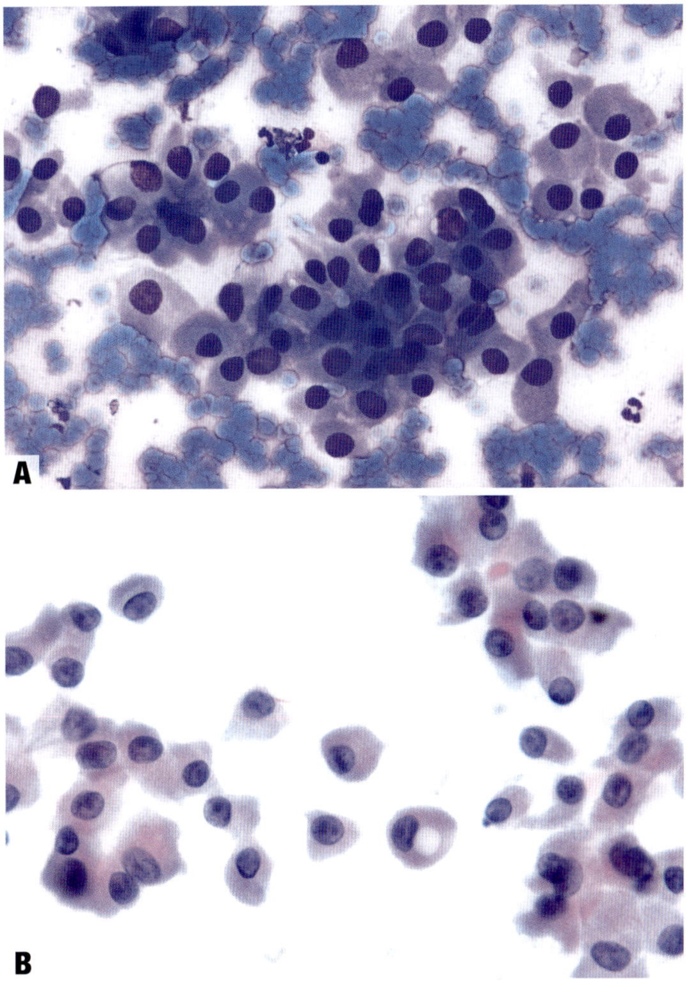

Fig. 3.62 Oncocytic carcinoma. Giemsa-stained air-dried smear (**A**) and Pap-stained alcohol-fixed smear (**B**) from an FNA specimen of oncocytic carcinoma showing a monotonous population of oncocytic cells arranged in loosely cohesive groups.

Diagnostic molecular pathology

Mutations typical of thyroid cancer genes, including RAS genes, *TSHR*, *EIF1AX*, *TP53*, *PTEN*, *BRAF*, *PAX8::PPARG*, and *MEN1* {1123,1293,1490,1492,1637,2212,2520,3261,3987,4835, 4913}, are generally uncommon in OCA, causing false negative molecular results in preoperative FNA samples. Alterations of chromatin regulatory genes are reported at low frequency {1490,1637,3480,3948}.

Essential and desirable diagnostic criteria

Essential: an invasive follicular cell–derived neoplasm consisting of oncocytic cells that account for ≥ 75% of the tumour; absence of PTC nuclei and high-grade features.

Staging

OCA is staged according to the Union for International Cancer Control (UICC) and American Joint Committee on Cancer (AJCC) staging systems, incorporating age at diagnosis.

Prognosis and prediction

The prognosis largely depends on the extent of vascular invasion: the more vessels invaded, the more guarded the prognosis (mortality rate: > 90% at 10 years) {2764}. There appear to be molecular changes associated with those OCAs having extensive vascular invasion; patients affected by such OCAs have a more aggressive clinical course {2764,4854,108,5175, 1491,2083,4919,3404}.

The overall survival rate for OCA ranges from almost 100% in minimally invasive cases (capsular invasion only) to 10% for widely invasive lesions. Tumours with high-grade features and oncocytic poorly differentiated thyroid carcinoma have a worse prognosis {266}. A small percentage of OCAs undergo transformation to anaplastic carcinoma. This may occur after a history of OCA with recurrence, or it may be noted in the initial diagnostic biopsy or surgery with a tumour showing anaplastic carcinoma intermixed with OCA {3660}.

High-grade follicular cell–derived non-anaplastic thyroid carcinoma

Tallini G
Asa SL
Barletta JA
Kondo T
Lam AK
Piana S

Definition

High-grade follicular cell–derived non-anaplastic thyroid carcinoma is a neoplasm of thyroid follicular cells with high-grade features as defined by mitotic count and tumour necrosis, without anaplastic histology. Such tumours may be poorly differentiated or may retain the distinctive morphology of other well-differentiated carcinomas of follicular cell derivation.

ICD-O coding

8337/3 Poorly differentiated thyroid carcinoma
8337/3 High-grade differentiated thyroid carcinoma

ICD-11 coding

2D10.Y & XH8VU6 Other specified malignant neoplasms of thyroid gland & Poorly differentiated thyroid carcinoma

Related terminology

Acceptable: poorly differentiated (insular) thyroid carcinoma; papillary thyroid carcinoma, high-grade; follicular thyroid carcinoma, high-grade; oncocytic follicular thyroid carcinoma, high-grade; follicular-derived carcinoma, non-anaplastic high-grade; high-grade differentiated thyroid carcinoma.

Not recommended: solid type follicular carcinoma; trabecular carcinoma; poorly differentiated thyroid carcinomas defined on the basis of mitosis and necrosis; high-risk thyroid carcinoma of follicular cell origin.

Subtype(s)

Poorly differentiated thyroid carcinoma (PDTC); high-grade differentiated thyroid carcinoma (HGDTC)

Localization

PDTC and HGDTC can develop at any site where thyroid parenchyma may be present, including the mediastinum {1135}, thyroglossal duct cysts {4915}, and ovary in the context of struma ovarii {2274}. Progression to high-grade carcinoma may occur in lymph node metastases or at other metastatic extrathyroidal sites {3547,4979}.

Clinical features

Tumours typically present as a large solitary mass that has grown over several months {650}. In some cases, they manifest as a rapidly growing mass in the background of multinodular goitre. At diagnosis, distant metastases are found in approximately 20–25% of patients {650,1610,2021,4915,4480}. Tumours are solid, heterogeneous, hypoechoic with irregular and indistinct borders by ultrasound, typically cold by scintigraphy, and positive on FDG PET {2021,56}. PDTC and other HGDTCs account for approximately 50% of thyroid tumours that are positive on FDG PET and lack radioactive iodide uptake {3755}. For patient follow-up, clinicians should rely on FDG PET imaging rather than only on serum thyroglobulin measurements and radioiodine scans {3755,2021,1727}.

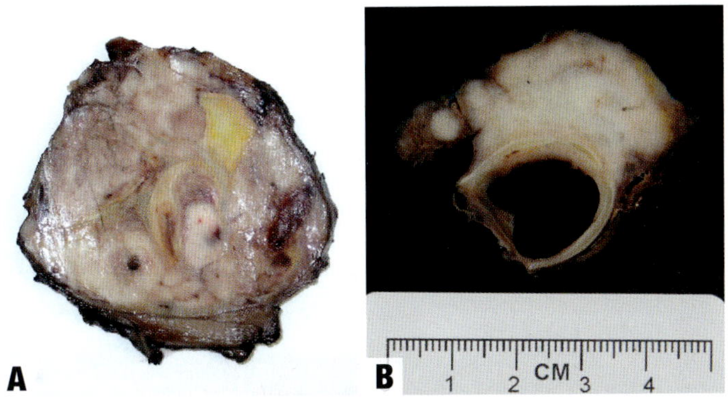

Fig. 3.63 High-grade follicular cell–derived non-anaplastic thyroid carcinoma. **A** Macroscopic appearance of a widely invasive poorly differentiated carcinoma showing a variegated cut surface with foci of haemorrhage and necrosis. **B** Macroscopic appearance of a high-grade differentiated thyroid carcinoma that infiltrates the trachea.

Epidemiology

PDTC and HGDTC are uncommon. The reported prevalence of PDTC varies from < 1% to 6.7% of all thyroid carcinomas {1610,4979,4915}; the incidence is higher in Europe (6.7%) and South America (4%) than in North America (1.8%) and Japan (0.3%) {650,228,1610,56,4480}. The mean age at diagnosis is 55–65 years for both PDTC and HGDTC {4726,1610,4919}. Cases in children and young patients are rare but well documented {1811,228,794}. Tumours show a slight female predilection (M:F ratio: 1:1.1–2.1) {650,4726,2246,1610,4979,4919,4915}.

Etiology

Genetic and environmental factors (iodide deficiency) may have an impact on tumour prevalence in different geographical regions, as indicated by the link of PDTC with longstanding goitre {4730}. There is no association with radiation exposure {2707}.

Pathogenesis

HGDTC and many PDTCs arise after synchronous or metachronous progression of well-differentiated forms of carcinoma of follicular cell derivation, of which they retain the driving molecular signatures {650,228,2520,4919,4915}.

The number of mutations per tumour is intermediate between well-differentiated and undifferentiated carcinomas {2520}. Consistent with a general model of multistep progression from well-differentiated to poorly differentiated to undifferentiated carcinoma, somatic genetic alterations include early and late events.

Early driver changes are mostly RAS and *BRAF* p.V600E mutations; thus, high-grade thyroid carcinomas retain *BRAF*

Table 3.04 Common driver mutations and somatic genetic alterations in high-grade follicular cell–derived non-anaplastic thyroid carcinoma compared with those in well-differentiated and undifferentiated (anaplastic) thyroid carcinomas

Well-differentiated thyroid carcinoma		High-grade follicular cell–derived non-anaplastic carcinoma	Anaplastic thyroid carcinoma
Follicular carcinoma[a]	**Papillary carcinoma**		
RAS: 30–50%[b] *TERT*: 10–35%[c] *PIK3CA*: 0–10% *PTEN*: 0–10% Gene fusions (mostly *PAX8::PPARG*): 10–50%	*BRAF* p.V600E: 40–80% *TERT*: 5–15%[c] *RAS*: 0–10%[b] Gene fusions (*RET*[d], *NTRK1*[e], *NTRK3*[e], *BRAF*, others): 5–25%	*RAS*: 20–50%[b] *TERT*: 20–50%[c] *TP53*: 10–35% *BRAF* p.V600E: 1–35%[h] *PTEN*: 5–20% *PIK3CA*: 0–15% *EIF1AX*: 5–15%f Gene fusions (*RET*, *ALK*, others): 5–25%	*TP53*: 40–80% *TERT*: 30–75%[c] *RAS*: 10–50%[b] *BRAF* p.V600E: 10–50% *PIK3CA*: 5–25% *PTEN*: 10–15% *EIF1AX*: 5–15%[f] Gene fusions (*RET*, others): 0–5% MMR genes: 10–15%
Can be genetically unstable and aneuploid, median number of mutations: ≤ 5[g]	Genetically stable, median number of mutations: 1 ± 1[g]	Genetically unstable, aneuploid, median number of mutations: 2 ± 3[g]	Genetically unstable, highly aneuploid, median number of mutations: 6 ± 5[g]
RAS-like TCGA molecular profile[h]	*BRAF* p.V600E–like TCGA molecular profile[h]	PDTC: *RAS*-like TCGA molecular profile[h] HGDTC: *BRAF* p.V600E–like TCGA molecular profile[h]	Mostly *BRAF* p.V600E–like TCGA molecular profile due to high MAPK transcriptional output regardless of the driver mutation[h]

HGDTC, high-grade differentiated thyroid carcinoma; MMR, mismatch repair; PDTC, poorly differentiated thyroid carcinoma; TCGA: The Cancer Genome Atlas.
[a]Encapsulated follicular-variant papillary thyroid carcinomas, with invasion or without invasion (non-invasive follicular thyroid neoplasm with papillary-like nuclear features), have molecular alterations similar to those of follicular carcinoma. [b]Mutations in *NRAS*, *HRAS*, and *KRAS*; *NRAS* is the gene most frequently mutated. [c]*TERT* promoter mutations: p.C228T (c.-124G>A) and p.C250T (c.-146G>A). [d]The prevalence of *RET*-rearranged cases is higher in children and young patients and in radiation-associated papillary carcinoma. [e]The prevalence of *NTRK* rearrangements is variably reported as 0–5% for *NTRK1* and *NTRK3* in most series from non–radiation-associated papillary carcinoma in adult patients; the prevalence is higher in children and young patients and in radiation-associated papillary carcinoma. [f]*EIF1AX* mutations occur in *RAS*-mutated tumours. [g]The mutation burden per tumour is estimated from TCGA Research Network, 2014 {622}; Landa et al., 2016 {2520}; and Pozdeyev et al., 2018 {3600}. [h]TCGA Research Network, 2014 {622}.
Note: The main molecular alterations are shown, with the estimated ranges of mutation prevalence.

p.V600E–like or RAS-like signatures {622,2520}. RAS-activating mutations are highly prevalent in poorly differentiated carcinoma, indicating that most develop from follicular carcinoma or from encapsulated follicular variant papillary carcinomas. *BRAF* p.V600E mutations predominate in HGDTC because most are high-grade papillary carcinoma. Gene fusions occur in as many as 25% of high-grade papillary carcinomas {2520,4915}.

The most frequent late changes are *TP53* and *TERT* promoter mutations or alterations of the PI3K/PTEN/AKT pathway. Other late alterations, such as those in SWI/SNF chromatin-remodelling complex genes, associate more frequently with anaplastic carcinoma than with non-anaplastic high-grade carcinomas {2520}. *TERT* promoter mutations are associated with a high risk of distant metastases {2520}. Chromosome 1q gain, typically found in aggressive/advanced papillary thyroid carcinomas (PTCs) that are histologically high-grade, is associated with an unfavourable outcome {2520,1488,4915}. *TP53* mutations occur in PDTC and HGDTC, but their prevalence is highest in anaplastic carcinoma {2520,1013}. See also Table 3.04 and Table 3.05.

Macroscopic appearance

PDTC and HGDTC are often large and usually measure 40–60 mm {650,4726,228,1610,4919,4915}, but small tumours may rarely occur. The cut surface is typically solid and light brown to grey, sometimes with grossly evident pale areas of necrosis. Most tumours are widely invasive, although some may be partially or even totally encapsulated {3757,4919}. Frequently, there are satellite nodules, and in some cases multinodular growth may simulate goitre.

Histopathology

There are two groups of high-grade follicular cell–derived non-anaplastic thyroid carcinoma. PDTC is a tumour that has lost architectural and cytological differentiation in the absence of anaplastic histology. HGDTC is a high-grade tumour that is still differentiated since it retains the distinctive architectural and/or cytological properties of well-differentiated histotypes of carcinoma of follicular cell derivation (e.g. nuclear features and/or architecture of papillary carcinoma, follicular growth pattern of follicular carcinoma or oncocytic thyroid carcinoma).

Table 3.05 Mutation profile of high-grade follicular cell–derived non-anaplastic thyroid carcinomas according to subtype {2520}

Subtype	*BRAF* p.V600E	*RAS*[a]	*TERT*	*TP53*	*EIF1AX*	*PTEN*	*PIK3CA*
PDTC	6%	44%	44%	15%	15%	6%	2%
HGDTC	81%	6%	39%	3%	3%	0%	3%

HGDTC, high-grade differentiated thyroid carcinoma; PDTC, poorly differentiated thyroid carcinoma.
[a]PDTC: *NRAS* 33%, *HRAS* 8%, *KRAS* 4%; HGDTC: *NRAS* 6%.

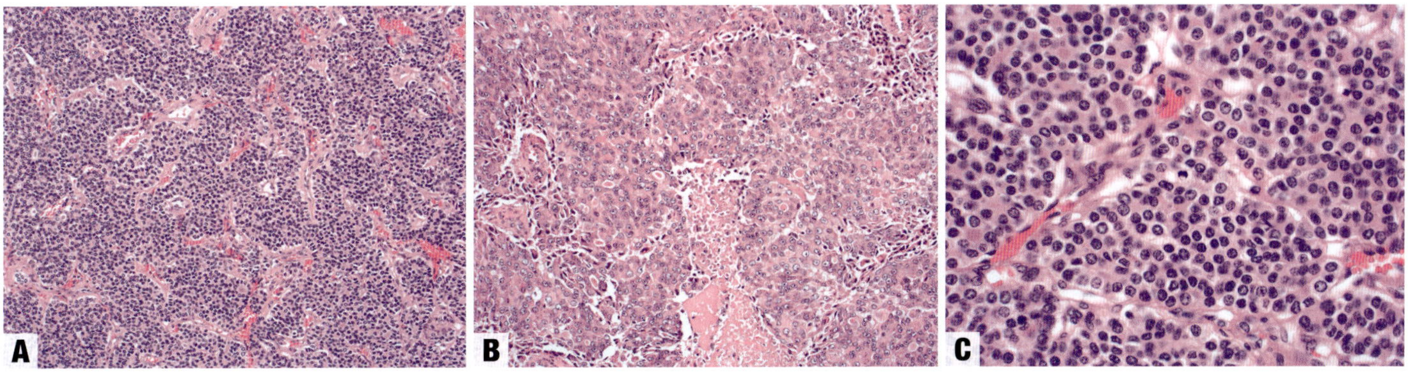

Fig. 3.64 Poorly differentiated thyroid carcinoma. **A** Solid growth pattern. **B** This carcinoma is composed of oncocytic cells growing in a solid pattern with tumour necrosis. **C** The tumour is composed of solid nests of cells with hyperchromatic round nuclei with mitoses (centre).

PDTC

PDTC represents the paradigm of histologically aggressive thyroid carcinomas that are both high-grade and histologically poorly differentiated {4391}. The diagnosis of PDTC is based on Turin consensus criteria {4726}: (1) the presence of a solid/trabecular/insular pattern of growth in a tumour diagnosed as malignant based on invasive properties; (2) an absence of conventional nuclear features of papillary carcinoma; (3) the presence of at least one of the following: convoluted nuclei, a mitotic count of ≥ 3 mitoses/2 mm^2, tumour necrosis {4726}. The prototype of PDTC is the tumour originally reported as insular carcinoma {650}, characterized by well-defined neoplastic cell nests (insulae). These nests are surrounded by thin fibrovascular septa, from which they can be separated by artefactual clefts. Tumour nests are predominantly solid or contain poorly differentiated microfollicles with minimal amounts of colloid. Tumour cells are small and uniform, with round hyperchromatic nuclei, indistinct nucleoli, and minimal pleomorphism. In some cases, nuclei are reminiscent of papillary carcinoma nuclei, showing convoluted and irregular (raisin-like) contours, but they have darker chromatin and no pseudoinclusions (so-called dedifferentiated papillary carcinoma nuclei). Mitoses are common, but proliferative activity may vary within the tumour. Necrosis can be found in small foci at the centre of insulae, as patches involving one or more insular clusters, or as large areas with residual surviving tumour cells grouped around blood vessels resulting in a peritheliomatous appearance.

Other PDTCs share high-grade features (mitoses and necrosis) with the prototypical insular carcinoma but are composed of larger, more pleomorphic cells. Colloid formation is minimal, like it is in solid papillary carcinoma. Some PDTCs are predominantly composed of oncocytic follicular cells {1105,266}.

Rare tumours are characterized by clear {866}, mucinous {2376}, signet-ring {1348}, or rhabdoid cells {84}. Angioinvasion is identified in most cases. Extrathyroidal extension is common {650,4726,228,1610,4919}.

Within a given tumour, PDTC areas can be associated with a heterogeneous group of thyroid carcinoma histotypes, which may or may not be of high grade, including areas of follicular variant papillary carcinoma or follicular carcinoma {4919} as well as areas of aggressive papillary carcinoma histotypes such as the hobnail subtype {122}. Foci of undifferentiated cells with marked nuclear pleomorphism indicate progression to anaplastic carcinoma {4918}. Progression to PDTC in metastatic lymph nodes or at distant sites can occur {3547,4979}.

HGDTC

HGDTCs are not poorly differentiated histologically but all have increased mitotic counts and/or tumour necrosis. The mitotic count must, by definition, be ≥ 5 mitoses/2 mm^2 after evaluation of the most mitotically active areas (hotspot mitotic counting) {1889,4480}. Tumour necrosis is defined by karyorrhectic nuclear debris or ghost contours of dead tumour cells: it must be distinguished from infarct-type necrosis resulting from FNA

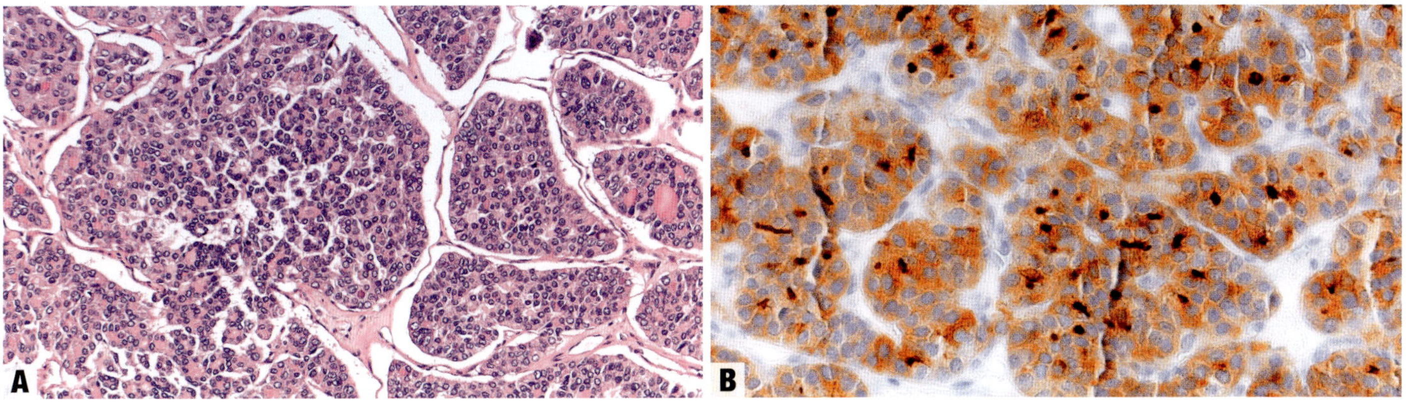

Fig. 3.65 Poorly differentiated thyroid carcinoma. **A** Insular growth pattern with tumour nests showing artefactual separation form the surrounding fibrovascular stroma. **B** Thyroglobulin expression is reduced and there is distinctive dot-like paranuclear immunoreactivity.

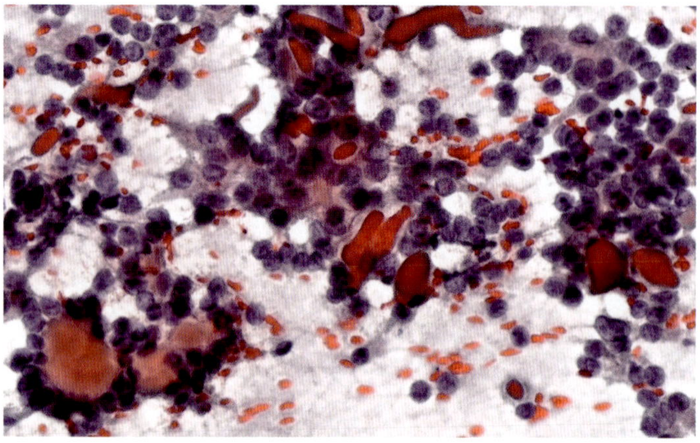

Fig. 3.66 Poorly differentiated thyroid carcinoma. Preoperative fine-needle aspirate showing uniform cells with round, hyperchromatic nuclei; scant, fragile, and poorly defined cytoplasm; and a few microfollicles (lower left).

or regressive changes as in the case of oncocytic tumours {1889}. Tumour necrosis may be obvious, sometimes comedo-like, but can also be very focal. HGDTCs should be subclassified according to their dominant histotype. Most are high-grade PTCs, often belonging to aggressive subtypes such as tall cell, hobnail, or columnar cell, but they can also be conventional or follicular-variant PTCs {1889,4391,1610,4979,4915}. High-grade follicular carcinomas are much less common and usually widely invasive {1610,4979}. Oncocytic thyroid carcinomas may have a poorly differentiated architecture (solid or trabecular growth), and therefore when mitotically active they usually fulfil the Turin consensus criteria for PDTC {1105,266}. Still, when there is no solid/trabecular/insular architecture, oncocytic thyroid carcinomas may fulfil the criteria for HGDTC. HGDTC may show poorly differentiated areas. HGDTC can progress to anaplastic thyroid carcinoma (with severe nuclear pleomorphism), and the presence of any anaplastic component should be reported {4918}.

Immunohistochemistry

Neoplastic cells are immunoreactive for keratins, thyroglobulin, thyroid transcription factor 1 (TTF1), and PAX8, and non-reactive for calcitonin and chromogranin. Thyroglobulin expression is typically reduced and focal in poorly differentiated areas, often with a peculiar dot-like paranuclear pattern. The proliferation rate is increased and the Ki-67 (MIB1) labelling index is elevated (usually 10–30%, depending on the tumour category) {4394,3918,3286,2164,56}.

Cytology

Highly cellular smears show crowded solid, insular, or trabecular tissue fragments and often plentiful single cells, which appear uniform, with scant cytoplasm and a high N:C ratio in the tissue fragments {464}. The dispersed cells may have plasmacytoid or oncocytic cytoplasm. Mitoses and necrosis are seen, but anaplastic nuclei are not present. Thin fibrovascular strands surround the insular tissue fragments. A specific diagnosis relies on surgical pathology, and most preoperative FNA diagnoses are malignant or suspicious for malignancy, but in 30–35% of cases the diagnosis is follicular neoplasm {3882,56}. Cytopathological features vary with HGDTC histopathological type and show necrosis and a high mitotic count without anaplasia, in a background of papillary nuclear features or microfollicles, and usually reflect the presence of aggressive papillary carcinoma subtypes {3828}.

Diagnostic molecular pathology

Molecular pathology is not required for diagnosis but may be indicated in some cases, according to the changes described above (see *Pathogenesis*).

Essential and desirable diagnostic criteria

See Table 3.06.

PDTC

Essential:

- Solid/trabecular/insular pattern of growth in a tumour diagnosed as malignant on the basis of the presence of invasion
- Absence of conventional papillary carcinoma nuclear alterations
- At least one of the following features: convoluted nuclei, mitotic count ≥ 3 mitoses/2 mm², tumour necrosis
- Retention of some (but not all) morphological and immunohistochemical biomarkers of thyroid follicular epithelial cells
- Poorly differentiated but lacking anaplastic cellular morphology

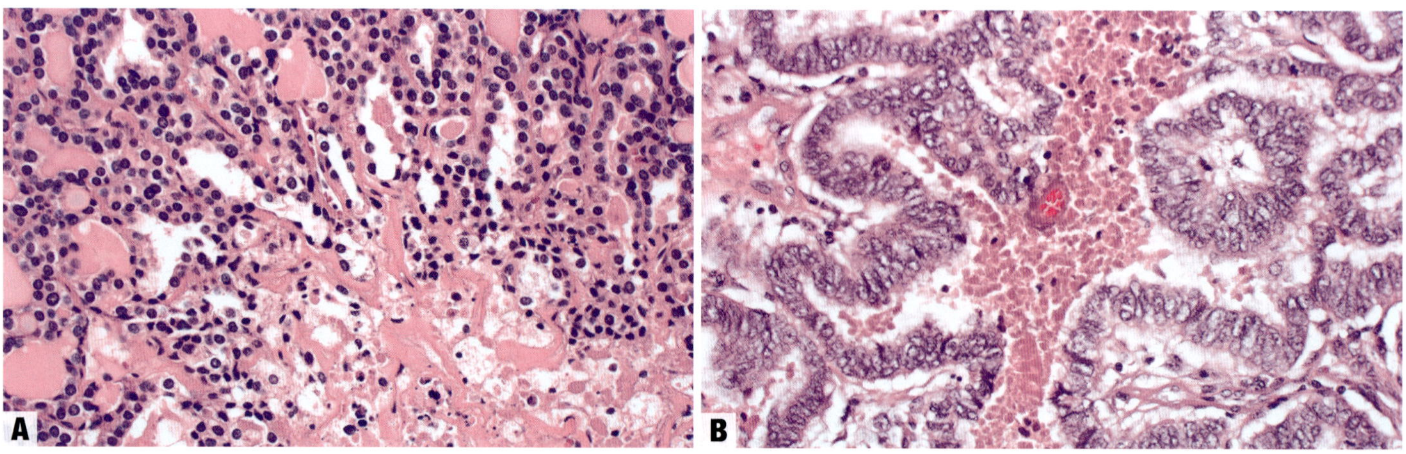

Fig. 3.67 High-grade differentiated thyroid carcinoma. **A** Tumour necrosis in the centre of a follicular tumour lacking the nuclear features of papillary carcinoma. **B** This papillary tumour shows papillae lined by cells with the nuclear alterations of papillary carcinoma and abundant tumour necrosis.

Table 3.06 Diagnostic criteria for high-grade follicular cell–derived thyroid carcinomas

	Poorly differentiated thyroid carcinoma (Turin proposal)	High-grade differentiated thyroid carcinoma
Architectural pattern	Solid/trabecular/insular growth required	Papillary, follicular, solid[a]
Nuclear features	Absence of nuclear features of PTC required	Any
Necrosis, mitosis, and convoluted nuclei	At least one of the following three features: • Mitotic count: ≥ 3 mitoses/2 mm^2 • Tumour necrosis • Convoluted nuclei	At least one of the following two features: • Mitotic count: ≥ 5 mitoses/2 mm^2 • Tumour necrosis
Anaplastic features	None	None

PTC, papillary thyroid carcinoma.
[a]Tumours with solid growth and PTC nuclear features are classified as high-grade differentiated thyroid carcinoma.

HGDTC

Essential:

- Presence of ≥ 5 mitoses/2 mm^2 and/or tumour necrosis, with invasion
- Retention of distinctive architectural and/or cytological features of well-differentiated histotypes of carcinoma of follicular cells (e.g. papillary, follicular, or oncocytic)
- Retention of some (but not all) morphological and immunohistochemical biomarkers of thyroid follicular epithelial cells
- Lacking anaplastic cellular morphology

Staging

Staging is according to the Union for International Cancer Control (UICC) and American Joint Committee on Cancer (AJCC) staging systems, incorporating age at diagnosis.

Prognosis and prediction

Tumours have aggressive clinicopathological features, and the prognosis is intermediate between well-differentiated carcinomas of follicular cells (papillary, follicular, and oncocytic thyroid carcinoma) and anaplastic carcinoma.

The mean disease-specific survival time is approximately 5 years after the original diagnosis {4726,4915}. The overall survival rate at 5 years in most series is 50–70% {1889,4726,228,1610, 2021,2514,4480}, with recurrences usually developing within the first 3 years {650,1889,1610}. Response to radioiodine treatment is poor in many patients {650,3755,2021}. Patient age ≥ 45 years {228}, gross extrathyroidal extension {2021}, tumour size ≥ 50 mm {1610}, and distant metastases at presentation {2021,4480} have been associated with a poor outcome by multivariate analysis.

High-grade follicular cell–derived non-anaplastic thyroid carcinomas have a higher postsurgical histopathological TNM (pTNM) stage and develop in older patients than conventional well-differentiated thyroid carcinomas {4730,2021,1610,4915}. Tumours are often widely invasive, extending into perithyroidal soft tissues in about 60–70% of cases {4730,1889}, with gross extrathyroidal extension that may be more common in high-grade PTC {4915}. Lymph node metastases are found in about 30–40% of cases at initial surgery and are more common in high-grade PTCs than in PDTC {2021,4915}. Distant metastases are identified in about 20–25% of cases at diagnosis {650,2021, 1610,4915}, but eventually develop in 40–70% of cases – typically to lung, followed by bone and other sites (including brain, liver, skin, spleen, and kidney) {650,1889,4726,228,1610,2021, 4480}. A few high-grade follicular cell–derived non-anaplastic thyroid carcinomas are fully encapsulated, with various degrees of invasion {3757,4979}. Encapsulated non-invasive neoplasms of follicular cells with high-grade features are very rare {3757} and usually show indolent behaviour, although 1 case was shown to develop bone metastasis {466}.

Anaplastic thyroid carcinoma

Erickson LA
Nosé V
Asa SL
Barletta JA
Kondo T
Lam AK
Piana S

Definition

Anaplastic thyroid carcinoma (ATC) is a highly aggressive thyroid malignancy composed of undifferentiated cells that may have focal features of thyroid follicular differentiation and/or a previous differentiated thyroid carcinoma.

ICD-O coding

8020/3 Anaplastic thyroid carcinoma

ICD-11 coding

2D10.3 Undifferentiated carcinoma of thyroid gland

Related terminology

Acceptable: undifferentiated thyroid carcinoma.

Subtype(s)

None

Localization

ATC arises in the thyroid but often shows extensive local invasion and regional lymph node and distant metastasis.

Clinical features

ATC often presents as a rapidly enlarging, fixed, and widely infiltrative neck mass that may be associated with compressive symptoms, pain, hoarseness, and dyspnoea. Paraneoplastic hypercalcaemia, leukocytosis, neutrophilia, or a maculopapular eruption may occur {5}. ATC usually affects older adults (mean age: 65–75 years) {1585,4958,1051,1036}. The M:F ratio is 1:1.4 {224,2660}. More than 50% of individuals present with lymph node metastases, and 30–40% present with distant metastasis, often to the lung, bone, and brain {2001}.

Epidemiology

ATC accounts for 1% of thyroid carcinomas in the USA {3515}. The incidence remains stable in the USA, but a study from the Netherlands suggests a slightly rising incidence over the past three decades {2660,3515,1036}. In other series, the incidence is decreasing with earlier detection of precursor well-differentiated carcinomas {5}. Overall, ATC represents 1–4% of thyroid cancers worldwide {5}.

Etiology

The causative factors for the development of ATC remain unknown. ATCs may arise de novo or from / in combination with well-differentiated thyroid carcinomas. ATCs are considered the end-point of follicular cell–derived carcinoma progression. Preceding or coexisting well-differentiated thyroid carcinomas were found in 0–75% of ATCs {2514,3679,4970}. In a study of 360 ATCs, 208 (58%) occurred with a differentiated thyroid carcinoma, the most common being papillary thyroid carcinoma

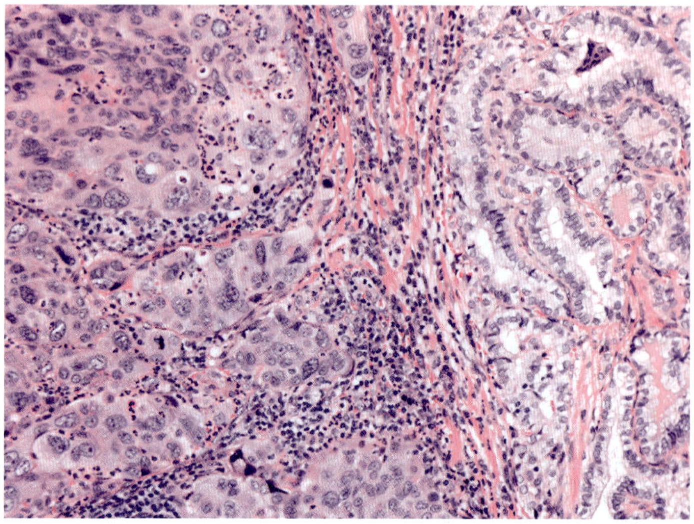

Fig. 3.68 Anaplastic thyroid carcinoma. An anaplastic thyroid carcinoma (left) consisting of markedly pleomorphic cells is identified in association with a papillary thyroid carcinoma (right). A heavy neutrophilic infiltrate is not uncommon in anaplastic thyroid carcinoma.

(*n* = 150) {4970}. A poorly differentiated thyroid carcinoma component was noted in 13% of cases in a study of 38 ATCs {2514}. The progression to ATC has been considered a multistep process with dedifferentiation of a pre-existing papillary or follicular thyroid cancer, as evidenced by frequent mutations in the RAS and *BRAF* genes associated with coexisting mutations in *TP53* {2375}. Whereas *BRAF* p.V600E and RAS mutations remain the main drivers in differentiated thyroid carcinoma, ATC gains additional mutations such as *TERT* promoter mutation and *TP53* mutation {4974}. Radiation exposure and iodine deficiency have also been associated with ATC, in 10% of cases each.

Pathogenesis

A multistep process in ATC development suggests early drivers and late events. Early driver events are mostly RAS and *BRAF* p.V600E mutations, whereas the late events include, above all, *TP53* and *TERT* promoter mutations, because *TP53* and *TERT* promoter mutations are frequently identified in ATC {4729}. Most ATCs with a component of papillary thyroid carcinoma harbour *BRAF* p.V600E mutations {1163,784}. Somatic mutations in known thyroid cancer genes detected in ATC {4974} include those in *BRAF*, RAS genes, *PIK3CA*, *PTEN*, *EIF1AX*, *TP53*, *ATM*, *TERT* promoter, *ATM*, *CDKN1B*, *CDKN2C*, and *CTNNB1* {2449,4357,2520}. Other mutated genes in ATC pathogenesis include *SWI/SNF*, *ALK*, and *CDKN2A*, and there are changes in the expression of different microRNAs {4}. ATCs may also have mutations in genes generally not mutated in thyroid cancer, including *NF1*, *NF2*, mismatch repair genes (*MLH1*, *MLH3*, *MSH5*, *MSH6*), and *USH2A* {2449}.

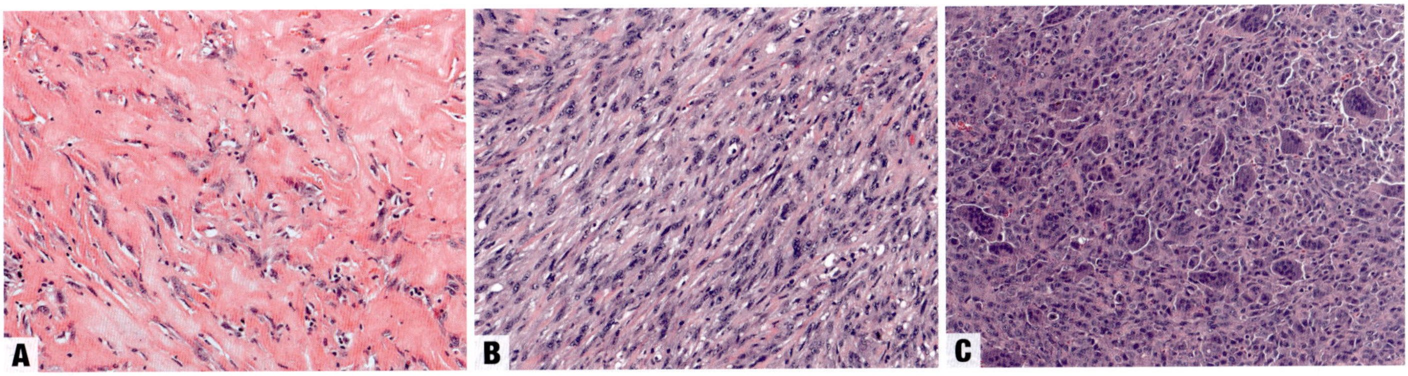

Fig. 3.69 Anaplastic thyroid carcinoma. **A** Paucicellular subtype. This paucicellular anaplastic thyroid carcinoma shows a prominent hyalinized/sclerotic background and could be mistaken for a reactive process such as Riedel thyroiditis. **B** Spindle subtype. This anaplastic thyroid carcinoma shows prominent spindling of markedly atypical cells. **C** This tumour is rich in osteoclast-like giant cells of probable monocytic lineage. The actual anaplastic cells are the mononuclear cells with monotonous oval nuclei.

Macroscopic appearance

ATCs are large (up to 150 mm), bulky tumours that can involve both lobes {2514,4970}. The tumours frequently show haemorrhage, necrosis, and extrathyroidal growth.

Histopathology

ATCs are highly infiltrative malignancies with frequent extrathyroidal growth, necrosis, prominent mitotic activity, atypical mitoses, significant nuclear pleomorphism, and angiolymphatic invasion. ATCs are high-grade tumours that may be epithelioid, spindle, giant cell, pleomorphic, paucicellular, rhabdoid, angiomatoid, or squamous; may show metaplastic chondroid or osteoid; and often have a neutrophilic infiltrate {4772,651,1051,4970, 2683}.

ATC, squamous cell carcinoma pattern

ATC can have focal squamous features or be completely squamous. Primary thyroid squamous cell carcinoma has a similarly poor overall survival to that of conventional ATC and is now considered a pattern of ATC {2509,4970}. ATC with a squamous cell carcinoma phenotype has a previous or concurrent differentiated thyroid carcinoma more frequently than does conventional ATC (76% vs 55%, $P = 0.004$), and it has frequent *BRAF* p.V600E mutations {4970}.

Immunohistochemistry

ATC usually shows some cytokeratin expression (75% of cases) {4970}. A minor subset of cases focally express thyroid transcription factor 1 (TTF1). Thyroglobulin is almost always negative, with very rare cases focally expressing thyroglobulin in epithelioid cells {1051,4970}. PAX8 (MRQ-50) is positive in half of ATCs, with expression correlating with epithelial morphology and a coexisting differentiated carcinoma component {2504}. p53 is expressed in > 50% of ATCs, and the Ki-67 proliferation index is usually high {1051}. ATC with a squamous cell carcinoma phenotype has a squamous immunophenotype and is positive for high-molecular-weight keratins, 34βE12, CK5/6, p63, p40, and occasionally TTF1 {4970}. ATC composed of pure squamous cell carcinoma shows a higher frequency of PAX8 and p53 immunopositivity than other forms of ATC {2509}.

Differential diagnosis

This includes primary thyroid sarcoma (synovial sarcoma, malignant peripheral nerve sheath tumour, angiosarcoma, leiomyosarcoma, and rhabdomyosarcoma), melanoma, medullary thyroid carcinoma, mucoepidermoid carcinoma, sclerosing mucoepidermoid carcinoma with eosinophilia, Riedel thyroiditis, NUT carcinoma, intrathyroid epithelial thymoma, and spindle epithelial tumour with thymus-like elements. ATC is distinguished from high-grade follicular-derived carcinomas by its marked pleomorphism,

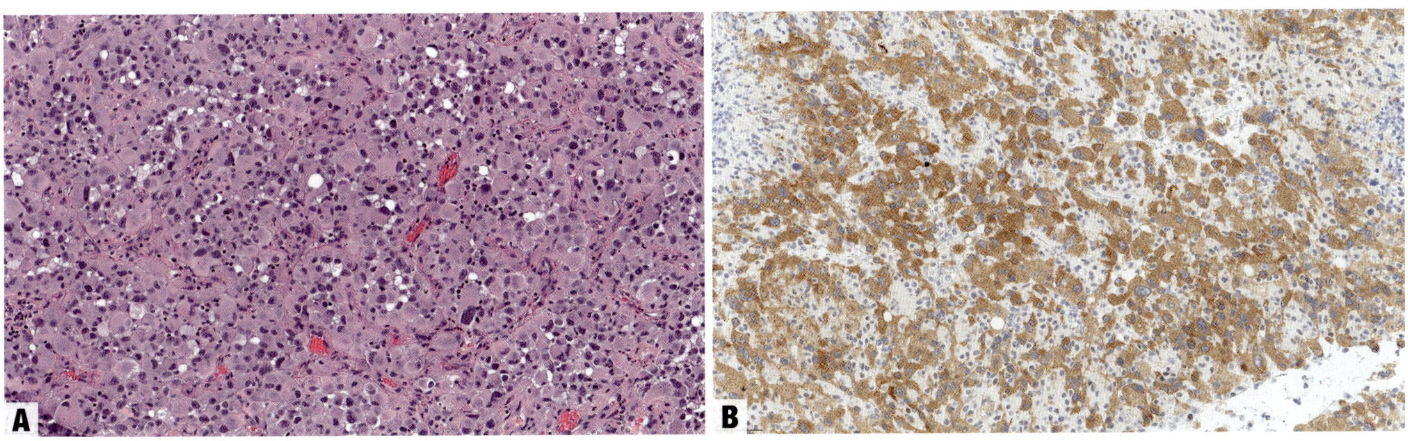

Fig. 3.70 Anaplastic thyroid carcinoma. **A** This tumour has a rhabdoid morphology characterized by cells with eccentric nuclei and abundant eosinophilic cytoplasm. **B** This tumour with rhabdoid morphology is immunopositive for BRAF p.V600E. This stain is currently used to stratify patients with anaplastic thyroid carcinoma for targeted therapy.

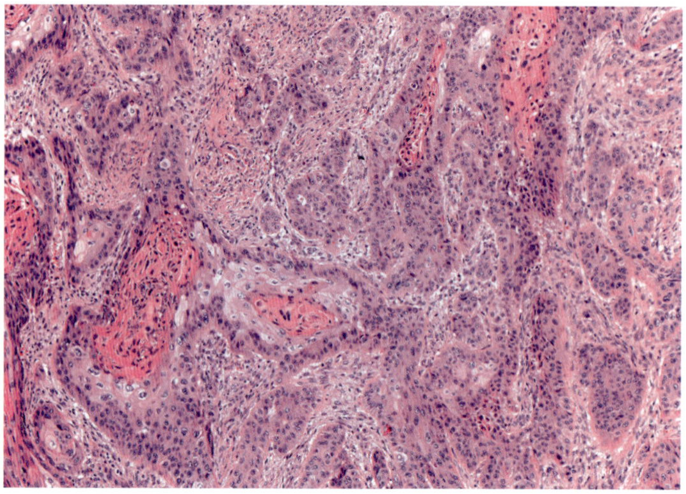

Fig. 3.71 Anaplastic thyroid carcinoma, squamous pattern. This anaplastic thyroid carcinoma has a squamous cell carcinoma phenotype. These tumours can be primary to the thyroid and must be differentiated from secondary involvement by a squamous cell carcinoma from another site.

lack of any organoid growth pattern, and absence of thyroglobulin immunoreactivity in almost all instances.

Cytology

Smears show variable (sparse to marked) cellularity, with frequent necrosis and neutrophils in the background. Individual polygonal, plasmacytoid, spindle, or rhabdoid tumour cells predominate, with a variable number of small tissue fragments. Nuclei are markedly pleomorphic and often enlarged, with coarse chromatin, prominent pleomorphic nucleoli, perinucleolar clearing, pseudoinclusions, multinucleation, and frequent mitoses. There may be an element of papillary or other carcinoma.

Diagnostic molecular pathology

ATC has more complex molecular changes than poorly differentiated carcinoma or well-differentiated (papillary and follicular) thyroid carcinomas. A wide variety of genetic alterations are found in ATCs. RAS (10–50%) and *BRAF* (10–50%) mutations are early molecular events. *TP53* (40–80%) and *TERT* (30–75%) promoter mutations and dysregulation of the PIK3CA/PTEN/AKT/mTOR pathway, as late events, are the most common genetic changes. Mutations in *PIK3CA* are present in 5–25% of cases, in *PTEN* in 10–25%, and in *EIF1AX* in 5–15% {4729}. Epigenetic modifications including non-coding RNAs are also involved in the pathogenesis.

Essential and desirable diagnostic criteria

Essential: a thyroid malignancy composed of undifferentiated cells with focal features of thyroid follicular differentiation and/or a previous differentiated thyroid carcinoma.

Desirable: exclusion of other undifferentiated malignancies in the differential diagnosis.

Staging

ATC is staged according to the Union for International Cancer Control (UICC) and American Joint Committee on Cancer (AJCC) staging systems.

Prognosis and prediction

ATCs are highly aggressive tumours, almost always lethal. Negative prognostic features are older age (> 60 or > 70 years), male sex, rapid tumour growth, leukocytosis, dyspnoea, extrathyroidal extension, large size (> 50 mm, > 60 mm, or > 70 mm), lymphocytic and neutrophilic infiltrate, incomplete resection, distant metastasis, RAS mutation, *PIK3CA* mutation, and concurrent mutations of RAS or *BRAF* with *TERT* {5053,4353,4322,260,2001,1163,4970,5025,2505,4225}. In a study of 360 cases, residual gross disease was the only independent predictor of lower survival in patients who underwent resection {4970}. In a SEER study of 719 ATCs (1998–2011), non-White patients had worse overall survival, and individuals in high-poverty areas had worse overall and disease-specific survival {3774}. Tumours with a minor anaplastic component and no extrathyroidal extension have a more favourable prognosis.

Historically, the mortality rate for ATC at 3–6 months was 90%. With treatment advances including multimodal therapy, extensive

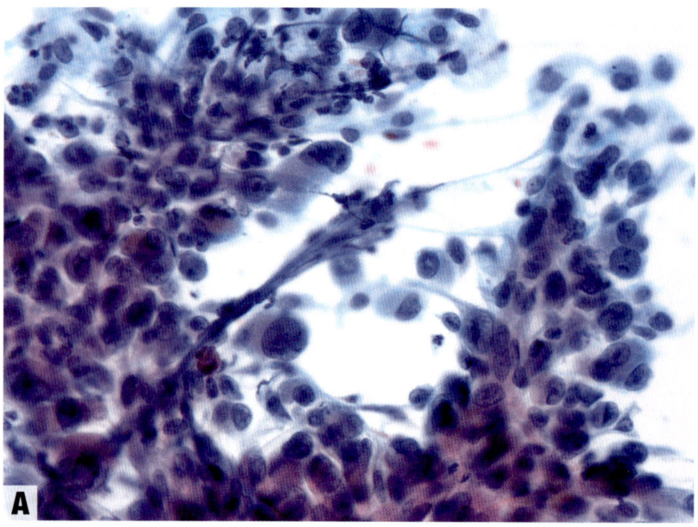

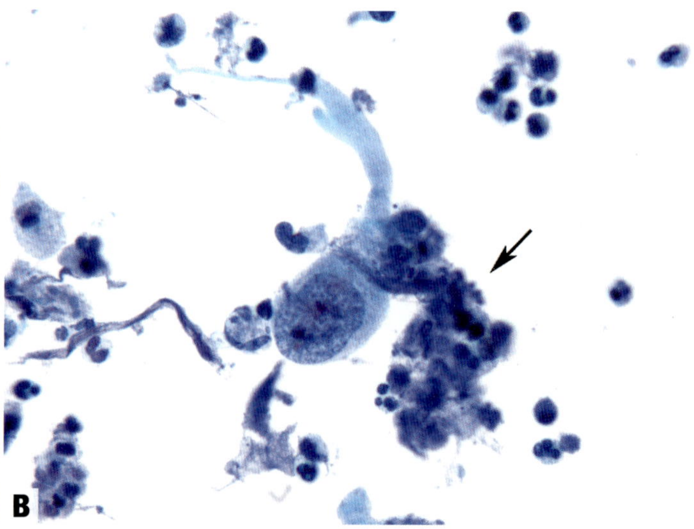

Fig. 3.72 Anaplastic thyroid carcinoma. **A** FNA specimen (alcohol-fixed, Pap-stained smear preparation) showing a cohesive tissue fragment of epithelioid and spindle-shaped cells with marked cellular pleomorphism and interspersed neutrophils. **B** FNA specimen (liquid-based cytology preparation) showing pleomorphic tumour cells with necrotic debris (arrow).

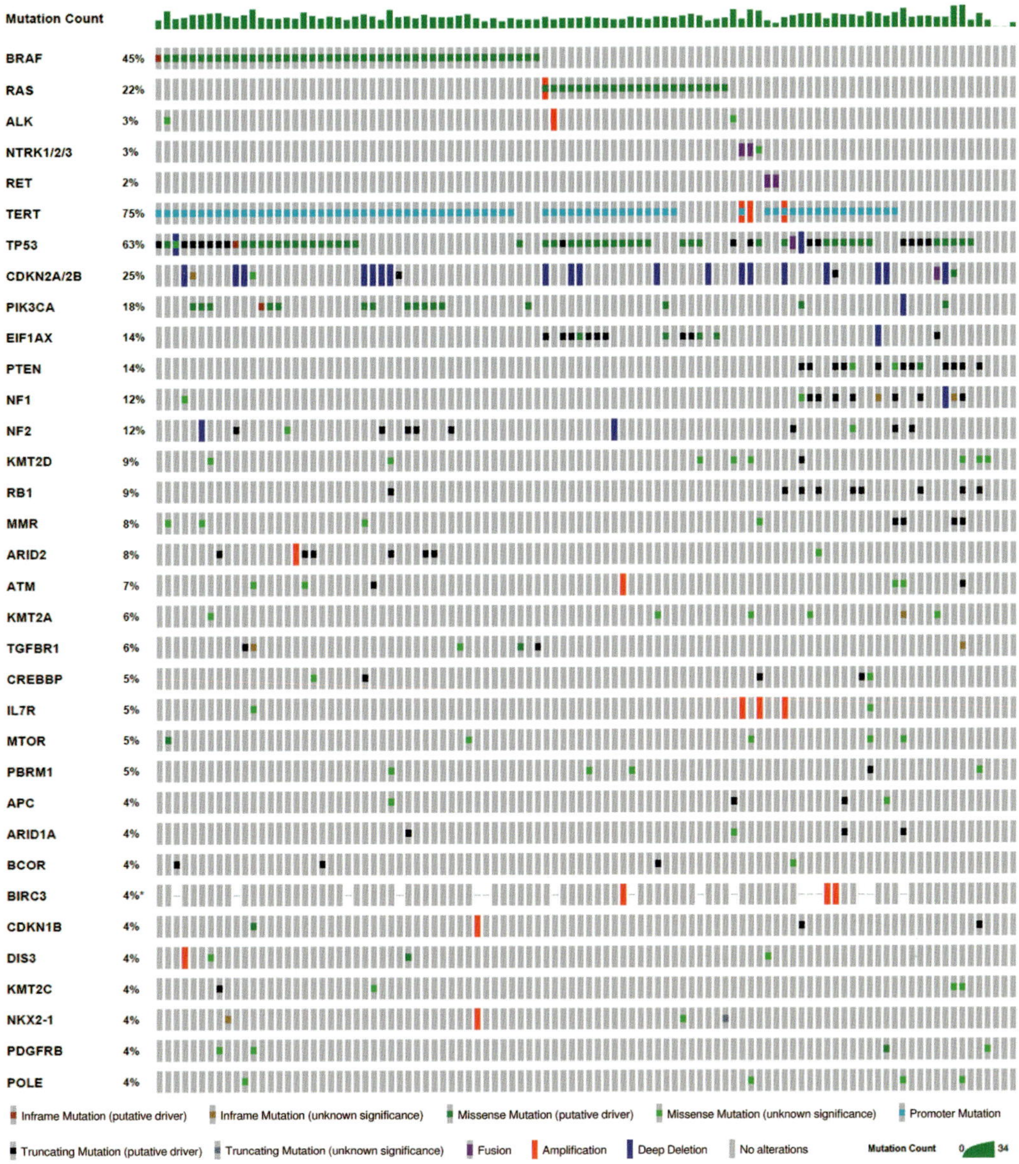

Fig. 3.73 Molecular profile of anaplastic thyroid carcinoma. Mutation count and frequency of genetic alterations in 102 anaplastic thyroid carcinomas sequenced using the Memorial Sloan Kettering Integrated Mutation Profiling of Actionable Cancer Targets (MSK-IMPACT) next-generation sequencing platform.

surgical resection, high-dose external beam radiation, and possibly chemotherapy, survival time may be increased, but it remains in most cases < 2 years {778,4353,4322,2469,4958,1036,3024,4225,2839}. Rare survival times of > 5 years have been reported {2675,5053,4353,4614,2183}. BRAF p.V600E immunostaining and/or genotyping is now mandatory, because BRAF and MEK inhibitors were shown to be clinically active in *BRAF* p.V600E–mutated ATC and approved by the United States Food and Drug Administration (FDA) {1069}. Other therapies targeting cell membrane kinases and downstream proteins, including EGFR, FGFR, VEGFR, KIT (c-KIT), PDGFR, RET, VEGF, and mTOR, are in clinical trials {4}. PDL1 immunostaining positivity (defined as a tumour proportion score of ≥ 1%) has been reported in 39–60% of ATCs {5197,602}. One study showed a better response to immunotherapy (directed against PD1) in PDL1-positive ATC compared with PDL1-negative tumours {631}.

Medullary thyroid carcinoma

Osamura RY
Bongiovanni M
Fuchs TL
Gill AJ
Tallini G
Volante M

Definition

Medullary thyroid carcinoma (MTC) is a malignant neuroendocrine tumour derived from the calcitonin-producing parafollicular C cells of the thyroid gland.

ICD-O coding

8345/3 Medullary thyroid carcinoma
8345/3 Medullary microcarcinoma

ICD-11 coding

2D10.4 Medullary carcinoma of thyroid gland

Related terminology

Acceptable: C-cell carcinoma.
Not recommended: parafollicular cell carcinoma.

Subtype(s)

Medullary microcarcinoma

Localization

Although MTCs may arise throughout the thyroid, they follow the distribution of normal C cells and so are most likely to arise in the region of highest C-cell density at the junction of the upper and middle thirds of the thyroid lobes.

Clinical features

MTC typically presents as a solitary palpable thyroid nodule in the upper to middle thirds of the lateral lobes {2879}. Invasion of surrounding structures may occur, resulting in dysphagia or respiratory difficulty. At diagnosis, lymph node metastases are present in 50–75% of patients {3851,4848} and distant metastasis in 10–15% {4152}. The most common sites for metastatic disease are the mediastinum, liver, lungs, and bone {3852}. The high levels of serum calcitonin secreted from these tumours can lead to symptoms such as flushing, diarrhoea, and/or weight loss {3852}. Rarely (< 1% of cases), these tumours can be nonsecretory {1485}. CEA is another useful serum tumour marker, found in > 50% of patients with MTC {3852}. An increasing CEA level in the presence of a stable calcitonin level can be a sign of dedifferentiation of the tumour and is associated with a worse prognosis. Conversely, a rapid decrease in serum CEA predicts cure by surgery {775,1597}. Some tumours secrete various other hormones such as serotonin, substance P, VIP, ACTH, CRH, and catecholamine metabolites {3852}. This may give rise to paraneoplastic Cushing syndrome {3574}.

Patients with hereditary MTC commonly present at a younger age and with multifocal and bilateral disease. They can present with diarrhoea, flushing, or weight loss caused by excessive calcitonin secretion by the tumour, or they can be diagnosed after presenting with an associated disease such as phaeochromocytoma or hyperparathyroidism {3852}. Currently, most patients with hereditary MTC are identified by genetic testing of at-risk family members, resulting in younger patient ages at diagnosis and earlier identification of tumours in appropriately screened individuals {4849}.

Imaging

Preoperative ultrasonography typically demonstrates nonspecific features of malignancy, including hypoechoic solid nodules with irregular borders and intranodular vascularization {4548}. Functional imaging modalities, primarily FDOPA and FDG PET-CT, play a crucial role in the evaluation of disease extent during the initial staging and postoperative follow-up of patients with MTC {2462}. FDOPA PET-CT is particularly sensitive for detecting occult metastatic disease and is typically followed by targeted imaging using alternative techniques depending on specific organ involvement {4545,2462}.

Epidemiology

MTC accounts for approximately 2% of thyroid malignancies and 8% of thyroid cancer–related deaths in the USA {318}. The average age at diagnosis of sporadic MTC is 45–55 years, and there is a slight female predominance {318}. As many as 25% of MTCs are hereditary, resulting from autosomal dominant germline gain-of-function mutations in the *RET* proto-oncogene, indicating multiple endocrine neoplasia type 2A (MEN2A) or type 2B (MEN2B) {2425,2538}. These patients typically present in the second and third decades of life {1617}. Hereditary isolated MTC, formerly known as familial MTC, is recognized as a subtype of MEN2A by the American Thyroid Association (ATA) guidelines on MTC published in 2015 {4848}.

Etiology

About 25% of cases of MTC are associated with germline *RET* mutation (i.e. MEN2 syndrome). The etiology of sporadic MTC is unknown. There is no evidence of an association with external ionizing radiation, occupational exposure, or cigarette smoking {2165}. A number of studies have demonstrated an association between sporadic MTC and goitre or thyroid nodules {3203,2165}. Some authors have also reported an association between MTC and Hashimoto thyroiditis in female patients, although this finding requires confirmation in larger prospective studies {5121}. Germline *MET* mutation is associated with familial MTC {4253}.

Pathogenesis

Activating *RET* mutations drive tumorigenesis via the activation of multiple pathways including the MAPK and PI3K pathways, which promotes cell growth, proliferation, survival, and differentiation {3794}. Alternate mechanisms of activating the MAPK pathway, including RAS mutations, drive many *RET*-wildtype MTCs {456,857,3116,46,4151,3700}. Epigenetic and other alterations, including somatic copy-number loss of *CDKN2C* {1681}, mTOR pathway activation {2770,4397}, increased expression of the histone methyltransferases EZH2 and SMYD3 {4254}, and *TERT* promoter methylation and copy-number gain {4797}, have also been reported to contribute to neoplastic progression.

Macroscopic appearance

Tumours range in size from < 1 mm in diameter to those that replace the entire thyroid lobe. Sporadic MTC is typically unilateral, whereas heritable MTC is often bilateral and multicentric {2879}. The tumours are typically well circumscribed but unencapsulated with a solid tan-yellow cut surface. Occasionally, they may appear infiltrative {1098}. Prophylactic thyroidectomies in patients with familial syndromes require complete examination of the thyroid, because gross tumours may not be seen.

Tumours measuring < 10 mm in diameter have been termed medullary microcarcinoma {2879}. Most of these tumours are found incidentally in thyroids removed for other reasons or have been detected on the basis of abnormal calcitonin levels in patients with nodular thyroid disease {2879}. Some authors have suggested that the term "microcarcinoma" should be reserved for tumours measuring < 5 mm, because tumours of this size have not been associated with any reports of nodal metastasis or postoperative hypercalcitoninaemia {3561,580,1346,1504}.

Histopathology

The morphological spectrum of MTC is broad and includes features that may mimic the entire spectrum of thyroid malignancies. Typically, tumours show solid, nested, insular, or trabecular growth patterns separated by varying amounts of fibrovascular stroma that give rise to an organoid architecture {1098,2879}. The cells are typically polygonal with granular amphophilic cytoplasm and fine nuclear chromatin {1098}. Nucleoli are usually inconspicuous. Various other cell types can also be seen, including plasmacytoid and spindle-shaped cells, with frequent admixtures of more than one cell type in a single tumour. There is typically a low to moderate degree of nuclear atypia, although some cases show scattered markedly pleomorphic cells with bizarre nuclei and sometimes multinucleated forms. Occasional nuclear pseudoinclusions may be present. Mitotic activity is usually low and tumour necrosis is uncommon {121,1450}. Calcification, including psammoma-like bodies and ossification, may be seen.

Stromal amyloid deposition is seen in 50–90% of cases and may be highlighted with Congo red histochemistry {2275,3114}. Spectrometric analyses have shown that calcitonin is the primary constituent of the amyloid in MTC, although a number of amyloid-associated proteins, such as katacalcin, apolipoprotein E, and vitronectin, have also been shown to colocalize with the deposits {2275,1272,4186}.

Electron microscopy reveals small (< 200 nm in diameter) and medium-sized (200–300 nm in diameter) secretory granules with round, uniform cores surrounded by a tight or loosely fitted membrane {1930}. Both granule types contain calcitonin {1066,1067}.

Tumours from patients with heritable forms of MTC are histologically indistinguishable from those occurring sporadically. An association with C-cell hyperplasia has been reported in inherited forms of MTC; however, this finding is not specific and is often reported in association with sporadic tumours and in thyroids removed for reasons other than MTC {1722,83,1448}.

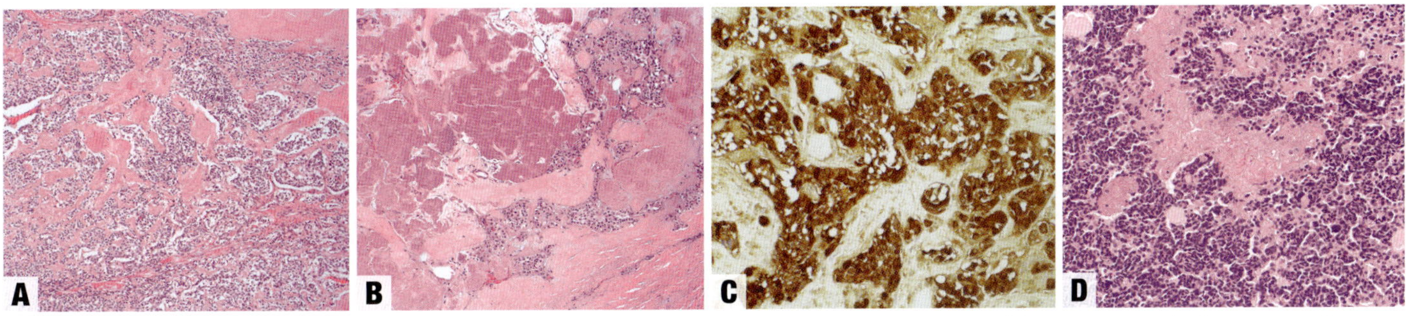

Fig. 3.74 Medullary thyroid carcinoma. **A** The tumour cells in this classic medullary thyroid carcinoma are arranged in solid nests separated by fibrous septa with stromal amyloid deposition. **B** This tumour shows extensive amyloid deposition with calcification. **C** The tumour is strongly and diffusely positive with calcitonin immunoperoxidase staining. **D** The small cell pattern of medullary thyroid carcinoma is composed of sheets of cells with round to ovoid nuclei and scant cytoplasm, reminiscent of small cell neuroendocrine carcinoma (SCNEC). Central tumour necrosis is also present.

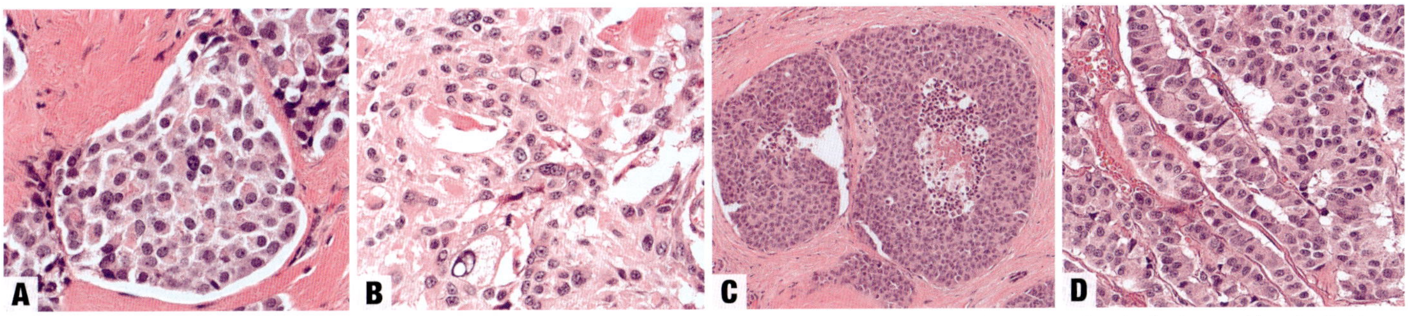

Fig. 3.75 Medullary thyroid carcinoma. **A** The tumour cells have a distinctive plasmacytoid morphology. **B** Some cases show scattered markedly pleomorphic cells with bizarre nuclei, multinucleated forms, and nuclear pseudoinclusions. **C** This tumour shows central tumour necrosis within nests of neoplastic cells. **D** This tumour has a predominantly trabecular growth pattern.

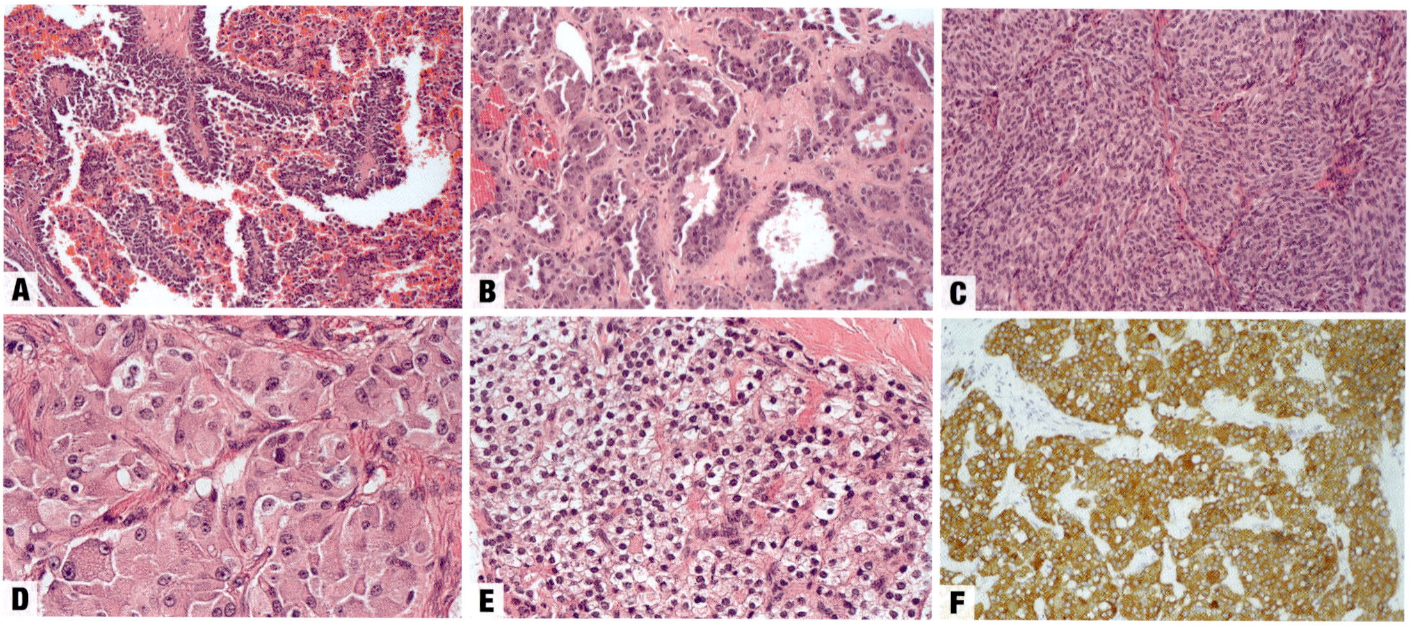

Fig. 3.76 Medullary thyroid carcinoma. **A** In the papillary pattern, tumour cells are aligned along true fibrovascular cores that are often hyalinized and contain amyloid deposits. **B** In the follicular (tubular/glandular) pattern, the tumour cells are arranged in follicular structures. **C** This tumour is composed of spindle cells arranged in short intersecting fascicles. **D** The oncocytic pattern of medullary thyroid carcinoma is composed of sheets of polygonal cells with abundant granular eosinophilic cytoplasm that may mimic oncocytic cells. **E** Clear cell pattern of medullary thyroid carcinoma. **F** Tumours show positive immunohistochemical expression of synaptophysin (and other neuroendocrine markers).

Immunohistochemistry

MTC is positive for calcitonin in 95% of cases, although the staining may be focal {2879}. Neuroendocrine markers, such as chromogranin A, synaptophysin, NSE, and INSM1, are positive. CGRP is also positive in a high proportion of cases, and occasional calcitonin-negative cases may express CGRP {3171, 1485}. CEA is expressed in most cases and may be expressed in the rare calcitonin-negative cases {2879}. Thyroid transcription factor 1 (TTF1) is expressed in most cases, although the intensity of staining is typically less than in normal follicular cells and their tumours {2232,370}. MTC is negative for thyroglobulin. However thyroglobulin from adjacent non-neoplastic follicles may leak over the neoplastic cells and cause difficulty in interpretation in small biopsies. Staining for polyclonal PAX8 is variable and weak {5142,3286}. However, MTC is negative for monoclonal PAX8 {1692}. SSTR2A and SSTR5 may be expressed {1277}. It is noteworthy that calcitonin can be expressed in a variety of extrathyroid neuroendocrine neoplasms (NENs) especially in intermediate-grade laryngeal neuroendocrine tumours (NETs) {1901}. The lack of diffuse and strong TTF1 in the latter can help separate it from MTC {1901}.

Histological patterns

Numerous histological patterns of MTC have been described. Although most of these patterns have no prognostic significance, their recognition is important to avoid confusion with other tumour types {2879}. In most instances, tumours show admixtures of conventional and variant cytoarchitectural morphologies, and the quantitative criteria used to define these patterns in heterogeneous tumours have yet to be established. The papillary and pseudopapillary patterns may be particularly challenging to distinguish from papillary thyroid carcinoma. In the papillary pattern, the tumour cells are aligned along true fibrovascular cores that are often hyalinized and contain amyloid deposits {3423,2241}. The tumour cells may also contain intranuclear pseudoinclusions, making the distinction from papillary thyroid carcinoma even more challenging {2006}. More commonly, there is a pseudopapillary pattern, in which groups of tumour cells are artifactually separated from the adjacent stroma owing to tissue fragmentation {2241,2006}.

In the follicular (tubular/glandular) pattern, the tumour cells are arranged in follicular structures that may contain luminal eosinophilic material that may represent secreted calcitonin and other proteins {593}. Unlike in follicular carcinoma, the tumour cells and these secretions are calcitonin-positive and thyroglobulin-negative {593}.

The spindle cell pattern is composed of elongated fusiform cells arranged in loose clusters or as single units {3635}. Some tumours may show a striking angiosarcoma-like appearance {2501}. Tumours may also contain a predominant population of plasmacytoid cells, squamous cells, giant cells, clear cells, or oncocytic cells {2879}. The oncocytic pattern of MTC often mimics oncocytic follicular cell neoplasms, featuring sheets of polygonal cells with abundant granular eosinophilic cytoplasm {4245}. The melanotic pattern is extremely rare and is characterized by variable amounts of melanin pigment in the cytoplasm of tumour and/or stromal cells {4774}. The amphicrine pattern is composed of cells containing both mucin and calcitonin {1623, 1136}.

The paraganglioma-like pattern resembles the classic growth pattern of paraganglioma/phaeochromocytoma with a Zellballen architecture and possible S100-positive sustentacular-like cells {2791,448,2096,3864,696,1666,1957}. The presence of cytokeratin and TTF1 distinguishes this MTC pattern from intrathyroidal paraganglioma, which lacks these markers.

The encapsulated pattern is characterized by a complete fibrous capsule, and these tumours may appear entirely cystic macroscopically {3380,36}.

The small cell pattern, reminiscent of small cell neuroendocrine carcinoma (SCNEC), is very rare. Diagnosis of this pattern should be made with caution, particularly when the tumour cells do not express calcitonin {4691}. Calcitonin can be normal or only slightly elevated in serum in this pattern {5065}. Some tumours initially interpreted as small cell MTC have since been shown to represent metastatic neuroendocrine carcinomas (NECs) originating in other locations {2881,3627}. It has also been suggested that some of these tumours may be related to the Ewing tumour family on the basis of *EWSR1::FLI1* rearrangements {1233}.

Cytology

Smears are usually highly cellular with single dispersed plasmacytoid, polygonal, round, or spindle cells usually predominating, with a variable number of loosely cohesive or syncytial tissue fragments and in some cases binucleated or giant cells {2926,3812}. Nuclei are round to oval with mixed fine and coarse, stippled chromatin, resembling neuroendocrine nuclei, with occasional nuclear pseudoinclusions and inconspicuous nucleoli. The eccentric cytoplasm varies in amount and may contain azurophilic/red (Giemsa) granules. Amyloid may be seen in variable amounts in the background as relatively dense and hard-edged, amorphous mauve (Giemsa) or pale-green to eosinophilic (Pap) material {2926}. When tumour cells are round or polyhedral with finely granular cytoplasm, the differential diagnosis is follicular cell–derived neoplasms {3080, 3927,36,2680}, but cellular dyscohesion is a hallmark of MTC {2680}. Metastatic NEC and melanoma can also mimic MTC. The FNAB diagnosis of MTC can be challenging, owing to its diverse appearances and morphological overlap with other thyroid neoplasms, and the diagnostic accuracy is less consistent than for follicular cell–derived neoplasms {4549}. In a meta-analysis of 641 MTCs, the overall sensitivity was found to be only 56.4% {4549}. Immunocytochemistry for calcitonin and neuroendocrine markers is helpful in making the correct diagnosis. Elevated serum calcitonin may aid in the identification of MTC in nodules that have a benign ultrasonographic appearance {2468,4466}. In a retrospective analysis of 140 patients with MTC, the sensitivities of FNAB and serum calcitonin for the diagnosis were 51.3% and 98.7%, respectively {4152}. Measurement of calcitonin levels in the washout fluid of thyroid FNAB in patients with borderline or elevated serum calcitonin values has been shown to have a high sensitivity {2865,4547}. Molecular testing provides another strategy for improving the diagnostic accuracy of FNAB {4937}.

Diagnostic molecular pathology

Approximately 25% of patients with MTC will have MEN2, and germline testing for *RET* mutations is recommended for all patients, regardless of family history {4848}. Depending on available resources, one approach is to first sequence mutation hotspots – the cysteine codons in exons 10 and 11 (codons 609, 611, 618, 620, 630, and 634), and additional *RET* codon mutations in exons 13, 14, 15, and 16 {1223}. Other institutions sequence the entire *RET* coding region or use a 2-tiered approach, beginning with hotspot exons.

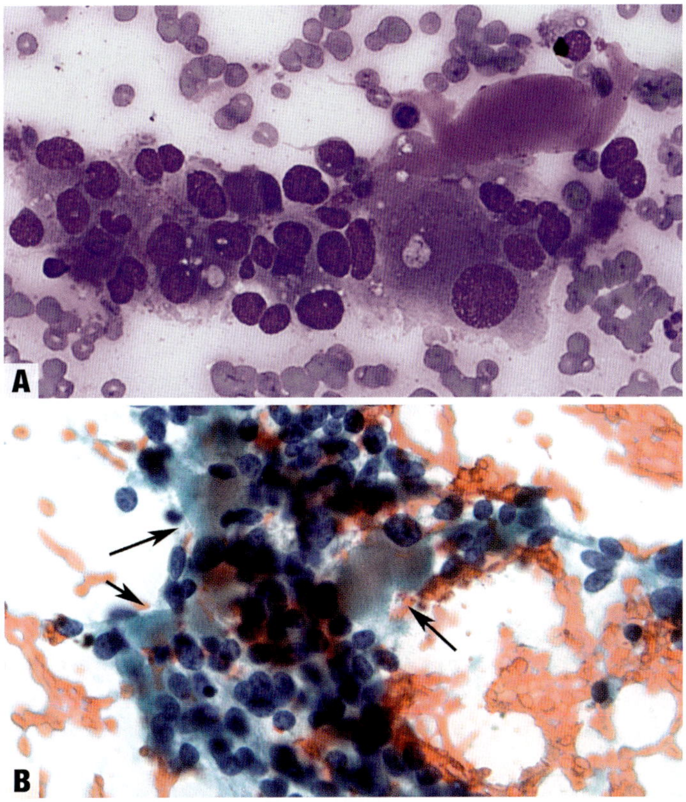

Fig. 3.77 Medullary thyroid carcinoma. **A** Amyloid is seen as amorphous eosinophilic material in the upper-right corner of this group of tumour cells (Giemsa). **B** The tumour cells are round to oval with salt-and-pepper chromatin. Amyloid (arrows) is also present (FNA, Pap-stained alcohol-fixed smear).

Somatic-only *RET* mutations have been reported in approximately half of all sporadic MTCs {1222,3115,2984,3797,456, 857} and are important to identify, because MTCs associated with either somatic or germline *RET* mutations are likely to respond to treatment with targeted *RET* inhibitors {4901}.

The most common somatic *RET* mutation in sporadic MTC is the *RET* p.M918T mutation, which accounts for as many as 80% of *RET* mutations in sporadic MTC {1222,3116,2984,3797,456, 857,4985}. Mutations at codon 634 account for approximately 15% of *RET* mutations {1222}. Interestingly, the prevalence of the p.M918T mutation is substantially lower in medullary thyroid microcarcinomas {3797}, and substantially higher in the setting of advanced disease {3793}, suggesting that *RET* mutations might be secondary events driving tumorigenesis rather than initiators of tumour development {1974}. In addition, aneuploidy (trisomy and tetrasomy) of chromosome 10 is seen in approximately one quarter of sporadic MTCs in a variable proportion of tumour cells, resulting in *RET* copy-number alterations, with a higher prevalence detected in *RET*-mutant MTC {856}.

A few non-*RET* molecular alterations have been reported in MTC. Approximately 70% of tumours that are wildtype for *RET* harbour RAS gene mutations, with *HRAS* mutations being the most common, followed by *KRAS* mutations, and rarely *NRAS* mutations {456,857,3116,46,4151,3700}. In a recent study, RAS alterations were found in 24% of sporadic MTCs, with 17% harbouring *HRAS* mutations, 7% having *KRAS* mutations, and < 1% having *NRAS* mutations {857}. *RET* and RAS mutations are virtually always mutually exclusive; however, rare tumours

Table 3.07 Grading scheme for medullary thyroid carcinoma

Mitoses/2 mm²		Ki-67 proliferation index		Tumour necrosis	Grade
< 5		< 5%		Absent	Low
≥ 5	and/or	≥ 5%	and/or	Present	High

harbouring both *RET* and RAS mutations have been reported {857,3116}. Fewer than 20% of sporadic MTCs are wildtype for both *RET* and RAS {857,46}, and sequencing studies have found that these tumours also lack other recurrent mutations {46,4151,1854,757,857}. There have been isolated reports of *RET* and *ALK* gene rearrangements {1680,2107}.

Essential and desirable diagnostic criteria

Essential: a primary non-follicular cell–derived thyroid tumour with morphological and immunohistochemical features of neuroendocrine derivation including expression of calcitonin and/or CEA.

Desirable: lack of expression of thyroglobulin.

Staging

MTC is staged according to the Union for International Cancer Control (UICC) and American Joint Committee on Cancer (AJCC) staging systems.

Prognosis and prediction

Among patients presenting with a palpable thyroid nodule, the rate of clinical cervical lymph node involvement at the time of diagnosis is as high as 75% in some series {3851}, and the rate of distant metastasis is as high as 15% {3066,2538,4152}. Nodal metastases most commonly involve central compartment nodes (affected in 50–75% of cases), the ipsilateral jugulocarotid chain (in 50–60%), and the contralateral jugulocarotid chain (in 25–50%) {3084,4040,5011}. Distant metastases occur most commonly in the liver, lungs, and bones, and less frequently in other sites such as the brain, skin, adrenal glands, and breast {3385,4848,2940}.

Reported 5-year and 10-year overall survival rates are 75–96% and 64–91%, respectively, depending primarily on disease stage {3789,3728,11,2876}. In cases of hereditary MTC, early detection of thyroid-confined disease through biochemical or genetic screening has resulted in significant improvements in prognosis {4848}, with some studies reporting overall survival rates comparable to those of the general population {2876}. It has also recently been reported that patients with early-stage disease and without regional lymph node metastasis have similar survival rates to the general population {2876}. Other factors known to influence survival include larger tumour size, older age, male sex, extrathyroidal extension, and serum calcitonin and CEA levels {2248,1222,1908,4848,2063,4593,3356}.

RET mutations have also been shown to be prognostically significant in MTC. In sporadic tumours, the presence of a *RET* mutation has been shown to correlate with higher disease stage at diagnosis, disease recurrence, and shorter survival {3997, 1222,3793,4752,4985}. Specifically, tumours harbouring *RET* mutations in exons 15 and 16 (which includes the *RET* p.M918T mutation) are associated with the worst outcome, whereas tumours with other *RET* mutations have the most indolent behaviour, and those with no *RET* mutations tend to have an intermediate prognosis {3115}. Thus, the poor prognosis associated with *RET*-mutant sporadic MTC is largely attributable to the high rate of the *RET* p.M918T mutation {318}. In patients with MEN2, the specific location of the inherited *RET* mutation also determines the timeline of disease manifestation and prognosis {318}. The vast majority of patients with MEN2B harbour the aggressive *RET* p.M918T mutation and, if this is unrecognized, they typically die by the age of 21 years {318}. Patients with MEN2A present with MTC between 25 and 35 years of age, with lymph node metastases present in > 70% {318}. The age of disease manifestation in MEN2A is determined by the specific mutation present, with tumours harbouring the exon 11 *RET* p.C634 mutation demonstrating an earlier onset than tumours with all other mutations (largely in exon 10) {318}. MTCs associated with both sporadic and germline *RET* mutations have demonstrated a good response with rationally designed *RET* inhibitors {4901}.

Until recently there has been no widely accepted histopathological grading scheme for MTC. Recently, histological grading schemes based on proliferative activity (mitotic count and Ki-67 proliferation index) and tumour necrosis {1450,121} have been validated. In the original studies {121,1450} and in a subsequent validation cohort {3158}, the grading systems had significant impacts on overall survival {1450}, disease-specific survival {121,3158}, local recurrence–free survival {121,1450}, and distant metastasis–free survival {121}. Subsequently, a 2-tiered consensus grading scheme has been developed {121,1450}. Using this grading system, high-grade MTCs are defined as tumours with at least one of the following three features: mitotic count ≥ 5 mitoses/2 mm², Ki-67 proliferation index ≥ 5%, and/or tumour necrosis {4971} (see Table 3.07). It is emphasized that the Ki-67 index and mitotic counts are continuous variables, so in addition to histological grade, the precise mitotic count and Ki-67 proliferation index and the presence or absence of tumour necrosis should be reported {4971}.

Mixed medullary and follicular cell–derived thyroid carcinoma

Osamura RY
Fuchs TL
Gill AJ
LiVolsi V
Papotti M
Volante M

Definition

Mixed medullary and follicular cell–derived thyroid carcinoma (MMFCC) is a primary malignant epithelial neoplasm of the thyroid gland showing morphological and immunophenotypic evidence of coexisting follicular and C cell–derived neuroendocrine tumour cell populations within the same lesion.

ICD-O coding

8346/3 Mixed medullary–follicular carcinoma
8347/3 Mixed medullary–papillary carcinoma
8346/3 Mixed medullary and oncocytic carcinoma
8346/3 Mixed medullary and poorly differentiated carcinoma
8346/3 Mixed medullary and anaplastic carcinoma

ICD-11 coding

2D10.Y & XH7DG7 Other specified malignant neoplasms of thyroid gland & Mixed medullary-follicular carcinoma

Related terminology

Acceptable: mixed follicular and C-cell carcinoma; composite medullary and follicular cell–derived carcinoma.

Not recommended: biphasic carcinoma; compound medullary–follicular carcinoma; concurrent medullary–follicular carcinoma; stem cell carcinoma.

Subtype(s)

Mixed medullary–follicular carcinoma; mixed medullary–papillary carcinoma; mixed medullary and oncocytic carcinoma; mixed medullary and poorly differentiated carcinoma; mixed medullary and high-grade differentiated carcinoma; mixed medullary and anaplastic carcinoma

Localization

MMFCC can occur anywhere in the thyroid gland.

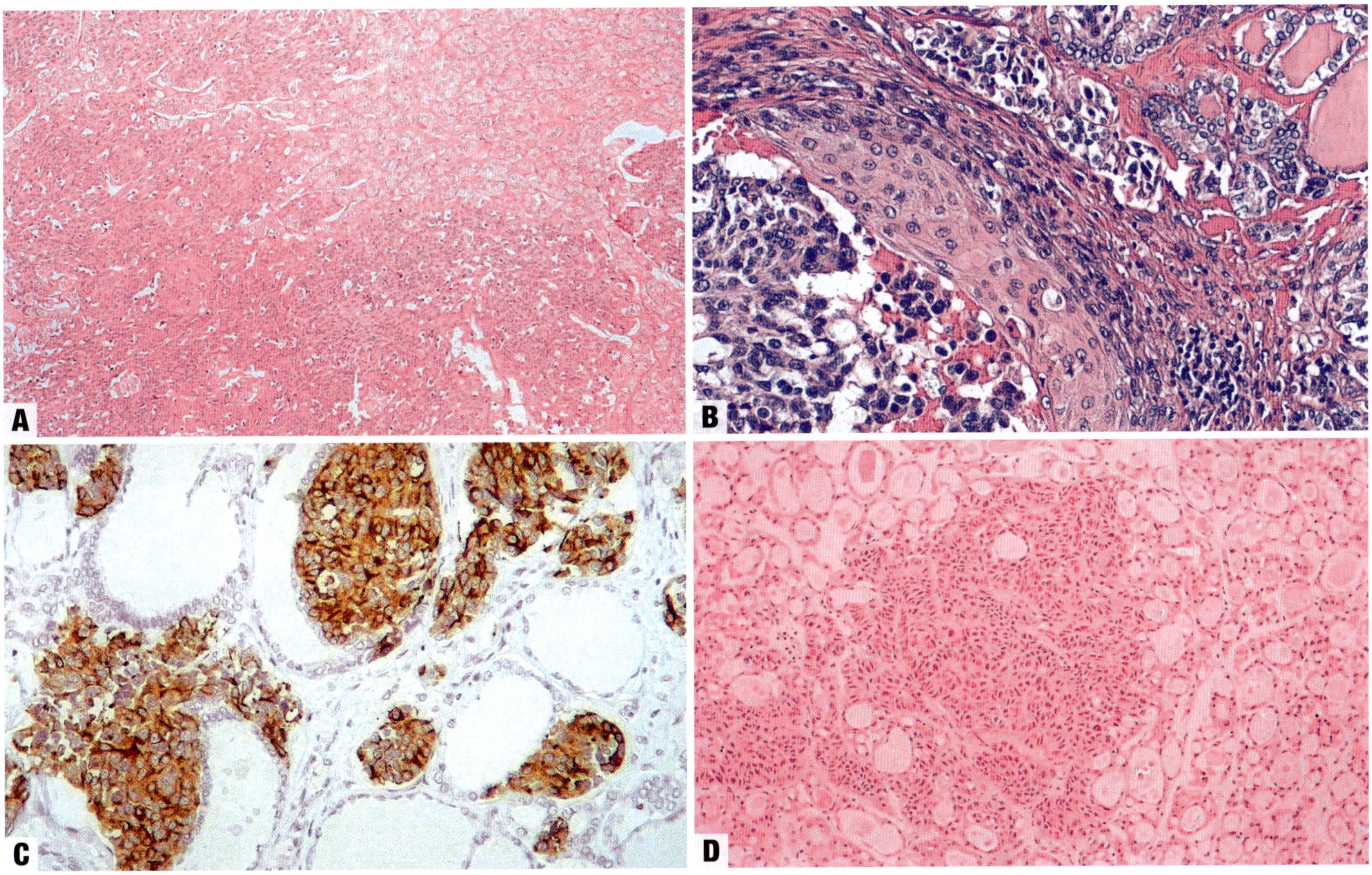

Fig. 3.78 Mixed medullary and follicular cell–derived thyroid carcinoma. **A** A medullary carcinoma component (predominant on the left) admixed with a papillary carcinoma component with solid growth (predominant at the upper right). **B** The papillary carcinoma component has follicular growth and shows squamous metaplasia. It is intimately admixed with the medullary carcinoma. **C** Calcitonin immunostaining highlights the intimate admixture between the two components. **D** A medullary carcinoma component (in the middle) growing in an otherwise oncocytic carcinoma.

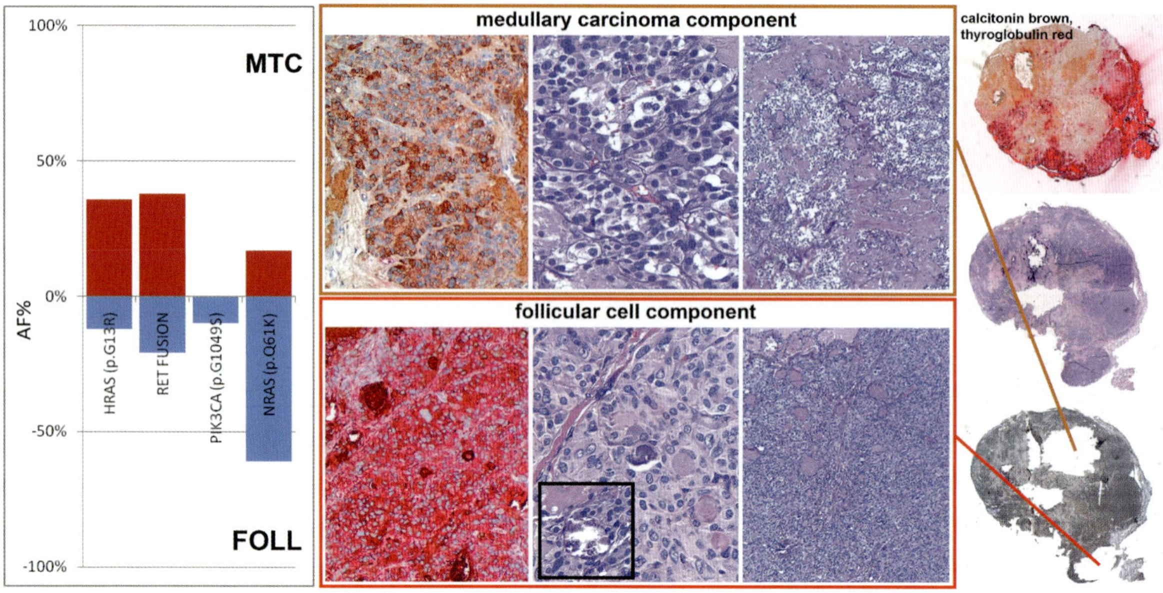

Fig. 3.79 Mixed medullary and follicular cell–derived thyroid carcinoma. Tumour analysed using targeted next-generation sequencing after manual microdissection of medullary carcinoma–predominant (MTC, brown box) and papillary carcinoma with follicular/solid growth–predominant (FOLL, red box) areas. The medullary carcinoma component showed *HRAS* mutation and *RET* fusion, whereas the papillary carcinoma component had an *NRAS* mutation associated with *PIK3CA* mutation with low allelic frequency (AF).

Clinical features

The clinical features are heterogeneous and mostly depend on the predominant C cell or follicular cell–derived tumour component. Most cases present with a palpable solitary nodule, although they may be discovered incidentally {4734,415}. Lymph node metastases are present in 25% of cases at diagnosis {738}. Serum calcitonin levels are often elevated, although they may be within the normal range {5194,2699}. Serum CEA and thyroglobulin may also be elevated {2407,3639}, and the latter may be associated with increased iodine-131 uptake {415}. Ultrasonography typically demonstrates nonspecific features of malignancy, including hypoechoic solid nodules with irregular borders and intranodular vascularization. Microcalcifications may be present in cases of mixed medullary–papillary carcinoma {3922}.

Epidemiology

MMFCC is extremely rare, accounting for < 0.1% of all thyroid malignancies {2679}, with an average age of 54 years and a slight female predominance {2679}. Exceptional cases have been described in children {1654}.

Etiology

MMFCC may occur sporadically or in the setting of hereditary multiple endocrine neoplasia types 2A and 2B {3046,4734, 1424,3639}. There is no association with any specific germline *RET* mutations. The etiology of sporadic medullary thyroid carcinoma (MTC) is unknown.

Pathogenesis

The medullary carcinoma component of MMFCC harbours similar molecular alterations to those seen in pure MTCs, including somatic *RET* mutations, *RET* fusions, and *HRAS* mutations {738, 1118}. In cases of mixed medullary–papillary carcinoma, *BRAF* mutations have been described in the papillary component {738}.

Clonality analyses have suggested that in some cases, the medullary and follicular cell–derived components are unrelated, and in some cases the follicular components have been shown to be polyclonal/oligoclonal {4734} and may represent collision tumours.

In terms of histogenesis, the stem cell theory (clonal evolution) suggests that the two cell populations are both derived from an uncommitted stem cell precursor that is capable of differentiating into divergent neoplastic cell populations {1262,3262}.

In contrast, the hostage theory suggests that the medullary carcinoma component sequesters normal thyroid tissue and subsequently triggers oncogenesis of the follicular cell–derived component {1719}.

Macroscopic appearance

MMFCC presents as a solid, firm, whitish unencapsulated nodule, with a mean size of 29 mm (range: 4–55 mm). The gross appearance of MMFCC is not specific and largely depends on the predominant tumour cell component.

Histopathology

The histopathological hallmark of MMFCC is the coexistence, in variable relative proportions, of two distinct tumour cell populations within a single thyroid nodule, showing features of both MTC and a follicular cell–derived neoplasm {2549, 81,3426,3871}. There is no recommendation on the amount of each component required for MMFCC diagnosis; however, focal expression of calcitonin or CEA in a tumour that otherwise shows typical morphological features of a follicular-derived neoplasm is insufficient to warrant the diagnosis of MMFCC. The medullary carcinoma component is morphologically identical to conventional forms. The follicular cell–derived component includes classic or follicular-variant papillary thyroid carcinoma (by far the most commonly reported); or follicular, oncocytic, poorly differentiated, high-grade differentiated, or (rarely) anaplastic carcinoma {3426,3447}. Lymph node metastases may show mixed histology {162,3048,4734,4130,4613} or may contain only one of the neoplastic components. Concurrent and synchronous medullary carcinoma and follicular cell–derived carcinomas that are anatomically separate, or that merge into one another but are clearly distinct lesions, should not be considered as MMFCC.

Immunohistochemistry

Immunohistochemistry is mandatory to prove the dual C-cell (positive for calcitonin) and follicular cell (positive for thyroglobulin, with the exception of the anaplastic component) differentiation, either in separate cell clusters or within individual cells. In situ hybridization for calcitonin and/or thyroglobulin mRNA may be useful to distinguish true expression from false immunohistochemical positivity due to nonspecific staining caused by cell entrapment {3422,4385}. Thyroid transcription factor 1 (TTF1) is expressed by both components. PAX8 expression patterns in MMFCC have not been described.

Differential diagnosis

The entities include the follicular pattern of medullary carcinoma (thyroglobulin-negative), medullary carcinoma with entrapped non-neoplastic follicles, and follicular carcinoma with neuroendocrine differentiation (chromogranin A–positive but calcitonin-negative) {609}.

Cytology

In most cases, preoperative fine-needle aspirates suggest a cytological diagnosis of MTC, follicular neoplasm (including oncocytic), or papillary carcinoma, depending on the relative proportions of the associated components {1767,2754,3186,1970,1808}. In rare instances, the presence of a clearly distinguishable dual component may lead to a preoperative diagnosis of MMFCC {2754,381,1191}.

Diagnostic molecular pathology

Like conventional MTC, all cases of MMFCC should be investigated for the presence of germline *RET* mutations. No clinical role has been established for molecular markers in sporadic MMFCC.

Essential and desirable diagnostic criteria

Essential: medullary carcinoma and follicular cell–derived carcinoma components should be intimately intermixed within the same lesion; the two components should be morphologically recognizable, and C-cell and follicular cell derivation should be proved by appropriate immunohistochemistry.

Staging

MMFCC is staged according to the MTC staging rules as applied by the Union for International Cancer Control (UICC) and American Joint Committee on Cancer (AJCC) staging systems.

Prognosis and prediction

Either or both components may recur or metastasize, but the clinical behaviour of MMFCC is more similar to that of conventional MTC. Response to radioactive iodine treatment has been documented in metastatic cases with elevated serum thyroglobulin levels {415}. Lymph node involvement and distant metastases (mostly in lung, liver, and bones) occur in as many as 25% of cases {2407,3278,3543,738}. Disease-related mortality is documented in approximately 20% of cases {2407}.

Mucoepidermoid carcinoma

Ghossein RA
Cameselle-Teijeiro JM
Kerr DA
LiVolsi V

Definition
Mucoepidermoid carcinoma is a salivary gland–type carcinoma characterized by mucous, intermediate, and epidermoid (squamoid) tumour cells forming cystic and solid growth patterns.

ICD-O coding
8430/3 Mucoepidermoid carcinoma
8480/3 Mucinous carcinoma

ICD-11 coding
2D10.Y & XH1J36 Other specified malignant neoplasms of thyroid gland & Mucoepidermoid carcinoma

Related terminology
None

Subtype(s)
Mucinous carcinoma (rare subtype)

Localization
It can occur anywhere in the thyroid gland {4852} and (extremely rarely) in a thyroglossal duct cyst {4820}.

Clinical features
Patients are typically euthyroid, with most presenting with a unilateral painless nodule {737}. These tumours are cold on radioiodine scan {4852,737}.

Epidemiology
Mucoepidermoid carcinoma of the thyroid is a very rare tumour, with approximately 48 cases reported to date {737}. It has a female predilection (M:F ratio: 1:1.5), and the mean age at diagnosis is 46 years (range: 10–91 years) {2554,737}. A history of previous neck irradiation in childhood has been reported in some cases {460,1331}. Associated chronic lymphocytic thyroiditis is common {4852}.

Etiology
Unknown

Pathogenesis
The histogenesis of this entity has been subject to significant controversy, with origins proposed from ectopic salivary gland, solid cell nests, and thyroglossal duct remnants {611,3613}. Inception from metaplastic follicular epithelium is now favoured, implicating metaplastic dedifferentiation of well-differentiated thyroid carcinoma {3613,737}.

The *CRTC1::MAML2* fusion transcript, which results from the t(11;19) translocation and is characteristic of salivary gland mucoepidermoid carcinoma, was found in 1 of 3 thyroid mucoepidermoid carcinomas tested {4506}. In 1 other tumour tested, the t(11;19) translocation was not detected, but an increased copy number of the *MAML2* gene was observed {4820}. *BRAF* p.V600E mutations were not present in any thyroid mucoepidermoid carcinomas analysed for that mutation {4563}.

Macroscopic appearance
Reported tumours range from 3 to 100 mm in dimension, with a mean size of 27 mm {737}. On cut section, the tumours are tan-brown to yellow-orange, solid/firm in consistency, with occasional cystic areas {4852}.

Histopathology
The tumours consists of large nests surrounded by a fibrotic stroma. The tumour islands are composed predominantly of epidermoid cells admixed with a smaller number of mucocytes that are easily highlighted by mucicarmine stain. The epidermoid cells are round to polygonal and have eosinophilic cytoplasm with round to oval nuclei and prominent central nucleoli {4852}. Keratin formation can occur, and ciliated epithelial cells have been reported in some instances {4852}. A cribriform pattern with lumina containing colloid-like material has been described {4126}. Cysts, extracellular mucin, and psammoma bodies can be found {4852,298,3198}. There is mild nuclear pleomorphism,

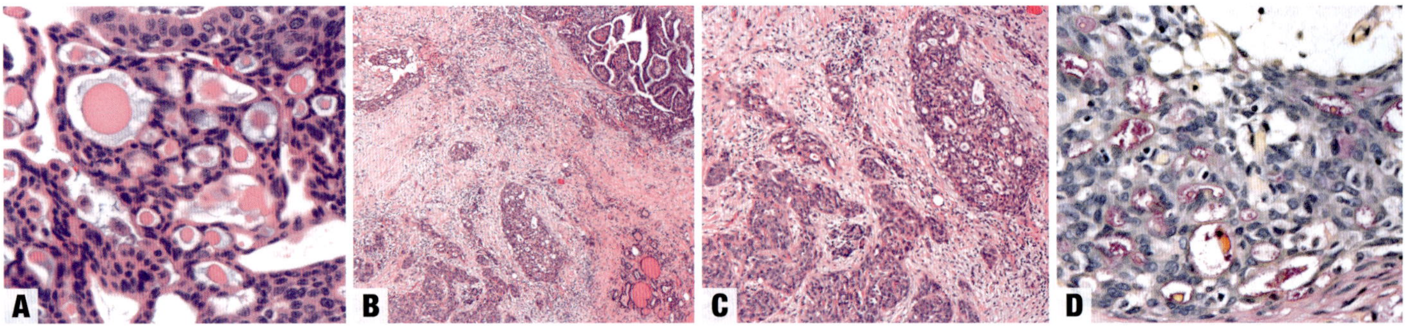

Fig. 3.80 Mucoepidermoid carcinoma of the thyroid. **A** Mucocytes and glandular spaces are intermixed with epidermoid cells. **B** A mucoepidermoid carcinoma (left and centre) associated with a papillary thyroid carcinoma (upper right). **C** Solid sheets of tumour cells composed of epidermoid cells, mucous cells, and glandular spaces. **D** Mucin is present in glandular spaces and mucocytes (goblet cells) (mucicarmine stain).

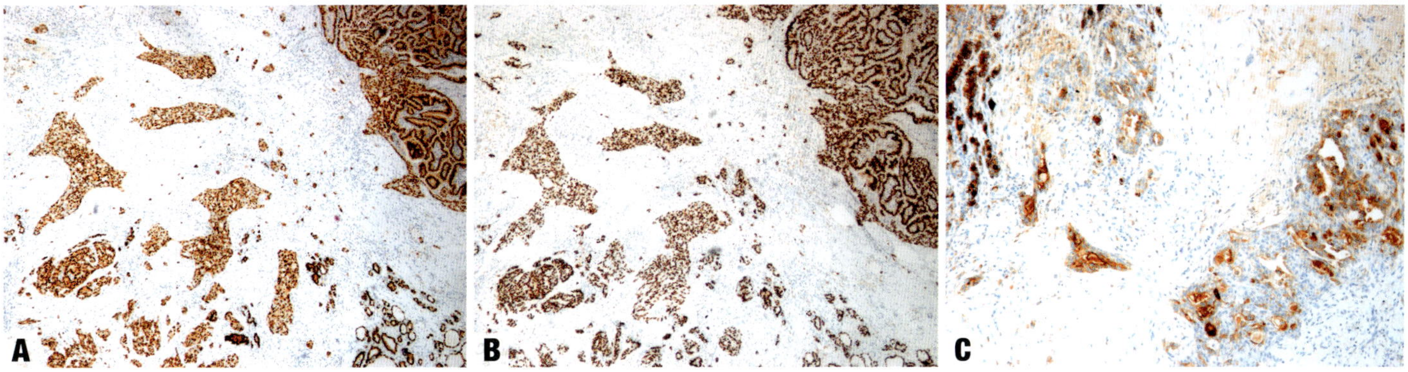

Fig. 3.81 Mucoepidermoid carcinoma of the thyroid. **A** PAX8 immunopositivity is seen in the mucoepidermoid carcinoma and in the concurrent papillary thyroid carcinoma. **B** Both the mucoepidermoid carcinoma and the concurrent papillary thyroid carcinoma are positive for thyroid transcription factor 1 (TTF1). **C** The tumour can express thyroglobulin.

and mitotic figures are rarely seen {4852}. Necrosis is seldom present. A concurrent papillary thyroid carcinoma is found in half of the cases {4852,298,737}. Rarely, there is a concomitant follicular or oncocytic cell carcinoma {3613}. Some mucoepidermoid carcinomas of the thyroid can transform into anaplastic thyroid carcinoma {1429,298}. Chronic lymphocytic thyroiditis is a common finding in the background thyroid {4852}. Mucoepidermoid carcinomas of the thyroid are immunopositive for cytokeratins and p63 and negative for calcitonin, chromogranin, and synaptophysin {737}. They can express PAX8, thyroid transcription factor 1 (TTF1), and thyroglobulin, whereas calcitonin and neuroendocrine markers are negative {298,1331,4346,737}.

Cytology

FNA smears contain predominantly epidermoid cells along with cells showing squamous differentiation with keratinization and intercellular bridges, as well as glandular cells with intracytoplasmic mucin {3198,4676}. A microcystic-like pattern containing small eosinophilic globules and/or amorphous material can be found {4676}. A third cellular component of papillary thyroid carcinoma cells can also be seen {3198}. Features of an associated anaplastic carcinoma can rarely be present {608}.

Diagnostic molecular pathology

Demonstration of *MAML2* rearrangement may be helpful in selected cases {4506}.

Essential and desirable diagnostic criteria

Essential: a tumour with mucous cells, intermediate cells, and squamoid cells.

Desirable: MAML2 rearrangement (in selected cases).

Staging

Staging is according to the Union for International Cancer Control (UICC) and American Joint Committee on Cancer (AJCC) staging systems.

Prognosis and prediction

Most patients have an excellent outcome, and mucoepidermoid carcinoma of the thyroid is considered to be an indolent tumour {737,4852,1331}. Metastases to the neck lymph nodes are common {1429,3044}, but distant metastases are unusual {4852,460,737}. Death from the disease occurs in a minority patients, often due to anaplastic transformation {1429,4676,298}.

Secretory carcinoma

Seethala R
Kerr DA
Mete O

Definition

Secretory carcinoma (SC) is a salivary gland–type carcinoma often composed of microcystic, tubular, and solid structures with abundant eosinophilic homogeneous or bubbly secretions. It is usually characterized by specific rearrangement of the *ETV6* gene.

ICD-O coding

8502/3 Secretory carcinoma

ICD-11 coding

2D10.Y & XH44J4 Other specified malignant neoplasms of thyroid gland & Secretory carcinoma

Related terminology

Acceptable: mammary analogue secretory carcinoma.

Subtype(s)

None

Localization

SC can occur in either lobe or in the isthmus.

Clinical features

SC usually presents as a uninodular mass. Compression or invasion of adjacent structures and nodal disease are more common than in salivary SC {1097,737}.

Epidemiology

Average age at presentation is slightly older than at salivary gland sites (61.5 years, range: 36–74 years). There appears to be a female predilection {1097,737}.

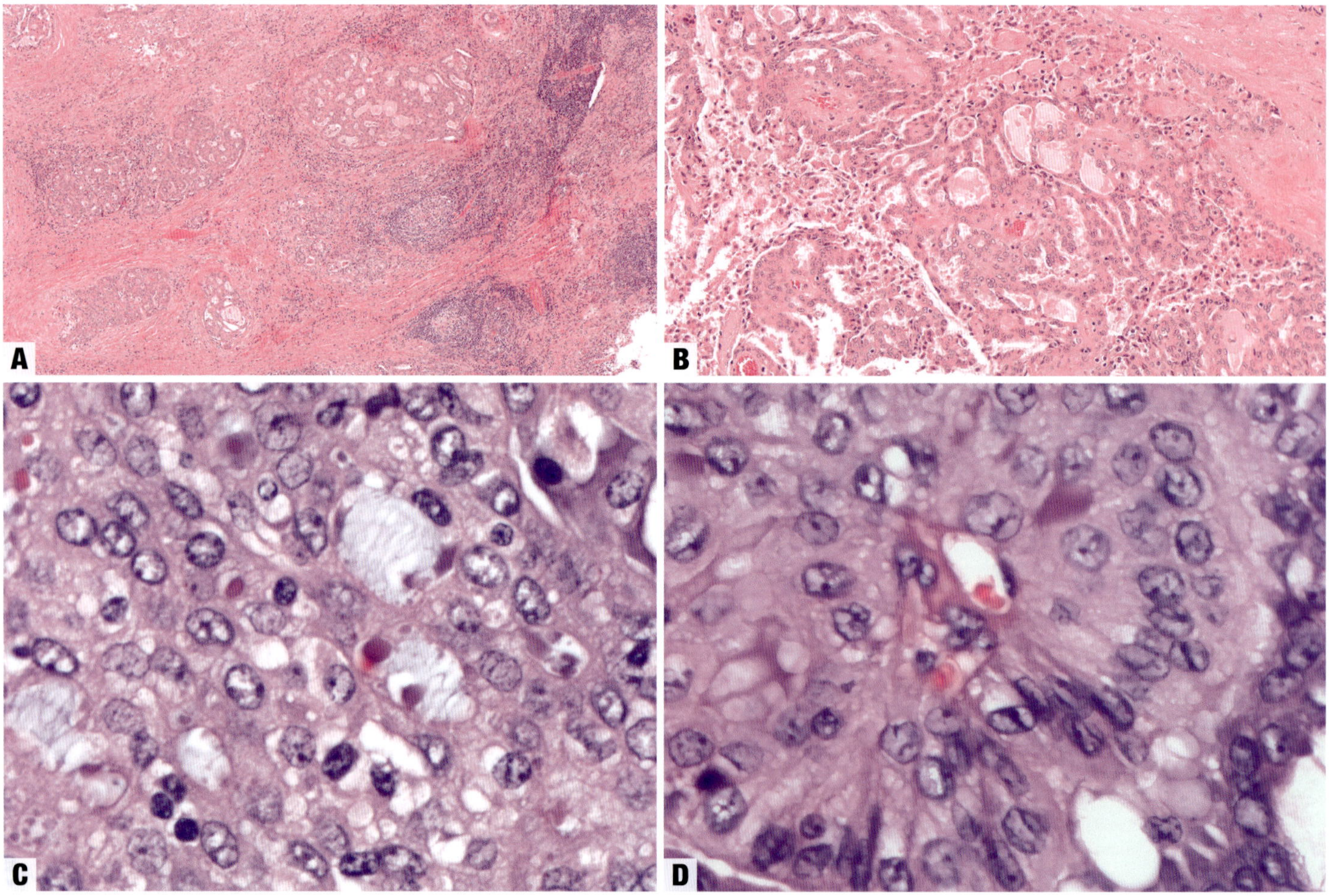

Fig. 3.82 Secretory carcinoma. **A** Sclerosis and infiltration of adjacent thyroid. **B** A mixture of cribriform and micropapillary growth patterns is common. **C,D** Eosinophilic to vacuolated cytoplasm with bubbly luminal secretions composed of a mixture of dense eosinophilic substance and mucin. Nuclei are often cleared and ovoid with prominent nucleoli (**C**), and foci with elongation and grooves reminiscent of papillary thyroid carcinoma may be noted (**D**).

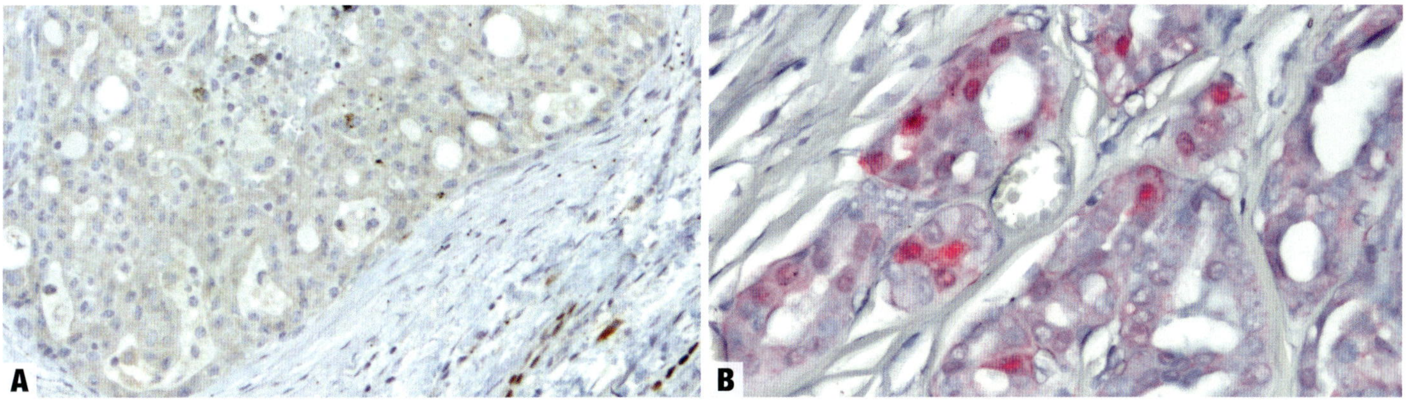

Fig. 3.83 Secretory carcinoma. **A** Thyroid transcription factor 1 (TTF1) negativity. **B** S100 positivity.

Etiology

The etiology is unclear. Occasional co-occurrence with papillary thyroid carcinoma, including rare cases with shared translocations, is noted {1125}, implying a possible follicular origin.

Pathogenesis

SCs are characterized by *ETV6* translocations, with *ETV6::NTRK3* exclusively seen in the thyroid to date {3915}.

Macroscopic appearance

The mean size of reported thyroid SCs is 44 mm (range: 24–76 mm). They show firm, white-tan, often infiltrative cut surfaces {1097,737}.

Histopathology

Thyroid SCs are morphologically similar to SCs at other sites and are composed of cells with eosinophilic, vacuolated cytoplasm, arranged in papillary, tubular, microcystic, and solid patterns. SC characteristically shows eosinophilic, bubbly luminal secretions. Rare cases show high-grade transformation {4944, 1097,3915}.

Immunohistochemistry

SCs characteristically stain for S100, mammaglobin, GATA3, and (often) GCDFP-15. Thyroglobulin and thyroid transcription factor 1 (TTF1) are typically negative, with weak, focal PAX8 staining {1104,737}. PAS and mucicarmine usually highlight the secretions.

Differential diagnosis

Architecture, nuclear features, and eosinophilic cytoplasm may raise consideration for oncocytic carcinoma, medullary carcinoma, and papillary thyroid carcinoma. However, the characteristic cytoplasm, secretions, and immunophenotype are highly unlikely to be seen outside of SC. Secondary involvement by a non-thyroid SC should be excluded clinicoradiologically.

Cytology

Aspirates show cohesive vaguely histiocytoid cells with eosinophilic vacuolar cytoplasm arranged in sheets or arborizing 3D structures. Nuclei have moderate size variation and may show clearing, prominent nucleoli, and membrane irregularities such as grooves or rare pseudoinclusions {3858}.

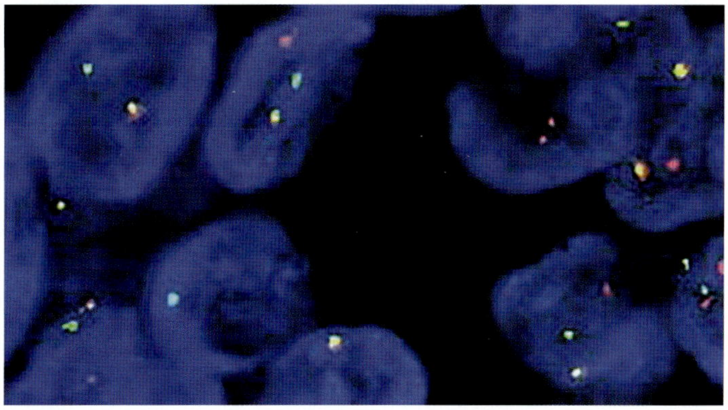

Fig. 3.84 Secretory carcinoma. Break-apart FISH for *ETV6* confirms the translocation status.

Diagnostic molecular pathology

ETV6 translocations confirm the diagnosis when present along with the typical morphology and immunophenotype.

Essential and desirable diagnostic criteria

Essential: eosinophilic vacuolar cells; bubbly secretions; microcystic, tubular, solid, and papillary architecture; S100/SOX10 (not well studied in thyroid SC) and mammaglobin expression; absent to weak thyroid differentiation marker expression.

Desirable: ETV6 translocation.

Staging

Staging is according to the Union for International Cancer Control (UICC) and American Joint Committee on Cancer (AJCC) staging systems.

Prognosis and prediction

Thyroid SCs appear more aggressive than their salivary counterparts. More than half of patients experience either locoregional recurrence or distant metastases. Positive margins and extrathyroidal extension may be associated with recurrence {1097,737}.

Sclerosing mucoepidermoid carcinoma with eosinophilia

Kerr DA
Cameselle-Teijeiro JM
LiVolsi V
Nosé V
Sadow PM

Definition

Sclerosing mucoepidermoid carcinoma with eosinophilia (SMECE) is a thyroid carcinoma composed of epidermoid and mucous cells in a background of marked stromal sclerosis with infiltration of eosinophils and lymphocytes.

ICD-O coding

8430/3 Sclerosing mucoepidermoid carcinoma with eosinophilia

ICD-11 coding

2D10.Y & XH1J36 Other specified malignant neoplasms of thyroid gland & Mucoepidermoid carcinoma

Related terminology

None

Subtype(s)

None

Localization

Unilateral thyroid lobe involvement is most common, although diffuse, bilateral involvement may occasionally be seen {4078}.

Clinical features

SMECE typically presents as a slow-growing, unilateral painless mass in euthyroid or hypothyroid patients, the latter presentation being more common. SMECE shows a female predilection (M:F ratio: 1:13). The average age at presentation is 55 years (range: 26–89 years) {3651,2025,31}.

Ultrasound imaging shows a smooth, isoechoic mass with possible coarse calcifications. The tumours are hypofunctioning (cold) on radioiodine scan {4097,2025,737}.

Epidemiology

SMECE is a rare tumour, with < 100 cases reported to date {2025, 4328,737,3173,2834,3288,31}. Women are almost exclusively affected (> 90% of cases) {1995,3651,4078,2025}. SMECE is nearly universally associated with chronic lymphocytic thyroiditis {4328,737}.

Etiology

Unknown

Pathogenesis

SMECE is likely to be of ultimobranchial body / solid cell nest origin {1995,4078,4880}. Genomic studies of SMECE have thus far been largely uninformative, generally showing a notable absence of alterations characteristic of mucoepidermoid carcinoma (*MAML2* rearrangements) or *BRAF* mutations {4078, 4880,31}. Isolated cases of SMECE have been reported to harbour several different alterations of thus far undetermined significance, including *MET* hyperploidy in the absence of amplification; point mutations in *APC*, *NTRK3*, and *NF1*; and NTRK1 overexpression without an associated translocation {4078, 4880,3288}. Very recently, *BRAF* p.V600E has been reported in tumours believed to represent combined SMECE with papillary or anaplastic carcinoma {4328,2834}.

Macroscopic appearance

The average tumour size is 43 mm in largest dimension, with reported sizes ranging from 5 to 130 mm {4078,737,459}. Cut surfaces are firm, solid, and white-yellow, and they may have cystic change {3651,4078}. Gross extrathyroidal extension is noted in 25% of cases {737}.

Histopathology

SMECE shows distinctive histology characterized by an admixture of squamoid/epidermoid cells and mucocytes set in a densely sclerotic stroma with lymphocytes, eosinophils, and plasma cells. The tumour cells form cords, strands, and nests with areas of cellular dyscohesion imparting a pseudoangiomatous pattern. Foci of clear cell change (glycogenation), mucus extravasation, and/or keratinization may be identified {82}.

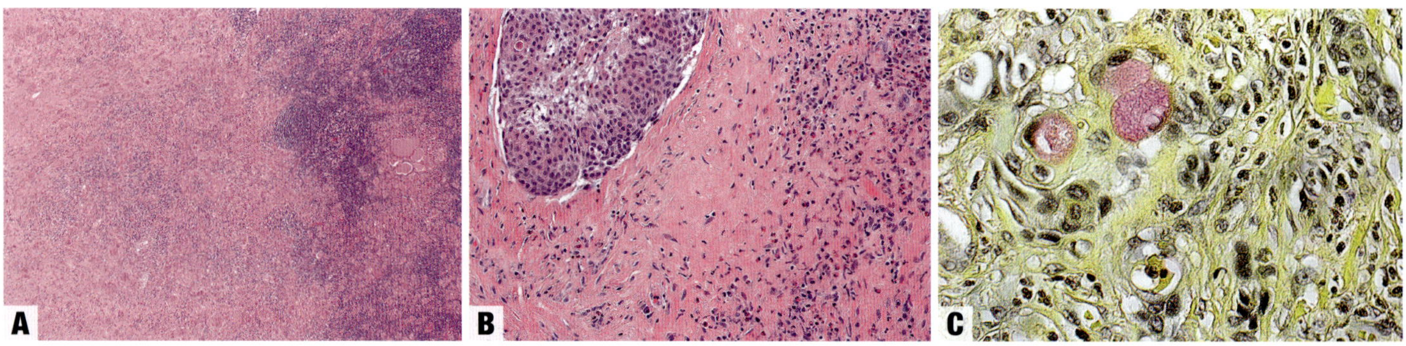

Fig. 3.85 Sclerosing mucoepidermoid carcinoma with eosinophilia. **A** The sclerotic tumour (left) appears to merge with associated underlying chronic lymphocytic thyroiditis (right). **B** The squamoid tumour cells are associated with a dense sclerotic stroma infiltrated by lymphocytes and eosinophils. **C** A mucicarmine special stain highlights intracellular mucin within the neoplastic mucocytes.

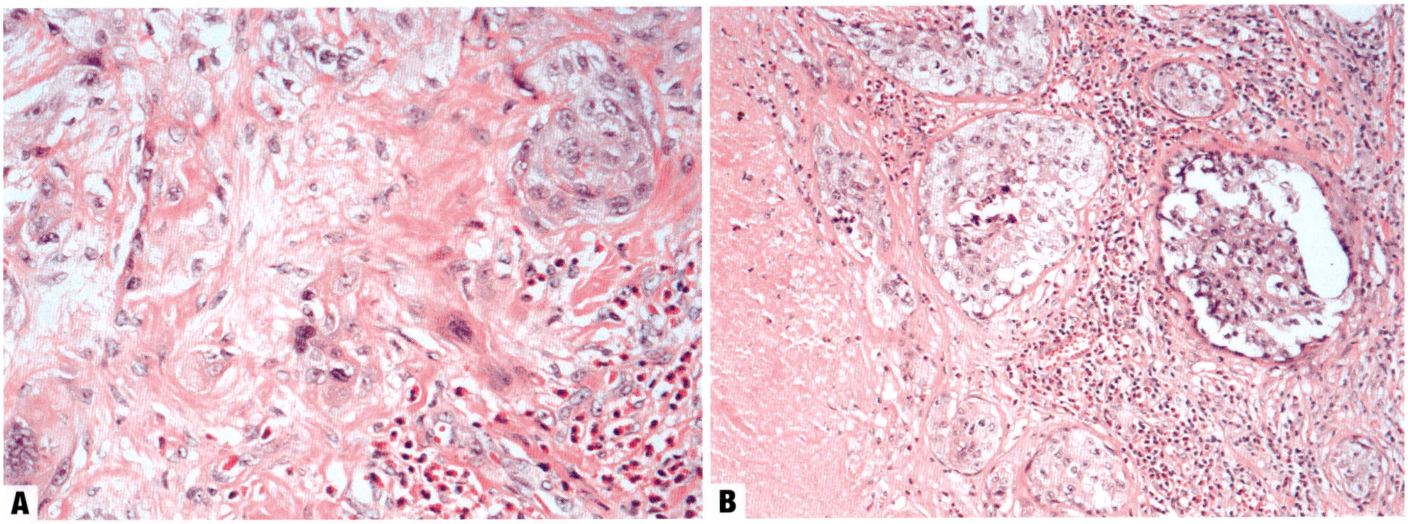

Fig. 3.86 Sclerosing mucoepidermoid carcinoma with eosinophilia. **A** Large malignant cells are within a sclerotic stroma with numerous eosinophils. **B** Nests of tumour cells intermixed with eosinophils with an adjacent area of tumour necrosis.

Lymphocytes often predominate within the stromal inflammatory component, and although eosinophils are always present, their quantity can range from limited to abundant. The tumour cells show mild to moderate nuclear atypia with small, distinct nucleoli. Nuclear irregularities may be seen, but well-developed nuclear features of papillary carcinoma are not present. Mitotic rate is variable, ranging from 0 to 6 mitoses/5 mm^2 (equating to 20 HPF of 0.25 mm^2). The background thyroid parenchyma invariably demonstrates chronic lymphocytic thyroiditis, often the fibrosing pattern of Hashimoto thyroiditis, and in areas, the associated squamous metaplasia may merge imperceptibly with foci of tumour {743,4078,3651}. A separate synchronous or metachronous focus of papillary carcinoma is identified in 20% of cases {4078,4880,737}. Rarely, SMECE has been reported to arise as a component of papillary or anaplastic thyroid carcinoma {2025,2834}.

Immunohistochemistry

By histochemistry, the mucus cells and foci of extracellular mucin are positive for mucicarmine and PAS. Immunohistochemistry shows consistent reactivity for p63 and cytokeratins in the squamoid tumour cells {1995,2025}. Differential staining between the luminal cell compartment (highlighted by CK7) and basal cell compartment (reactive for CK5/6) may be seen {2834,31}. Focal and weak expression of thyroid transcription factor 1 (TTF1) is present in approximately 50% of cases {82, 4078,4328,737}. Thyroglobulin and PAX8 are typically negative, whereas calcitonin, chromogranin, and S100 are consistently negative {3651,2025,737}.

Differential diagnosis

The differential diagnosis includes conventional mucoepidermoid carcinoma, metastatic squamous cell carcinoma, anaplastic thyroid carcinoma, diffuse sclerosing papillary thyroid carcinoma, and intrathyroidal thymic carcinoma {3651,3689, 4880}. Particularly within a lymph node metastasis, Hodgkin lymphoma enters the differential diagnosis {4220,82,3651}, as does IgG4-related disease.

Cytology

Cytological features are frequently nonspecific. Fine-needle aspirates are usually highly cellular, and the tumour cells have variable amounts of cytoplasm with ovoid nuclei, small nucleoli, and rare grooves or pseudoinclusions. Squamoid cells, keratin pearls, and rare intracytoplasmic vacuoles have been reported. The background commonly shows lymphocytes; eosinophils and mucinous or keratinaceous material may be present. Fine-needle aspirates are most commonly diagnosed as atypia of undetermined significance, with few cases reported as positive for malignancy but without a specific diagnosis of SMECE rendered {459,1900,129,4880,3173,3288}.

Diagnostic molecular pathology

Not relevant

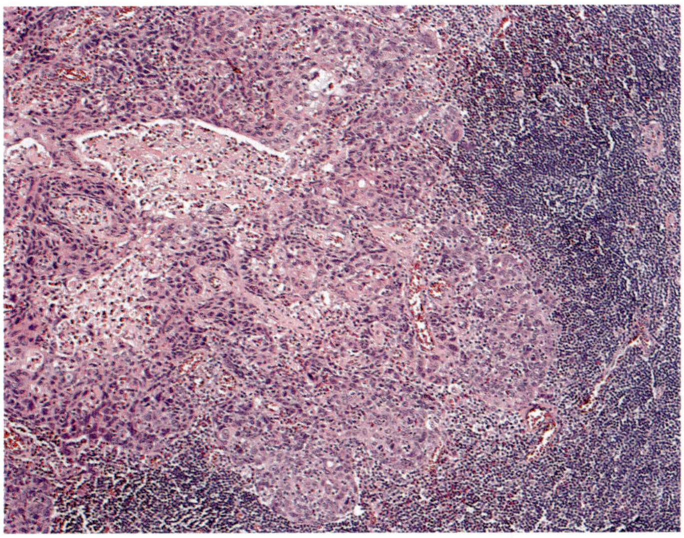

Fig. 3.87 Sclerosing mucoepidermoid carcinoma with eosinophilia. A lymph node metastasis recapitulates the morphological features characteristic of the primary tumour.

Essential and desirable diagnostic criteria

Essential: primary thyroid carcinoma showing epidermoid/squamoid and mucous cells in a background of stromal sclerosis with a rich inflammatory infiltrate containing eosinophils.

Desirable: a background of chronic lymphocytic thyroiditis; thyroglobulin and PAX8 are typically negative.

Staging

No staging is available.

Prognosis and prediction

As many as 40% of patients have regional lymph node metastases {4328,737}. In some series, upon clinical follow-up, two thirds of patients were reported to be alive without disease {2025,4328,2834,31}. Occasional instances (< 15% of cases) of distant metastases to lung, bone, liver, mediastinum, or kidney have been documented {4078,4328}. Long-term follow-up is needed because recurrences and/or metastases may appear as long as 20 years after the original surgery. Reliable prognostic or predictive indicators have not been developed.

Cribriform morular thyroid carcinoma

Erickson LA
Cameselle-Teijeiro JM
Jung CK
LiVolsi V
Mete O
Nosé V
Sobrinho-Simoes M

Definition

Cribriform-morular thyroid carcinoma (CMTC) is a malignant thyroid tumour with a particular growth pattern secondary to constitutive activation of the WNT/β-catenin pathway that can occur with familial adenomatous polyposis or sporadically.

ICD-O coding

8201/3 Cribriform morular thyroid carcinoma

ICD-11 coding

2D10.Y & XH1YZ3 Other specified malignant neoplasms of thyroid gland & Cribriform carcinoma, NOS

Related terminology

Not recommended: cribriform-morular variant of papillary thyroid carcinoma.

Subtype(s)

None

Localization

Cribriform-morular thyroid carcinoma (CMTC) is usually multifocal and/or bilateral in familial adenomatous polyposis (FAP), whereas sporadic cases appear as a solitary nodule {606, 3295,3297,1703}.

Clinical features

CMTC almost exclusively occurs in young women (97%) with 89% occurring in individuals aged < 40 years (mean age: 28 years, range: 8–69 years) {2510}. The M:F ratio is 1:31–61 {2510,615}. As many as 53% of CMTCs are associated with FAP {2510}. Tumours may present as a painless mass, hoarseness, or dysphagia, or they may be incidentally discovered on ultrasound.

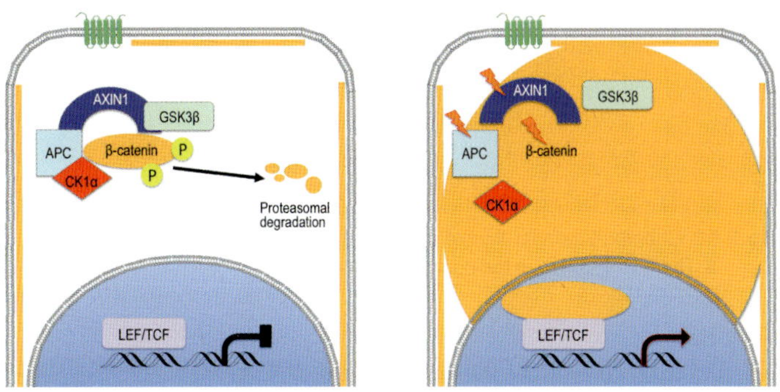

Fig. 3.88 Pathogenesis of cribriform-morular thyroid carcinoma. Under normal conditions, in the absence of WNT binding to Frizzled receptors, β-catenin interacts with the destruction complex (CK1, GSK3B, APC, and AXIN1), resulting in its phosphorylation by CK1 and GSK3B and its subsequent degradation by the proteasome. In sporadic cribriform-morular thyroid carcinoma, somatic mutations in *APC*, *CTNNB1*, and/or *AXIN1* alter the destruction complex, impairing β-catenin phosphorylation and degradation. β-Catenin accumulates in the cytoplasm and subsequently translocates to the nucleus, where it acts as an activator of TCF/LEF proteins that lead to the constitutive expression of WNT target genes. In cribriform-morular thyroid carcinomas associated with familial adenomatous polyposis, there are germline *APC* mutations.

CMTCs are circumscribed and hypoechoic with a heterogeneous echotexture, and they lack a halo and calcifications by ultrasonography {838}.

Epidemiology

In a review of 129 CMTCs in the English literature, 63% of reported cases were from Asia, 26% were from America, and 11% were from Europe {2510}. The frequency of thyroid carcinoma in FAP has increased with screening ultrasound and FNAB {615}. Ultrasonographic screening of 129 Japanese individuals with FAP identified CMTCs in 6.2% {4608}.

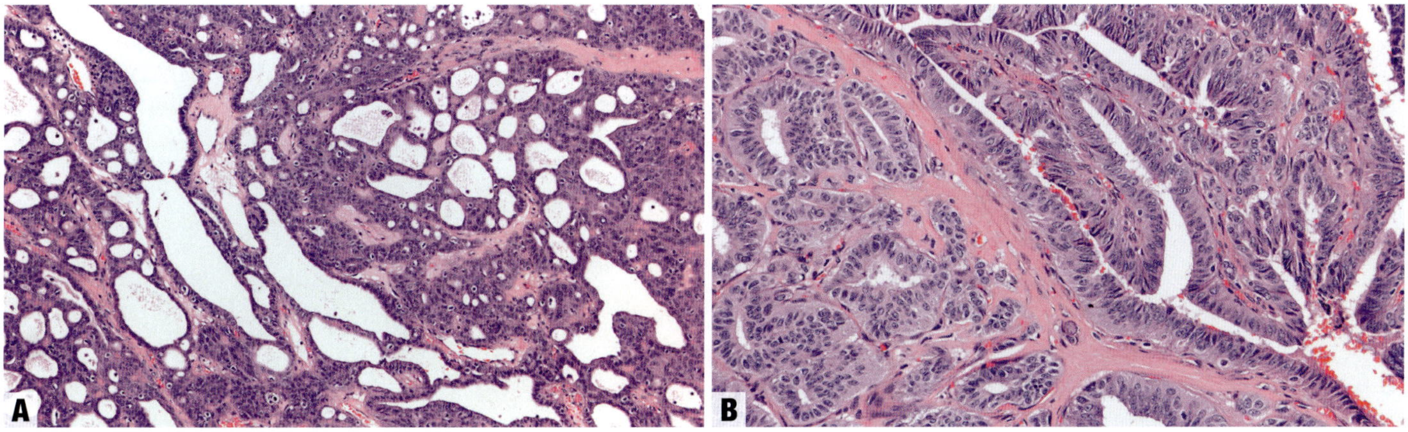

Fig. 3.89 Cribriform-morular thyroid carcinoma. **A** The cribriform structures lack intervening fibrous stroma and merge with tubular follicles that lack colloid. **B** Papillae and pseudopapillae are lined by tall, cuboidal or pseudostratified columnar cells. Tubular follicles lacking colloid are seen.

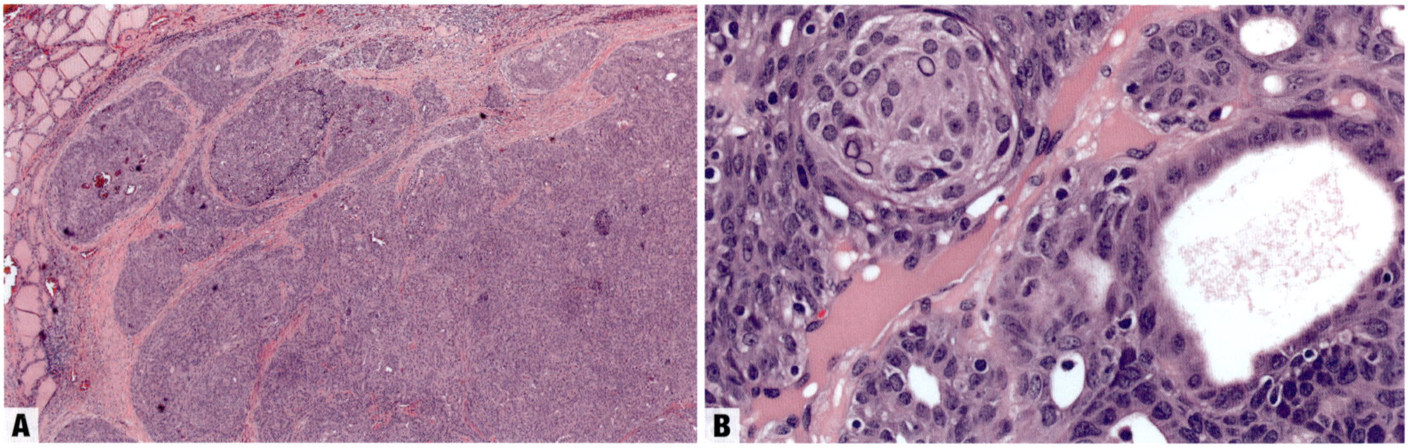

Fig. 3.90 Cribriform-morular thyroid carcinoma. **A** These tumours are usually circumscribed or encapsulated but can have fibrous bands imparting a multilobulated appearance. **B** There is a morule in the upper-left corner and cribriform tubular growth in the lower-right corner.

Etiology

In patients with FAP, CMTC is secondary to germline *APC* mutations. Somatic mutations resulting in permanent activation of the WNT/β-catenin signalling pathway are responsible for sporadic tumours {615}. Female sex is a risk factor {726,615}.

Pathogenesis

Most germline *APC* mutations in FAP with thyroid tumours occur in exon 15 (codons 463–1387), whereas codon 1061 is a hotspot for hepatoblastoma and CMTC {725}. *APC* mutations lead to a truncated APC protein, which is unable to contribute to β-catenin proteasomal degradation. Stabilized β-catenin is translocated into the nucleus and binds TCF/LEF proteins, leading to the constitutive expression of WNT target genes involved in proliferation and loss of differentiation {615}. In FAP with multiple CMTCs, each tumour has a different somatic *APC* mutation (second hit) {3041}. A second-hit somatic mutation in *KMT2C* and *KMT2D* was described in some familial CMTCs {3242}.

Somatic *APC* mutation in exon 15 (codon 1309) has been detected in a sporadic CMTC {612}. Somatic mutations in functionally equivalent genes, such as *CTNNB1* (exon 3) {4987, 507} and *AXIN1* (exons 1 and 7) {615} are reported in sporadic CMTCs. Somatic alterations involving *RET* (in the form of rearrangements) {4233,724}, *PIK3CA* {2471}, and *KRAS* {1560},

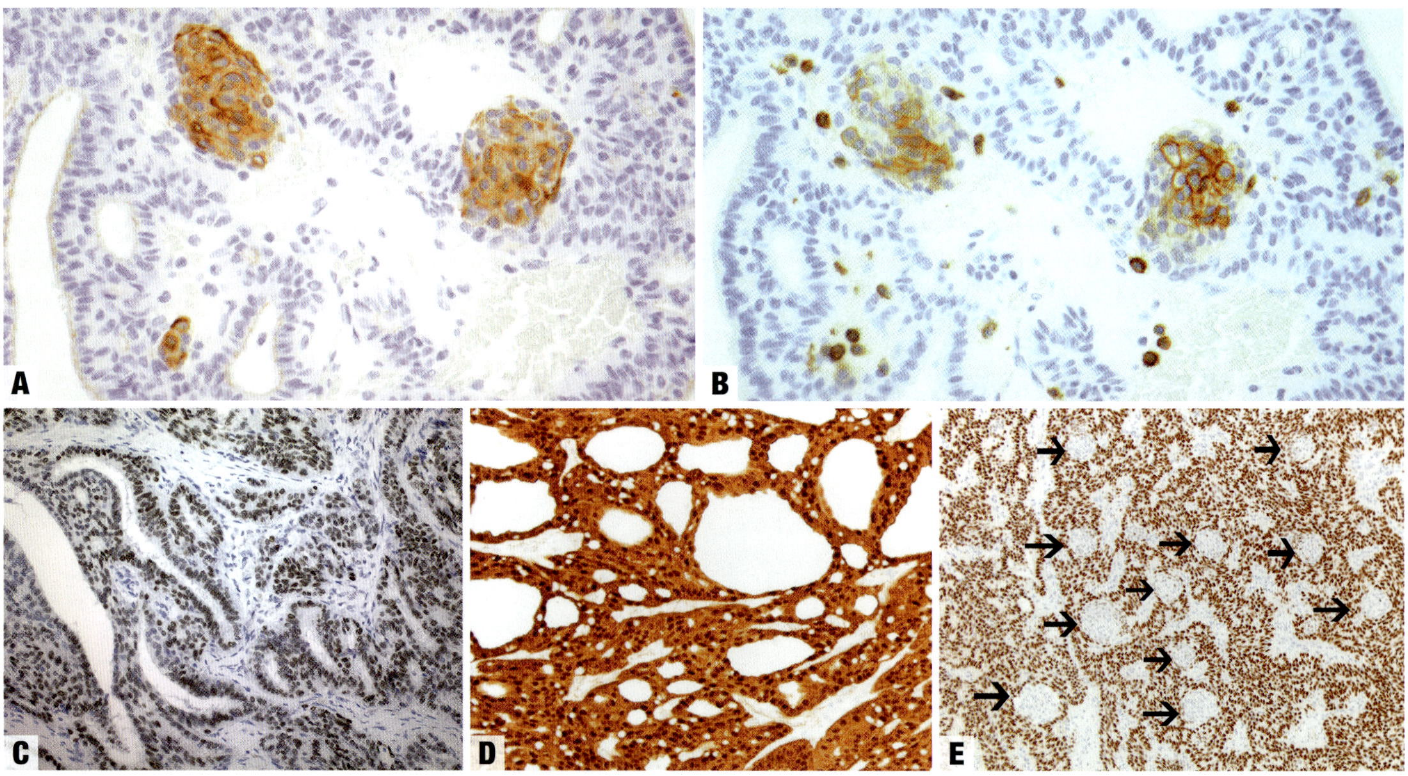

Fig. 3.91 Cribriform-morular thyroid carcinoma. **A** The morular component is positive for CK5. **B** Immunostaining for CD5 highlights the morular component of these tumours, as well as scattered CD5+ T lymphocytes. **C** This tumour is diffusely positive for ER. **D** β-Catenin immunostaining shows characteristic aberrant positivity in the nuclei and in the cytoplasm of the tumour cells. **E** The tumour is immunopositive for thyroid transcription factor 1 (TTF1) except in the morules (arrows).

as well as *TERT* promoter mutations {3320}, could be additional effectors of the WNT/β-catenin pathway in familial and sporadic CMTC {615}.

Macroscopic appearance

CMTCs in FAP are often multifocal (4–13 foci), bilateral, and small, whereas sporadic tumours are larger (mean: 30 mm) single nodules {507,1783,606,3297,615,3435}. CMTCs are well circumscribed or encapsulated, solid but may be cystic, and white-tan {615}.

Histopathology

CMTCs are circumscribed or encapsulated and may have a lobulated appearance due to fibrous septa {3295,615,1783}. Angioinvasion occurs in 30% of cases and capsular invasion in 40% {615}. CMTCs have an admixture of growth patterns not seen in other thyroid carcinomas {3295,1783}. As originally described, CMTCs display "an intricate blending of cribriform, follicular, papillary, trabecular, and solid patterns of growth, with morular (squamoid) areas" {606}. The cribriform structures are composed of anastomosing bars and arches without intervening fibrous stroma that merge with tubular follicles that lack colloid {606,615}. Papillae and pseudopapillae are lined by tall, cuboidal or pseudostratified cells, and trabecular areas show spindle cells reminiscent of hyalinizing trabecular tumour {606, 3297,615}. Squamoid morulae are whorls of spindle to ovoid cells that lack keratinization and show nuclear clearing due to biotin accumulation {606,1703,615}. Psammoma bodies are rare {2510,615}. With these distinctive features, the tumour was initially named "cribriform-morular variant of papillary thyroid carcinoma" {606}. Correlation between the morphological features of the tumour and recently understood molecular alterations brought about the name change to "cribriform-morular thyroid carcinoma" {3299,3297,615,617,507}.

Immunohistochemistry

Aberrant strong nuclear and cytoplasmic β-catenin staining is the hallmark of this thyroid tumour {3297,1703,615}. CMTC is positive for thyroid transcription factor 1 (TTF1) (clones SPT24 and 8G3G7/1), various keratins, EMA, ER, and PR; it is negative for CK20, calcitonin, and WT1 {604,605,1560,2471,1703,615}. Thyroglobulin expression is typically negative; however, focal nonspecific diffusion-type staining can occur due to entrapped non-tumorous thyroid follicles {507}. PAX8 immunohistochemistry using either the monoclonal BC12 or polyclonal antisera shows no or focal weak staining in these tumours {507}. Morulae are negative for keratin 34βE12, thyroglobulin, TTF1, PAX8, ER, PR, and E-cadherin, but stain for CDX2, CD10, CD5, and CK5 {604,605,1560,2471,615,507}. The Ki-67 index is usually < 5%. High-grade CMTCs have increased mitotic activity, necrosis, and Ki-67 indexes of 15–60%; they may have neuroendocrine differentiation, and can occur in sporadic and familial settings {609,3172,911,4576}. In a study of 33 CMTCs, high-grade features were present in 2 sporadic CMTCs and in none of the FAP-associated CMTCs {507}.

Cytology

Smears are hypercellular, with predominantly large complex tissue fragments that show a papillary arrangement of tall columnar cells, and a cribriform pattern due to slit-like spaces, with swirling of nuclei representing morulae, and in some cases hyaline strands. There are spindle cells and haemosiderin-laden macrophages and histiocytes, but no colloid in the background. Nuclei can show peculiar nuclear clearing with thick membranes, as well as grooves and pseudoinclusions. Nuclear β-catenin immunocytochemistry on cell blocks is helpful in the differential diagnosis with other thyroid gland tumours, including the aggressive tall cell papillary thyroid carcinoma {2156,1897}.

Diagnostic molecular pathology

Evaluation for germline *APC* mutations is desirable in patients with CMTC. About 85% of germline *APC* mutations are in exon 15, usually outside the mutation cluster region {725,615}. In familial and sporadic cases, constitutive WNT/β-catenin pathway activation is evidenced by strong nuclear β-catenin immunostaining – a hallmark of CMTC and an important diagnostic criterion. *BRAF* mutations are absent.

Essential and desirable diagnostic criteria

Essential: a well-circumscribed or locally invasive TTF1-positive thyroid neoplasm; diffuse nuclear β-catenin expression; predominant complex architecture including cribriform and squamoid morulae, with no colloid formation.

Desirable:

- Cribriform areas: positive for pancytokeratin, ER, and PR; negative (or focal weak) reactivity for PAX8; negative for thyroglobulin.
- Morulae: positive for CD10, CDX2, CD5, and CK5; negative for TTF1, PAX8, thyroglobulin, ER, and PR.

Staging

Staging is according to the Union for International Cancer Control (UICC) and American Joint Committee on Cancer (AJCC) staging systems.

Prognosis and prediction

CMTC is associated with lymph node metastases at presentation in 12% of cases and distant metastases in 3%, with an overall mortality rate of 2% {2510}. High-grade CMTCs behave aggressively {3172,3320,4576}.

Thymoma

Cameselle-Teijeiro JM
Chan JKC
Jain D
LiVolsi V
Papotti M

Definition

Intrathyroidal thymoma is an organotypic thymic epithelial tumour occurring within or attached to the thyroid gland.

ICD-O coding

8580/3 Thymoma, NOS
8581/3 Thymoma, type A
8582/3 Thymoma, type AB
8583/3 Thymoma, type B1
8584/3 Thymoma, type B2
8585/3 Thymoma, type B3
8580/1 Micronodular thymoma with lymphoid stroma
8580/3 Metaplastic thymoma

ICD-11 coding

2C27.2 & XH6WN9 Malignant thymoma & Thymoma, type A
2C27.2 & XH0JH0 Malignant thymoma & Thymoma, type AB
2C27.2 & XH66U8 Malignant thymoma & Thymoma, type B1
2C27.2 & XH2G89 Malignant thymoma & Thymoma, type B2
2C27.2 & XH4EW9 Malignant thymoma & Thymoma, type B3
4B40.Y & XH56K5 Other specified diseases of thymus & Micronodular thymoma with lymphoid stroma
2C27.2 & XH3DX0 Malignant thymoma & Metaplastic thymoma

Related terminology

Acceptable: ectopic thymoma.

Subtype(s)

Types A {1541,4447}, AB {880,3280}, B1 {2475,3280,2593,4845, 1890}, B2 {2475,4845,1890}, and B3 {3004,4431,3280,1890}, according to the WHO classification of thoracic tumours {4871}; micronodular thymoma with lymphoid stroma; metaplastic thymoma

Localization

Intrathyroidal thymoma occurs within or attached to the thyroid gland, more commonly in the lower pole of the left lobe (anterolateral neck, deep to the sternocleidomastoid muscle) {744, 5006,3323,4431,3280}.

Clinical features

This tumour usually presents as an asymptomatic euthyroid mass that often has been present for years {744,3589,880,4845}; however, some cases may be associated with pain {4845}, compressive symptoms (dysphagia and/or dyspnoea) {1890,1541}, and tracheal deviation {2593}. Intrathyroidal thymomas are hypofunctioning on radionuclide scan {3016}. Myasthenia gravis and other paraneoplastic disorders have not been reported {2593,4845}.

Epidemiology

Intrathyroidal thymomas are very rare. Most occur in the fifth to sixth decade of life (mean: 53 years, range: 28–81 years), with a female predominance (M:F ratio: 1:3) {880,1541,2475,4431, 2593,4845,1890}.

Etiology

Unknown

Pathogenesis

These tumours are thought to arise from thymic or branchial pouch remnants displaced during embryological development {744,4845}. There is no association with EBV {2475}.

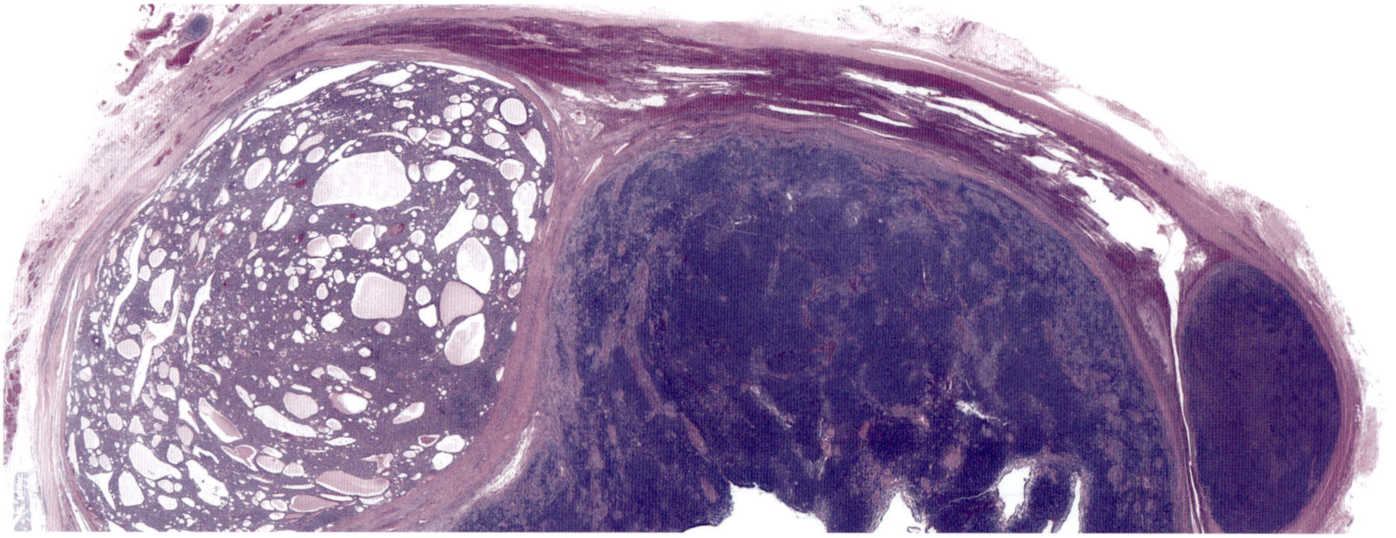

Fig. 3.92 Intrathyroidal thymoma. Residual compressed thyroid tissue is seen in the left field. The tumour exhibits a lobulated architecture, and the various tumour lobules exhibit different morphologies.

Macroscopic appearance

They are encapsulated and/or well circumscribed, with a nodular, yellow-tan cut surface interspersed with fibrous septa {4845, 2593,1541,880}. Tumours vary in size from 10 to 80 mm in diameter {744,2623,4845,4447,756,3589,3004}.

Histopathology

Intrathyroidal thymoma displays similar histopathological appearances/subtypes to those seen in mediastinal thymoma {744, 5006,1890}. The prototypical morphology is that of an encapsulated or well-delimited tumour forming jigsaw puzzle–like lobules separated by sclerotic septa. There are polygonal to spindled, occasionally squamoid, epithelial cells interspersed with variable numbers of small lymphocytes {5006}. Some cases can show entrapment of thyroid follicles within the tumour {4845}, dystrophic calcifications {1541}, and/or residual ectopic thymus tissue at the periphery {744}. Intrathyroidal thymomas are usually non-invasive, but invasion through the tumour capsule or into the surrounding fatty tissue has also been reported {4431,3280}.

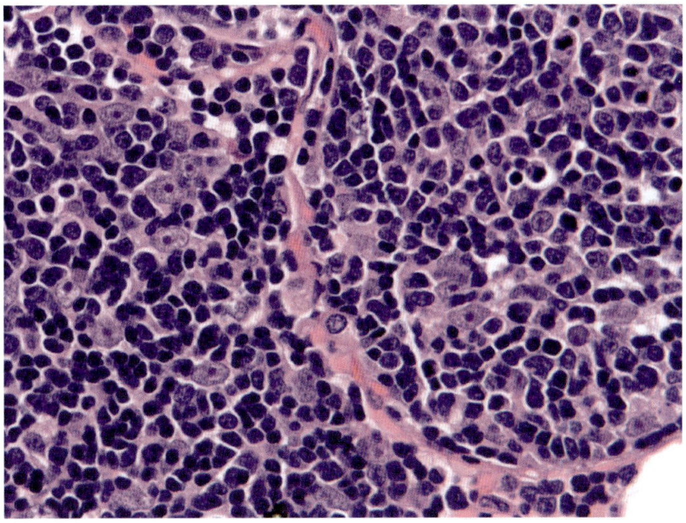

Fig. 3.93 Intrathyroidal thymoma. High-power view of an ectopic thymoma in the thyroid, featuring scattered single or grouped epithelial cells in a background of small lymphoid cells.

Immunohistochemistry

The neoplastic epithelial cells are diffusely positive for pancytokeratin and CK5/6 {1541,4845}, and negative for thyroid transcription factor 1 (TTF1) {2475} and monoclonal PAX8 {4845, 4347}. The lymphocytic component consists of immature T cells characteristically positive for TdT {1541,4447,4431,2593,4845}.

Differential diagnosis

Intrathyroidal thymoma should be distinguished from ectopic thymic tissue {4845}, mediastinal thymoma with cervical extension {744}, branchioma (ectopic hamartomatous thymoma), anaplastic carcinoma {880}, medullary carcinoma {2475}, intrathyroidal thymic carcinoma {4845}, and the spindle cell subtype of papillary thyroid carcinoma. Branchioma is not a true thymoma; it selectively occurs in the sternoclavicular region, lacks a lobulated pattern, and is characterized by a fascicular or lattice-like pattern with bland-looking spindle cells interspersed with fat. This lesion often includes squamoid islands, syringoma-like tubules, simple glands, and squamous cysts {744,4481}.

Cytology

FNA smears show variable proportions of lymphocytic and epithelial cells {1541}, which might lead to misdiagnosis as Hashimoto thyroiditis {4845,3004,4681}, lymphoproliferative disorders {4681,3323,3589,880,2593,1890}, or carcinoma {4431} (mainly papillary thyroid carcinoma {4447,4431}). If the lymphocytic component is prevalent, flow cytometry immunophenotyping may help in diagnosis {3589}.

Diagnostic molecular pathology

None

Essential and desirable diagnostic criteria

Essential: jigsaw puzzle–like tumour lobules separated by sclerotic septa; a variable mixture of bland-looking epithelial cells and TdT-positive lymphocytes.

Staging

Not applicable

Prognosis and prediction

The vast majority of patients do not show recurrence or metastasis after surgical excision. Two patients with lymph node metastases {1890,2475} and another with lung metastases {4431} had tumours with extensive infiltration of the thyroid gland, venous invasion, and/or infiltration of the adjacent connective tissue.

Spindle epithelial tumour with thymus-like elements

LiVolsi V
Cameselle-Teijeiro JM
Erickson LA
Folpe AL
Papotti M

Definition

Spindle epithelial tumour with thymus-like elements (SETTLE) is a malignant intrathyroidal tumour arising from intrathyroidal thymic tissue, also occurring in the mediastinum, characterized by a lobulated architecture and biphasic cellular composition, with spindle epithelial cells that merge into glandular structures.

ICD-O coding

8588/3 Spindle epithelial tumour with thymus-like elements

ICD-11 coding

2D10.Y & XH6ZG8 Other specified malignant neoplasms of thyroid gland & Spindle epithelial tumour with thymus-like element

Related terminology

Acceptable: spindle epithelial tumour with thymus-like differentiation.

Subtype(s)

None

Localization

Intrathyroidal, arising from intrathyroidal thymic tissue

Clinical features

The usual presentation is a painless thyroid mass of variable duration. Less common presentations include a rapidly enlarging neck mass, local tenderness, and diffuse thyroid enlargement. The tumour appears cold on thyroid scan, and it displays heterogeneous solid and cystic density on CT. Approximately 10% of patients have cervical lymph node metastasis at presentation {3702,2040,3175}.

Epidemiology

SETTLE is very rare. It predominantly affects children and young adults, with a median age of 19 years (range: 2–70 years) and a male predilection (M:F ratio: 1.5:1) {3702,2040,2581}.

Etiology

Unknown

Pathogenesis

Single cases have been reported to show mutation of *KRAS*, *NRAS*, *SMYD1* (*KMT3D*), or *KMT2C* {4977,4283}.

Macroscopic appearance

SETTLE is grossly encapsulated, partially circumscribed, or infiltrative, with an average size of 42 mm (range: 11–120 mm) {2040}. The cut surface is firm, predominantly solid, greyish-white to tan, and vaguely lobulated {744,1399}.

Histopathology

SETTLE is a highly cellular tumour, vaguely lobulated by thick or thin fibrous septa {744,1399}. Although most cases are biphasic, occasional cases (also referred to as the monophasic pattern) consist almost exclusively of spindled cells or glandular structures {801,13}. Compact admixtures of reticulated, microcystic, and/or hyalinized long fascicles of spindle cells merge imperceptibly with areas showing an epithelial appearance, with tubulopapillary, glomeruloid, cystic, and glandular structures. Cleft-like spaces containing grey-blue mucin are common. The spindle cells have scant cytoplasm and elongated nuclei with fine chromatin and inconspicuous nucleoli; ultrastructurally the spindle cells have an epithelial nature (tonofilaments, desmosomes, and basal lamina) {2067,744}. Mitotic figures are rare, although prominent mitotic activity and focal necrosis may be found in isolated cases {2318}. The epithelial component is composed of cuboidal to columnar cells sometimes containing mucin or cilia. Their nuclei are similar to those of spindled cells except for their oval or round shape. Infrequently, there are foci of abrupt squamous differentiation {744}. Few lymphocytes and rare calcifications may be seen {21,3185}. Vascular invasion may be detected {4283}.

Immunohistochemistry

Both spindled and glandular cells express pancytokeratins, with a higher reactivity for high-molecular-weight (versus

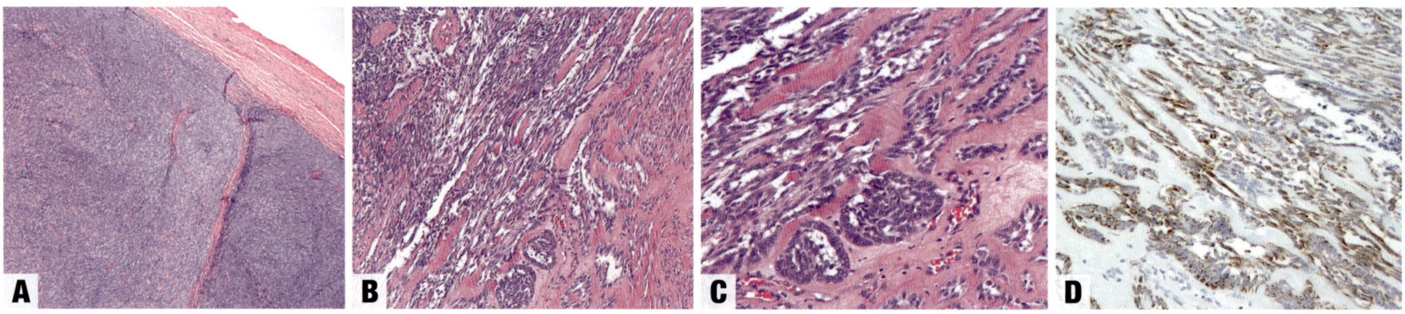

Fig. 3.94 Spindle epithelial tumour with thymus-like elements. **A** Note the lobulated growth pattern with a dominance of spindle cells. The capsule of the tumour at the right shows no invasion. **B** Epithelial nests appear near spindle cell bundles. **C** Epithelial nest resembling a glomeruloid body. **D** Immunohistochemistry for cytokeratin (CAM5.2) shows staining of spindle cells.

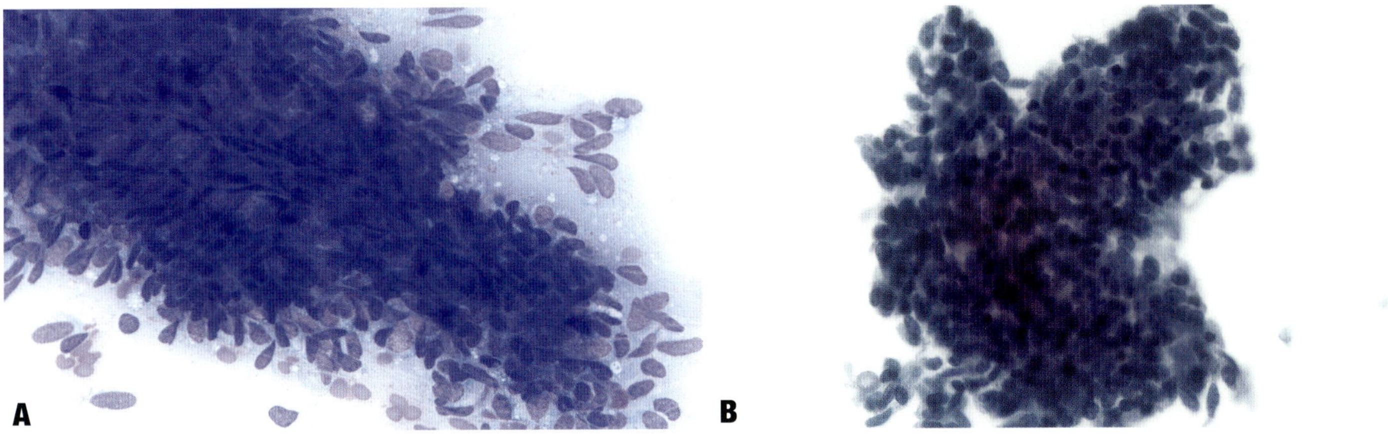

Fig. 3.95 Spindle epithelial tumour with thymus-like elements, FNAC. **A** Air-dried, Giemsa-stained smear showing a tissue fragment of spindle cells, some with an epithelioid appearance. **B** Liquid-based cytology preparation showing spindle cells with mild nuclear pleomorphism arranged in cohesive tissue fragments.

low-molecular-weight) types, including CK7 {1399,2873}. Myoepithelial markers (SMA and MSA) may be found in the spindle cell component {4312,4977,2873}. Vimentin and EMA are also expressed {5067,3033,4283}, as are p40/p63 {3175, 2581,4283}, CD99, BCL2, KIT (CD117), SMARCB1 (INI1), and TLE1 {1399,3175,2198}, as well as (focally) D2-40 and MOC31 {4283}. No reactivity was found for CK20, thyroglobulin, calcitonin, CEA, thyroid transcription factor 1 (TTF1), CD5, TdT, S100, desmin, CD34, calretinin, or WT1 {4283,335,1399,2873}. The Ki-67 proliferation index is low (3–5%) {3318,3175}, although it has been reported to be as high as 25% in metastatic tumour tissue {3650}.

Differential diagnosis

SETTLE can be distinguished from synovial sarcoma by the lobulated growth pattern, lower overall nuclear grade, glomeruloid glandular structures, absence of intraglandular necrotic debris, stromal hyalinization, paucity of mast cells, and diffuse expression of high-molecular-weight cytokeratin and p63/p40, as well as the absence of *SS18::SSX1*, *SS18::SSX2*, or *SS18::SSX4* gene fusion {1399,4871}. SETTLE should also be distinguished from sarcomatoid anaplastic thyroid carcinoma, intrathyroidal thymoma, and spindle cell medullary thyroid carcinoma. Anaplastic carcinoma does not usually present in young people and is an infiltrative high-grade pleomorphic tumour with necrosis and high mitotic activity. Thymoma has more jigsaw puzzle–like lobulation and is accompanied by a variable number of immature TdT-positive lymphocytes. In medullary carcinoma, the stroma may show amyloid and the cell nuclei have coarser chromatin; calcitonin and CEA immunostains are also positive.

Cytology

Aspirates are highly or moderately cellular, including cohesive and single dissociated spindle cells with bland oval nuclei. Occasional groups of epithelioid and columnar cells can be seen. Mitotic figures are rare or absent. Extracellular metachromatic material should not be misinterpreted as amyloid and therefore lead to a false diagnosis of medullary carcinoma {2873,4522,2234,335,21}.

Diagnostic molecular pathology

SETTLE lacks *SS18::SSX1*, *SS18::SSX2*, or *SS18::SSX4* gene fusion. *KRAS* {4977}, *NRAS*, *KMT2D*, or *KMT2C* {4283} somatic mutations have been reported in single cases.

Essential and desirable diagnostic criteria

Essential: a biphasic tumour with fascicles of spindled cells merging into complex glandular elements; a reticulated or sieve-like pattern in some areas; diffuse immunoreactivity for keratins (especially high-molecular-weight keratins).

Desirable: no *SS18::SSX1*, *SS18::SSX2*, or *SS18::SSX4* gene fusion (in selected cases).

Staging

Not applicable

Prognosis and prediction

SETTLE is a slow-growing tumour, with an overall survival rate of 86% (median follow-up: 6.3 years) {3702}. The metastatic rate is 26%, but this increases to 40% when follow-up exceeds 5 years {3702,803}. The time from diagnosis of the primary tumour to metastasis is highly variable (2–25 years), with a median of 10 years {2040}. The presence of cervical lymph node metastasis is associated with a high risk of subsequent development of distant metastasis {3702}. The tumour can metastasize to lymph node, bone, and kidney, but the most common site of metastasis is lung {2040}. Metastatic disease can still be compatible with long survival after treatment {803}. In a review of 42 cases, 5 of the 37 patients with follow-up information available died of delayed distant metastasis or treatment complications {2040}.

Intrathyroidal thymic carcinoma

Cameselle-Teijeiro JM
Chan JKC
Jain D
LiVolsi V
Papotti M

Definition

Intrathyroidal thymic carcinoma (ITC) is a malignant epithelial tumour with thymic differentiation occurring within the thyroid gland.

ICD-O coding

8589/3 Intrathyroidal thymic carcinoma

ICD-11 coding

2C27.0 Carcinoma of thymus

Related terminology

Acceptable: thymic carcinoma.

Not recommended: CD5-positive thyroid carcinoma; lymphoepithelioma-like carcinoma of the thyroid; intrathyroidal epithelial thymoma; primary thyroid thymoma; thyroid carcinoma showing thymus-like differentiation; intrathyroidal carcinoma showing thymus-like elements.

Subtype(s)

None

Localization

ITC occurs within the thyroid (mainly in the lower pole of both thyroid lobes) or attached to the thyroid gland {3715,2064,4334,1898,4942,893,4871}.

Clinical features

Presentation is typically with a firm, painless neck mass in euthyroid patients, sometimes accompanied by hoarseness and/or dysphagia {4942,2847,1138,1495,793,3341}. The tumour appears as a cold nodule on thyroid scan, and ultrasound, CT, PET-CT, and MRI findings are nonspecific {4942,893,1495}. At presentation, lymph node metastases occur in as many as 50% of cases {3715,2064,4334,4372}. Fever of unknown origin has been attributed to ITC in 1 case {854}, but neither myasthenia gravis nor polymyositis has been reported.

Epidemiology

ITC is a rare neoplasm, accounting for up to 0.15% of all malignant thyroid tumours {844,893,1138}. Most published cases have occurred in Asian people {844,2064,4334,1896,1898,4579,3280,893,1138,1495,4372,3341}. This tumour typically

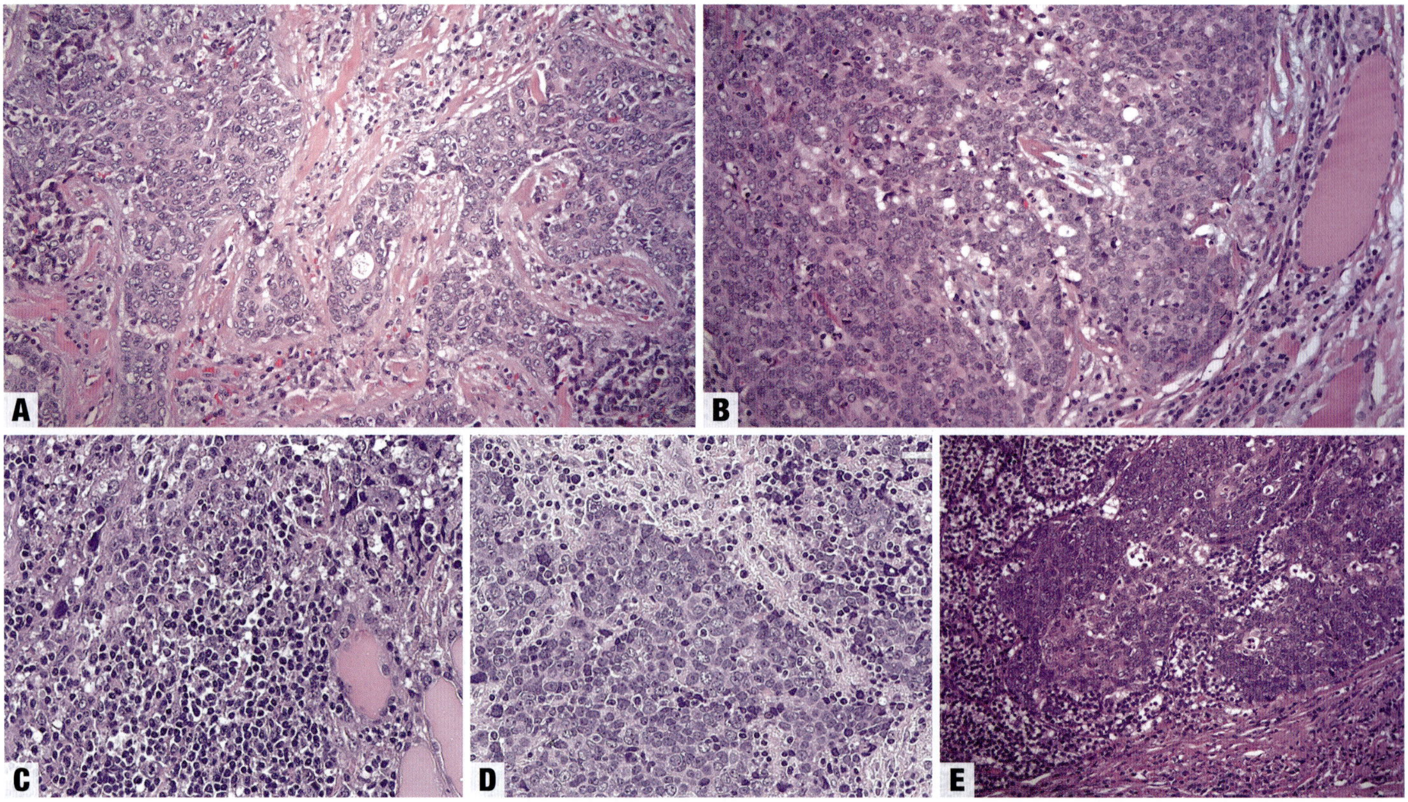

Fig. 3.96 Intrathyroidal thymic carcinoma. **A** Anastomosing islands of tumour cells surrounded by fibrous stroma. **B** Well-circumscribed but unencapsulated tumour with the surrounding thyroid parenchyma. **C** Stromal infiltration by atypical tumour cells accompanied by numerous lymphocytes and plasma cells. **D** The nuclear chromatin is vesicular, with small and easily identifiable nucleoli. **E** Tumour islands invade into an adjacent parathyroid gland.

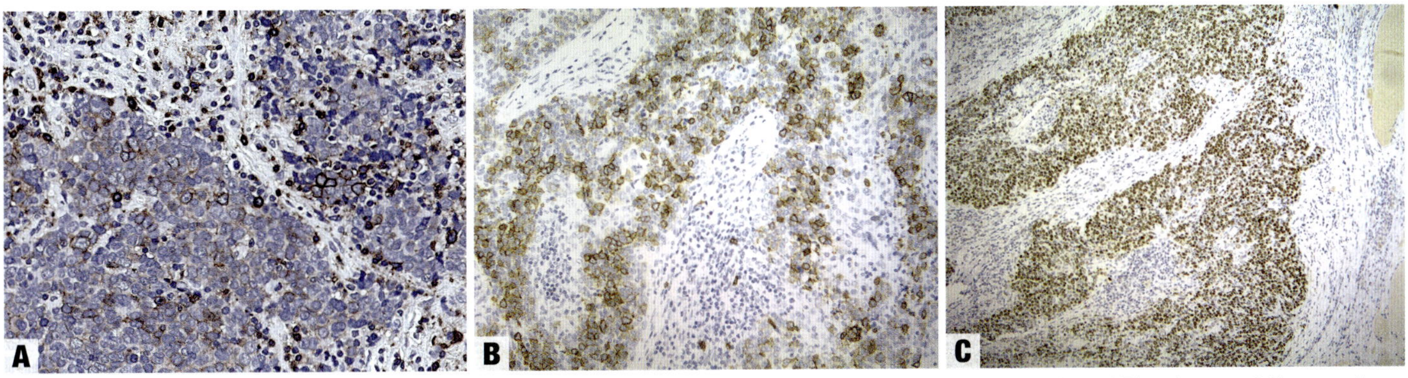

Fig. 3.97 Intrathyroidal thymic carcinoma. **A** Immunostaining for CD5 shows membrane positivity in tumour cells and in the cytoplasm of T lymphocytes. **B** Tumour cells are positive for KIT (CD117). **C** Nuclear positivity for p63.

occurs in middle-aged patients (median age: 52 years, range: 25–79 years), with a slight female predilection (M:F ratio: 1:1.2).

Etiology

The higher prevalence of ITC in Asian countries suggests that genetic, ethnic, and/or environmental factors may contribute to tumorigenesis {1522}.

Pathogenesis

ITC is thought to arise in or adjacent to the thyroid from intrathyroidal or perithyroidal thymic tissue, vestiges of the thymopharyngeal duct, or branchial pouch remnants (including solid cell nests) {744,3715,5064}. Gains on chromosome arm 1q, as well as losses on 6p, 6q, and 16q, are frequent chromosomal imbalances {4679} and are similar to those found in thymomas and thymic carcinomas, thus indicating analogous tumorigenesis. Although KIT (also called c-KIT and CD117) is immunohistochemically expressed in all ITCs, no activating mutations of *KIT* have been detected {4680,4372}. Somatic *EGFR* mutations in exon 20 (p.T790M) {3667} and exon 21 (p.R841K) {4372} have been found in isolated cases {4680,4372}. *TERT* promoter mutation has been identified in some ITCs {4372}. *BRAF* p.V600E {4372}, *KRAS* {4680}, and *PDGFRA* {4680} mutations have not been detected. There is no association with EBV {4372}.

Macroscopic appearance

ITC is a hard, pink-white, solid, lobulated tumour, usually lacking calcifications or cysts on its cut surfaces.

Histopathology

ITC displays histopathological features similar to those of thymic squamous cell carcinoma {744,3042,3715,2064}. There are expansile irregular lobules and cords of epithelial tumour cells, accompanied by sclerohyaline to desmoplastic stroma that is variably infiltrated by lymphocytes and plasma cells. The tumour cells are squamoid or syncytial-appearing, with occasional single-cell keratinization. They are oval or spindled with large oval nucleus, pale to vesicular chromatin, and distinct nucleoli. Nuclear atypia is usually mild to moderate, and mitotic figures are rare (< 3 mitoses/2 mm^2) {3042}. Some cases have obvious keratinization; others have basaloid features or prominent lymphoplasmacytic infiltration similar to that seen in nasopharyngeal non-keratinizing squamous cell carcinoma (basaloid squamous cell carcinoma or lymphoepithelial carcinoma, respectively) {744}. In some cases there are rosette-like arrangements and expression of neuroendocrine markers in addition to CD5 {3042,5009,3725,4871}. Focal glandular structures can be seen exceptionally {5077,5009}.

Immunophenotype

Tumour cells are immunoreactive for pancytokeratin, CK19, p63, and p40. Like mediastinal thymic carcinomas, they express CD5 and KIT (also called c-KIT and CD117). They also commonly express BCL2, calretinin, CEA, and p53 {194,1143,1142,1898}. Scattered cells positive for chromogranin A and/or synaptophysin can be detected in some cases {1898,1979}. ITCs are negative for thyroid transcription factor 1 (TTF1), thyroglobulin, calcitonin {4334,1898,1522}, and monoclonal PAX8 {4347}. The Ki-67 index usually varies from 2% to 40% {1898,4579,4680}.

Differential diagnosis

Because of its better prognosis, it is important to distinguish ITC from metastatic squamous cell carcinoma and from anaplastic thyroid carcinoma (including the squamous cell carcinoma pattern). Squamous cell carcinoma usually displays more keratinization and invasiveness and is negative for CD5 {3715,2509}. Anaplastic thyroid carcinoma is also negative for CD5 and typically has more pleomorphism, atypical mitoses, and necrosis {2062}. ITC contains a small number of S100A9-expressing cells in a scattered pattern, whereas both squamous cell carcinoma and anaplastic thyroid carcinoma have diffuse and laminated positivity for S100A9 {194,2062}. Immunohistochemical data useful for differential diagnosis are shown in Table 3.08 (p. 198).

Cytology

Cytological features consistent with ITC are 3D tissue fragments without a papillary or follicular pattern, basaloid structures, loosely arranged clusters of round or spindly tumour cells, hyperchromatic to vesicular chromatin, distinct nucleoli, lymphocytic background, few keratinized cells, and occasional mitotic figures {1896,3725}. Because the cytomorphological features overlap with those of other tumours, a diagnosis not more specific than that of carcinoma is usually made {3222, 893,3725}. Immunohistochemical positivity for CD5 and KIT (CD117) in paraffin-embedded cell-block material can aid in a more specific diagnosis {3222,893,3725}.

Table 3.08 The main immunohistochemical and in situ hybridization features in the differential diagnosis of intrathyroidal thymic carcinoma (ITC)

Markers	ITC	HGFDC	ATC	MTC	MLCNEC	MNPC	FDCS
CD5	+	–	–	–	–	–	–
KIT (CD117)	+	+/–	–	+ (~25%)	+ (> 70%)	+ (~33%)	–
p63, p40	+	–	+/–	–	–/+	–	–
Pancytokeratin	+	+	+	+	+	+	–
Thyroglobulin	–	+	–	–	–	–	–
PAX8 (monoclonal)[a]	–	+	+/–	–	–	–	–
Calcitonin	–	–	–	+	Rare	–	–
Synaptophysin, chromogranin A	+/–	–	–	+	+	–	–
p53	+ (~78%)	+/–	+ (~80%)	–	+	+	–
CD21, CD35	–	–	–	–	–	–	+
EBER[b]	–	–	–	–	–	+	–

ATC, anaplastic thyroid carcinoma; EBER, EBV-encoded small RNA; FDCS, follicular dendritic cell sarcoma; HGFDC, high-grade follicular cell–derived carcinoma (including poorly differentiated thyroid carcinoma); MLCNEC, metastatic large cell neuroendocrine carcinoma; MNPC, metastatic nasopharyngeal carcinoma; MTC, medullary thyroid carcinoma.
[a]ITCs and MTCs are negative for PAX8 using monoclonal antibodies, but positivity has been reported with polyclonal antibodies in both tumours {4347,4372,1692}. [b]In situ hybridization.

Diagnostic molecular pathology

Not relevant

Essential and desirable diagnostic criteria

Essential: invasive squamoid or syncytial epithelial lobules delimited by lymphoplasmacytic-rich fibrous septa; mild to moderate nuclear atypia and generally low mitotic activity; immunohistochemical demonstration of thymic origin.

Staging

Currently, no staging system is available for ITC.

Prognosis and prediction

ITC has a more favourable clinical outcome than eutopic thymic carcinoma and anaplastic thyroid carcinoma {744,4334,1138, 4372,3341,1630}. The 5- and 10-year survival rates are 90% and 82%, respectively {2064}. Only occasional fatalities have been reported {2163,1522,1495}. Unfavourable pathological findings are venous invasion, laryngeal nerve invasion {3341, 2064}, a high proliferation index {3341}, and extrathyroidal extension including tracheal invasion {1143,5077,844,2064, 4579,2847,1495}. Lymph node metastases are found at initial surgery in 40–50% of cases {2064,4579}. PDL1 expression has been detected in ITCs and may predict response to anti-PD1 treatment {4372,2733}. The roles of COX-2 and EGFR, and of *TERT* promoter mutations, remain to be determined {4680,4372}.

Surgery is the mainstay of treatment {2064,747}. Postoperative radiotherapy may improve locoregional control of the tumour and may even improve survival {3732,2378}.

Thyroblastoma

Agaimy A
Nosé V
Sobrinho-Simoes M

Definition

Thyroblastoma is an embryonal high-grade thyroid neoplasm composed of primitive thyroid-like follicular cells surrounded by a primitive small-cell component and mesenchymal stroma with variable differentiation.

ICD-O coding

8970/3 Thyroblastoma

ICD-11 coding

2D10.Y Other specified malignant neoplasms of thyroid gland

Related terminology

Not recommended: malignant thyroid teratoma; immature teratoma; carcinosarcoma; teratocarcinosarcoma; malignant teratoid tumour.

Subtype(s)

None

Localization

One or both thyroid lobes

Clinical features

Thyroblastoma presents as a rapidly growing mid-cervical thyroid mass diffusely infiltrating one or both thyroid lobes and extending into perithyroid tissue {32}. There is a striking female predilection (M:F ratio: 1:3) and a median age of 43 years (range: 17–65 years) {32}.

Epidemiology

Thyroblastoma is a rare tumour that is likely underrecognized, with 8 recently reported and molecularly verified cases; most of these were initially diagnosed as malignant teratoma {3655, 5026,3809,32}. Most thyroblastoma cases would previously have been classified as malignant (grade 3) teratoma of the thyroid gland {4474,3743,4705}, and some as carcinosarcoma {5026}. No epidemiological data are available, because of the lack of standard terminology in earlier series.

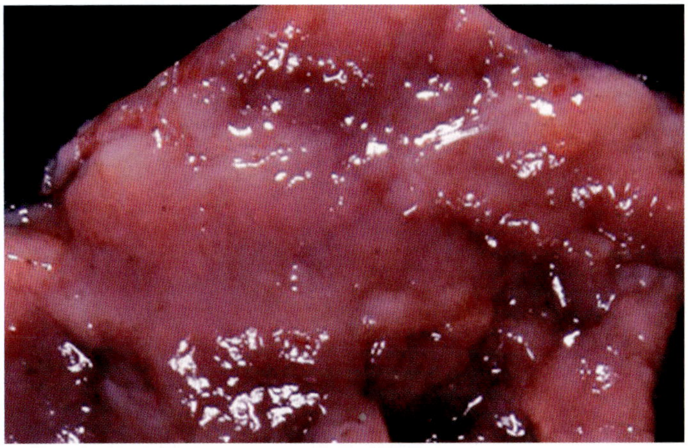

Fig. 3.98 Thyroblastoma. The thyroid lobe is replaced by a friable, soft pink tumour mass. The gross cut surface shows the features of this aggressive tumour with complete replacement of the thyroid.

Etiology

Etiological factors other than *DICER1* mutations are not known. Pre-existent nodular goitre was present in 1 case {32}. Older age at presentation and a lack of personal or family history argue for a sporadic neoplasm unrelated to the hereditary *DICER1* syndrome.

Pathogenesis

Thyroblastomas are probably due to somatic mutations in *DICER1*, which encodes an enzyme involved in microRNA processing. *DICER1* mutations have been detected in all tested thyroblastoma cases {3655,32,3809}.

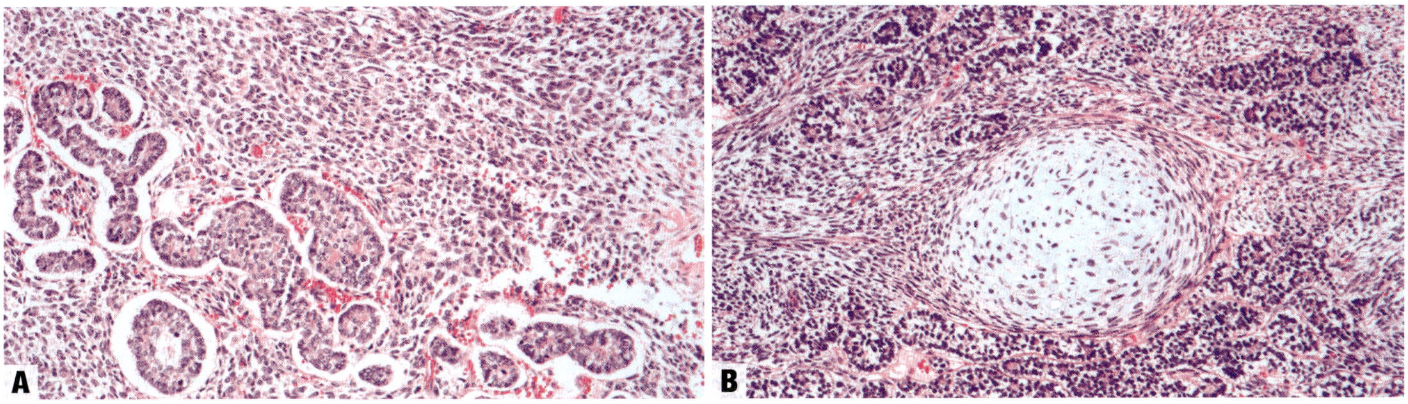

Fig. 3.99 Thyroblastoma. **A** This primitive tumour has a biphasic growth pattern composed of nests and cords of primitive epithelial cells intermixed with primitive spindle stromal cells. **B** Lung metastasis from a thyroblastoma showing cartilage foci (cartilage was not detected in the primary tumour).

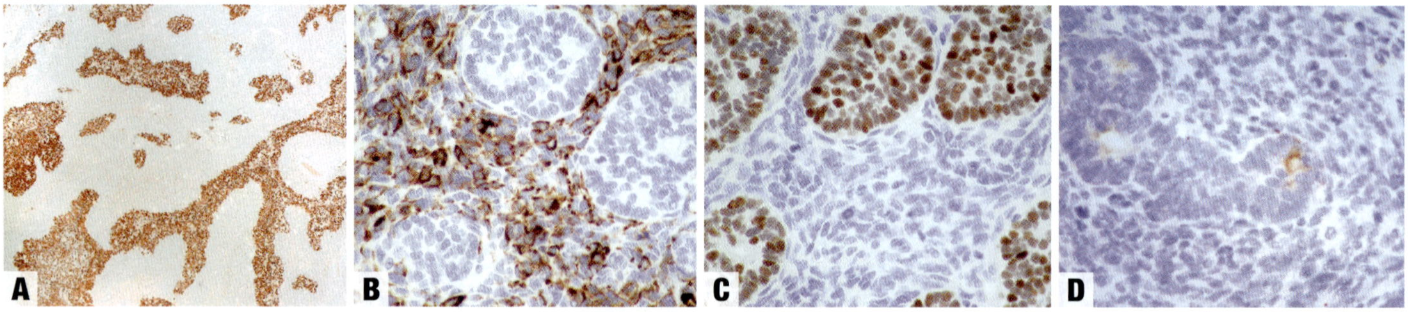

Fig. 3.100 Thyroblastoma. **A** SALL4 is strongly positive in the primitive solid nests. **B** The primitive stromal cells stain for desmin, whereas the primitive follicles are negative. **C** The primitive follicles stain for thyroid transcription factor 1 (TTF1) and PAX8. The stroma is negative. **D** Thyroglobulin in a few primitive follicles.

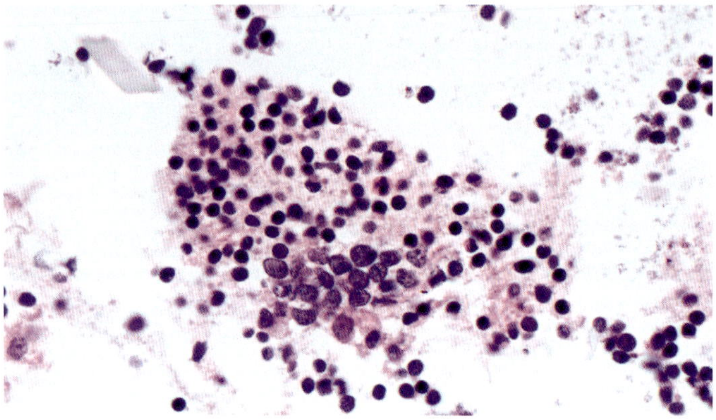

Fig. 3.101 Thyroblastoma cytology. Mixed cell population.

Macroscopic appearance

On cut surface, a soft, friable, grey-whitish to pink tan-yellow mass infiltrating the entire lobe or both lobes and extending to margins and soft tissues, measuring 17–100 mm, is noted.

Histopathology

Histologically, thyroblastoma is an embryonal neoplasm that mostly resembles thyroid parenchyma within the first trimester of prenatal development. Thyroblastoma comprises three cellular components: (1) a component of embryonal-type thyroid transcription factor 1 (TTF1)+ / PAX8+ / focal thyroglobulin+ primitive-appearing thyroid follicles and fetal-type glands, (2) primitive small round to oval cells arranged into irregularly communicating solid aggregates and sheets with foci of necrosis and brisk mitotic activity that may form focal periglandular cuffs, and (3) a primitive spindle cell stroma of variable cellularity arranged into fascicles, usually positive for SMA and (focally) for desmin and myogenin. Foci of cartilage are seen in half of all cases, but well-differentiated adult-type organoid structures, pilosebaceous elements, and other skin adnexa as seen in genuine teratomas are absent. However, mature skin, skeletal muscle, and smooth muscle tissue have been identified focally in 1 case.

Immunohistochemistry

The primitive small cells and the stroma show frequent rhabdomyoblastic differentiation, with desmin and myogenin immunoreactivity, but they are negative for TTF1, PAX8, and thyroglobulin. The primitive small-cell component expresses SALL4 but not OCT3/4 or PLAP. SMARCA4 expression is retained in the different tumour components {5026,3809,32,3294}.

Differential diagnosis

The entities include thyroid teratoma (benign or immature), carcinosarcoma, teratocarcinosarcoma, poorly differentiated thyroid carcinoma, and metastatic sarcoma or poorly differentiated carcinoma.

Cytology

Smears show marked hypercellularity, epithelial proliferations, absence of colloid, and predominance of immature spindle cells in the small number of cases reported, and represent a challenge to FNAB diagnosis {3012}.

Diagnostic molecular pathology

Pathogenic somatic *DICER1* variants are present in all tested cases and help to distinguish them from teratomas {3655,32, 3809}. Thyroblastoma lacks isochromosome 12p, a characteristic of genuine germ cell neoplasms {4270}.

Tumours with an immature phenotype are a feature of *DICER1* syndrome (due to germline *DICER1* pathogenic variants), and the syndrome is also associated with frequent thyroid abnormalities: usually multinodular hyperplasia, but sometimes well-differentiated carcinoma (both papillary and follicular) {3028}. Because it is possible that some thyroblastoma cases may be hereditary, germline *DICER1* testing should be considered {32}.

Essential and desirable diagnostic criteria

Essential: primitive thyroid epithelium; small-cell blastemal component; mesenchymal stroma with or without rhabdomyoblastic differentiation; absence of conventional thyroid carcinoma and conventional germ cell components; expression of specific germ cell markers.

Desirable: thyroid transcription factor 1 (TTF1)/PAX8/thyroglobulin expression within primitive follicles; minute foci of cartilage.

Staging

No staging system is currently available.

Prognosis and prediction

Thyroblastoma pursues a highly aggressive course, with > 50% of patients dying at a median follow-up time of 11.5 months.

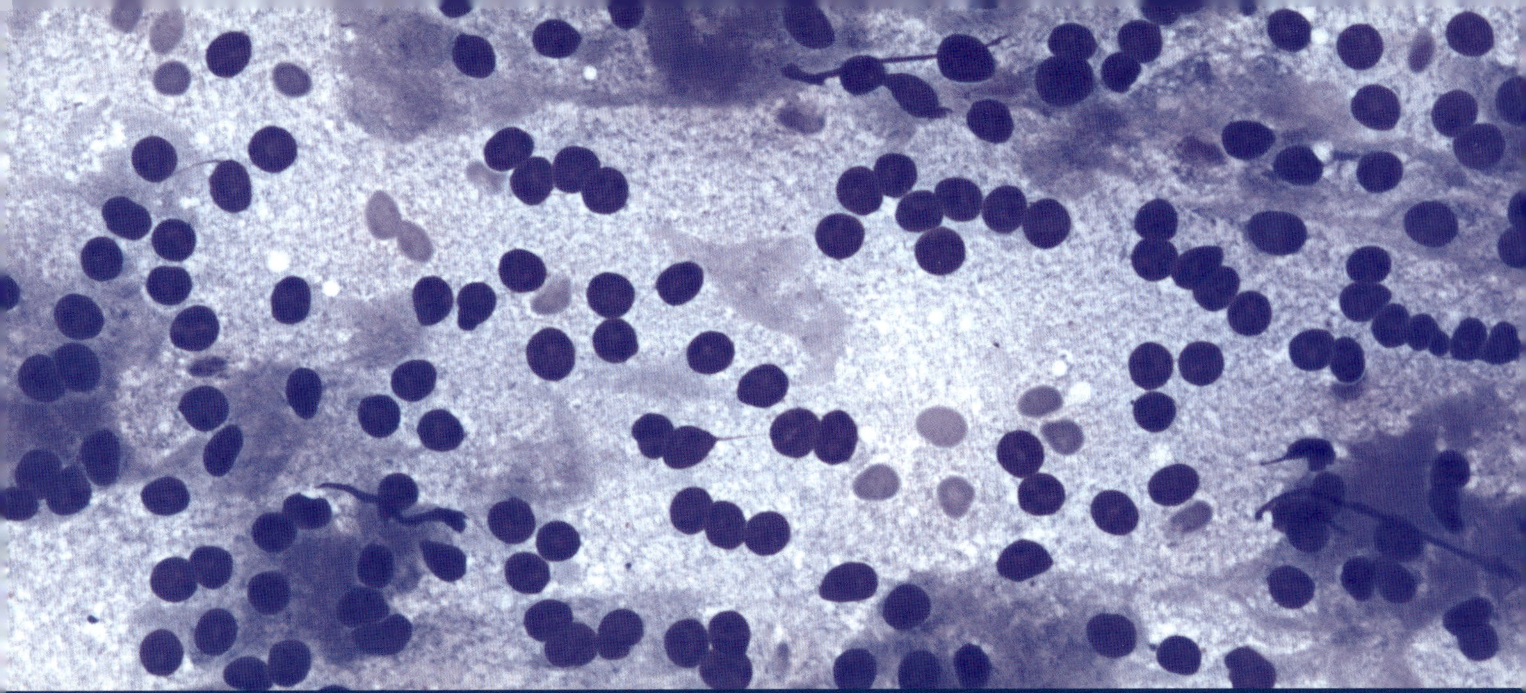

4

Parathyroid tumours

Edited by: Erickson LA, Gill AJ, Mete O

Parathyroid tumours: Introduction

Erickson LA
Asa SL
Mete O

The morphological correlates of hyperparathyroidism include parathyroid hyperplasia, parathyroid adenoma, and carcinoma. Accurate diagnosis of parathyroid disorders relies on clinical, laboratory, and genetic findings, along with detailed morphological assessment.

In this edition, for the first time, parathyroid hyperplasia is discussed. By definition, hyperplasia is a potentially reversible condition that is caused by a known stimulus. From such a perspective, secondary hyperplasia (most commonly attributable to chronic renal failure) represents the only true parathyroid hyperplasia. In tertiary hyperparathyroidism, autonomous hyperparathyroidism occurs as a result of hyperplasia-to-neoplasia progression. Despite evidence of neoplastic transformation, because tertiary hyperplasia is by definition always associated with pre-existing secondary hyperplasia and appears to represent a morphological and biological continuum, this is also discussed in the section on hyperplasia.

The individual parathyroid glands in the setting of advanced hyperplasia, particularly tertiary hyperparathyroidism due to chronic renal failure, may show highly atypical architectural features that can mimic carcinoma, including the presence of pseudoinvasion and a high proliferation index {4886}. Although there is a risk of local recurrence or diffuse recurrence in the neck (parathyromatosis), distant metastasis is exceptional in the setting of renal failure–induced hyperparathyroidism {3572, 4886}. Therefore it is emphasized that the diagnosis of parathyroid carcinoma should not be made in the setting of chronic renal failure in disease confined to the neck unless there is unequivocal vascular space invasion or very marked invasive growth – for example, unequivocal extension into adjacent organs such as the thyroid, oesophagus, or skeletal muscle {4886}.

Despite the historical use of the term "hyperplasia" for the multiple endocrine neoplasia syndromes, hyperparathyroidism in these syndromes is almost always due to multiglandular/multinodular adenomas {516,1168,4589}. For this reason these are discussed in the section on parathyroid adenoma. In the context of multiple endocrine neoplasia type 1 it is again noted that although there is a high risk of local recurrence in the neck, distant metastasis is extremely rare, warranting similar strict criteria for malignancy to those applied in secondary/tertiary hyperplasia {4886}.

An abnormal parathyroid gland is often enlarged and cellular, usually exceeding 8 mm and 60 mg {1168}. The distinction between parathyroid adenoma and hyperplasia may not always be possible with certainty and a descriptive diagnosis such as "pathologically enlarged cellular (fat-depleted) parathyroid gland consistent with..." is often appropriate. The importance of proper macroscopic assessment and sampling of the specimen to ensure sectioning through the hilum of the gland is emphasized, because that is where the non-neoplastic tissue, used to support the diagnosis of adenoma over hyperplasia, is usually found.

The molecular genetics of parathyroid neoplasms (adenomas and carcinomas) have been elucidated, and although there is no need for routine immunohistochemistry in the majority of these tumours, there is a need to recognize the morphological features of inherited disease. Parafibromin-deficient tumours (those associated with *CDC73* mutations) exhibit eosinophilic cytoplasm with perinuclear clearing, nuclear enlargement, microcystic change, and a sheet-like growth pattern {1580}. The presence of multinodular multiglandular disease is a feature of inherited disease, and the role of molecular immunohistochemistry for parafibromin, menin, and p27 in facilitating the screening of *CDC73*-related, *MEN1*-related, and *CDKN1B*-related pathogenesis is discussed {1271}.

Parathyroid lipoadenoma is discussed as an individual entity, unlike in previous editions, where it was included as a variant of parathyroid adenoma. The term "lipoadenoma" is only appropriate when there is an unequivocal increase in parenchymal parathyroid tissue as well as abundant adipose tissue, so parathyroid glands that are enlarged solely because of an increase in adipose tissue are not considered lipoadenomas {2431}. The general rule that > 50% of the volume of the gland should be adipose tissue to warrant the diagnosis of lipoadenoma is recommended so that otherwise typical adenomas with only a small increase in fat are not considered lipoadenomas {2005, 2431,2144}.

The term "atypical parathyroid tumour", defined as a parathyroid neoplasm of uncertain malignant potential that demonstrates atypical cytological and architectural features but lacks unequivocal features of malignancy, is introduced to replace previous terms such as "atypical parathyroid adenoma". It is unclear how much cytological or architectural atypia is required to separate atypical parathyroid tumour from usual parathyroid adenoma. For instance, small areas of fibrosis, an occasional mitotic figure (< 5 mitoses/10 mm^2), extension into but not through a thickened capsule, and a little contour irregularity not worrying for invasive growth are not uncommon in parathyroid adenomas and are insufficient to warrant designation as atypical parathyroid tumour, particularly if there has been previous manipulation or trauma of the gland {118,2285,1899}. Immunohistochemistry for various biomarkers associated with parathyroid carcinoma (e.g. parafibromin, PGP9.5, RB1, p53, galectin-3, E-cadherin, APC, 5-hydroxymethylcytosine, MDM2, and BCL2) is often informative in the differential diagnosis. Although extremely rare, cases initially categorized as atypical parathyroid tumour with subsequent metastasis have been reported. However, current data on atypical parathyroid tumours suggest that they may be followed similarly to usual parathyroid adenomas in the absence of concerning clinical features or parafibromin deficiency {4886,722}. Therefore, although this diagnostic category should not be an excuse to avoid appropriate assessment, the only clinically relevant differential diagnosis for atypical parathyroid tumour is parathyroid carcinoma.

Reviews of the epidemiological data identified an increase in the worldwide incidence of parathyroid carcinoma {2578,552, 3863,4799,2380}. The rigid pathological criteria for parathyroid carcinoma remain unchanged, requiring the presence of vascular invasion (angioinvasion), lymphatic invasion, perineural invasion, unequivocal invasion into adjacent structures or organs, or metastatic disease. The role of biomarkers in the diagnostic workup of parathyroid carcinoma is reviewed, along with the differential diagnosis. It is desirable to perform biomarker analysis routinely in parathyroid carcinomas. Among these biomarkers, parafibromin stands out as the most reliable biomarker of malignancy and also has the utility to inform germline screening for pathogenic *CDC73* variants. Other somatic mutations identified in parathyroid carcinomas are discussed {2143}. The prognostic role of angioinvasion characterized by tumour cells invading a vessel wall and intravascular tumour cells admixed with thrombus is emphasized {1276, 65}. Like for other neuroendocrine neoplasms (NENs), assessment of the proliferative activity of all parathyroid carcinomas by recording a formal Ki-67 proliferation index and mitotic count using standardized approaches is now recommended {4886,943}.

Parathyroid hyperplasia

Perren A
Johnson SJ
Juhlin CC
Mete O
Williams MD

Definition
Parathyroid hyperplasia is defined as an absolute increase in non-neoplastic parathyroid parenchymal cells in multiple parathyroid glands.

ICD-O coding
None

ICD-11 coding
5A51.0 Primary hyperparathyroidism

Related terminology
None

Subtype(s)
Primary hyperplasia; secondary hyperplasia; tertiary hyperplasia

Localization
Hyperplasia may occur in both eutopic and ectopic parathyroid glands.

Clinical features
Primary hyperplasia is where hyperplasia occurs in the absence of a physiological stimulus. Because multiple endocrine neoplasia (MEN) and many other forms of hereditary hyperparathyroidism are now recognized as usually being due to multiple adenomas, this is extremely rare.

Secondary hyperplasia is where physiological stimuli (e.g. high serum phosphate, low serum calcium, and/or vitamin D deficiency) lead to a compensatory hyperplasia. Parathyroid hyperplasia in secondary hyperparathyroidism is characterized by the underlying disease leading to decreased calcium or 1,25D3. Chronic renal disease is the most common cause, followed by chronic malabsorption or vitamin D deficiency {957}. Hyperparathyroidism is associated with poor outcomes in chronic renal disease {444}. Cardiovascular disease and bone disorders with an increased risk of fractures are the most common clinical complications {444}.

Tertiary hyperparathyroidism is defined as a progression of secondary hyperparathyroidism, where the glands acquire the ability to autonomously secrete PTH despite elevated serum PTH and calcium levels. Untreated, this is associated with increased renal transplant rejection and decreased survival {1179}.

By definition, hyperplasia is a potentially reversible condition that is caused by a known stimulus. Most instances of multiglandular parathyroid disease associated with a genetic predisposition (e.g. the MEN syndromes) that were previously classified as primary hyperplasia are now recognized as multiple, sometimes coalescing, parathyroid adenomas and should be classified as such. These are therefore now discussed in the subsequent section on parathyroid adenoma.

Epidemiology
Historically, about 5–10% of cases of primary hyperparathyroidism were reported to be due to hyperplasia {2843}. However, this figure dates from a time when MEN and other causes of hereditary hyperparathyroidism were considered hyperplasias rather than being recognized as multiglandular adenomas. Now, particularly with the increased availability of germline testing, true primary hyperplasia is very rare. Water-clear cell hyperplasia is exceedingly rare and to date has not been associated with a specific genetic predisposition. Chronic renal disease is a worldwide public health problem, and secondary hyperparathyroidism is a very frequent complication {2626}.

Etiology
True primary hyperplasia not associated with a genetic predisposition to multifocal parathyroid neoplasia remains to be fully characterized.

In secondary hyperparathyroidism due to renal insufficiency, the three factors of hypocalcaemia, hyperphosphataemia, and low 1,25D3 levels lead to an increased secretion of PTH. In the early phases of renal insufficiency, phosphate is retained by the kidney. The increase in PTH and FGF23 counteracts the phosphate accumulation but reduces the serum concentration of 1,25D3. The binding of calcium to phosphate leads to hypocalcaemia, stimulating PTH secretion indirectly. Hypocalcaemia increases parathyroid chief-cell proliferation, supported by the absence of the antiproliferative 1,25D3 {3784}. External radiation and long-term lithium therapy (> 10 years) can lead to parathyroid adenomas and (rarely) to four-gland hyperplasia {245, 4362,2176}.

Over time, the accumulation of additional genetic alterations {182,2033,1938} in combination with a progressive reduction in the expression of PTH receptors {3784} occurs in parathyroids showing secondary hyperplasia. This leads to the development of tertiary hyperparathyroidism, where the gland is refractory to the action of its natural inhibitors.

Pathogenesis
In patients with renal failure on dialysis, hyperphosphataemia directly stimulates PTH secretion and maintains a persistent stimulus for parathyroid hyperplasia. High phosphate levels prevent activation of CaSR and thereby stimulate PTH secretion despite normal serum calcium levels {716}. Phosphate also generates skeletal resistance to the calcaemic effect of PTH {3781}, further contributing to hypocalcaemia and stimulating parathyroid hyperplasia. In renal insufficiency, the production of 1,25D3 is reduced in the kidney, additionally contributing to hypocalcaemia and parathyroid hyperplasia. FGF23 is able to reduce PTH secretion by binding to the FGFR1–Klotho receptor complex {4623}. In patients with secondary hyperparathyroidism, the downregulation of Klotho and FGFR1 is often observed,

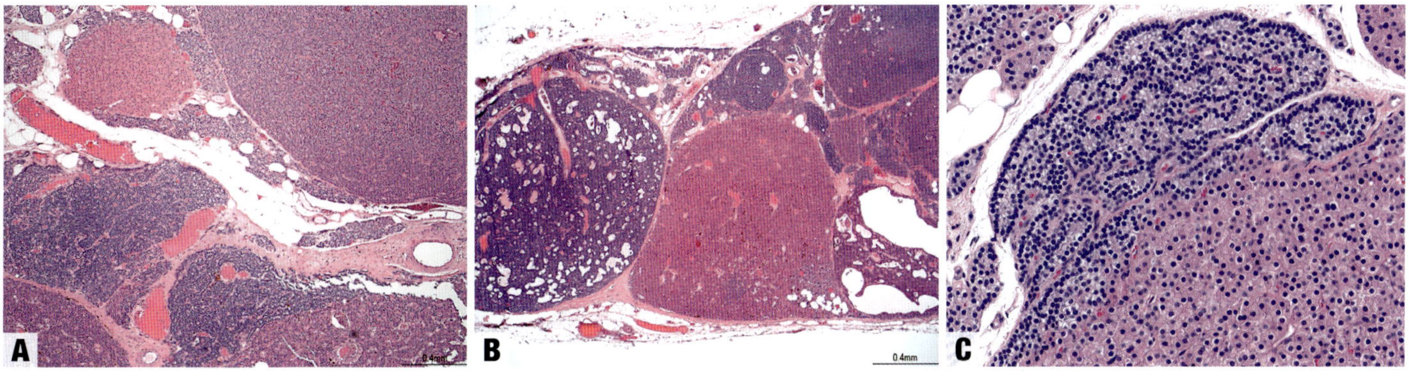

Fig. 4.01 Parathyroid hyperplasia. **A** Hyperplasia in tertiary hyperparathyroidism. Medium magnification of left superior gland. **B** Hyperplasia in tertiary hyperparathyroidism. Low-power view of the right superior gland (patient after renal transplantation) showing multiple nodules and parathyroid parenchyma with remaining fat cells. **C** Secondary parathyroid gland hyperplasia. The patient had a long history of dialysis due to renal failure. Note the numerous nodules and increased cellularity of chief, oncocytic, and clear parathyroid parenchymal cells, with a decrease in stromal adipose tissue.

and FGF23 thereby loses the ability to suppress PTH secretion {2239}. A progressive reduction of parathyroid receptors contributes to the transformation to nodular hyperplasia and tertiary hyperparathyroidism.

Clonality studies have demonstrated that 38% of cases of secondary/tertiary hyperparathyroidism are monoclonal {182} and 24% of cases of tertiary hyperparathyroidism demonstrate clonal chromosomal aberrations using comparative genomic hybridization analysis {2033}. Therefore, although most of the somatic mutations identified in chronic renal failure–related secondary/tertiary hyperparathyroidism are different to those identified in usual adenomas {1938}, many cases of secondary/tertiary hyperparathyroidism actually represent true neoplasms progressing via a hyperplasia-to-neoplasia sequence.

Macroscopic appearance

Primary chief-cell hyperplasia or multiglandular disease in the absence of a genetic predisposition is so rare it remains to be fully characterized. In primary water-clear cell hyperplasia, the hyperplastic parathyroids weigh 1000–6000 mg; the upper glands tend to be larger than the lower glands {1065}. In secondary hyperplasia, the weight varies with the stage of the disease, with weights of 120–6000 mg reported {3841}. In tertiary hyperplasia, nodularity is seen in > 50% of cases {2427}.

Histopathology

For all parathyroids with hyperplastic changes, close clinicopathological correlation is important. Histologically, primary chief-cell hyperplasia is characterized by an increased number of chief cells as compared with stromal fat cells {1168} in multiple parathyroids. Hyperplasia may be diffuse, nodular, or mixed {1168}. Primary nodular disease is almost always associated with germline predisposition syndromes and represents multifocal adenomas; therefore, this is discussed in *Parathyroid adenoma* (p. 207). Immunohistochemistry may be useful in the differential diagnosis. For example, loss of menin immunostaining is found more frequently in patients with MEN type 1 (MEN1), but it can also occur in sporadic disease {1000,1271}. Water-clear cell hyperplasia is a diffuse proliferation composed entirely of clear cells with distinct cell borders {2441}.

Hyperplasia in secondary and tertiary hyperparathyroidism involves multiple glands asymmetrically and is characterized by an increase in parenchymal cells and a decrease in stromal and intracellular fat {60}. The growth pattern can be diffuse, trabecular, acinar, pseudofollicular, or cord-like. Increasing severity of hyperparathyroidism correlates with a more nodular growth pattern, and advanced cases may show areas of haemorrhage, cyst formation, fibrosis, and chronic inflammation {1168}. Particularly in the setting of tertiary hyperparathyroidism, the individual glands may show highly atypical architectural features that can mimic carcinoma, including the presence of pseudoinvasion and a high proliferation index {4886}. Although these patients may be at high risk of local recurrence or diffuse recurrence in the neck (parathyromatosis), distant metastasis is exceptional in renal failure–induced hyperparathyroidism {3572,1168}. Therefore, in the setting of established chronic renal failure, the diagnosis of parathyroid carcinoma should not be made in disease confined to the neck unless there is unequivocal vascular space invasion or very marked invasive growth – for example, unequivocal extension into adjacent organs such as the thyroid, oesophagus, or skeletal muscle {65,4886}. Parathyromatosis (defined as local recurrence throughout the neck and/or mediastinum due to mechanical displacement or hyperplasia of rests of parathyroid tissue) may show fibrosis and pseudoinvasion of fat in a buckshot pattern that can be impossible to distinguish from parathyroid carcinoma without the history of hyperplasia

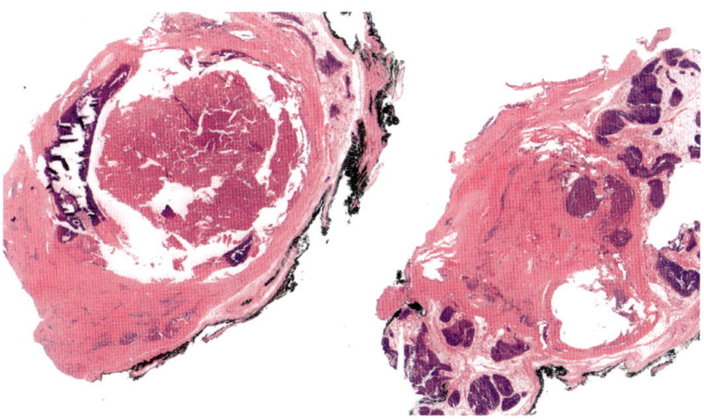

Fig. 4.02 Parathyroid hyperplasia in secondary hyperparathyroidism. Secondary parathyroid hyperplasia with abundant fibrosis and irregular growth (low magnification). Additional gland with hyperplasia was also submitted.

and close clinicopathological correlation. Although biomarker studies are useful in the distinction of parathyroid carcinoma from parathyromatosis {1172}, vascular invasion, perineural invasion, and distant spread are absent in parathyromatosis and always warrant the diagnosis of carcinoma {4886,4027}.

Differential diagnosis

Although multinodularity and the absence of a rim of non-tumorous parathyroid tissue are clues to hyperplasia, in the absence of clinical correlation (e.g. knowledge that the other glands are normal or that PTH has normalized after removal), the distinction between adenoma and hyperplasia is not possible with certainty and a descriptive diagnosis such as "pathologically enlarged cellular (fat-depleted) parathyroid gland consistent with..." may be appropriate.

Cytology

There are no cytological criteria described for the diagnosis of parathyroid hyperplasia.

Diagnostic molecular pathology

No diagnostic molecular tests are indicated in parathyroid hyperplasias caused by secondary or tertiary hyperparathyroidism. In the setting of apparently primary hyperplasia or multiglandular disease, screening for an underlying germline abnormality is recommended. If an underlying genetic predisposition (e.g. MEN1) is identified, reclassification as multiglandular/multinodular parathyroid adenomas is usually appropriate.

Essential and desirable diagnostic criteria

Essential: clinical or pathological evidence of involvement of more than one parathyroid gland.

Desirable: the presence of a clinical disorder known to cause secondary or tertiary hyperparathyroidism, or the exclusion of a genetic syndrome known to cause multiglandular adenomatous disease.

Staging

Not relevant

Prognosis and prediction

The prognosis depends on the underlying disease. Secondary hyperparathyroidism and (especially) tertiary hyperparathyroidism are treated by surgery when they are refractory to conservative medical therapy {3784}. Local recurrence may occur after surgery, a condition termed parathyromatosis if it occurs diffusely in several foci. Patients with parathyroid hyperplasia that demonstrates marked nodularity, an elevated proliferation index, or redevelopment of chronic renal failure are at higher risk of recurrence {3572}.

Parathyroid adenoma

Perren A
Johnson SJ
Juhlin CC
Mete O
Williams MD

Definition

Parathyroid adenoma is a benign parathyroid neoplasm composed of chief, transitional oncocytic, oncocytic, or clear cells, or a mixture of cell types.

ICD-O coding

8140/0 Parathyroid adenoma
8290/0 Oncocytic (oxyphil cell) parathyroid adenoma
8322/0 Water-clear cell parathyroid adenoma

ICD-11 coding

2F37.Y & XH3DV3 Other specified benign neoplasm of endocrine glands & Adenoma, NOS

Related terminology

None

Subtype(s)

Oncocytic (oxyphil cell) parathyroid adenoma; water-clear cell parathyroid adenoma

Localization

Parathyroid adenomas arise in parathyroid glands, with the inferior glands affected slightly more frequently than the superior glands. Parathyroid adenomas can also occur in supernumerary parathyroid tissue or in ectopic regions related to embryonic parathyroid development (thyroid, retro-oesophageal space, hypoglossal nerve, thymus, mediastinum, carotid sheaths, and pericardium) {4490,2211}. Atypical and ectopic localization may be a source of disease recurrence, especially in multiglandular disease including multiple endocrine neoplasia (MEN) type 1 (MEN1)-related multiglandular multiple adenomas. As many as 15% of patients have double adenomas, which show a predilection for the superior parathyroid glands (fourth pouch disease) {3003}. Inferior parathyroid glands/adenomas may be intrathyroidal.

Clinical features

Parathyroid adenomas account for > 85% of primary hyperparathyroidism. Historically, relapsing renal stones and bone pain due to bone loss and osteitis fibrosa cystica were more common before the implementation of serum calcium screening {1431}. Hypercalcaemic crisis with nephrogenic diabetes insipidus and dehydration and acute pancreatitis occurred when calcium levels were > 3 mmol/L. Since the introduction of automated calcium measurements, the detection of primary hyperparathyroidism has risen by a factor of 4–5 {1431}, and patients are relatively asymptomatic or have weakness, fatigue, or anxiety {1431}. The relative proportion of patients presenting with symptomatic versus asymptomatic disease is dependent on the level of population screening for serum calcium {2667}. The deranged trabecular bone mineralization/organization is

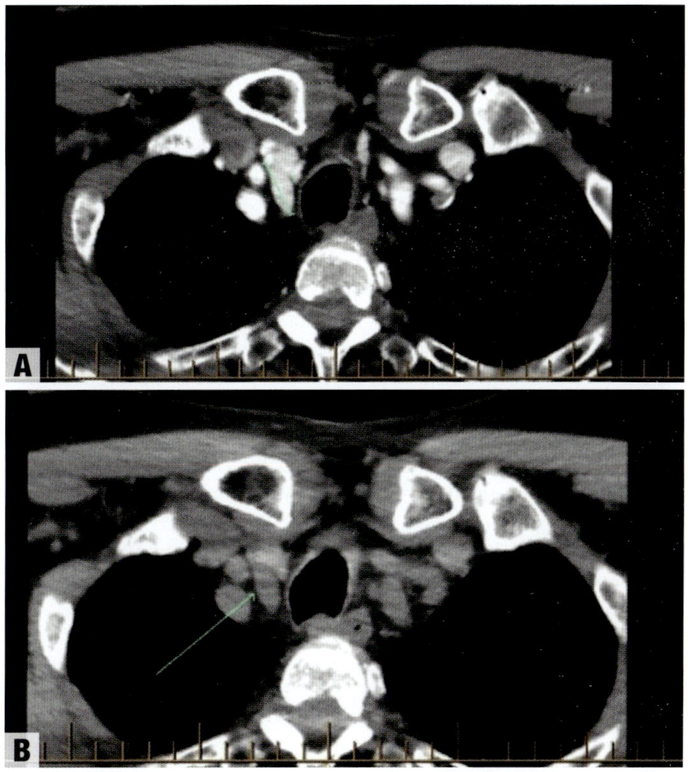

Fig. 4.03 Ectopic parathyroid adenoma. **A** Contrast CT with enhancement of ectopic parathyroid adenoma. **B** CT of ectopic parathyroid adenoma (arrow).

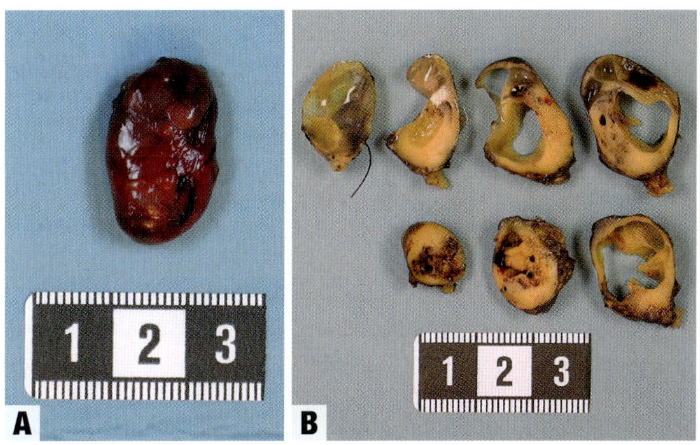

Fig. 4.04 Parathyroid adenoma. **A** Macroscopy of parathyroid adenoma. **B** Cystic parathyroid adenoma. More than 50% of the volume of the adenoma is cystic.

linked to an increase in sometimes asymptomatic vertebral fractures {864}. Between 12% and 50% of patients have nephrolithiasis on imaging studies {864,1216}.

In clinical settings that predispose to secondary/tertiary hyperparathyroidism (e.g. chronic renal failure), the finding of multiple abnormal parathyroid glands generally results in the diagnosis of parathyroid hyperplasia rather than adenoma. However in the absence of predisposing conditions, the overwhelming majority of cases of primary hyperparathyroidism associated with multiglandular parathyroid disease (previously classified as primary hyperplasia) are now recognized as multiglandular adenomas. For instance, MEN1-related multiglandular parathyroid lesions are composed of multiple clonal proliferations, constituting multiple multiglandular adenomas {1438, 516,1168}. In MEN1 syndrome, hyperparathyroidism is the first manifestation in approximately two thirds of patients {1645} and affects > 93% of patients {110}. About 20–30% of patients with MEN type 2A will develop hyperparathyroidism. Hyperparathyroidism is not found in patients with MEN type 2B or isolated familial medullary thyroid carcinoma (a clinical subtype of MEN type 2A) {4667}. Hyperparathyroidism is a leading symptom of MEN type 4 {51}.

There is a correlation between adenoma size and calcium and PTH levels. Parathyroid adenomas measuring > 10 mm are more frequently associated with bone disease and hypercalcaemic crisis {3902}. Oncocytic parathyroid adenomas are more frequently symptomatic and are associated with slightly higher preoperative serum calcium (10.8 vs 10.4 mg/dL) than are age- and sex-matched non-oncocytic adenomas {1967}. Another study found oncocytic adenomas to be larger than non-oncocytic adenomas (1011 vs 557 mg) {1267}. As PTH is now more frequently measured in the absence of elevated calcium levels, normocalcaemic primary hyperparathyroidism is increasingly detected. Although these patients seem to benefit from surgery, with a reported postoperative reduction of renal and bone disease, this is still debated and an individualized approach is suggested {1008}.

Preoperative localization studies include ultrasonography, 99mTc sestamibi (MIBI) scintigraphy/SPECT, four-dimensional parathyroid CT (4DPCT), MRI, and (most recently) 18F-fluorocholine PET-CT. Although the combinations of ultrasound and scintigraphy or ultrasound and 4DPCT are still standard, choline PET-CT shows the highest sensitivity and specificity and may become the method of choice, especially in persistent/recurrent primary hyperparathyroidism {1595}.

A significant drop in intraoperative PTH (often > 50% within 10–15 min) after the removal of an enlarged cellular gland with no features of malignancy can be used to confirm the removal of the adenoma responsible for causing clinical hyperparathyroidism {1168}.

Epidemiology

Although primary hyperparathyroidism was historically considered an uncommon disease, the implementation of serum calcium screening has led to an increase in the reported incidence. In 90% of all patients, chronic hypercalcaemia is attributable to primary hyperparathyroidism {5058}. Incidence rates varying from 16 cases per 100 000 person-years in Denmark {9} to 50 cases per 100 000 person-years in the USA {5058} have been reported. The M:F ratio is 1:2–3 for sporadic cases. In a population-based study from California (1995–2019), the prevalence of primary hyperparathyroidism increased from 76 cases to 233 cases per 100 000 person-years in the female

Table 4.01 Syndromic and non-syndromic inherited forms of primary hyperparathyroidism

Inherited disease	Gene involved	Chromosomal location	Pathology (lifetime risk of development)
MEN1	*MEN1*	11q23	Multiglandular parathyroid disease (multiglandular parathyroid adenomas) (95%) PanNET (40%) PitNET/adenoma (30%) Duodenal NET, gastric NET (20%) Meningiomas Facial angiofibromas
MEN2/3	*RET*	10q11.2	Medullary thyroid carcinoma (99%) Phaeochromocytoma (50%) Multiglandular parathyroid disease (multiglandular parathyroid adenomas) (20%) Ganglioneuromatosis
MEN4	*CDKN1B* (*P27*)	12p13	Multiglandular parathyroid disease (multiglandular parathyroid adenomas) PitNET/adenoma Adrenocortical tumours Meningiomas
HPT-JT	*CDC73* (*PARAFIBROMIN*)	1q25	Parathyroid carcinoma Atypical parathyroid tumour Jaw tumours
FHH1	*CASR* (dominant)	3q21	Normal parathyroids
NS-PHPT	*CASR* (recessive)	3q21.1	Multiglandular parathyroid disease (multiglandular parathyroid adenomas)
FHH2	*GNA11*	19p13	Normal parathyroids
FHH3	*AP2S1*	19q13	Normal parathyroids

FHH1–3, familial hypocalciuric hypercalcaemia types 1–3; HPT-JT, hyperparathyroidism–jaw tumour syndrome; MEN1–4, multiple endocrine neoplasia types 1–4; NET, neuroendocrine tumour; NS-PHPT, non-syndromic primary hyperparathyroidism; PanNET, pancreatic neuroendocrine tumour; PitNET, pituitary neuroendocrine tumour.

population and from 30 cases to 85 cases per 100 000 person-years in the male population. The incidence was highest among Black people, followed by White people, Asian people, Hispanic people, and people from other ethnic groups {5058}. The incidence increases with age in all ethnic groups, and is as high as > 300 cases per 100 000 person-years in Black women aged > 80 years {5058}. About 1.5 of 1000 parathyroid adenomas are composed of almost entirely clear (water-clear) cells (clear cell parathyroid adenomas) {2149}. The epidemiology of normocalcaemic primary hyperparathyroidism is still unclear. A Swedish study reported 230 cases in 5771 postmenopausal women (3.4%) {2761}.

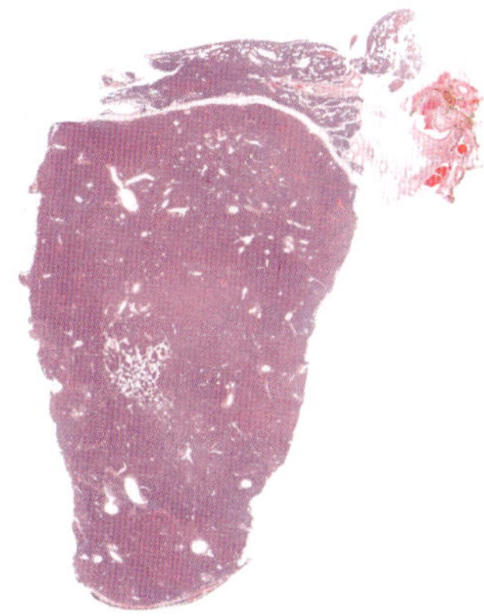

Fig. 4.05 Parathyroid adenoma. Cut section. Note the normal parathyroid (superior) with associated adipose tissue.

Etiology

The etiology of most sporadic parathyroid adenomas is unknown. As many as 10% of parathyroid adenomas are hereditary, either as part of a syndrome or non-syndromic {4443}. MEN1 syndrome–related parathyroids show multiglandular parathyroid disease that is characterized by multiple multiclonal adenomas (although this is often mislabelled clinically as hyperplasia in MEN1 syndrome) {516,4589}, and this disorder and other related genetic susceptibility syndromes are more accurately classified as multiglandular adenomas. In tertiary hyperparathyroidism, autonomous hyperparathyroidism occurs as a result of the hyperplasia-to-neoplasia progression sequence in the background of longstanding chronic renal failure {2956}.

Genetic susceptibility

The syndromes in which parathyroid adenomas occur are MEN types 1, 2, and 4, as well as *CDC73*-related disorders including hyperparathyroidism–jaw tumour syndrome. Pathogenic *MAX* mutations (MEN type 5) have also expanded the spectrum of multiglandular parathyroid adenomas {4047}. Non-syndromic inherited forms are summarized as familial isolated hyperparathyroidism (see respective syndromes). Age < 45 years, male sex, and multiglandular disease are risk factors for an underlying germline mutation {1218}.

Environmental carcinogens

Neck irradiation is a recognized risk factor for parathyroid adenomas, especially in children, occurring after a longer latency than thyroid disease {4278}. External ionizing radiation exposure is also a risk factor, as observed in external therapeutic ionizing radiation to the head and neck and in survivors of the atomic bombing of Hiroshima and the Chernobyl nuclear power plant accident {1452,2176}. An increased rate of parathyroid hyperplasia (with a strong background of vitamin D deficiency) was described 27–32 years after exposure to radiation in the Chernobyl accident {2176}. Long-term lithium therapy (> 10 years) can lead to parathyroid adenomas and (rarely) to four-gland hyperplasia {245,4362}.

Pathogenesis

The mode of inheritance and the genes involved in familial hyperparathyroidism are reported in Table 4.01. In sporadic parathyroid adenomas, the most frequent somatic alterations are loss of heterozygosity of 11q13 (35%) and biallelic *MEN1* inactivation (20%) {528}. Although *CCND1* (encoding cyclin D1) only rarely undergoes rearrangements with *PTH* (detected in up to 8% of parathyroid adenomas), cyclin D1 overexpression is detected in 18–40% of cases, which in turn might be influenced by aberrant promoter hypermethylation of various CDK inhibitors {189}. The causal link between tumour development and *MEN1*/*CCND1* dysregulation is strengthened by the observation of hypercellular parathyroids with hyperparathyroidism in aberrant *MEN1* and *CCND1* mouse models.

Other somatic mutations in parathyroid adenomas are rare and have mostly been described in *CDKN1B* (encoding p27)

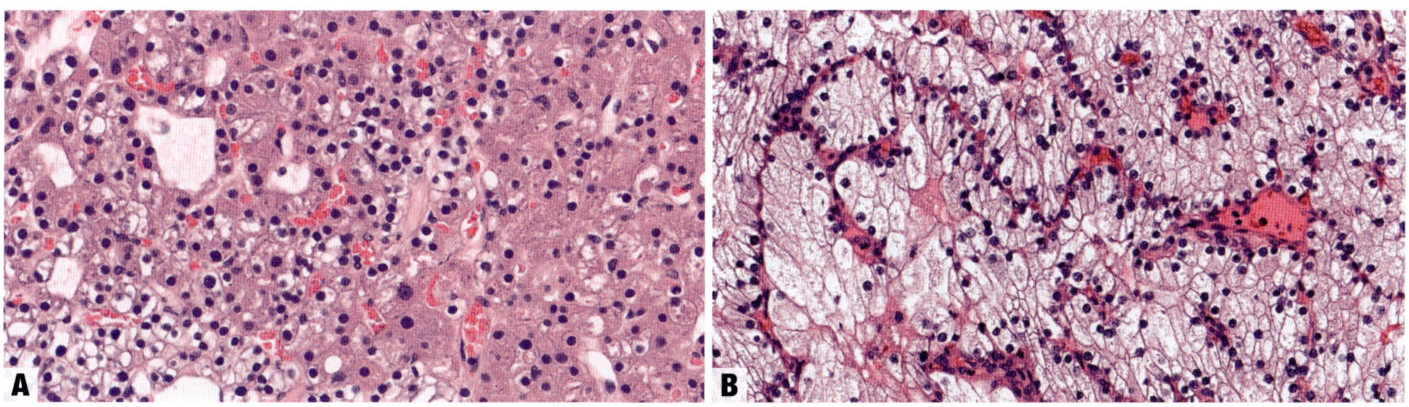

Fig. 4.06 Parathyroid adenoma. **A** Like hyperplasia, parathyroid adenoma is commonly composed of a mixture of cell types, including chief cells, clear cells, and oxyphils. **B** Water-clear cell parathyroid adenoma. This parathyroid adenoma is composed of large cells with abundant clear cytoplasm that displaces the nuclei to the cell periphery.

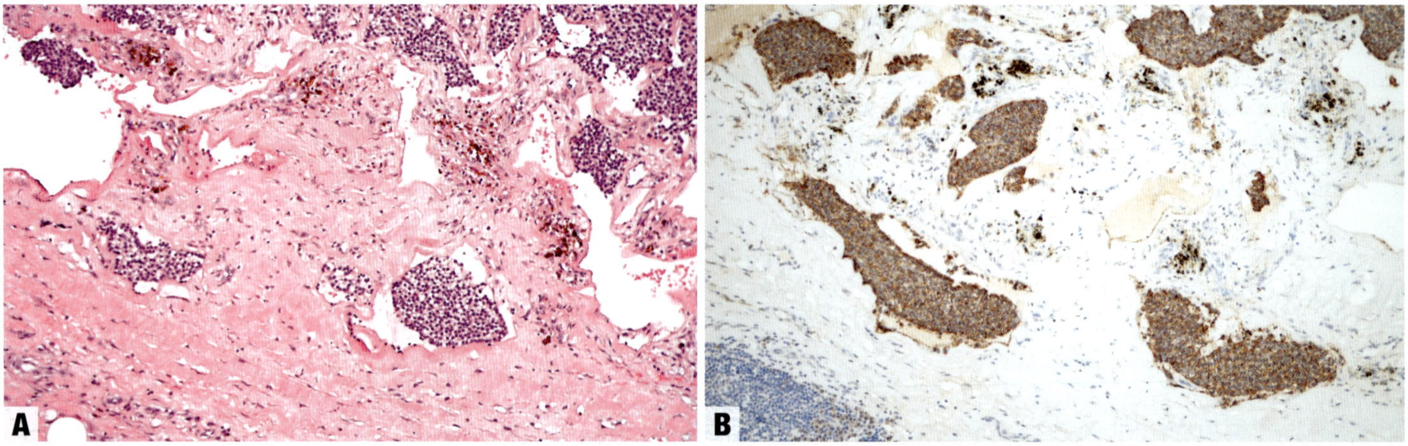

Fig. 4.07 Parathyroid adenoma. Degenerative changes including fibrosis and haemosiderin deposition. **A** Note the pseudovascular spaces, devoid of endothelial cell lining, not to be confused with vascular invasion. **B** Medium magnification. Immunohistochemistry for PTH showing cytoplasmic remnants lining pseudovascular spaces.

{929}, the epigenetic modifier *EZH2* {944,1938}, *ZFX* (encoding a transcription factor with a role in self-renewal) {4232}, and the transcriptional regulator *ASXL3* {4837,1938} and *MTOR* {1938}. In chronic renal failure–related secondary/tertiary hyperparathyroidism, the nodular parathyroid tissue demonstrates different somatic alterations than adenomas identified in primary hyperparathyroidism {1938}. Somatic mutations of other familial drivers (*CDKN1A*, *CDKN1B*, *CDKN2A*, *CDKN2B*, *CDKN2C*, and *GCM2*) are very rare in parathyroid adenomas. *CDC73* mutations are mostly restricted to atypical parathyroid tumours and parathyroid carcinomas, as well as adenomas occurring in hyperparathyroidism–jaw tumour syndrome, although small subsets of clinically recurrence-free adenomas with cystic features have been found to carry this aberration {2138}. *CDC73*-mutated parathyroid adenomas also display a unique cytogenetic profile compared with *CDC73*-wildtype cases {4329}. Although no somatic mutations in *RET*, *CASR*, or *VDR* are found in sporadic parathyroid adenomas, expressional dysregulation of the calcium sensor and vitamin D receptors may play a role in the hyperparathyroidism phenotype {528}. On the epigenetic level, aberrant methylation of tumour-related genes, including *WT1*, *PRDM2* (*RIZ1*), and *RASSF1* (*RASSF1A*), has also been reported in parathyroid adenomas {4269,660,2148}.

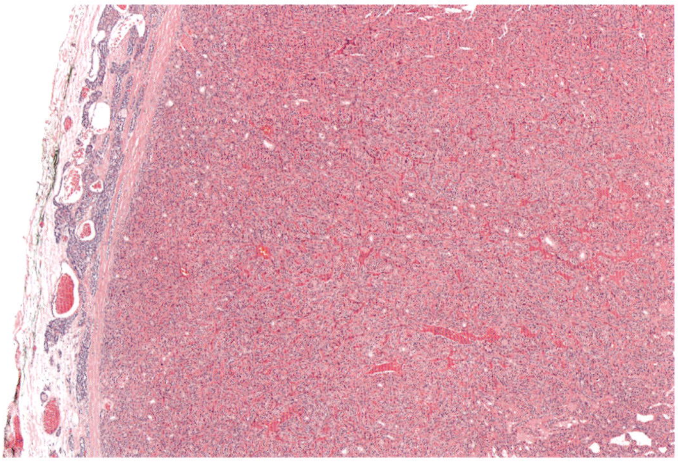

Fig. 4.08 Oncocytic parathyroid adenoma. The tumour is composed entirely of oncocytes. Note the rim of non-neoplastic parathyroid.

Macroscopic appearance

Parathyroid adenomas are ovoid, pink or tan tumours surrounded by a delicate pseudocapsule. A rim of atrophic parathyroid tissue is often identifiable at the vascular pole of a gland {1168}. Sectioning the gland horizontally through the vascular hilum often demonstrates this rim of suppressed non-neoplastic tissue {1168}. A normal gland measures up to 6–8 mm and weighs up to 40–60 mg {1168}. Tumours weighing < 100 mg and with a diameter < 6 mm {1613} may correspond to microadenomas and may be incidental findings rather than the cause of clinical hyperparathyroidism. One definition of a giant parathyroid adenoma is a tumour weighing > 2 g {2981}, but adenomas may measure several centimetres and weigh tens if not hundreds of grams {2832}. Some parathyroid adenomas can be bilobated or multilobulated. Parathyroid adenomas may contain fluid-filled cysts and can be termed cystic parathyroid adenomas if cysts make up > 50% of the tumour volume. Cystic adenomas tend to be larger, with higher calcium and PTH levels, and they may be confused with thyroid cysts because subsets are negative on 99mTc sestamibi (MIBI) scintigraphy {1976}. Cystic changes may be accompanied by prominent areas of fibrosis or foci of calcification {749}. Spontaneous infarction or haemorrhage in parathyroid adenomas may occur, sometimes leading to adherence to surrounding structures and rarely leading to spontaneous remission of hyperparathyroidism {2223}.

Histopathology

Parathyroid adenomas are histologically well circumscribed or encapsulated by a thin fibrous pseudocapsule. Stromal fat is usually absent or sparse. A rim of atrophic parathyroid tissue is observed in more than half of the adenomas, but it is detected less frequently in larger tumours {59}. Rim-like areas can also occasionally be identified in parathyroid hyperplasia. It is therefore necessary to correlate the morphological features with clinical findings (e.g. absence of secondary/tertiary hyperparathyroidism), radiographic findings, and laboratory findings (e.g. significant drop of intraoperative PTH or postoperative biochemical cure) {1168}. A slightly cellular rim may be seen in the setting of underlying vitamin D deficiency.

Parathyroid adenomas are usually composed of chief cells with a round nucleus and scant cytoplasm, but they can be composed of a mixture of parenchymal cell types including chief,

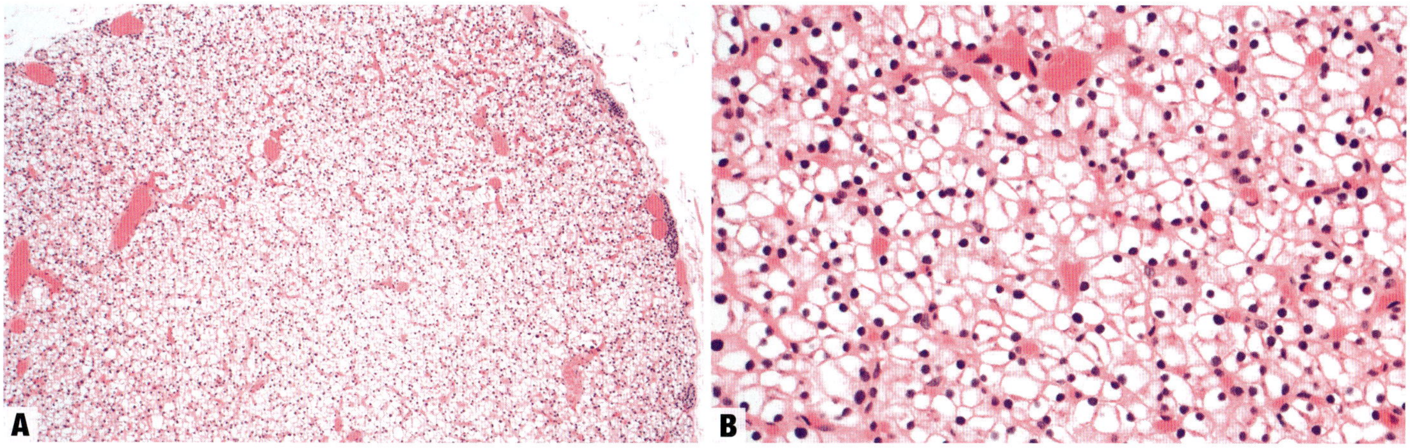

Fig. 4.09 Water-clear cell parathyroid adenoma. **A,B** This subtype is characterized by neoplastic cells with strikingly clear cytoplasm.

transitional, oncocytic, and clear cells. There may be lobules or nodules within the adenoma. Oncocytic change may occur focally. When oncocytic cells constitute > 75% of the adenoma, it is termed oncocytic/oxyphilic parathyroid adenoma.

The tumour cells in parathyroid adenomas are arranged in sheets or nests in a delicate capillary network. The tumour cells may have a palisaded appearance around blood vessels. The tumour cell nuclei are slightly larger than those of the adjacent parathyroid tissue. Formation of follicular structures is not uncommon, and a few adenomas demonstrate a predominantly follicular growth. In such cases, the absence of birefringent calcium oxalate crystals and the presence of well-defined cell membranes can help in the differentiation from thyroid tissue. Papillary growth is rare {3886}. Chief cells are polygonal with clear or slightly eosinophilic cytoplasm. The nuclei are lymphocyte-like and centrally located and have well-defined cell membranes. Multinucleated tumour cells and patchy endocrine nuclear atypia may occur. Occasional mitotic figures (< 5 mitoses/10 mm^2) can be identified.

Most parathyroid adenomas are composed predominantly of chief cells, often with a mixture of oncocytic (oxyphil) and clear cells. Oncocytic (oxyphil cell) parathyroid adenomas account for about 3–6% of parathyroid adenomas {1967}. Water-clear cell parathyroid adenomas are uncommon {267,2149}.

In large and giant adenomas, fibrosis, cholesterol clefts, contour irregularity, and/or haemorrhage with haemosiderin deposition and cyst formation are more frequent. In cases with broad fibrous bands, necrosis, or elevated mitotic counts in the absence of invasive growth, the diagnosis of atypical parathyroid tumour (see *Atypical parathyroid tumour*, p. 215) should be considered. Adenomas and atypical parathyroid tumours are distinguished from parathyroid carcinomas by the absence of unequivocal invasive growth. The rim of non-neoplastic parathyroid tissue adjacent to parathyroid adenoma is often indistinguishable from normal parathyroid tissue, although this tissue may be considered suppressed because the proliferation rate and secretory set point are often decreased {3430}. Confident separation of adenoma from nodular chief-cell hyperplasia, including in asymmetrical and asynchronous cases, is not possible by morphological criteria alone in a single gland. However, pathologists and clinicians encounter this issue less often with more extensive radiographic assessments and with the utilization of rapid intraoperative PTH testing {1168}.

Immunohistochemistry

Immunohistochemically, parathyroid adenomas are positive for PTH and GATA3, and for the neuroendocrine markers chromogranin A and synaptophysin {1271}. Thyroglobulin, thyroid transcription factor 1 (TTF1), and monoclonal PAX8 stains are negative. The vast majority of sporadic parathyroid adenomas show nuclear parafibromin expression {2138,1578,2151}. Morphological clues to tumours associated with *CDC73* mutations, termed parafibromin-deficient parathyroid tumours, include eosinophilic

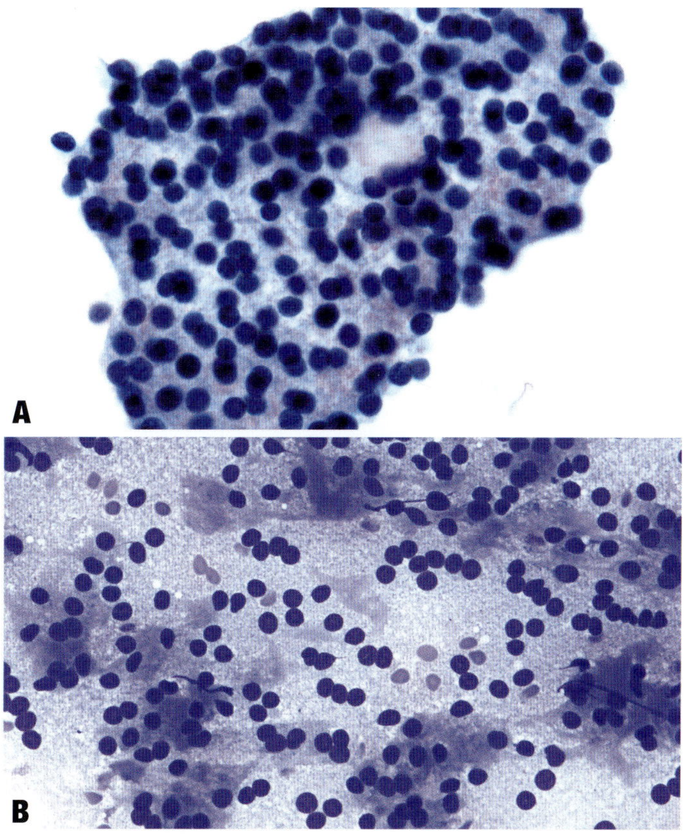

Fig. 4.10 Parathyroid adenoma. **A** FNA specimen showing a tissue fragment with a monotonous population of lesional cells with round nuclei, evenly dispersed nuclear chromatin, and delicate cytoplasm with sharp cytoplasmic borders (ThinPrep preparation). **B** FNA specimen showing a monotonous population of lesional cells with round nuclei and delicate cytoplasm (air-dried smear preparation, Diff-Quik stain).

cytoplasm with perinuclear clearing, nuclear enlargement, microcystic change, and a sheet-like growth pattern {1580}.

Differential diagnosis

On the pathological examination of only one parathyroid gland in the absence of clinical information, the distinction between adenoma and different types of hyperplasia is not possible with certainty and a descriptive diagnosis such as "pathologically enlarged fat-depleted parathyroid gland consistent with..." may be preferable.

Cytology

Smears show low to moderate cellularity with variable patterns including cohesive sheets and more complex papilliform (with thin fibrovascular cores) and microfollicular tissue fragments {14}. The nuclei are regular in arrangement, small, central, and round to oval, with a regular membrane and even fine chromatin {4340,1726}. The scant cytoplasm is pale, finely granular, and eosinophilic (Pap), and it can be oxyphilic or vacuolated {4340}. There is no thin colloid in the clean background where stripped nuclei may be present. Without clinical information, parathyroid adenoma may be misdiagnosed as a thyroid lesion, when the FNAB target is a thyroid nodule or a lesion that may be in ectopic parathyroid tissue; but with clinical and ultrasound correlation the diagnosis can be suggested, and immunocytochemical studies for PTH on cell blocks and PTH measurements using needle washouts can confirm the diagnosis {596,4345}.

Diagnostic molecular pathology

No diagnostic molecular tests are indicated in sporadic parathyroid adenomas. Screening for an underlying germline abnormality is recommended for individuals with primary hyperparathyroidism if any of the following features are present: (1) age at disease onset < 45 years, (2) a family history of primary hyperparathyroidism or other tumours that can occur in inherited syndromes, (3) a personal history of a neuroendocrine neoplasm (NEN; e.g. pituitary, pancreas) or other tumours that can feature primary hyperparathyroidism, (4) primary hyperparathyroidism due to multiglandular parathyroid disease (e.g. MEN1-related multiple multiglandular adenomas), and (5) histological findings of a possible *CDC73*-associated tumour or mutation-associated immunohistochemistry findings (e.g. loss of menin, parafibromin, and p27) suggestive of inherited disease {653,2143}.

Essential and desirable diagnostic criteria

Essential: an enlarged cellular gland (> 6–8 mm and > 40–60 mg) consisting of a benign parathyroid cell proliferation, often surrounded by a rim of atrophic parathyroid parenchyma.

Desirable: a significant drop in intraoperative PTH; postoperative biochemical cure; additional parathyroid gland(s) with no pathological diagnosis.

Staging

Not relevant

Prognosis and prediction

Parathyroid adenomas are benign. Recurrent hyperparathyroidism develops in < 2% of patients {2048}. In the setting of multiglandular disease the prognosis is dependent on the underlying clinical or genetic syndrome {4589}.

Parathyroid lipoadenoma

Juhlin CC
Johnson SJ
Perren A
Williams MD

Chapter 4

Definition

Parathyroid lipoadenoma is a benign parathyroid neoplasm characterized by an unequivocal increase in parenchymal parathyroid tissue associated with abundant adipose tissue.

ICD-O coding

8324/0 Parathyroid lipoadenoma

ICD-11 coding

2F37.Y & XH8P28 Other specified benign neoplasm of endocrine glands & Lipoadenoma

Related terminology

Not recommended: parathyroid hamartoma.

Subtype(s)

None

Localization

Parathyroid lipoadenomas can arise in normally positioned glands, predominantly in left-sided locations {2005}. Ectopic sites have also been reported, most commonly the mediastinum {1788,4911,2005}. Subsets of patients develop multiglandular disease with two or more enlarged glands exhibiting abundant fat, termed lipohyperplasia {4302,4054,2144}.

Clinical features

Most parathyroid lipoadenomas are functioning, and patients usually exhibit mild biochemical evidence of hyperparathyroidism with classic symptomatology {2005,2144,2431}.

Epidemiology

Fewer than 100 cases have been reported in the literature {2144}. A slight female predominance and a mean age of 56 years are noted {2005}.

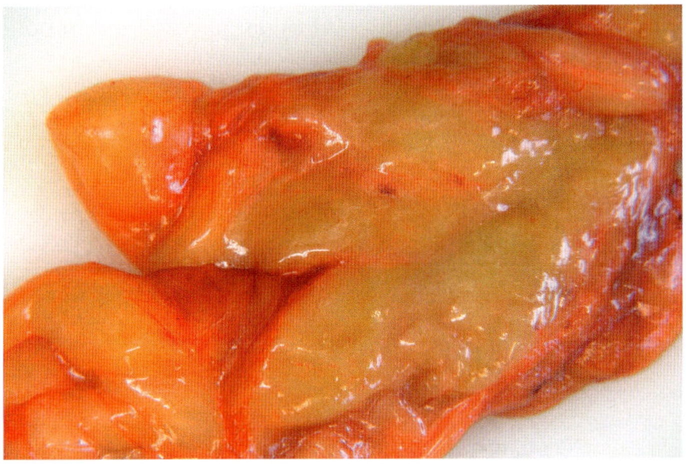

Fig. 4.11 Parathyroid lipoadenoma. Gross appearance of a parathyroid lipoadenoma.

Etiology

The etiology is unknown. There is no known hereditary predisposition. An association with hypertension has been suggested {2144}.

Pathogenesis

The underlying molecular events are unknown.

Macroscopic appearance

The reported size and glandular weights vary, and parathyroid lipoadenomas tend to be larger than parathyroid adenomas {2005}, with mean weights > 1 g reported in some case series {4054}. Tumours are often encapsulated and display a yellow cut surface.

Histopathology

The diagnosis should be restricted to adenomas with a significant increase in both adipose and parenchymal tissue {2431}.

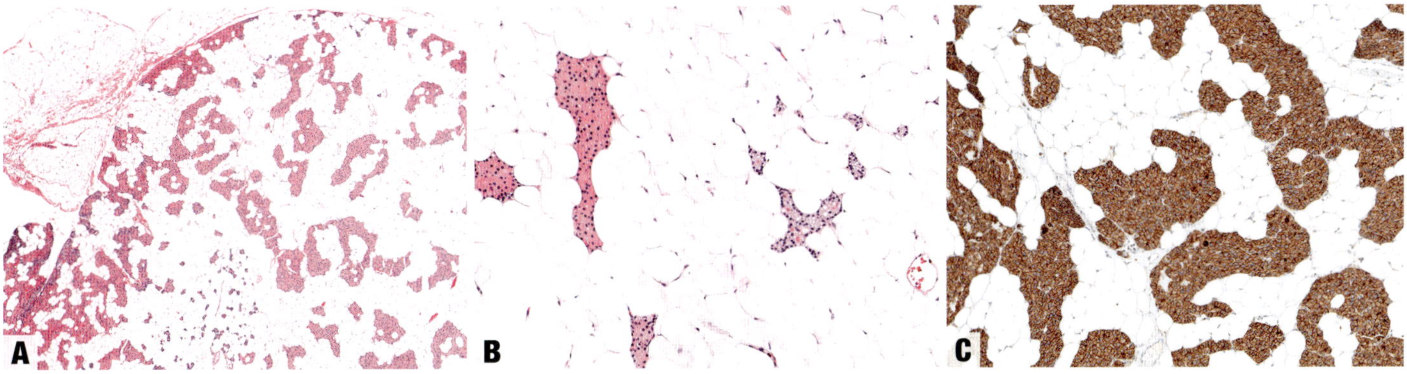

Fig. 4.12 Parathyroid lipoadenoma. **A** Parathyroid lipoadenoma composed of increased amounts of both acinar and adipose tissue. The glandular component grows in branching cords. **B** High-magnification view revealing a mixture of both chief cells and oncocytic cells. **C** Strong and diffuse PTH immunoreactivity in the acinar component.

Parathyroids that are enlarged solely because of an accumulation of adipose tissue but without an increase in parenchymal content should not be considered lipoadenoma {2431}. Similarly, the presence of some adipose tissue in an otherwise typical parathyroid adenoma should not warrant the diagnosis {2144}. A useful general rule is that > 50% of the volume of the gland should be adipose tissue to warrant the diagnosis {2144}. The stromal component may include brown fat and myxoid or fibrous differentiation {2005,2144}. A rim of compressed non-tumorous parathyroid tissue is usually present.

Cytology

Not relevant

Diagnostic molecular pathology

Not relevant

Essential and desirable diagnostic criteria

Essential: a definite increase in both parenchymal and adipose tissue in a parathyroid tumour; > 50% of the glandular volume is adipose tissue.

Desirable: a significant drop in intraoperative PTH or evidence of postoperative biochemical cure, or additional parathyroid gland(s) without a pathological diagnosis.

Staging

Not relevant

Prognosis and prediction

Lipoadenomas are benign. A series from Sweden suggested that patients with hyperparathyroidism treated by removal of lipoadenoma may have a lower initial biochemical cure rate and higher recurrence rate than those treated by removal of usual adenoma; however, this observation requires further validation {2144}.

Atypical parathyroid tumour

Erickson LA
Gill AJ
Johnson SJ
Juhlin CC
Perren A
Williams MD

Definition

Atypical parathyroid tumour (APT) is a parathyroid neoplasm that demonstrates atypical cytological and architectural features but lacks unequivocal capsular, vascular, or perineural invasion or invasion into adjacent structures or metastases.

ICD-O coding

8140/1 Atypical parathyroid tumour

ICD-11 coding

2F9A Neoplasms of unknown behaviour of endocrine glands

Related terminology

Acceptable: atypical parathyroid neoplasm; parathyroid tumour of low/uncertain malignant potential.
Not recommended: atypical parathyroid adenoma.

Subtype(s)

None

Localization

APT can involve any parathyroid gland.

Clinical features

APTs usually occur sporadically, but they can occur in familial isolated hyperparathyroidism, hyperparathyroidism–jaw tumour syndrome, and in multiple endocrine neoplasia type 1 {722}. In a review of 672 APTs, all but 24 occurred sporadically {722}. Patients may be asymptomatic or have fatigue, weakness, weight loss, nausea, polyuria, or polydipsia. Clinically, APTs may be indistinguishable from parathyroid carcinomas, but a palpable neck mass is much less common in APT (3%) than in carcinoma (13%) {4014}. Serum calcium is elevated (< 13.5 mg/dL) but is generally lower than in carcinoma and often intermediate between that of adenoma and carcinoma.

Preoperative localization may include ultrasound, scintigraphic studies, dual-phase SPECT, MRI, 18F-fluorocholine PET-CT. Choline PET-CT shows the highest sensitivity and specificity and may become the method of choice in persistent/recurrent primary hyperparathyroidism {1595}.

Epidemiology

The incidence of APT may be dependent on the pathological criteria used and ranges from 0.5% to 4.4% in individuals undergoing surgery for primary hyperparathyroidism {722}. Most cases occur sporadically, but APT can occur in familial isolated hyperparathyroidism, hyperparathyroidism–jaw tumour syndrome, and multiple endocrine neoplasia type 1. Sporadic cases are more common in women, with an M:F ratio of approximately 1:1.5 and a mean age of 48.2 years (± 18.5 years, range: 16–80 years) {722}. Familial cases show an equal sex distribution and on average occur two decades earlier {722}.

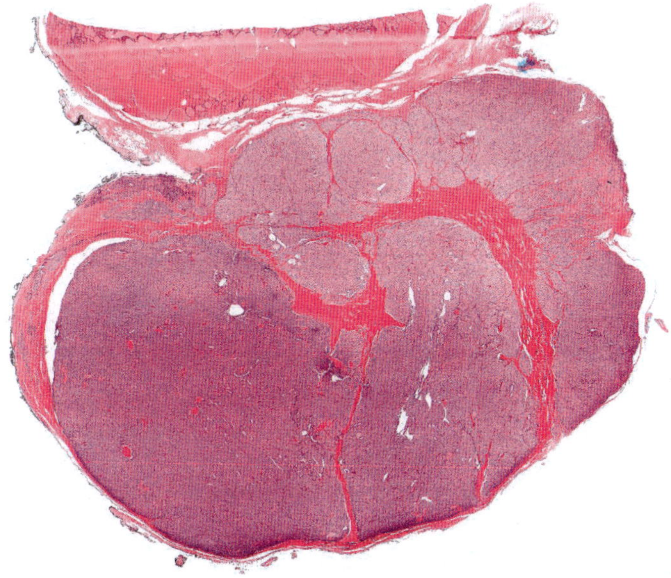

Fig. 4.13 Atypical parathyroid tumour. An example with fibrosis adjacent to the thyroid gland, but not invading it.

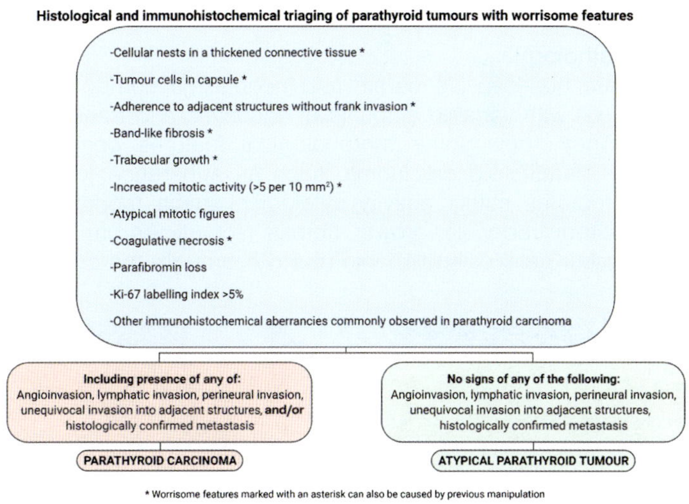

Fig. 4.14 Parathyroid neoplasms. Diagnostic algorithm.

Etiology

The etiology of APT is unknown. A minority of cases occur in familial disease.

Pathogenesis

It is unclear whether there is true progression from benign to malignant in parathyroid lesions, including in hyperparathyroidism–jaw tumour syndrome, in which the prevalence of parathyroid carcinoma is high. APTs rarely have somatic *MEN1* mutations {863}. In a study of 38 APTs, 25 (66%) showed loss

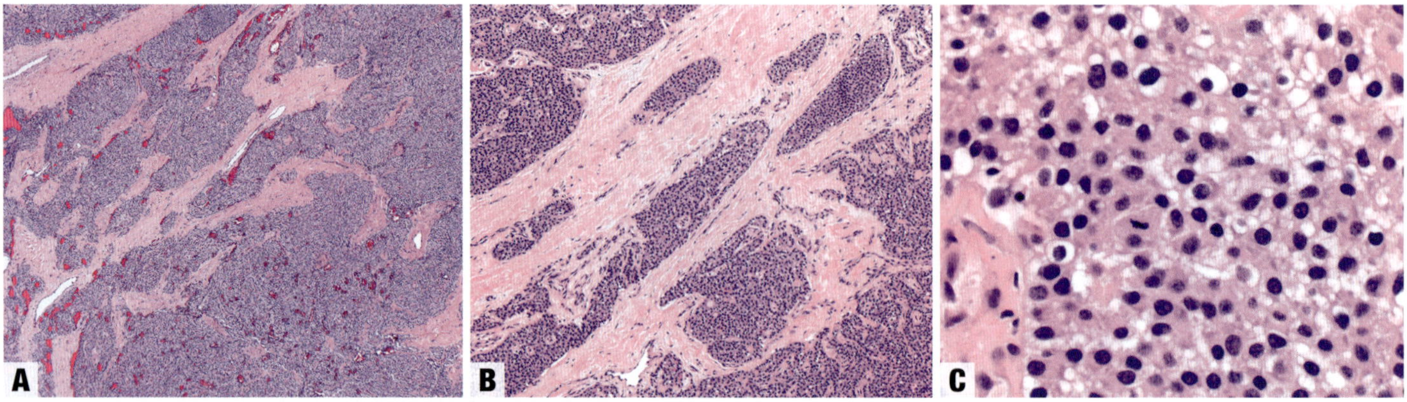

Fig. 4.15 Atypical parathyroid tumour. **A** This tumour shows irregular growth with prominent areas of fibrosis but does not show definitive capsular or vascular invasion or invasion into adjacent structures. **B** These tumours may show fibrosis including thick fibrous bands, but they do not show definitive invasion. **C** Mitotic activity can be seen in any parathyroid lesion, whether benign or malignant. Although prominent mitotic activity is a worrisome feature, the presence of mitotic activity is insufficient for a diagnosis of parathyroid carcinoma.

of heterozygosity (at the *CDKN1A* [*P21*] locus in 9 cases, at *CDC73* and *PTEN* in 6 cases, and at *RB1* in 4 cases) {2915}. Targeted sequence analysis of 50 APTs for 15 tumour-related genes showed that 16 (32%) had least one alteration (*CDC73* in 12 cases [24%], *EZH2* in 4 cases [8%], *HIC1* in 1 case [2%], and *CDKN2A* in 1 case [2%]) and suggested that the genetic profile of APTs more closely resembles that of parathyroid carcinoma than adenoma {2835}.

Macroscopic appearance

APTs are usually solid but can be cystic, with a median size of 30 mm (10–72 mm), and are adherent to adjacent structures in half of the cases {722}.

Histopathology

APTs are non-invasive parathyroid neoplasms composed of chief cells with variable amounts of oncocytic and transitional cells. They show some morphological features commonly seen in parathyroid carcinoma, such as adherence to adjacent structures, mitotic activity, cytological atypia, monotonous sheet-like or trabecular growth, fibrosis (sometimes band-like), and tumour cells extending into (but not through) the capsule. They are distinguished from parathyroid carcinoma by the lack of unequivocal full-thickness capsular invasion with clear-cut extension into soft tissue, vascular or perineural invasion, or invasion into adjacent structures.

Conventional parathyroid adenomas (particularly if large) commonly demonstrate focal fibrosis, an occasional mitotic figure, or focal capsular thickening. However, the diagnosis of APT is reserved for parathyroid neoplasms with significantly atypical features that are worrisome for a parathyroid carcinoma but for which definitive invasion cannot be documented. This diagnosis should be based on the constellation of features and the clinical context.

APTs may show monotonous, solid growth of sheets of cells or closely packed nests, similar to that seen in parathyroid carcinoma. Fibrosis can be identified in secondary/tertiary hyperparathyroidism and with prior manipulation (e.g. FNAB) and is insufficient to warrant the diagnosis of APT if it can be confidently attributed to posttraumatic regenerative change. The association of fat necrosis and haemosiderin deposition with fibrosis or contour irregularity is a useful clue to posttraumatic regenerative change {118,1168,2285,1899}. Mitotic activity is seen in benign and malignant disease. A mitotic rate

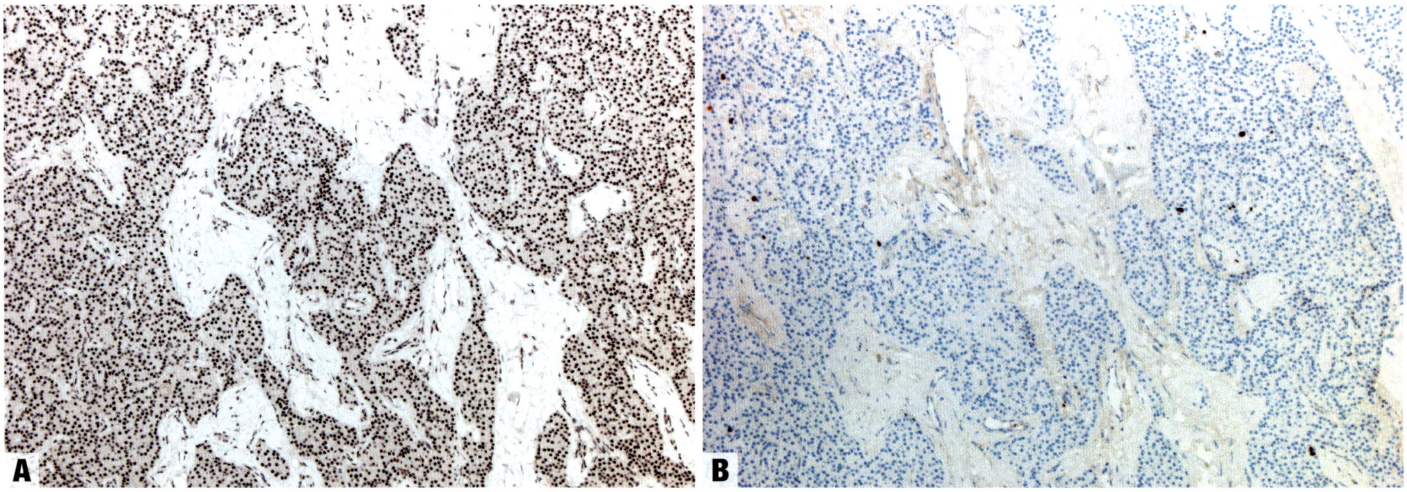

Fig. 4.16 Atypical parathyroid tumour. **A** Parafibromin shows retained nuclear immunostaining in this atypical parathyroid tumour. **B** Ki-67 immunostain shows only scattered positive cells in this atypical parathyroid tumour with a low proliferation index.

of > 5 mitoses/10 mm^2 or a Ki-67 proliferation index of > 5%, necrosis, macronucleoli, or atypical mitoses are more common in malignancy {461,2712,722}. However, a definitive diagnosis of carcinoma requires invasive growth or metastasis.

Immunohistochemistry

APTs show positivity for PTH, GATA3, and chromogranin A. Numerous biomarkers, including combinations, have been evaluated in parathyroid neoplasms, including Ki-67, cyclin D1, p27, RB1, BCL2, MDM2, p53, galectin-3, E-cadherin, and PGP9.5 {1268,1267,188,4289,1364,1276,4014,1953,1271,4144}. All show some utility, but they do not consistently differentiate benign from malignant parathyroid neoplasms.

Parafibromin is encoded by *CDC73*. Absent nuclear parafibromin immunoreactivity in the presence of an internal control (termed parafibromin deficiency) indicates biallelic *CDC73* inactivation, which is commonly associated with germline mutation {2143,1578,1580,2151}. Parafibromin has shown utility in predicting outcome in APTs {2150,2438}. Given the association of somatic *CDC73* mutations and sporadic parathyroid carcinoma, and the increased risk of carcinoma and metachronous tumours in individuals with germline *CDC73* mutation, long-term follow-up is recommended with parafibromin-deficient tumours {1578,1953,1271,2143}.

Cytology

APTs have not been extensively studied cytopathologically, but the distinction from parathyroid adenoma and carcinoma is reported as not possible {596}. Parathyroid must be differentiated from thyroid, and immunostains can be performed or PTH evaluated with needle washout fluid {4345}.

Diagnostic molecular pathology

Germline *CDC73* mutation testing is recommended in parafibromin-deficient APT {4886,1580,2151}, but otherwise molecular testing is usually not performed unless there is a suspicion of hereditary disease.

Essential and desirable diagnostic criteria

Essential: atypical cytological or architectural features; absence of invasive growth.

Desirable: large size; marked hypercalcaemia.

Staging

According to American Joint Committee on Cancer (AJCC) eighth-edition staging, APT is staged as Tis.

Prognosis and prediction

Although APTs are considered an intermediate type of parathyroid neoplasm of uncertain malignant potential and metastases have been reported, the great majority do not recur after simple excision, and some suggest they may be followed similarly to adenomas in the absence of concerning clinical or immunohistochemical features (e.g. parafibromin deficiency) {722,4886}. APTs with parafibromin deficiency have an increased risk of recurrence, predominantly as metachronous disease in other glands but occasionally as true recurrence, and warrant long-term follow-up {2150,2438,1580,2151}.

Parathyroid carcinoma

Mete O
Johnson SJ
Juhlin CC
Perren A
Williams MD

Definition

Parathyroid carcinoma is a malignant neoplasm originating from parathyroid parenchymal cells.

ICD-O coding

8140/3 Parathyroid carcinoma

ICD-11 coding

2D12.1 & XH7JQ0 Adenocarcinoma of other endocrine glands or related structures & Parathyroid carcinoma

Related terminology

None

Subtype(s)

None

Localization

Parathyroid carcinoma can arise in any of the normal anatomical locations of parathyroid glands or in anatomical sites where developmental parathyroid tissue may be identified, including the neck, thyroid, retro-oesophageal space, thymus, mediastinum, and pericardium {627,96,4964,382}.

Clinical features

Most patients with parathyroid carcinomas present with symptomatic primary hyperparathyroidism {4951,575,1275,221,65}; however, extremely rare examples have been reported in the setting of chronic renal failure–related tertiary hyperparathyroidism {4517,2997,2267,2231,2280,1369}. Symptomatic patients have renal disease with nephrolithiasis and/or bone disease {1168}. Other signs and symptoms of hypercalcaemia (including weakness, vomiting, constipation, nausea, polyuria, polydipsia, pancreatitis, arrhythmias, and neurological manifestations) can also occur {1172,65}. Patients with hyperparathyroidism–jaw tumour syndrome (HPT-JT) can also manifest associated characteristics features (see *Hyperparathyroidism–jaw tumour syndrome*, p. 448).

Biochemical investigations

Laboratory tests usually show significantly elevated levels of PTH (usually > 3 times and often 10 times the upper limit of normal) and calcium (> 3 mmol/L or > 12 mg/dL, or 3–4 mg above the upper limit of normal) {4951,575,3980,1785,1275,221}. Rare examples of biochemically non-functioning parathyroid carcinomas {1362,1785,721,4316,1625,4252} have been reported, occurring in up to 3% of parathyroid carcinomas in clinical series {1785}. A third-to-second generation PTH assay ratio > 1 has been shown to help predict the risk of malignancy with a high sensitivity (~83%) and specificity (range: 97–100%) {674,710,709}. Symptomatic hyperparathyroidism in association with a palpable neck mass (often > 30 mm) requires exclusion of parathyroid carcinoma {3980,1172}.

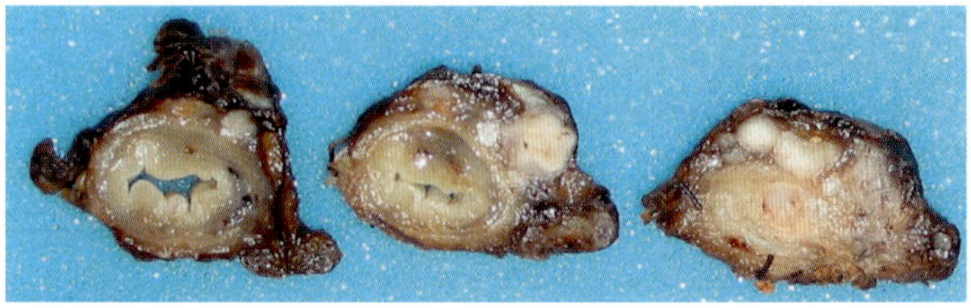

Fig. 4.17 Parathyroid carcinoma. Gross image of a tumour infiltrating the oesophagus.

Imaging

Structural (e.g. ultrasonography, CT) and functional (e.g. 99mTc sestamibi scan) imaging studies are often used in the preoperative workup of any patients with hyperparathyroidism. Imaging findings concerning for parathyroid carcinoma include the presence of invasive growth and/or calcification on ultrasound, or the suspicion of metastatic disease on 99mTc sestamibi scan or CT) {1172}. However, most parathyroid carcinomas are diagnosed by histopathological examination of a parathyroidectomy specimen or during the workup of a metastatic carcinoma. However, a fraction of patients with parathyroid carcinoma can manifest with recurrent laryngeal nerve paralysis with vocal cord dysfunction and hoarseness, invasion into adjacent anatomical structures (either on imaging studies or intraoperative documentation), or distant metastasis at the time of their clinical workup {3493,1785,4799,65}.

Epidemiology

Parathyroid carcinoma accounts for < 1% of primary hyperparathyroidism. The reported incidence of parathyroid carcinoma has increased in parallel to the increasing rate of parathyroid surgery in North America {2578}, Finland {3863}, Australia {552}, China {4799}, and the Republic of Korea {2380} over the past decade(s). Epidemiological data indicate that these tumours affect 5.73 (USA, 2000–2003), 6.6 (Republic of Korea, 2016), and 10.4 (Finland, 2010–2013) individuals per 10 million population per year {2578,2380,3863}. It is unclear whether increased laboratory screening for hypercalcaemia {1168} and the integration of ancillary biomarker studies {552} have contributed to this observation.

Parathyroid carcinoma can occur at any age, including in the paediatric population {4951,1785,1275,222,221,65,395,2380,3663}. The mean age at the time of diagnosis is 51–57 years in most clinical series {4951,1785,1275,3869,222,221,65,2380}. Compared with people in other ethnic groups, non-Hispanic White people in the USA had a disproportionately higher incidence of parathyroid carcinoma in the National Cancer Database (NCDB) {3869}. Although an equal or not significantly different sex distribution is reported in most cohorts {1988,4951,

222,4799,221}, a slightly decreased M:F ratio has been noted in some studies {1275,3863,65,2380,3663,1785}. Parafibromin-deficient parathyroid carcinomas are reported to have a male predilection {2151,5180} and are more frequent in younger patients {1580,5180}.

Etiology

CDC73 mutation, associated with HPT-JT, dramatically increases the lifetime risk of parathyroid carcinoma {1574,4589}. Given its rarity, there are few studies on the etiology of sporadic parathyroid carcinoma. An association with previous irradiation to the head and neck region has been reported, although this phenomenon is also reported for parathyroid adenomas {848}.

Pathogenesis

Parathyroid carcinoma can occur sporadically, but it is also a feature of familial hyperparathyroidism syndromes, most notably occurring in 10–15% of patients with HPT-JT as well as in rare forms of familial isolated hyperparathyroidism {677,3956,2011, 530,2401,2928,1580}. When parathyroid carcinomas arise in the setting of HPT-JT, inactivating germline mutations or deletions of *CDC73* are found in the majority of kindreds {677,4094,4154}. Moreover, 40–80% of sporadic parathyroid carcinomas harbour inactivating *CDC73* mutations in addition to frequent loss of heterozygosity of the *CDC73* locus at chromosome 1q25-q31 {1961,4094,1821,723,1994,720}. The *CDC73* mutations are frequently germline, indicative of de novo mutations or undetected HPT-JT {4094,723,707}.

CDC73 encodes parafibromin, a nuclear tumour suppressor belonging to PAF1C (a multiprotein unit that interacts with RNA polymerase II to facilitate mRNA elongation and post-transcriptional processing) {3854,5048,1330}. Parafibromin exhibits antiproliferative and proapoptotic properties, partly through the epigenetic regulation of the oncogenes *CCND1* (encoding cyclin D1) and *MYC* (*c-myc*) oncogenes and partly through interactions with the WNT pathway effector β-catenin {3104,2663,5036}. The majority of *CDC73* mutations in parathyroid carcinomas are truncating or frameshift alterations (or alternatively, missense mutations in conserved regions), and loss of parafibromin immunoreactivity is observed in *CDC73*-mutated cases {4094,4406,1578,2153}. Premature truncating mutations often lead to an abolished nuclear localization signal, providing an explanation for the absence of nuclear parafibromin expression in *CDC73*-mutated parathyroid carcinomas {1744,1578,510}. Moreover, *CDC73* mutations abolishing the nucleolar localization signal have also been reported, and these rare cases might display an exclusive loss of parafibromin nucleolar expression, suggesting a nucleolar tumour-suppressor role for parafibromin in addition to the established nuclear properties {1745,3405,2146,2864}. *CDC73*-mutated parathyroid carcinomas may display an increase in genomic instability, highlighted by augmented levels of copy-number alterations, an increased tumour mutation burden, and poorer patient outcomes, as compared with *CDC73*-wildtype cases {1977}.

Other reported genomic alterations in sporadic parathyroid carcinomas include loss of *TP53* and *RB1* alleles, although mutations in these genes are rarely found {952,951,873}. Amplifications of *CCND1* (encoding cyclin D1) have been demonstrated in subsets of cases {3402}. Unlike in parathyroid adenoma, *MEN1* mutations are only rarely reported in parathyroid carcinoma {1822,873,2465}. *TERT* promoter mutations are also rarely reported in parathyroid carcinoma {1742,2465}. Parathyroid carcinomas recurrently have mutations in genes with potential implications for targeted molecular therapies, including *PTEN*, *NF1*, *KDR*, and *PIK3CA* {2189,2465}. Previously unrecognized *DICER1* mutations were recently reported in a series of advanced parathyroid carcinomas {2465}.

From an epigenetic standpoint, parathyroid carcinomas display aberrant methylation of several cancer-specific genes, including the WNT pathway regulator *APC* and the cell-cycle regulators *CDKN2A* and *CDKN2B* {4269,4352}. Levels of 5-hydroxymethylcytosine have been found to be extensively reduced in parathyroid carcinomas, suggestive of a universal reduction in demethylation events across the genome in parathyroid carcinoma {310}.

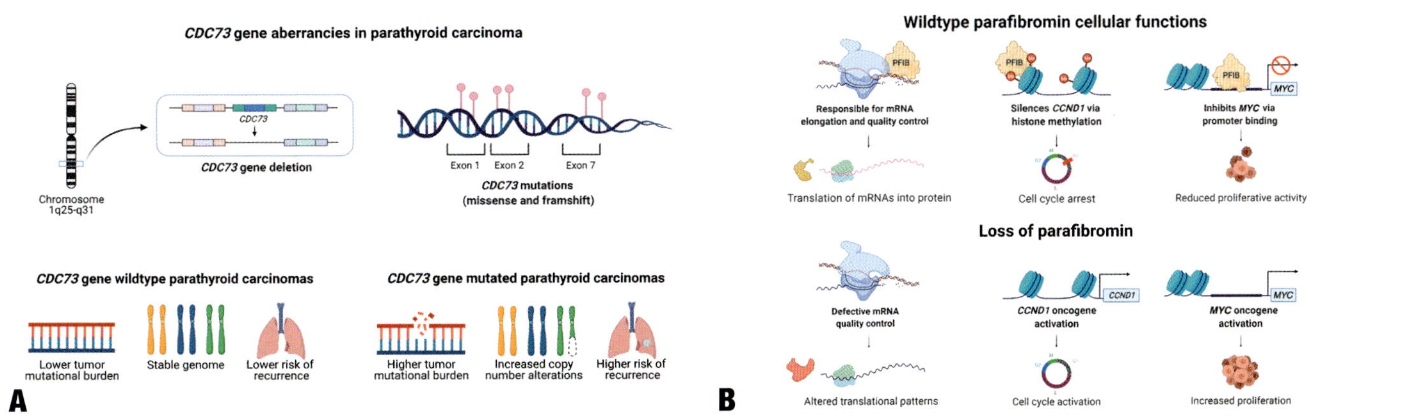

Fig. 4.18 Parathyroid carcinoma. **A** Schematic overview of *CDC73* gene aberrancies and associated genomic hallmarks in parathyroid carcinoma. Positioned at chromosome 1q25-q31, the *CDC73* gene locus recurrently exhibits loss of heterozygosity in parathyroid carcinoma, in addition to gene mutations occurring most frequently in exons 1, 2, and 7. At the pangenomic level, *CDC73*-mutated parathyroid carcinomas display a higher mutation burden, more copy-number alterations, and poorer patient outcomes than *CDC73*-wildtype cases. **B** Parafibromin (PFIB) exhibits numerous tumour-suppressor functions in the cell. As a member of the RNA polymerase II–associated factor (PAF) complex, parafibromin is required for mRNA elongation and quality control processes, and it also controls the expression of the proto-oncogenes *CCND1* (encoding cyclin D1) and *MYC* via epigenetic mechanisms. Upon loss of parafibromin, these processes are dysregulated, which in turn has been associated with cell-cycle activation and increased proliferative ability.

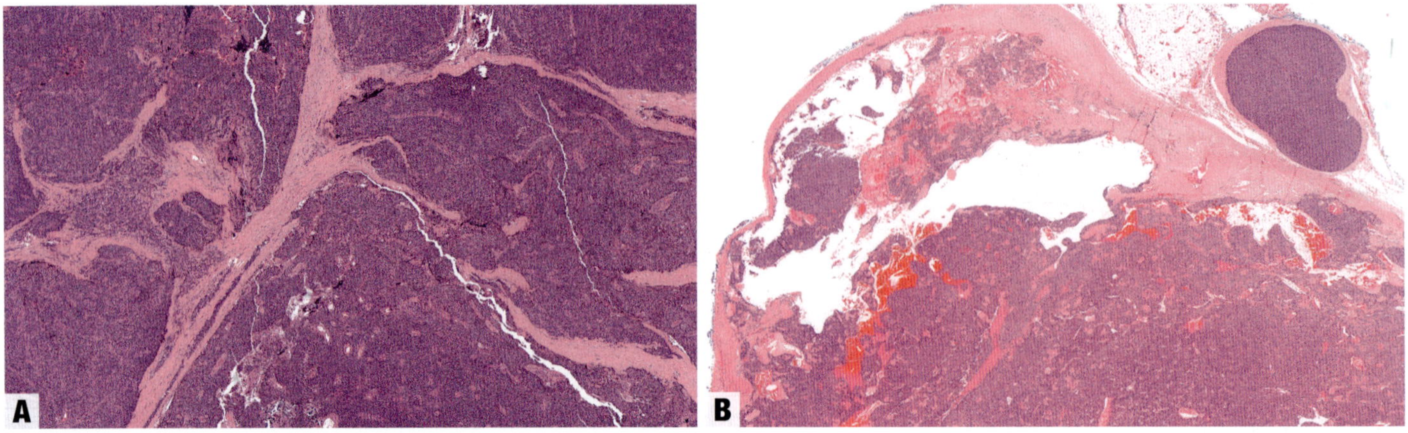

Fig. 4.19 Parathyroid carcinoma. **A** Fibrous bands in parathyroid carcinoma. However, this finding alone does not warrant the diagnosis of malignancy. **B** Local gross nodular invasion into the adjacent soft tissue. The tumour also showed angioinvasion (not shown here).

Macroscopic appearance

The gross examination findings vary considerably among tumours. Smaller tumours may be indistinguishable from parathyroid adenomas. However, most parathyroid carcinomas are large, poorly circumscribed masses and are variably encapsulated, weighing 1.5 g to > 50 g {440}. The mean tumour size range is 30–49 mm {1275,3863,65}, but smaller tumours (e.g. 11 mm) have been reported {4144}. Tumours may be grossly adherent to the thyroid gland and/or adjacent structures. The cut section of the tumours is often firm and tan to pink, with a lobular appearance attributable to band-forming fibrosis {3985, 1172,1168}.

Histopathology

The histopathological diagnosis of a parathyroid carcinoma is restricted to parathyroid tumours that show at least one of the following findings: (1) angioinvasion (vascular invasion), (2) lymphatic invasion, (3) perineural invasion, (4) local malignant invasion into the adjacent structures/organs, or (5) regional or distant metastasis. The submission of a complete parathyroidectomy specimen is required in the diagnostic workup of a parathyroid neoplasm. Evaluation of multiple levels and the use of ancillary tools can assist the diagnostic assessment.

Like in other endocrine neoplasms, angioinvasion is typically assessed at the tumour periphery or the tumour capsule, but not within the tumour substance. The demonstration of angioinvasion is a highly reliable criterion of malignancy {4388,1275, 4028,1276,1172,4144} and has prognostic significance {4388, 1275,4028,3863,65}. Angioinvasion often involves small veins and is characterized by tumour cells invading through a vessel wall and/or intravascular tumour cells admixed with thrombus/fibrin {1276,1275,1172}. When the latter is subtle, the fibrin–platelet complex can be highlighted using CD61 or Martius Scarlet Blue histochemistry. Vascular endothelium can be highlighted using ERG, CD34, and CD31. Lymphatic invasion can be highlighted using D2-40. Perineural invasion is often a microscopic finding, but gross invasion into large nerve bundles (e.g. recurrent laryngeal nerve invasion) can also occur and can be noted in intraoperative findings.

Most parathyroid carcinomas lack a true fibrous capsule. The tumours are variably cellular and are often subdivided by broad bands of fibrous connective tissue extending from the peritumoural pseudocapsule. Fibrous bands are present in most parathyroid carcinomas {3985,1172,96}; however, their presence alone is not diagnostic of malignancy {461,118,1172, 2285,1899}. In addition, focal extension into a fibrotic band or cellular nests in a connective tissue component overlying the external border of the lesion does not qualify for malignancy. The latter becomes critical in parathyroidectomy specimens that were subjected to previous manipulations (e.g. FNAB, PTH washout, ethanol injection) or in parathyroids from patients with longstanding secondary/tertiary hyperparathyroidism {843,118, 3289,1172,2285,65,1899}. The upper parathyroid glands in particular may be embedded in the pseudocapsule or parenchyma of the thyroid gland, and this should not be mistaken for true invasive growth {2439,96,65}.

Cytological atypia can be variable in parathyroid carcinomas. Some tumours may show marked pleomorphism with coarse chromatin and prominent macronucleoli, but others that are enriched in chief cells with micronucleoli and no marked atypia are indistinguishable from their benign counterparts with the exception of their invasive growth. *CDC73*-mutated parathyroid carcinomas commonly have eosinophilic cytoplasm with perinuclear clearing {1580}. Other morphological correlates of *CDC73*-mutant parathyroid neoplasms include larger tumours with encapsulation, diffuse sheet-like growth, nuclear enlargement, arborizing vasculature, and microcystic change {1580}, as well as high proliferative rates {2151}.

In the parathyroid, an increased mitotic count is defined as > 5 mitoses/10 mm² {461}. Increased mitotic count can occur in secondary/tertiary hyperparathyroidism–related multiglandular parathyroid disease and in parathyroid adenomas with degenerative changes {3985,4196,1172}. However, the identification of even a single atypical mitotic figure and/or coagulative tumour necrosis should alert the pathologist to the possibility of parathyroid carcinoma. A triad of coagulative necrosis in association with increased mitotic activity (> 5 mitoses/10 mm²) and prominent macronucleoli is worrisome for malignancy {461}. It is desirable to assess such tumours using ancillary biomarkers and to evaluate multiple levels to help identify invasive growth.

Like for other neuroendocrine neoplasms (NENs), assessment of the proliferative activity of all parathyroid carcinomas by recording a formal Ki-67 proliferation index and mitotic count using standardized approaches is now recommended {4886}.

Immunohistochemistry

Unlike parathyroid adenomas, carcinomas are associated with immunohistochemical loss of expression of parafibromin, APC, E-cadherin, p27, BCL2, MDM2, and 5-hydroxymethylcytosine; positivity for PGP9.5, galectin-3, and TERT; p53 overexpression; and an increased Ki-67 labelling index (often > 5%) {1268,4289, 396,1578,1960,3364,2150,1275,1276,4567,1172,1953,311,1271, 2151,65}. Among these, loss of nuclear parafibromin expression has been regarded as a reliable biomarker of malignancy in the appropriate morphological setting {1578,2153,1276,2196, 2151,4144,2143}. Loss of parafibromin expression, termed parafibromin deficiency, can be seen in any tumour, benign or malignant, in the setting of germline *CDC73* mutation (HPT-JT) {1580}. However, it has been proposed that a lower threshold for invasive growth may be appropriate in parafibromin-deficient parathyroid tumours {1580}. Nucleolar loss of parafibromin has also been reported in some parathyroid carcinomas {2146, 1918,2151}, and the significance of this finding requires further somatic/germline *CDC73* mutation analysis in individual cases. A panel approach and diagnostic nomograms combining multiple biomarkers (e.g. parafibromin, PGP9.5, Ki-67, and galectin-3) have also been suggested to be helpful {4289,396,1960, 4567,1953,1271,4144,1003}.

Differential diagnosis

The main differential diagnoses of parathyroid carcinoma include parathyroid adenoma with postbiopsy reactive changes {118,3289,2285,1899}, secondary/tertiary parathyroid hyperplasia with increased proliferative activity and fibrosis (discussed in *Parathyroid hyperplasia*, p. 204), atypical parathyroid tumour (see *Atypical parathyroid tumour*, p. 215), and parathyromatosis {1363,4027}.

Parathyromatosis represents foci of parathyroid tissue that often grow around the site of a former surgery or biopsy due to an inadvertent implantation of lesional parathyroid tissue, and can also be related to the persistence of developmental remnants {1417,1387,4027,1899}. The locally infiltrative growth of parathyromatosis may make it indistinguishable from parathyroid carcinoma; however, biomarker studies, markedly elevated serum calcium and PTH levels, a palpable neck mass, and (more importantly) the presence of vascular or perineural invasion can help distinguish parathyroid carcinoma {1363,1172, 4027}.

Atypical parathyroid tumours that show coagulative tumour necrosis, atypical mitotic figures, or loss of parafibromin may represent parathyroid carcinomas that are not captured using the conventional strict criteria. Therefore, it may be helpful to perform parafibromin immunohistochemistry in atypical parathyroid tumours, because parafibromin-deficient atypical parathyroid tumours have an increased risk of recurrence or metachronous disease in other glands and would warrant long-term follow-up {1580}.

Some parathyroid carcinomas display follicular growth with variable luminal proteinaceous material that can simulate a

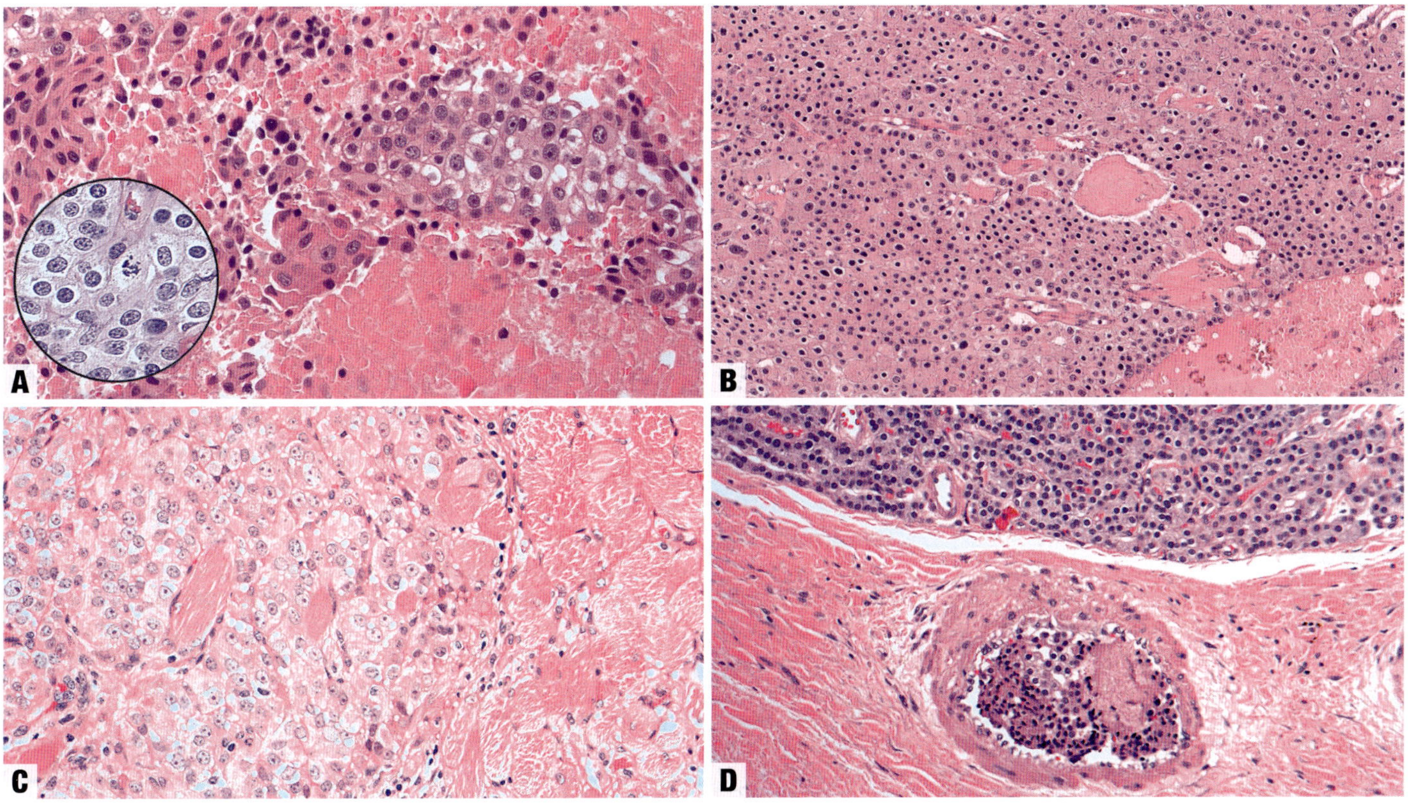

Fig. 4.20 Parathyroid carcinoma. **A** The triad of high-risk histopathological features comprises foci of coagulative tumour necrosis in association with prominent macronucleoli and increased mitotic activity (> 5 mitoses/10 mm^2). **Inset:** High magnification showing mitosis. **B** Cytomorphological features of a parafibromin-immunodeficient tumour. The tumour is enriched in oncocytic cells with perinuclear clearing. This morphology is not specific to parathyroid carcinoma; the identification of invasive growth is required to render the morphological diagnosis of parathyroid carcinoma. **C** Locally invasive tumour with strap muscle invasion. **D** A focus of angioinvasion characterized by intravascular tumour cells admixed with fibrin/thrombus. Vascular invasion (angioinvasion) is typically assessed at the tumour periphery or at the tumour capsule, but not within the tumour substance.

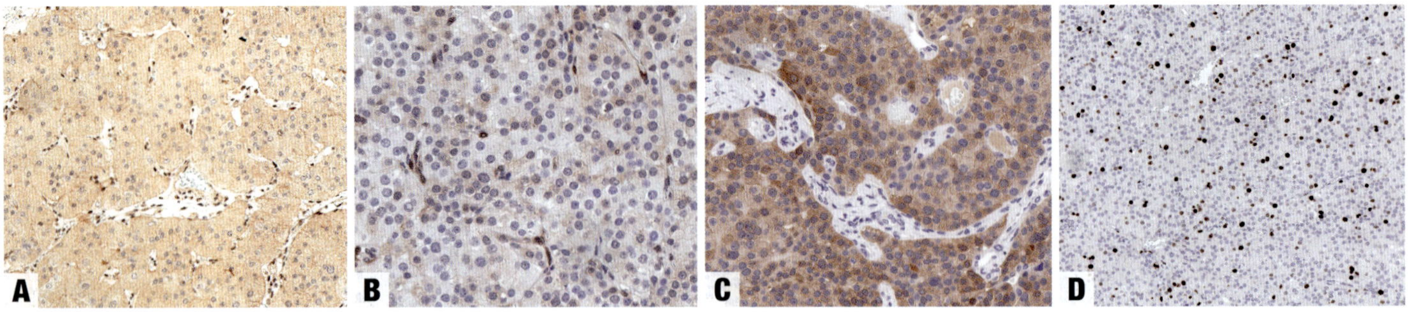

Fig. 4.21 Parathyroid carcinoma. **A** Parafibromin immunohistochemistry. Loss of nuclear parafibromin expression has been regarded as a reliable biomarker of malignancy in the appropriate morphological setting. This photomicrograph shows loss of nuclear parafibromin expression in a morphologically diagnosed parathyroid carcinoma. Note that the intratumoural endothelial cells, which serve as an internal control, show retained nuclear parafibromin reactivity. **B** P27 immunohistochemistry. Parathyroid carcinoma with loss of nuclear expression of p27. Note that the endothelial cells retain nuclear p27 expression. **C** Galectin-3 immunohistochemistry. Unlike adenomas, parathyroid carcinomas can feature galectin-3 expression. **D** Ki-67 immunohistochemistry. Most parathyroid carcinomas show a Ki-67 labelling index > 5%. This photomicrograph illustrates an increased Ki-67 proliferation index from a parathyroid carcinoma.

follicular thyroid neoplasm. Rarely, the tumours can demonstrate a carcinosarcomatous growth {4370} that can mimic various other neoplasms. Most parathyroid carcinomas show diffuse sheet-like or trabecular (rather than acinar) growth. The trabecular pattern may be mistaken for a poorly differentiated thyroid carcinoma or medullary thyroid carcinoma, especially when parathyroid carcinomas involve the thyroid gland {96,65,5012}. In addition, parathyroid carcinomas composed exclusively of oncocytic cells can mimic an oncocytic thyroid carcinoma. In difficult cases, immunohistochemical markers to confirm parathyroid origin are usually definitive {1271}.

With the exception of non-functioning disease, PTH is often expressed in parathyroid carcinomas. However, PTH expression alone is not specific for parathyroid neoplasms, because other NENs can (rarely) show aberrant PTH expression {1271}. The latter may be of significance when assessing biopsy specimens from metastatic tumours {1170}. Parathyroid carcinomas are positive for the transcription factors GCM2 {3283} and GATA3 {3357}. As GCM2 immunohistochemistry is not widely used in most laboratories, positivity for PTH and GATA3 can be used to confirm parathyroid origin {1271}.

Rare paragangliomas {2619} and metastases (especially of breast origin) {348} have been identified in parathyroids and can be mistaken for parathyroid neoplasms. GATA3 alone is also not specific to parathyroid, because NENs (including paragangliomas and pituitary neuroendocrine tumours [PitNETs] and other carcinomas (notably from the breast) can be positive for GATA3 {3358,2971,4592,2305}.

Calcitonin and CGRP reactivity should not be relied upon completely to distinguish medullary thyroid carcinoma from parathyroid, because these proteins can also be expressed in parathyroid proliferations, including parathyroid carcinomas {1918}. Thyroid transcription factor 1 (TTF1) reactivity and diffuse monoclonal CEA expression can help identify medullary thyroid carcinoma {284}. It is important to recognize that C-terminus–specific PAX8 antibodies are negative in NENs; however, polyclonal PAX8 can show variable staining in parathyroid tumours {1271}.

Parathyroid carcinomas are typically positive for cytokeratins and chromogranins, like other epithelial NENs {1271}, but often lack INSM1 {2154}.

Cytology

Smears show the same features as those of parathyroid adenoma, although it has been suggested that more prominent nucleoli, mitoses, and (possibly) a papillary-solid pattern may suggest a carcinoma, whereas nuclear atypia is seen in both lesions {596}.

Diagnostic molecular pathology

Molecular profiling of a parathyroid neoplasm may be used to assist the diagnosis of malignancy {4269,1402,4330,2143}. Screening for germline *CDC73* variants should be considered for all parathyroid carcinomas, particularly parafibromin-deficient tumours {4093}. Patients with advanced disease may benefit from somatic mutation analyses to search for personalized actionable targets {2465}.

Essential and desirable diagnostic criteria

Essential: a parathyroid neoplasm with one of the following features: (1) angioinvasion (vascular invasion), (2) lymphatic invasion, (3) perineural invasion, (4) local invasion into adjacent structures/organs, (5) histologically confirmed metastasis.

Desirable: ancillary biomarkers including but not limited to Ki-67 (MIB1), parafibromin, and galectin-3 immunohistochemistry; germline and somatic genotyping.

Staging

Staging of parathyroid carcinoma is based on the eighth edition of the Union for International Cancer Control (UICC) / American Joint Committee on Cancer (AJCC) system.

Prognosis and prediction

Older age, tumour size > 32 mm, completeness of tumour excision, high-risk clinicopathological findings (angioinvasion, local gross invasion into neck organs, nodal and distant metastases), loss of parafibromin expression, and galectin-3 positivity have been considered risk factors in parathyroid carcinomas {4082, 2171,4388,1785,4028,221,65,4144,5180}.

Locoregional recurrence and/or distant metastasis (e.g. to lung, liver, bone) occurs in 25–60% of parathyroid carcinomas {4388,4709,1275,221,65,4144}. Late distant metastasis (after 10 years) has been reported {221}. The 20-year cumulative incidence of distant metastasis is reported to be about 40% in a large series from MD Anderson Cancer Center {221}.

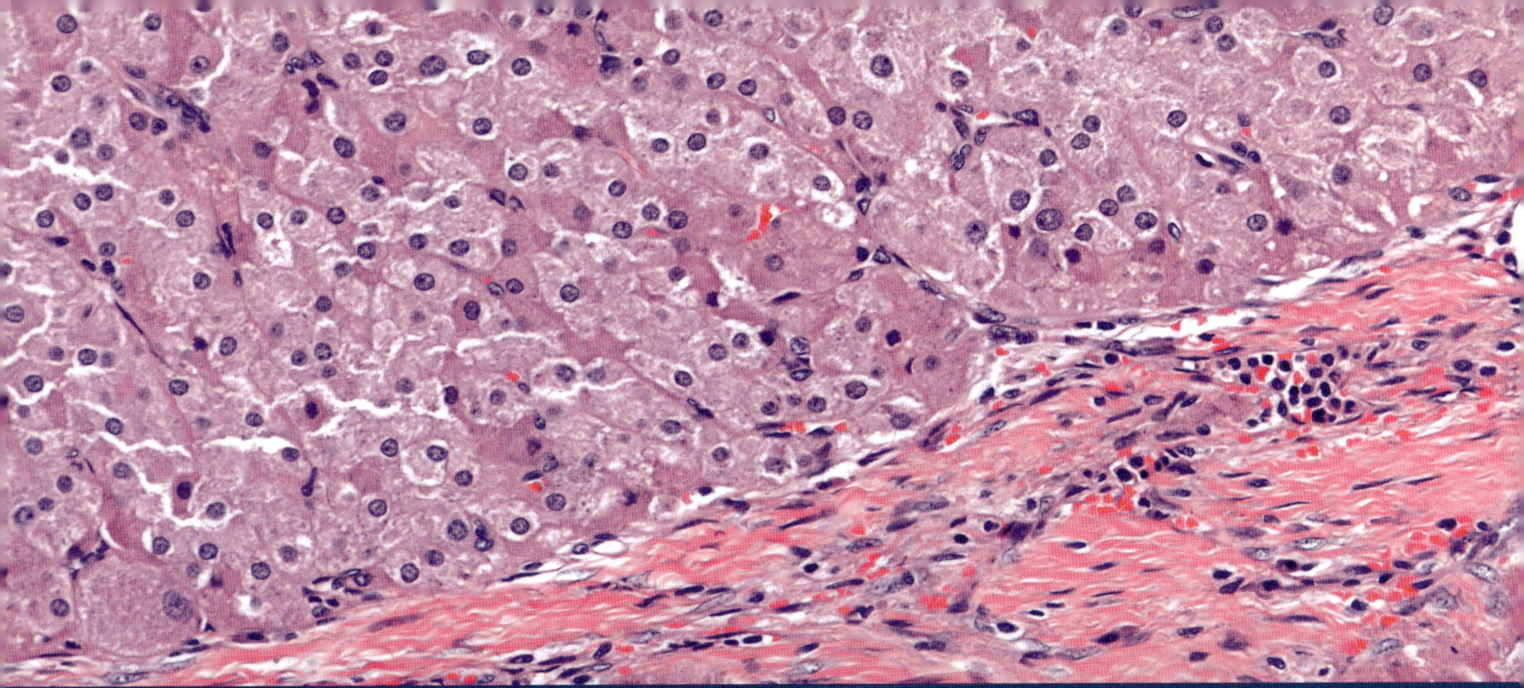

5

Adrenal gland tumours

Edited by: de Krijger RR, Erickson LA, Mete O, Papotti M

Adrenal gland tumours: Introduction

Erickson LA
de Krijger RR
Gill AJ
Papotti M

Although some entities in the classification of adrenal cortical diseases are quite classic, the classification of some others has changed greatly in recent years. The importance of a classic entity, such as adrenal rests, centres on the adrenal cortical tumours that can arise in them as well as the hyperplasia that can occur, such as in Nelson syndrome. Adrenal rests may also stimulate other steroid cell, Leydig cell, and renal cell tumours. Adrenal pseudocysts are encountered by most pathologists, whereas true adrenal cysts (endothelial or epithelial) are rare {1270}. Endothelialization of pseudocysts can be mistaken for an endothelial cyst or a vascular neoplasm. Most grossly cystic adrenal glands are adrenal cortical neoplasms, usually adenomas (rarely carcinomas) or phaeochromocytomas with prominent cystic degeneration or pseudocysts {1270}. Pseudocysts can be mistaken for necrosis, which would be an ominous finding for an adrenal cortical neoplasm.

Adrenal myelolipomas are non-functioning, usually asymptomatic, incidental findings; they are usually unilateral, although they are more frequently bilateral in congenital adrenal hyperplasia (CAH), where they occur more often than in the general population {3210}. CAH, an autosomal recessive disorder caused by mutations in genes involved in the adrenal cortical enzymatic steps of steroid production resulting in the proliferation of adrenal cortical cells, remains a significant issue clinically, with the classic type being most severe and usually identified by neonatal screening. Non-classic CAH is more common and milder than classic salt-wasting or classic simple virilizing CAH. If untreated, the adrenal glands show marked bilateral cortical hyperplasia, with lipid depletion imparting a dark colour to the adrenal glands. Testicular adrenal rest tumours occur in 14–86% of patients with CAH and can be mistaken for Leydig cell tumours if the clinical situation is not known {1252}.

Sporadic subcentimetre adrenal cortical nodules may be clonal {4663,2141}, and so the term "sporadic nodular adrenal cortical disease" has replaced "cortical nodular hyperplasia" for incidental non-functioning cortical nodules {3390,2141}. Primary bilateral nodular adrenal cortical disease consists of multiple independent clonal proliferations, and therefore older terms such as "primary bilateral micronodular" or "macronodular adrenal cortical 'hyperplasia'" are no longer appropriate {2141}. However, the term "diffuse hyperplasia" is appropriate for adrenal glands affected by excess pituitary ACTH production. Virtually all cases of bilateral micronodular adrenal cortical disease and a significant fraction of cases of bilateral macronodular adrenal cortical disease are caused by genetic susceptibility {2141,2963,2175}. In bilateral nodular adrenocortical disease, germline susceptibility is followed by a somatic second hit involving the other allele. Bilateral micronodular adrenocortical disease is linked to pathogenic germline variants leading to the activation of the PKA pathway, including *PRKAR1A*, *PRKACA*, *PDE11A*, *PDE8B*, and 2p16 *CNC2* locus alterations {2141,2175,2963}. Bilateral macronodular adrenal cortical disease has been linked to several germline alterations, including *ARMC5*, *MEN1*, *FH*, and *APC* alterations; somatic *GNAS* mosaicism; and rare *PDE11A*, *PDE8B*, and *EDNRA* variants {238,1283,4683,1969,1518,4633,2963,5178}.

The understanding and classification of primary aldosteronism has advanced greatly in recent years. Bilateral adrenal gland involvement occurs in 60–70% of cases of primary aldosteronism with bilateral diffuse zona glomerulosa hyperplasia and bilateral aldosterone-producing microadenomas (< 10 mm) {1171,1916,2141,5125}. The distinction of bilateral aldosterone excess from unilateral disease (often due to adenoma or microadenoma) is important in deciding surgical intervention {557,1916}. Aldosterone-producing cortical lesions can be unifocal or multifocal and unilateral or bilateral, and they may include microscopic clonal nodular proliferations. Aldosterone-producing microtumours can be difficult to identify. Therefore, CYP11B2 immunohistochemistry is helpful in the evaluation of adrenal gland(s) in individuals with primary aldosteronism, to identify functional sites of aldosterone {2959,4887,2141}. The recent histopathology of primary aldosteronism (HISTALDO) consensus classification combines the histological evaluation of an adrenal gland with the CYP11B2 staining pattern to identify adrenal nodules and standardize nomenclature to provide a clinically relevant diagnostic approach to reporting unilateral primary aldosteronism specimens {4887}.

The confirmation of the adrenal cortical origin of any non-functioning adrenal neoplasm should be considered routinely. SF1 is the most specific biomarker for confirming adrenal cortical origin {2959}.

The distinction of adrenal cortical carcinoma from adenoma in organ-confined tumours may be difficult and a number of different approaches are used, with some being more appropriate in specific settings {1591}. The classic pathological criteria proposed for adrenal cortical carcinoma described by Dr Weiss in 1984 and 1989 continue to be widely used. Because the Weiss system may lead to the overdiagnosis of some oncocytic adrenal tumours as malignant, the Lin–Weiss–Bisceglia system is used for pure (> 90%) oncocytic adrenal cortical tumours. In myxoid carcinomas, some Weiss parameters may be absent or difficult to assess, thus increasing the risk of an underdiagnosis of malignancy. More recent classification systems, including the reticulin algorithm and the Helsinki score, have been helpful in conventional adrenal cortical neoplasms as well as in myxoid and oncocytic cortical neoplasms {3510,1183,1184,1591}. Paediatric adrenal cortical tumours continue to be primarily classified with the system described by Dr Wieneke in 2003 {4876}.

Adrenal cortical carcinomas with invasive growth or high-grade features do not usually pose a challenge for diagnosticians; however, biomarkers may help in the distinction of low-grade adrenal cortical carcinomas confined to the adrenal gland and carcinomas with adenoma-like regions {2967,2959, 2141,1591}. Rare cases with equivocal features may sometimes be diagnosed as adrenal cortical neoplasm of uncertain malignant potential. Although an increased Ki-67 proliferation index (often > 5%, and > 15% usually malignant) and p53 overexpression can be helpful in some cases {2959,2967}, IGF2 paranuclear immunoreactivity has been shown to be the most reliable translational biomarker in the distinction of adrenal cortical carcinoma from adenoma {2967,4006,4230}. Molecular studies can also help in the distinction of carcinoma {1592,1594,1035, 5160,236}. There is now clear evidence for grading adrenal cortical carcinoma on the basis of the mitotic count and Ki-67 proliferation index, and although precise cut-off points are still debated, the provision of a formal mitotic count and Ki-67 proliferation index in all cases is now recommended {413,1185,3092, 3727,1591}.

Adrenal rests

Papotti M
Falhammar H
Sasano H

Definition

Adrenal rests represent isolated benign adrenocortical tissue outside orthotopic adrenal glands and may be associated with adrenomedullary (chromaffin) cells.

ICD-O coding

None

ICD-11 coding

LC8Y & XH9RV1 Other specified structural developmental anomalies of the adrenal glands & Adrenal rest tumour

Related terminology

Acceptable: adrenal ectopia; adrenal heterotopia; adrenal choristoma; adrenal remnants.
Not recommended: adrenal rest tumour.

Subtype(s)

None

Localization

Adrenal rests occur in anatomical locations that are aligned with their embryogenesis, and in unusual locations (choristomas) that cannot be explained by embryogenesis (see Box 5.01).

Box 5.01 Reported locations of adrenal rests

- Spermatic cord {1319}
- Rete testis {2771,1252,2723}
- Epididymis {914}
- Ovary and paraovarian locations {572,4631,495,4173,811,776,1319,4504}
- Streak gonads {1653}
- Fallopian tube and parasalpinx {2271,4503,1319}
- Liver {1253,4323,252,169,253}
- Kidney {597,2570,5092}
- Broad ligament {3960,2216,1319}
- Retroperitoneum {67,5075}
- Pelvic (between urinary bladder and prostate) {916}
- Groin {4064,2265}
- Pituitary {4586,2974}
- Choroid plexus {1158}
- Spine and spinal nerves {2807,1587,3036}
- Placenta {3988}
- Lung {177,2841}

Clinical features

Adrenal rests are generally incidental findings in organs resected for other diseases {1319}. In the testis, they can be identified within specific screening for congenital adrenal hyperplasia {1252,2723}, other endocrinological disorders {3624}, or subfertility due to impaired rete testis blood flow and seminiferous tubule function {2105,870}.

Rests can become hyperplastic in the presence of Nelson syndrome {4894,4685,2128}.

Tumours arising in adrenal rests may be endocrinologically functional {252}. Rarely, a mass as seen in adrenocortical rest tumours may be the presenting symptom. Imaging characteristics are dependent on adrenal rest location and size. Adrenal choristomas in the pituitary are seen in association with corticotroph pituitary neuroendocrine tumours (PitNETs) {4586, 2974}. In the testis, key ultrasonographic features include bilateral lesions, well-circumscribed nodules, and a homogeneous hypoechoic texture {2771,4815}. Precise radiological criteria for ovarian and other organ adrenal rests have not been developed {495}. Functional imaging studies (11C-metomidate PET-CT) may help localize adrenal rest tumours {572}.

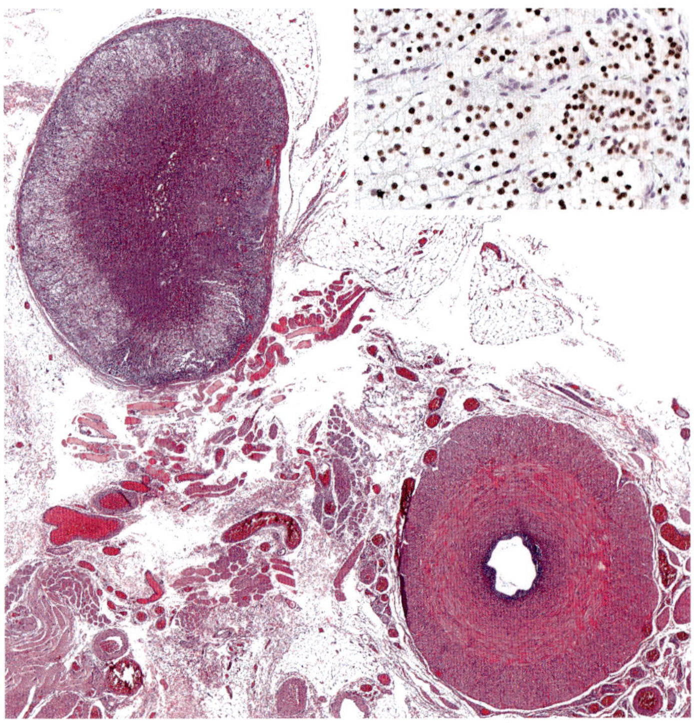

Fig. 5.01 Adrenal rests. A nodule of adrenocortical cells is embedded in the fibrofatty tissue of the spermatic cord. **Inset:** Ectopic adrenocortical cells in the fibrofatty tissue of the spermatic cord show SF1 immunoreactivity.

Epidemiology

The exact prevalence of adrenal rests is not known, being reported in as many as 20% of autopsies {5092,597}. In congenital adrenal hyperplasia, testicular adrenal rests occur in 14–86% of cases depending on patient age, disease severity, and detection modalities {1252,1322}.

Etiology

Most adrenal rests are explained with misplaced developmental tissues; however, the etiology is unknown in unusual locations.

Pathogenesis

Developmental defects {2257,4966} in the delamination of the adrenogonadal primordia or failure in the encapsulation of SF1-expressing precursor cells of the fetal adrenal zone may be the source of embryogenesis-related adrenal rests. Differentiation of uncommitted mesenchymal stem cells in usual anatomical locations has also been suggested {2974,3334}. A prolonged ACTH stimulation of pluripotent cells has also been suggested in testes {1252,4185}. An association of adrenal rests with Beckwith–Wiedemann syndrome remains to be clarified {1158,652, 1757}.

Macroscopic appearance

Most adrenal rests are not grossly evident, measuring only a few millimetres {3615,811,2271}. Adrenocortical tumours can arise in adrenal rests {2570,916,3029,169,253,3960,5075,252, 67,2216}.

Histopathology

Adrenal rests appear as aggregates of large polygonal cells with eosinophilic or clear cytoplasm, a uniform round nucleus, and finely dispersed chromatin, resembling orthotopic adrenocortical cells {1252,5092,2723,1319}. Adrenomedullary cells are rarely present. Cortical cells may be intermingled with other parenchymal cells or located in the fibroadipose tissue surrounding the organ. Like orthotopic cortical cells, SF1 and melan-A are positive in adrenal rests {253,169,1319,2974}. Adrenal rest tumours may simulate steroid cell tumours, Leydig cell tumours, or renal cell carcinoma in some anatomical locations {1252,597,5092,2723,2740}. Adrenocortical-specific steroidogenic enzymes (CYP11B1, CYP11B2) may be helpful in the distinction of adrenal rest–related tumours {5075,2740}.

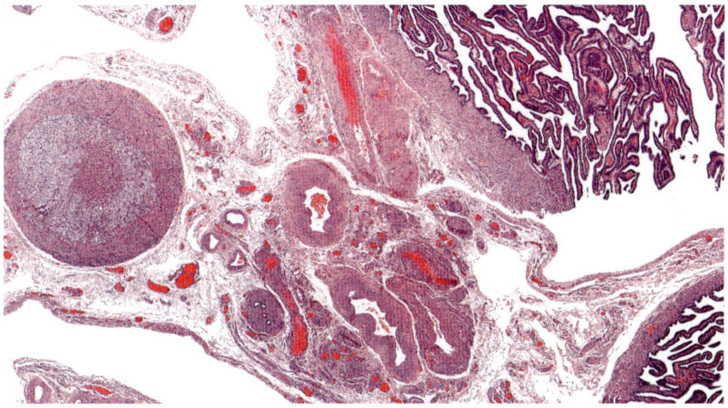

Fig. 5.02 Adrenal rests. A nodule of adrenocortical cells is embedded in the fibrofatty parasalpingeal tissue.

Cytology

Not applicable

Diagnostic molecular pathology

None

Essential and desirable diagnostic criteria

Essential: clusters or nodules composed of large polygonal adrenal cortical cells with no sign of malignancy; may have associated adrenomedullary (chromaffin) cells; immunohistochemical confirmation of adrenocortical cell differentiation.

Desirable: SF1 positivity; adrenocortical steroidogenic enzyme positivity in the distinction of selected adrenal rest–related tumours.

Staging

Not applicable

Prognosis and prediction

Most adrenal rests have no clinical significance; however, patients with congenital adrenal hyperplasia with poor hormonal control may present with large testicular adrenal rest–related tumours that can cause infertility {3787}.

Adrenal cysts

Papotti M
Falhammar H

Definition
Adrenal cysts are benign, circumscribed, fluid-containing, tumour-like lesions.

ICD-O coding
None

ICD-11 coding
LC8Y Other specified structural developmental anomalies of the adrenal glands

Related terminology
Not recommended: cystic adrenal tumour.

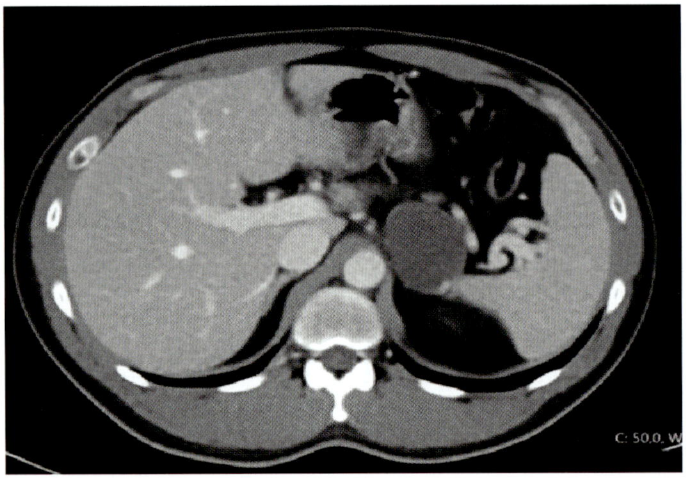

Fig. 5.03 Adrenal cyst. A 50 mm cyst in the left adrenal is visualized on CT.

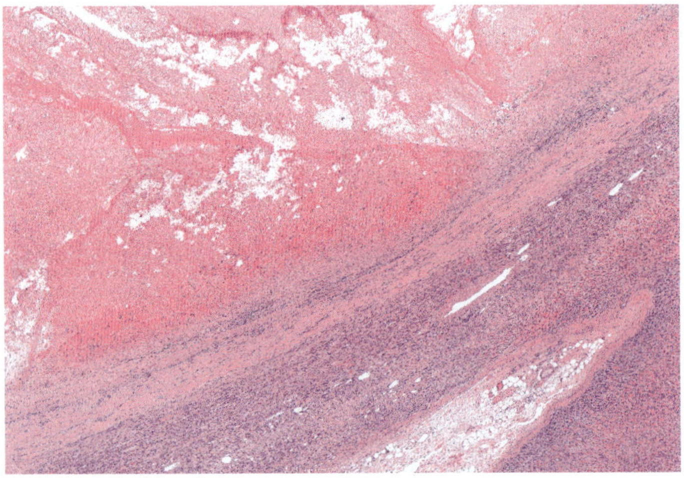

Fig. 5.04 Adrenal pseudocyst. These are often demarcated by dense fibrous tissue, lack a cellular lining, and contain fibrinous/haemorrhagic material.

Subtype(s)
Endothelial (vascular) cyst; epithelial (mesothelial) cyst; parasitic cyst; pseudocyst

Localization
They occur in adrenal glands and may show retroperitoneal extension.

Clinical features
Adrenal cysts occur mainly in the third to sixth decade of life {1270,711}. They are often detected as incidentalomas but may also present with mass-related nonspecific symptoms (e.g. abdominal pain, vena cava compression). Ultrasonography, CT, and MRI are useful in recognizing cystic lesions but are often inadequate for their subtyping {1270,1475,1629}. Large cysts and pseudocysts may simulate malignancy {1614,5161, 1166}.

Epidemiology
Adrenal cysts represent approximately 4% of adrenal masses {5161}, with a prevalence rate of 0.06–0.18% in autopsy series {1270,173,711}. Pseudocysts (39–78%) are the most common primary adrenal cysts followed by endothelial, epithelial, and parasitic cysts {1258,1410,1614,374,818,1270}.

Etiology
Depending on the subtype, cysts can be developmental, infectious, post-haemorrhagic, or traumatic.

Pathogenesis
Endothelial cysts are postulated to result from dilated and thrombosed vessels, whereas pseudocysts are thought to be post-haemorrhagic or traumatic {1166} or may be related to vascular cysts with repeated haemorrhage. Epithelial cysts are related to mesothelial rests. *Echinococcus* infestations cause parasitic cysts {1258,488,5196}.

Macroscopic appearance
Cysts are often unilocular, and they have a thin fibrous wall with clear or haemorrhagic/fibrinous content {1270,818}.

Histopathology
Cysts have a thin wall. Endothelial cysts more commonly arise from the lymphatic endothelium and may show papillary protrusions into the lumen. Epithelial cysts are lined by mesothelial cells {5161}. Immunohistochemistry for epithelial and endothelial markers helps in the distinction between endothelial and epithelial cysts {4325}. Parasitic (hydatid) cysts are uniloculated or multiloculated, with a fibrous wall, calcifications, and clear fluid content {57,5196,488}. Pseudocysts are often demarcated by dense fibrous tissue, lack a

cellular lining, and contain fibrinous/haemorrhagic material with cholesterol clefts and haemosiderin-laden macrophages {5161}. The differential diagnosis includes cystic degeneration in adrenocortical neoplasms, cystic phaeochromocytoma, vascular tumours or malformations, cystic renal cell carcinoma, and ectopic thyroid {4048,818,1614,1270,3799, 5161}.

Cytology

Pseudocysts on FNAB can yield nonspecific proteinaceous material, whereas vascular tumours generally yield blood and are usually sampled in the workup of adrenal masses {2229, 2106}.

Diagnostic molecular pathology

Not clinically relevant

Essential and desirable diagnostic criteria

Pseudocyst

Essential: no cyst lining or parasitic infestation; haemorrhagic/ fibrinous cyst content.

Epithelial (mesothelial) cyst

Essential: a cyst lined by epithelial cells; often positive for mesothelial markers.

Endothelial (vascular) cyst

Essential: a cyst lined by endothelium; positive for at least one endothelial marker (D2-40, ERG, CD34, CD31).

Parasitic cyst

Essential: a cyst related to a parasitic (*Echinococcus*) infestation.

Staging

Not applicable

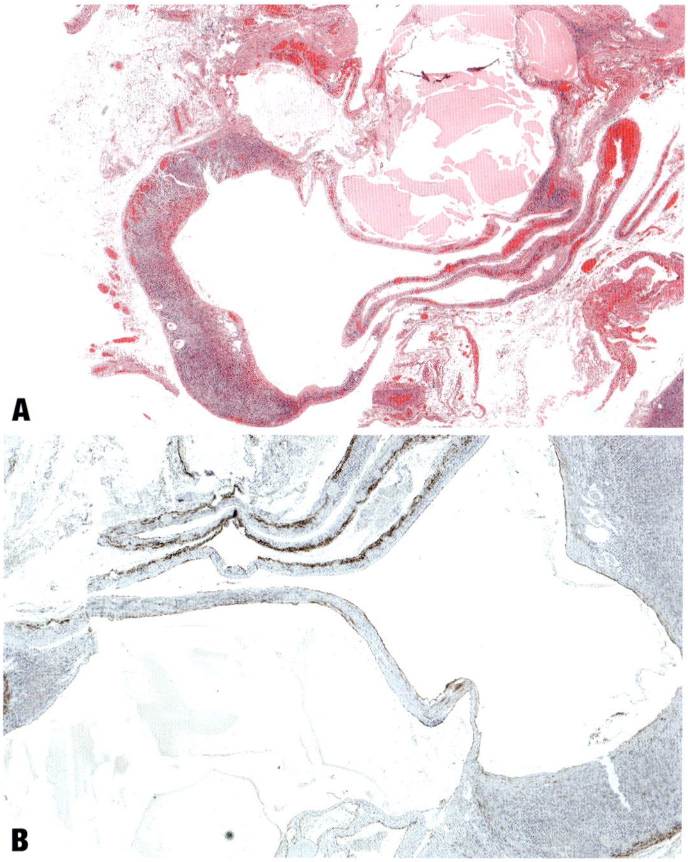

Fig. 5.05 Vascular adrenal cyst. **A** These cysts are lined by endothelial cells. **B** Vascular cysts are more commonly of lymphatic endothelium. This photomicrograph illustrates D2-40 immunoreactivity in the cyst lining of a vascular adrenal cyst.

Prognosis and prediction

Compression of surrounding organs, rupture, and haemorrhage are potential complications.

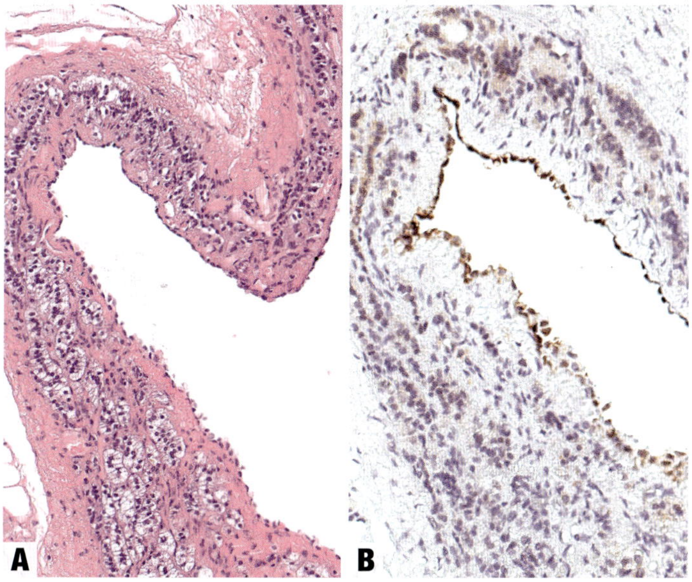

Fig. 5.06 Epithelial (mesothelial) adrenal cyst. **A** A cyst with a fibrous wall and mesothelial lining is shown here. **B** This cyst is lined by calretinin-positive mesothelial cells.

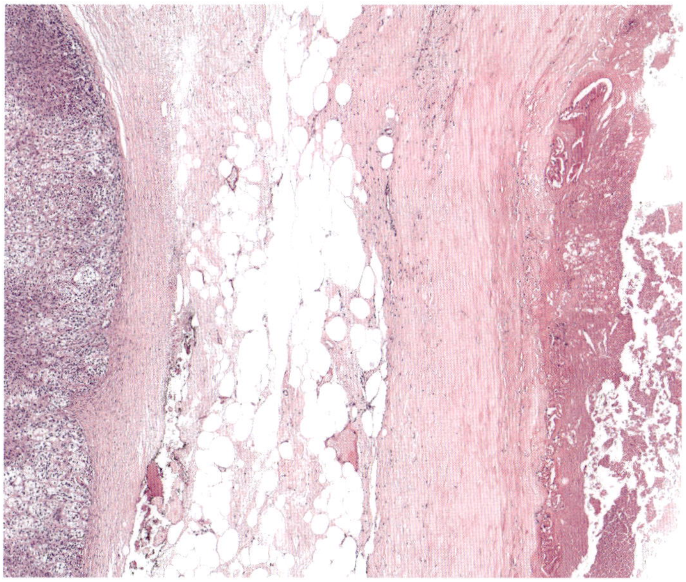

Fig. 5.07 Parasitic adrenal cyst. A cyst in the periadrenal fat with PAS-positive laminar membranes in the wall.

Adrenal myelolipoma

Papotti M
Falhammar H

Definition

Adrenal myelolipoma is a benign tumour made of mature adipose tissue and haematopoietic cells.

ICD-O coding

8870/0 Adrenal myelolipoma

ICD-11 coding

2F37.Y & XH17C5 Other specified benign neoplasm of endocrine glands & Myelolipoma

Related terminology

None

Subtype(s)

None

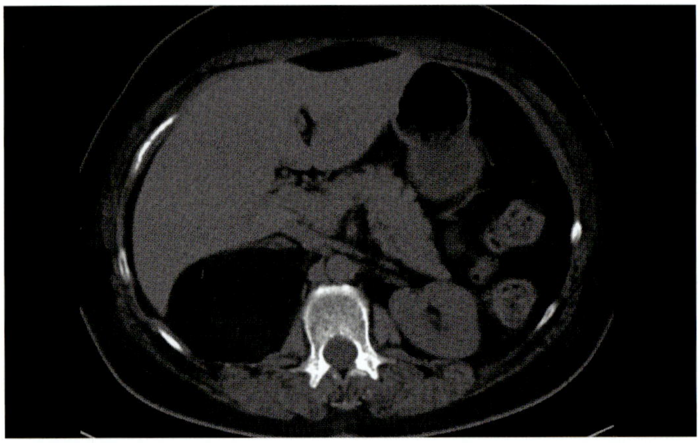

Fig. 5.08 Adrenal myelolipoma. CT demonstrates a well-demarcated, fat-containing, 90 mm large lesion in the right adrenal.

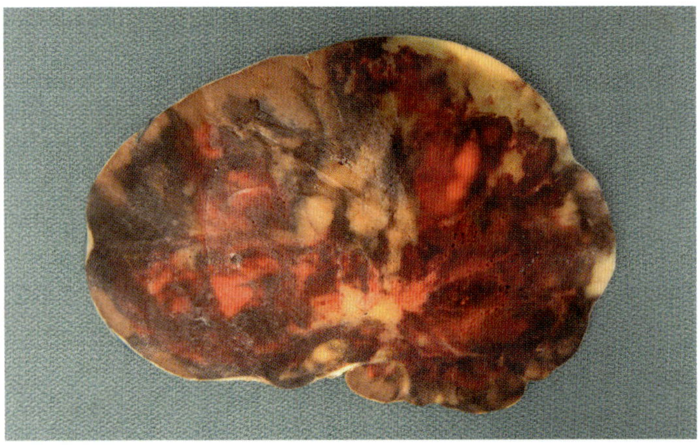

Fig. 5.09 Adrenal myelolipoma. Macroscopic appearance of a 245 mm myelolipoma replacing almost the entire adrenal gland.

Localization

Most adrenal myelolipomas occur in one gland, and bilaterality accounts for about 5% of cases {1758}. Rare examples occur in adrenal rests {1050}.

Clinical features

Myelolipoma often manifests with asymptomatic incidental adrenal lesions that may be detected as a result of nonspecific abdominal discomfort or pain {427}. Large myelolipomas, especially giant myelolipomas (> 100 mm), can cause compression, rupture, or haemorrhage {4102,4157}. They are hormonally inactive unless combined with a functioning adrenocortical tumour or occurring in the setting of congenital adrenal hyperplasia (CAH) {1050,2508,3210}. In CAH, myelolipomas are more frequently bilateral {3210}. Most are hypoechoic on ultrasound and are well-demarcated heterogeneous lesions on CT {825,1629}.

Epidemiology

Adrenal myelolipomas account for 3.3–6.5% of all primary adrenal tumours, with no sex bias and an average age of 50–60 years {1050}. In patients with CAH, myelolipomas account for 25% of CAH-related adrenal tumours {3210}.

Etiology

Unknown

Pathogenesis

Several hypotheses have been suggested, including (1) interactions between two stem cell progenitors of adipocytes and bone marrow cells; (2) inflammation- or stress-induced metaplastic changes of blood capillary reticuloendothelial cells; (3) chromosomal translocation t(3;21)(q25;p11) or non-random X-chromosome inactivation {753,432}; and (4) hormonal factors, mostly linked to ACTH overexpression or an androgen-mediated stimulus, as well as overexpression of MC2R and AR {1050,2508,5177,733,106}.

Macroscopic appearance

Adrenal myelolipoma is a well-demarcated yellow or red nodule with a mean size of 100 mm (range: 5–430 mm) {1050} and a median size of 23 mm {1758}. The weight of giant myelolipomas can exceed 11 kg {100}.

Histopathology

Myelolipoma is composed of mature adipocytes and all three haematopoietic cell lineages. Calcifications and osseous metaplasia can occur. Myelolipoma can develop in combination with adrenocortical tumours, ganglioneuroma, hibernoma, bilateral macronodular adrenocortical disease, and CAH-related compact cell adrenocortical hyperplasia {1050,2508,1188}.

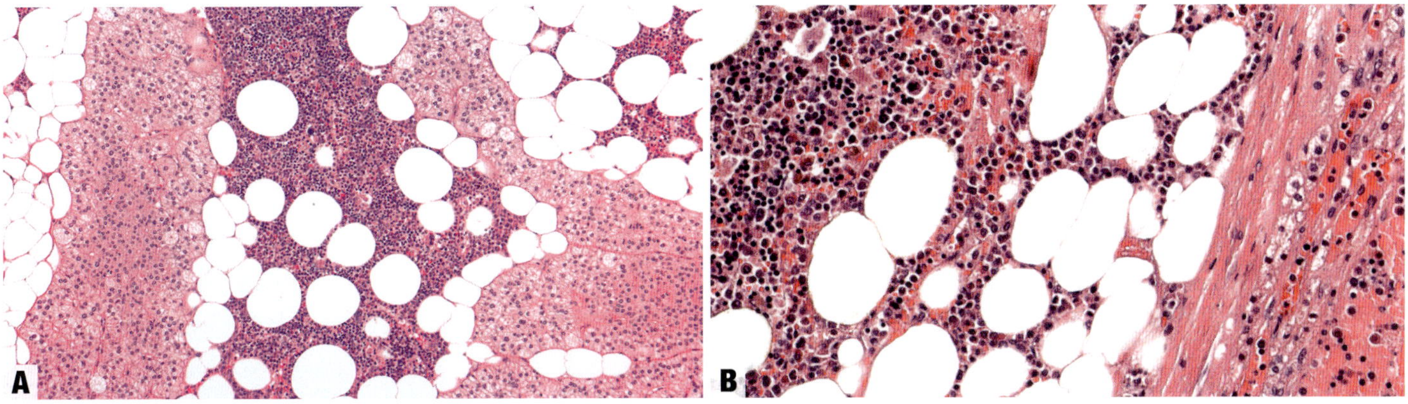

Fig. 5.10 Adrenal myelolipoma. **A** An example composed of mature adipocytes and haematopoietic cells including megakaryocytes that are admixed with adrenal cortical cells. **B** Haematopoietic cells representing the three bone marrow lineages are evident adjacent to fat cells.

Myelolipomas with extensive haemorrhage can be mistaken for an adrenal haematoma or malignancy. The differential diagnosis includes adrenal lipoma, angiomyolipoma, and liposarcoma {1050,2508}.

Cytology

Smears show scattered haematopoietic cells admixed with mature fat cells in a lipid-rich background, to suggest myelolipoma {1804,4073,3578,2106}.

Diagnostic molecular pathology

Not clinically relevant

Essential and desirable diagnostic criteria

Essential: a circumscribed adrenal tumour composed of mature adipocytes and haematopoietic cells.

Staging

Not applicable

Prognosis and prediction

No malignant progression has been reported. Acute haemorrhage and tumour rupture can (rarely) occur in large myelolipomas, usually those > 80 mm. Therefore, surgery can be considered for large and/or symptomatic tumours, with complete recovery expected.

Congenital adrenal hyperplasia

Erickson LA
Falhammar H
Jarzembowski JA
Juhlin CC
Mete O

Definition

Congenital adrenal hyperplasia (CAH) is a proliferation of adrenal cortical cells caused by mutations in genes involved in the enzymatic steps of steroid production in the adrenal cortex.

ICD-O coding

None

ICD-11 coding

5A71.01 Congenital adrenal hyperplasia

Related terminology

Not recommended: adrenogenital syndrome.

Subtype(s)

21-hydroxylase deficiency (classic type and non-classic type); 11β-hydroxylase deficiency; 17α-hydroxylase deficiency; 3β-hydroxysteroid dehydrogenase deficiency; P450 oxidoreductase deficiency; congenital lipoid adrenal hyperplasia; P450 cholesterol side-chain cleavage enzyme deficiency

Localization

Adrenal glands become enlarged if untreated. Adrenal cortical neoplasms and myelolipomas may also occur. Testes can become enlarged by adrenal cortical rest–related proliferations. In rare instances, adrenal rests occur in the ovaries or retroperitoneum, and other unusual places along the adrenal embryonic and gonadal pathways may be affected {1319,776, 4598}.

Clinical features

Infants with classic CAH, the most severe form of CAH, are usually identified by neonatal screening (elevated 17-hydroxyprogesterone) and may have ambiguous genitalia (female), enlarged genitalia (male), virilization, poor feeding, weight loss, dehydration, hyponatraemia, and hyperkalaemia {2946,1230, 4861}. Because of the complexity of the *CYP21A2* locus, genotyping is not used for first-line screening {3557,2946}.

Mutations in *CYP21A2*, which encodes the enzyme 21-hydroxylase, cause 95–99% of cases of CAH, resulting in hypocortisolism and (in 75% of cases) hypoaldosteronism. Hypoaldosteronism results in the inability to retain water and salt (salt wasting), which can result in hypotension, shock, and even death due to adrenal crisis. A variable degree of hyperandrogenism is present in all patients and can result in ambiguous external genitalia in female patients and normal or enlarged genitalia in male patients. The simple virilizing form of CAH is generally not associated with overt salt wasting.

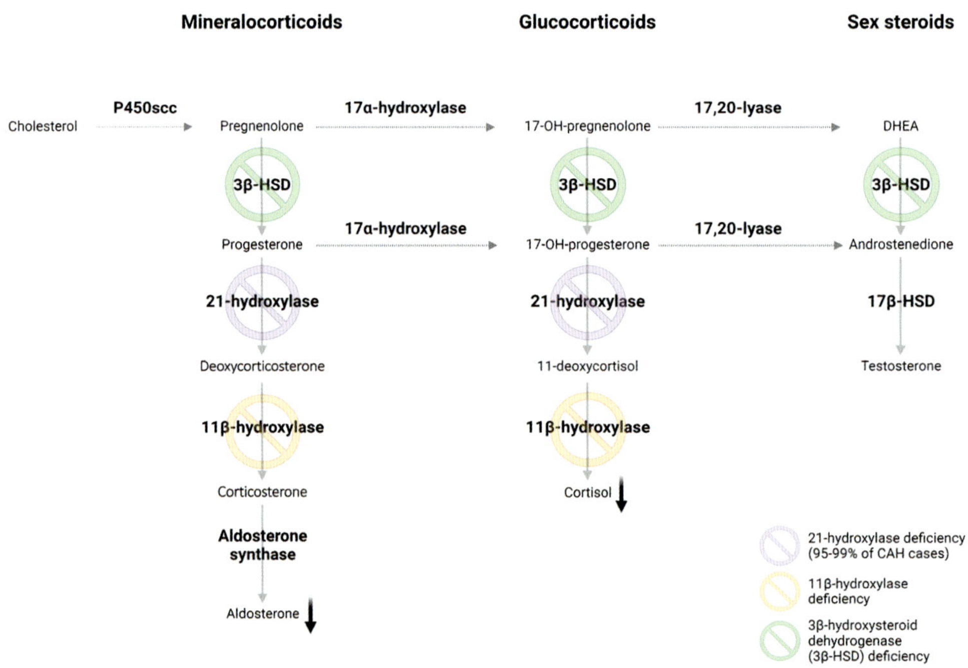

Fig. 5.11 Schematic overview of adrenal cortical hormone biosynthesis and aberrant enzyme expression in various congenital adrenal hyperplasia (CAH) subtypes. By far the most common cause of CAH is 21-hydroxylase deficiency. Note that patients are unable to produce aldosterone and cortisol irrespectively of the subtype of CAH. Although patients with 21-hydroxylase and 11β-hydroxylase–deficient CAH often display signs of virilization due to an excess of androgens, patients with 3β-hydroxysteroid deficiency also display decreased levels of sex hormones.

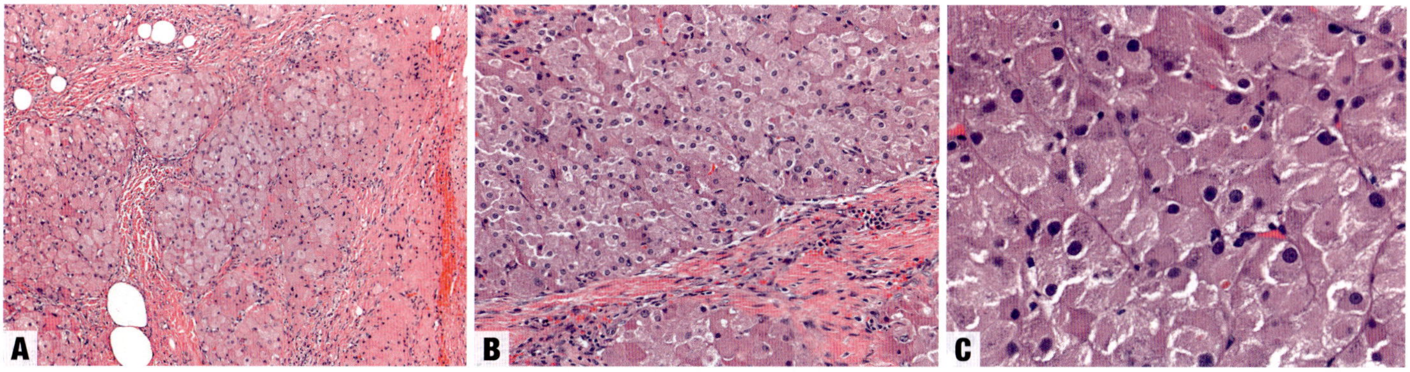

Fig. 5.12 Congenital adrenal hyperplasia. **A** Trophic stimulation by ACTH results in hyperplasia of the zona fasciculata. **B** Expansion of the zona fasciculata in congenital adrenal hyperplasia. Enlarged hyperplastic accessory cortical nodules are also present. **C** Congenital adrenal hyperplasia has cells with marked eosinophilic cytoplasm due to ACTH stimulation, rather than the lipid-rich, pale-staining cells of normal zona fasciculata.

The prevalence of adrenal cortical tumours and myelolipomas in CAH is approximately 30% {3210,3209}. Of the adrenal tumours, 25% are myelolipomas, and > 90% of individuals with these have undiagnosed or poorly managed CAH {3210}. The overall prevalence of myelolipomas in CAH may be increased, and they tend to occur at a younger age {3210}. Testicular adrenal rest tumours (TARTs) occur in a subset of patients and vary based on the severity of the underlying *CYP21A2* mutation {3787}. A recent summary of 33 original articles reported that the prevalence of TARTs ranges from 14% to 86%, depending on genotype. The prevalence of TARTs was related to the severity of disease, with the highest prevalence in the most severely affected individuals, and with the overall prevalence of TARTs being 37% of male patients with CAH {1252}. Only a few TARTs are reported in non-classic CAH {1252}.

Non-classic CAH is much more common and milder than classic salt-wasting CAH or classic simple virilizing CAH. Classic CAH is identified in infants, whereas individuals with non-classic CAH may not be symptomatic until childhood or adulthood, if ever. Those presenting in childhood may have precocious puberty and an increased growth rate, and those presenting later may have amenorrhoea or oligomenorrhoea, hirsutism, and decreased fertility {2946}. Gynaecomastia can be the first presentation in male patients with non-classic CAH {661}.

In 10% of individuals with CAH, there is disruption of *CYP21A2* and *TNXB*, resulting in CAH-X syndrome, in which features of both CAH and Ehlers–Danlos syndrome may be present, because *TNXB* encodes tenascin X {2370,3015,2527}.

Epidemiology

Classic CAH occurs in 1 in 14 000–18 000 people, with a ratio of salt-wasting to simple virilizing types of 2.7:1 {4454}, whereas non-classic CAH occurs in 1 in 200 people {4247,1770}.

Etiology

CAH is an autosomal recessive disorder caused by inactivating germline mutations in genes encoding enzymes in the adrenal cortical steroidogenesis pathway {4248,869}.

Pathogenesis

In CAH, the disruption of adrenal cortical steroidogenesis due to enzyme defects results in the aberrant production of adrenal cortical hormones (see Table 5.01). The most commonly affected gene is *CYP21A2*, located on chromosome 6p21.33 {869}, and it accounts for 95–99% of mutations in all patients with CAH {4248,869}. Mutations in this gene are most

Table 5.01 Subtypes of congenital adrenal hyperplasia (CAH) {1230,300,75,563,4454,4247,1770,4862}

Subtype of CAH	Gene	Clinical
21-hydroxylase deficiency	*CYP21A2*	*Classic:* Incidence 1:14 000–18 000; salt wasting; ambiguous genitalia in 46,XX; virilization *Non-classic:* Incidence 1:200; hypertension; virilization
11β-hydroxylase deficiency	*CYP11B1*	*Classic:* Incidence 1:100 000; hypertension; virilization; disorder of sex development in 46,XX *Non-classic:* Rare; possible hypertension; virilization
17α-hydroxylase/17,20-lyase deficiency	*CYP17A1*	Incidence 1:50 000; hypertension; sexual infantilism and puberty failure with female external genitalia in both 46,XX and 46,XY
3β-hydroxysteroid dehydrogenase deficiency	*HSD3B2*	Rare; salt wasting; ambiguous genitalia in male patients; rarely virilization in 46,XX
P450 oxidoreductase deficiency	*POR*	Rare; hypertension; atypical genitalia in female and male patients; sex steroid deficiency; skeletal abnormalities similar to those in Antley–Bixler syndrome
Congenital lipoid adrenal hyperplasia	*STAR*	Rare; most severe form of CAH; deficiency of all steroid hormones; salt wasting in classic type; female external genitalia in 46,XX and 46,XY infants; sex steroid deficiency; lipid droplets may accumulate in tissues
P450 cholesterol side-chain cleavage enzyme deficiency	*CYP11A1*	Rare; salt wasting in classic type; female external genitalia in 46,XX and 46,XY infants; sex steroid deficiency

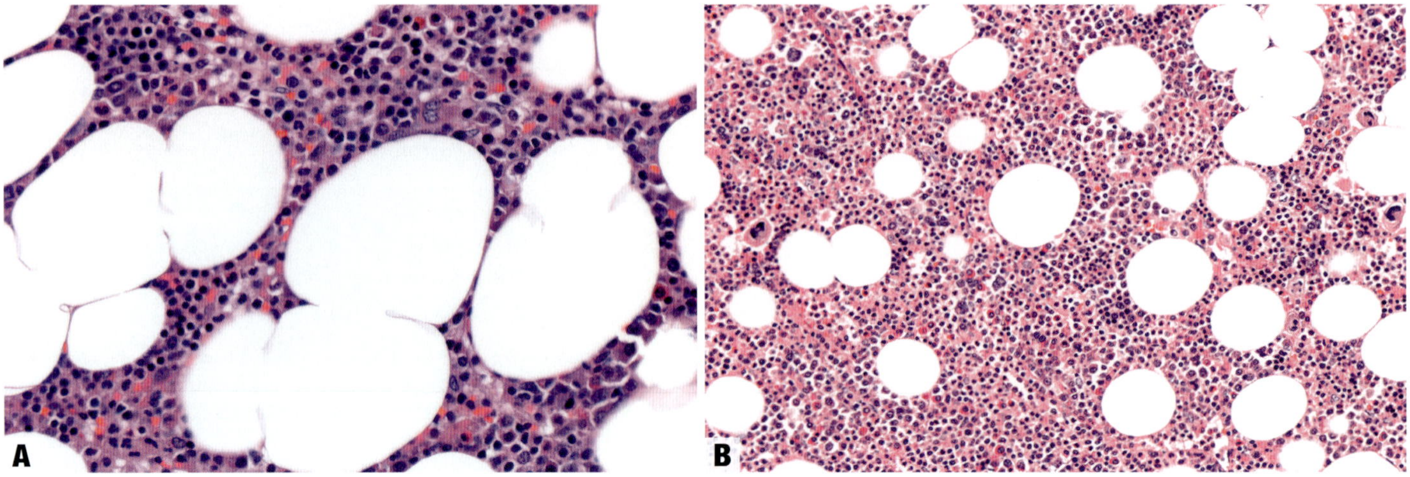

Fig. 5.13 Congenital adrenal hyperplasia. **A** This myelolipoma was identified in an individual with congenital adrenal hyperplasia. The lesion is composed of mature adipose tissue admixed with haematopoietic elements. **B** In congenital adrenal hyperplasia, adrenal myelolipomas are identified more frequently in individuals with undiagnosed or poorly managed congenital adrenal hyperplasia.

commonly caused by complex intergenic recombinations involving misalignments with the closely positioned *CYP21A1P* pseudogene {869,4596}. *CYP21A2* encodes 21-hydroxylase, an enzyme responsible for the conversion of progesterone to deoxycorticosterone in the mineralocorticoid synthesis chain as well as the formation of 11-deoxycortisol from 17-hydroxyprogesterone in the glucocorticoid production chain. Biallelic mutations will therefore severely affect the adrenal production of both aldosterone and cortisol, and an accumulation of 17-hydroxyprogesterone will lead to an increase in the production of androgens, causing virilization. The reduction in cortisol causes an impeded negative feedback at the pituitary level, leading to a compensatory rise of ACTH and hyperplastic adrenals. Other genes associated with CAH are rare and include several other genes in the cortisol production chain, such as *CYP11B1* (encoding 11β-hydroxylase), *HSD3B2* (encoding 3β-hydroxysteroid dehydrogenase), and *CYP17A1* (encoding 17α-hydroxylase) {869}.

Increased screening may contribute to the increased detection of adrenal tumours in people with CAH compared with the general population; however, the stimulatory effects of ACTH have been hypothesized, given the fact that many of these tumours arise in the background of severe cases with poor hormonal control {869,3209,3211}.

Macroscopic appearance

The adrenal glands are enlarged (10–15 g in children, 30–35 g in adults) and may have a cerebriform or convoluted surface due to cortical hyperplasia from trophic stimulation by ACTH {1816}. CAH-associated adrenal cortical tumours appear similar to sporadic tumours but the background adrenal cortex may be hyperplastic. TARTs appear as yellow, firm, round to oval, sharply delineated nodules, often multinodular with fibrous bands, frequently located near or in the mediastinum testis, and bilateral {1252}.

Histopathology

The adrenal glands (and accessory adrenal cortical tissue) may show varying histological features depending on whether or not the patient was treated with exogenous corticosteroids. If untreated, the adrenal glands show marked bilateral cortical compact cell hyperplasia characterized by expansion of

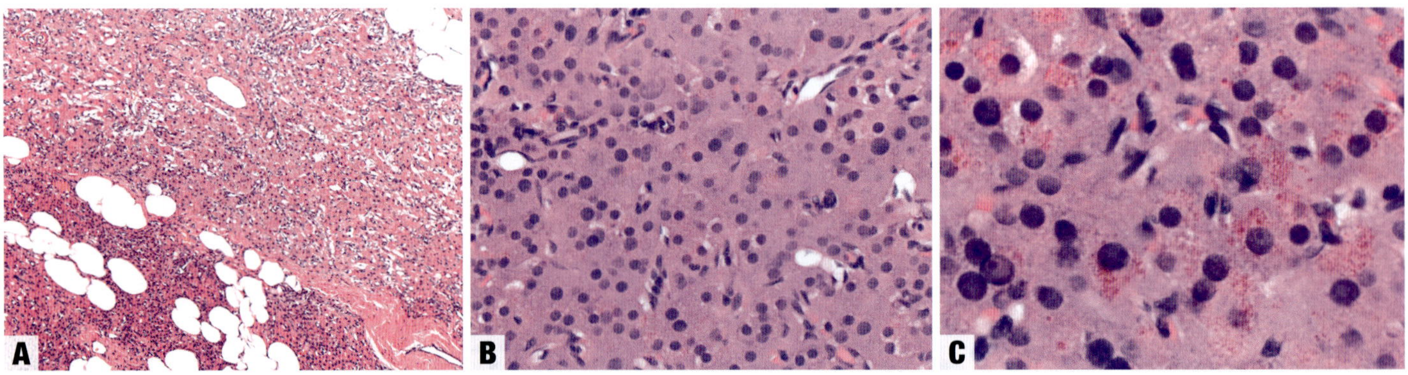

Fig. 5.14 Testicular adrenal rest tumour in the setting of congenital adrenal hyperplasia. **A** Testicular adrenal rest tumours are usually identified in the mediastinum (hilum) of the testis and are often bilateral. They must be differentiated from Leydig cell tumours, which they closely resemble. **B** Testicular adrenal rest tumours are composed of nests and sheets of cells with granular pink cytoplasm. The tumour cells resemble Leydig cells. The presence of bilateral disease and the knowledge that the lesion is occurring in the setting of congenital adrenal hyperplasia are helpful in differentiating testicular adrenal rest tumour from Leydig cell tumour. **C** The cells have fairly uniform round to oval nuclei and granular pink cytoplasm. Most tumour cells contain prominent lipofuscin (lipochrome pigment).

the adrenal cortex with a lipid depletion pattern due to a zona reticularis–like compact cell predominance that imparts a dark colour to the adrenal glands {2496}. Incomplete steroid replacement may result in a mixture of columns of zona fasciculata–like lipid-rich cells intermixed with lipid-depleted compact cell glands {2496}.

TARTs are composed of sheets and nests of large vacuolated cells with granular pink cytoplasm, often containing lipofuscin pigment, with round to oval nuclei and small nucleoli similar in appearance to those of Leydig cells {869,1322,2723,1252}. TARTs and Leydig cell tumours cannot be reliably differentiated by histomorphology, although Reinke crystalloids, which may be seen in Leydig cell tumours, are absent in TARTs {1252}. TARTs are more often bilateral than testicular Leydig cell tumours are (77% vs < 10%) {1252}. In addition to the expression of adrenal cortical steroidogenesis enzymes (CYP11B1 and CYP21A2), an absence of INSL3 expression and an abundance of DLK1 may help distinguish TART from Leydig cell tumours {2740}; however, these biomarkers are not widely available in most clinical laboratories. Therefore, a clinical history of CAH and assessment of the testicular parenchyma may be helpful.

Cytology

Not applicable

Diagnostic molecular pathology

Genetic testing is considered to accurately determine the specific mutation in affected individuals.

Essential and desirable diagnostic criteria

Essential:

- Clinical: physical and laboratory findings confirming the diagnosis of CAH, including hypocortisolism and hypoaldosteronism in association with elevated 17-hydroxyprogesterone for classic 21-hydroxylase deficiency, and cosyntropin stimulation test for non-classic or milder subtypes (see Table 5.01, p. 233).
- Pathological: adrenal gland enlargement with variable degrees of compact cell hyperplasia in the appropriate clinical context and with the typical laboratory findings.

Desirable: genetic testing for pathogenic variants of genes encoding steroidogenic enzymes.

Staging

Not applicable

Prognosis and prediction

Neonatal screening has decreased infant mortality and morbidity in CAH. CAH is treated to replace deficient hormones, reduce excessive androgens, and prevent adrenal crisis (commonly triggered by an infection). Exogenous glucocorticoids may result in a complication of iatrogenic Cushing syndrome {1169}. Bilateral adrenalectomy with glucocorticoid and mineralocorticoid replacement has been proposed as a therapeutic strategy, most often used to control hyperandrogenism/virilization and/or Cushing syndrome {2782}. Deaths may occur due to adrenal crisis. Non-classic CAH is comparatively mild, not life-threatening, and treated symptomatically as required.

Adrenocortical nodular disease

Erickson LA
Gill AJ
Jarzembowski JA
Juhlin CC
Mete O
Sasano H

Definition

Adrenocortical nodular disease comprises a group of distinct pathological entities characterized by benign adrenal cortical nodular proliferations.

ICD-O coding

None

ICD-11 coding

5A70.Y Other specified Cushing syndrome

Related terminology

Acceptable: adrenal cortical nodular disease; cortical nodular disease; nodular adrenocortical disease.

Not recommended: cortical nodular hyperplasia; adrenocortical nodular hyperplasia; micronodular adrenocortical hyperplasia; macronodular adrenocortical hyperplasia.

Subtype(s)

Sporadic nodular adrenocortical disease; bilateral micronodular adrenocortical disease (isolated micronodular adrenocortical disease [i-MAD] and primary pigmented nodular adrenocortical disease [PPNAD]); bilateral macronodular adrenocortical disease

Localization

The micronodular and macronodular forms of adrenocortical nodular disease involve both adrenal glands, whereas sporadic nodular adrenocortical disease may manifest as unilateral or bilateral adrenal gland involvement {1916,2141}.

Clinical features

Sporadic nodular adrenocortical disease often consists of one or more incidentally discovered non-functioning adrenocortical nodule(s) that measure < 10 mm and can occur in all age groups {1916,2141,1166}. They may be found on imaging, at autopsy, or during the histopathological examination of adrenalectomy specimens for other reasons {1760,1916}.

Individuals with bilateral micronodular or macronodular adrenocortical disease usually have variable degrees of endogenous Cushing syndrome {1167,2963,1916,2141,2175,116}. Bilateral micronodular adrenocortical nodular disease occurs in children and young adults (often in those aged < 30 years) {2175,1285}, with a female predominance {407,2797}. PPNAD, a distinct subtype of bilateral micronodular adrenocortical disease, is a characteristic endocrine manifestation of Carney complex {667,1285} and has been reported in about 57% of patients with Carney complex {1285}. Because PPNAD can occur in the absence of Carney complex (isolated PPNAD [i-PPNAD]) {1677,2141,1167}, the term "c-PPNAD" has been applied to PPNAD associated with Carney complex {2175,1167,2963}. i-MAD is a very rare subtype of bilateral micronodular adrenocortical disease that is distinguished from i-PPNAD on the basis of histopathological characteristics {1167,2963,2175,490}. Both PPNAD and i-MAD show variable degrees of hypercortisolism, including cyclic Cushing syndrome, and may exhibit a paradoxical response to a dexamethasone suppression (Liddle test) with an increase in 17-hydroxycorticosteroid and urinary free cortisol levels {2742, 2175,1285,2963}. Unlike children with Cushing syndrome due to other causes {1167}, children with PPNAD may exhibit normal growth {2797,4297}.

Bilateral macronodular adrenocortical disease (formerly known as primary bilateral macronodular adrenal cortical

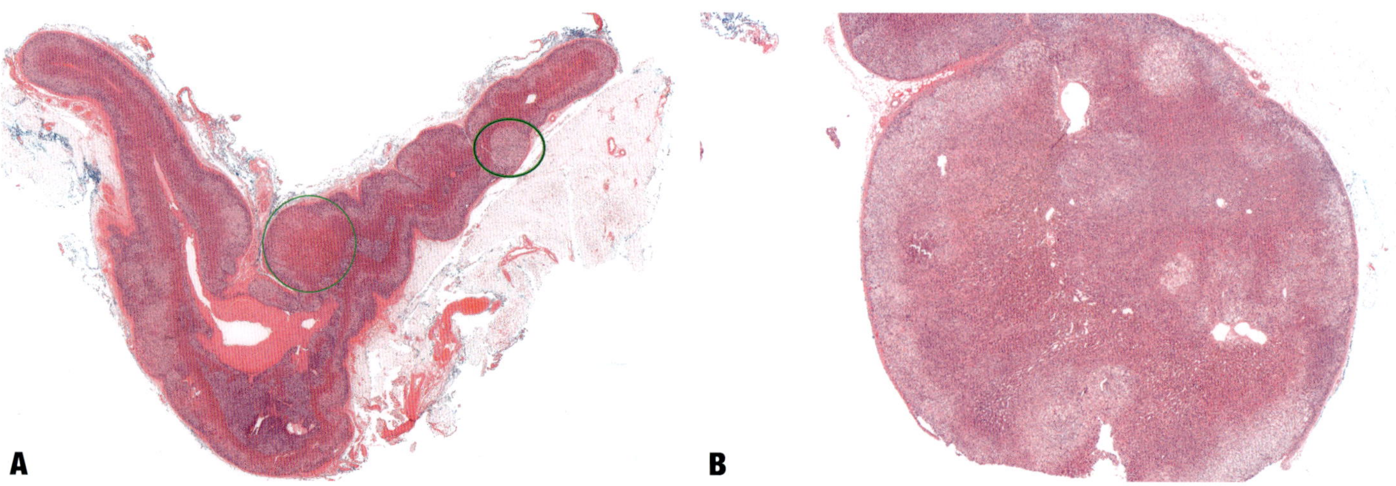

Fig. 5.15 Sporadic nodular adrenocortical disease. **A** Two foci of randomly distributed sporadic nodular adrenocortical disease that ranged in size from 1.5 to 3 mm are seen. The large focus is enriched in compact cells with variable pigment deposition, whereas the small focus is enriched in lipid-rich clear cells. **B** Sporadic nodular adrenocortical disease with a nodule measuring 7 mm. With the exception of its size (< 10 mm), sporadic nodular adrenocortical disease is indistinguishable from other non-functioning adenomas.

hyperplasia or ACTH-independent macronodular adrenocortical hyperplasia) is more frequent in adults; however, paediatric manifestations also exist {2175,1167,2963,2141}. In a large series, the age at onset in adults ranged from 30 to 75 years (mean: 53 years) and there was a female predominance {1283}. *ARMC5*-related macronodular disease has no sex predominance {1283}. Fewer than about 10% of individuals with bilateral macronodular adrenocortical disease may have biochemically non-functioning disease, and the remainder show a variable degree of Cushing syndrome {1283}. *ARMC5*-related bilateral macronodular adrenocortical disease often has a significantly higher level of cortisol secretion than *ARMC5*-wildtype disease and an absence of non-functional manifestations {1283}. Childhood-onset bilateral macronodular adrenocortical disease often shows more pronounced Cushing syndrome {2963,1167}.

Imaging

On imaging studies, massive bilateral adrenal gland enlargement is the hallmark of bilateral macronodular adrenocortical disease {1140,3776,1916}. CT and MRI findings in bilateral micronodular adrenocortical disease are variable and may underestimate the presence of bilateral adrenal gland involvement {1285,1916}. Half of all affected patients may have an abnormal imaging finding {1285}, including multiple bilateral small bead-like nodules {3776}. Functional imaging studies using iodocholesterol (NP-59) scintigraphy/PET help identify the bilateral nature of the disease in ACTH-independent Cushing disease with normal CT {4695}.

Epidemiology

Adrenal incidentalomas are reported in about 5% of people who undergo imaging studies {3148,496,1760}. Although not all adrenal incidentalomas are of cortical origin, they may be underreported {1760}. Therefore, the prevalence of sporadic nodular adrenocortical disease in surgical and radiological series with complete endocrine workup remains to be determined. Nevertheless, sporadic nodular adrenocortical disease is more frequent than bilateral micronodular and macronodular adrenocortical disease. Bilateral micronodular and macronodular subtypes of adrenocortical disease account for up to 2% of cases of endogenous Cushing syndrome {2797,2175}.

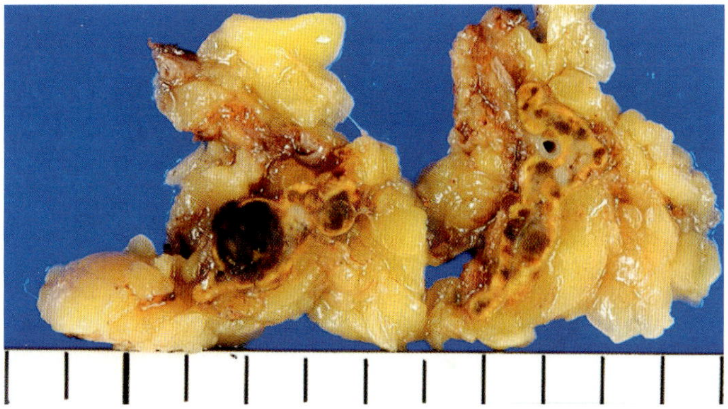

Fig. 5.16 Primary pigmented nodular adrenocortical disease. Gross examination of primary pigmented nodular adrenocortical disease identifies bilateral small pigmented cortical nodules (< 10 mm, often ≤ 5 mm).

Etiology

The etiology of sporadic nodular adrenocortical disease is largely unknown. However, cigarette smoking may be a risk factor, because the prevalence of both benign and malignant adrenocortical neoplasms is higher in individuals with a history of tobacco use {5090}. Virtually all cases of bilateral micronodular adrenocortical disease and a significant fraction of cases of bilateral macronodular adrenocortical disease are caused by genetic susceptibility (see *Pathogenesis*) {2141,2963,2175}.

Pathogenesis

Sporadic small adrenocortical nodules (as small as 3–5 mm) may be clonal {4663,2956}. Therefore, the term "sporadic nodular adrenocortical disease" has replaced "cortical nodular hyperplasia" for incidental non-functioning cortical nodules measuring < 10 mm {2141,3390}

In bilateral nodular adrenocortical disease, germline susceptibility is followed by a somatic second hit involving the other allele. Bilateral micronodular adrenocortical disease is linked to pathogenic germline variants leading to the activation of the PKA pathway {2141,2963}, including *PRKAR1A* (the most frequent alteration in c-PPNAD and i-PPNAD), *PRKACA* alterations (i-PPNAD and i-MAD), *PDE11A* (i-MAD), *PDE8B* (i-MAD), and 2p16 *CNC2* locus alterations (*PRKAR1A*-wildtype c-PPNAD) {2175,2963}. The discovery of a pathogenic germline *MYH8*

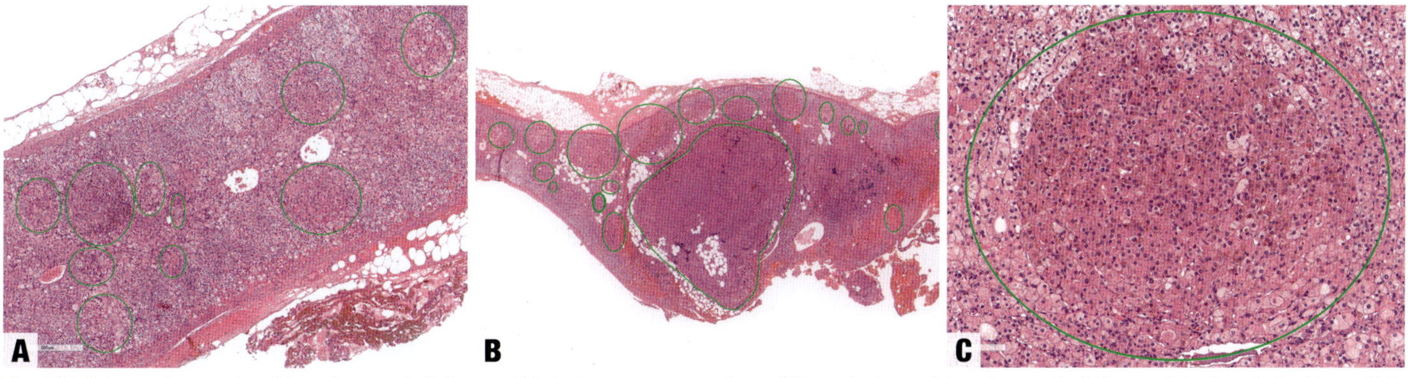

Fig. 5.17 Primary pigmented nodular adrenocortical disease. This is the most common form of bilateral micronodular adrenocortical disease. It is characterized by multiple pigmented small nodules (< 10 mm) that often range in size from 1 to 4 mm; cortical micronodules are enriched in compact (lipid-poor) adrenocortical cells (**A–C**). Internodular cortical atrophy with reduced cortical thickness can be noted (**A,B**).

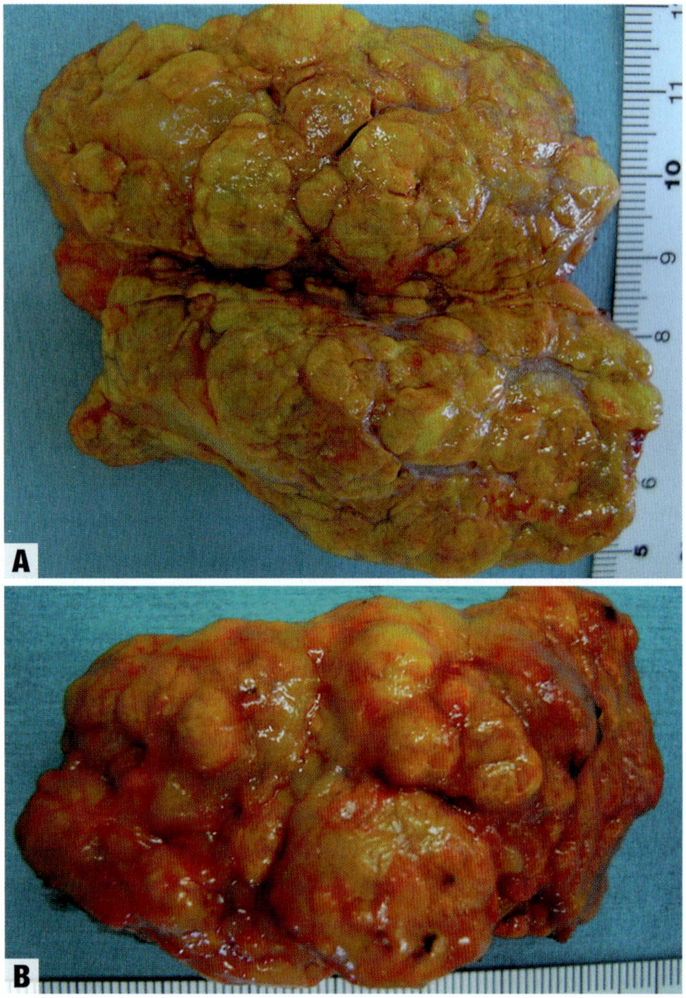

Fig. 5.18 Bilateral macronodular adrenocortical disease. Irregular adrenal gland enlargement due to multiple adrenal cortical nodules, each > 10 mm. **A** Right adrenal gland. **B** Left adrenal gland.

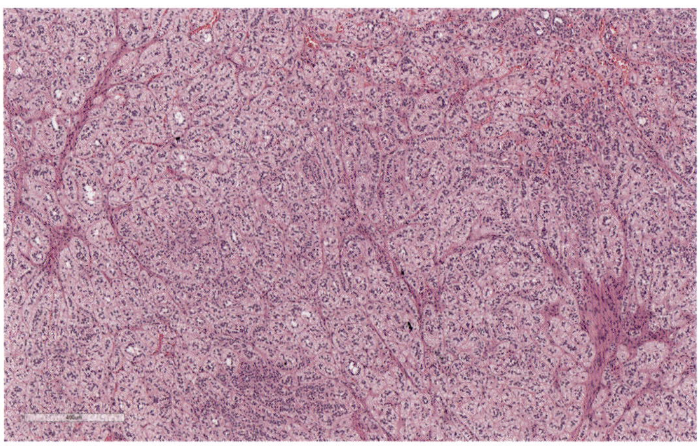

Fig. 5.19 Bilateral macronodular adrenocortical disease. The disease is characterized by bilateral multiple clear cell–rich nodules, each measuring > 10 mm.

variant has also expanded the spectrum of isolated bilateral micronodular adrenocortical disease in early infancy {2802}.

Because bilateral macronodular adrenocortical disease consists of multiple independent clonal proliferations {2141,2963,238, 1318}, the traditional terminology of "primary bilateral macronodular adrenal cortical hyperplasia" is no longer appropriate {2141, 2963,1916}. The pathogenesis of bilateral macronodular adrenocortical disease has been linked to several alterations, including germline pathogenic *ARMC5* variants (most frequent cause, 25–55% of cases) {238,1283}, *MEN1* (in multiple endocrine neoplasia type 1) {566,4683,4633}, *FH* (in hereditary leiomyomatosis and renal cell cancer) {2892,1969}, *APC* (in familial adenomatous polyposis) {1518,1969}, and somatic *GNAS* mosaicism (in McCune–Albright syndrome) {4710,4633,2963}, as well as rare *PDE11A* {1969,1769,2963}, *PDE8B* {1769,2963}, and *EDNRA* {5178} variants. In addition, several additional complex mechanisms including aberrant G protein–coupled receptor expression {2497,2498}, dysregulation of ectopic hormone receptors or their expression {2498,2499,2904,2537}, aberrant intra-adrenal ACTH production {2741,2596,2963}, and increased *PRKAR2B* expression are described in a subset of cases of bilateral macronodular adrenocortical disease {489}.

Pangenomic characterization of benign adrenocortical lesions identified an ovarian gene expression signature (*FOXL2*, *CYP19A1*, *PTHLH*) and global CpG hypermethylation in *ARMC5*-related bilateral macronodular adrenocortical disease {1318}. Specific microRNA signatures also distinguish PPNAD from cortisol-secreting adenomas {1318}.

Macroscopic appearance

Sporadic nodular adrenocortical disease appears as randomly distributed small (< 10 mm) yellow to brown cortical nodules {1916}. Adrenal glands show no significant enlargement in bilateral micronodular adrenocortical disease. Gross examination can identify bilateral small cortical nodules (often < 5 mm) that are pigmented in PPNAD and non-pigmented in i-MAD {1167,2963}. Bilateral irregular adrenal gland enlargement due to multiple cortical nodules is a characteristic finding of bilateral macronodular adrenocortical disease {1916}. In adults, the mean weight for both adrenal glands has been reported as 81 g; however, an individual adrenal gland can weigh > 120 g in individuals with bilateral macronodular adrenocortical disease {1283}. *ARMC5*-driven macronodular disease is associated with an increased number of nodules (> 5 nodules in 75%), leading to a significantly increased adrenal size and weight compared with *ARMC5*-wildtype macronodular disease {1283}.

Histopathology

With the exception of size, sporadic nodular adrenocortical disease is indistinguishable from non-functioning adrenocortical adenomas. There can be more than one nodule per gland, and both adrenal glands may be involved. When they occur in adrenals from patients with functioning adenomas, their distinction from subcentimetre functioning adrenal cortical adenomas requires the use of steroidogenic enzyme immunohistochemistry (e.g. CYP11B2, CYP11B1, CYP17) {2959,3959} (see *Adrenal cortical adenoma*, p. 240).

Bilateral micronodular adrenocortical disease (PPNAD and i-MAD) is characterized by multiple small nodules (< 10 mm) that often range in size from 1 to 4 mm {1916,2963}. Cortical micronodules are composed of compact (lipid-poor) adrenocortical cells and are typically located in the zona fasciculata or in the intersection of the zona reticularis and zona fasciculata {2963}. PPNAD is distinguished from i-MAD by the presence of pigmented nodules and internodular cortical atrophy in PPNAD {2141,2175,490}. Rarely, myelolipomas {2744}, adrenal cortical adenomas (> 10 mm) {5082,2744}, and adrenal cortical carcinomas {3094,161} have been described in c-PPNAD.

Bilateral macronodular adrenocortical disease is characterized by bilateral multiple clear cell–rich nodules, each > 10 mm with small lipid-poor cortical cells dispersed among large clear cells {2141,2963,1167,3961}. Internodular cortical atrophy is identified in some adrenal glands {2175}. Patients with McCune–Albright syndrome–related Cushing syndrome can have diffuse and/or macronodular adrenocortical hyperplasia. A subset of infants with McCune–Albright syndrome may present with adrenal glands that have a bimorphic pattern of diffuse and nodular adrenocortical hyperplasia with alternating areas of cortical hyperplasia and atrophy (also known as primary bimorphic adrenocortical disease; see *McCune–Albright syndrome*, p. 471) {673}.

Cytology

Not applicable

Diagnostic molecular pathology

Germline testing for pathogenic variants is considered in light of clinicopathological findings.

Essential and desirable diagnostic criteria

Essential:

- For sporadic nodular adrenocortical disease: non-functioning benign adrenal cortical nodules measuring < 10 mm
- For bilateral micronodular adrenocortical disease: bilateral multiple pigmented (PPNAD) or non-pigmented (i-MAD) compact cell adrenocortical nodules measuring < 10 mm (often < 5 mm); internodular cortical atrophy (in PPNAD); Cushing syndrome
- For bilateral macronodular adrenocortical disease: bilateral marked adrenal gland enlargement with multiple benign clear cell–rich adrenocortical nodules measuring > 10 mm; Cushing syndrome

Staging

Not applicable

Prognosis and prediction

Although adrenocortical nodular disease is a benign disorder, uncontrolled hypercortisolism due to bilateral nodular forms of adrenocortical disease (especially in infants/neonates) and additional pathologies associated with genetic tumour syndromes are important prognostic factors.

Adrenal cortical adenoma

Erickson LA
Assié G
Juhlin CC
Mete O
Sasano H
Volante M

Definition

Adrenal cortical adenoma is a benign epithelial neoplasm of adrenal cortical cells.

ICD-O coding

8370/0 Adrenal cortical adenoma

ICD-11 coding

2F37.Y & XH3DV3 Other specified benign neoplasm of endocrine glands & Adenoma, NOS

Related terminology

Acceptable: adrenocortical adenoma.
Not recommended: oncocytoma.

Subtype(s)

None

Localization

Adrenal cortical adenoma is usually a unilateral and solitary mass arising in the adrenal gland; however, bilateral and multifocal adenomas can occur {2141}. Ectopic tumours also occur {1147,3207}.

Clinical features

Adrenal cortical adenomas may be hormonally active with associated clinical manifestations, or they may be non-functioning (silent) and may be discovered incidentally on imaging studies performed for other reasons {1916}.

Primary aldosteronism (Conn syndrome) is primarily a laboratory diagnosis that requires confirmation of the plasma aldosterone-to-renin ratio followed by aldosterone suppression testing {1171,2963,1989}. It is the most common cause of secondary hypertension {1171}. Not all affected patients have hypokalaemia. Affected patients may present with headaches, palpitations, weakness, polydipsia, and polyuria with hypertension and hypokalaemia/normokalaemia, and they have an increased risk of cardiovascular disease {1171}. Bilateral adrenal gland involvement occurs in 60–70% of cases of primary aldosteronism {1171,1916}. Bilateral manifestations are enriched in bilateral diffuse zona glomerulosa hyperplasia and bilateral aldosterone-producing microadenomas (< 10 mm) {2141,5125}. The distinction of bilateral aldosterone excess from unilateral disease (often due to adenoma or microadenoma) is important in deciding on surgical intervention {557,1916,1461}. Adrenal venous sampling is the historical standard in the lateralization of aldosterone excess {1461}, but the optimal approach is still debated {557}. Some patients may have concurrent primary aldosteronism and Cushing syndrome {2035,4995,4411}. Mild autonomous cortisol secretion in adrenal cortical adenomas may pose diagnostic challenges, and a subset of these can simulate a non-functioning cortical adenoma {1916,4416,3967}. Therefore, dynamic endocrine tests {1916,3967,1167} and functional imaging studies (including but not limited to iodocholesterol [NP-59] studies) {3161,3335} are useful in this distinction.

In patients with cortisol-producing adrenal cortical adenomas, clinical features of cortisol excess include central obesity, rounded facies, hirsutism, poor wound healing, skin striae, weight gain, proximal muscle weakness, hypertension, hyperglycaemia, osteoporosis, and susceptibility to infections {1167}. Growth failure is an important paediatric manifestation {1167}.

Virilization or feminization is extremely rare in adrenal cortical adenomas {1968,280,1937,69,5174}. This diagnosis requires exclusion of an adrenal cortical carcinoma. The diagnosis of adenoma is made with caution in this functional group. These tumours may also cosecrete glucocorticoids, similarly to some adrenal cortical carcinomas {1937}. Testosterone-producing adrenal cortical adenomas are more common in children {1968, 280,1937,69}, but rare examples have been reported in adults {5174}. Oncocytic adrenal cortical adenomas may cosecrete testosterone and cortisol {69,1937}.

Non-functioning adrenal cortical adenomas are often discovered incidentally, with the increased use of imaging studies. Large tumour size, invasiveness, heterogeneity, lipid content, and the rate of washout after intravenous contrast on CT

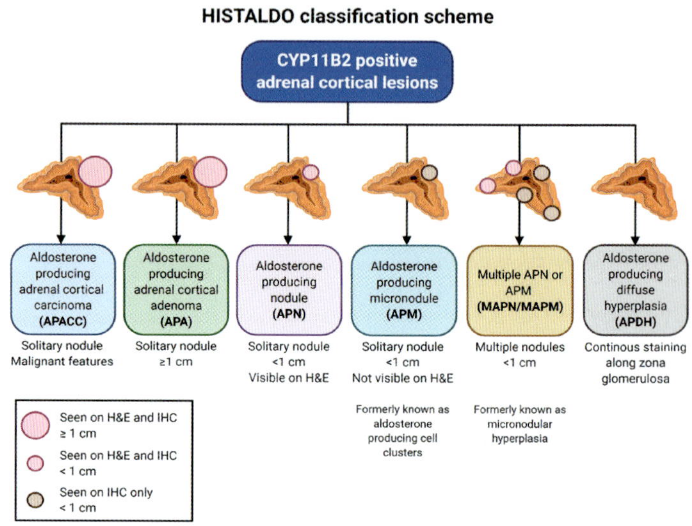

Fig. 5.20 Histopathology of primary aldosteronism (HISTALDO) classification. Aldosterone-producing adrenal cortical carcinoma and adenoma are solitary lesions clearly visible by both routine H&E and immunohistochemical staining for CYP11B2 (aldosterone synthase). Smaller (subcentimetre) solitary lesions visible by H&E and immunohistochemistry (IHC) are designated as aldosterone-producing nodules (APNs), whereas their counterparts that may be hard to distinguish using H&E but are always visualized on IHC are called aldosterone-producing micronodules (APMs; formerly known as aldosterone-producing cell clusters). When multifocal, these entities are termed multiple APN and multiple APM, respectively (formerly known as micronodular hyperplasia). Aldosterone-producing diffuse hyperplasia is characterized by continuous CYP11B2 staining along the zona glomerulosa.

imaging studies are important factors that are considered in the surgical management of a non-functioning adrenal cortical neoplasm {1916}. For instance, lipid-rich adrenal cortical neoplasms discovered incidentally are less worrisome and may be observed; however, large (> 40 mm) and lipid-poor tumours or those with heterogeneous radiographic features are of greater concern and are therefore subjected to surgery. FDG PET-CT imaging has been suggested to discriminate benign from malignant adrenal lesions, with a maximum standardized uptake value of ≥ 4.6 being suggestive of malignancy. However, lower values are not specific for adenoma {4742}, and false positive or inconclusive results have been observed in some cases including black adenomas {2888}.

Epidemiology

Approximately 5% of the general population have one or more adrenal cortical nodule(s) that are usually solitary and unilateral but can be multifocal or bilateral {3148,496,1760}. Adrenal cortical adenomas are the most common adrenal cortical tumour.

Etiology

Genetic factors and environmental factors contribute to the etiology of adrenal cortical neoplasms. Tobacco use has been shown to be associated with an increased risk of benign and malignant adrenal cortical neoplasms {5090}.

Pathogenesis

Genetic predisposition occurs in a small fraction of adrenal cortical neoplasms {2141,1916}. The past decade has seen significant progress in the understanding of genomic correlates of aldosterone- and cortisol-producing adrenal cortical adenomas and the pathways responsible for the physiological regulation of these hormones, which has facilitated a better understanding of the tumorigenesis of functional adrenal cortical disorders {1171, 2141}.

Aldosterone-producing adrenal cortical adenomas

Mutations in various genes encoding ion channels are pathognomonic of this disease, because depolarization of the membrane in a zona glomerulosa cell will stimulate aldosterone production irrespective of whether the depolarization event is caused by angiotensin II stimulation or a dysfunctional ion channel {2141}. The normal regulation of aldosterone production in the zona glomerulosa via the renin–angiotensin system is primarily governed by the membrane potential. In the resting state, K+ channels in the zona glomerulosa cells are open constitutively, thus maintaining a hyperpolarized state in which voltage-dependent Ca2+ channels remain closed. Upon renin–angiotensin activation, K+ channels will close, leading to depolarization and the opening of voltage-dependent Ca2+ channels. The influx of Ca2+ will stimulate the transcription of *CYP11B2* (encoding aldosterone synthase) {2141}. Intriguingly, mutations in genes encoding various ion channels expressed in the zona glomerulosa mimic this physiological response, thus causing cell-cycle activation and aldosterone excess. To date, mutually exclusive somatic mutations in *KCNJ5* (encoding a K+ channel) {831,4888}, *ATP1A1* (Na+/K+ channel) {411,250,4888}, *ATP2B3* (Ca2+ channel) {411, 4888}, *CACNA1D* (Ca2+ channel) {250,4017,3183}, *CACNA1H* (Ca2+ channel) {4018,3183,3179}, and *CLCN2* (Cl– channel) {4019,1357,3708} have been described for the vast majority of

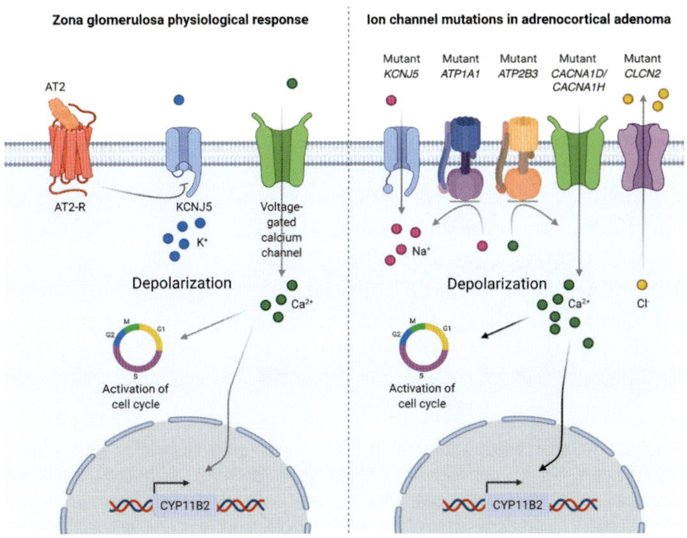

Fig. 5.21 Ion channel. Physiological regulation of proliferation and aldosterone production is intimately coupled to depolarization of the membrane potential in the zona glomerulosa (left). Mutations in various membrane-bound ion channels (right) mimic the stimulatory role of angiotensin II, causing depolarization either through the increased influx of sodium (mutant *KCNJ5*) or calcium (mutant *CACNA1H/CACNA1D*), or through the inhibition of extracellular transportation of sodium (mutant *ATP1A1*) or calcium (mutant *ATP2B3*), or through the increased efflux of chloride ions (mutant *CLCN2*).

tumours, including reports of mutations in as many as 90% of patients in American series and 96% of patients in Japanese series {3181,3180,3183}. Of note, *KCNJ5* mutations are found in approximately 40% of aldosterone-producing adrenal cortical adenomas, and they seem to be overrepresented in younger female patients with pronounced hormonal activity {2606}. Additional genotype–phenotype correlates have been proposed, including differences in steroidogenic enzyme expression, cytomorphology, and clinical aspects such as the adrenal vein sampling lateralization index {249,4817}. Of clinical interest,

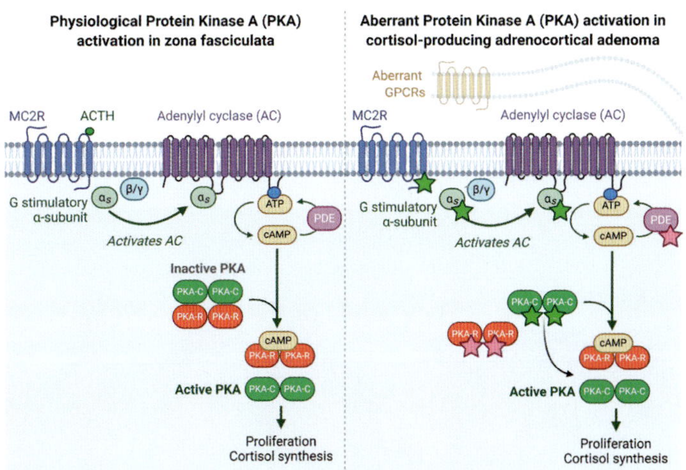

Fig. 5.22 PKA signalling pathway. The PKA signalling pathway mediates the zona fasciculata response to ACTH binding the ACTH receptor (MC2R) and activating adenylyl cyclase (AC). The increasing levels of cAMP will release the inhibition of the catalytic PKA subunits (PKA-C) by the regulatory PKA subunit (PKA-R), stimulating cell growth and cortisol production. Aberrant PKA signalling is a recurrent theme in cortisol-secreting adrenal cortical lesions and might stem from activating mutations (green stars) as well as inactivating events (pink stars). GPCR, G protein–coupled receptor; PDE, phosphodiesterase.

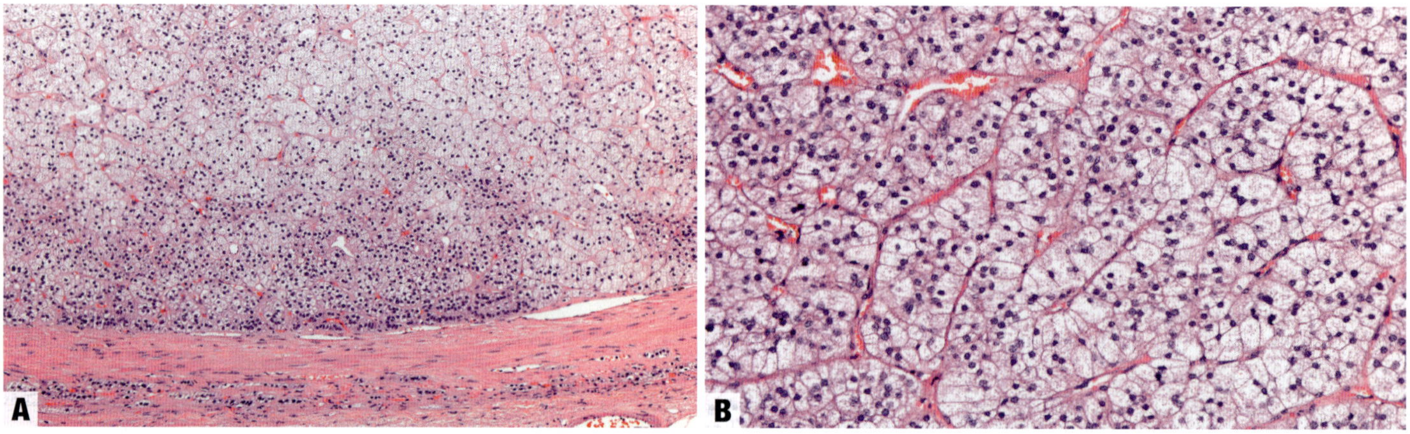

Fig. 5.23 Adrenal cortical adenoma. **A** Cushing syndrome–associated adrenal cortical adenomas are usually composed of predominantly pale-staining, lipid-rich, zona fasciculata–like cells, but they can have variable cell types. **B** Cortisol-secreting adrenal cortical adenomas are often composed of zona fasciculata–like cells with markedly vacuolated cytoplasm, giving the lesion a clear appearance at low magnification. These lesions often have a nesting pattern of growth, or they may have trabeculae, cords of cells, or mixtures of cell types. The predominance of lipid-rich cells gives the tumour a yellow appearance on cut section grossly.

subsets of patients may also display pathogenic germline mutations in *KCNJ5*, *CACNA1H*, *CACNA1D*, or *CLCN2*, leading to familial forms of primary aldosteronism with early-onset hypertension {2141}. In addition to ion-channel aberrancies, subsets of aldosterone-producing adrenal cortical adenomas display activating somatic mutations in *CTNNB1* (encoding the WNT pathway effector β-catenin), thus reinforcing the importance of this signalling network also in benign adrenal cortical tumours {4948,61}. These patients are often female, with a delayed age of disease onset.

Cortisol-producing adrenal cortical adenomas

Mutations are congregated in genes regulating the PKA pathway {2141}. In the normal physiological regulation of cortisol secretion from the zona fasciculata, ACTH binds MC2R, in turn activating adenylyl cyclase, which triggers the conversion of ATP to cAMP. When cAMP levels rise, the regulatory subunits of PKA are inhibited, thereby freeing catalytic subunits to enter the nucleus, in turn leading to the transcription of target genes stimulating cell growth and cortisol production. Therefore, cortisol-producing tumours often display mutations or deletions in genes regulating this process, including *PRKACA* (the most common alteration, identified in ~40% of cases), *PRKAR1A*, *GNAS*, or *PRKACB* {3969,4461,412,1618,1111,406,1284}. The discovery of the rare *AKAP13*::*PDE8A* fusion also expands the spectrum of cortisol-producing adrenal cortical adenomas {1110}. Moreover, activating *CTNNB1* mutations can occur in a subset of cortisol-producing adenomas {4461,1618}. Cortisol-producing adenomas with *PRKACA* and *PRKAR1A* aberrancies are often associated with smaller tumours and overt Cushing syndrome, whereas *CTNNB1*-mutated cortisol-producing adenomas are associated with mild autonomous cortisol secretion {2963,3969,1318}.

The observation of somatic *KCNJ5* mutations in cortisol- and aldosterone-producing adenomas has been recorded {4995, 4411}. Similarly, the identification of germline *ARMC5* variants in *KCNJ5*-mutant sporadic aldosterone-producing adenomas {5187,3126} and germline *PDE2A* and *PDE3B* variants in patients with primary aldosteronism {3685} challenge the occurrence of a potential crosslink between functional pathways. Nevertheless, current observations are that PKA-driven (overt adrenal Cushing syndrome) and WNT pathway (non-functioning adenomas or adenomas causing mild autonomous cortisol secretion) dysregulated tumours are often genetically and clinically distinct. These observations have also been reproduced using a pangenomic classifying algorithm, in which PKA-aberrant

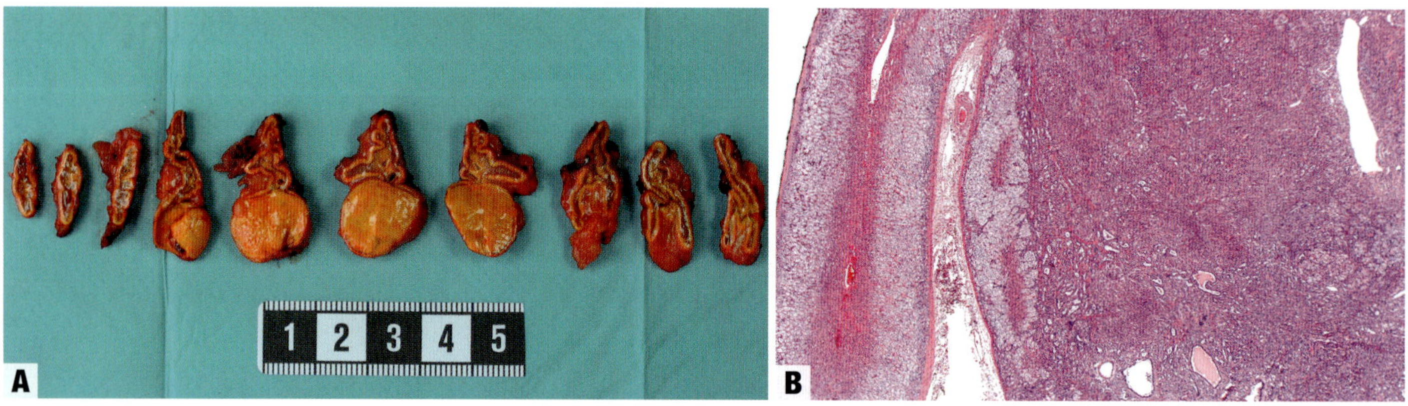

Fig. 5.24 Adrenal cortical adenoma. **A** A 23 mm aldosterone-producing adrenal cortical adenoma. The golden-yellow colour reflects the high lipid content. **B** Adrenal cortical adenomas with primary hyperaldosteronism (Conn syndrome) are not associated with atrophy of the associated adrenal cortex, as is seen in cortisol-producing adrenal cortical adenomas.

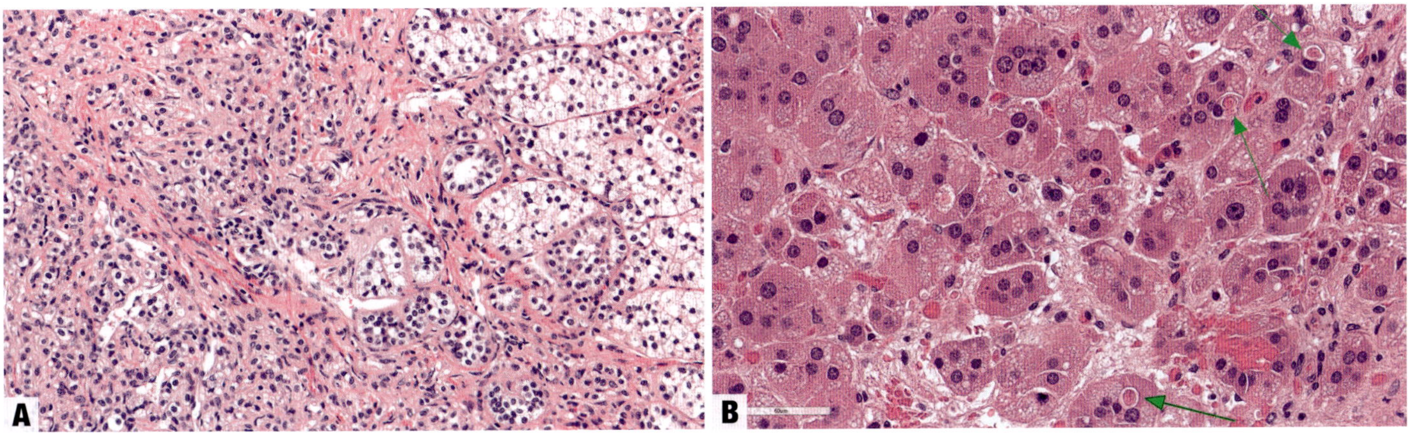

Fig. 5.25 Adrenal cortical adenoma. **A** Aldosterone-secreting adrenal cortical adenomas often have lipid-rich clear cells centrally, with compact cells and zona glomerulosa–type cells at the peripheral aspect of the lesion. **B** An aldosterone-producing adenoma enriched in lipid-poor (compact) cells with variable spironolactone bodies (arrows).

tumours also clustered separately from *CTNNB1*-driven lesions in terms of global mRNA profiles {1318}. In terms of molecular backgrounds, the bulk of evidence argues in favour of distinct chromosome, mutation, expression, and epigenetic patterns in adrenal cortical adenomas versus carcinomas {2141}. Therefore, future multiomics-based algorithms might be of potential clinical utility in separating these entities.

Non-functioning adrenal cortical adenomas

Evidence suggests that most non-functioning adrenal cortical adenomas, especially larger ones, are enriched in *CTNNB1* mutations {1318,2963,3969}.

Sex steroid–producing adrenal cortical adenomas

The molecular pathogenesis of exceptional cases of sex steroid–producing adrenal cortical adenomas is unknown.

Macroscopic appearance

Adrenal cortical adenomas, including non-functioning adenomas, are more commonly unilateral and solitary; however, bilateral multiple tumours occur. Adrenal cortical adenomas are usually solitary, well-circumscribed tumours, measuring ≤ 50 mm and weighing less than 50–100 g {2446,1089}. Aldosterone-producing adrenal cortical adenomas usually have a yellow-gold colour on gross examination due to the prominent lipid-rich zona fasciculata–type clear cells {1916}. Aldosterone-producing adrenal cortical adenomas usually measure ≥ 10 mm, an arbitrary size cut-off point that has been used in the distinction of adenoma from sporadic nodular adrenocortical disease {1916}. Functioning adenomas can be < 10 mm, especially in patients with primary aldosteronism {4887}. Cortisol-producing adrenal cortical adenomas are usually solitary, unilateral, and tan in colour, with atrophy (≤ 2 mm cortical thickness) due to suppression by glucocorticoid excess {1916,3390}. Some adenomas are pigmented (black adenoma) {1916}. Adrenal cortical adenomas with extensive oncocytic change appear orange-brown on cut section {1916}.

Histopathology

Adrenal cortical adenomas are composed of lipid-rich cells resembling the zona fasciculata and compact lipid-poor cells resembling the zona reticularis. Adrenal cortical adenomas are circumscribed and cellular with abundant vasculature. The cells are organized in nests or cords. Reticulin histochemistry often shows a preserved framework {2967}. The tumours can have variable amounts of large oncocytic cells with intensely eosinophilic cytoplasm, with some nearly completely oncocytic, which can be functional but are often non-functional {2951}. Mitotic activity is absent or low, and atypical mitotic figures are generally not seen. Histological features characteristic of malignancy, such as necrosis, high nuclear grade, prominent mitotic activity, atypical mitoses, angioinvasion (venous invasion), lymphatic invasion, and invasive growth (see *Adrenal cortical carcinoma*, p. 246), are not seen. Myelolipomatous and lipomatous change can be seen in adrenal cortical adenomas and is rather frequent in cortisol-producing adenomas, thought to occur as a result of cell senescence by cortisol excess {2325}, without clinical significance. In addition to prominent oncocytic change, myxoid change can be seen in adrenal cortical adenomas {545}. Myxoid change is a concerning feature {545}, and the behaviour of adrenal cortical neoplasms with myxoid change can be difficult to predict with Weiss classification systems {3424}. Pigmented (black) adenomas are composed predominantly or entirely of cells with compact eosinophilic cytoplasm that are similar to, but larger than, cells of the zona reticularis. There is a variable amount of brown or golden-brown pigment (lipofuscin) in the cytoplasm {1916}.

Aldosterone-producing adrenal cortical adenomas are composed of lipid-rich zona fasciculata–type clear cells or compact zona reticularis–like and/or zona glomerulosa–like cells {2963, 2141}. Oncocytic change can be seen in aldosterone-producing adenomas, although oncocytic adrenal cortical adenomas are usually non-functioning {2951}. Spironolactone bodies with concentric laminated concretions are often seen in the zona glomerulosa of aldosterone-producing adenomas in individuals treated with spironolactone {1006,1171,1916}. Confirming the source of aldosterone excess in adrenalectomy specimens can be complicated. Aldosterone-producing cortical lesions can be unifocal or multifocal and unilateral or bilateral, and they may include microscopic clonal nodular proliferations {2141}. Not detected on imaging studies, aldosterone-producing microtumours may be difficult to identify. Therefore, CYP11B2 immunohistochemistry is helpful in the evaluation of the adrenal gland(s) in individuals with primary aldosteronism to identify functional sites of aldosterone production {4887,1171,2141,2963,2959}. *CYP11B2*

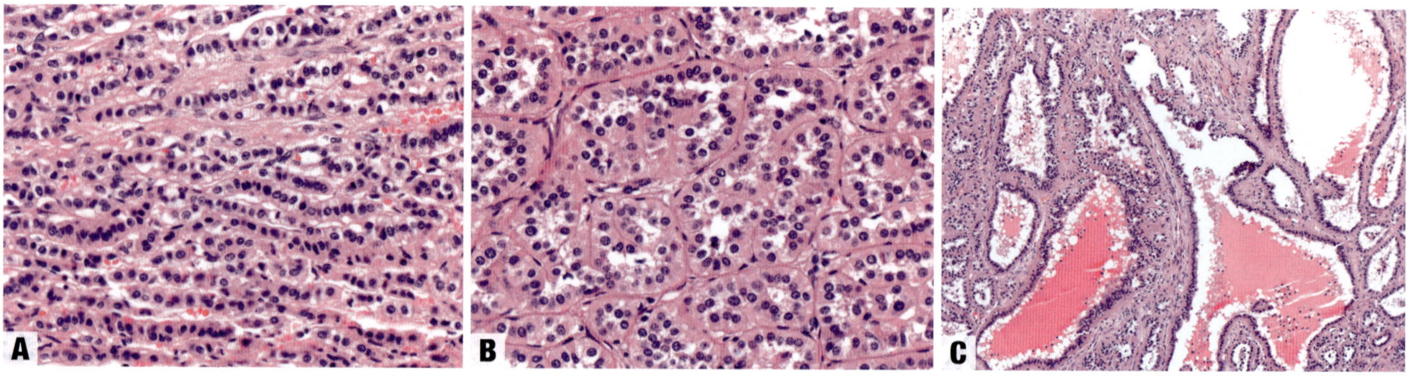

Fig. 5.26 Adrenal cortical adenoma. **A** Although nesting is a very common architectural pattern in aldosterone-secreting adenomas, a variety of patterns can be seen. This lesion has a very prominent pattern of growth of linear cords of cells. **B** This aldosterone-producing adrenal cortical adenoma has a pseudoglandular growth pattern. A variety of patterns and mixtures of patterns can be seen in adrenal cortical adenomas. **C** This aldosterone-producing adrenal cortical adenoma has prominent areas of glandular-like growth.

encodes aldosterone synthase, and ion-channel mutations result in depolarization and subsequent *CYP11B2* transcription {2141,2963,1171,2959,4887}. The recent histopathology of primary aldosteronism (HISTALDO) consensus classification combines the histological evaluation of an adrenal gland with the CYP11B2 staining pattern to identify adrenal nodules and standardize nomenclature to provide a clinically relevant diagnostic approach to reporting unilateral primary aldosteronism specimens {4887}. For instance, a solitary CYP11B2-expressing adenoma or nodule is referred to as classic histology, whereas CYP11B2-positive diffuse hyperplasia and multifocal CYP11B2-positive (micro)nodules are regarded as non-classic histology {4887}. Lack of postoperative biochemical improvement was reported in 42% of patients with non-classic histology, compared with 4.5% of patients with classic histology {4887}. The histological and clinical features of aldosterone-producing adrenal cortical adenomas may correlate with underlying somatic mutations {2141,2963}. Adenomas with wildtype *KCNJ5* are more frequent in male patients and are often small, multifocal, and composed of compact cells, whereas those with *KCNJ5* somatic mutations are more frequent in female patients, usually larger and solitary, and are composed of lipid-rich zona fasciculata–type cells {2141,2963}.

Cortisol-secreting adrenal cortical adenomas are usually solitary, unilateral neoplasms composed of lipid-rich zona fasciculata–like clear cells, but they can have variable amounts of compact cells, oncocytic change, or pigment {1171,2963, 4634}. It is important to recognize the adjacent adrenal cortical atrophy, indicative of autonomous cortisol secretion or exogenous glucocorticoid treatment {2953}.

Differential diagnosis and immunohistochemistry

The main differential diagnosis of adrenal cortical adenomas is with adrenal cortical carcinoma (see *Adrenal cortical carcinoma*, p. 246) and phaeochromocytoma. In the presence of predominant compact or oncocytic cells, the differential diagnosis also includes perivascular epithelioid cell tumours (PEComas; angiomyolipomas) {2978,4528}.

The standard diagnostic classification for distinguishing adrenal cortical adenoma from carcinoma is the Weiss system {4843,4844}, with the Lin–Weiss–Bisceglia system {431} used for neoplasms with > 90% oncocytic cells, and a separate US Armed Forces Institute of Pathology (AFIP) system {4876} used for paediatric adrenal cortical neoplasms. Additional classification systems include the reticulin algorithm {1184,4724} and the Helsinki score {3510,1183} as discussed in *Adrenal cortical carcinoma* (p. 246). Myxoid adrenal cortical neoplasms may be very difficult to classify with the standard Weiss system, and so the possibility of malignant behaviour is difficult to exclude in these neoplasms {3424}.

SF1 is the most reliable biomarker for confirming the cortical origin of an adrenal neoplasm {2959}. Several less specific

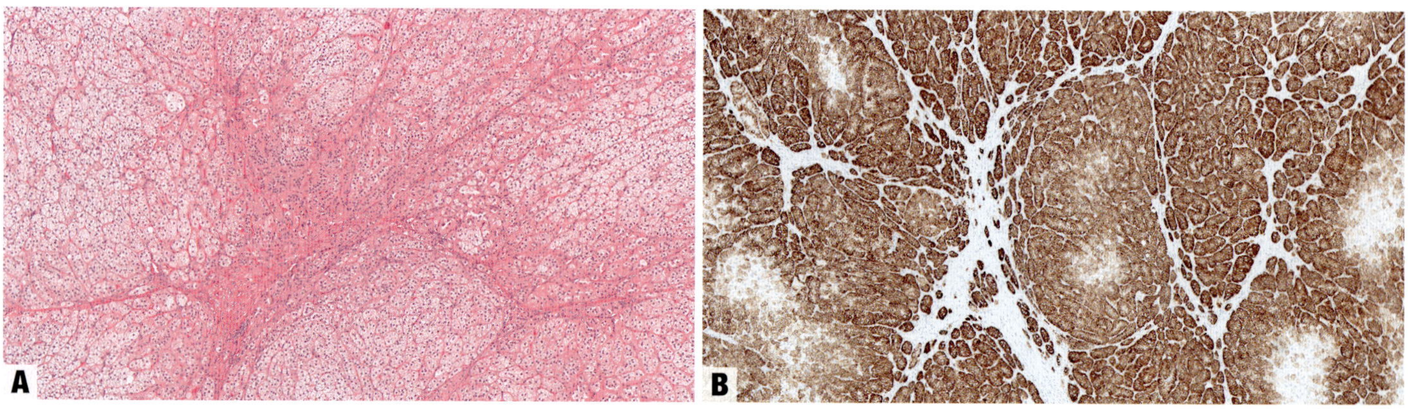

Fig. 5.27 Aldosterone-producing adrenal cortical adenoma. A clear cell–rich aldosterone-producing adrenal cortical adenoma (**A**) with diffuse CYP11B2 expression (**B**). The tumour measured 12 mm grossly.

biomarkers (e.g. melan-A, synaptophysin, α-inhibin, calretinin) may be used in a panel approach, but staining for these markers is also variable {2959}. Synaptophysin {2959} and α-inhibin {2975} can be expressed in phaeochromocytomas. Unlike cortical neoplasms, phaeochromocytomas are positive for INSM1 and/or chromogranin A.

When PEComas/angiomyolipomas are considered, melan-A positivity is often misleading and should be integrated with other PEComa-specific markers, such as HMB45 and SMA {2978}. Clear cell tumours, notably renal cell carcinoma, may metastasize to the adrenal and simulate cytological and architectural features of adrenal cortical adenoma. Immunohistochemistry should be interpreted with caution, because the non-specific renal cell carcinoma marker CD10 may be positive in adrenal cortical adenomas {2970}, and Xp11-translocation renal cell carcinomas can also express melan-A {4959}.

Functional steroidogenic enzyme immunohistochemistry is useful in the assessment of adrenal cortical neoplasms {2959, 1916}; among these, CYP11B2 immunostaining has shown a particular benefit in identifying functional sites in primary aldosteronism {4887,4737,3165,2959,3182,4736}.

Cytology

Smears show small sheets and tissue fragments that may include thin fibrovascular strands, and predominantly single uniform polygonal cells with delicate, granular, or vacuolated cytoplasm; uniform, round nuclei with inconspicuous nucleoli; and occasional variations in cell size and enlarged pleomorphic nuclei consistent with endocrine organ atypia. The cells are fragile, and naked nuclei and lipid vacuoles are prominent in the background. Adrenal gland hyperplasia / benign cortical nodule and adrenal adenoma cannot be distinguished on FNA cytopathology {2106}. The role of FNA in adrenal incidentalomas is contentious {2776}, but FNA (including EUS-FNAB) offers a minimally invasive biopsy of adrenal lesions found in the workup of patients with possible metastatic carcinomas, including lung and pancreas primaries, and can provide material for molecular studies {2229,2106,3578,302}.

Diagnostic molecular pathology

Germline testing for pathogenic variants is considered in the context of clinicopathological findings.

Essential and desirable diagnostic criteria

Essential: an adrenal cortical neoplasm without morphological features of malignancy; non-tumorous cortical atrophy is diagnostic of autonomous cortisol secretion in the absence of exogenous cortisol intake; immunohistochemical confirmation of adrenal cortical origin in all non-functioning adenomas with oncocytic or compact cell changes.

Desirable: CYP11B2 immunohistochemistry in patients with primary aldosteronism.

Staging

Not applicable

Prognosis and prediction

Adrenal cortical adenomas are benign and associated with an excellent prognosis. The evaluation of aldosterone-producing adrenal cortical neoplasms can be more complicated, and CYP11B2 immunostaining is helpful in identifying functional sites in primary aldosteronism and predicting possible biochemical recurrence. Uncontrolled Cushing syndrome is associated with significant mortality and morbidity.

Adrenal cortical carcinoma

Mete O
Assié G
Gill AJ
Juhlin CC
Papotti M
Sasano H
Volante M

Definition

Adrenal cortical carcinoma is a malignant epithelial tumour originating from adrenal cortical cells.

ICD-O coding

8370/3 Adrenal cortical carcinoma
8370/3 Conventional adrenal cortical carcinoma
8370/3 Oncocytic adrenal cortical carcinoma
8370/3 Myxoid adrenal cortical carcinoma
8370/3 Sarcomatoid adrenal cortical carcinoma

ICD-11 coding

XH4KH2 Adrenal cortical carcinoma

Related terminology

Acceptable: adrenocortical carcinoma.

Subtype(s)

Conventional adrenal cortical carcinoma; oncocytic adrenal cortical carcinoma; myxoid adrenal cortical carcinoma; sarcomatoid adrenal cortical carcinoma

Localization

Most adrenal cortical carcinomas manifest with unilateral adrenal gland involvement; however, exceptional examples can occur in heterotopic/ectopic locations such as the retroperitoneum, pelvic region (between the urinary bladder and prostate), and ovary {4939,67,5075,916,3916,4570}. Adrenohepatic fusion/adhesion or heterotopia/ectopia may explain the occurrence of odd examples of hepatic adrenal cortical carcinomas {3524}. For unknown reasons, left adrenal gland involvement has been recorded more frequently {1340,1184}.

Clinical features

Approximately 10–15% of adrenal cortical carcinomas are incidentally detected during imaging studies for unrelated causes {1339}; however, most patients become clinically apparent because of symptoms related to autonomous hormone secretion and/or an abdominal mass {1339,1916}. Hormone secretion occurs in nearly half of the patients {101,1339}. In adults, adrenal virilization/feminization syndrome due to an adrenal mass is generally considered a sign of malignancy {1916}. Autonomous glucocorticoid secretion (adrenal Cushing syndrome) or synchronous glucocorticoid and sex-steroid secretion (Cushing syndrome and virilization/feminization syndrome) accounts for the vast majority of functioning adrenal cortical carcinomas; however, isolated sex-steroid production (often androgen, less frequently estrogen) occurs less frequently than the former functional states {1916,1339}. Primary aldosteronism due to aldosterone-producing adrenal cortical carcinomas is rare {1669,3113,3095,4887}.

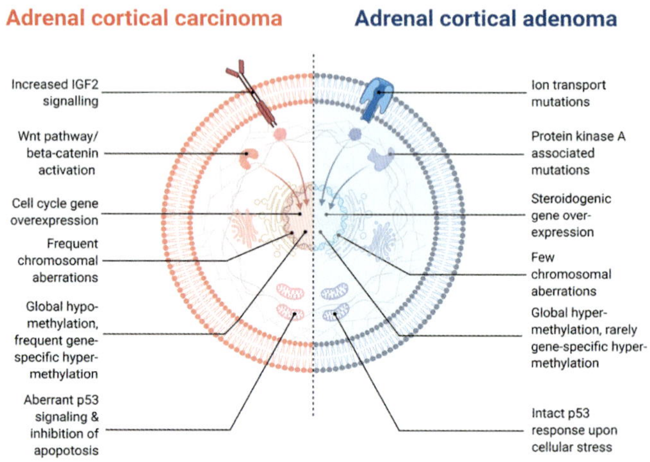

Fig. 5.28 Molecular attributes of adrenal cortical carcinoma and adenoma. Mechanisms underlying the development of adrenal cortical carcinomas (depicted to the left, in red) include overexpression of IGF2 and mutations in the WNT and p53 signalling pathways. Cell cycle–related genes are often upregulated, and chromosomal aberrations (usually deletions) are plentiful. Adrenal cortical carcinomas are furthermore characterized by global hypomethylation but increased promoter-specific hypermethylation, as opposed to adrenal cortical adenoma (right, in blue). In turn, adrenal cortical adenomas often lack WNT and p53 pathway mutations but instead exhibit mutations in genes encoding various ion channels (*KCNJ5*, *ATP1A1*, *ATP2B3*, *CACNA1D*, and *CACNA1H*) and in genes regulating PKA-related pathways (*PRKACA* and *PRKAR1A*). The transcriptome is overrepresented in genes associated with steroidogenesis, and chromosomal aberrations are few.

Patients with hypercortisolism often develop several signs of Cushing syndrome, including central obesity, muscle weakness, easy bruising, fatigue, and depression {52,1167}, but mild autonomous glucocorticoid secretion (subclinical Cushing syndrome) can also occur in adrenal cortical carcinomas {3825}. Also, related clinical signs such as hypertension, osteoporosis, metabolic syndrome, and diabetes mellitus may exist. Many possible clinicopathological conditions must be taken into consideration in the clinical workup of patients with Cushing syndrome {1167, 2141}, but markedly rapid-onset symptoms with accentuated hypertension and poorly regulated blood glucose with increased precursor steroids (e.g. DHEAS) may be clues to an underlying cortisol-producing adrenal cortical carcinoma {1001}. Female patients with androgen-secreting adrenal cortical carcinomas may exhibit clinical signs of virilization, whereas the hormonal excess might be masked in men (but not in children) because of the higher testosterone levels produced from the testes {1220}. In rare instances of estrogen production, the inverse might be true, with male patients having gynaecomastia and adult female patients being relatively asymptomatic {4947,3090}.

Apart from symptoms related to hormone excess, the second most common presentation is attributable to nonspecific signs of mass effect, when the tumour growth compresses nearby

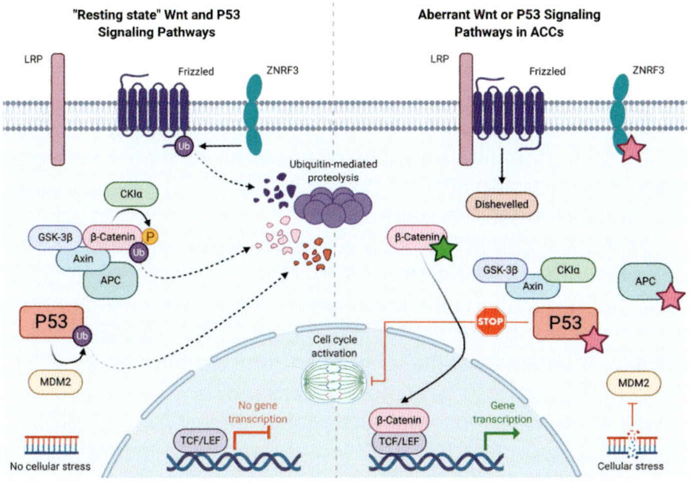

Fig. 5.29 WNT and p53 pathways in adrenal cortical carcinoma. Schematic representation of the WNT and p53 pathways in resting states and in adrenal cortical carcinoma. In its idle state, the WNT pathway main effector β-catenin is sent for ubiquitin-mediated proteolysis by a trimolecular complex (APC, GSK3β, and AXIN), and the p53 protein is regulated negatively in a similar manner by MDM2 (left). Adrenal cortical carcinomas recurrently demonstrate activating *CTNNB1* (β-catenin) mutations (green star), which allows β-catenin to escape degradation and instead transport to the nucleus, where it will initiate transcription of WNT target genes, in turn promoting proliferation. This can also be achieved by inactivating mutations or deletions of the negative WNT regulators *ZNRF3* and *APC* (pink stars). Upon cellular stress (e.g. extensive DNA damage), MDM2-mediated inhibition of p53 is lifted, leading to the activation of p53, which will promote DNA repair and apoptosis. However, in adrenal cortical carcinoma with inactivating *TP53* gene mutations (pink star), this process is inhibited, leading to inhibited proliferation and accumulation of additional DNA damage.

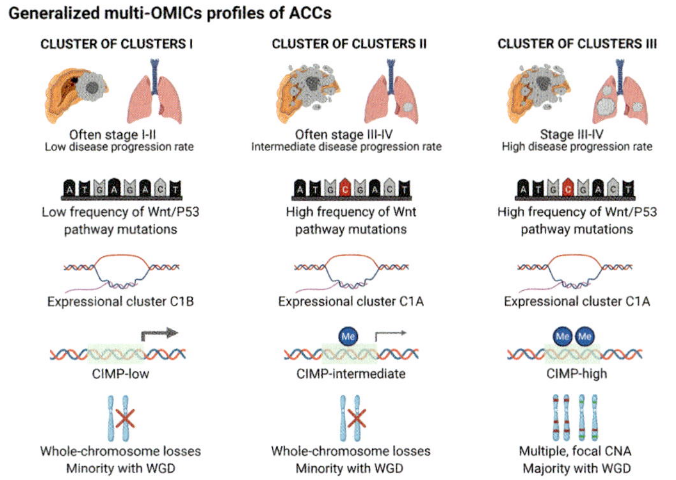

Fig. 5.30 Generalized multiomics profiles of adrenal cortical carcinoma (ACC). Via the pangenomic characterization of the mutational, chromosomal, expressional, and epigenetic landscapes of ACC, three main clusters have emerged, called cluster of clusters I–III (CoC I–III). CoC I ACCs exhibit the best prognosis of the three and are regularly associated with lower TNM stages. These tumours are characterized by a low frequency of mutations in WNT and p53 signalling pathway genes and associate to the mRNA expressional cluster C1B enriched for genes regulating immune response mechanisms. Furthermore, CoC I ACCs exhibit low levels of gene-specific methylation and are therefore characterized as CpG island methylator phenotype – low. Amplifications and whole-chromosome deletions are commonly seen, but whole-genome doubling (WGD) is rare. CoC II ACCs are considered an intermediate group of tumours in terms of prognosis and genetic aberrancies. CoC III ACCs exhibit the worst prognosis and the most advanced genetic imbalances; they are characterized by frequent mutations in WNT and p53 pathway gene members, expression of genes primarily associated to mitotic regulation (cluster C1A), and a high CpG island methylator phenotype. Chromosomal aberrations are frequent and scattered across the genome (noisy), and WGD is evident in the majority of CoC III ACCs.

structures {1338,1339}. Abdominal and/or flank pain are commonly encountered. Especially in non-functioning tumours, metastasis-related symptoms may be the initial finding at the time of diagnosis.

Most adrenal cortical carcinomas are distinguished from adenomas on CT because the former usually show a higher Hounsfield density (often > 10 Hounsfield units), heterogeneous CT contrast washout, a larger tumour size (often > 40 mm), and the presence of heterogenic appearances suggestive of necrosis and/or haemorrhage {2321,1916}. In addition, a heterogeneous signal drop on chemical-shift MRI can be useful. Functional imaging studies with FDG PET can provide additional value for the prediction of malignancy risk in adrenal cortical neoplasms (e.g. tumour-to-liver maximum standardized uptake value ratio: > 1.5), because in general most carcinomas have a higher uptake of glucose {3912}, but exceptions such as oncocytic adenomas exist.

Adrenal cortical carcinomas are usually larger than their benign counterparts, with median sizes ranging from 80 to 100 mm {102,2657,2406}. Because the clinical diagnosis of hormonally inactive carcinomas may be delayed {2831}, they might occasionally reach impressive proportions (380 mm) {1183}. Adrenal cortical carcinoma may infiltrate the periadrenal fat and adjacent organs (e.g. kidney, liver, spleen, large veins) {2845}. Regional lymph node metastases are common, and distant metastatic sites include the lungs, bone, liver, and brain {4241}.

Epidemiology

Adrenal cortical carcinoma accounts for the majority of deaths attributable to primary adrenal neoplasia. The annual incidence is 0.7–2 cases per 1 million USA inhabitants, affecting mostly female patients, with a broad age span (peaking in the fifth and sixth decades of life) {2650,4936}. In the paediatric population, girls are also more frequently affected, and age at the time of diagnosis ranges from 1.5 to 16 years {5113}. In adult patients, although the vast majority of cases are sporadic, with no known family history, subsets of affected patients are associated with one of several germline susceptibility syndromes (see *Pathogenesis*) {1237}. For instance, the prevalence of germline *TP53* p.R337H variants in 0.3% of the general population in southern Brazil may explain the higher frequency of adrenal cortical carcinoma in that geographical area with more frequent paediatric manifestations {1557}.

Etiology

Besides the well-established genetic susceptibility syndromes (see *Pathogenesis*) {2141}, cigarette smoking {5160, 5090,1730,1972} and oral contraceptive use (especially before the age of 25 years) {1972} have been suggested as risk factors for these tumours. A recent review of SEER Program data from 2001 to 2016 underscored the association between tobacco use and adrenal cortical neoplasia {5090}. Another study showed that a family history of cancer in general was associated with a risk of adrenal cortical carcinoma in both sexes, whereas alcohol consumption was associated with reduced risk in men {1730}.

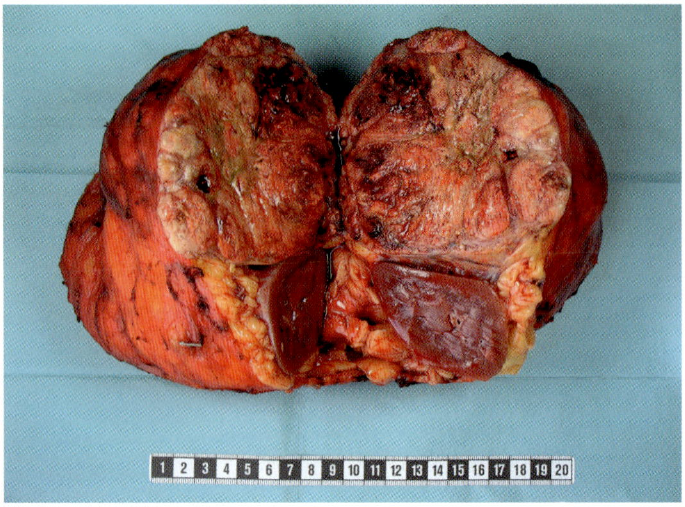

Fig. 5.31 Adrenal cortical carcinoma. The cut surface of the tumour shows a yellowish-tan variegated appearance with necrosis and haemorrhage. The tumour shows no direct invasion into the kidney.

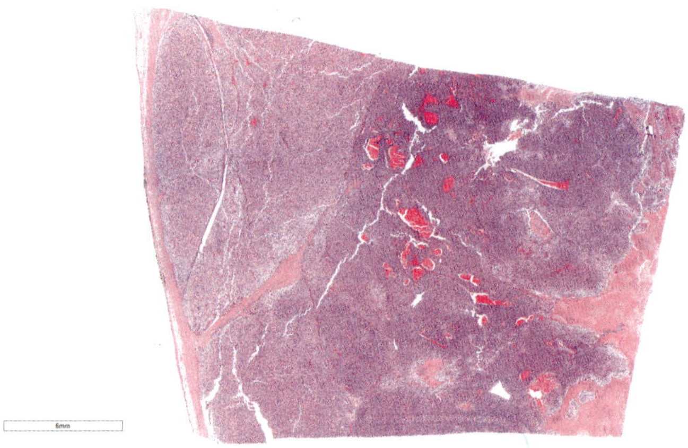

Fig. 5.32 Adrenal cortical carcinoma. An example with diffuse solid and broad trabecular growth with tumour necrosis.

Pathogenesis

Adrenal cortical carcinoma mainly develops through the somatic acquisition of genetic alterations, leading to the activation of certain signalling pathways that promote proliferation {2141, 4721}. In adults, 90% of cases are sporadic, and the remainder are related to genetic susceptibility (see below).

Pathways and processes affected by common driver alterations in adrenal cortical carcinoma include (1) the WNT signalling pathway (e.g. *CTNNB1* mutations and *ZNRF3* deletions), (2) cell-cycle regulation (e.g. *TP53*, *RB1*, *MDM2*, *CDK4*, and *CDKN2A* mutations), (3) chromosome maintenance / chromatin remodelling (*DAXX*, *ATRX*, *MEN1*, and *TERT* mutations, as well as *TERF2* amplifications), and (4) the PKA pathway (*PRKAR1A* mutation) {5160,1061,3390}. Aldosterone-producing adrenal cortical carcinomas lack the aldosterone-driver mutations identified in aldosterone-producing adenomas {3113}.

Inactivating *TP53* mutations are reported in approximately one fifth of all adrenal cortical carcinomas, thus constituting the most common mutational event {2141}. *TP53* encodes p53, an established tumour suppressor that induces apoptosis when triggered by environmental stress and DNA damage, and the importance of this signalling network is further accentuated by the finding of mutations in *RB1* and *CDKN2A* in additional cases {237}. Somatic mutations in other genes traditionally associated with the development of hereditary syndromes, such as *PRKAR1A*, *MSH2*, *APC*, *MEN1*, and *NF1*, are also reported {237}. Apart from the regulation of apoptosis and cell-cycle progression described above, genetic alterations in genes regulating the WNT signalling pathway are commonly noted in adrenal cortical carcinomas, not least *CTNNB1* mutations and *ZNRF3* mutations and deletions {4510,237,2145}. Interestingly, *TP53* or WNT pathway alterations are often mutually exclusive, but both are enriched in poor-prognostic tumours {237,2145,5160}. Additionally, mutations in the chromatin-remodelling genes *ATRX* and *DAXX* have also been established {237}.

Regarding chromosomal alterations, three types of profiles have been reported: (1) extended chromosome losses reflecting uniparental isodisomy (50% of tumours; variable outcome), with potential duplication of the remaining genome; (2) numerous non-recurrent alterations, with various levels of ploidy (50% of tumours; poorer outcome); (3) almost normal chromosomal structure, with a limited number of alterations (rare; better outcome). Beyond these general profiles, loss of the maternal 11p15 allele is one of the most common findings in these tumours {1863,1569}. This genomic region contains the imprinted tumour suppressor gene *H19* and oncogene *IGF2*, which are expressed from maternal and paternal alleles respectively.

Epigenetically, these tumours show various levels of DNA methylation in CpG islands of gene promoter regions. Hypermethylation in these regions is associated with a poorer outcome {2134,323,3059}.

The past few decades have seen extensive genomic studies including transcriptome and next-generation sequencing analyses on adrenal cortical carcinoma that yielded several molecular subclasses/clusters with prognostic relevance {5160,1592, 1594,1017,1035,323,237,2145}. The most validated algorithm to date divides tumours into two principal classes, based upon the mutation signatures, mRNA expression profiles, DNA methylation patterns, and copy-number landscape {237,5160,236}. By these stratifications, a group of tumours are characterized by a low disease-progression rate. These cases seldom exhibit *TP53* or WNT pathway mutations, adhere to an mRNA expression cluster traditionally associated with a more indolent disease that exhibits low levels of gene-specific methylation (low CpG island methylator phenotype), and do not display whole-genome doubling. On the other hand, the other subgroup of adrenal cortical carcinomas represent high-risk cases with frequent *TP53* and WNT pathway gene mutations, an expression pattern often associated with a worse outcome, recurrent CpG island methylation (high CpG island methylator phenotype), and numerous non-recurrent alterations with (potentially) whole-genome doubling.

The identification of mutation signatures of smoking and mismatch repair deficiency in some cases further linked these tumours to tobacco use and Lynch syndrome {5160}.

Genetic susceptibility

Li–Fraumeni syndrome is caused by germline inactivating *TP53* gene mutations, and this alteration is noted in 50–80% of paediatric cases of adrenal cortical carcinoma, as well as in 3–5% of adult cases {1237,2141,4758,4824,2924,3699}. Adrenal cortical carcinoma is also represented in patients with Lynch syndrome {2924,3699,1132}, Carney complex {405,1282,3094}, familial adenomatous polyposis {1518,2840,4193}, Beckwith–Wiedemann syndrome {408,1863}, multiple endocrine neoplasia type 1 {566,1517,2523,4181,4760,4180}, neurofibromatosis type 1 {2943,4757}, and possibly subsets of the familial paraganglioma phaeochromocytoma syndromes {1236}. Isolated reports have expanded the association of adrenal cortical carcinoma with germline pathogenic variants of *ATM* {4529}, *CHEK2* {4962}, *MUTYH* {3558}, *FH* (hereditary leiomyomatosis and renal cell carcinoma syndrome) {1710}, *FLCN* {1926}, and *EGFR* (especially in adolescents and young adults) {62}, as well as synchronous *MSH2* and *RET* variants (without multiple endocrine neoplasia type 2) {3697}.

Macroscopic appearance

Adrenal cortical carcinomas are often large, solitary, heterogeneous tumours that weigh > 100 g. However, smaller tumours (≤ 20 mm) can occur {1184,1183}. The cut surface shows a yellowish-tan variegated appearance, with nodularity that may reflect intratumoural heterogeneity. Necrosis and haemorrhage are frequent in high-grade tumours. Gross extension into large veins, extra-adrenal adipose tissue, and adjacent organs is a feature of stage III and stage IV disease.

Histopathology

The diagnosis of adrenal cortical carcinoma is based on invasive growth (e.g. angioinvasion, capsular invasion, local gross invasion), increased proliferative activity, and a combination of cytological and architectural features. The histological features are usually assessed with one of several multifactorial algorithms / scoring systems {4843,243,431,1184,4724,3510}. No single system has been shown to be completely sensitive or specific in all settings.

Unlike adenomas, adrenal cortical carcinomas often show solid, broad trabecular, or large nested growth. The latter is reflected in a loss of reticulin framework on Gordon–Sweet silver histochemistry {1184,2967}, which is also a requirement of the reticulin algorithm {1184,1404}. Variable qualitative reticulin alterations (e.g. pericellular mesh-like staining) can feature in benign and malignant adrenal cortical neoplasms; however, qualitative reticulin alterations in association with a loss of the reticulin framework is a feature of adrenal cortical carcinoma {2967}. It is important to recognize sites of degeneration or haemorrhage that may show a disrupted reticulin framework {1916}.

Tumour invasion (e.g. capsular invasion, lymphatic invasion, vascular invasion) is assessed at the tumour periphery, in and around the tumour capsule {1591,2967,1916}. The demonstration of bona fide vascular invasion is a highly reliable criterion of malignancy and stands out as one of the diagnostic criteria that is of prognostic significance {2967}. Vascular invasion often involves veins and is characterized by tumour cells invading through a vessel wall and/or intravascular tumour cells admixed with thrombus/fibrin {2967,1591}; however, gross invasion into a large vessel can occur in advanced-stage disease.

Adrenal cortical carcinoma is a proliferation-driven malignancy, a finding that has been supported on numerous genomic studies. Therefore, the assessment of proliferative activity using both mitotic count {4844,2967,4843,243,431,1184,3510,3420,

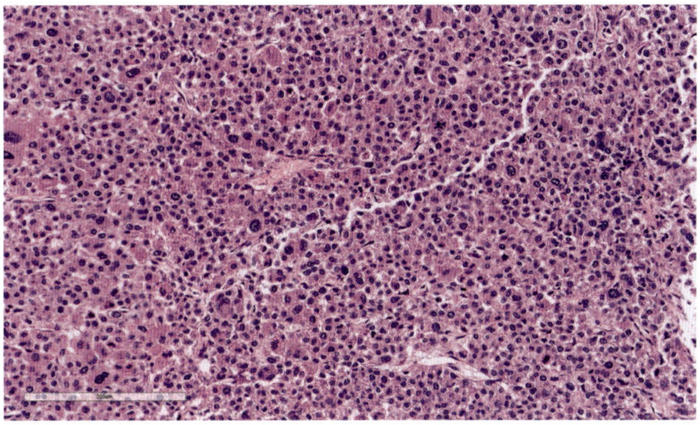

Fig. 5.33 Adrenal cortical carcinoma. A conventional adrenal cortical carcinoma enriched in compact tumour cells with diffuse growth, variable cytological atypia, and an atypical mitotic figure.

4656} and Ki-67 immunohistochemistry {2861,3548,2967,4288, 184,4230,4755} is important for the diagnostic workup and prognostication of these tumours {1591,1916,2962}.

An increased mitotic activity, defined as > 5 mitoses/10 mm^2 (50 HPF of 0.2 mm^2), has been incorporated in all diagnostic algorithms {1958,3420,3510,4656,4843}. Proliferative heterogeneity can occur in these tumours; therefore, the mitotic count is assessed in 10 mm^2 from areas with highest mitotic density. Phosphohistone H3 immunohistochemistry may help highlight mitoses in carcinomas with a low mitotic count {1185}. Atypical

Table 5.02 Weiss scoring system

Parameter	Score
High Fuhrman nuclear grade (III or IV)	1
Mitotic count: > 5 mitoses/10 mm^2 (50 HPF of 0.2 mm^2)	1
Atypical mitosis	1
Necrosis	1
Diffuse architecture > 30% of tumour volume	1
Clear cells ≤ 25% of tumour volume	1
Capsular invasion	1
Venous invasion (vascular invasion)	1
Sinusoidal (lymphatic) invasion	1
Total score[a]	**9**

[a]A total score of ≥ 3 indicates malignancy.

Table 5.03 Modified Weiss system

Parameter	Score
Mitotic count: > 5 mitoses/10 mm^2 (50 HPF of 0.2 mm^2)	2
Clear cells in ≤ 25%	2
Atypical mitosis	1
Necrosis	1
Capsular invasion	1
Total score[a]	**7**

[a]A total score of ≥ 3 indicates malignancy.

Box 5.02 Lin–Weiss–Bisceglia criteria for oncocytic adrenal cortical neoplasms

Major criteria:
Mitotic count: > 5 mitoses/10 mm^2 (50 HPF of 0.2 mm^2)
Atypical mitosis
Venous invasion

Minor criteria:
Large size (> 100 mm and/or > 200 g)
Necrosis
Capsular invasion
Sinusoidal invasion

Malignant: At least one major criterion

Uncertain malignant potential: At least one minor criterion

Benign: Absence of major and minor criteria

Box 5.03 Reticulin algorithm

Criteria:

Altered reticulin framework in association with one of the following features indicates malignancy:

- Mitotic count: > 5 mitoses/10 mm^2 (50 HPF of 0.2 mm^2)
- Tumour necrosis
- Vascular invasion

mitotic figures are also important findings suggestive of abnormal chromosome content (aneuploidy) {3951}.

Traditionally, adrenal cortical carcinomas are subdivided on the basis of mitotic activity into low-grade (≤ 20 mitoses/10 mm^2) and high-grade (> 20 mitoses/10 mm^2) {1590,4844}, and this approach has shown prognostic value {4844,2967}. The optimal cut-off point for paediatric adrenal cortical carcinomas remains to be validated {2962}.

Studies assessing Ki-67 immunohistochemistry in adrenal cortical carcinomas have shown that most carcinomas have a Ki-67 labelling index > 5% {3548,2861,2967,4288,184,4230,4755}. In adrenal cortical carcinomas, the Ki-67 index has been regarded as a prognostic biomarker {2861,2967,3548,1185,413}, and it can also help rationalize the need for adjuvant mitotane therapy {1339,2959}. Given the critical value of this biomarker, manual counting or automated image analysis algorithms should be applied in the assessment of the Ki-67 proliferation index {2959,1591,2746,3414,5010}.

Punctate/comedo-type or geographical necrosis is frequently seen in high-grade carcinomas. In fact, the most recently proposed Helsinki scoring system weighted the importance of this finding by combining with increased mitosis and Ki-67 labelling index {3510}.

The well-recognized histological subtypes, in decreasing order of frequency, are oncocytic, myxoid, and sarcomatoid carcinomas {1062}. Oncocytic carcinomas require > 90% of the tumour to be composed of oncocytic cells {431,1591} and should not be assessed with the Weiss system because of their eosinophilic cytoplasm, diffuse growth pattern, and high-grade nuclei (see Table 5.02 and Table 5.03, p. 249). The Lin–Weiss–Bisceglia system has been applied to these tumours {431} (see Box 5.02), but the Helsinki score and reticulin algorithm can also be used {3510,1183,1184,1591} (see Box 5.03 and Table 5.04).

Myxoid carcinomas have abundant extracellular connective tissue mucin {1971,3424,2103}. In myxoid carcinomas, some Weiss parameters (e.g. diffuse growth pattern, lymphatic invasion, and

Table 5.04 Helsinki scoring system

Parameter	Score[a]
Mitotic count: > 5 mitoses/10 mm^2 (50 HPF of 0.2 mm^2)	3
Necrosis	5
Ki-67 proliferation index (%)	Numerical value of the Ki-67 index from the highest proliferative area

[a]Score of 0–8.5: benign; > 8.5: malignant; > 17: adverse prognosis.

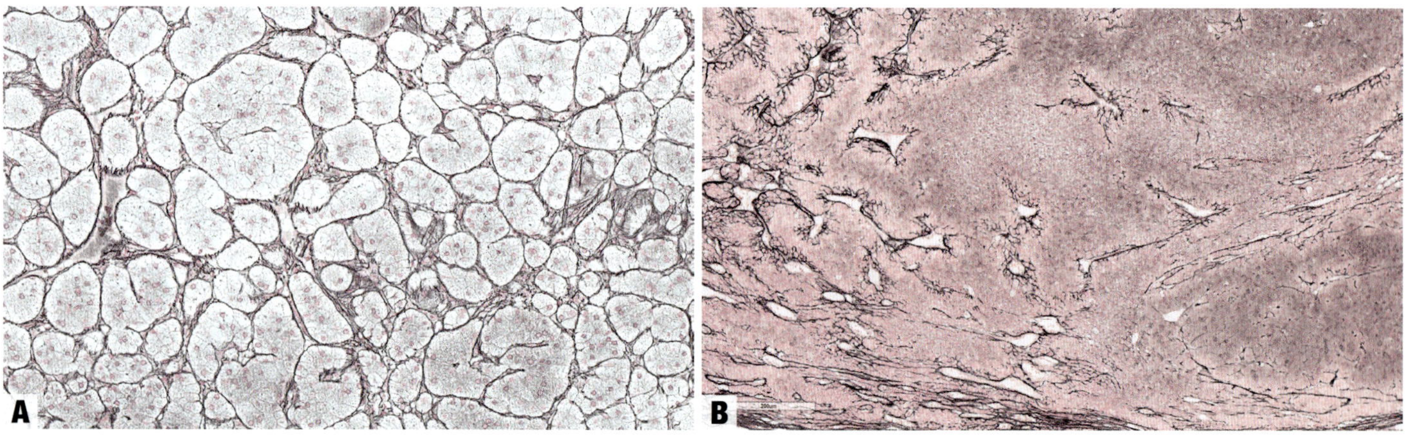

Fig. 5.34 Reticulin histochemistry in adrenal cortical tumours. **A** Adrenal cortical adenomas show a preserved nested reticulin framework (Gordon–Sweet silver). **B** Unlike adrenal cortical adenomas, adrenal cortical carcinomas show a loss of reticulin framework (Gordon–Sweet silver).

nuclear atypia) may be absent or difficult to assess, thus increasing the risk of an underdiagnosis of malignancy.

Sarcomatoid carcinomas show loss of cortical differentiation {3409,5160} and can be biphasic with typical differentiated areas; when monophasic, these tumours can be indistinguishable from true sarcomas of the adrenal {1831} and retroperitoneal sarcomas involving the adrenal gland {5160}.

The classification of paediatric tumours is a common challenge {1057} and requires the application of the US Armed Forces Institute of Pathology (AFIP) criteria {4876} (see Table 5.05, p. 252). The application of Ki-67 with a cut-off point of 15% has been suggested in the workup of paediatric adrenal cortical tumours {2861,3548}.

Diagnostic biomarker studies

The differential diagnosis of adrenal cortical carcinoma includes adrenal cortical adenoma (including oncocytic adenomas), phaeochromocytoma, renal cell carcinoma, hepatocellular carcinoma, sarcoma, metastatic melanoma, and other metastases (lung, colorectal, and bladder). The confirmation of the cortical origin of a non-functioning adrenal neoplasm is usually considered {2959}. SF1 is the most reliable biomarker for confirming the cortical origin {2959}. Several less specific biomarkers (e.g. melan-A, synaptophysin, α-inhibin, and calretinin) may be used in a panel approach, but staining for these markers is also variable {2959}. Synaptophysin {2959} and α-inhibin {2975} can be expressed in phaeochromocytomas. EMA, CEA, and other common transcription factors are generally negative, and variable keratin expression can occur.

Adrenal cortical carcinomas with invasive growth or high-grade features often do not pose a diagnostic challenge; however, the distinction of low-grade adrenal cortical carcinomas confined to the adrenal gland and carcinomas with adenoma-like regions may require the use of ancillary biomarkers in addition to the accepted multifactorial systems {2967,2959,2141}. Rare cases with equivocal features may sometimes be diagnosed as adrenal cortical neoplasm of uncertain malignant potential. Although an increased Ki-67 index (often > 5%) and overexpression of p53 can be helpful in some cases {2959, 2967}, IGF2 paranuclear immunoreactivity has been shown to be the most reliable translational biomarker in the distinction of adrenal cortical carcinomas from adenomas {2967,4006,4230}.

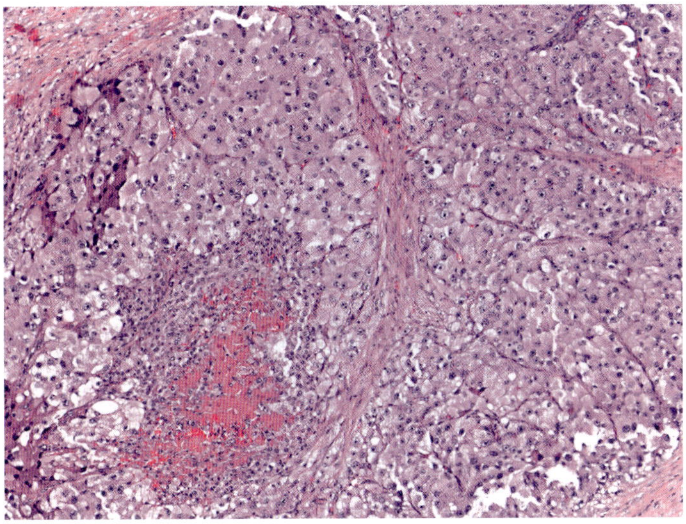

Fig. 5.35 Oncocytic adrenal cortical carcinoma. An oncocytic adrenal cortical carcinoma with focal comedonecrosis.

Molecular studies can also help in the distinction of carcinoma {1592,1594,1035,5160,236}.

Cytology

Cytological assessment may be considered in the distinction of metastatic disease from an adrenal cortical neoplasm. Smears are usually cellular, with well-differentiated carcinomas indistinguishable from adenomas, whereas high-grade carcinomas show necrosis, marked nuclear pleomorphism and hyperchromasia, macronucleoli, and mitoses {3723}. FNAB including EUS-FNAB offers a minimally invasive biopsy of adrenal lesions found in the workup of patients with possible metastatic carcinomas, including lung and pancreas primaries, and can provide material for molecular studies {2229, 2106,3578,302}.

Diagnostic molecular pathology

The diagnosis of malignancy can be rendered using molecular testing of an adrenal cortical neoplasm {1592,1594,1035, 5160,236}; however, molecular tests are not used in standard clinical practice. Molecular characterization of adrenal

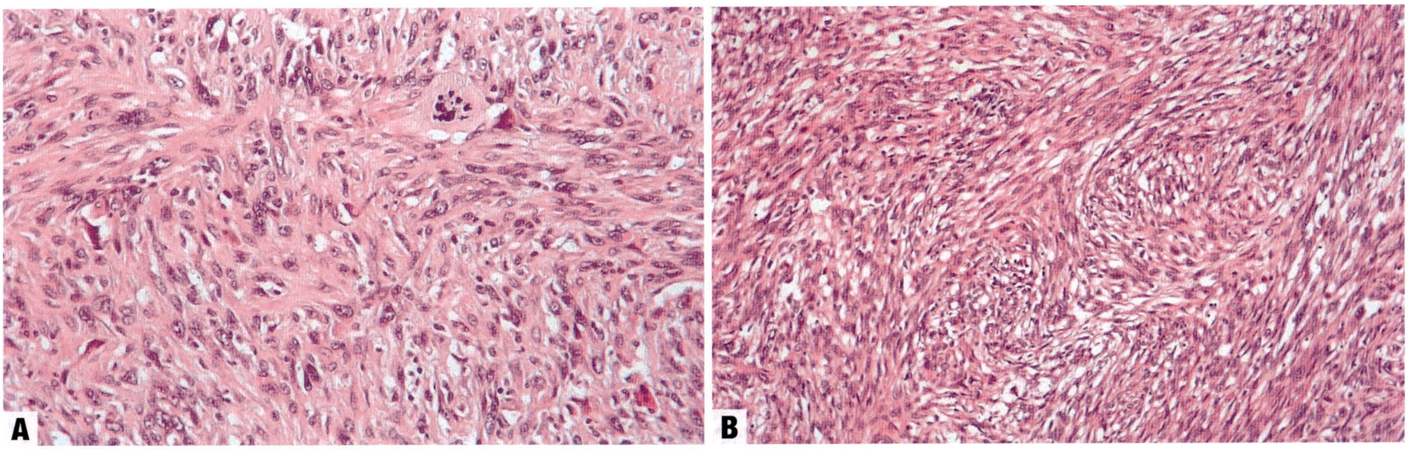

Fig. 5.36 Sarcomatoid adrenal cortical carcinoma. These can be biphasic with typical differentiated areas (**A**), or they can have a monophasic appearance that can simulate a sarcoma (**B**).

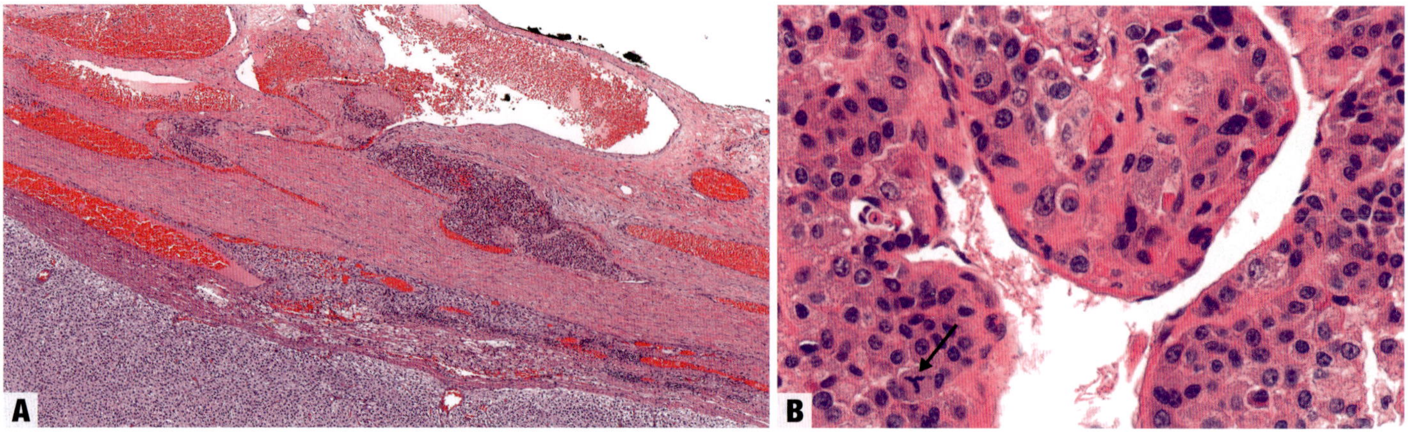

Fig. 5.37 Adrenal cortical carcinoma. **A** Foci of venous angioinvasion (vascular invasion) in adrenal cortical carcinoma are characterized by intravascular tumour cells admixed with fibrin/thrombus. **B** In adrenal cortical carcinomas, atypical mitotic figures (arrow) are important findings suggestive of abnormal chromosome content.

cortical carcinomas has shown promise in the prognostication of patients with adrenal cortical carcinomas (see *Pathogenesis* and *Prognosis and prediction*) {236,2141,5160,3059,2134}.

Essential and desirable diagnostic criteria

Essential: morphological and/or immunohistochemical evidence of adrenal cortical differentiation, and evidence of malignancy usually based on a multiparameter scoring system (see note below); mitotic tumour grading and Ki-67 immunohistochemistry.

Desirable: confirmation of adrenal cortical differentiation using SF1; application of prognostic biomarkers.

Note: fulfils one of the established multiparameter scoring systems for malignancy, including:

- Conventional adrenal cortical neoplasms in adults (one of the following): Weiss score ≥ 3, modified Weiss score ≥ 3, Helsinki score > 8.5, reticulin algorithm
- Oncocytic adrenal cortical neoplasms (one of the following): Lin–Weiss–Bisceglia (any major criterion), Helsinki score > 8.5, reticulin algorithm
- Paediatric adrenal cortical neoplasms: AFIP criteria score ≥ 4

Table 5.05 US Armed Forces Institute of Pathology (AFIP) criteria for paediatric adrenal cortical neoplasms

Parameter	Score
Tumour weight > 400 g	1
Tumour size > 105 mm	1
Extension into periadrenal soft tissue or adjacent organs	1
Invasion into vena cava	1
Vascular invasion	1
Capsular invasion	1
Presence of tumour necrosis	1
Mitotic count > 15 mitoses/4 mm^2 (20 HPF of 0.2 mm^2)	1
Presence of atypical mitosis	1
Total score[a]	**9**

[a]A total score of ≥ 4 indicates malignancy / poor clinical outcome; 3, uncertain malignant potential; ≤ 2; benign behaviour.

Staging

Tumour staging is based on the American Joint Committee on Cancer (AJCC) / Union for International Cancer Control (UICC) TNM system or the European Network for the Study of Adrenal Tumours (ENSAT) staging system.

Prognosis and prediction

Advanced tumour stage, lack of completeness of tumour excision, tumour functionality, angioinvasion, high mitotic tumour grade, high Ki-67 proliferation index (see below), and molecular characteristics (e.g. methylome, microRNAome, transcriptome profiling) of an adrenal cortical carcinoma are considered important dynamic risk factors {2406,2321,1339,2967,4844, 2959,3510,2861,3548,1185,413,1035,1592,236}.

Angioinvasion is a well-recognized adverse feature, and it also stands as the best predictor of disease-free survival in patients with low-grade adrenal cortical carcinomas {2967}. In terms of the Ki-67 labelling index, some clinical series have considered risk categorization based on 3-tiered Ki-67 cut-off points such as < 10%, 10–19%, and ≥ 20%; or < 20%, 20–50%, and > 50% {1185,413}; however, recent evidence suggests that a Ki-67 index of > 15% is a reliable biomarker for predicting a poor outcome in adult and paediatric tumours {2861,3548}. A Helsinki score of > 17 also correlates with a poor prognosis {3510}.

Molecular studies have underscored the role of p53 and β-catenin as prognostic biomarkers, because most carcinomas with adverse molecular clusters tend to show nuclear β-catenin expression and/or aberrant p53 staining (overexpression or global loss) {2141,2959}. For this reason, the application of both p53 and β-catenin immunohistochemistry may help risk stratification, in addition to Ki-67 and mitotic count. Besides the mitotic count and Ki-67 index, other cell cycle–related biomarkers (e.g. BUB1B, HURP, and NEK2) showed correlation with adrenal cortical carcinomas {2967}. Other correlates of a poorer clinical outcome include a high expression of SF1 {1187,3975} and loss of *ATRX* and *ZNRF3* expression {540}.

Mismatch repair immunohistochemistry is considered to screen for the possibility of Lynch syndrome–related adrenal cortical carcinomas {3699,1132,2959,2141}; however, the combination of mismatch repair and PDL1 immunohistochemistry also helps determine eligibility for immunotherapy in select patients {172,1532}.

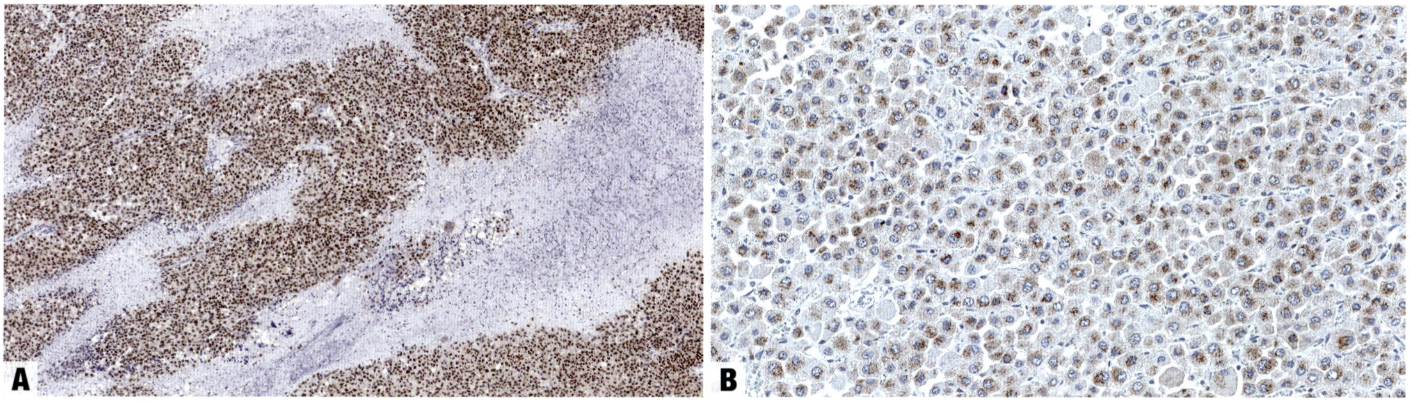

Fig. 5.38 Adrenal cortical carcinoma. **A** SF1 is the most reliable biomarker for confirming the cortical origin. Diffuse nuclear SF1 expression is seen here in an adrenal cortical carcinoma. Note the absence of nuclear reactivity at sites of necrosis. **B** IGF2 paranuclear immunoreactivity has been shown as the most reliable translational biomarker in the distinction of adrenal cortical carcinoma from adenomas.

Several candidate biomarkers (e.g. RRM1 and CYP2W1) for mitotane response have been identified {4735,3807}, but none of these have been validated for clinical practice at this time.

Transcriptome {1035,1592} and pangenomic {237} studies clearly underscored the role of molecular risk stratification in adrenal cortical carcinomas {236}. The expression of two genes, *BUB1B* and *PINK1*, predicted prognosis {1035}. A specific methylation signature has been established in adrenal cortical carcinoma with a particularly poor prognosis, suggesting that methylation patterns may predict clinical outcomes {323}. There is also evidence suggesting a role for the dysregulation of microRNA in adrenal cortical carcinoma, for example the downregulation of miR-195 and overexpression of miR-483-5p, which were identified in cases with increased mortality {4231}. Moreover, low and high circulating levels of miR-195 and miR-483-5p, respectively, have been detected in adrenal cortical carcinoma patients with shorter survival times {730}. Although not yet easily translated into the clinical routine workup of adrenal cortical carcinomas, hypermethylation of *G0S2* is strongly associated with the high CpG island methylator phenotype group of poor-prognostic and fatal carcinomas that are designated as cluster-of-clusters (CoC) III tumours {3059}. Moreover, although *TERT* promoter mutations are rare in adrenal cortical carcinomas, aberrant *TERT* promoter methylation could constitute a helpful marker to pinpoint subsets of cases at risk of disease dissemination {2692,3413,4350}.

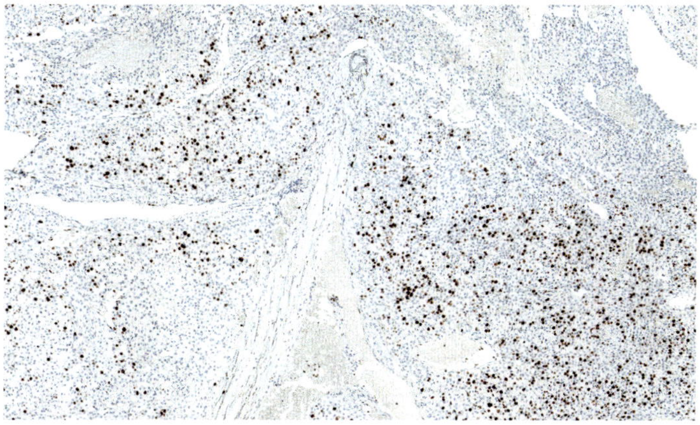

Fig. 5.39 Adrenal cortical carcinoma. An example with intratumoural proliferative heterogeneity demonstrated using Ki-67 immunohistochemistry. Most adrenal cortical carcinomas show a Ki-67 labelling index > 5%.

The 5-year overall survival rate is 37–47% in adrenal cortical carcinoma {1235,1340}. Although completely excised localized disease with no angioinvasion is potentially curable, the numbers for patients with disseminated (stage IV) adrenal cortical carcinoma are dismal, with few patients surviving the 5-year mark {2650,2406}. Current recommendations are that all patients with adrenal cortical carcinoma are followed by tertiary centre experts {2321}.

Adrenal sex cord stromal tumour

Cheng L
Asa SL
Ezzat S
Tischler AS

Definition
Adrenal sex cord stromal tumour is a tumour with sex cord stromal differentiation arising in the adrenal cortex.

ICD-O coding
8590/1 Sex cord stromal tumour
8650/1 Leydig cell tumour
8620/3 Granulosa cell tumour

ICD-11 coding
2F9A & XH0667 Neoplasms of unknown behaviour of endocrine glands & Sex cord-stromal tumour, unclassified

Related terminology
None

Subtype(s)
Leydig cell tumour; granulosa cell tumour

Localization
These tumours arise in the adrenal cortex.

Clinical features
Patients with adrenal granulosa cell tumour present with irregular uterine bleeding and/or an abdominal mass {3362,888}. In contrast, patients with adrenal Leydig cell tumour typically present with virilization and have elevated serum testosterone and DHEAS, with pituitary suppression of LH.

Epidemiology
Few cases have been reported {3362,888,789,4556,4674, 3586}; all occurred in postmenopausal women (median age: 60 years).

Etiology
Unknown

Pathogenesis
The histogenesis is uncertain {3362,888,789,4556,4674, 3586}. An origin from ectopic gonadal stroma is suggested by the close embryological origin of gonads and adrenals {2251, 3772,4534} and from reports of non-neoplastic Leydig cells in the adrenal cortex and within adrenal ganglioneuromas {2787,

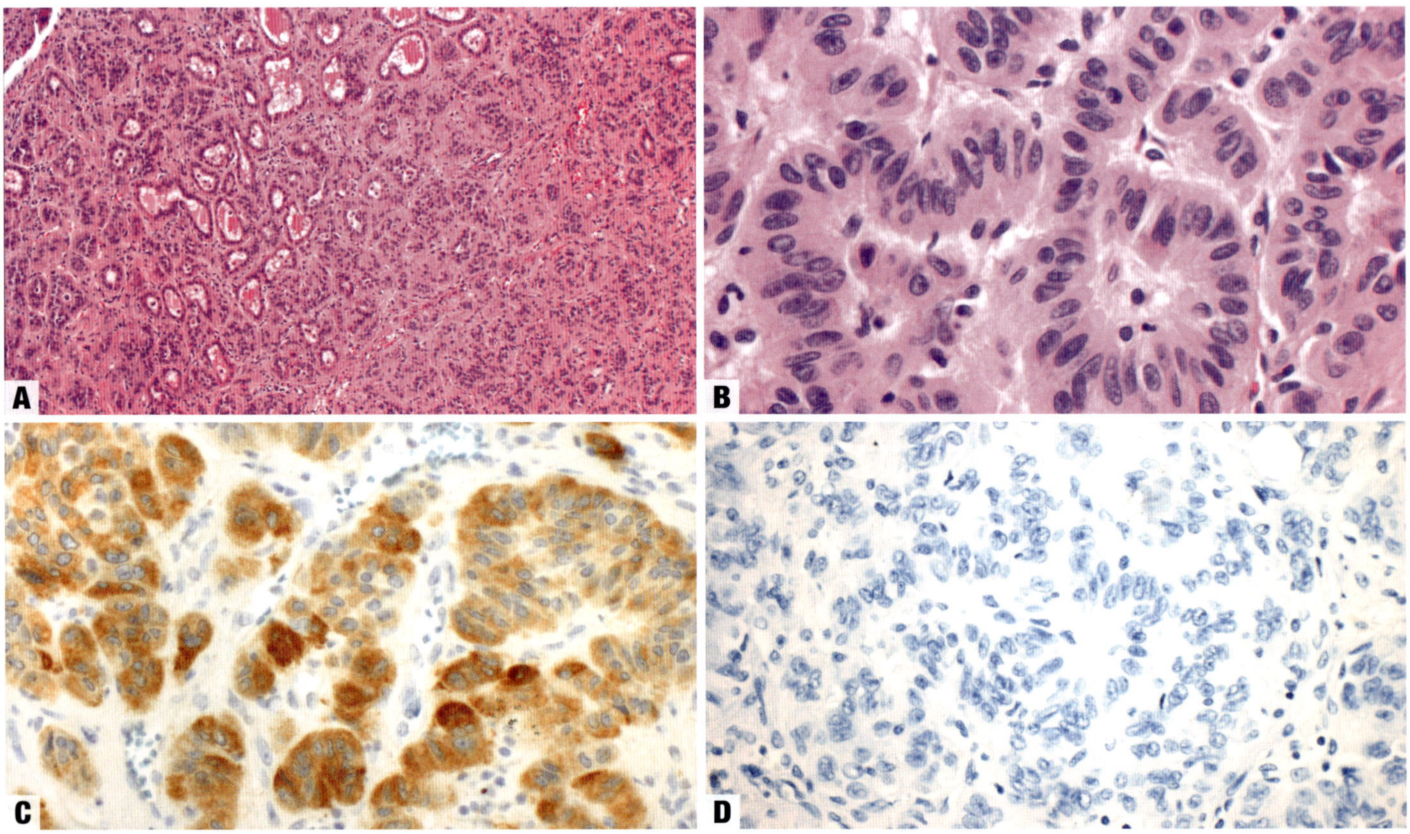

Fig. 5.40 Adrenal granulosa cell tumour. **A,B** Tumour cells are arranged in nests, cords, and tubules. **C** Inhibin staining is positive. **D** Chromogranin A is negative.

1943,47,4045}. Alternatively, they may arise from pluripotential mesenchymal cells exposed to high levels of gonadotropins or adrenocorticotropin {1943}. Primitive spindle cells with Reinke-like crystals have been described in the adrenal cortex, supporting this hypothesis {2787}. So-called ovarian thecal metaplasia in the adrenal supports this mechanism {664,4927,1379, 2976}.

Macroscopic appearance

These solitary unilateral solid tumours are well circumscribed, often encapsulated, and only occasionally cystic. Tumour sizes range from 19 to 90 mm. The cut surface is yellow, white, or brown {47}.

Histopathology

Like their ovarian adult granulosa cell counterparts, granulosa cell tumours display a microfollicular architecture with Call–Exner bodies and with macrofollicular, solid, and sarcomatoid patterns {5086,3362,888,789}. Tumour cells are round to oval with scant cytoplasm and pale nuclei. Nuclear grooves are variably seen.

Leydig cell tumour is composed of closely packed cell nests with a prominent intervening capillary network. Trabeculae or cords interrupted by oedema cause small cysts or pseudoglands. Tumour cells have abundant eosinophilic cytoplasm and round to oval nuclei with small to moderate-sized nucleoli. Brown cytoplasmic lipochrome pigment is common. Reinke crystals are necessary for classification as Leydig cell tumour {4556,4674,3586}.

Sex cord tumours express SF1, α-inhibin, calretinin, and melan-A, but not adrenocortical-specific steroidogenic enzymes (CYP11B1, CYP11B2) {3654,5152}.

Cytology

Not applicable

Diagnostic molecular pathology

Not clinically relevant

Essential and desirable diagnostic criteria

Essential:

- For granulosa cell tumour: a neoplasm composed of microfollicular architecture, large neoplastic cells, Call–Exner bodies, and round nuclei with irregular nuclear membranes and grooves
- Leydig cell tumour: a neoplasm composed of bland steroid-producing cells in closely packed nests, showing cytoplasmic Reinke crystals

Desirable: positivity for inhibin, calretinin, SF1, and melan-A (MART1), and negativity for EMA and other keratins, in selected cases.

Staging

Not applicable

Prognosis and prediction

Surgical resection results in hormone normalization, with a good prognosis for the limited cases reported {789}.

Adenomatoid tumour

Karpathiou G
Hiroshima K

Definition

Adenomatoid tumour is a benign tumour of mesothelial differentiation arising in the adrenal gland.

ICD-O coding

9054/0 Adenomatoid tumour, NOS

ICD-11 coding

2F10 & XH6BY3 Benign neoplasm of mesothelial tissue & Adenomatoid tumour, NOS

Related terminology

None

Subtype(s)

None

Localization

The left and right adrenal glands are equally affected.

Clinical features

Most cases are diagnosed incidentally during imaging or surgical procedures, or found at autopsy. Some cases are diagnosed during hypertension workup {4501,1509,855}, but this association needs further investigation.

Epidemiology

Adenomatoid tumour is a rare entity, with about 50 cases published to date. The age at diagnosis is 22–65 years (median: 40 years). There is a marked male predominance (> 90% of cases are in men) {430,2209}.

Etiology

Unknown

Pathogenesis

Adenomatoid tumours have not yet been evaluated in the adrenal gland, but in the genital tract they harbour somatic missense mutations in *TRAF7* {1635} and do not show alterations in *BAP1*, *NF2*, or *CDKN2A* {1635,4383}. Despite well-documented mesothelial differentiation, tissue origin is unknown given the absence of adrenal gland mesothelial lining. Proposed theories include an origin from mesothelial inclusions or from pluripotent mesenchyme associated with the Müllerian tract {2051}.

Macroscopic appearance

The tumour is usually well circumscribed, grey-tan, and solid, but in almost half of the cases a cystic component is reported; this is usually in the form of multiple small cystic spaces, giving a spongy appearance, but rarely, macroscopic cystic tumours are reported {430,3652}. The tumours measure 5–180 mm (median: 38 mm) in greatest dimension. Haemorrhage is also reported in some cases {4501}.

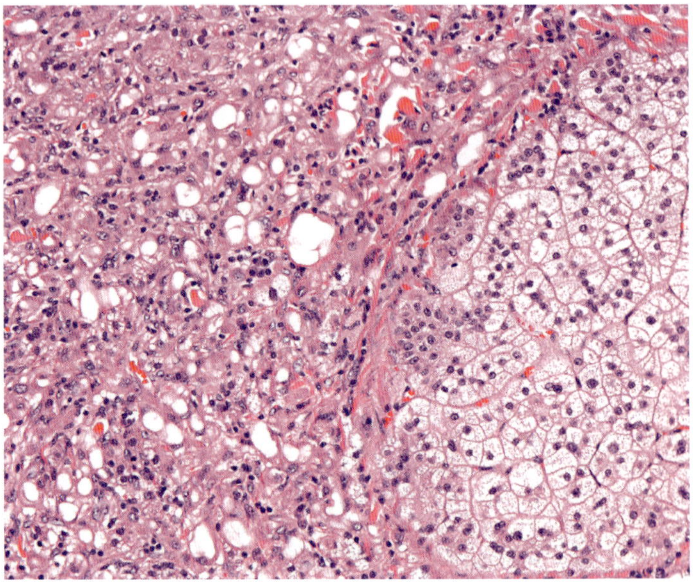

Fig. 5.41 Adenomatoid tumour of the adrenal gland. An example showing channels and microcysts lined by flattened cells in a delicate fibrous stroma.

Histopathology

The tumours usually show variably sized interanastomosing tubules, channels, and cystic spaces lined by flat to cuboidal cells with scant epithelioid cytoplasm or cytoplasmic vacuoles, often giving a signet ring–like appearance {2051,1509,3652}. Some tumours harbour papillary formations {564,1608,3881,3652}. The tumours often reveal infiltrative margins. No atypia, mitosis, or necrosis is found. The stroma is fibrous and often harbours lymphoid aggregates. Other adrenal lesions are occasionally reported in conjunction with adenomatoid tumours, such as nodular cortical hyperplasia {855,1188}, myelolipoma {1188,4501}, ganglioneuroma {1188}, vascular cyst {1509}, and cortical adenoma {4425}.

The tumour stains for cytokeratins and mesothelial cell markers such as calretinin, D2-40, and WT1 {2051,1509,1188}. Adenomatoid tumours should have intact BAP1 expression {2133,1257}.

The main differential diagnoses include lymphangioma, angiosarcoma, mesothelioma, and metastatic adenocarcinoma, which should be excluded by immunohistochemistry {2209}. Adenomatoid tumours show retained BAP1 expression {2133,1257} and frequent L1CAM expression {1635,2052,2208}. They harbour somatic missense mutations in *TRAF7* {1635}, and they do not show alterations in *BAP1*, *NF2*, or *CDKN2A* {1635,4383}.

Cytology
Not clinically relevant

Diagnostic molecular pathology
Not clinically relevant

Essential and desirable diagnostic criteria
Essential: a proliferation composed of tubular and cystic spaces lined by flattened or cuboidal cells in a fibrous stroma often harbouring lymphoid aggregates; expression of mesothelial markers.
Desirable: expression of BAP1 in selected cases.

Staging
Not relevant

Prognosis and prediction
Tumours follow a benign clinical course after complete excision.

Adrenal melanoma

Scolyer RA
de la Fouchardière A

Definition

Adrenal melanoma is a malignant melanocytic neoplasm arising within the adrenal gland.

ICD-O coding

8720/3 Adrenal melanoma, NOS

ICD-11 coding

2D11.Y & XH4846 Other specified malignant neoplasms of adrenal gland & Melanoma

Related terminology

Acceptable: melanoma of the adrenal gland.

Subtype(s)

None

Localization

There is unilateral involvement of the adrenal gland. Bilateral adrenal gland involvement strongly favours metastatic disease originating from an extra-adrenal primary melanoma {683}.

Clinical features

Primary adrenal melanoma usually occurs as a unilateral suprarenal mass. Patients may present with constitutional symptoms, flank pain, or symptoms related to mass effect, or cases may be detected incidentally on radiological imaging performed for other reasons {1634,4978,5112,3446}. Most cases show no hormonal abnormalities {4978,2622,1113}, but rare patients have elevated serum and urine catecholamines {319,2783,1663}. Tumour thrombus and extension into the inferior vena cava has also been described {244}. Adrenal melanomas are usually avid on FDG PET-CT {3665,1155,404,4424}.

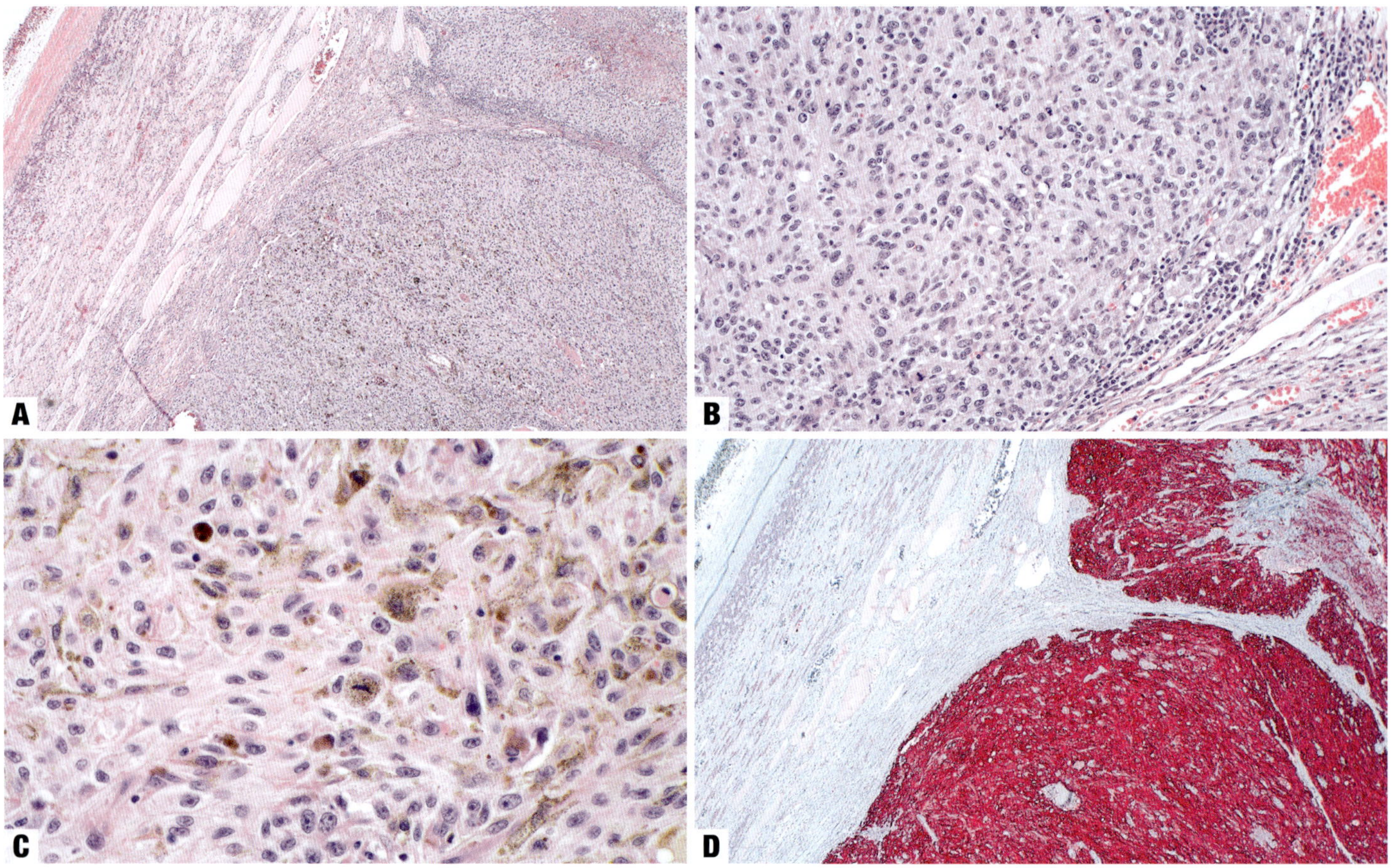

Fig. 5.42 Primary adrenal melanoma. **A** The focally pigmented tumour has a nodular architecture and is circumscribed. Adjacent adrenal cortical tissue is present (upper left). **B** The tumour is formed by pleomorphic polygonal and epithelioid cells. A lymphoid infiltrate is present at the periphery and focally within the tumour. **C** Many of the melanoma cells include intracytoplasmic melanin pigment. Occasional mitoses are present. **D** Melan-A immunostain showing strong positive staining of the melanoma cells. Weak positive staining is present in the adjacent adrenal cortex (upper left).

Epidemiology

Primary melanoma involving the adrenal gland is extremely rare (< 30 reported cases) and accounts for < 0.1% of all adrenal malignancies {1634,4978,5112,319,1663,244,3621,2649, 336,128,987,3962,2352,1117}. The median age at diagnosis is 50 years (range: 24–78 years), and there is no racial or sex predisposition {1634}.

Etiology

Unknown

Pathogenesis

Melanocytes are not a normal cell population of the adrenal gland. However, adrenal medullary chromaffin cells and melanocytes share a common embryological origin through neuroectodermal progenitor cells of the neural crest {2507,2558}. Therefore, it is hypothesized that ectopic melanocytes can exist within the adrenal gland and can undergo metaplastic and neoplastic transformation {4424}. Nevertheless, it has been questioned whether the condition actually exists. The difficulty arises because an unrecognized primary cutaneous melanoma can occasionally undergo complete regression and disappear without a trace, whereas an adrenal metastasis that has arisen from it may continue to grow and eventually be detected as an apparently isolated focus of melanoma. Molecular analysis of carefully selected cases may address this hypothesis {5016}.

Isolated cases with documented mutation testing showed a wildtype *BRAF* genotype {4978,319,3621}.

Macroscopic appearance

Tumours are often large (60–170 mm), with attenuation of the surrounding adrenal gland. The cut surface often shows areas of dark-brown discolouration, haemorrhage, and cystic necrosis {1634,4978,1215}. The tumour may involve adjacent structures, including large vessels {244}.

Histopathology

Adrenal melanoma is typically formed by sheets of pleomorphic epithelioid and fusiform cells and may contain multinucleated tumour cells {4978}. The nuclei have irregular nuclear membranes, vesicular chromatin, intranuclear inclusions, and prominent nucleoli. Immunohistochemical stains for S100, SOX10, melan-A, and HMB45 are often positive, and the tumour is consistently negative for cytokeratins, synaptophysin, and chromogranin {1634}. The presence of melanosomes can be detected on ultrastructural examination {128}.

Cytology

Cytological preparations of aspirate samples from melanoma (including of primary or metastatic origin) typically demonstrate loosely cohesive large pleomorphic epithelioid to plasmacytoid cells with irregular nuclear membranes and prominent nucleoli. Pigment, if present, can also be detected within tumour cells or histocytes {305}.

Diagnostic molecular pathology

Not clinically relevant

Essential and desirable diagnostic criteria

Essential: demonstration of malignant and melanocytic differentiation; identification of adjacent adrenal tissue; absence of evidence for previous or synchronous melanoma outside of the adrenal gland.

Staging

There are no Union for International Cancer Control (UICC) staging criteria for primary adrenal melanoma.

Prognosis and prediction

There is limited information from case reports about the prognosis of primary adrenal melanoma, but the prognosis is generally poor in the absence of intervention {987}. Patients may progress rapidly to disseminated peritoneal disease, and distant metastasis to lymph nodes, lung, liver, spleen, brain, and bone has been described {4978,1663}.

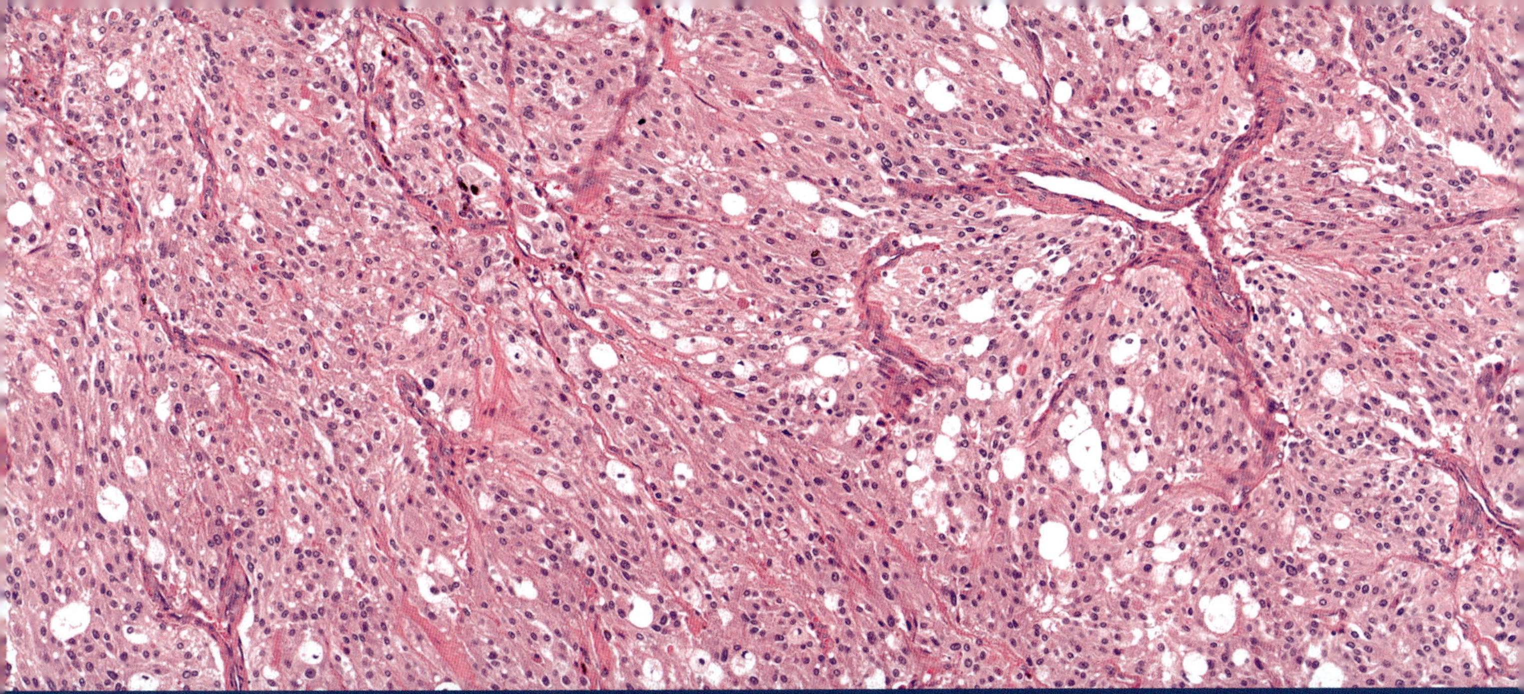

6

Adrenal medulla and extra-adrenal paraganglia tumours

Edited by: de Krijger RR, Erickson LA, Gill AJ

- Neuroblastic tumours
  - Neuroblastoma
  - Ganglioneuroblastoma, intermixed
  - Ganglioneuroblastoma, nodular
  - Ganglioneuroma
- Paraganglioma and phaeochromocytoma
  - Phaeochromocytoma
  - Sympathetic paraganglioma
  - Parasympathetic paraganglioma
- Composite paraganglion tumours
  - Composite phaeochromocytomas and paragangliomas

Adrenal medulla and extra-adrenal paraganglia tumours: Introduction

de Krijger RR
Asa SL
Erickson LA
Mete O
Shimada H
Tischler AS

Two groups of tumours with complementary but overlapping epidemiology occur in the adrenal medulla and extra-adrenal paraganglia: neuroblastic tumours (mostly neuroblastoma and ganglioneuroblastomas), usually in infants and children; and paragangliomas, usually in adults. Phaeochromocytomas are part of the paraganglioma family of tumours and can therefore be addressed as adrenal (sympathetic) or intra-adrenal paraganglioma. Although a neural crest origin for both groups of tumours has long been accepted, advances in developmental biology, including single-cell RNA sequencing and lineage tracing, have provided a new understanding of the derivation of normal chromaffin cells and sympathetic neurons. New developmental concepts may help to explain distinct characteristics associated with tumour location for both paragangliomas and neuroblastomas, as well as age and genotype associations and the existence of composite tumours {2170}. A study performed in 2017 in mice showed that while sympathetic ganglia were populated predominantly by direct migration of progenitors from the neural crest, the chromaffin cells of the adrenal medulla {1463} and extra-adrenal paraganglia {2221} arose from nerve-associated progenitors termed Schwann cell precursors. These Schwann cell precursors

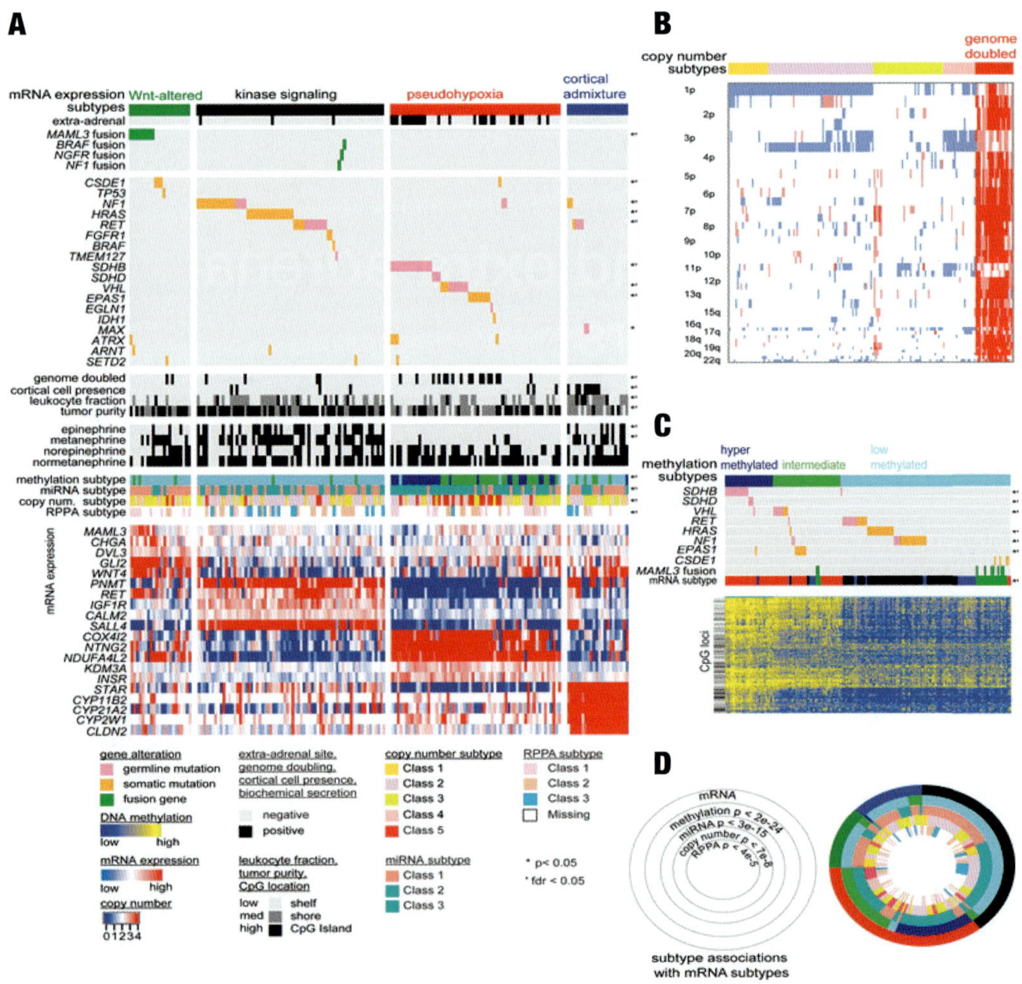

Fig. 6.01 Integrated molecular subtypes of phaeochromocytoma and paraganglioma. **A** mRNA subtypes. Primary tumours (n = 173) are displayed in columns, and clinical and genomic features are displayed in rows. Categorical features were analysed using the Fisher exact test; continuous features were analysed using the Kruskal–Wallis test. Select differentially expressed genes are displayed below each subtype. **B** DNA copy-number clustering {22544022}. Primary tumours (n = 173) are displayed in columns. **C** DNA methylation clustering. Primary tumours (n = 173) are displayed in columns. Features were tested for association with methylation subtypes by same methods as in **A**. **D** Ring plot displaying cross-platform subtype association. p refers to the chi-squared test on platform subtype versus mRNA expression subtype.

Table 6.01 Categories and subtypes of peripheral neuroblastic tumours as defined in the International Neuroblastoma Pathology Classification (INPC)

Category	Definition	Subtype	Remarks
Neuroblastoma (Schwannian stroma–poor)	Cellular neuroblastic tumour without prominent Schwannian stroma	Undifferentiated	No clearly identifiable neuropil formation Supplementary diagnostic techniques required
		Poorly differentiated	Diagnosis can be made by pure morphological criteria Characteristic neuropil is present Differentiating neuroblasts < 5%
		Differentiating	Usually with abundant neuropil Differentiating neuroblasts > 5%
Ganglioneuroblastoma, intermixed (Schwannian stroma–rich)	Intermingled microscopic foci of neuroblastic elements in an expanding Schwannian stroma, constituting > 50% of the tumour volume		Neuroblastic foci are microscopic, without grossly visible nodular formation Neuroblastic foci are composed of a mixture of neuroblastic cells in various stages of differentiation, in a background of naked neuropil
Ganglioneuroblastoma, nodular (composite Schwannian stroma–rich/ dominant and Schwannian stroma–poor)	A grossly visible neuroblastic nodular (stroma-poor) component coexisting with an intermixed ganglioneuroblastoma (stroma-rich) or ganglioneuroma (stroma-dominant) component		The proportion of the components varies The stroma-poor component is usually haemorrhagic and/or necrotic
Ganglioneuroma (Schwannian stroma–dominant)	Predominantly composed of Schwannian stroma, with individually distributed neuronal elements No detectable naked neuropil	Maturing	Contains both maturing and mature ganglion cells
		Mature	Contains exclusively mature ganglion cells surrounded by satellite cells

are derived from neural crest cells that remain in place near the dorsal root ganglia and then reach their destinations by migrating along nerves. Subsequent studies in 2021 showed a more complex situation in humans, with a variety of bridge cells and developmental transitions between neuronal and chromaffin cell precursors {2170}. In both species, Schwann cell precursors provide a source of neural crest–like cells for the expansion and diversification of sympathoadrenal tissues after direct migration is no longer possible because of body enlargement and the fact that the neural crest itself no longer exists.

The morphological classification of neuroblastomas, ganglioneuroblastomas (nodular and intermixed), and ganglioneuromas has not changed since the previous edition (see Table 6.01). Advances with regard to prognostically and therapeutically relevant molecular abnormalities continue to be achieved. Notably, mechanisms of telomere maintenance have been studied and partly elucidated, including TERT overexpression and alternative lengthening of telomeres {18, 1803}.

The previous edition of the WHO classification of tumours of endocrine organs addressed the fact that all phaeochromocytomas and paragangliomas should be considered malignant. This is continued in the new edition. Consequently, the adjectives "benign" and "malignant" are no longer recommended and can be replaced by a concept of risk stratification. Although several systems have been proposed to predict the risk of metastasis, no individual system is endorsed for routine use. The previous edition also noted that small adrenal medullary lesions historically known as hyperplastic nodules should be considered neoplasms, because they have

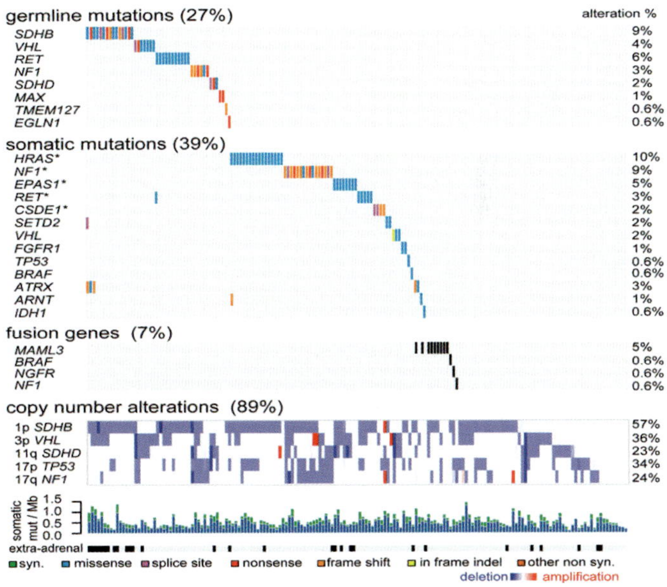

Fig. 6.02 Germline and somatic genome alterations in phaeochromocytoma and paraganglioma. Genomic features are in rows and primary tumours (n = 173) are in columns; shading indicates the effect of a mutation on the protein sequence. Significant somatically mutated genes (MutSig2, $q < 0.05$) are indicated by asterisks.

been shown to carry the same clonal molecular abnormalities as larger tumours {2956,2400}. As a result, the term "microphaeochromocytoma" has been put forward, analogous to microtumours elsewhere in the body, such as the thyroid and pancreas.

The new edition places increased emphasis on the importance of biomarkers. Given the complexity of neuroendocrine neoplasms (NENs), it is often not sufficient to classify a lesion using chromogranin and S100 immunohistochemistry alone. The recognition that paragangliomas can occur in unusual locations, including primary lesions in lung and liver, makes this even more critical {203}. The importance of applying stains for GATA3 and tyrosine hydroxylase in diagnosis is emphasized, and the value of Ki-67 in predicting metastasis is now recognized.

Emphasis on hereditary disease has also increased. Paragangliomas are characterized by a very high incidence of genetic predisposition {1385,4587,3415}. Awareness of this phenomenon has led to the discovery of new genes implicated in their tumorigenesis and new syndromes with novel associated neoplasms {1385}. The concept of molecular immunohistochemistry provides the pathologist with tools for predicting the genetic basis of these neoplasms and for avoiding the pitfall of diagnosing multifocal primary tumours as metastatic disease {4587,3415,2139}.

Neuroblastoma

Shimada H
Fischer M
Jarzembowski JA
Tonini GP
Tornóczky T

Definition

Neuroblastoma is a peripheral neuroblastic tumour of neural crest origin containing proliferating neoplastic cells of various grades of neuroblastic differentiation with < 50% Schwannian stromal content.

ICD-O coding

9500/3 Neuroblastoma
9500/3 Undifferentiated neuroblastoma
9500/3 Poorly differentiated neuroblastoma
9500/3 Differentiating neuroblastoma

ICD-11 coding

2D11 & XH85Z0 Malignant neoplasm of adrenal gland, neuroblastoma & Neuroblastoma, NOS

Related terminology

None

Subtype(s)

Undifferentiated neuroblastoma; poorly differentiated neuroblastoma; differentiating neuroblastoma

Localization

The adrenal gland is the most common primary site of neuroblastoma, and > 40% of tumours are found in the adrenal medulla and periadrenal locations. Other primary sites include the abdomen (25%), posterior mediastinum (15%), pelvic cavity (5%), and neck (~3–5%). Rare tumours are found in the paratesticular region, and 1% of patients are recorded to have metastatic disease with no detectable primary tumours {550,1729, 2464,68,4719}.

Clinical features

A large primary adrenal neuroblastoma may cause abdominal distension. Adrenal neuroblastoma can also be detected before birth, by ultrasound scans during prenatal care. Metastases can cause lymphadenopathy, hepatomegaly, bone pain, and raccoon eyes (exophthalmia associated with distinct bruising and swelling around the eyes). Metastatic dissemination to the lung and brain is rare {1174,2253}. CNS involvement, when present, often shows diffuse spreading along the meningeal surfaces.

Several paraneoplastic syndromes are associated with adrenal neuroblastoma. They include (1) WDHA syndrome (watery diarrhoea, hypokalaemia, and achlorhydria; also called Verner–Morrison syndrome) caused by the tumour secreting VIP {491}, (2) opsoclonus-myoclonus-ataxia syndrome (dancing eyes and acute cerebellar ataxia, possibly via an autoimmune mechanism) {3842}, (3) hypertension (due to catecholamine secretion or renal artery compression by the tumour) {4050,4127}. Rare cases with constitutional mutations of *PHOX2B* have also been documented with congenital central hypoventilation and

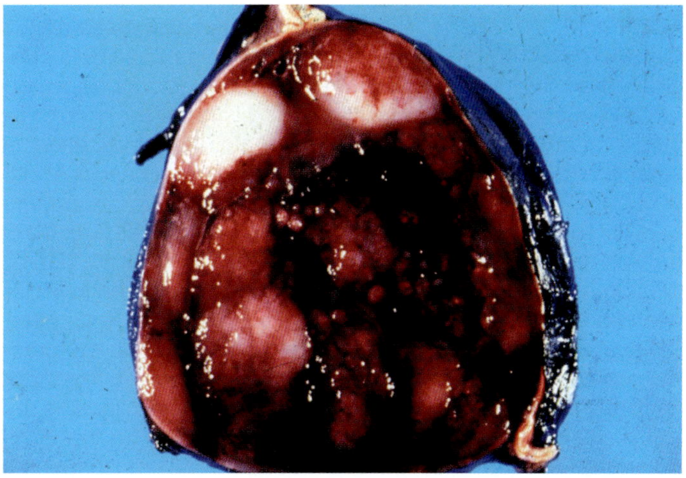

Fig. 6.03 Adrenal neuroblastoma. Gross appearance of adrenal neuroblastoma. The tumour has a haemorrhagic appearance with focal necrosis and calcification.

Hirschsprung disease {1853,130}. *PHOX2B* encodes a homeodomain transcription factor that promotes cell-cycle exit and neuronal differentiation; therefore, it plays a crucial part in the development of neural crest–derived autonomic neurons.

Epidemiology

Peripheral neuroblastic tumours are the third most common childhood neoplasm after leukaemias and brain tumours, and 80% of them are in the neuroblastoma category. They are the most common neoplasms during the first year of life, and the most common extracranial solid tumours in the first 2 years of life. In the USA, the prevalence of this disease is 1 case per 7 000 live births, and nearly 90% are diagnosed before 5 years of age (median age: 17.3 months). The disease is slightly more common in boys than in girls (M:F ratio: 1.2:1) {1966}. A similar frequency has been observed in Europe {2758}, China {1848, 308}, and Japan {3160,3169}. Familial neuroblastoma occurs as an autosomal dominant disorder with incomplete penetration {2172} and seems to constitute approximately 1–2% of all neuroblastomas {4131}. Neuroblastomas in patients with a hereditary predisposition are usually diagnosed at an earlier age (mean age: 9 months) than are sporadic cases (mean age: 17.3 months), and ≥ 20% of these patients have bilateral adrenal or multifocal primaries. A substantial fraction of familial neuroblastoma is caused by pathogenic germline variants in *ALK* {4515}. *PHOX2B* pathogenic variants are also identified in a small number of inherited cases {1853}.

Etiology

Neuroblastoma is caused by the transformation of neural crest cells due to genetic or epigenetic events during pre-migration, migration, and/or postmigration. Although a great deal has been discovered about the genetic and transcriptional regulation of neural crest development, the events leading to tumorigenesis remain poorly understood. The early age at onset of disease as well as the concept of in situ neuroblastoma {4117} suggests that the tumour develops during fetal life. To date, however, there are no definite preconceptional or gestational factors accepted as consistently increasing the incidence of neuroblastoma.

Pathogenesis

MYC-family oncogene (MYCN and MYC) overexpression

The *MYCN* oncogene, located on chromosome 2p24.3, is considered a major oncogenic driver of neuroblastoma. Elevated *LIN28B* expression enhanced by *MYCN* is reported to contribute to neuroblastoma tumorigenesis. *MYCN* amplification is seen in approximately 20–25% of neuroblastoma cases. About 90% of *MYCN*-amplified tumours overexpress MYCN protein {3241}. There are also neuroblastomas overexpressing MYC (c-myc) protein. In contrast to MYCN-overexpressing neuroblastoma, it is extremely rare to see gene amplification in MYC-overexpressing neuroblastoma {2890}. In this regard, other molecular mechanisms for a higher level of MYC protein expression independent of genomic amplification have been reported, such as oncogene activation through enhancer hijacking by translocations, focal enhancer amplification near to the *MYC* coding region (8q24), or MK2-mediated OCT4 transcriptional activation of *MYC* {5188,4836}. Tumours overexpressing MYC-family proteins (MYCN or MYC) are collectively named MYC-driven neuroblastomas {4795}.

Abnormal maintenance/elongation of telomeres

Two mechanisms associated with telomere abnormalities that provide the tumour cells with infinite proliferating capability are reported in neuroblastoma: TERT overexpression and the alternative-lengthening-of-telomeres (ALT) phenotype. TERT is the protein component of telomerase, and higher levels of expression are observed in both MYC-driven and non–MYC-driven neuroblastomas. In the former, *TERT* is the direct transcriptional target of MYC-family proteins {2365}. In the latter, it is likely a result of long-range genomic rearrangements of *TERT*. *TERT* promoter hypermethylation may also be involved in its activating mechanism {2671,2672,2579,4638}, whereas most of the tumours with ATRX loss due to *ATRX* mutation show the ALT phenotype {3760}. The ALT phenotype is characterized by low *TERT* expression levels, and *ATRX* mutations occur almost mutually exclusively with genomic alterations of *MYCN* and *TERT*. Patients with ALT-positive neuroblastomas are significantly older at diagnosis than those with ALT-negative tumours {807,1803}. The ALT phenotype is also reported in rare neuroblastomas with loss of DAXX due to the gene mutation {2455}.

ALK gene overexpression

As mentioned above, constitutive activating germline pathogenic variants in the oncogene *ALK*, located on chromosome 2p23, seem to account for most cases of hereditary neuroblastoma {3110,2089}. About 6–10% of sporadic neuroblastomas carry somatic *ALK*-activating pathogenic variants, and an additional

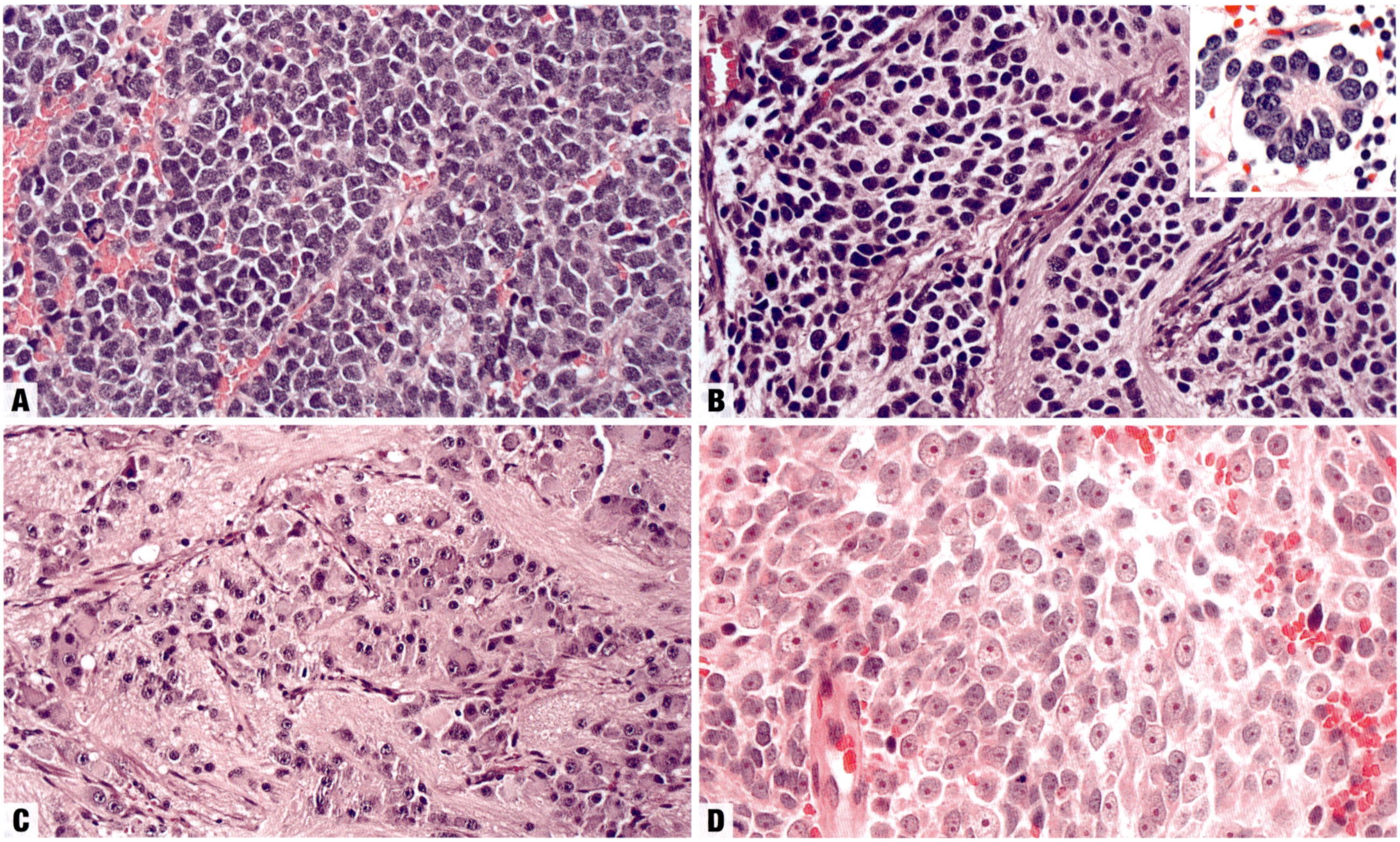

Fig. 6.04 Histopathology of tumours in the neuroblastoma (Schwannian stroma–poor) category. **A** Neuroblastoma, undifferentiated subtype. **B** Neuroblastoma, poorly differentiated subtype (**inset:** Homer Wright rosette). **C** Neuroblastoma, differentiating subtype. **D** Large cell neuroblastoma with uniquely enlarged and euchromatin-rich nuclei and nucleolar hypertrophy.

3–4% have *ALK* amplification. Genomic rearrangements or amplification of *ALK* are observed in sporadic neuroblastoma only and have not been found in familial neuroblastoma thus far. ALK is a receptor tyrosine kinase with expression that is physiologically restricted mainly to the developing central and peripheral nervous system {2089}. *ALK* mutations at hotspots (e.g. R1275, F1174, and F1245) lead to the activation of multiple signalling pathways, including the RAS/MAPK pathway and the PI3K/AKT pathway {2089}. *ALK* mutations are single-nucleotide variants in the tyrosine kinase domain (TKD)-encoding region of the gene {2172}. The *ALK* p.R1275Q variant occurs most frequently in familial neuroblastoma and is also one of the most prevalent pathogenic variants in sporadic neuroblastic tumours {2172,527}. By contrast, substitutions at F1174 and F1245, which are frequent mutations in sporadic neuroblastoma, have been detected rarely in familial cases and only in the context of severe neurocognitive defects and brainstem abnormalities {1033}. ALK protein overexpression as a result of *ALK* mutation/rearrangement/amplification seems to be responsible for its oncogenic activity {3109}. However, in mouse and zebrafish models, activated *ALK* has been shown to efficiently induce neuroblastoma development in combination with *MYCN* overexpression {1879,403,5181,712}. By contrast, neuroblastoma did not develop or rarely developed in these models when activated *ALK* was expressed in the absence of a *MYCN* transgene. It is noted that the development of ALK-driven malignancies other than neuroblastoma has not been reported in children with germline *ALK* pathogenic variants.

Macroscopic appearance

Neuroblastomas can reach 100 mm in diameter and form a soft, grey-tan mass (often haemorrhagic), with or without foci of necrosis and calcification. The tumour mass can be well encapsulated or show invasive growth into the surrounding tissue. Biologically favourable primary neuroblastoma of the adrenal often pushes down the kidney without invasive growth. In contrast, biologically unfavourable neuroblastoma, especially with amplified *MYCN* oncogene, demonstrates direct invasion into the renal parenchyma.

Histopathology

Tumours in the neuroblastoma category are composed of neuroblastic cells forming groups or nests that are demarcated by thin fibrovascular septa with no or limited Schwannian proliferation {4118}. The International Neuroblastoma Pathology Classification (INPC) defines three subtypes based on the grades of neuroblastic differentiation.

Neuroblastoma, undifferentiated subtype, is rare and requires supplementary studies such as immunohistochemistry and/or molecular tests to establish the diagnosis, because the proliferating cells have a uniformly primitive small blue round cell appearance without clearly recognizable neurite formation.

Neuroblastoma, poorly differentiated subtype, is defined as a tumour with a background of readily detectable neurites with or without Homer Wright rosette formation. Fewer than 5% of neuroblasts have cytomorphological features of differentiation towards mature neurons. This is the most common histological subtype in the neuroblastoma category. The conventional nuclear morphology of the neuroblasts in this subtype is often described as a salt-and-pepper appearance.

Neuroblastoma, differentiating subtype, is a tumour with usually abundant neurites, and where > 5% of tumour cells have the appearance of differentiating neuroblasts, characterized by synchronous differentiation of the nucleus (enlarged and eccentrically located, with a vesicular chromatin pattern and usually a single prominent nucleolus) and of the cytoplasm (eosinophilic/amphophilic and with a diameter at least twice that of the nucleus).

There are tumours with transitional histology between that of the differentiating subtype of neuroblastoma (Schwannian stroma–poor) and that of intermixed ganglioneuroblastoma (Schwannian stroma–rich; > 50% of the tumour tissue is composed of Schwannian stroma, presenting a ganglioneuromatous appearance). It is noted that undifferentiated / poorly differentiated tumours infrequently show unusual histological features (large, pleomorphic, fusiform, spindle, and pseudorhabdoid) focally or diffusely.

According to the INPC, mitotic and karyorrhectic activities are also evaluated, and the mitosis-karyorrhexis index (MKI; i.e. low, < 100/5000 cells; intermediate, 100–200/5000 cells; or high, > 200/5000 cells), is determined for the individual tumours. It is reported that *MYCN*-amplified neuroblastoma shows the characteristic histology of either the undifferentiated subtype or the poorly differentiated subtype with a high MKI. It is also reported that MYC-driven neuroblastoma overexpressing MYC-family protein (either MYCN or MYC) often demonstrates prominent nucleolar formation (nucleolar hypertrophy) that is considered a putative site of MYCN/MYC RNA synthesis and accumulation {3241, 4317,4794,4795,2358}. The histologically defined, rare, and very aggressive large cell neuroblastoma (LCN) is also included in this MYC-driven neuroblastoma group {4525}. Although the nuclear morphology of LCN cells is often similar to that of differentiating neuroblasts, these two cell types should be strictly distinguished. The tumour cells in LCN have larger nuclei than conventional neuroblasts and their cytoplasm is similarly scant. In contrast, differentiating neuroblasts have abundant cytoplasm with a diameter at least twice that of the nucleus {4526}.

Immunophenotype

An immunohistochemistry panel including neuronal markers (synaptophysin, chromogranin, PGP9.5, CD56, and neurofilament), so-called neuroblastoma marker (NB84) {2991}, and neural crest markers (tyrosine hydroxylase and PHOX2B) {420,1813} is usually advised. Among these markers, PHOX2B is the most reliable for supporting a neuroblastoma diagnosis, even for the undifferentiated subtype {4821}. Tyrosine hydroxylase immunostaining for metastatic neuroblastoma often fades after decalcification on bone marrow biopsy samples. Generally, a combination of positive staining for these markers along with negative staining for markers of other small round cell tumours is suggested. Certain MYC-driven neuroblastomas, especially those of LCNs, are reported to express the intermediate filaments of desmin {2890}. S100 immunohistochemistry can stain some Schwannian stromal cells and putative Schwann cells (Schwannian blasts) in the fibrovascular septal tissue, especially in biologically favourable tumours in the neuroblastoma category {4120}.

International Neuroblastoma Pathology Classification

The INPC was established in 1999 by adapting the original Shimada classification {4121} with minor modifications {4119}, and it was then revised in 2003 {3541}. According to the INPC, tumours

Table 6.02 Prognostic distinction of tumours in the neuroblastoma category according to the International Neuroblastoma Pathology Classification (INPC) {4119}

Age at diagnosis	Subtype (grade of neuroblastic differentiation)	Mitosis-karyorrhexis index	Prognostic group
< 18 months	Undifferentiated	Any	Unfavourable histology
	Poorly differentiated	Low or intermediate	Favourable histology
	Differentiating	Low or intermediate	Favourable histology
	Any	High	Unfavourable histology
18 months to 5 years	Undifferentiated	Any	Unfavourable histology
	Poorly differentiated	Any	Unfavourable histology
	Differentiating	Low	Favourable histology
	Differentiating	Low or intermediate	Unfavourable histology
	Any	High	Unfavourable histology
> 5 years	Any	Any	Unfavourable histology

in the neuroblastoma category are classified into favourable or unfavourable histology groups on the basis of age-dependent evaluation of the grade of neuroblastic differentiation (i.e. undifferentiated, poorly differentiated, or differentiating subtype) and mitotic and karyorrhectic activity (i.e. low, intermediate, or high MKI; see Table 6.02). Tumours in the favourable histology group are within a framework of age-appropriate differentiation/maturation sequence and age-appropriate MKI class. As shown in Table 6.02, two age cut-off points – 18 months (548 days) and 60 months (5 years) – are introduced in the INPC. Prognostic classification by this system should only be performed on primary or metastatic tumours before treatment (chemotherapy, radiation). It is noted that MKI determination is not feasible or reliable on metastatic neuroblastoma in bone marrow biopsy samples.

Subgrouping of unfavourable-histology neuroblastomas

Recent advances in neuroblastoma research demonstrate that unfavourable-histology neuroblastomas are heterogeneous. Based on a molecular approach, four subgroups are proposed in the unfavourable-histology neuroblastomas: the MYC subgroup (overexpressing MYCN or MYC protein), the TERT subgroup (TERT overexpression due to genomic abnormalities), the ALT subgroup (ALT phenotype due to ATRX loss), and the null subgroup. These subgroups are molecularly and immunohistochemically identified by their protein markers, which could be potential targets for future precision therapy {2029}.

Cytology

FNA or other cytopathological evaluation may not be representative and requires ancillary testing for a definitive diagnosis. Smears are highly cellular and show predominantly single cells along with discohesive tissue fragments showing moulding and occasionally a rosette-like architecture with pale, pink (H&E stain) or blue to grey (Giemsa stain) central fibrillary neuropil, which is diagnostic when present. The cells have high N:C ratios and oval to irregular nuclei with evenly dispersed granular salt-and-pepper chromatin and inconspicuous to small nucleoli, and they may show wispy cytoplasmic extensions. Apoptotic necrosis and chromatinic smearing are frequently present, and neuropil may be seen in the background with variable Schwannian stroma. Larger binucleated or multinucleated ganglion cells may be present. In the absence of the rosettes, immunohistochemistry is required to differentiate other tumours, including lymphomas, Ewing sarcoma, rhabdomyosarcoma, and nephroblastoma {2405,4158}.

Diagnostic molecular pathology

Genomic/molecular characteristics significantly associated with tumorigenesis and/or the clinical behaviour of neuroblastomas include tumour DNA content and segmental chromosomal aberrations, *MYCN* oncogene amplification and MYC-family protein overexpression, abnormal maintenance/elongation of telomeres, and *ALK* gene abnormalities and protein overexpression (see *Prognosis and prediction*).

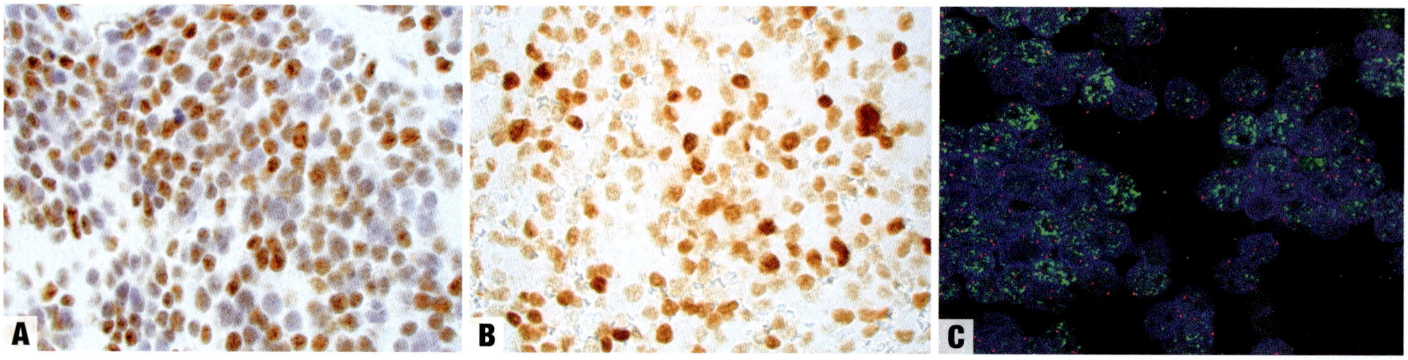

Fig. 6.05 Molecular and immunohistochemical features of neuroblastoma. **A** MYC protein–positive neuroblastoma. MYC-driven neuroblastoma. MYC (c-myc) immunostaining with haematoxylin counterstaining. **B** MYCN protein positivity in neuroblastoma MYC-driven neuroblastoma. MYC protein immunostaining without haematoxylin counterstaining. **C** *MYCN* amplification in neuroblastoma as determined by FISH. Multiple *MYCN* signals (green), along with two control signals (red), in neuroblastoma interphase nuclei, counterstained with DAPI (blue).

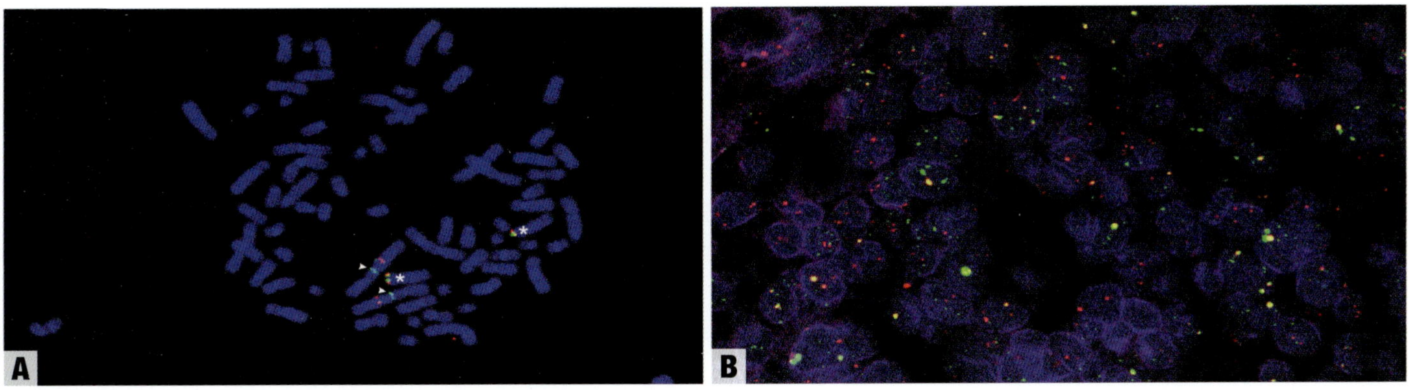

Fig. 6.06 Molecular features of neuroblastoma. **A** *TERT* rearrangement in neuroblastoma. Break-apart FISH of *TERT* in metaphase, with split *TERT* (green) and control (red) signals in two derivative chromosomes, indicating rearrangement of the *TERT* locus (arrowheads), in addition to the colocalization of the signals in two normal copies of chromosome 5 (asterisks). **B** Alternative-lengthening-of-telomeres phenotype in neuroblastoma cells, as indicated by alternative lengthening of telomeres–associated promyelocytic leukaemia (PML) nuclear bodies (APBs) in interphase nuclei. Telomeric FISH (green) and PML immunofluorescence (red) were combined, and APB was identified by the colocalization of bright telomere and PML signals.

Essential and desirable diagnostic criteria

Essential:

- Confirming the diagnosis of neuroblastoma: histologically, the tumour is composed of neuroblastic cells forming groups/nests irregularly demarcating thin fibrovascular septa with no or limited Schwannian stromal development; tumour nuclei typically show a salt-and-pepper appearance, whereas MYC-driven neuroblastoma characteristically demonstrates nucleolar hypertrophy; diagnosis is supported by immunohistochemistry using neuronal markers (synaptophysin, chromogranin, CD56, etc.) and neural crest markers (PHOX2B, tyrosine hydroxylase)
- Distinguishing favourable- and unfavourable-histology tumours according to the INPC: the prognostic distinction is made by age-linked evaluation of histological factors – the grade of neuroblastic differentiation (undifferentiated, poorly differentiated, or differentiating) and the MKI (low, intermediate, or high)

Desirable (as available): molecular/genomic testing including *MYCN* oncogene status and MYC-family protein expression (immunohistochemistry), telomere maintenance–associated gene (*TERT, ATRX*) status, and *ALK* oncogene status; DNA index and segmental chromosomal aberrations for prognostic prediction.

Staging

There are two widely used clinical staging systems: the International Neuroblastoma Staging System (INSS; stages 1, 2A, 2B, 3, 4, and 4S) {538,537} and the International Neuroblastoma Risk Group Staging System (INRGSS; stages L1, L2, M, and MS) {3072}. The INSS is based on the postsurgical evaluation of the disease status, whereas the INRGSS depends on the presurgical determination of the presence or absence of image-defined risk factors. Many collaborative and independent clinical studies have started using INRGSS, which eliminates the surgical approach for determining clinical staging (see Table 6.03, p. 270).

Prognosis and prediction

Besides clinical stage, age at diagnosis {3438,884,2043}, and histopathology (INPC), the genomic/molecular properties of the individual tumours have significant prognostic effects for patients with neuroblastomas. They are summarized below.

Tumour DNA content and segmental chromosomal aberrations

Tumours presenting with numerical whole-chromosome copy-number gains without structural abnormalities (hyperdiploid, DNA index > 1) are associated with an excellent prognosis {2729,1537}. Hyperdiploidy presumably results from chromosome-segregation failure during mitosis. In contrast, tumours in the diploid range (DNA index = 1) are associated with a poor clinical outcome. Flow cytometric analysis for the determination of the DNA index has been used as a simple and semi-automated method of measuring total cell DNA in neuroblastomas. However, the prognostic significance of ploidy determined by flow cytometry seems to be lost in children aged > 2 years, possibly because tumours with a DNA index > 1 in older children typically have a number of structural abnormalities.

Various segmental chromosomal aberrations are reported as indicators of a poor clinical outcome in neuroblastomas {4000,242,655,2849,499,3542,1121}. Loss of heterozygosity of chromosome 1p has been reported in 25–35% of cases, and most of the deletions are located distal to 1p36. Distal 1p likely harbours tumour suppressor genes or genes controlling differentiation of neuroblastic cells. A relationship between loss of heterozygosity of chromosome 1p and *MYCN* amplification has been described. Loss of heterozygosity of chromosome 11q has been identified in 35–45% of cases; 11q23 is the most common site for deletion. Chromosome 11q deletions are often associated with older patients and rarely occur in combination with *MYCN* amplification. Trisomy 17q (17q gain) may be the most prevalent genetic abnormality in neuroblastomas, and it has been detected in about 60% of cases. Although the gain can occur independently, it frequently occurs as part of an unbalanced translocation between chromosomes 1 and 17. The 17q breakpoints vary but most frequently occur at 17q22-qter. Chromosome 1q gain is also reported in neuroblastomas.

The prognostic effects of the segmental chromosomal alterations (i.e. 1p deletion, 11q deletion, and 17q gain) were tested in neuroblastomas without *MYCN* amplification; 11q deletion and 17q gain were associated with poor survival in a univariate analysis. A segmental profile (i.e. the presence of 1p deletion and/or 11q deletion and/or 17q gain, rather than a single

Table 6.03 International Neuroblastoma Risk Group Staging System (INRGSS)

Stage	Description
L1	Localized tumour not involving vital structures as defined by the list of image-defined risk factors and confined to one body compartment
L2	Locoregional tumour with presence of one or more image-defined risk factors
M	Distant metastatic disease (except stage MS)
MS	Metastatic disease in children aged < 18 months with metastases confined to skin, liver, and/or bone marrow

Note: See Monclair et al., 2009 {3072}, for detailed criteria. Multifocal primary tumours should be staged according to the greatest extent of disease as defined above.

and specific genetic alteration) adds prognostic information to patient age and clinical stage, according to a multivariate analysis {4001}.

MYCN oncogene amplification and MYC-family (MYCN/MYC) protein overexpression

It is well known that *MYCN* amplification is associated with advanced-stage disease and aggressive clinical behaviour {2849,539,4051}. A large region including the *MYCN* locus becomes amplified as extrachromosomal double minutes, and it may be linearly integrated into a chromosome as homogeneously staining regions. By FISH, *MYCN* status is determined as amplified (> 4-fold increase in the *MYCN* signal number compared with the reference probe located chromosome 2), gain (with increased signals but < 4 times as many vs reference signals of chromosome 2), or non-amplified. It is recommended to report the extent of amplification (i.e. > 4–10 times, > 10–30 times, or > 30 times), and on the type of amplification (i.e. double minutes or homogeneously staining regions). In the past few years, heterogeneous *MYCN* intratumoural amplification has been appreciated in association with a diverse aggressive phenotype {391}.

Recent studies support the notion that MYCN protein overexpression, rather than gene amplification, is critical for determining aggressive tumour behaviour {4317}. There are also neuroblastomas overexpressing MYC (c-myc) protein. As mentioned above, it is extremely rare to see gene amplification in MYC-overexpressing neuroblastoma {2890}.

Tumours overexpressing MYC-family protein (MYCN overexpression detected in ~20% or MYC overexpression detected in ~10% of neuroblastomas of the undifferentiated or poorly differentiated subtypes) are collectively named MYC-driven neuroblastomas {4795}. Those MYC-driven neuroblastomas are highly aggressive {4794} and histologically characterized by prominent nucleolar formation (nucleolar hypertrophy). Because of the presence of prominent nucleoli, MYC-driven neuroblastoma can be morphologically distinguished from other conventional neuroblastomas, which have salt-and-pepper nuclei.

Abnormal maintenance/elongation of telomeres

Abnormalities of telomere maintenance have been suggested to be the hallmark of high-risk neuroblastoma, discriminating these cases from spontaneously regressing low-risk tumours {18}. Both TERT overexpression and the ALT phenotype are reported to be predictive of reduced patient survival {806,3487,18}. Elevated levels of TERT expression and enzymatic activity are associated with either *MYCN* amplification or rearrangements of the *TERT* locus {2671,2579,4638}. Most of the ALT phenotype is associated with ATRX protein loss, which is due to *ATRX* gene mutations leading to recombinogenic telomeres {807,18,1803}.

ALK gene abnormalities and protein overexpression

Genomic *ALK* alterations causing protein overexpression {3110, 2088,787,5164} have been reported to be associated with a poor prognosis in patients with neuroblastoma {675,3109}. However, the prognostic significance of *ALK* overexpression has been controversial. For example, the clinical outcomes of patients within the same family bearing a germline *ALK* mutation are different and not always poor {2172}, and spontaneous regression has been documented in *ALK*-mutated neuroblastomas {18}. It is therefore likely that, in addition to *ALK* mutations, further genomic alterations (e.g. *MYCN* amplification, *TERT* rearrangement, or *ATRX* mutation) might be required for oncogenic development and full malignant transformation of neuroblastoma cells in both familial and sporadic tumours {18}. Regairaz et al. reported that the expression of ALK and its active form, phosphorylated ALK, was immunohistochemically detected in many neuroblastomas, independently of *ALK* mutations/amplification {3707}. The therapeutic effect of ALK inhibitors in *ALK*-mutated neuroblastoma is currently under investigation in clinical trials {4026}.

Risk grouping system

Historically, there have been several risk grouping systems proposed by different cooperative groups, such as the International Society of Paediatric Oncology Europe Neuroblastoma Group (SIOPEN), the Society for Paediatric Oncology and Haematology (GPOH), and the Children's Oncology Group (COG). Currently, two systems – the International Neuroblastoma Risk Group Staging System (INRGSS) and the COG risk grouping system – are widely accepted; both are based on a combination of predictive factors, such as clinical stage, patient age at diagnosis, histopathology, and genetic and genomic/molecular properties. The COG risk grouping system has been used for the purpose of patient stratification and protocol assignment in clinical trials {3438,4839}. Patients in the low-risk group are often followed by observation (with no chemotherapy or radiation) after surgery or even biopsy alone. Patients in the intermediate-risk group are treated with surgery or biopsy followed by non-aggressive chemotherapy. Patients in the high-risk group are treated with intensive chemotherapy, surgery, radiation therapy, bone marrow / haematopoietic stem cell transplantation, and biologically based therapies. The reported 5-year survival rates for non–high-risk and high-risk patients are 90% and 50%, respectively {3438,2043}.

The INRGSS has been designed to facilitate the comparison of risk-based clinical trials conducted in different regions and countries, and it distinguishes very low-risk (> 85% event-free survival), low-risk (75–85% event-free survival), intermediate-risk (50–75% event-free survival), and high-risk (< 50% event-free survival) patients {884}.

Ganglioneuroblastoma, intermixed

Beiske KH
Irwin MS
Jarzembowski JA
Navarro S
Peuchmaur M
Sartelet H

Definition
Intermixed ganglioneuroblastoma (GNBi) is a form of peripheral neuroblastic tumour transitional between neuroblastoma and ganglioneuroma, composed of Schwannian stroma containing scattered well-defined foci of neuroblastic cells at various stages of maturation.

ICD-O coding
9490/3 Ganglioneuroblastoma, intermixed

ICD-11 coding
2A00.21 & XH0RB7 Mixed neuronal-glial tumours & Ganglioneuroblastoma, intermixed

Related terminology
Acceptable: Schwannian stroma–rich intermixed tumour.

Subtype(s)
None

Localization
GNBi occurs most frequently in the abdominal cavity / retroperitoneum (usually adrenal), but also in the mediastinum, cervical region, and pelvis {1840}.

Clinical features
GNBi often presents as an asymptomatic mass {1047,91,3336}, generally lacking the elevated urine catecholamines seen in neuroblastoma. Imaging shows an encapsulated, well-circumscribed mass. MRI diffusion-weighting characteristics may help distinguish ganglioneuroma/GNBi from neuroblastoma {1479, 3475}. Tumours are less likely to be MIBG-avid than neuroblastomas {1047,91}.

Epidemiology
Ganglioneuroma and GNBi together account for approximately 25% of peripheral neuroblastic tumours {1047,91,3336}. Compared with neuroblastoma, GNBi tumours occur in older children (median age: 4–7 years) and patients are less likely to have elevated urine catecholamines {1047,91}.

Etiology
Unknown

Pathogenesis
Peripheral neuroblastic tumours originate from neural crest cells that give rise to adrenal medulla and sympathetic ganglia.

Histologically and genetically low-risk neuroblastomas (see *Neuroblastoma*, p. 265) may spontaneously mature into GNBi {4118,125}. *MYCN* oncogene amplification is rare (< 1%) {3336, 4317}. Segmental chromosomal aberrations are infrequent, but neuroblastic cells may harbour numerical chromosomal aberrations. DNA content is frequently diploid {3336} because of an abundance of stromal cells.

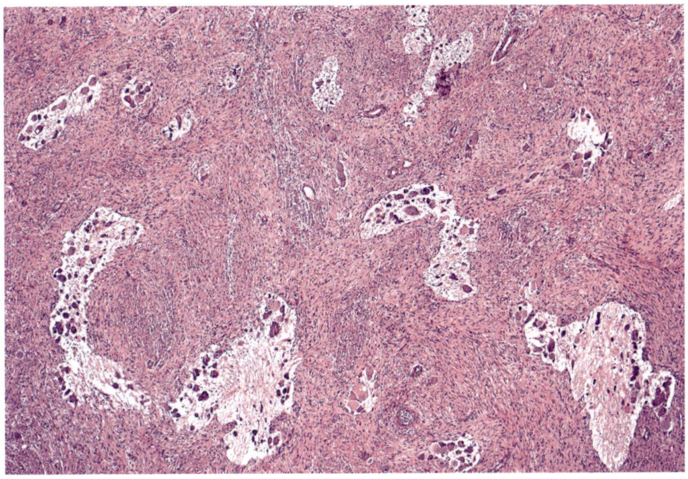

Fig. 6.07 Ganglioneuroblastoma, intermixed. Hallmarks of intermixed ganglioneuroblastoma are well-demarcated microscopic foci containing neuroblastic cells embedded in neuropil. The foci are randomly distributed in ganglioneuromatous tissue composed of Schwannian cells and maturing/mature ganglionic cells. The ganglioneuromatous component exceeds 50% of the section.

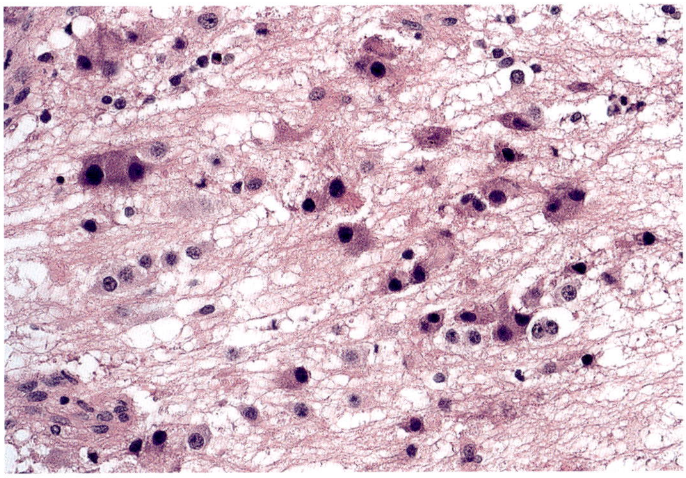

Fig. 6.08 Ganglioneuroblastoma, intermixed. The neuroblastic cells are at various stages of differentiation and are dominated by differentiating neuroblasts.

Macroscopic appearance
GNBi is a solid, well-defined mass displaying a homogeneous pale-grey cut surface.

Histopathology
Well-circumscribed lacunar areas of neuroblastic cells embedded in neuropil are randomly distributed in ganglioneuromatous tissue composed of Schwannian cells and maturing/mature

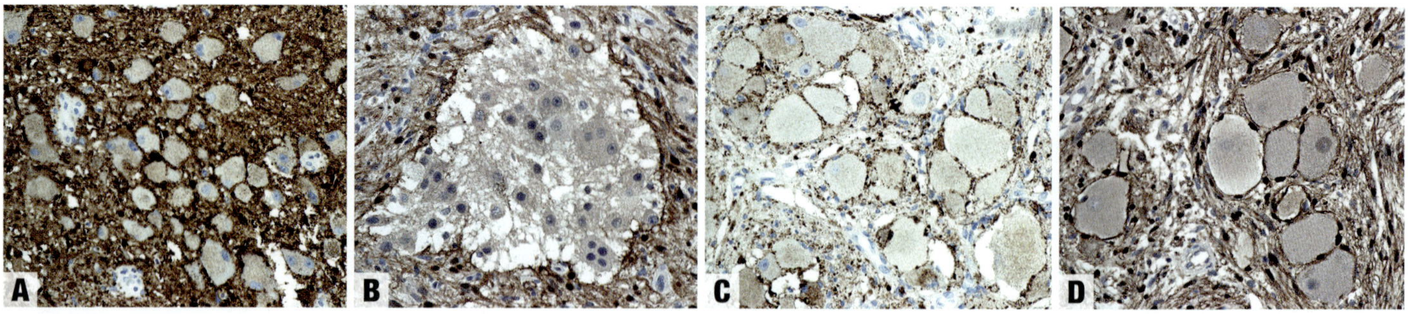

Fig. 6.09 Ganglioneuroblastoma, intermixed (GNBi). Immunohistochemical staining for synaptophysin (**A,C**) and S100 (**B,D**). The presence of neuropil in tumour foci is a prerequisite for the diagnosis of GNBi. Neuropil strongly expresses synaptophysin (**A**) but is negative for S100 (**B**). In addition to neuropil-containing tumour foci, GNBi may show clusters of ganglionic cells that do not include appreciable amounts of synaptophysin-positive neuropil (**C**), but do show S100-positive Schwannian cells (**D**), typically found in maturing and mature ganglioneuroma, thus demonstrating the ongoing differentiation from a stroma-rich to a stroma-dominant tumour. Immunostaining for synaptophysin might aid the identification of neuropil in the differential diagnosis between GNBi and ganglioneuroma.

ganglionic cells. The neuroblastic cells comprise various stages of differentiation. No pushing borders are encountered between areas of neuroblastic cells and the ganglioneuromatous component {4118}.

Cytology

Smears and touch imprints show a heterogeneous population of larger ganglionic cells with large round to mildly irregular nuclei; prominent single nucleoli; considerable coarsely granular, dark blue (Giemsa), usually eccentric cytoplasm; a variable number of smaller neuroblasts with the same features as those seen in neuroblastoma; and a variable amount of Schwannian stroma {2405}.

Diagnostic molecular pathology

Not clinically relevant

Essential and desirable diagnostic criteria

Essential: a Schwannian stroma–prominent tumour; well-demarcated microscopic foci of neuropil and mainly differentiating neuroblastic cells; a ganglioneuromatous component constituting > 50% of the tumour volume.

Desirable: immunohistochemistry for synaptophysin and S100 aids in distinguishing neuropil and Schwann cells.

Staging

All neuroblastic tumours are staged according to the International Neuroblastoma Risk Group Staging System (INRGSS) {3072}.

Prognosis and prediction

According to the INRGSS, GNBi is usually a locoregional tumour, classified as low risk with extremely rare metastatic spread {1047, 91,1479}. GNBi is usually chemotherapy-insensitive {1047}.

Ganglioneuroblastoma, nodular

Cullinane C
Beiske KH
Jarzembowski JA
Peuchmaur M
Shimada H

Definition
Nodular ganglioneuroblastoma (GNBn; composite Schwannian stroma–rich/dominant and Schwannian stroma–poor) is composed of distinct histologies (clones): intermixed ganglioneuroblastoma (GNBi) or ganglioneuroma and neuroblastoma.

ICD-O coding
9490/3 Ganglioneuroblastoma, nodular

ICD-11 coding
2A00.21 & XH77W7 Mixed neuronal-glial tumours & Ganglioneuroblastoma

Related terminology
None

Subtype(s)
None

Localization
Primary GNBn occurs in sites associated with neural crest migration, including the adrenal medulla {3541,4620}.

Clinical features
Adrenal GNBn is detected as a suprarenal mass {147,1840}. Occasionally, metastatic disease leads to the diagnosis {3541}.

Epidemiology
GNBn is uncommon, accounting for 8% of all peripheral neuroblastic tumours filed at the Children's Oncology Group (COG) Neuroblastoma Pathology Reference Laboratory. It is rare in infancy, and the majority of cases are diagnosed in children aged > 18 months {147}.

Etiology
Unknown

Pathogenesis
GNBn has multiple components, i.e. GNBi or ganglioneuroma (biologically favourable with advanced tumour maturation) and neuroblastoma (either biologically favourable or unfavourable with less tumour maturation) in a single mass. These are considered to represent different clones rather than focal maturation or dedifferentiation {3541,4620}.

Macroscopic appearance
The neuroblastoma component, often haemorrhagic and necrotic, is typically a discrete nodule in a background of GNBi/ganglioneuroma that is solid/firm and white/yellow. Multiple nodules may be present. Sampling of all nodules for histopathological and molecular evaluation is critical for case management.

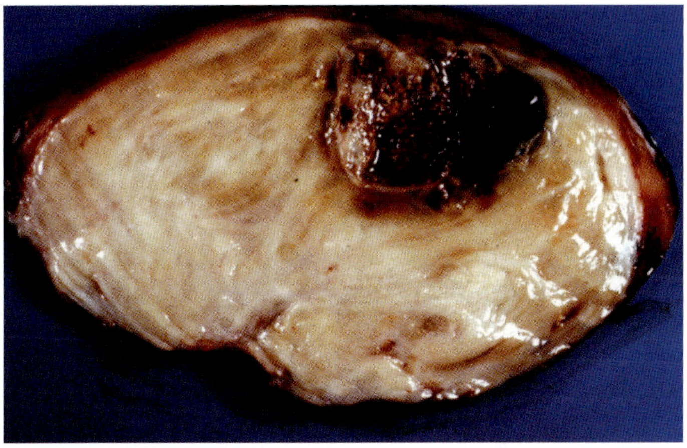

Fig. 6.10 Ganglioneuroblastoma, nodular. Composite Schwannian stroma–rich/dominant tumour with a discrete haemorrhagic neuroblastoma (Schwannian stroma–poor) nodule.

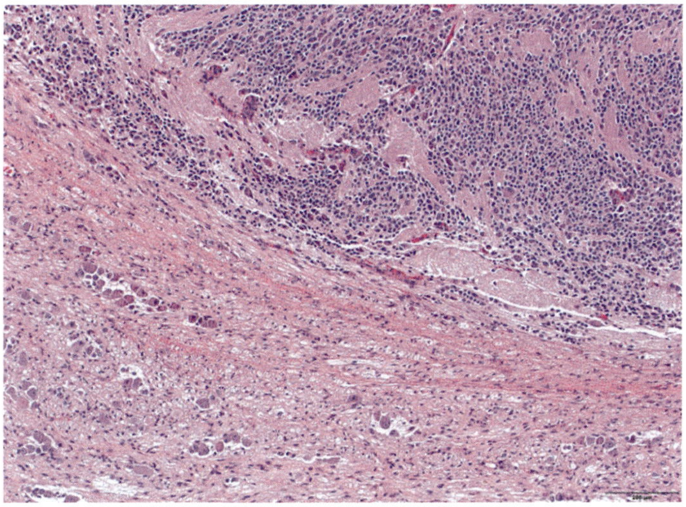

Fig. 6.11 Ganglioneuroblastoma nodular. Neuroblastoma (Schwannian stroma–poor, poorly differentiated) nodule with a pushing margin at the junction with ganglioneuroblastoma, intermixed (Schwannian stroma–rich).

The proportion of neuroblastoma and GNBi/ganglioneuroma in an individual tumour varies case by case.

Histopathology
Diagnosis requires the identification of GNBi/ganglioneuroma and neuroblastoma in a single tumour. The neuroblastoma nodule is separated from the GNBi/ganglioneuroma by a fibrous capsule, a pushing border without a definite capsule, or an infiltrative margin. Rarely, a primary site biopsy shows GNBi/ganglioneuroma with neuroblastoma detected in a metastatic

site. The neuroblastic differentiation, grade, and mitosis-karyorrhexis index of each neuroblastoma nodule is essential, with categorization as "favourable histology" or "unfavourable histology" according to the International Neuroblastoma Pathology Classification (INPC; see *Neuroblastoma*, p. 265).

Cytology

Cytopathological smears are similar to those of GNBi {2405}.

Diagnostic molecular pathology

Genomic/molecular investigation is focused on the neuroblastoma component (see *Neuroblastoma*, p. 265). *MYCN* amplification is rare (2%) {147}.

Essential and desirable diagnostic criteria

Essential: distinct histologies (clones) of GNBi/ganglioneuroma and neuroblastoma; assessment of the neuroblastoma component as per the INPC criteria.

Desirable: genomic/molecular testing of the neuroblastoma component.

Staging

The International Neuroblastoma Risk Group Staging System (INRGSS) is recommended for clinical staging based on the presence or absence of image-defined risk factors {3072}.

Prognosis and prediction

The prognosis for patients with GNBn is determined by the clinical, histopathological, and molecular characteristics of the neuroblastoma component {3541,147,1840} (see *Neuroblastoma*, p. 265).

Ganglioneuroma

Cullinane C
Jarzembowski JA
Shimada H

Definition

Ganglioneuroma (Schwannian stroma–dominant) is the final stage of maturation of peripheral neuroblastic tumours of neural crest origin.

ICD-O coding

9490/0 Ganglioneuroma
9490/0 Maturing ganglioneuroma
9490/0 Mature ganglioneuroma

ICD-11 coding

2A00.21 & XH03L9 Mixed neuronal-glial tumours & Ganglioneuroma

Related terminology

None

Subtype(s)

Maturing ganglioneuroma; mature ganglioneuroma

Localization

Ganglioneuroma occurs in sites associated with the development of the sympathetic nervous system {1531,1047,91}.

Clinical features

Most ganglioneuromas are incidental discoveries during imaging for unrelated events {4250} and are usually non-functioning {1047,1011}.

Epidemiology

Ganglioneuroma is a rare tumour; its incidence is unknown. In paediatric series, older children and adolescents are affected {91,1011,3336}. Adrenal ganglioneuroma is a rare incidentaloma in adults {4250,2012}.

Etiology

Unknown

Pathogenesis

Maturation from neuroblastoma to ganglioneuroma is supported by cross-talk between neural crest–derived neuroblastic tumour cells and Schwannian stromal cells. The latter are recruited by biologically favourable neuroblasts that release factors promoting Schwann cell proliferation and development {4118,2691}. In return, Schwann cells may secrete antiproliferation and differentiation factors that are critical for neuronal differentiation {2467}.

Macroscopic appearance

Adrenal ganglioneuroma is a localized, firm, yellow mass without haemorrhagic or necrotic areas. Focal calcification may be present. It can encase large vessels and may compress but not invade other vital structures {2012}.

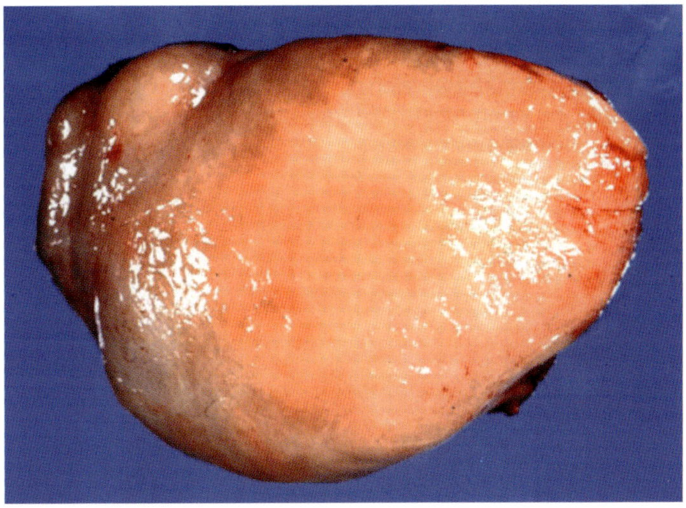

Fig. 6.12 Ganglioneuroma. Schwannian stroma–dominant.

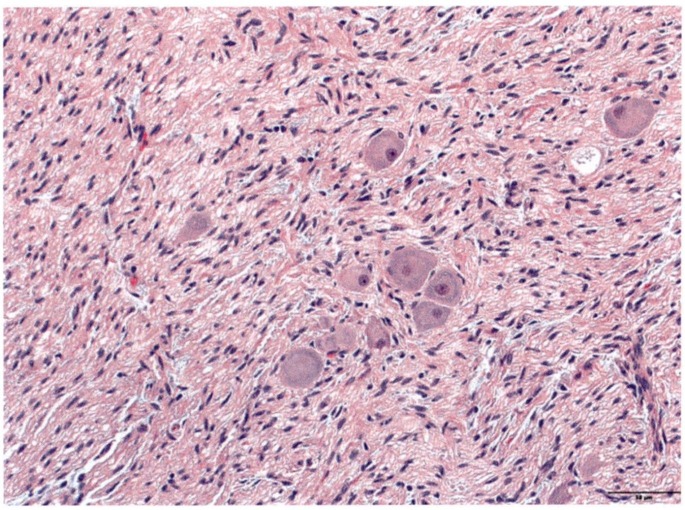

Fig. 6.13 Ganglioneuroma. Maturing subtype, composed of mature Schwannian stroma and ganglion cells, some of which are not completely mature.

Histopathology

Ganglioneuroma contains abundant Schwann cells in sheets and fascicles organized and bundled by perineurial cells. Variable numbers of mature and maturing ganglion cells that differ in size and shape and may be multinucleated are distributed individually or in small clusters in the maturing subtype of ganglioneuroma. In the mature subtype of ganglioneuroma, all ganglion cells are mature and covered with satellite cells. In both subtypes, naked neuritic processes (neuropil) are not detected around the ganglion cells because they are immediately incorporated into the cytoplasm of Schwann cells {4118}.

Cytology

Smears show a variable number of ganglion cells admixed with considerable cellular fibrillary Schwannian stroma {2405}. There is no neuroblastoma.

Diagnostic molecular pathology

Not clinically relevant

Essential and desirable diagnostic criteria

Essential: a dominant Schwannian stromal component; maturing and/or mature ganglion cells.

Desirable: no neuroblast clusters in neuropil (naked neurites); no neuroblastoma nodules.

Staging

In the International Neuroblastoma Risk Group Staging System (INRGSS), ganglioneuromas are typically locoregional tumours of stage L1 or L2 {3072,3336,1047,91}.

Prognosis and prediction

The International Neuroblastoma Pathology Classification (INPC) classifies both ganglioneuroma subtypes into the favourable histology group {4122}. The prognosis is excellent, even if excision is incomplete {4250,1047,91}. Rarely, biopsy may miss a coexisting neuroblastoma nodule whose biological characteristics may alter behaviour (see *Ganglioneuroblastoma, nodular*, p. 273), and therefore a disclaimer, such as "Favourable histology based on review of limited material", should be added.

Phaeochromocytoma

Tischler AS
Assié G
Erickson LA
Lam AK
Mete O
Osamura RY
Oudijk L

Definition

Phaeochromocytoma is a neuroendocrine neoplasm (NEN) that originates from chromaffin cells of the adrenal medulla and is an intra-adrenal paraganglioma.

ICD-O coding

8700/3 Phaeochromocytoma

ICD-11 coding

2D11.1 & XH3854 Malignant phaeochromocytoma of adrenal gland & Phaeochromocytoma, NOS

Related terminology

Acceptable: intra-adrenal paraganglioma; adrenal sympathetic paraganglioma.

Not recommended: chromaffin cell tumour; chromaffinoma; benign phaeochromocytoma; malignant phaeochromocytoma.

Subtype(s)

None

Localization

Phaeochromocytoma is an adrenal medullary tumour. These tumours may rarely occur in ectopic adrenal tissue {3331}. Neoplasms with similar cytomorphological, immunohistochemical, and functional features that arise from dispersed extra-adrenal paraganglia are termed paragangliomas.

Clinical features

Clinical and biochemical features

Most phaeochromocytomas can synthesize catecholamines, and patients with this tumour classically present with signs and symptoms related to catecholamine excess. However, a widening clinical spectrum is now recognized, reflecting differences in patients' nationalities {2108}, geographical locations, age groups, and genetic background {1198}. In contrast to the classic presentation, the majority of phaeochromocytomas are now discovered during the workup of adrenal incidentalomas, in cancer imaging studies, or during the screening of patients with genetic susceptibility syndromes {1198} (see *SDH-deficient tumour syndromes*, p. 457). Many patients with phaeochromocytomas discovered by these routes have few or no symptoms {1198}, but the tumours are almost always biochemically functional and amenable to biochemical testing {1210}. In patients with paraganglioma syndromes, associated neoplasms may present before phaeochromocytomas and can be the first clue to the presence of disease.

In symptomatic patients, the most frequent manifestation is hypertension, most often paroxysmal in adults and sustained in children {3478}. Classic symptoms are headache, palpitations, and diaphoresis; however, < 25% of patients exhibit this

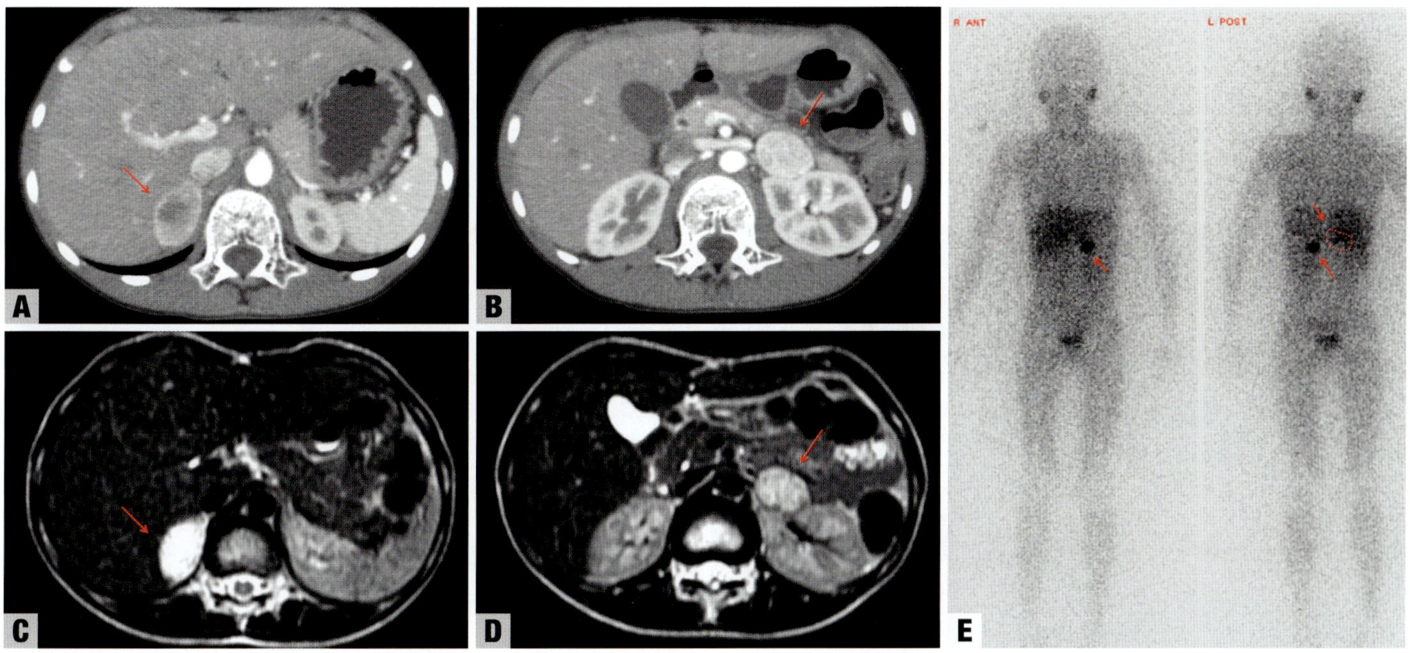

Fig. 6.14 Imaging studies in a patient with paediatric-onset bilateral phaeochromocytoma. CT (**A,B**) and MRI (**C,D**) show bilateral adrenal tumours (arrows) in this patient with a family history of von Hippel–Lindau syndrome. Hyperintense tumours are identified by T2-weighted MRI (**C,D**). **E** 123I-MIBG scintigraphy shows bilateral uptake in both adrenal tumours.

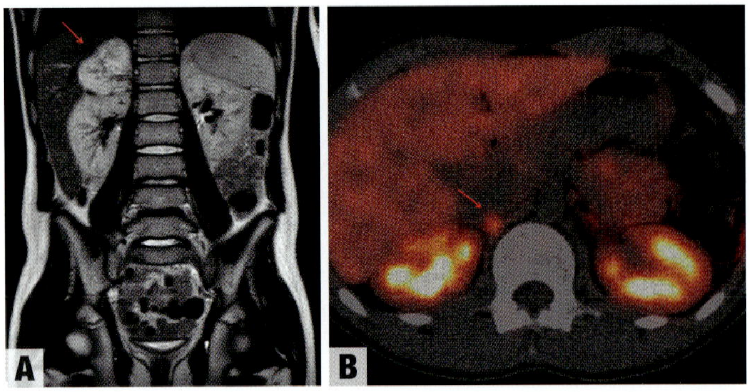

Fig. 6.15 Imaging studies in a patient with paediatric-onset phaeochromocytoma with recurrent hypertension. The patient initially presented with hypertension and was found to have elevated catecholamine levels. **A** MRI showed a heterogeneous adrenal tumour (arrow). The adrenalectomy specimen confirmed the diagnosis of phaeochromocytoma. Subsequent genetic analysis identified a pathogenic *SDHB* variant. **B** During the follow-up period, an additional functioning tumour (arrow) was noted on imaging studies using 68Ga-DOTATOC PET-CT. The tumour was not in the former surgery site, and histopathological examination confirmed this lesion as a metachronous primary paraganglioma.

classic triad, and some patients have no symptoms {1198}. High levels of catecholamines may result in chronic and acute myocardial injury mimicking ischaemic injury, including dilated cardiomyopathy and takotsubo cardiomyopathy, which may present as life-threatening emergencies {5169}. Other signs and symptoms may include abdominal pain and constipation {4492}, weight loss, tremor, facial pallor, panic attacks, asthenia, hypertensive crises, and seizures {4715,1040}. Some patients experience (groups of) symptoms as recurrent self-limited spells, which are diagnostically useful but nonspecific to phaeochromocytoma {5088}. Factors contributing to an absence of symptoms in some patients include small tumour size, intratumoural O-methylation of catecholamines to produce metanephrines {1209,1211}, or a low expression of catecholamine biosynthesizing enzymes associated with some hereditary genotypes {4499}.

Occasionally, phaeochromocytomas cause endocrine paraneoplastic syndromes by producing ectopic regulatory peptides. The most common is Cushing syndrome, caused by ACTH {3247} or (rarely) CRH {355} secretion. Others include WDHA syndrome (watery diarrhoea, hypokalaemia, and achlorhydria; also called Verner–Morrison syndrome) caused by VIP {2719} and most often associated with composite phaeochromocytomas {2109,4507}. Secretion of various other hormones has been reported, with or without accompanying symptoms {151,816}. Examples with accompanying symptoms include β-hCG (hyperandrogenism) {816}, vasopressin (haemodynamic instability) {447}, growth hormone / GHRH (acromegaly) {447}, and calcitonin (hypercalcaemia) {1845}. In addition, inflammatory paraneoplastic symptoms have been reported in association with IL-6 production {2931}.

Biochemical testing generally precedes imaging studies during clinical workup. Measuring 24 h fractionated urine or plasma free catecholamine metabolites (metanephrine, normetanephrine, 3-methoxytyramine) is often preferable to measuring parent catecholamines, because the metabolites are generated intratumourally {1211} from parent amines that leak into the tumour cell cytoplasm from secretory granules. These are therefore more sensitive biomarkers than catecholamines per se, which are also produced by sympathetic neurons {1210}. The serum chromogranin A level is often elevated but is a less sensitive marker than metanephrines {424}. New testing approaches aim to identify succinate or other markers associated with specific gene mutations {1210,1449}.

Phaeochromocytomas exhibit a strong correlation between genotype and biochemical phenotype, and accordingly sort into multiple genomic clusters {1385,1343,966,1210}. Cluster 1 (the pseudohypoxia cluster) consists of tumours with mutations of genes that affect hypoxic signalling, principally *VHL* and the SDH genes {2349,966}, and manifests with dopaminergic, noradrenergic, mixed dopaminergic and noradrenergic, or non-functioning tumours; cluster 2 {966} (the tyrosine kinase cluster) is characterized by mutations of *RET*, *NF1*, and other genes that affect kinase signalling; and the recently described cluster 3 (the WNT-altered pathway cluster) {1385} tends to manifest with either adrenergic or mixed adrenergic and noradrenergic tumours {1210}. In Europe and North America, metanephrine elevation points both to specific genes and to intra-adrenal tumour location, which has led to the belief that extra-adrenal paragangliomas generally cannot produce epinephrine {1210}. Although this is consistent with the fact

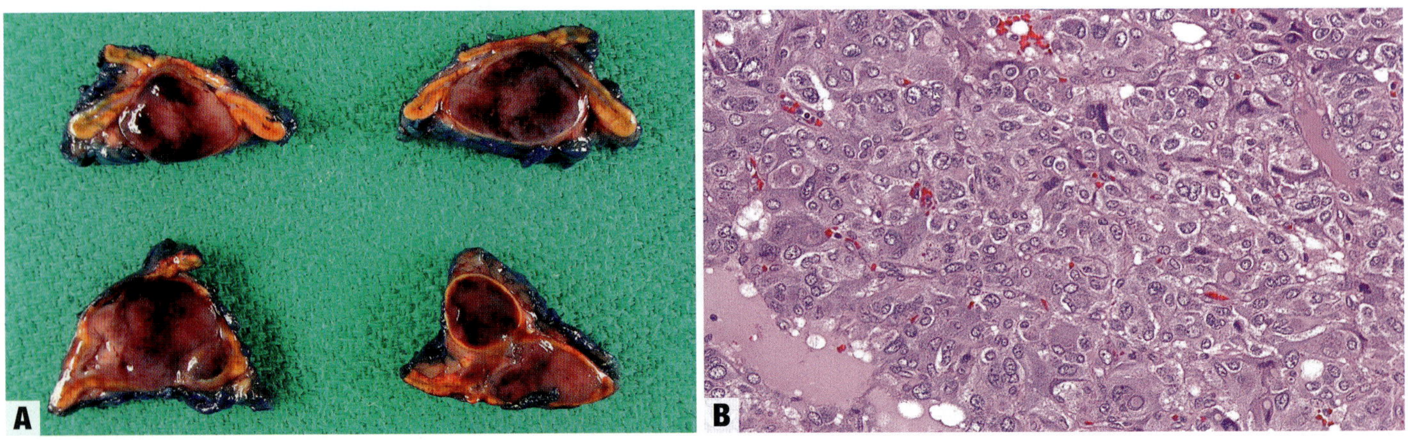

Fig. 6.16 Paediatric phaeochromocytoma. **A** Gross findings. The cut surface of the adrenal gland shows a phaeochromocytoma. **B** Conventional cytomorphology. Like in adults, conventional phaeochromocytomas in children consist of tumour cells resembling normal chromaffin cells that display basophilic to amphophilic cytoplasmic granularity. The cells here show mild nuclear pleomorphism and occasional nuclear pseudoinclusions, which can also be seen in adrenal cortical carcinomas.

that the normal adrenal medulla is essentially the body's only source of circulating epinephrine {1210}, a large study from China shows a different genetic and phenotypic landscape from North America and Europe, including fewer germline mutations and multiple epinephrine-producing paragangliomas caused by somatic *HRAS* and *FGFR1* mutations {2108}. These findings suggest that underlying mutations are the main determinant of biochemical phenotype and that the rarity of epinephrine-producing paragangliomas in populations of European descent is caused by a predominance of cluster 1 mutations {2108}.

Imaging

Of the structural/anatomical imaging modalities, CT and MRI are equally considered the first choice for defining tumour size and extent {78}. Because of CT-related radiation concerns, MRI is often employed in paediatric age groups {3478,4921}. Ultrasound is considered for children aged < 10 years who cannot tolerate MRI {4921,4583}. Most phaeochromocytomas demonstrate a characteristic delineated hyperintense appearance (the radiological lightbulb sign) on T2-weighted MRI {78}. However, heterogeneous or lower intensity may also occur {1763}. Whole-body MRI provides additional value in the detection of bilateral and extra-adrenal tumours in patients harbouring germline mutations {1763}.

Functional imaging studies are used for purposes including the workup of patients with an adrenal mass and inconclusive biochemical results, assessment of multifocal disease, and staging/screening for metastatic and locoregional tumour spread. In addition, theragnostic imaging, defined as the use of a tracer molecule labelled with one radioisotope for imaging followed by the same tracer with a different isotope for treatment, is increasingly employed. The sensitivity of a functional imaging modality is influenced by tumour location, tumour mutation status, and the transporters or receptors that the tumour may express {4374,1240}. A long-established use of this approach is imaging with iobenguane (metaiodobenzylguanidine; 123I-MIBG), which binds to the norepinephrine transporter, followed by 131I-MIBG for radiotherapy of unresectable or metastatic disease if high signal intensity indicates that the transporter is highly expressed {4374}. Similarly, SSTR imaging using 68Ga-DOTATATE PET-CT may determine eligibility for peptide receptor radionuclide therapy (PRRT) with 177Lu- or 90Y-DOTATATE {4374,1240,3964}. 64Cu has recently been proposed as an effective substitute for 68Ga {644}.

Epidemiology

The estimated incidence of phaeochromocytomas ranges from 0.4 to 9.5 cases per 1 million person-years, with national and regional differences resulting in part from different founder mutations causing varied prevalence rates and types of hereditary tumours {1198,2108}. Nationwide population studies show that the incidence of phaeochromocytoma has increased approximately 5-fold since the 1970s {1198}, mostly due to an increase in small incidentalomas in older patients with few or no symptoms {1198}. Most phaeochromocytomas are diagnosed in patients in their fifth or sixth decade of life, with a roughly equal sex distribution or a slight female predominance {1198}. As many as 20% occur in children {417}, who may be as young as 2.7 years {4242}.

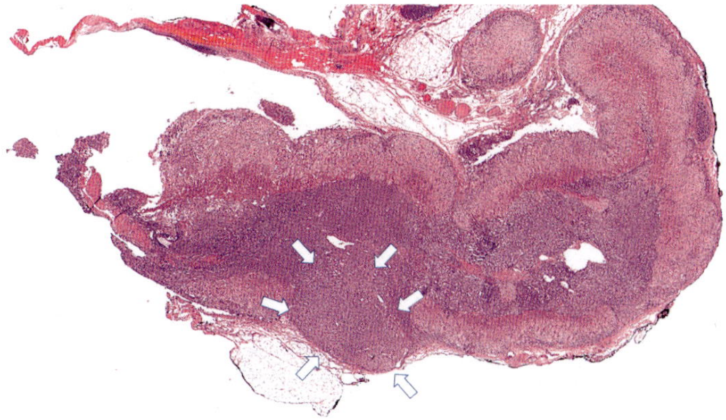

Fig. 6.17 Adrenal gland from a patient with paediatric-onset multiple endocrine neoplasia type 2 with a microphaeochromocytoma arising in the background of adrenal medullary hyperplasia. Arrows indicate a microtumour in the background of expanded (hyperplastic) adrenal medulla.

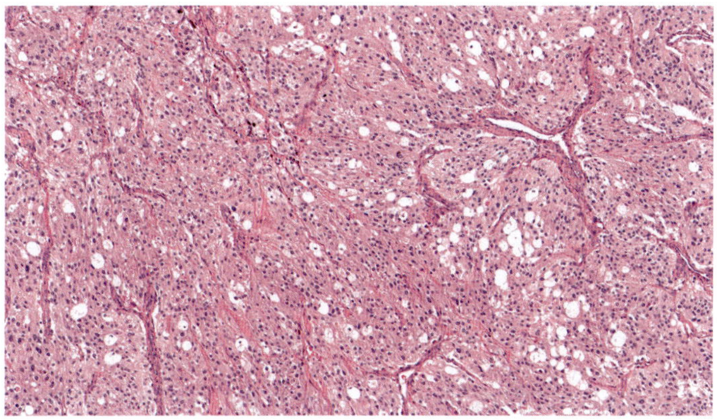

Fig. 6.18 SDH-related paediatric phaeochromocytoma. Cytoplasmic eosinophilia and/or intracytoplasmic vacuoles are variably noted in SDH-related phaeochromocytomas.

As many as 40% of phaeochromocytomas overall and as many as 80% in children {255,3395} are associated with germline mutations in hereditary susceptibility genes. The risk of metastasis varies according to the genotype and guides recommendations for screening {3478,417}. Multifocal tumours, including phaeochromocytomas with synchronous or metachronous paragangliomas, are more frequent in children than in adults {3395} and are suggestive of hereditary disease. However, hereditary disease can also manifest in elderly patients as an apparently sporadic tumour {4838}.

Etiology

Genetic factors

Genetic and/or epigenetic alterations of ≥ 23 mutually exclusive genes are responsible for tumour development. At least 17 are hereditary susceptibility genes, including *RET*, *NF1*, *VHL*, *TMEM127*, *SDHA*, *SDHB*, *SDHC*, *SDHD*, *SDHAF2*, *FH*, *MAX*, *EPAS1*, *DLST*, *MDH2*, *GOT2*, *SLC25A11*, and *DNMT3A*. Other genes that are not implicated in heredity but are somatically mutated in sporadic tumours include *HRAS*, *BRAF*, *SETD2*, *FGFR1*, *TP53*, *ATRX*, *ARNT*, *IDH1*, *H3-3A* (*H3F3A*), *MET*, and *CSDE1* {692}. Some mutated genes, especially *NF1*, *RET*, and *VHL*, are associated with both hereditary and sporadic tumours, whereas others, especially SDH genes, are exclusively hereditary {692}.

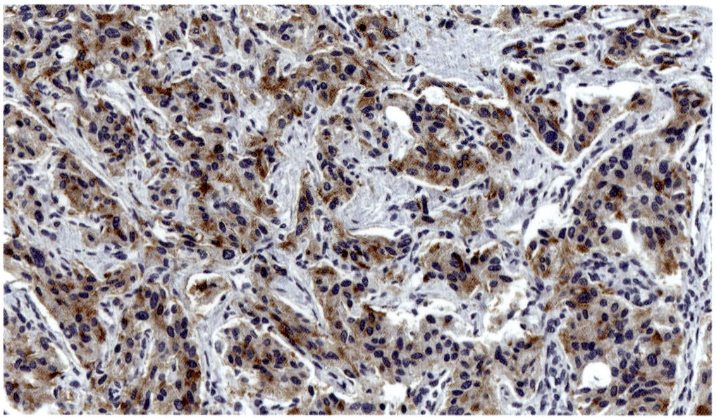

Fig. 6.19 SDH-related paraganglioma. Paragangliomas associated with a pseudohypoxia pathway alteration express inhibin; this can be misleading in the adrenal, where inhibin is often thought to indicate cortical differentiation.

Risk factors

The environmental factors triggering tumour development are largely unknown. Chronic hypoxia due to cyanotic congenital heart disease has been proposed as a risk factor {38}. Some of the patients described have underlying genetic susceptibility, suggesting that hypoxia is a phenotype modifier affecting penetrance, and the majority of them harbour *VHL* or SDH gene mutations, which drive hypoxic signalling {255}. Other patients have no detected underlying genetic abnormality {4830}.

Pathogenesis

According to transcriptional profiling, most alterations cluster to either hypoxia signalling (cluster 1) or kinase signalling (cluster 2) pathways {1385,1343,966}. In cluster 1 tumours, different cellular mechanisms cause stabilization of hypoxia-inducible transcription factors and consequent upregulation of hypoxia signalling target genes. Additional features of tumours caused by mutations in Krebs cycle genes (e.g. SDH genes, *FH*) are metabolic rewiring and inhibition of demethylases and deacetylases by oncometabolites, resulting in a hypermethylator phenotype and altered gene expression profiles {1343,2349} including hypoxia-related microRNAs (e.g. miR-210) {4573}. Mutations in cluster 2 tumours (e.g. *RET*, *NF1*, *TMEM127*) result in the activation of kinase signalling pathways via different mechanisms involving the MAPK and PI3K/AKT/mTOR pathways {3281}. The Cancer Genome Atlas (TCGA) project on the genomic characterization of phaeochromocytomas and paragangliomas also revealed rare somatic *MAML3* oncogene fusions and *CSDE1* mutations that defined the WNT-altered pathway (cluster 3 disease) in sporadic adult phaeochromocytomas {1385}.

Macroscopic appearance

Phaeochromocytomas originate from the adrenal medulla and may extend into adjacent structures. They are circumscribed but usually unencapsulated. As they expand, they compress the adrenal cortex, and the capsule of the adrenal becomes the apparent capsule of the tumour. A tumour pseudocapsule may be present. However, a thick vascularized capsule in association with degenerative vascular stroma raises the possibility of von Hippel–Lindau syndrome {695}. The tumour diameter is usually about 30–50 mm but may exceed 100 mm. In small tumours, the cut surface is pink-grey to tan (in contrast to yellow adrenal cortical neoplasms), but it may become slightly yellow after exposure to air or formalin. As tumours enlarge, haemorrhage, cystic change, and fibrosis are variably present. Sampling of the non-tumorous adrenal tissue is required in order to search for additional adrenal medullary micronodules indicative of a hereditary disease, especially multiple endocrine neoplasia type 2, or more rarely *VHL*-related, SDH-related, or *MAX*-related genetic disease {2400,1674,3790}. The tumour periphery should also be searched for residual adrenal cortex to confirm an origin within rather than adjacent to the adrenal, which would have different genetic and clinical implications.

Molecular profiling has shown that distinct medullary nodules usually represent synchronous microphaeochromocytomas rather than adrenal medullary hyperplasia {2956,2400}, making the latter terminology no longer tenable. In the absence of medullary nodules, diffuse hyperplasia can be recognized if

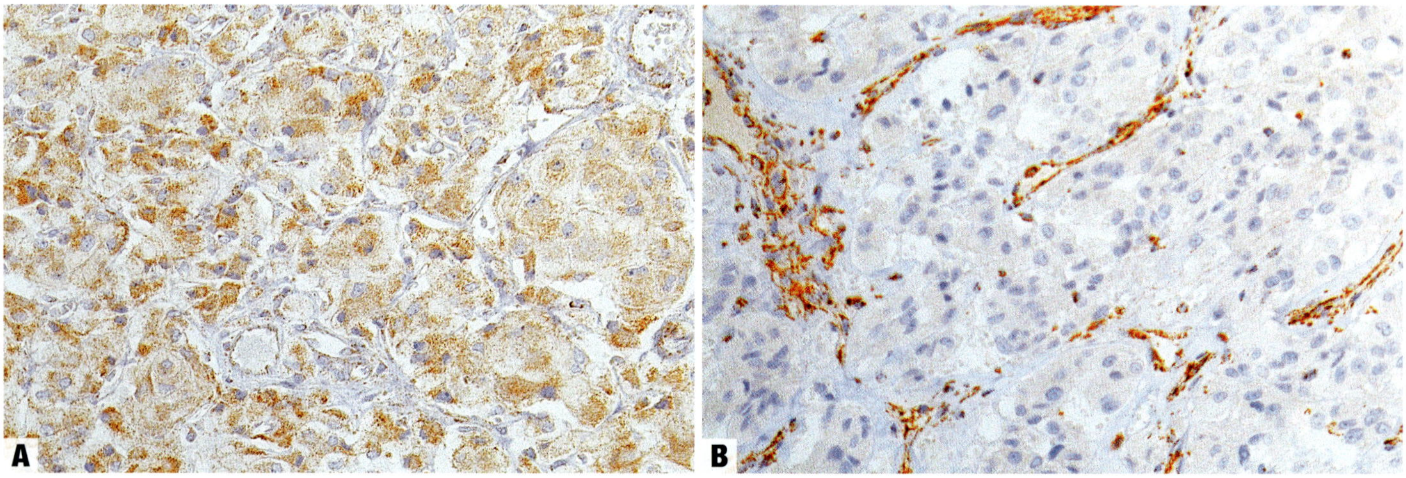

Fig. 6.20 SDHB is a crucial molecular immunohistochemistry biomarker in the detection of SDH-related pathogenesis. **A** Normal staining is characterized by the presence of intracytoplasmic granular reactivity in the neoplastic cells as well as in the non-neoplastic elements including endothelial cells and inflammatory cells. The granularity corresponds to the mitochondrial localization of SDHB. **B** Loss of cytoplasmic granular staining is a sign of succinate dehydrogenase immunodeficiency and requires germline testing to confirm underlying pathogenic *SDHA*, *SDHB*, *SDHC*, *SDHD*, and *SDHAF2* variants. The presence of positive staining in endothelial cells is an obligatory endogenous control.

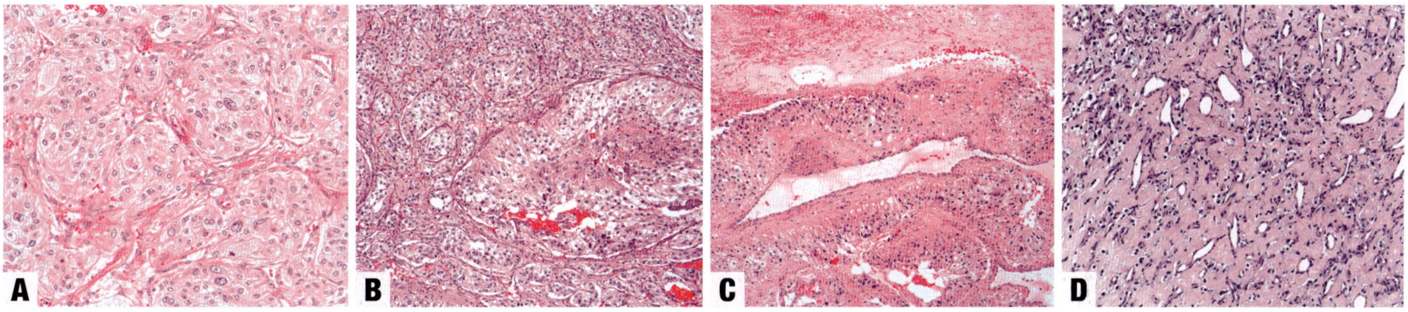

Fig. 6.21 Spectrum of morphological changes in a von Hippel–Lindau syndrome–related paediatric phaeochromocytoma. A range of cytological and architectural variations are identified in these phaeochromocytomas. **A** Like in conventional phaeochromocytomas, a nested Zellballen pattern can be identified. However, trabecular or diffuse growth with large confluent nests (**B**) and/or pseudorosettes (**C**) can also occur. The illustrated case also shows comedonecrosis. Von Hippel–Lindau syndrome–related phaeochromocytomas display variable degrees of clear cell change (**A–D**). Increased stromal vascularity and degenerative changes can feature in these tumours (**D**).

medullary tissue, which is normally confined to the head and body of the adrenal, extends prominently into the alae and tail {1068}. However, normal anatomical variation should be kept in mind, and mild diffuse hyperplasia is not reliably detectable without morphometric analysis {1068}.

Histopathology

Phaeochromocytomas exhibit wide architectural and cytological variation, sometimes in a single tumour {4472}. A Zellballen pattern is most common, consisting of nests of tumour cells separated by peripheral capillaries. Trabecular or diffuse growth with large confluent nests and/or pseudorosettes variably occurs. Conventional tumours consist of cells resembling normal chromaffin cells that display basophilic to amphophilic granular cytoplasm. In some tumours, the cells may be smaller or larger than normal, the latter often with vesicular nuclei and conspicuous nucleoli. PAS-positive hyaline globules and nuclear pseudoinclusions are often present. Nuclear atypia and cellular pleomorphism are sometimes conspicuous, but mitoses are rare {4307}. Less common features are spindle cells, clear cells (lipid degeneration), focal or extensive oncocytic cells {2218}, and lipofuscin or cutaneous-type melanin {2159}. Scattered ganglion cells may be present but are not sufficient for a diagnosis of composite phaeochromocytoma, which requires complete architectural features of ganglioneuroma or ganglioneuroblastoma (see *Composite phaeochromocytomas and paragangliomas*, p. 292).

Immunohistochemistry

Most phaeochromocytomas are positive for tyrosine hydroxylase, DBH {2303}, GATA3, and general neuroendocrine biomarkers (chromogranin A, synaptophysin, INSM1 {2794}), and are negative for keratins {4482,1170}. S100 and SOX10 immunohistochemistry stains intratumoural sustentacular cells. Tyrosine hydroxylase expression can be focal or, rarely, negative in nonfunctioning tumours {4499}. Immunohistochemistry is sometimes required, to distinguish between a phaeochromocytoma and an adrenocortical neoplasm, particularly in cases with predominant clear or oncocytic cell change. Positivity for melan-A and SF1 and negativity for chromogranin A, GATA3, and tyrosine hydroxylase are characteristic of adrenal cortical tumours {2959}. Synaptophysin and inhibin {2975} can be expressed in both phaeochromocytoma and adrenal cortical tumours and should not be used to distinguish the two.

Like in other NENs, the tumour proliferation rate should be routinely assessed {4482} by performing a formal mitotic count from areas with a high mitotic density and determining the Ki-67 (MIB1) labelling index (by counting ≥ 1000 tumour cells

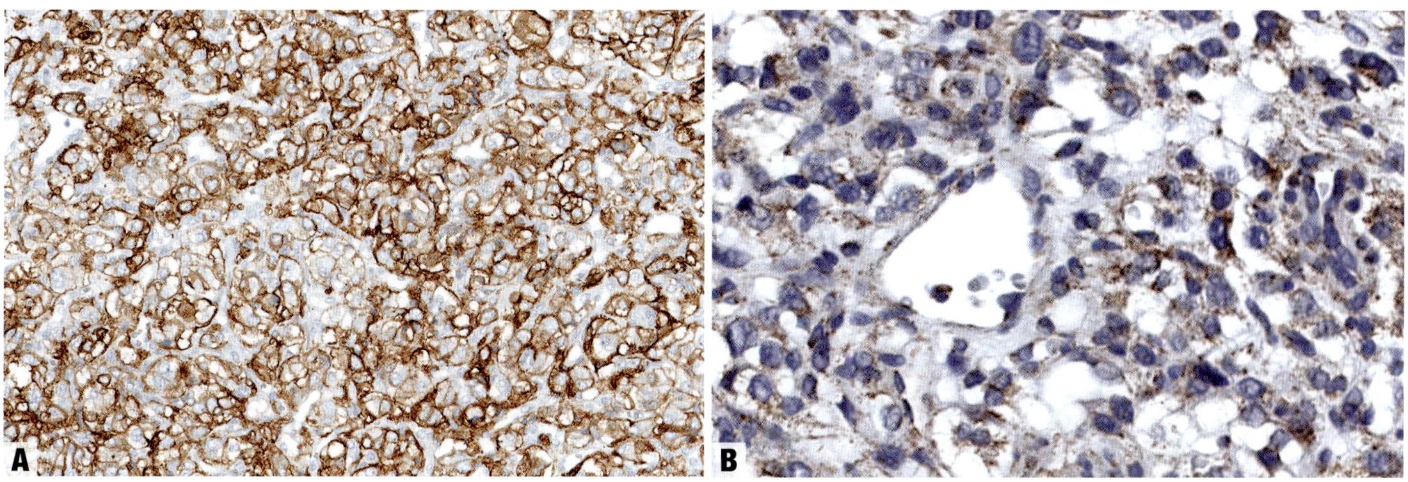

Fig. 6.22 CAIX as a molecular immunohistochemistry biomarker for *VHL*-related pathogenesis. **A** Membranous CAIX reactivity is illustrated in a *VHL*-related phaeochromocytoma. Note that negative staining does not exclude the possibility of von Hippel–Lindau syndrome. However, given the high frequency of *VHL*-related paediatric-onset phaeochromocytomas, pathologists can use this ancillary biomarker to facilitate germline screening in patients with no family history. **B** Note that the same tumour shows no loss of SDHB immunoreactivity.

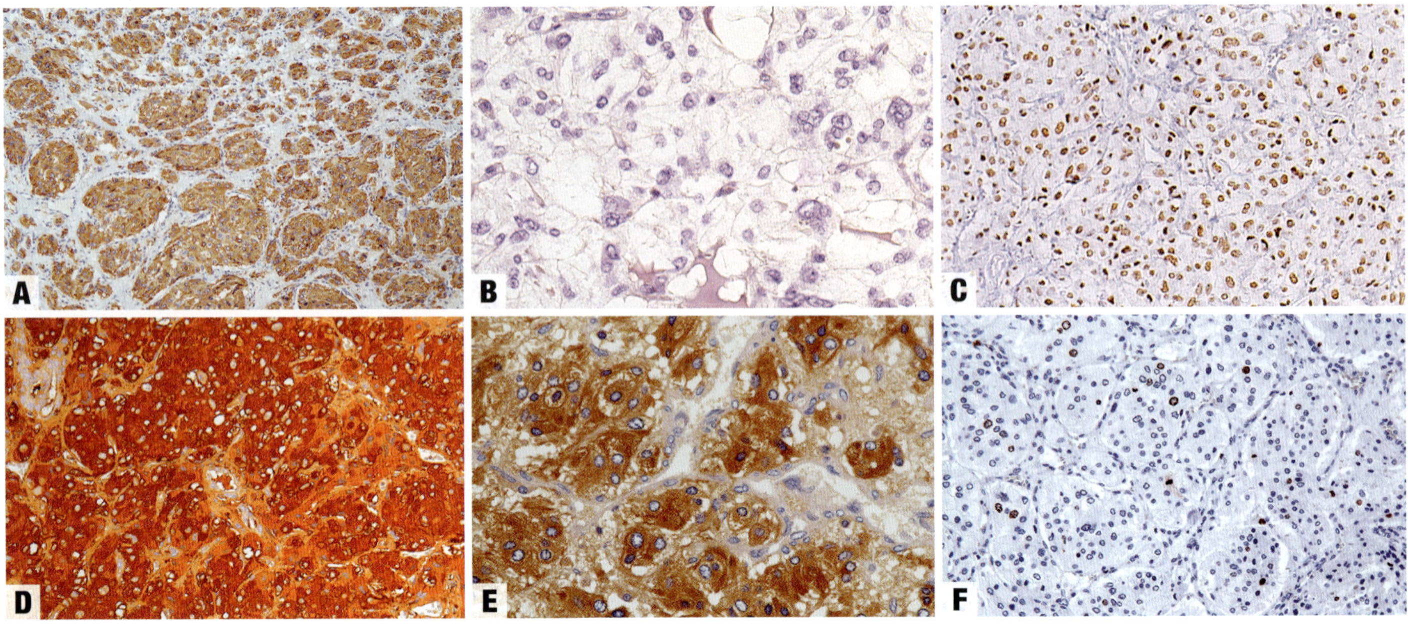

Fig. 6.23 Biomarkers of phaeochromocytomas. Several immunohistochemical biomarkers can be used to confirm the diagnosis of phaeochromocytoma. The tumour cells are strongly and diffusely positive for chromogranin A (**A**) and negative for cytokeratins (AE1/AE3; **B**). Positivity for GATA3 is variably reported (**C**). Immunohistochemistry for tyrosine hydroxylase (the rate-limiting enzyme in catecholamine synthesis) is very useful for confirming the diagnosis of phaeochromocytoma (**D**). DBH, which converts dopamine into norepinephrine (noradrenaline), has also been found useful in supporting the diagnosis (**E**). Like in other epithelial neuroendocrine neoplasms (NENs), Ki-67 (MIB1) labelling (**F**) is assessed by counting ≥ 1000 tumour cells from hotspots, either by automated image analysis or in a printed image. Markers not shown here are synaptophysin and INSM1. Although synaptophysin is positive in phaeochromocytomas, it is also expressed in adrenal cortical tumours and should not be used to distinguish the two tumour types. Because expression of GATA3 and INSM1 is not specific to paraganglial NENs, it should be assessed along with other biomarkers and correlated to the clinical context.

from hotspots, either using an automated nuclear algorithm or by image-captured counting). Mitoses are often very rare or absent, and the Ki-67 index is usually less than about 10% {4472}. A high proliferative fraction should raise the suspicion that a tumour is not a phaeochromocytoma.

Histological features are not a reliable indicator of tumour genotype but can be suggestive in some cases. Cytoplasmic eosinophilia and/or intracytoplasmic vacuoles and clearing, as well as tight, well-formed, rounded nests of neoplastic cells, may be seen more commonly in SDH-related tumours {1170, 4587,4590}. Clear cell change, especially in association with other morphological findings (e.g. a thick vascular tumour capsule, a myxoid and hyalinized stroma, a rich vascular network intermixed with tumour cells displaying variable clear and amphophilic cytoplasm, an absence of cytoplasmic hyaline globules) raises the suspicion of von Hippel–Lindau syndrome {2361,695,4587}. However, molecular immunohistochemistry is a complement to genetic testing and can predict or validate test results {3415}. Loss of SDHB expression serves as a surrogate biomarker for tumours caused by *SDHA*, *SDHB*, *SDHC*, *SDHD*, or *SDHAF2* alterations {3412,1575,4654}. In addition to loss of SDHB, loss of SDHA expression is found in

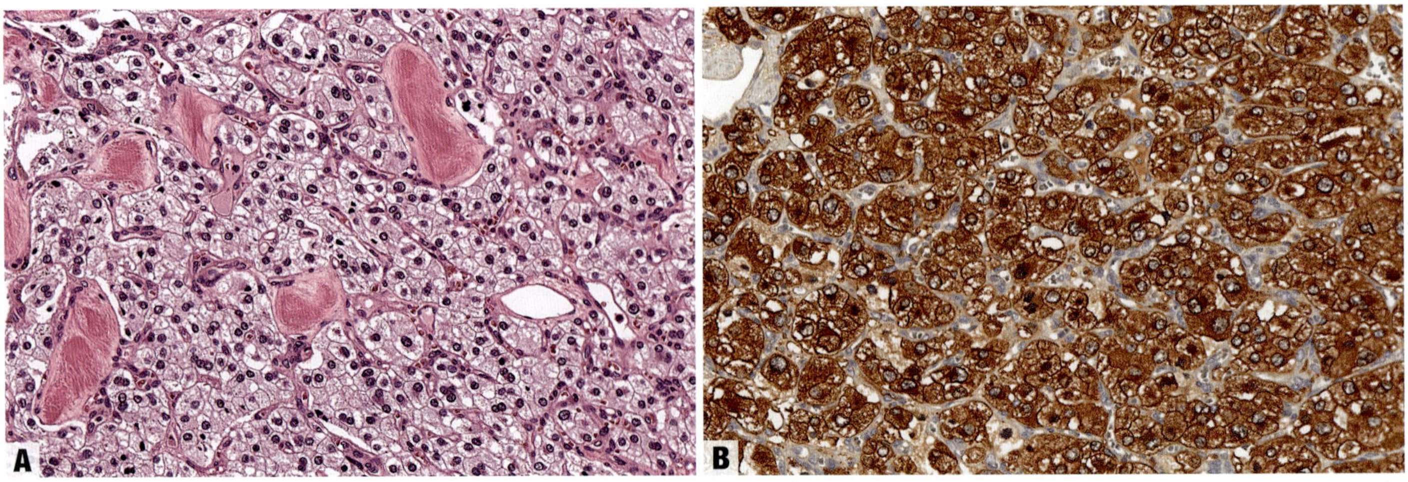

Fig. 6.24 Clear cell change in a phaeochromocytoma. Clear cell change in a phaeochromocytoma should not be mistaken for an adrenal cortical neoplasm. The spectrum of clear cell change varies in phaeochromocytomas. This composite photomicrograph shows an example of diffuse zona fasciculata–like clear cell change in a von Hippel–Lindau syndrome–related phaeochromocytoma (**A**). The tumour was negative for SF1 (not shown) and diffusely positive for tyrosine hydroxylase (**B**), GATA3 (not shown), and chromogranin A (not shown).

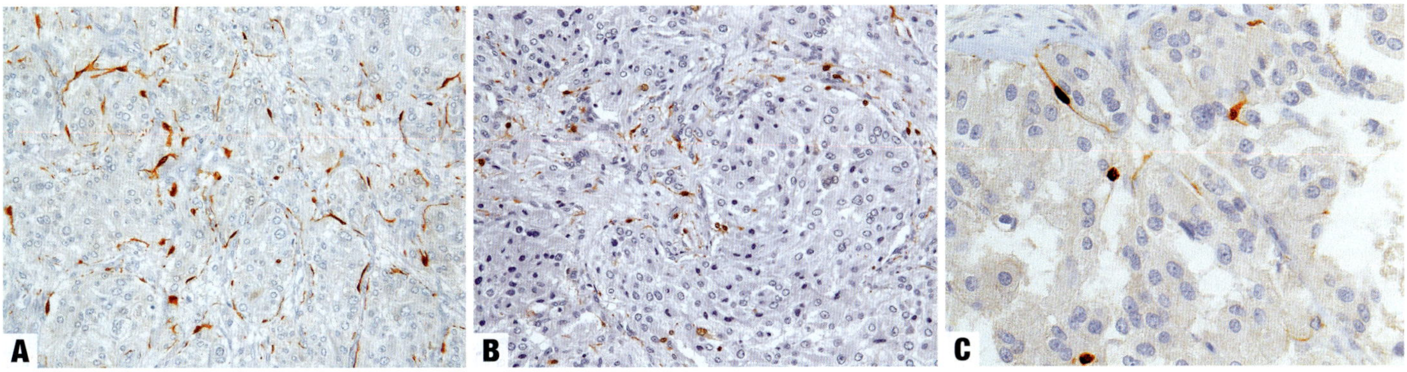

Fig. 6.25 Intratumoural sustentacular cells in paediatric phaeochromocytoma. Tumours show intertumoural and intratumoural variations in sustentacular cells, ranging from a well-developed sustentacular cell network (**A**) to a reduced or disorganized sustentacular cell network (**B,C**). Evidence suggests that sustentacular cells are non-neoplastic in nature. S100 (**A,B**) and SOX10 (**C**) stain sustentacular cells. The use of sustentacular cell biomarkers is not required for the diagnosis of phaeochromocytoma.

tumours driven by *SDHA* mutations {3412,2398}. Loss of MAX expression may be a clue to *MAX* mutation (multiple endocrine neoplasia type 5), but its sensitivity and specificity have been questioned {4047,808,2399}. Loss of fumarate hydratase together with the presence of 2-succinocysteine {4611,4587, 4177,1449} can facilitate screening for *FH*-related tumours. Membranous CAIX supports a diagnosis of von Hippel–Lindau syndrome but can also be found in some SDH-related tumours {3563,2975}. Recently, α-inhibin was suggested as a novel immunohistochemical biomarker of pseudohypoxia-related tumours {2975}.

Diagnosis of metastases

Multifocal primary paragangliomas in various sites should not be mistaken for the metastatic spread of phaeochromocytoma {203}. Metastasis is defined by a tumour identified at sites where normal paraganglia do not occur (i.e. histologically confirmed lymph node or bone). Familiarity with the normal anatomical distribution of autonomic nervous system elements is essential when diagnosing metastatic disease {203}. Involvement of the lungs or liver is not always a sign of metastatic disease, because primary paragangliomas can occur, rarely, in those locations {203}. The absence of sustentacular cells (positive for SOX10 and S100) may favour metastatic disease {4622}.

Cytology

FNAB of phaeochromocytomas is not advised because of potential bleeding or catecholamine release with possible life-threatening hypertensive crisis {4661}. When FNAB is used to assess an adrenal or other intra-abdominal mass where phaeochromocytoma is suspected, preprocedural biochemical testing for plasma fractionated metanephrines or 24 h urine fractionated metanephrines and catecholamines is required in order to exclude a phaeochromocytoma. When it is inadvertently undertaken, complications may occur, although FNAB and core needle biopsy may have different rates of individual complications {2113}. The smears are often highly cellular and bloody, with discohesive syncytial tissue fragments and dispersed single cells that vary from small to large and have abundant round to spindle cytoplasm that may contain red granules (on Giemsa stain) or hyaline intracytoplasmic bodies (on Pap) and oval to pleomorphic nuclei with fine speckled chromatin. Scattered large, highly pleomorphic nuclei with variably prominent nucleoli, binucleation, and intranuclear pseudoinclusions are usually present {2113}. Mitoses may be seen, along with necrosis.

Diagnostic molecular pathology

Molecular pathology is not required to render the diagnosis of a phaeochromocytoma. However, all patients should be offered some degree of germline screening, taking into consideration the clinical and pathological findings as well as the local resources.

Essential and desirable diagnostic criteria

Essential: a NEN arising from the adrenal medulla with consistent morphology and immunohistochemical confirmation in relevant cases.

Desirable:

- Succinate dehydrogenase immunohistochemistry to guide subsequent genetic testing
- Routine assessment of cell proliferation (mitotic count, Ki-67/MIB1 labelling index)
- Molecular immunohistochemistry biomarkers relevant to tumour pathogenesis
- Documentation of elevated levels of plasma free metanephrines or urine fractionated metanephrines (at least metanephrine and normetanephrine)
- Functional imaging studies and routine germline testing; measurement of all three metabolites of parent catecholamines (3-methoxytyramine, metanephrine, and normetanephrine)

Staging

The eighth edition of the American Joint Committee on Cancer (AJCC) / Union for International Cancer Control (UICC) TNM staging system is applied to these tumours. Multidisciplinary international expert pathology reporting templates with integrated clinicopathological data are available {2977,4482}. A recent international pathology-standardized reporting guide was introduced by the International Collaboration on Cancer Reporting (ICCR) {4482}. Tumour size ≥ 50 mm and the presence of invasion into surrounding tissues including extra-adrenal adipose increase tumour stage in the AJCC system {3792}.

Prognosis and prediction

All patients with phaeochromocytomas are currently considered to have a lifelong risk of metastases, and therefore, conceptually, all phaeochromocytomas are considered malignant. The risk of metastasis ranges from ~5 to 15%. There is no single histological finding or biomarker to reliably predict metastatic disease, and multiparameter scoring systems have been proposed. The most readily accepted adverse histological findings common to most systems are a high proliferative fraction, comedonecrosis, a diffuse growth pattern, and high cellularity {4482}. Four systems currently exist: the phaeochromocytoma of the adrenal gland scaled score (PASS) {4472}, the grading system for adrenal phaeochromocytoma and paraganglioma (GAPP) {2306}, the modified GAPP {2367}, and the recently proposed composite phaeochromocytoma/paraganglioma prognostic score (COPPS) {3551}. Validation studies have confirmed that both PASS and GAPP have predictive value to varying degrees, especially as a rule-out rather than a rule-in approach for risk stratification {4756,4277}. Both systems also may overestimate risk if the rule-in approach is used {4276}. The use of scoring systems is neither endorsed nor discouraged, but it is generally agreed that histological parameters are best interpreted in conjunction with clinical and molecular data {4482}. The prognosis also depends on complete tumour resection. One approach is to suggest, on the basis of all clinical, molecular, and pathogenic findings, that a tumour may be of "low to average" or of "higher than average" risk of metastasis.

From a molecular perspective, germline *SDHB* mutations confer the highest risk of metastasis {2121}. Somatic mutations in *ATRX* or *SETD2*, a high total somatic mutation burden, *MAML3* fusions, the WNT-altered pathway, and *TERT* activation have also been associated with increased risk {1385,2119}.

Sympathetic paraganglioma

Tischler AS
Assié G
Hicks MJ
Jarzembowski JA
Kimura N
Mete O

Definition

Sympathetic paraganglioma is a neuroendocrine neoplasm (NEN) that develops from neural crest–derived progenitors in paraganglia associated with the prevertebral and paravertebral sympathetic chains, sympathetic nerve plexuses, and sympathetic nerve fibres.

ICD-O coding

8681/3 Sympathetic paraganglioma
8693/3 Composite paraganglioma

ICD-11 coding

2F7A.Y & XH4G21 Other specified neoplasms of uncertain behaviour of endocrine glands & Sympathetic paraganglioma

Related terminology

Acceptable: extra-adrenal paraganglioma.

Not recommended: extra-adrenal phaeochromocytoma; phaeochromocytoma.

Subtype(s)

Composite paraganglioma

Localization

Sympathetic paragangliomas occur predominantly in the abdomen, retroperitoneum, pelvis, and thorax, and occasionally in or near the cervical sympathetic ganglia.

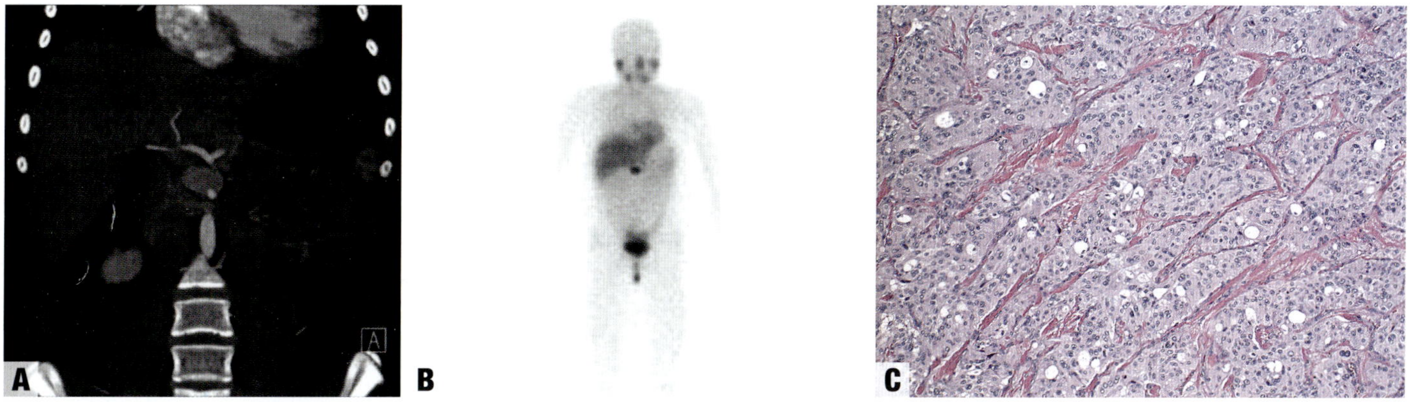

Fig. 6.26 Anatomical and functional imaging in a patient with an abdominal paraganglioma. The patient was a 13-year-old girl in a family with a known *SDHB* mutation. Two older family members had already developed paragangliomas. Genetic testing confirmed that she was also a mutation carrier. Biochemical testing for metanephrines was negative. CT (**A**) and whole-body MIBG scan (**B**) showed a small midline paraganglioma with varied histological patterns, including irregular nests and cords of cells with prominent intervening sclerosis (**C**). Intratumoural heterogeneity was also observed with respect to several immunohistochemical markers.

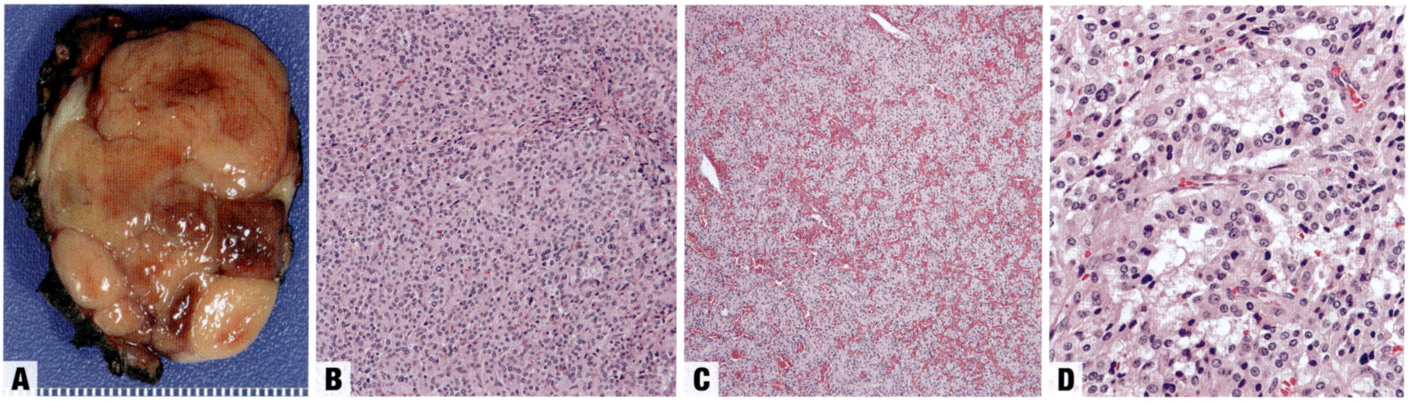

Fig. 6.27 Multicentric paragangliomas. **A** A paraganglioma from a patient with a hereditary *SDHB* mutation, who was screened for tumours in her early twenties. At that time, she had already developed three paragangliomas (34–47 mm) adjacent to her lumbar vertebrae, each with a somewhat different gross appearance. **B** Multiple histological patterns can be found in synchronous paragangliomas with the same genetic background. This solid growth pattern with a high cellularity was associated with tumour necrosis and coarse nodularity (not shown); all of these are putative risk factors for metastasis. Other morphological features included sharply defined tumour cell nests (Zellballen pattern) (**C**) and clear cells with patchy degenerative changes (**D**).

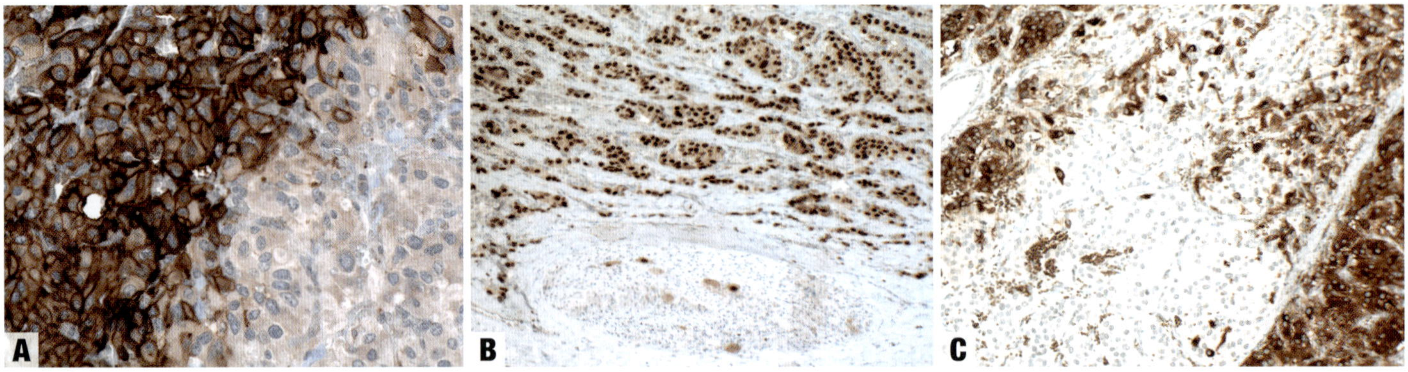

Fig. 6.28 Biomarker expression in an abdominal paraganglioma. **A** Staining of a resected paraganglioma for SSTR2A can be useful as a preliminary test to assess whether functional imaging or treatment with radiolabelled somatostatin analogues would be suitable to screen for or treat metastases. Most sympathetic paragangliomas express SSTR2A; however, intratumoural heterogeneity can be marked, like in this example. **B** Sympathetic paragangliomas can show intratumoural heterogeneity with respect to biomarker expression, varying with both the type of marker and individual tumour. Transcription factors are often diffusely expressed, whereas expression of functional markers can be focal and weak. Shown here is a uniformly positive immunohistochemical stain for GATA3, showing characteristic nuclear staining in a paraganglioma and in two neurons in an adjacent normal ganglion at the bottom. **C** Highly variable staining for tyrosine hydroxylase.

Clinical features

See *Phaeochromocytoma* (p. 277). Some may be biochemically non-functioning, especially those with *SDHB* mutations. Surveillance of patients with hereditary predisposition should not rely solely on biochemical testing {4499}.

Epidemiology

Paragangliomas and phaeochromocytomas (PPGLs) are developmentally and functionally related {2170,1463,1915,2221}, and because of their commonalities they are often grouped together in epidemiological studies. Sympathetic paragangliomas account for 10–18% of all PPGLs in population-wide studies consisting mostly of adult patients {393}. In the Netherlands {393} and the Republic of Korea {2287}, which have national registries, the incidence rates are approximately 0.5 and 0.18 cases per 100 000 person-years, respectively. The overall prevalence of PPGL in the Republic of Korea was 2.13 cases per 100 000 population {2287}. Patients typically present in their fifth or sixth decade of life (age range: 0–88 years) {393}. A slight female predominance {393} and an equal sex distribution {2287} have both been reported.

Approximately 10–20% of phaeochromocytomas and paragangliomas occur in paediatric patients {1040}. In a 2020 French registry series of 81 patients aged < 18 years, there were 41 patients with phaeochromocytomas and 40 with paragangliomas. The median patient age in that cohort was 13.3 years (range: 4.6–18 years), and the M:F ratio was 1:1. Sixty-two per cent of tumours were in the abdomen, 12.5% were in the thorax, and a single tumour was in the pelvis {1040}. In a comparable 2020 Italian registry series there were 28 patients with phaeochromocytoma and 22 with paraganglioma. The median patient age was 11.6 years, and the M:F ratio was 1.7:1. Tumour locations were the abdomen (72.2%), pelvis (13.6%), and mediastinum (4.5%) {4715}. Both series also included tumours in the head and neck (22.5% and 9.1%, respectively), without specific indication of their precise locations or characteristics.

Etiology

Genetic factors

It is extremely likely that paediatric paragangliomas have a hereditary basis. In the 2020 French and Italian series, pathogenic variants were found in 78% and 59% of patients who underwent genetic testing, with the most common mutations being in *SDHB* or *VHL* {1040,4715}.

Risk factors

There are no proven factors for sympathetic paragangliomas other than familial.

Pathogenesis

See *Phaeochromocytoma* (p. 277).

Macroscopic appearance

Sympathetic paragangliomas can appear identical to phaeochromocytomas and can be located close to the adrenal. Care should be taken during gross and microscopic examination to ascertain that their location is extra-adrenal, because a diagnosis of phaeochromocytoma would have different genetic and clinical implications {1212}.

Histopathology

Paragangliomas are often indistinguishable from phaeochromocytomas microscopically. Some have cells with particularly clear cytoplasm, resembling head and neck paraganglioma, which can cause them to be mistaken for urinary bladder {5172}, prostate {4783}, or kidney {1859} carcinomas. Immunohistochemical markers are the same as for phaeochromocytomas.

Cytology

FNAB is generally not advised {4661}, but occasionally it is performed during the workup for other tumours, including those in the head and neck. Smears show a bloody background with single cells and discohesive small tissue fragments that can be acinar and resemble follicular cells of the thyroid. The cells have eccentric, sometimes spindle, cytoplasm that may contain fine red granules (Giemsa stain) and round to oval pleomorphic nuclei with prominent anisonucleosis and even, finely granular, speckled, neuroendocrine-type chromatin. Nucleoli can be prominent. Hyperchromatic nuclei and nuclear grooves may be seen {1386}.

Diagnostic molecular pathology

See *Phaeochromocytoma* (p. 277).

Essential and desirable diagnostic criteria

Essential:

- Clinical: biochemical testing for metanephrines; structural imaging
- Pathology: diagnosis based on morphological criteria and immunohistochemistry as required, with no "benign" or "malignant" subcategories; all paragangliomas are considered to have metastatic potential

Desirable:

- Clinical: biochemical testing including 3-methoxytyramine; structural imaging accompanied by functional imaging in appropriate clinical settings; routine genetic testing in all affected patients
- Pathology: routine use of immunohistochemistry for SDHB and other relevant biomarkers (see *Phaeochromocytoma*, p. 277)

Staging

See *Phaeochromocytoma* (p. 277).

Prognosis and prediction

For individual tumours, the prognostic and risk factors are the same as for phaeochromocytoma. However, location is itself considered a risk factor. Approximately 30% of abdominal paragangliomas may ultimately metastasize, versus about 8% of phaeochromocytomas {945}. It is difficult to ascertain the contributions of genotype versus anatomical site. Extra-adrenal abdominal paragangliomas often harbour *SDHB* mutations, which may be the major cause of their aggressive behaviour {945}.

Parasympathetic paraganglioma

Tischler AS
Assié G
Hicks MJ
Jarzembowski JA
Kimura N
Mete O

Definition

Parasympathetic paraganglioma is a well-differentiated non-epithelial neoplasm derived from paraganglion cells of the autonomic nervous system.

ICD-O coding

8682/3 Parasympathetic paraganglioma (head and neck paraganglioma)
8693/3 Composite paraganglioma

ICD-11 coding

2F7A.Y & XH5LK3 Other specified neoplasms of uncertain behaviour of endocrine glands & Parasympathetic paraganglioma

Related terminology

Acceptable: head and neck paraganglioma.
Not recommended: glomus tumour; carotid body tumour; glomus caroticum; glomus jugulare; glomus tympanicum; chemodectoma.

Subtype(s)

Composite paraganglioma

Localization

Tumours are typically associated with the vagus and glossopharyngeal nerves. Although "parasympathetic" and "head and neck" are generally considered synonyms, head and neck lesions may include sympathetic paragangliomas associated with the cervical sympathetic chains {2193,587,4071,979} or arise from paraganglia with mixed sympathetic and parasympathetic innervation {3075}.

Tumours develop around the carotid body (40–60%), middle ear (jugulotympanic paraganglia; 30%), vagal nerve trunk in or near the nodose ganglion (10%), sympathetic chain (4%), and (rarely) in the larynx, thyroid gland, parathyroid gland, mandible, parotid gland, nasopharynx and paranasal sinuses, sella turcica, orbit, and clivus {2502,1470,203,3862}. Bilateral/multifocal paragangliomas account for 10–40% of cases {1385,4885}.

Clinical features

Carotid body paragangliomas usually present as asymptomatic mass lesions. Middle ear paragangliomas present with pulsatile tinnitus, hearing abnormalities, or a sensation of aural fullness. Large or infiltrative tumours and most vagal paragangliomas are associated with cranial nerve symptoms {1627}. Horner syndrome and first bite syndrome are associated with sympathetic paragangliomas {979,4071,2193}. Increasingly, tumours are discovered by screening families with known genetic predisposition syndromes. These patients require lifelong surveillance and management tailored to specific genotypes.

Only about 4% of head and neck paragangliomas are biochemically functional, producing predominantly dopamine and/or 3-methoxytyramine. Occasionally, norepinephrine or normetanephrine is elevated {3155,2524}, but elevated metanephrine/epinephrine levels usually indicate a concurrent sympathetic paraganglioma/phaeochromocytoma {4188}.

Paragangliomas are detected with the highest sensitivity by PET-CT. 68Ga-DOTATATE PET-CT is most commonly available in North America, and other methods use 68Ga-DOTATOC or 68Ga-DOTANOC. This technique has the added advantage of predicting the efficacy of somatostatin-based therapies, including peptide receptor radionuclide therapy (PRRT) {1240,4374}. Other techniques, such as iobenguane

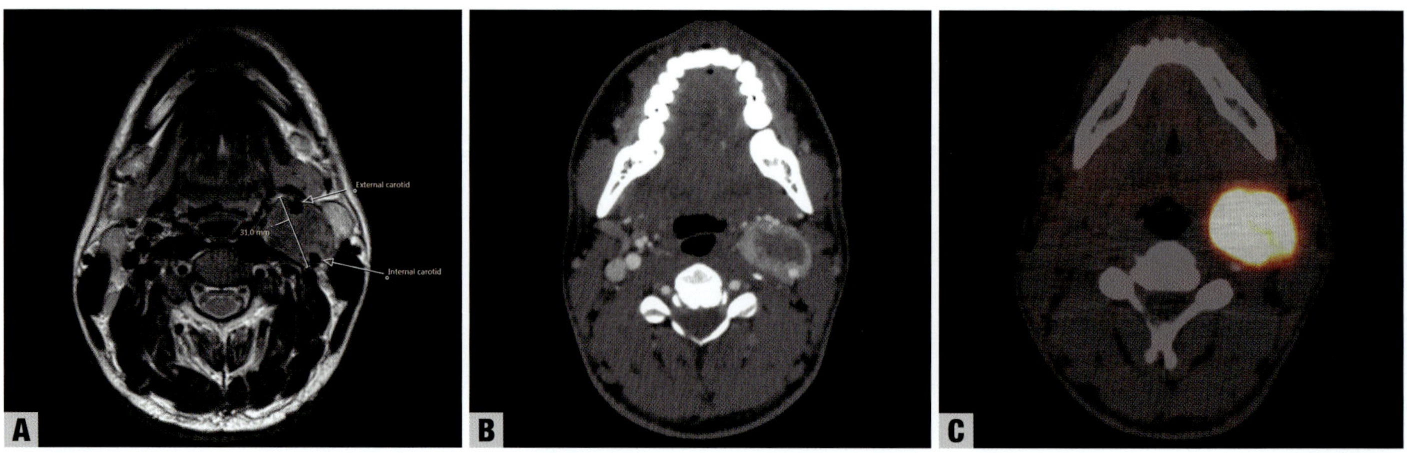

Fig. 6.29 Structural and functional imaging studies in a carotid body paraganglioma. Classic anatomical and functional imaging characteristics in a patient imaged at 19 years of age. **A** T2-weighted MRI showed a hypervascular tumour in the bifurcation of the carotid artery. **B** To assess potential surgical options, CT angiography was performed, further demarcating the lesion, which was deemed unresectable because of encasement of the internal and external carotid. **C** To exclude metastases, 68Ga-DOTATOC PET-CT was performed, showing bright labelling consistent with intense expression of SSTR. Genetic testing showed a germline *SDHD* mutation.

(metaiodobenzylguanidine; 131I-MIBG) scan and SSTR scintigraphy with 111In-pentetreotide, have significant limitations but may be useful if other studies are unavailable {4500,2392}.

Epidemiology

Paragangliomas represent < 0.5% of head and neck tumours, with an estimated incidence of 1 case per 30 000–100 000 person-years {4188}. They can occur at any age, from childhood to old age, with a mean in the sixth decade of life {4188}. In contrast to their sympathetic counterparts, there is a definite female predominance (M:F ratio: 1:1.7) {1263}. Paediatric cases are very rare, mostly reported in the teenage years. About 9–23% of paragangliomas in this population are found in the head and neck {1040, 4715}.

Etiology

Genetic factors

Head and neck paragangliomas have a hereditary predisposition of ≥ 40%, approaching 85% of patients of all ages tested in some series {4188,3953}. As many as two thirds of carotid body paragangliomas may be associated with SDH mutations {3953}. Consequently, there is a high probability of synchronous or metachronous multicentric paragangliomas, which may be confined to the head and neck or occasionally include sympathetic paragangliomas and phaeochromocytomas {4188,985}. The most common mutations in paragangliomas are in *SDHD* (46.5%), followed by *SDHB* (30.2%), and *SDHC* (16.3%) {4188}. *SDHD* mutation is associated predominantly with single or multifocal tumours in the head and neck, with a lower probability of phaeochromocytomas and thoracoabdominal sympathoadrenal paragangliomas. *SDHB* is more often associated with thoracoabdominal tumours {3316}. Paragangliomas in the head and neck are rarely associated with mutations of *VHL*, *RET*, or *NF1* {3316}. A rare, non-hereditary, genetic association is Carney triad. Most cases of Carney triad show downregulation of succinate dehydrogenase (SDH) through site-specific hypermethylation of *SDHC* {4074}, which has recently also been reported in both parasympathetic and sympathetic paragangliomas without other components of the triad {400}. Carney–Stratakis dyad, consisting of hereditary SDH-deficient paraganglioma and gastrointestinal stromal tumour, is a component of multiple paraganglioma syndromes caused by germline mutations within one of the genes encoding SDH subunits {4074} and is not a distinct diagnostic entity.

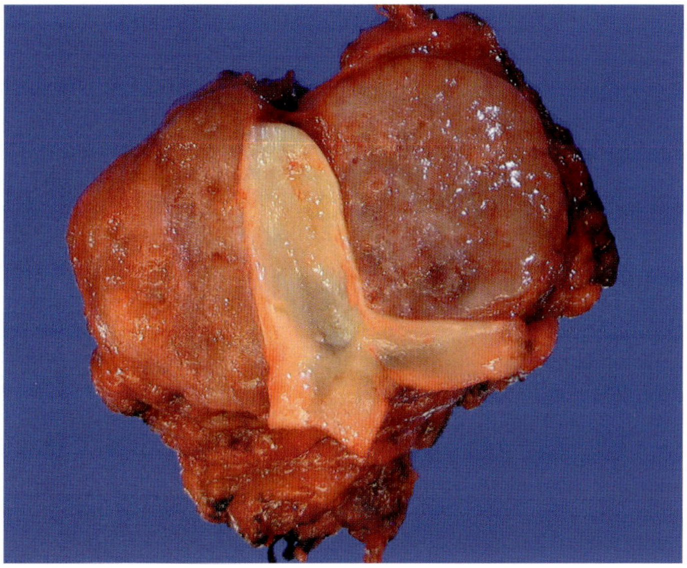

Fig. 6.30 Carotid body paraganglioma. This paraganglioma encircles the carotid bulb and partially surrounds the internal carotid artery.

Chapter 6

Risk factors

For carotid body paragangliomas in particular, tumour incidence is increased and the M:F ratio is as high as 1:9 in some populations living at high altitudes, probably reflecting effects of hypoxia as a phenotypic modifier in patients with *SDHD* {240, 1255} or *SDHB* {718} mutations. An association with congenital cyanotic heart disease has also been reported {2804}. Although the *SDHD* mutation can be transmitted by either a male or female carrier, tumours usually occur only after paternal transmission, causing skipped generations {1920}.

Pathogenesis

Familial paragangliomas are autosomal dominant disorders in which a germline mutation is followed by a second hit inactivating the wildtype allele {692}.

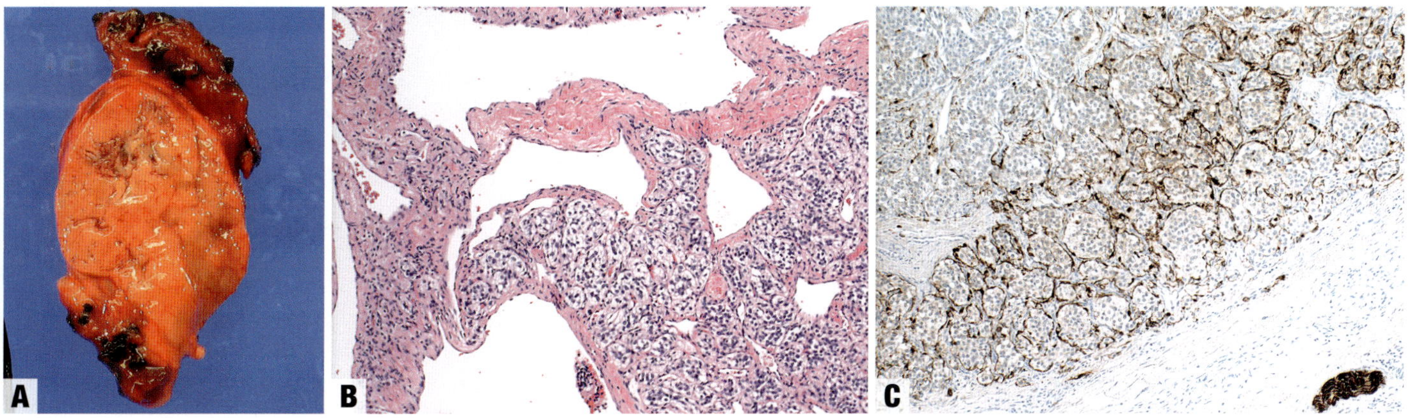

Fig. 6.31 The spongy cut surface of this sporadic paraganglioma (**A**) corresponds histologically to cavernous blood vessels (**B**) that communicate with vessels in the tumour capsule. Prominent, well-formed nests of clear tumour cells are highlighted by immunohistochemical stains for S100 (nuclear and cytoplasmic; **C**) and SOX10 (nuclear; not shown). Note the intratumoural variation in density of sustentacular cells, with a gradient in this case from the periphery to the centre. A small nerve outside the tumour is present at the lower right.

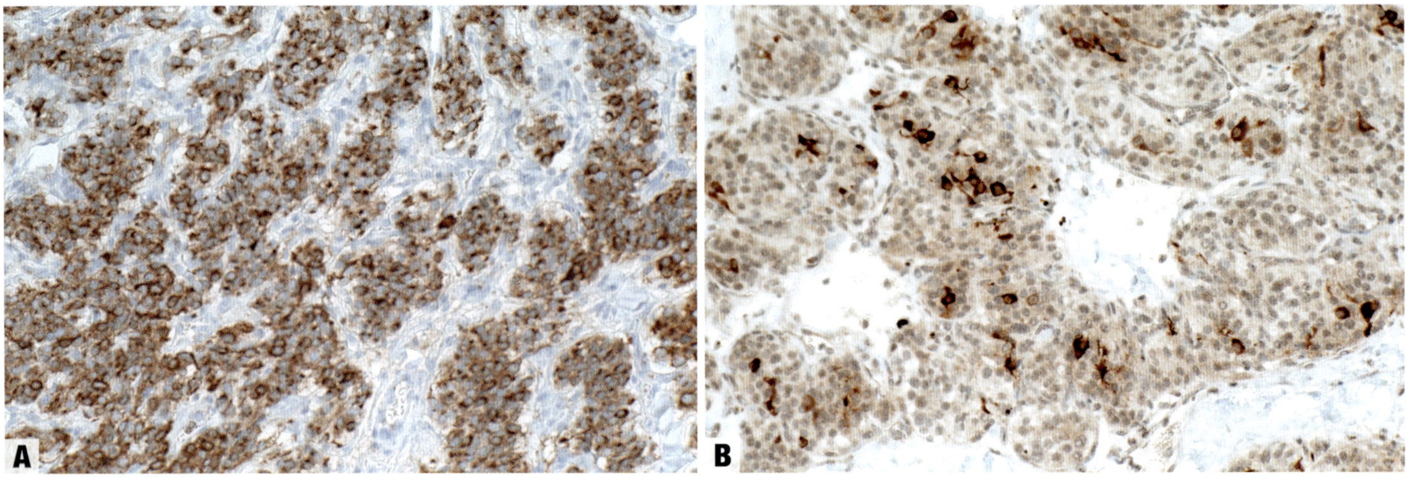

Fig. 6.32 Carotid body paraganglioma. The relative levels of expression of neuroendocrine markers in this apparently sporadic carotid body paraganglioma are those generally seen in other head and neck parasympathetic paragangliomas, including chromogranin A (**A**) and tyrosine hydroxylase (**B**). Chromogranin A can be expressed in a patchy pattern, and often in only a dot-like cytoplasmic distribution. Tyrosine hydroxylase is often absent or focal.

Macroscopic appearance

Parasympathetic paragangliomas are typically encapsulated, pink to tan, firm nodules. There may be areas of haemorrhage, especially after preoperative embolization, which is frequently employed in head and neck sites.

Histopathology

Tumours exhibit a variable Zellballen architecture composed of chief cells with abundant pale eosinophilic cytoplasm with slightly to moderately atypical nuclei, and peripherally located sustentacular cells, usually difficult to detect in H&E sections. The stroma is highly vascular. Mitotic figures are usually rare.

Composite paraganglioma, composed of paraganglioma admixed with ganglioneuroma, is at most very rare in the head and neck. Only one case has been reported and in that example ganglion cells retained immunoreactivity for SDHB, which was lost in the paraganglioma. The pathogenesis was therefore unclear {1071}.

Chief cells express markers of neuroendocrine differentiation, including INSM1 {2435}, synaptophysin, and chromogranin A, as well as nuclear GATA3. Catecholamine-synthesizing enzymes, tyrosine hydroxylase and DBH, are expressed in 32% and 11%, respectively, of head and neck paragangliomas, including tumours considered non-functioning because of undetectable catecholamine metabolites {3367}. Chief cells are almost always non-reactive for keratins {1092}. Sustentacular cells express S100, SOX10, and (uncommonly) GFAP {5176}. Loss of reactivity for SDHB is associated with mutations of *SDHA*, *SDHB*, *SDHC*, *SDHD*, and *SDHAF2* {4654}. Ancillary markers of pseudohypoxic tumours are imperfect, but α-inhibin is expressed more commonly in SDH- related and *VHL*-related tumours {2975} and CAIX is expressed strongly in *VHL*-associated tumours {1344,3563}. Paragangliomas express SSTRs {1175}, and SDH-deficient paragangliomas have been reported to demonstrate stronger staining for SSTR2A and SSTR3 {2307,1240}.

Numerous primary and metastatic tumours constitute the differential diagnosis in head and neck regions, including epithelial neuroendocrine neoplasms (NENs) of the larynx {4885}, parathyroids {4671}, pituitary {54}, middle ear and temporal bone, and thyroid (medullary carcinoma) {2964}. Olfactory neuroblastoma, Merkel cell carcinoma, and rhabdomyosarcoma may also need consideration.

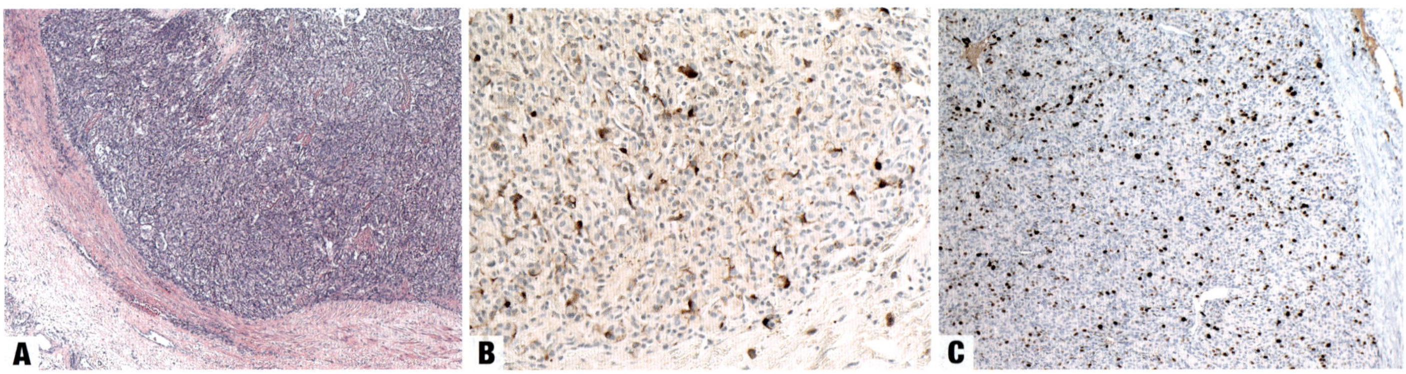

Fig. 6.33 Local recurrence of a carotid body paraganglioma. This neck mass was discovered on follow-up scanning in a patient with a germline *SDHB* mutation who had an ipsilateral sclerotic infiltrating paraganglioma resected 4 years earlier. **A** The lesion was 4–8 mm in diameter and protruded from the lumen of a vein. **B** In contrast to the initial tumour, which for the most part was highly cellular and consisted of small cells with infiltrative and solid growth patterns and extremely rare sustentacular cells, this tumour consists of larger cells with relatively well-formed nests and readily identified sustentacular cells (immunohistochemical stain for S100). The tumour was initially suspected of being a lymph node metastasis. Because no lymph node was present, it was considered to be a local recurrence, most likely from peripheral areas of the original neoplasm. **C** The Ki-67 proliferation index was comparable in solid areas of the initial tumour.

Negativity for keratins distinguishes paragangliomas from most but not all epithelial NENs and depends in part on antibody selection, because some epithelial tumours possess a limited repertoire of keratins {208}. Conversely, focal aberrant keratin expression can occur, very rarely, in paragangliomas {1092,2129}. Such cases must be approached with particular caution, using a battery of markers. Although GATA3 is a useful biomarker of paragangliomas, it is also expressed in normal and neoplastic parathyroid and pituitary {203,2305,1170,2992, 4592}. Paragangliomas can also express peptide hormones including calcitonin {2964,1170,284}. Although medullary thyroid carcinomas can also focally stain for tyrosine hydroxylase, they are typically negative for GATA3 and positive for CEA and thyroid transcription factor 1 (TTF1) {2964,284}. Sustentacular cells, identified by S100 or SOX10, are not specific for paraganglioma {1170,4238}.

Cytology

Smears usually show isolated tumour cells and small tissue fragments suggestive of microfollicles. The cells are often large, polygonal, and ovoid or elongated, with abundant granular, often eccentric, cytoplasm that is eosinophilic (H&E stain) or pale (Pap) or which may contain fine red granules (Giemsa stain). The nuclei are round to oval, with speckled chromatin typical of neuroendocrine differentiation and inconspicuous nucleoli. Nuclear grooves and intranuclear pseudoinclusions may be seen. Scattered cells may have larger, pleomorphic nuclei with prominent nucleoli and clumped chromatin, and similar stripped nuclei can be seen. The differential diagnosis includes medullary carcinoma of the thyroid. Cell-block material can be used for immunohistochemistry and shows neuroendocrine markers {3155,5109,3187}.

Diagnostic molecular pathology

Not clinically relevant

Essential and desirable diagnostic criteria

Essential: a nested/Zellballen pattern by histology, with round, hyperchromatic nuclei with stippled chromatin; SDHB immunohistochemistry to assess hereditary risk.

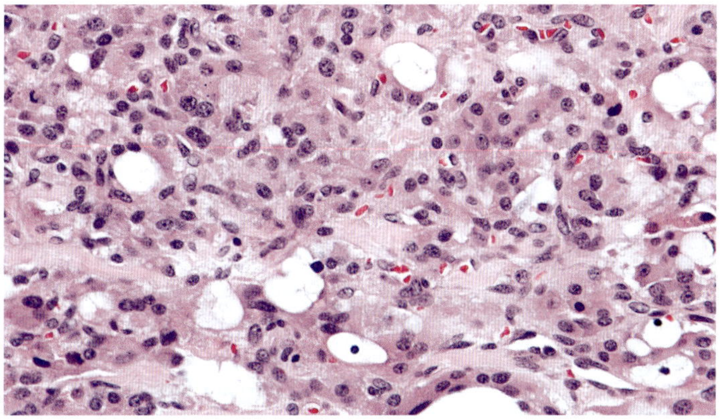

Fig. 6.34 *SDHB*-related paraganglioma in the neck. This neck paraganglioma from an adolescent boy with an *SDHB* mutation and a history of gastrointestinal stromal tumour has prominent vacuoles and slightly eosinophilic cytoplasm, which is often seen in association with *SDHB* mutation. In this case there is abundant cytoplasm, but the Zellballen pattern is poorly formed.

Desirable: neuroendocrine differentiation by immunohistochemistry, GATA3 expression, and negative keratins; relevant germline genetic evaluation.

Staging

There is no TNM system as published by the Union for International Cancer Control (UICC), but International Collaboration on Cancer Reporting (ICCR) and other expert-initiated reporting guidelines have been introduced {2977,4482}.

Prognosis and prediction

Head and neck paragangliomas have a low metastatic potential, with only a 4–6% risk of metastasis for those in the carotid body and 2% for those in the middle ear {4885}. The main putative risk factor for metastasis is hereditary mutation of *SDHB* {1227,2916}. Metastases can occur after many years, especially in patients harbouring *SDHB* mutations, where they may be difficult to distinguish from metachronous disease {2916}. However, locally invasive tumours can have a very aggressive course if unresectable {5176}. Patients with familial paragangliomas require lifelong surveillance for multicentric disease.

Composite phaeochromocytomas and paragangliomas

Lam AK
Gill AJ
Jarzembowski JA
Oudijk L

Definition

Composite phaeochromocytomas and paragangliomas are tumours with combined features of phaeochromocytoma or paraganglioma and a developmentally related neurogenic tumour such as ganglioneuroma, ganglioneuroblastoma, neuroblastoma, schwannoma, neurofibroma, or malignant peripheral nerve sheath tumour (MPNST).

ICD-O coding

Composite phaeochromocytoma

8700/3 Composite phaeochromocytoma-ganglioneuroma
8700/3 Composite phaeochromocytoma-ganglioneuroblastoma
8700/3 Composite phaeochromocytoma-neuroblastoma
8700/3 Composite phaeochromocytoma–malignant peripheral nerve sheath tumour

Composite paraganglioma

8693/3 Composite paraganglioma-ganglioneuroma
8693/3 Composite paraganglioma-ganglioneuroblastoma
8693/3 Composite paraganglioma-neuroblastoma

ICD-11 coding

2D11.1 & XH9K97 Malignant phaeochromocytoma of adrenal gland & Composite phaeochromocytoma

Related terminology

Not recommended: composite neuroendocrine-neuroblastic tumour; composite adrenal medullary tumour; compound adrenal medullary tumour; composite extra-adrenal phaeochromocytoma; compound paraganglioma; mixed extra-adrenal neuroendocrine–neural tumour; ganglioneuromatous paraganglioma.

Subtype(s)

Composite phaeochromocytoma

Composite phaeochromocytoma-ganglioneuroma; composite phaeochromocytoma-ganglioneuroblastoma; composite phaeochromocytoma-neuroblastoma; composite phaeochromocytoma–malignant peripheral nerve sheath tumour

Composite paraganglioma

Composite paraganglioma-ganglioneuroma; composite paraganglioma-ganglioneuroblastoma; composite paraganglioma-neuroblastoma

Localization

Composite phaeochromocytoma is more common in the right adrenal gland, with a right-to-left ratio of 1.4:1. Four bilateral tumours have been reported, accounting for 3.6% of all composite phaeochromocytomas. These comprise 3 composite phaeochromocytoma-ganglioneuromas {2308,799,2513} and

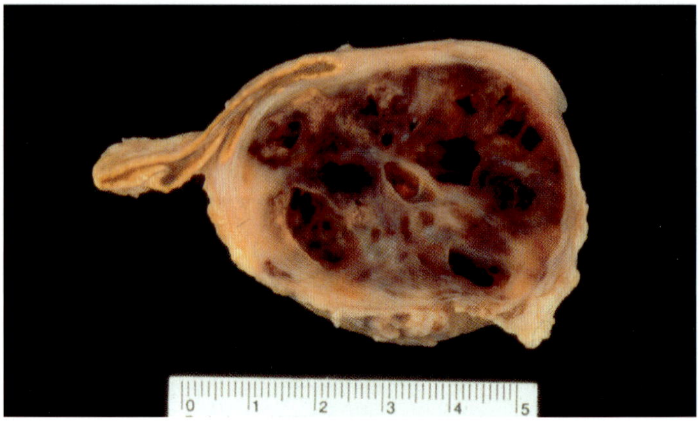

Fig. 6.35 Composite phaeochromocytoma. Adrenal gland with a mixture of a cystic brownish phaeochromocytoma region and a whitish ganglioneuroma region.

a composite phaeochromocytoma-MPNST {3893}; 3 of these 4 patients had neurofibromatosis type 1 {3893,799,2513}.

Composite paragangliomas are most often found in the retroperitoneum (accounting for nearly half of the cases) {1717, 5004,1973,3333,2803,1628,2053,1893,2037,4514,4410,1443, 179,2304,5083} and the urinary bladder {770,4629,1181, 2515,2495,1975}. Other reported sites include the spinal cord region {3638,4010,4085,2613,1527}, sacrum {4943}, mediastinum {1031}, and carotid body {1071}.

Clinical features

A quarter of composite phaeochromocytomas are incidental findings on radiological investigations (CT or MRI). Nevertheless, > 80% of composite phaeochromocytomas show increased catecholamine metabolites in serum or urine. About three quarters of patients with composite phaeochromocytomas are symptomatic, most often with signs and symptoms of catecholamine excess, such as paroxysmal hypertension, palpitations, headache, or sweating {2277,2793}. There are also patients with abdominal pain due to mass effect or haemorrhage of the tumour, and patients presenting with a palpable mass {4095}. About 10% of patients have WDHA syndrome (watery diarrhoea, hypokalaemia, and achlorhydria) due to VIP production {1247,2277,2793,1534,3355}. All cases were phaeochromocytoma-ganglioneuroma with secretion of VIP from the ganglioneuroma component.

More than half of the composite paragangliomas arising from the retroperitoneum or urinary bladder are associated with signs caused by catecholamine excess, such as increased catecholamine metabolites in urine, and paroxysmal hypertension, palpitation, headache, etc. In contrast, composite paragangliomas arising from the carotid body, spinal cord region, or sacrum are rarely hormone-producing. Patients with composite paraganglioma of the urinary bladder commonly have urinary symptoms including haematuria, dysuria, and micturition-induced hypertensive crises {770,4629,1181,2515,2495,1975}. A quarter of composite paragangliomas are incidental findings on radiological investigations (CT or MRI). One patient presented with WDHA syndrome due to VIP production {1973}.

Epidemiology

Composite phaeochromocytomas are uncommon, with > 130 cases reported in the literature. Approximately 75% of the composite tumours are phaeochromocytoma-ganglioneuromas, which has a female predilection (M:F ratio: 1:1.5). They are more commonly seen in the sixth decade of life, with a median age of 53 years (range: 12–86 years) {2277,1717}. The other types are composite phaeochromocytoma-ganglioneuroblastoma and composite phaeochromocytoma-neuroblastoma, each accounting for slightly more than 10% of cases of composite phaeochromocytoma. Both have a male predilection (M:F ratios: 2:1 and 3:1, respectively). Composite phaeochromocytoma-ganglioneuroblastoma occurs in patients with a median age of 37 years (range: 14–73 years) {3159,3466}, whereas composite phaeochromocytoma-neuroblastoma is seen in patients with a median age of 42 years (range: 5–59 years) {4536,3963}. Rarely, composite phaeochromocytoma-MPNST is noted; reported in 6 patients with a median age of 39 years (range: 13–48 years) {823,2550} and no sex predilection. In addition, a composite phaeochromocytoma–neuroendocrine carcinoma has been reported {2136}.

Composite paragangliomas are rare, with 35 cases reported. There is no sex predilection. More than 75% are composite paraganglioma-ganglioneuromas, which are usually seen in adult patients (median age: 51 years, range: 29–81 years). Half of the composite paraganglioma-neuroblastomas occurred in the paediatric age group {179}. The 3 cases of composite paraganglioma-ganglioneuroblastoma were in adult patients {1975, 2304,1527}.

Etiology

Most composite phaeochromocytomas are sporadic, with no known predisposing factors. In approximately 20% of tumours there are underlying hereditary syndromes. The most common genetic predisposition is neurofibromatosis type 1, accounting for approximately 70% of the hereditary cases {1108}. Other than this, 3 composite phaeochromocytoma-ganglioneuromas and 1 composite phaeochromocytoma-ganglioneuroblastoma were noted in multiple endocrine neoplasia type 2A {1203,4095,513, 2880}. In addition, 3 composite phaeochromocytoma-ganglioneuromas associated with von Hippel–Lindau syndrome {900, 1259,401} and 1 associated with multiple endocrine neoplasia type 2B have been reported {762}.

Most composite paragangliomas are sporadic, with no known predisposing factors. However, 2 retroperitoneal composite paragangliomas associated with neurofibromatosis {1717,2803} have been reported, as well as 1 associated with multiple endocrine neoplasia type 2B {5004} and 1 with *SDHB* deletion {179}.

Pathogenesis

Because of the rarity of composite phaeochromocytoma, the pathogenesis is largely unknown. However, it is known that both composing tumour types ultimately derive from neural crest progenitor cells, for which developmental plasticity has been shown {1463,2170}.

Both components of composite paraganglioma also have a common embryogenic origin in the neural crest.

Macroscopic appearance

The phaeochromocytoma component is brown with variable haemorrhage, fibrosis, central degenerative changes, or cystic change. The ganglioneuroma component is often white and firm, and the ganglioneuroblastoma or neuroblastoma components may reveal necrotic or haemorrhagic areas {2513,1534}.

The paraganglioma component is brown, haemorrhagic, and cystic, whereas the neural component is white and solid {1443, 1071}.

Histopathology

The diagnosis of composite phaeochromocytoma requires the presence of well-developed cytological and architectural features of both phaeochromocytoma and another neuroblastic tumour type. A reasonable guide is that ≥ 5% of the tumour should be composed of each tumour type, so the presence of scattered neuron-like cells or a little Schwannian stroma is not sufficient.

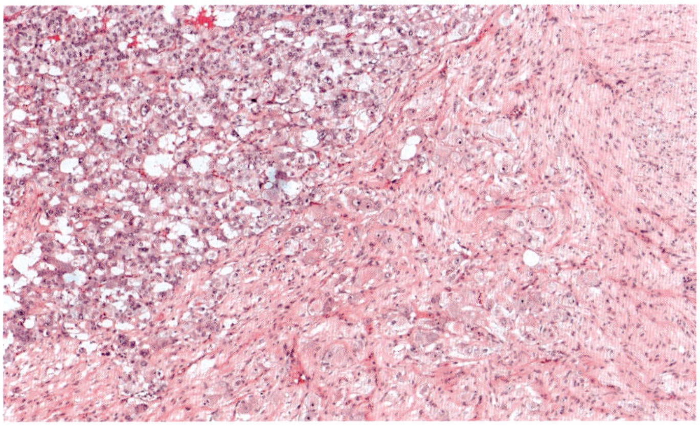

Fig. 6.36 Composite phaeochromocytoma. Histology showing a phaeochromocytoma composed of chromaffin tumour cells with basophilic granular cytoplasm (left) and ganglioneuroma with mature ganglion cells in a fibrillary Schwannian stroma–rich background (right).

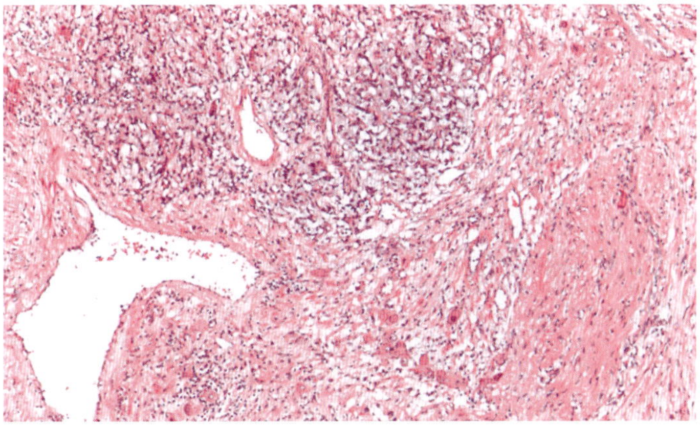

Fig. 6.37 Bladder composite paraganglioma. A composite paraganglioma of the urinary bladder with chromaffin tumour cells that have basophilic granular cytoplasm (right) and ganglioneuroma with mature ganglion cells in a fibrillary Schwannian stroma–rich background (left).

Chapter 6

The phaeochromocytoma component is composed of chromaffin tumour cells with basophilic granular cytoplasm. The most common non-phaeochromocytoma component is ganglioneuroma, characterized by mature ganglion cells in a fibrillary Schwannian stroma–rich background {1711}. The ganglion cells stain positive for NFP (which is negative in chromaffin cells). VIP immunohistochemical staining may be identified in the ganglioneuroma component in patients with WDHA syndrome {2793,2277}. Schwann cells stain for S100.

The other neurogenic components are neuroblastoma, ganglioneuroblastoma, or MPNST. A neuroblastoma component shows neuropil-type stroma with small blue round cells. This component is positive for PGP9.5 (phaeochromocytoma is negative for PGP9.5) {4536}. A ganglioneuroblastoma component shows a mixture of immature and maturing neurons, neuropil, and Schwann cells. No *MYCN* amplification was detected in composite phaeochromocytoma-ganglioneuroblastoma {900,4315}. An MPNST component contains a malignant spindle cell component with nuclear hyperchromasia, which forms fascicles in a myxoid stroma and shows frequent mitotic figures. Compact cellular nodules are also present. The spindle cells are positive for S100. Rhabdomyosarcomatous differentiation has been identified {1713}.

The diagnosis of composite paraganglioma requires the presence of well-developed cytological and architectural features of both paraganglioma and another neuroblastic tumour type. The presence of a few isolated ganglion cells or a small amount of Schwannian stroma in an otherwise typical paraganglioma does not warrant classification as a composite tumour. Again, a reasonable guide is that ≥ 5% of the tumour should be composed of each tumour type. The most common non-paraganglioma component is ganglioneuroma, followed by neuroblastoma {2495,1443,179}. Paraganglioma-ganglioneuroblastoma has been reported {1975,2304}. A case with melanin pigmentation has been reported {1181}. VIP immunohistochemical staining may be identified in the ganglioneuroma component {4410}.

Cytology

FNA has been reported in a composite phaeochromocytoma-ganglioneuroma showing the expected mixture of phaeochromocytoma (cells with granular cytoplasm) and ganglioneuroma (spindle cells with elongated nuclei and ganglion-like cells with Nissl granules) {2550}.

FNA has been reported in a retroperitoneal tumour showing the expected mixture of paraganglioma (cells with granular cytoplasm) and ganglioneuroma (spindle cells with elongated nuclei and ganglion-like cells with Nissl granules) {4410}.

Diagnostic molecular pathology

Most cases of composite phaeochromocytoma are sporadic, but clinical or molecular screening for *NF1* {1108}, *RET* {1203, 4095,513,2880,762}, *VHL* {762}, or *MAX* {3601} mutations may be appropriate in selected cases.

Most cases of composite paraganglioma are also sporadic, but clinical or molecular screening for *NF1*, *RET*, or SDH gene mutations may be appropriate in selected cases {1717,2803, 1071,179,5004}.

Essential and desirable diagnostic criteria

Composite phaeochromocytoma

Essential: the presence of ≥ 5% of histologically recognizable components of phaeochromocytoma and neurogenic tumour(s) such as ganglioneuroma, ganglioneuroblastoma, neuroblastoma, or MPNST.

Composite paraganglioma

Essential: the presence of ≥ 5% of histologically recognizable components of paraganglioma and neuroblastic tumour(s) such as ganglioneuroma, ganglioneuroblastoma, or neuroblastoma.

Staging

Not applicable

Prognosis and prediction

The prognosis of composite phaeochromocytoma is dependent on the highest-grade component present. Approximately 13% of composite phaeochromocytomas metastasize. Overall, 60% of these patients died of the disease, with a median survival time of 2 years. In composite phaeochromocytoma-ganglioneuroma, 6% of cases metastasize, whereas in composite phaeochromocytoma-ganglioneuroblastoma/neuroblastoma, metastases are more common and present in a quarter of cases. Composite phaeochromocytoma-MPNSTs are high risk and often metastatic at presentation. Common sites of metastases include lymph nodes {2513,823}, the retroperitoneum {2994,823}, and the contralateral adrenal gland {2513}. Distant metastases have been reported in the liver {2513,3244}, bones {3963,1428,823}, and lung {3963,823}.

Approximately 10% of composite paragangliomas metastasize. To date, all metastatic tumours have arisen in male patients with composite paraganglioma-neuroblastoma {2495,1443}. The sites of metastases were lymph nodes, bones, liver, lung, and skin.

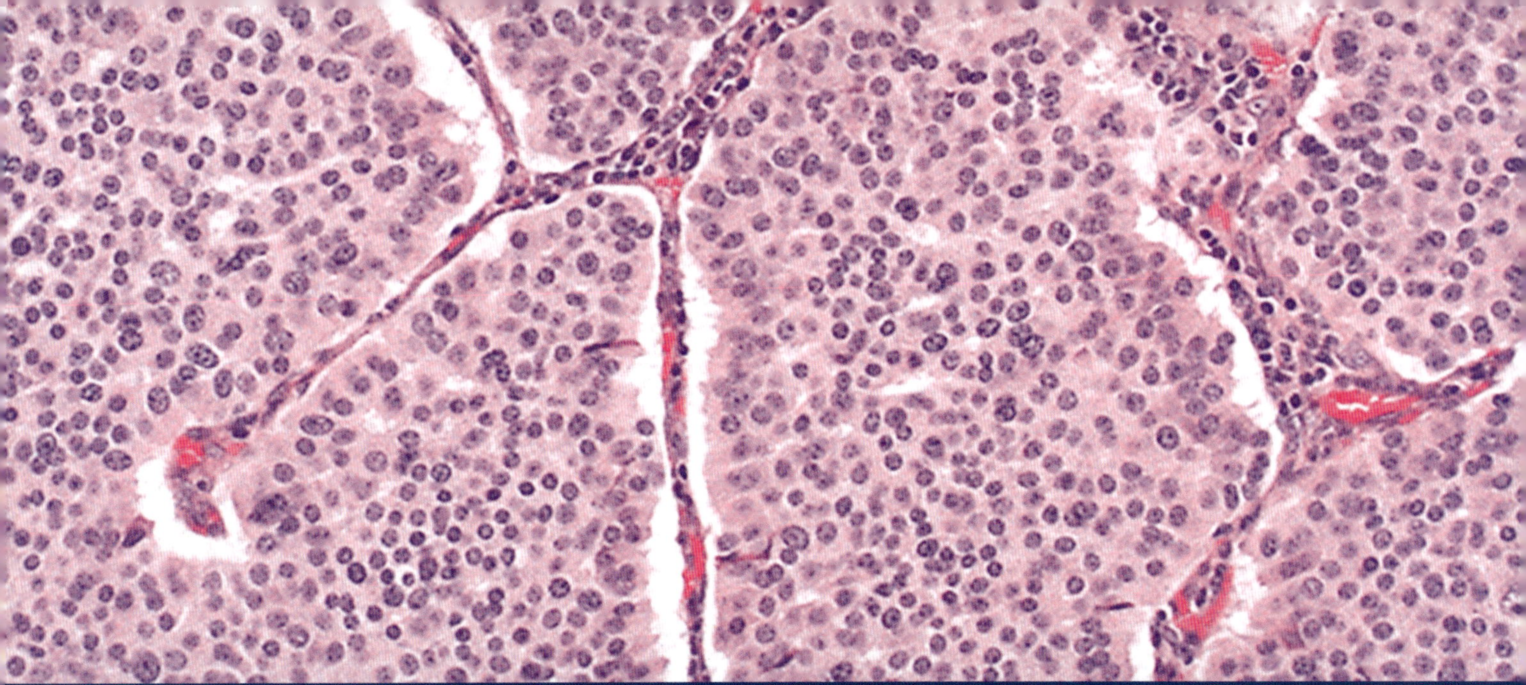

7

Pancreatic neuroendocrine neoplasms

Edited by: Klimstra DS, Mete O, Osamura RY, Washington MK

- Neuroendocrine neoplasms
  - Neuroendocrine tumours
    - Non-functioning (non-syndromic) pancreatic neuroendocrine tumours
    - Insulinoma
    - Glucagonoma
    - Somatostatinoma
    - Gastrinoma
    - VIPoma
    - Serotonin-producing tumours with and without carcinoid syndrome
    - Other pancreatic neuroendocrine tumours with ectopic hormone production
  - Neuroendocrine carcinomas
    - Pancreatic neuroendocrine carcinoma
  - Mixed neuroendocrine–non-neuroendocrine neoplasms
    - Mixed ductal adenocarcinoma–neuroendocrine neoplasms
    - Mixed acinar–neuroendocrine carcinoma

Pancreatic neuroendocrine neoplasms: Introduction

Klimstra DS
Asa SL
Gill AJ
Klöppel G
Rindi G

Terminology

Like other neuroendocrine neoplasms (NENs), pancreatic NENs (PanNENs) express synaptophysin and usually chromogranin A. PanNENs are malignant and are separated into well-differentiated epithelial NENs, called pancreatic neuroendocrine tumours (PanNETs), and poorly differentiated epithelial NENs, designated pancreatic neuroendocrine carcinomas (PanNECs), which can be either small cell or large cell type. PanNETs measuring < 5 mm, previously called neuroendocrine microadenomas, are now called neuroendocrine microtumours, in recognition that, very rarely, they may exhibit lymph node metastases. Neoplasms composed of a neuroendocrine component combined with a non-neuroendocrine component are called mixed neuroendocrine–non-neuroendocrine neoplasms (MiNENs).

Epidemiology

The relative frequency of NENs among all pancreatic neoplasms is 2–5%, and their estimated incidence is < 1 case per 100 000 person-years {1423,1752}. Autopsy studies that consider microtumours show a higher incidence {2310} (see *Non-functioning (non-syndromic) pancreatic neuroendocrine tumours*, p. 300). PanNETs make up 11% of all well-differentiated neuroendocrine tumours (NETs) throughout the body {1751,1423}. Risk factors include a family history of NENs, smoking, alcohol consumption, obesity, and diabetes {2609}.

Clinical features

PanNETs show no substantial sex difference and occur over a wide age range, with the highest incidence found in patients aged 30–60 years. PanNECs tend to affect older patients, overlapping with the prevalence of pancreatic ductal adenocarcinoma. The incidence of PanNETs has steadily increased over the past 40 years {1423,1844,500}, probably as a result of the increasing use of cross-sectional abdominal imaging.

PanNETs have traditionally been separated on the basis of hormonally mediated symptoms, into functioning and non-functioning types. Functioning PanNETs present with characteristic hormonal paraneoplastic syndromes, and the names of the corresponding neoplasms reflect this clinical functionality, such as insulinoma, glucagonoma, gastrinoma, and VIPoma. Less common functioning PanNETs produce syndromes due to serotonin, ACTH, GHRH, PTHrP, or CCK secretion {1502,3710,2180}. Clinically non-functioning PanNETs (NF-PanNETs) may also produce various peptide hormones and bioamines, such as PP, somatostatin, and chromogranins, which either are secreted at levels insufficient to cause symptoms or by themselves do not give rise to a clinical syndrome. These substances can be detected in serum assays or by immunohistochemistry. In some cases, production of these hormones may explain clinical symptoms that are not classic for the defined functioning PanNET types. Thus, "functionality" is somewhat difficult to define precisely. To standardize the approach, the current WHO classification of endocrine and neuroendocrine tumours retains the notion of clinical functionality to define the functioning PanNET types, with presenting symptoms aligning with those well recognized to reflect the abnormal secretion of specific hormones by the neoplasm.

Patients with NF-PanNETs usually have nonspecific symptoms such as abdominal pain or nausea. PanNETs in the head of the pancreas may cause jaundice due to biliary compression. In ≥ 15% of patients, NF-PanNETs are identified incidentally on abdominal imaging studies performed for other reasons {2259}. Finally, 40% of patients are asymptomatic until they develop metastases, and even then the symptoms may be relatively mild. Like other digestive NENs, larger PanNETs have a higher risk of metastasis {3751}.

In the past, functioning PanNETs accounted for 60–85% of all PanNETs, with insulinomas being the most frequent type (accounting for as many as 70% of cases), followed by gastrinomas, glucagonomas, VIPomas, and other functioning PanNETs. Recent data show that NF-PanNETs outnumber functioning NETs and account for > 60% of all cases {1320,1321}.

PanNECs and MiNENs are only exceptionally associated with a hormonal syndrome and present similarly to exocrine carcinomas of the pancreas, including commonly with manifestations of metastatic disease.

Genetic syndromes

In 10–20% of cases, PanNETs arise in the context of hereditary syndromes, including (in order of decreasing frequency) multiple endocrine neoplasia type 1, von Hippel–Lindau syndrome, tuberous sclerosis, neurofibromatosis type 1, glucagon cell hyperplasia and neoplasm syndrome (Mahvash disease), *MAFA*-related familial insulinomatosis, Lynch syndrome, and familial atypical mole–malignant melanoma syndrome (see the dedicated chapter on inherited tumour syndromes) {4169,1287}. Germline mutations in DNA repair genes (*MUTYH*, *CHEK2*, and *BRCA2*) have been described in patients with apparently sporadic PanNETs {4992,3977,207}. PanNECs and MiNENs do not show these associations {3977}.

Updated WHO classification

PanNENs are classified according to their degree of differentiation (well-differentiated vs poorly differentiated), and they are graded according to the mitotic rate and Ki-67 labelling index as grade 1 (G1), grade 2 (G2), or grade 3 (G3) (see Table 7.01). Despite sharing neuroendocrine differentiation, the well-differentiated and poorly differentiated groups are not closely related and represent genetically distinct categories of neoplasms. The 2010 WHO classification {484}, using the parameters above, effectively stratified groups predictive of patient survival. In the years since its publication, however, it became clear that some PanNENs with the histological features of PanNET (i.e. well differentiated) have a Ki-67 proliferation index > 20%. This is particularly common in liver metastases developing in the course of the disease.

Table 7.01 Comparison of the WHO classification of pancreatic neuroendocrine neoplasms (PanNENs) across editions

WHO 1980	WHO 2000/2004	WHO 2010	WHO 2017
Islet cell tumour (adenoma/carcinoma)	Well-differentiated endocrine tumour/ carcinoma (WDET/WDEC)	G1/G2 NET	G1/G2/G3 NET (well-differentiated NEN)
Poorly differentiated endocrine carcinoma	Poorly differentiated endocrine carcinoma / small cell carcinoma (PDEC)	NEC (G3), large cell or small cell type	NEC (G3), large cell or small cell type (poorly differentiated NEN)
	Mixed exocrine–endocrine carcinoma (MEEC)	Mixed adenoneuroendocrine carcinoma (MANEC)	Mixed neuroendocrine–non-neuroendocrine neoplasm (MiNEN)
Pseudotumour lesions	Tumour-like lesions (TLLs)	Hyperplastic and preneoplastic lesions	

NEC, neuroendocrine carcinoma; NEN, neuroendocrine neoplasm; NET, neuroendocrine tumour.

According to the 2010 WHO criteria, these histologically bland but more proliferative tumours would be classified as PanNECs. Although these tumours have a worse prognosis than G2 PanNETs, their behaviour is less aggressive than that of PanNECs {340,1850}. They show features associated with PanNETs (i.e. hormone expression, and association with hormonal and genetic syndromes) and usually lack the genetic abnormalities found in poorly differentiated PanNENs (e.g. changes in expression and mutation of *TP53* and *RB1*) {4992,339}. They can also retain the mutations characteristic of PanNETs (e.g. *MEN1*, *DAXX*, or *ATRX*). Finally, histological progression from G1 or G2 PanNETs to high-grade epithelial NENs was observed, strongly suggesting that the high-grade neoplasms are closely related to their lower-grade predecessors. From a clinical perspective, patients with high-grade PanNENs as defined by the 2010 WHO classification whose neoplasms had a Ki-67 proliferation index < 55% had a lower response rate but better survival than patients with neoplasms that had a Ki-67 proliferation index > 55% when treated with first-line platinum-based chemotherapy as used for the treatment of poorly differentiated epithelial NENs {4234}. Therefore, a novel tumour category, called G3 PanNET, was included in the 2017 WHO classification of tumours of endocrine organs. These tumours retain a well-differentiated histological pattern and have a Ki-67 proliferation index > 20% and usually (but not always) < 55% (see Table 7.02, p. 298). In the fifth-edition WHO classification of digestive system tumours, the G3 designation applied to PanNECs was dropped, because these neoplasms are high-grade by definition {4866}. This updated classification has been validated on a large surgical series {3748}.

The phenomenon of grade progression in PanNETs is increasingly recognized and is associated with poor patient outcome {486}. Higher-grade regions can occur within primary PanNETs, between the primary and the metastases, or among different metastases. In essentially all reported case, the higher-grade (G2 or G3) component is well differentiated. There is a possibility that bona fide poorly differentiated PanNECs could arise through progression of a well-differentiated PanNET, but this phenomenon has yet to be convincingly reported. Instead, PanNECs often have associated exocrine precursors (e.g. pancreatic intraepithelial neoplasia) or a component of exocrine carcinomas.

No upper limit has been defined for the mitotic count or the Ki-67 proliferation index of a G3 PanNET, but the lower limits, respectively, are > 20 mitoses/2 mm^2 or Ki-67 > 20%, by definition. In many G3 PanNETs, it is only the Ki-67 index that exceeds this threshold. The Ki-67 proliferation index of PanNECs is by definition > 20%, and most also have > 20 mitoses/2 mm^2. Primary G3 PanNETs have intact *TP53* and *RB1* in 96% and > 99% of cases, respectively. Occasionally, however, G3 PanNETs can develop a *TP53* mutation during progression {2388}.

PanNECs have poorly differentiated histological features (of either small cell or large cell type), often show p53 nuclear accumulation, lose RB1 expression, lack insulin gene enhancer protein ISL1 expression, and retain expression of DAXX and ATRX {4992,28}. Genetically, PanNECs may show similarities to ductal adenocarcinomas, because PanNECs frequently harbour *KRAS* mutations, which characterize ductal adenocarcinomas {2309, 2388}. In the absence of non-neuroendocrine tumour morphology, they may also express ductal lineage markers such as EMA (MUC1) and CEA {2388}.

Studies in large PanNET cohorts have shown that patients with G2 tumours have a significantly higher risk of progression when 5% is used as the Ki-67 proliferation index cut-off point, instead of 3% {3497,3978,3747}. However, the evidence of differences in clinical management based on this higher cut-off point is insufficient to justify changing it at this time. It is important to recognize that Ki-67 is a continuous variable in PanNETs, with higher rates predicting an increasingly poor prognosis regardless of the cut-off points used to place tumours into large groups. Therefore, establishing a single cut-off point to dichotomize the prognosis is inherently problematic. Reporting the actual Ki-67 index in the pathology report is critical for clinical management.

The terminology for mixed neoplasms was changed in the 2017 (fourth) edition of the WHO classification of tumours of endocrine organs and the 2019 (fifth) edition of the WHO classification of digestive system tumours, from mixed adenoneuroendocrine carcinoma (MANEC) to MiNEN, which is retained in the current edition. There are two reasons for this change. First, the complex neoplasms that are usually poorly differentiated in both components may occasionally be well differentiated; and second, they may contain a non-neuroendocrine component other than adenocarcinoma. The term "neuroendocrine" is the only one maintained from the previous terminology, because the neuroendocrine component is the constant of these mixed tumours.

The category of hyperplastic and preneoplastic lesions included in the 2010 (fourth) edition of the WHO classification of digestive system tumours was abolished in the 2017 (fourth) edition of the WHO classification of tumours of endocrine organs because PanNEN precursor changes have not been clearly identified in association with sporadic neoplasms. They are described in the settings of multiple endocrine neoplasia type 1, von Hippel–Lindau syndrome {4249}, and glucagon cell hyperplasia and neoplasia {2342,4169,1287}.

Table 7.02 2017 WHO classification and grading of pancreatic neuroendocrine neoplasms (PanNENs)

Classification/grade	Ki-67 proliferation index[a]	Mitotic count[a]
Well-differentiated PanNENs: pancreatic neuroendocrine tumours (PanNETs)		
G1 PanNET	< 3%	< 2
G2 PanNET	3–20%	2–20
G3 PanNET	> 20%	> 20
Poorly differentiated PanNENs: pancreatic neuroendocrine carcinomas (PanNECs)		
PanNEC (G3)	> 20%	> 20
Small cell type		
Large cell type		
Mixed neuroendocrine–non-neuroendocrine neoplasm (MiNEN)		

[a]The Ki-67 proliferation index is based on the evaluation of ≥ 500 cells in areas of higher nuclear labelling (hotspots). The mitotic count is based on the evaluation of mitoses in 50 HPF (0.2 mm² each) in areas of higher density and is expressed as the number of mitoses per 10 HPF (2.0 mm²). The final grade is determined on the basis of whichever index (Ki-67 or mitotic) places the tumour in the highest grade category. For assessing Ki-67, casual visual estimation (eyeballing) is not recommended; manual counting using printed images is advocated instead {3713}.

Definition of PanNET

PanNET is a well-differentiated NEN of low, intermediate, or high grade, composed of cells with minimal to moderate atypia, displaying organoid patterns, often lacking necrosis, and expressing general markers of neuroendocrine differentiation (diffuse/intense chromogranin A and synaptophysin staining) and hormones (usually intense but not necessarily diffuse), either orthotopic or ectopic to the pancreas. Immunoexpression of keratins is usually present and can help distinguish PanNETs from paragangliomas. Most PanNETs express peptide hormones or bioamines in highly variable proportions. Functioning PanNETs generally demonstrate expression of the hormone responsible for the clinical syndrome. Although routine staining of NF-PanNETs for hormones is not mandated, it can be helpful in some clinical situations to explain less specific hormone-mediated symptoms. Based on their proliferative activity, PanNETs are graded as G1 (< 2 mitoses/2 mm² or a Ki-67 proliferation index < 3%), G2 (2–20 mitoses/2 mm² or a Ki-67 proliferation index of 3–20%), or G3 (> 20 mitoses/2 mm² or a Ki-67 proliferation index > 20%) (see Table 7.02). In cases associated with a clinical hormonal syndrome, PanNETs are categorized as insulinoma, glucagonoma, somatostatinoma, gastrinoma, VIPoma, serotonin-producing tumour (with or without carcinoid syndrome), ACTH-producing PanNET, etc.

Definition of PanNEC

PanNEC is a poorly differentiated, high-grade epithelial NEN, composed of highly atypical small cells or intermediate to large cells expressing markers of neuroendocrine differentiation (diffuse/faint synaptophysin staining as well as faint/focal chromogranin A staining) and usually no hormones. PanNECs lack expression of acinar cell markers such as trypsin, chymotrypsin, or carboxyl ester hydrolase (detected by BCL10). Based on their proliferative activity (> 20 mitoses/2 mm² or a Ki-67 proliferation index > 20%), PanNECs are considered high-grade neoplasms but are not specifically graded (see Table 7.02).

Definition of MiNEN

MiNEN is not a specific diagnostic entity; rather, it is a conceptual category to encompass mixed neoplasms with a neuroendocrine component combined with a non-neuroendocrine component (typically ductal adenocarcinoma or acinar cell carcinoma). Each component should be histologically and immunohistochemically recognizable and account for ≥ 30% of the tumour cell population. This admittedly arbitrary threshold is intended to avoid including exocrine carcinomas with scattered neuroendocrine cells, or NENs with scattered exocrine marker expression, in the MiNEN category, on the basis that this minor extent of divergent differentiation is not thought to have an impact on the clinical behaviour of the neoplasm. When a minor cell population does not exceed the 30% threshold, its presence can be mentioned but does not affect the diagnostic categorization. One potential exception is the occurrence of a minor component of small cell neuroendocrine carcinoma (SCNEC) within an exocrine carcinoma. Given the potential for SCNEC to dictate the prognosis, even when present only focally, it is suggested that this component be mentioned whenever it is recognized.

The requirement that both components are morphologically recognizable excludes some carcinomas from the MiNEN category. For instance, many mixed acinar–neuroendocrine carcinomas have relatively uniform morphology, and the presence of both acinar and neuroendocrine differentiation can only be demonstrated by immunohistochemistry. Only rarely do mixed acinar–neuroendocrine carcinomas demonstrate morphologically separate components, qualifying as MiNENs.

Both components of MiNENs are usually high-grade (G3), but occasionally one or both components may be G1 or G2. Therefore, each component should be graded on the basis of the respective grading system for that component. Of particular importance is the grading of the neuroendocrine component, because it seems that the Ki-67 proliferation index of this component drives the prognosis of the MiNEN {3008}. Because MiNEN is a conceptual category rather than a discrete entity, individual diagnoses indicating the specific cellular components should be applied (i.e. mixed acinar–neuroendocrine carcinoma, mixed ductal–neuroendocrine carcinoma, etc.; see *Mixed ductal adenocarcinoma–neuroendocrine neoplasms*, p. 328, and *Mixed acinar–neuroendocrine carcinoma*, p. 330).

Reporting of PanNENs

PanNENs could be NET or neuroendocrine carcinoma (NEC) based on histology and immunohistochemistry. PanNETs are graded as G1, G2, or G3. PanNECs are defined as small cell or large cell type. Hormone expression assessment by immunohistochemistry should be provided upon clinical request. See the sections that follow for the tumour type–specific requirements.

Cytology

The features of PanNET are similar to those of NETs of other organs. Smears usually show a high cellularity, with plentiful dispersed cells and a variable number of loosely cohesive sheets and tissue fragments consisting of thin branching capillaries associated with similar cells. The cells are round or (often) plasmacytoid with low N:C ratios and abundant pale granular cytoplasm, which may contain granules (Giemsa stain), and they have uniform round to oval nuclei with coarse, granular chromatin and inconspicuous nucleoli (salt-and-pepper nuclei). There may be a granular background, and acinar or pseudorosette architecture may be present. Necrosis may suggest a higher-grade NET, but distinction requires cell-block or biopsy material. Mitotic figures are usually not identified. Grading of NF-PanNETs in cytological specimens can underestimate the true grade because of limited material {1336,4712,4139}.

Molecular genetics

MEN1 is somatically inactivated in about 40% of PanNETs. This gene codes for menin, a tumour suppressor protein with diverse functions. In addition, approximately 45% of PanNETs showed mutation in either *DAXX* or *ATRX*. The function of DAXX and ATRX proteins is to maintain chromatin remodelling at telomeric and pericentromeric regions. *DAXX* and *ATRX* mutations are strongly associated with the alternative-lengthening-of-telomeres pathway for telomere maintenance, as well as with chromosomal instability. *DAXX* and *ATRX* mutations and the alternative-lengthening-of-telomeres status are strong indicators of a poor prognosis in PanNET {2755}. About 15% of PanNETs have alterations in mTOR pathway genes, such as *TSC2* and *PTEN*. The mTOR pathway is important because it is a potential therapeutic target. There are also PanNETs with *HIF1A* and *VHL* alterations {4009, 2110, 4109, 4169, 1152, 1287, 3477, 3977}. Germline alterations affecting *MEN1*, *VHL*, *NF1*, *GCGR*, and *MAFA* are found in PanNETs associated with multiple endocrine neoplasia type 1, von Hippel–Lindau syndrome, neurofibromatosis type 1, glucagon cell hyperplasia and neoplasia, and insulinomatosis, respectively {2016}. Some of these PanNETs have distinctive morphologies. Mutations in *VHL* result in dysregulation of the HIF pathway, and PanNETs that arise in patients with von Hippel–Lindau syndrome often have clear cell morphology {1913}. Mutations in *GCGR* alter glucagon receptor signalling and lead to glucagon cell hyperplasia and subsequent neoplasia, but the mechanism through which these alterations occur is not yet clear {4169}. Missense mutations of *MAFA* in familial insulinomatosis cause the development of familial multifocal trabecular insulin-producing PanNETs {2016}. PanNETs usually lack mutations in the genes most commonly altered in pancreatic ductal adenocarcinoma, such as *KRAS*, *TP53*, and *SMAD4*. Mutations in *RB1* are nearly absent in PanNETs. The mutation status of PanNETs does not relate to PanNET Ki-67 grades. By contrast, recent evidence indicates that expression profiling and LINE1 methylation status of PanNETs correlate with Ki-67 grade, the switch from G1/G2 to G3 associating with profound transcriptome changes {4149}.

In PanNECs, only somatic genetic alterations have been identified. These include mutations of cell-cycle regulatory genes, such as *TP53*, *RB1*, and *CDKN2A*, whereas mutations in chromatin-remodelling genes, such as *MEN1*, *ATRX*, and *DAXX*, do not occur {4992,2388}. In addition, PanNECs may show *KRAS* mutations identical to those that occur in conventional ductal adenocarcinomas {4992,1887,2388}, suggesting a relationship with ductal neoplasia that also accounts for mixed ductal–neuroendocrine carcinoma, a type of MiNEN.

The molecular genetic features of MiNENs have not been thoroughly characterized but appear to correlate with each specific neoplastic component.

Staging (TNM)

Epithelial PanNEN staging, which is presented in *TNM staging of endocrine and neuroendocrine tumours* (p. 18), follows the eighth (2017) editions of the Union for International Cancer Control (UICC) TNM classification {532} and the American Joint Committee on Cancer (AJCC) cancer staging manual {132}, which rely on macroscopic assessment of site, tumour size, and metastases. This approach largely corresponds to that of the European Neuroendocrine Tumor Society (ENETS) classification {3747}.

Prognosis and prediction

In contrast to pancreatic ductal adenocarcinoma and NECs, PanNETs are low-grade malignancies with 10-year survival rates of about 40–50% {1377,2290,840}. Surgical resection markedly improves survival rates (see *Non-functioning (non-syndromic) pancreatic neuroendocrine tumours*, p. 300). In contrast, patients with PanNECs, which are fast-growing, rarely survive 1 year {339}. The prognosis of MiNENs is also usually poor, because most cases include a component of poorly differentiated NEC.

The WHO classification (PanNET vs PanNEC) and grading scheme for PanNETs (G1–G3) are highly useful for predicting prognosis, both for primary neoplasms and for metastases. Given the potential for grade progression in PanNETs, reassessment of the grade of metastases is important to predict the time to progression. The criteria that predict the risk of tumour progression of PanNENs are summarized in the TNM staging table at the beginning of this volume. The listed criteria (in particular the Ki-67 index {3497,3747}) significantly correlate with the behaviour of a given epithelial PanNEN {4007}. However, predicting the outcome of a PanNET often requires long clinical follow-up because metastasis may occur many years after resection of the primary.

Prognostic immunohistochemical markers other than Ki-67 (e.g. CK19, KIT, CD99, CD44, and p27) have been reported {1102,4007} (see also *Non-functioning (non-syndromic) pancreatic neuroendocrine tumours*, p. 300), but these have not been validated in large cohorts and are not in routine diagnostic use. Recent genetic studies in PanNETs showed that cases with *DAXX* or *ATRX* mutations, particularly G2 PanNETs, had a worse clinical outcome than those with wildtype *DAXX* and *ATRX* {4163,2290,3977,4660,3437}. Furthermore, primary PanNETs with loss of H3 p.K36me3, loss of ARID1A expression, and/or *CDKN2A* deletion reportedly have a poorer prognosis {3853}, but further investigations are required in order to confirm the clinical relevance of these genetic abnormalities.

Non-functioning (non-syndromic) pancreatic neuroendocrine tumours

Kasajima A
Basturk O
de Herder WW
Hong SM
La Rosa S

Definition

Non-functioning (non-syndromic) pancreatic neuroendocrine tumours (NF-PanNETs) are well-differentiated epithelial pancreatic neuroendocrine neoplasms (PanNENs) that measure ≥ 5 mm, without a distinct hormonal syndrome. A microtumour is an NF-PanNET measuring < 5 mm. "Microadenomatosis" is the former term for what is now classified as the multifocal occurrence of pancreatic neuroendocrine microtumours.

ICD-O coding

8150/3 Neuroendocrine tumour, non-functioning, pancreatic
8150/3 Oncocytic non-functioning (non-syndromic) pancreatic neuroendocrine tumour
8150/3 Clear cell non-functioning (non-syndromic) pancreatic neuroendocrine tumour
8150/3 Pleomorphic non-functioning (non-syndromic) pancreatic neuroendocrine tumour
8150/3 Cystic non-functioning (non-syndromic) pancreatic neuroendocrine tumour
8150/1 Pancreatic neuroendocrine microtumour

ICD-11 coding

2C10.1 & XH3709 Neuroendocrine neoplasms of pancreas & Pancreatic endocrine tumour, non-functioning

Related terminology

Acceptable: non-functioning pancreatic endocrine tumour.
Not recommended: low-grade endocrine carcinoma of the pancreas; islet cell tumour; microadenoma.

Subtype(s)

Oncocytic non-functioning (non-syndromic) PanNET; clear cell non-functioning (non-syndromic) PanNET; pleomorphic non-functioning (non-syndromic) PanNET; cystic non-functioning (non-syndromic) PanNET

Localization

NF-PanNETs have no specific site predilection {429,259}.

Clinical features

Sporadic NF-PanNETs can be diagnosed at any age between 10 and 80 years {4682,4133,1376,3978,1759,3747,3748}. Increasing numbers of NF-PanNETs are being diagnosed incidentally, and the optimal management of small (< 20 mm), asymptomatic, incidentally detected tumours is controversial and the subject of ongoing follow-up studies (e.g. ASPEN {878}) {2098,3449,3735}. The remaining NF-PanNETs present with symptoms due to local or metastatic tumour spread {2445}. As many as half of patients present with metastatic disease {5045,3747,3748}.

Metastases occur both to regional lymph nodes and to the liver. Other metastatic sites are mainly found in lung and bone {4682,2445,1321}.

Biochemical investigations

Specific NF-PanNET blood markers are not available at present, but general neuroendocrine neoplasm (NEN) serological markers (chromogranin A, pancreastatin, or vasostatin-1) can be used, and levels have been correlated with tumour size and aggressiveness {2098,1924}.

Imaging

NF-PanNETs and their metastatic spread can be diagnosed using EUS and CT-guided FNA, CT, MRI, and SSTR imaging (111In-pentetreotide [Octreoscan] and 68Ga-DOTATOC/DOTANOC PET) {3750,2445,1321,127}.

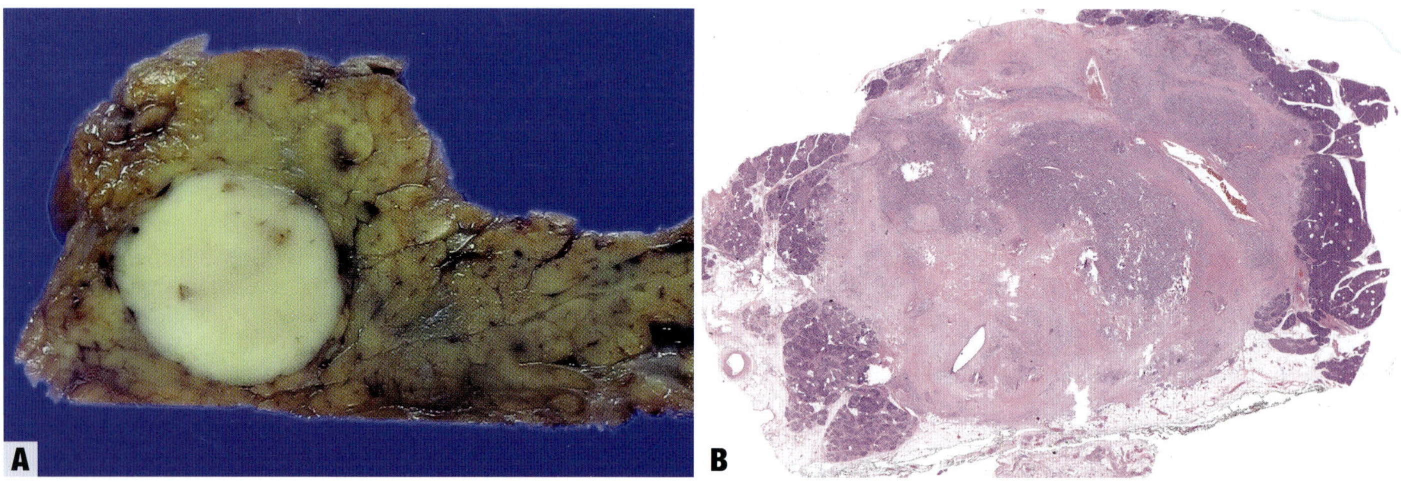

Fig. 7.01 Non-functioning pancreatic neuroendocrine tumour (PanNET). **A** Small (14 mm), solid, well-demarcated tumour in the pancreatic body. **B** Well-circumscribed tumour with conspicuous stromal sclerosis.

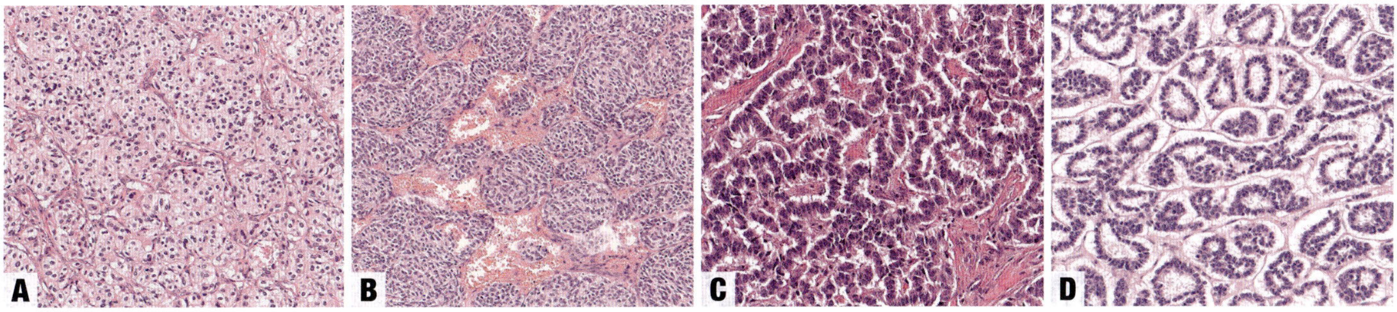

Fig. 7.02 Non-functioning pancreatic neuroendocrine tumour (PanNET). **A** Solid-nested pattern. **B** Solid-paraganglioma-like pattern. **C** Trabecular-reticulated pattern. **D** Trabecular-glandular pattern.

Epidemiology

The prevalence of clinically diagnosed PanNETs is increasing over time and currently amounts to 0.4 cases per 1 million person-years {1415}. However, this reflects a historical underestimation of the prevalence of this disorder, because autopsy studies show that the prevalence of PanNETs is between 3% and 10% {2310,2547,995}. Two to three decades ago, NF-PanNETs were reported to constitute only one third of all PanNETs {542,2345}, but in a recently published large international cohort study, NF-PanNETs represented two thirds of cases {1376,3978,3747,3748}. In multiple endocrine neoplasia type 1, 30–75% of patients are diagnosed with a PanNET, but at autopsy there is nearly 100% pancreatic involvement {4164, 902,3236,515}. In these patients, a high percentage of separate tumours are NF-PanNETs {1707,157,3555}, but the majority have at least one functioning PanNET, or a functioning duodenal gastrinoma {2346,2552,3236,515}. In von Hippel–Lindau syndrome (VHL), PanNETs are observed in 11–17% of patients {1761,442,3739,2428}; functioning lesions have not been reported {442,3522,2428}.

Etiology

Familial NF-PanNETs are found in several hereditary syndromes such as multiple endocrine neoplasia type 1, VHL, tuberous sclerosis, and neurofibromatosis type 1, and rarely in other syndromes (see *Pancreatic neuroendocrine neoplasms: Introduction*, p. 296).

Pathogenesis

The pathogenesis of NF-PanNETs is largely unknown, and precursors in both the ducts and the islets have been suggested. During disease progression, accumulation of additional genomic alterations accompanies the grade progression that may occur.

The genetic features of NF-PanNETs are similar to those described for PanNETs in general (see *Pancreatic neuroendocrine neoplasms: Introduction*, p. 296).

The most frequent recurring genetic features are inactivation of the genes *MEN1*, *DAXX* or *ATRX*, *SETD2*, *PTEN*, and *TSC1/TSC2*; hyperactivation of the PI3K/mTOR pathway; and alternative lengthening of telomeres {2110}. Epigenomic and transcriptomic profiles of most NF-PanNETs fall into either a group with A-cell lineage or a group with islet B-cell lineage features {713}. *MEN1/DAXX/ATRX* mutations are frequently detected in the A-cell group {740,1732}.

Macroscopic appearance

The majority of NF-PanNETs are well circumscribed and range from 20 to 50 mm in greatest dimension {2445}. Some large tumours are lobulated, with a nodular-infiltrative appearance. NF-PanNETs vary in consistency from soft and fleshy to hard and fibrous, and from red-tan to brown-yellow. Cystic change may occur, usually with a unilocular cyst filled with serous fluid surrounded by a rim of neoplastic tissue {2654,2387,4162}. Necrosis is uncommon.

Rarely, NF-PanNETs in the head of the gland narrow the common bile duct and infiltrate the duodenum; tumours in the tail of the gland extend into peripancreatic soft tissues and spleen. Tumour thrombi within large veins may be found.

Histopathology

NF-PanNETs are characterized by organoid growth patterns that do not differ from those of most types of functioning PanNETs {4412}. The two main growth patterns are solid and trabecular. The former can be subtyped into solid-nested and solid-paraganglioma-like and the latter into trabecular NOS, trabecular-reticulated, trabecular-gyriform, and trabecular-glandular patterns {2390,2213}. In some tumours, different patterns coexist {2344,2345}. Necrosis is uncommon and generally focal. The stroma can vary from a delicate fibrovascular network to broad areas of dense, hyalinized collagen. Some tumours may exhibit stromal calcifications and psammoma bodies.

The neoplastic cells are usually cuboidal, with eosinophilic to amphophilic, finely granular cytoplasm. The nuclei are round to oval, with minimal atypia and coarsely clumped (salt-and-pepper) chromatin. They are centrally located in tumours with a solid pattern, or polarized in trabecular tumours. Uncommon are eccentric nuclei associated with a rhabdoid or clear cell appearance {3517}, enlarged nuclei, irregular nuclear membranes, and prominent nucleoli. Mitoses are generally sparse (nearly always < 20 mitoses/2 mm^2). Some NF-PanNETs contain small non-neoplastic ductules, acini, and islets intermingled with the neoplastic cells {4649,2195}.

Subtypes

A number of NF-PanNETs have distinctive cytological features. Oncocytic NF-PanNETs are composed of large cells with eosinophilic cytoplasm (due to abundant mitochondria) and large nuclei frequently containing prominent nucleoli {4728}. Pleomorphic NF-PanNETs are characterized by marked nuclear pleomorphism, but these pleomorphic nuclei have no adverse prognostic significance, because they are associated with

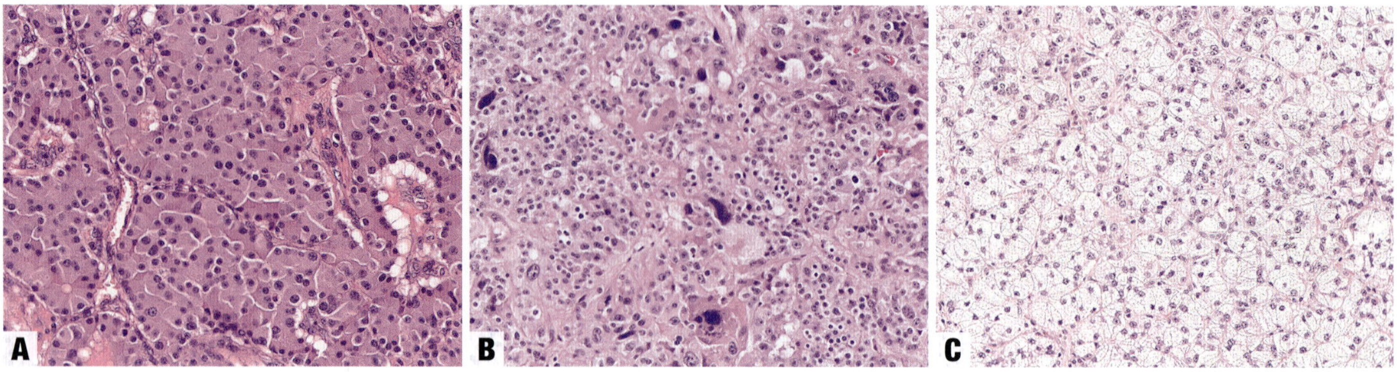

Fig. 7.03 Non-functioning pancreatic neuroendocrine tumour (PanNET). **A** Oncocytic cytological features. **B** Pleomorphic cytological features. **C** Clear cell cytological features.

a normal N:C ratio and no increased proliferation rate {5122}. Clear cell NF-PanNETs have innumerable lipid vacuoles in the cytoplasm, scalloping the nucleus. Although these tumours were first reported in patients with VHL, cases also occur outside the setting of VHL {1913,4161}.

Immunohistochemistry

The epithelial and neuroendocrine nature of NF-PanNETs is best recognized by cytokeratin, synaptophysin, chromogranin A, and INSM1 immunolabelling {4418,4604}. Many NF-PanNETs, although clinically non-functioning, immunolabel for peptide hormones in highly variable proportions of the tumour cells. About 40% of the tumours are multihormonal {2195,2292}. The hormones most often expressed are glucagon, PP, and somatostatin {1914,2195,2390}, although immunoreactivity for ectopic hormones (i.e. calcitonin, ACTH, α-hCG, neurotensin, etc.) can be detected as well {2488,4601}. Rarely, the entire tumour fails to label for any hormone. In some tumours, in which one hormone predominates, distinctive histological patterns may occur. Glucagon-positive NF-PanNETs frequently demonstrate cystic changes and the trabecular-reticulated pattern {2387}. Somatostatin-positive NF-PanNETs may show a nested, paraganglioma-like pattern and/or glandular structures with psammoma bodies {1501,2390}. Serotonin-positive NF-PanNETs often display small cell nests and tubules embedded in dense stromal sclerosis, and they frequently arise adjacent to the main duct, causing duct obstruction and dilatation (see *Serotonin-producing tumours with and without carcinoid syndrome*, p. 320) {2480,2906}. Pancreatic neuroendocrine microtumours generally show diffuse expression of a single peptide, most often glucagon, followed by PP {157}.

NF-PanNETs express the transcription factor insulin gene enhancer protein ISL1, which may be useful to support a pancreatic origin for a metastatic NET of unknown primary {1660, 28}. The intestinal marker CDX2 is expressed in about 10% of NF-PanNETs {1660}. Immunolabelling for DAXX and ATRX reveals loss of expression in as many as 45% of NF-PanNETs {2110,4841,2848}. Overexpression of p53 may be rarely seen in high-grade PanNETs (G3 NETs) {2388,2214}. Strong membranous expression of SSTR2A is usually seen in NF-PanNETs and correlates with molecular imaging {4725}. Occasionally, NF-PanNETs immunolabel for CEA and CA19-9 {5043,2178}.

Immunolabelling for Ki-67 reveals that most NF-PanNETs show low-grade (G1) to intermediate-grade (G2) proliferative features, and as many as 9% of these tumours show a Ki-67 labelling index > 20% {157,3748,2214}.

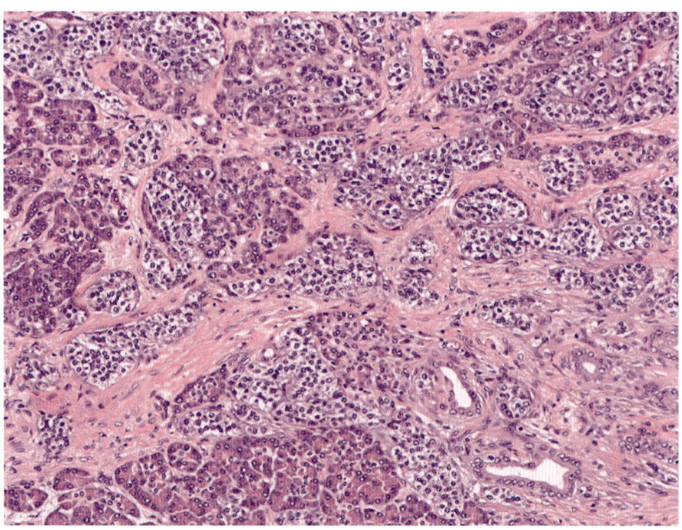

Fig. 7.04 Non-functioning pancreatic neuroendocrine tumour (PanNET). Entrapped ducts and acinar cells between solid tumour nests.

Ultrastructure

NF-PanNETs are characterized by variable numbers of membrane-bound electron-dense neurosecretory granules, either non-polarized within the cytoplasm or oriented near the basal surfaces facing the capillaries. The granule morphology is often nonspecific. The characteristic granule types of islet A or B cells sometimes found in functioning PanNETs are absent.

Differential diagnosis

The main entities include pancreatic neuroendocrine carcinoma (PanNEC), paraganglioma, acinar cell carcinoma, solid pseudopapillary neoplasm, pancreatoblastoma, and ductal adenocarcinoma. Metastasis from renal cell carcinoma may resemble a clear cell PanNET, particularly in patients with VHL, whereas metastases from hepatocellular carcinoma or adrenal cortical carcinoma may resemble oncocytic PanNETs {1913, 4728}. Mesenchymal neoplasms may also mimic PanNENs {2215}. Microtumours can be distinguished from enlarged islets by immunohistochemical staining for islet peptides, because

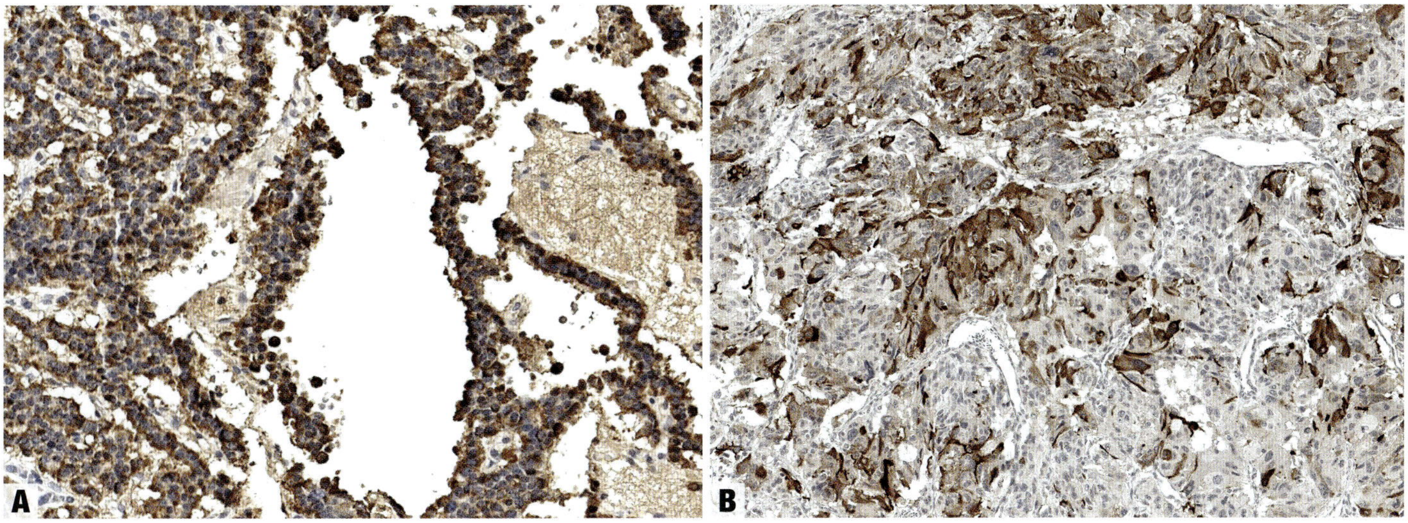

Fig. 7.05 Non-functioning pan-creatic neuroendocrine tumour (PanNET). **A** Glucagon-immunopositive cells forming a trabecular-reticulated pattern. **B** Somatostatin-immunopositive cells forming a paraganglioma-like pattern.

microtumours lose the normal proportions and non-random distribution of peptide cell types that characterize islets {157}.

Cytology

FNA specimens from PanNETs are usually highly cellular with a clean background. The neoplastic cells are found in loosely cohesive clusters and individually. A plasmacytoid configuration is characteristic. The nuclei are uniform and round to oval, and contain coarsely granular chromatin. Mitotic figures are usually not identified. Grading of NF-PanNETs in cytological specimens can underestimate the true grade because of limited material {1336,4712,4139}.

Diagnostic molecular pathology

Not clinically relevant

Essential and desirable diagnostic criteria

Essential: a keratin-positive PanNEN (PanNET); expression of general neuroendocrine markers (e.g. chromogranin A, INSM1, and synaptophysin); Ki-67 immunohistochemistry.

Desirable: positive immunohistochemistry for selected hormone products associated with special growth patterns; positive immunohistochemistry for cytokeratins (in selected cases).

Staging

The staging of NF-PanNETs, like that of all PanNENs, follows the eighth editions (2017) of the Union for International Cancer Control (UICC) TNM classification {532} and the American Joint Committee on Cancer (AJCC) cancer staging manual {132,850}, which rely on macroscopic assessment of site, tumour size, and metastases. This approach largely corresponds to that of the European Neuroendocrine Tumor Society (ENETS) classification {3747,3748}. The staging of well-differentiated PanNENs is presented in *TNM staging of endocrine and neuroendocrine tumours* (p. 18).

Prognosis and prediction

All NF-PanNETs are considered to be malignant. Neuroendocrine microtumours almost always have benign behaviour, but rare lymph node metastases have been reported {2470}. Approximately 55–75% of NF-PanNETs are diagnosed with extrapancreatic spread, metastases (predominantly in liver, bones, and distant lymph nodes), or recurrence {4682,3747, 3748}. After R0 resection of the primary PanNET (and synchronous metastases, if present), the recurrence rate is 26% {741}. This recurrence rate seems to be dependent on the Ki-67 index and varies from 14% in patients with a Ki-67 index of 0–5%, to 41% in patients with a Ki-67 index of 6–20% (indicating the need for closer follow-up of patients with tumours with a higher Ki-67 index). As a consequence, the 10-year disease-specific survival rates are 91% for a Ki-67 index of 0–5%, and 26% for a Ki-67 index of 6–20% {1528}.

A number of factors have been shown to predict the prognosis of PanNETs. The most important histological factor predictive of outcome is proliferative rate, based on mitotic count and Ki-67 proliferation index {1528} (see *Pancreatic neuroendocrine neoplasms: Introduction*, p. 296). Abundant data demonstrate the prognostic stratification of G1 and G2 NF-PanNETs, both

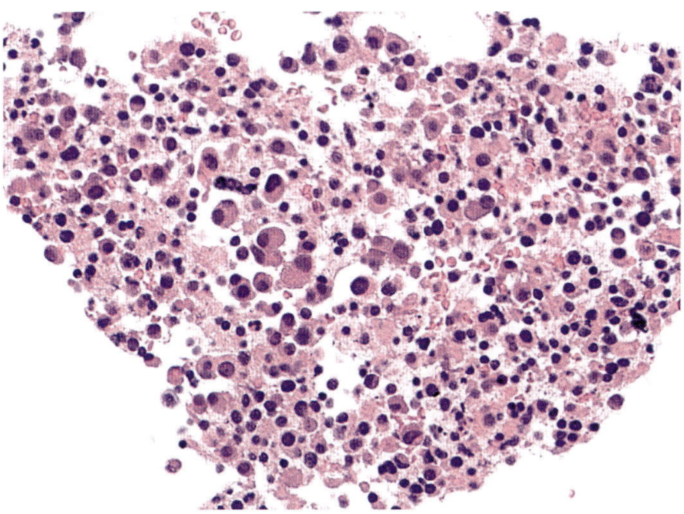

Fig. 7.06 Non-functioning pancreatic neuroendocrine tumour (PanNET). Cell-block cytology showing plasmacytoid cells with oncocytic cytoplasm and round nuclei.

Chapter 7

in the setting of a resected primary tumour and for metastatic disease. In biopsies of metastases, the Ki-67 proliferation index may be difficult to assess accurately because of the limited tissue available or tumour heterogeneity regarding highest proliferative activity {5039}. Both G1 and G2 PanNETs are prognostically separated from PanNECs {3009}. This is also true for the G3 PanNET group (see also *Pancreatic neuroendocrine neoplasms: Introduction*, p. 296), which is somewhat more aggressive than G2 PanNET but not as rapidly progressive as PanNEC {3748}. The 5-year survival rate is 62% for G2 PanNETs, 29% for G3 PanNETs, and 16% for PanNECs {340}.

Another predictor of outcome is tumour size. Tumours < 20 mm uncommonly demonstrate clinical aggressiveness, whereas tumours > 30 mm have a higher risk of metastasis {1707,2445}. Small (< 20 mm), low-grade NF-PanNETs have very indolent biology. Therefore, it has been suggested that asymptomatic cases may be closely monitored radiographically rather than resected {1321}. The likelihood of metastasis also increases with the extent of invasive growth (especially vascular invasion), necrosis, and the status of regional lymph nodes {4007}.

Immunolabelling for a peptide in the absence of a clinical syndrome has no prognostic relevance. The histological patterns of NF-PanNETs are not prognostically distinctive in general. Cystic PanNETs frequently lack adverse prognostic factors and often present at a lower stage {2654,2387}. Oncocytic NF-PanNETs appear to be more aggressive {4728}. Other immunohistochemical markers such as PTEN loss, loss of DAXX or ATRX expression, alternative-lengthening-of-telomeres activation, as well as the A-cell lineage subtype with alternative lengthening of telomeres were reported as adverse prognostic factors {2848,1289, 4163,713,1732}.

Insulinoma

La Rosa S
Brosens LAA
de Herder WW
Hong SM
Mete O
Ohike N

Definition

Insulinoma is a functioning well-differentiated neuroendocrine tumour (NET) composed of insulin-producing cells, causing a hypoglycaemic syndrome due to uncontrolled insulin secretion.

ICD-O coding

8151/3 Neuroendocrine tumour, insulin-producing (insulinoma)

ICD-11 coding

2C10.1 & XH3UK0 Neuroendocrine neoplasms of pancreas & Insulinoma, malignant

Related terminology

None

Subtype(s)

None

Localization

Insulinomas are evenly distributed in the pancreas {2927}. Extremely rare extrapancreatic insulinomas have been described in the lung, duodenum, ileum, jejunum, hilum of the spleen, and gastric antrum {4083,19,3495,2486,5148}.

Clinical features

Insulinomas are more frequently diagnosed in adults and the peak of incidence is in the sixth decade of life, although individuals of any age can be affected {2927}. Women are slightly more affected than men. About 10% of insulinomas develop metastases, which occur more frequently in men with tumours larger than 20 mm {4068,3248}. Multiple insulinomas are seen in about 10% of patients, most often in the setting of multiple endocrine neoplasia type 1 or, more rarely, *MAFA*-related familial insulinomatosis {153,2016}.

Hyperinsulinaemic hypoglycaemia is the clinical hallmark, characterized by autonomic and neuroglycopenic symptoms. Adrenergic symptoms include palpitations and tremor, while cholinergic symptoms include sweating, hunger, and/or paraesthesia. The neuroglycopenic symptoms include severe weakness and a variety of psychiatric and neurological manifestations. Other common signs and symptoms include confusion, agitation, blurred vision, seizures, transient loss of consciousness, and hypoglycaemic coma {950}. The diagnosis is based on the presence of hypoglycaemic symptoms and low plasma glucose levels, which resolve after glucose administration (the Whipple triad).

Biochemical investigations

The best diagnostic test is prolonged fasting (48–72 h) with measurement of blood glucose, serum insulin, C-peptide, and proinsulin {1019}. Biologically aggressive and metastatic insulinomas can change hormone production and, consequently, clinical syndrome during the course of the disease {1029,946}.

Chapter 7

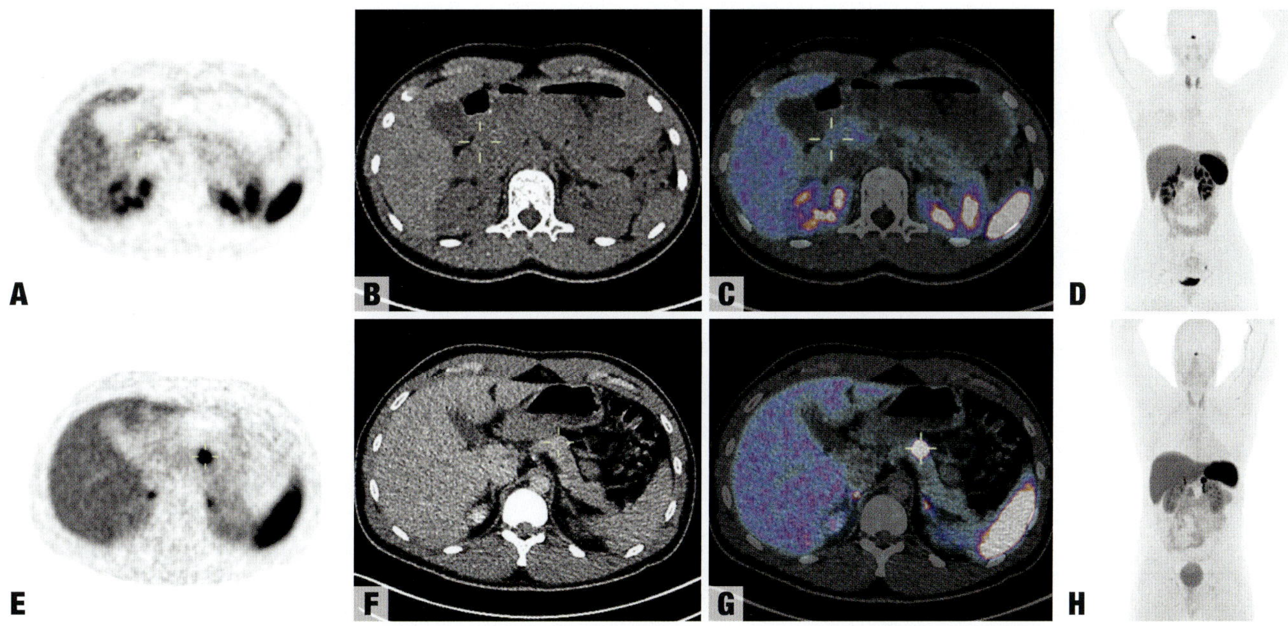

Fig. 7.07 Pancreatic insulinoma. **A–D** PET-CT 68Ga-DOTATOC axial images showing low uptake on PET (**A**), low-dose CT (**B**), fused PET-CT (**C**), and maximum intensity projection image (standardized uptake value scale: 0–15) (**D**). **E–H** PET-CT 68Ga-DOTATOC axial images showing high uptake (maximum standardized uptake value: 114) on PET (**E**), low-dose CT (**F**), fused PET-CT (**G**), and maximum intensity projection image (standardized uptake value scale: 0–20) (**H**).

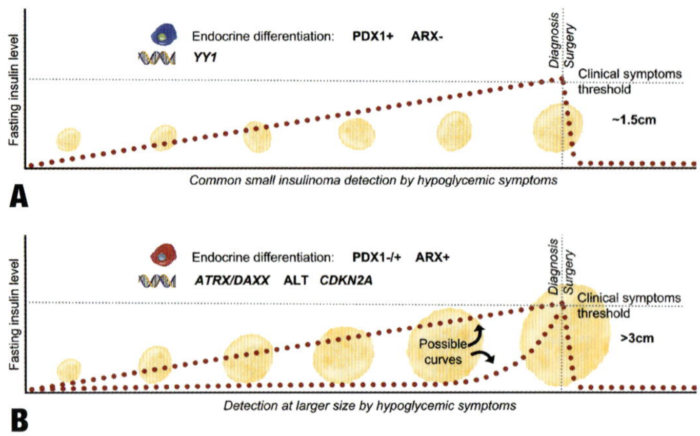

Fig. 7.08 Tumorigenic mechanisms in clinically defined insulinomas. **A** Indolent small insulinomas are characterized by recurrent *YY1* mutations (25%), neutral or amplified chromosomal copy numbers, and endocrine transcription factor expression consistent with normal islet B-cell differentiation (PDX1+/ARX–). **B** Large insulinomas show distinct tumorigenic mechanisms often seen in non-functioning PanNETs, and endocrine transcription factor expression inconsistent with normal islet B-cell differentiation (ARX+). ALT, alternative lengthening of telomeres.

Imaging

Insulinomas are detected by CT, MRI, EUS, 68Ga-DOTATOC/DOTATATE PET, and radiolabelled GLP analogue scintigraphy {1273,2343,4339,846}. 68Ga-DOTATOC/DOTATATE PET may show variable uptake and has a sensitivity of 25% in detecting insulinomas {594}.

Epidemiology

Insulinoma is the most common functioning pancreatic NET (PanNET), accounting for 42% of functioning PanNETs and 4–20% of resected PanNETs {5044,2054}. The incidence in a well-defined population (Olmsted County, south-eastern Minnesota, USA) was estimated to be 0.4 cases per 100 000 person-years {4068}, whereas in less well defined populations the incidence was found to range from 0.07 to 0.12 cases per 100 000 person-years {1752}.

Etiology

There are no known etiological factors for sporadic solitary insulinomas. Pathogenic germline *MEN1* variants can cause insulinomas. There may be an association with diabetes {1750}. Rare cases of insulinoma have also been observed in patients with tuberous sclerosis {71} and neurofibromatosis type 1 {3527}. Familial insulinomatosis has recently been attributed to pathogenic *MAFA* variants {2016}.

Pathogenesis

Recent molecular findings suggest that sporadic small and indolent insulinomas show a different molecular profile than aggressive insulinomas and other sporadic PanNETs {1734}. Indeed, indolent insulinomas show a lower tumour mutation burden than non-functioning PanNETs (NF-PanNETs). In addition, the genes that are frequently altered in NF-PanNETs (e.g. *MEN1*, *DAXX*, *ATRX*, *CDKN2A*, *PTEN*, and *TSC2*) are rarely mutated in sporadic indolent insulinomas {1935,1734}. Conversely, *YY1* mutation (p.T372R mutation), which is extremely rare in other PanNETs, is found in about 30% of cases and is considered a specific driver mutation, associated with older age and lower serum glucose level {629,2652,1935}. Although *YY1* mutation was not found to be associated with YY1 protein loss, strong YY1 immunoreactivity is thought to correlate with a better prognosis {629,4227}. Accordingly with the gene mutation profile, insulinomas cluster separately from other PanNET types at the RNA level {3867}. Alternative-lengthening-of-telomeres phenotype, *ATRX*/*DAXX* loss, and *CDKN2A* loss have been observed in some insulinomas that are associated with metastatic disease and ARX expression, suggesting that cellular differentiation and tumorigenic mechanisms in aggressive insulinomas are more closely related to NF-PanNETs than to small indolent insulinomas {1734,5097}.

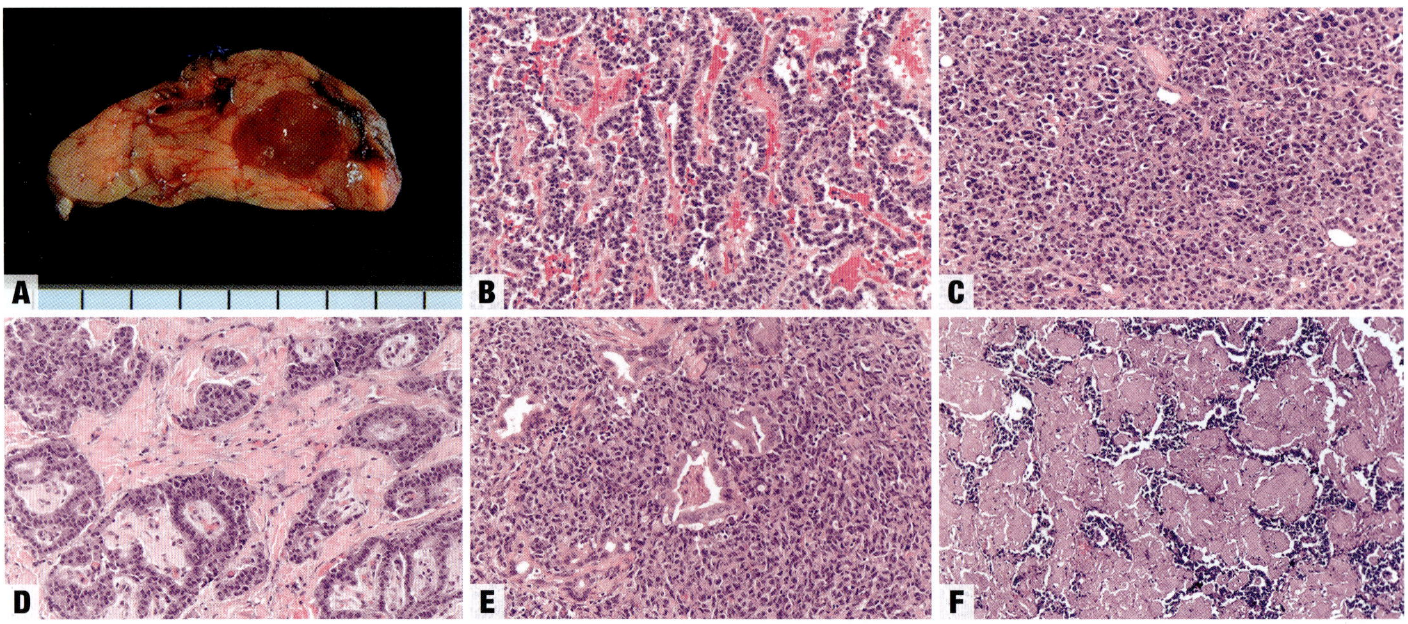

Fig. 7.09 Pancreatic insulinoma, indolent small. **A** Gross appearance of a well-circumscribed tumour showing a reddish-tan cut surface. **B** Trabecular architecture. **C** Solid architecture. **D** Tubuloacinar architecture with hyalinized stroma. **E** In this case, entrapped non-neoplastic ducts are observed. **F** Typical morphology with trabecular architecture and amyloid deposits.

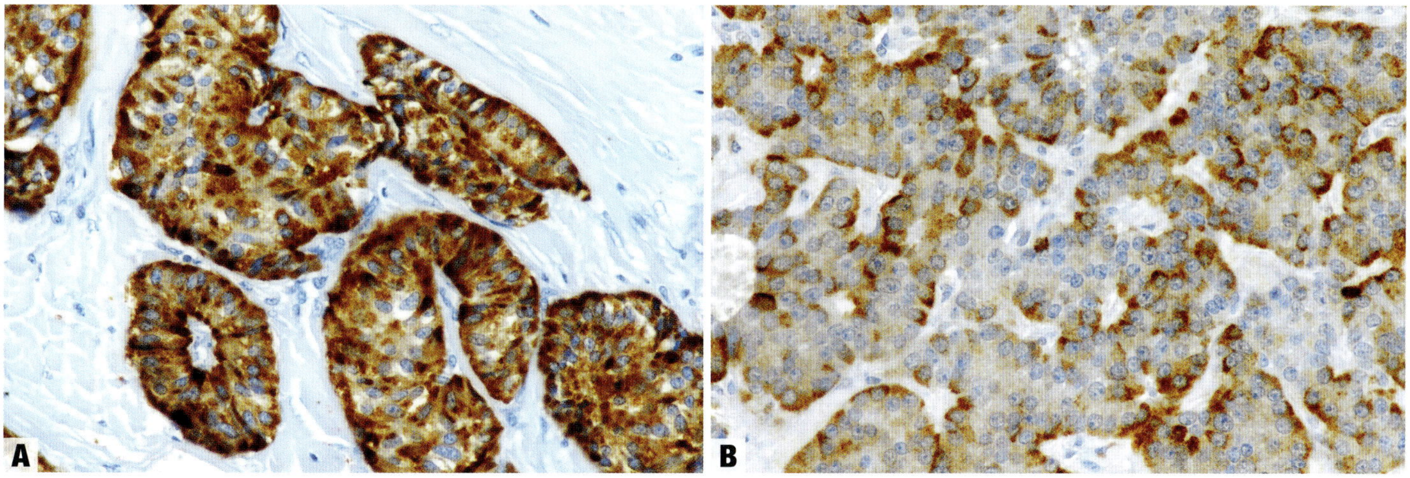

Fig. 7.10 Pancreatic insulinoma. **A** Insulin expression is intense and observed in most cells. **B** Sometimes, insulin expression is not observed in all neoplastic cells.

Macroscopic appearance

Insulinomas showing indolent behaviour are small (10–20 mm in diameter), solitary, and well-demarcated PanNETs, generally not associated with metastatic dissemination. Sometimes they can be haemorrhagic and (very rarely) cystic {2409}. Biologically aggressive insulinomas are typically larger than 30 mm and have a higher risk of metastatic dissemination {1734}.

Histopathology

Insulinomas are composed of well-differentiated neuroendocrine cells forming trabecular, solid, or (more rarely) tubuloacinar structures, sometimes entrapping non-neoplastic ductules. In some cases, prominent hyalinized sclerosis can be observed. Stromal amyloid deposits determined by the accumulation of islet amyloid polypeptide (IAPP; also called amylin) can be found in about 5% of cases and represents a quite specific morphological feature. However, amyloid deposition has also been described in extremely rare IAPP-secreting PanNETs not showing insulin expression {1486}.

Grading

Most insulinoma are G1, with a Ki-67 labelling index < 3%. Metastatic and aggressive insulinomas are more frequently G2. Very rare G3 cases (Ki-67 index > 20%) have been described {4792}.

Immunohistochemistry

Like in other PanNETs, tumour cells are positive for general neuroendocrine markers including synaptophysin, chromogranin A, and INSM1. They are also immunoreactive for insulin, proinsulin, and IAPP; IAPP is also positive in extracellular amyloid deposits. Insulin expression may vary in intensity among tumour cells and in some cases shows an apical cytoplasmic distribution, whereas proinsulin shows a perinuclear pattern reflecting Golgi localization. In patients with hyperinsulinaemic hypoglycaemia and multiple PanNETs, immunohistochemistry for insulin is required in order to distinguish insulinoma from other PanNETs, because the largest tumour is not always the one that is responsible for the clinical syndrome {157}. About half of insulinomas contain scattered cells positive for glucagon, PP, somatostatin, and/or other hormones. Small indolent insulinomas are strongly positive for PDX1 (an islet B-cell marker) and negative for ARX (an A-cell marker), whereas aggressive insulinomas are ARX-positive and show variable PDX1 expression {1734}.

Cytology

The cytological features are identical to those of other PanNETs.

Diagnostic molecular pathology

Not clinically relevant

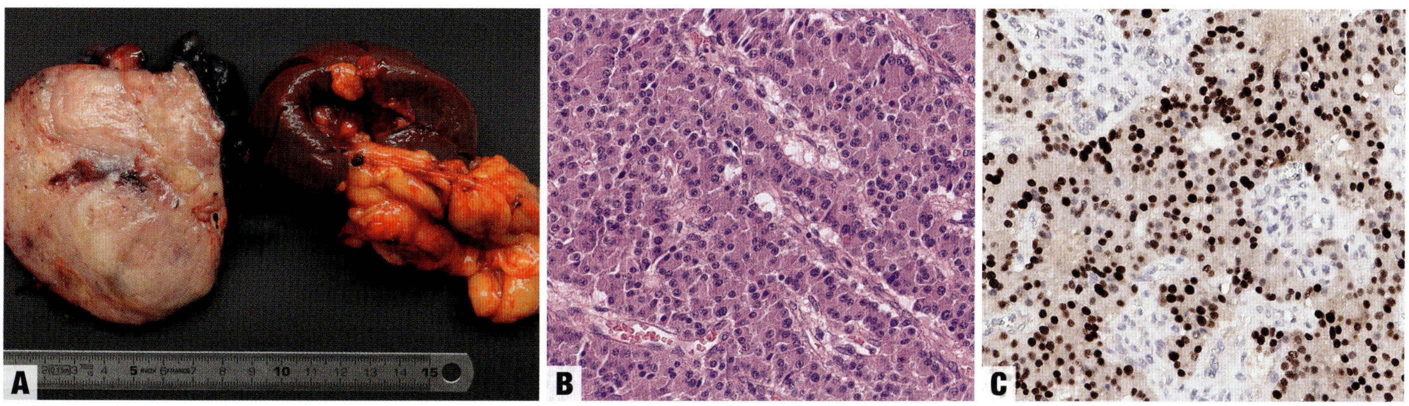

Fig. 7.11 Pancreatic insulinoma, aggressive. **A** Distal pancreatectomy and splenectomy revealing a 90 mm tumour. Histologically, this tumour shows well-differentiated neuroendocrine morphology (**B**) and ARX-positive tumour cells (**C**).

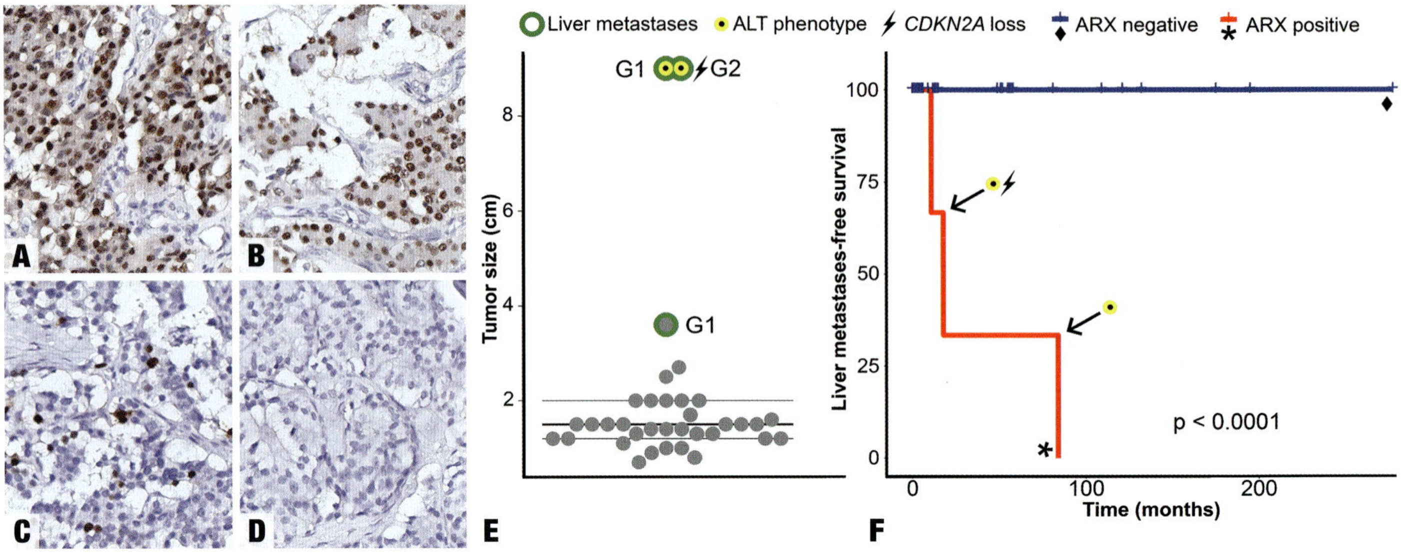

Fig. 7.12 Pancreatic insulinoma. ARX expression, tumour size, and liver metastasis–free survival in primary insulinomas. **A–C** Positive ARX expression in 3 metastatic primary insulinomas. **D** No ARX expression in a non-metastatic insulinoma. **E** Tumour size plot. Cases with liver metastases in the size plot are circled (green); WHO grade is given. **F** Kaplan–Meier curve of liver metastasis–free survival for ARX expression in the primary insulinoma cohort. The *P* value was calculated with the log-rank test.

Essential and desirable diagnostic criteria

Essential: clinical findings of hyperinsulinaemic hypoglycaemia associated with a keratin-positive PanNEN (PanNET); Ki-67 immunohistochemistry.

Staging

The staging of insulinomas is the same as for other PanNETs.

Prognosis and prediction

Stage is an important prognostic factor, whereas grade seems to have less prognostic impact in insulinomas, because it does not predict the prognosis between G1 and G2 cases {4792}. Insulinomas < 20 mm are associated with a 10-year survival rate close to 100%, whereas insulinomas > 20 mm and with *ALT* and *ATRX*/*DAXX* loss have an increased risk of metastasis and are associated with a 10-year survival rate of about 30% {2848,4792,3977,3853,740}. Recently, ARX protein expression was found to be associated with metastatic dissemination and worse survival, suggesting a distinct tumorigenic mechanism in aggressive insulinomas, with similarities to NF-PanNETs, compared with indolent ARX-negative / PDX1-positive insulinomas {1734}.

Glucagonoma

La Rosa S
Basturk O
Brosens LAA
de Herder WW
Hong SM
Mete O
Ohike N

Definition

Glucagonoma is a well-differentiated functioning pancreatic neuroendocrine tumour (PanNET) composed of cells producing glucagon and preproglucagon-derived peptide, with uncontrolled glucagon secretion, causing glucagonoma syndrome.

ICD-O coding

8152/3 Neuroendocrine tumour, glucagon-producing (glucagonoma)

ICD-11 coding

2C10.1 & XH87C1 Neuroendocrine neoplasms of pancreas & Glucagonoma, malignant

Related terminology

None

Subtype(s)

None

Localization

Glucagonoma predominantly involves the pancreatic tail {4226}.

Clinical features

Glucagonomas are characterized by glucagonoma syndrome, which includes a characteristic necrolytic migratory erythema (occurring in approximately 80% of patients); painful glossitis, cheilitis, and angular stomatitis (in ~41% of patients); onychodystrophy (in female patients); significant weight loss (in ~60% of patients); deep vein thrombosis; depression; new-onset or worsening diabetes mellitus (in ~70% of patients); normochromic normocytic anaemia (in ~50% of patients); hypoaminoacidaemia; and low zinc levels. In rare cases, glucagonomas are associated with dilated cardiomyopathy. The average time from symptom onset to final diagnosis is 31.4 months {4226}.

Almost invariably, the necrolytic migratory erythema and cardiomyopathy resolve after successful removal of the tumour. Patients who cannot undergo curative resection can be treated with surgical and non-surgical debulking therapies, somatostatin analogues, everolimus, peptide receptor radionuclide therapy (PRRT), or cytotoxic chemotherapy like for other PanNETs.

A second (rare) syndrome associated with hyperglucagonaemia, but not the clinical glucagonoma syndrome, is the autosomal recessive inherited glucagon cell hyperplasia and neoplasia syndrome (also known as Mahvash disease), in which numerous glucagon-producing PanNETs and microtumours are present, but the clinical syndrome is not present because of germline mutations in *GCGR* {5096} (see *Glucagon cell hyperplasia and neoplasia*, p. 478).

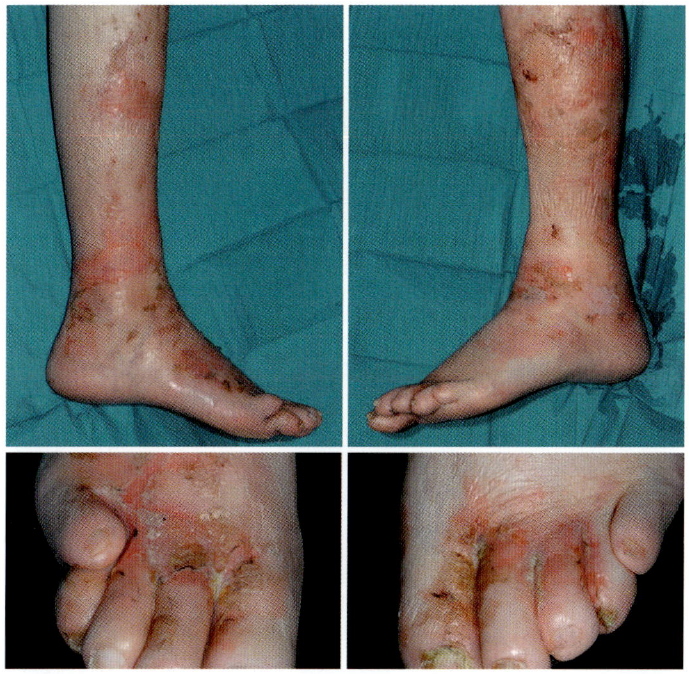

Fig. 7.13 Glucagonoma. Necrolytic migratory erythema in a patient with pancreatic glucagonoma.

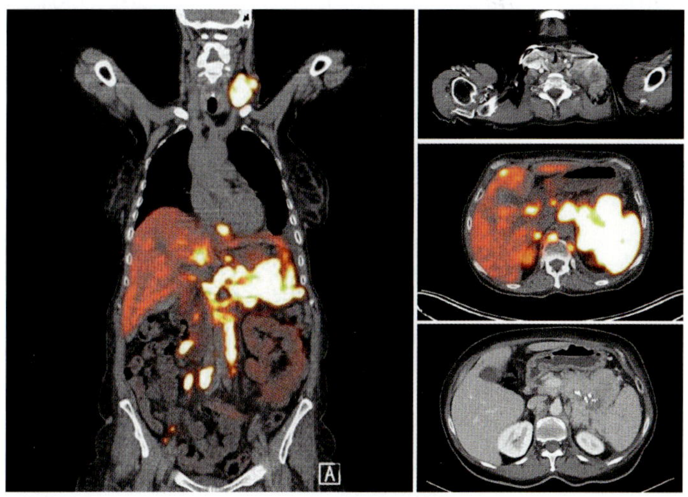

Fig. 7.14 Glucagonoma. 68Ga-DOTATATE PET-CT and 3-phase CT images (arterial phase) of a 54-year-old woman with an 84 mm glucagonoma of the pancreatic tail, with multilobar metastases in the liver, periaortic and pericaval lymph node metastases, a left adrenal metastasis (31 mm), and a 49 mm supraclavicular lymph node metastasis at the left side.

Biochemical investigations

The diagnosis of glucagonoma syndrome is based on the combination of elevated plasma glucagon levels and symptoms

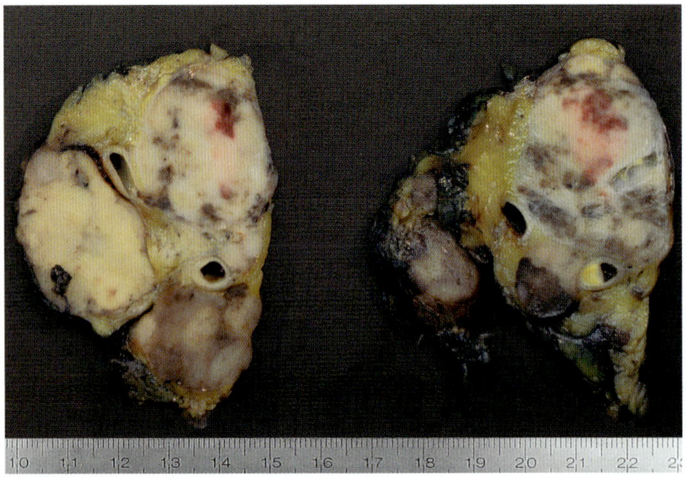

Fig. 7.15 Glucagonoma. Macroscopic appearance of a pancreatic glucagonoma measuring 80 mm located in the distal pancreas and involving peripancreatic lymph nodes.

previously described. Mildly elevated glucagon levels may be associated with several other diseases like cirrhosis, chronic renal failure, sepsis, acute or chronic pancreatitis, chronic hepatic failure, Cushing syndrome, acute trauma, diabetes mellitus, diabetic ketoacidosis, stress, burns, portocaval shunting, and familial hyperglucagonaemia. However, a fasting plasma glucagon level > 500 pg/mL (reference range: 70–160 pg/mL) is diagnostic for glucagonoma {4265}.

Imaging

Glucagonomas and their metastases highly express SSTR subtypes (97%) and therefore can be identified using SSTR PET with 68Ga-DOTA–labelled somatostatin analogues (DOTATATE, DOTANOC, and DOTATOC). Other imaging modalities include CT, MRI, and EUS {3849}.

Epidemiology

Glucagonoma is rare, accounting for 1–2% of all PanNETs, with an estimated annual incidence of about 1 case per 20 million people. It is the fourth most common functioning PanNET after insulinoma, gastrinoma, and VIPoma {5044,2099}. The average age of patients at diagnosis is 52.5 years, and there is a slight female predilection {4210}.

Etiology

There are not known etiological factors for sporadic glucagonomas. Approximately 10% of glucagonomas are associated with multiple endocrine neoplasia type 1 (MEN1) (see *Multiple endocrine neoplasia type 1*, p. 429) {4210,758,1084,4226,1924}.

Autosomal recessive inherited glucagon cell hyperplasia and neoplasia syndrome (also known as Mahvash disease) is covered separately (see *Glucagon cell hyperplasia and neoplasia*, p. 478).

Pathogenesis

Unknown

Macroscopic appearance

Glucagonomas are solitary, well-demarcated, large tumours, ranging from 30 to 70 mm in size {4856,4226}. Rarely, they are cystic {547,2387}.

Histopathology

Glucagonomas are composed of well-differentiated cells, which form densely packed trabecular structures in a scant fibrous stroma. The cytological appearance of tumour cells overlaps that of cells of other PanNETs. Mitotic figures are rare, as is necrosis.

Grading

Most glucagonomas are G1 or G2, but some may progress to G3.

Immunohistochemistry

Tumour cells are positive for keratin, general neuroendocrine markers, glucagon, and SSTR2A {4856}. Some cells may also be positive for PP.

Differential diagnosis

It is worth noting that PanNETs composed of glucagon-immunoreactive cells but lacking symptoms of glucagonoma syndrome are defined as non-functioning glucagon-producing PanNETs or A-cell PanNETs. They are frequently small and indolent tumours (or microtumours) associated with an excellent prognosis, whereas glucagonomas are larger and more frequently metastatic neoplasms.

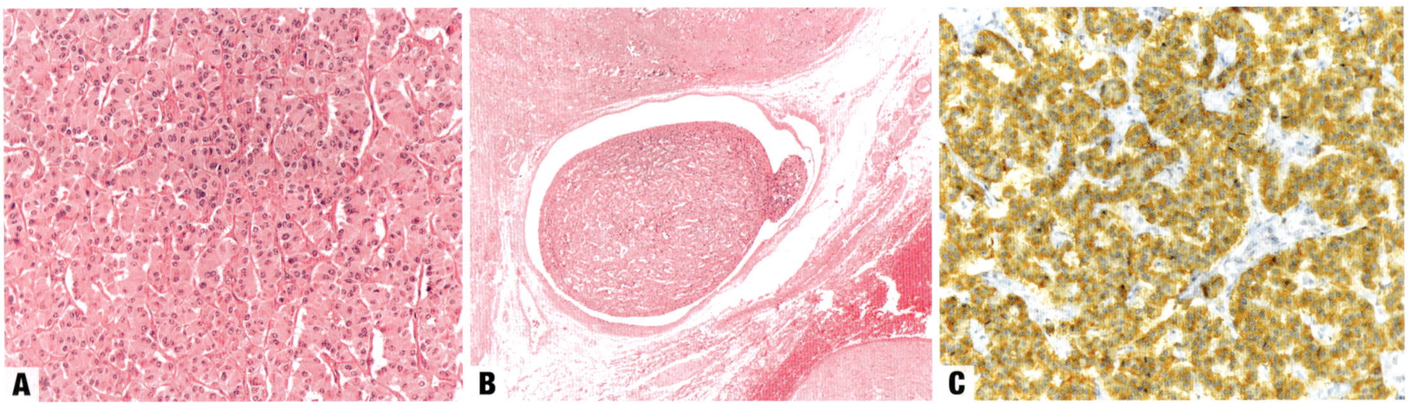

Fig. 7.16 Glucagonoma. **A** The tumour is composed of well-differentiated cells and shows a trabecular architecture. **B** A venous thrombus is present. **C** Tumour cells are positive for glucagon.

MEN1-related glucagon-secreting PanNETs are distinguished from sporadic manifestations by the presence of the islet dysplasia–neoplasia progression sequence as well as the presence of a plurihormonal immunohistochemical profile in tumours (see *Multiple endocrine neoplasia type 1*, p. 429).

Patients with Mahvash disease develop a multifocal glucagon cell–lineage hyperplasia–dysplasia–neoplasia sequence, characterized by multifocal glucagon-expressing neuroendocrine microtumours and PanNETs that do not cause glucagonoma syndrome. The latter should not be mistaken for a pancreatic glucagonoma (see *Glucagon cell hyperplasia and neoplasia*, p. 478).

Cytology

The cytology is the same as that of other PanNETs.

Diagnostic molecular pathology

Rarely, glucagonoma occurs in MEN1 {2099,4210}. FOXA2, which plays a crucial role in islet development, is reported to be deregulated in MEN1-associated glucagonomas {469}. In addition, biallelic inactivation of *DAXX* was reported in a sporadic glucagonoma {4401}.

Essential and desirable diagnostic criteria

Essential: a keratin-positive PanNEN (PanNET) with elevated plasma glucagon levels causing glucagonoma syndrome; Ki-67 immunohistochemistry.

Desirable: glucagon immunoreactivity.

Staging

The staging of glucagonomas is the same as for other PanNETs.

Prognosis and prediction

The prognosis mainly depends on stage {5044,2292}. Metastatic disease at initial diagnosis is common in patients with glucagonomas, most commonly affecting the liver, followed by the lymph nodes, mesentery/peritoneum, bone, lung, and spleen {4226}. The Ki-67 proliferation index was not found to have a prognostic impact in one study {2311}. The overall 5-year survival rate has been estimated as close to 70%, and the mean survival time is > 6 years {4856,1219,1704,4832}, although in a retrospective study, the average survival time was 32.1 months {4226}. Death is usually related to tumour growth rather than tumour-related functional complications {4856,2311}.

Somatostatinoma

Brosens LAA
Basturk O
de Herder WW
Hong SM
La Rosa S
Mete O
Singhi AD

Definition
Somatostatinoma is a functioning, well-differentiated pancreatic neuroendocrine tumour (PanNET) associated with clinical manifestations of inappropriate somatostatin secretion (somatostatinoma syndrome).

ICD-O coding
8156/3 Neuroendocrine tumour, somatostatin-producing (somatostatinoma)

ICD-11 coding
2C10.1 & XH9Z82 Neuroendocrine neoplasms of pancreas & Somatostatinoma, malignant

Related terminology
None

Subtype(s)
None

Localization
Somatostatinomas can arise throughout the pancreas, but approximately two thirds involve the head of the gland {2539, 2381,145,4211,3213,3091}.

Clinical features
The clinical findings indicative of excess somatostatin secretion are not as dramatic or distinctive as the features of other functioning PanNETs {2539,2381,145,4211,3213,3091,2760}. Tumours that demonstrate D-cell differentiation based on immunohistochemical labelling with somatostatin but lack symptoms of somatostatinoma syndrome, such as those observed within the ampulla and duodenum, should be designated as somatostatin-producing well-differentiated neuroendocrine tumours (NETs) and are not considered somatostatinomas.

The classic triad of somatostatinoma syndrome comprises diabetes mellitus / glucose intolerance, cholelithiasis, and diarrhoea/steatorrhoea as a result of hormonal suppression of insulin, exocrine pancreatic function, and CCK due to the elevated plasma somatostatin levels. Many patients with somatostatinomas also have gastric hypochlorhydria due to decreased gastric secretion. However, this classic triad is rare. These tumours usually progress asymptomatically and present with obstructive symptoms secondary to regional lymph node or hepatic metastases.

Biochemical investigations
Somatostatinoma syndrome can be confirmed by a fasting plasma somatostatin level > 25 pmol/L (> 60 pg/mL) {2381}.

Imaging
The initial diagnosis of a PanNET is usually based on imaging studies such as CT, MRI, and EUS. Adjunct tests include SSTR scintigraphy (111In-pentetreotide [Octreoscan]) and functional PET: 68Ga-DOTATOC, 68Ga-DOTATATE, FDOPA, and 11C-5-HTP PET {146,2429,1924}.

Epidemiology
Somatostatinomas are rare pancreatic neoplasms, with an incidence of 1 case per 40 million person-years, and they account for < 1% of functioning PanNETs {3213}. The mean patient age at diagnosis is 55 years (range: 30–74 years), and patients are more commonly female {4211,4714}.

Etiology
The etiology and pathogenesis of pancreatic somatostatinoma are unknown. Ampullary and duodenal somatostatinomas are often associated with a history of neurofibromatosis type 1,

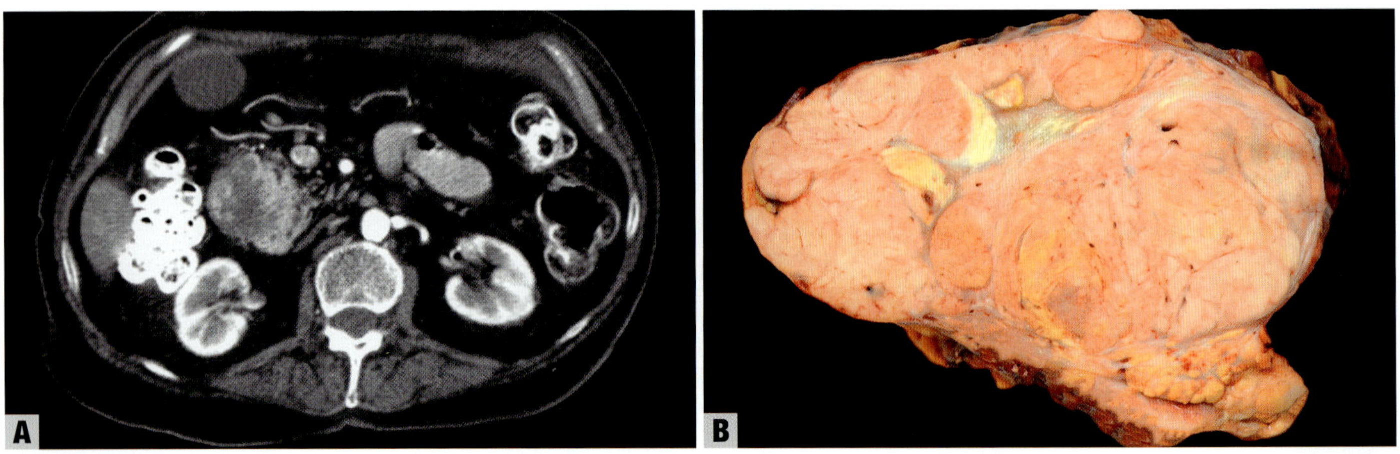

Fig. 7.17 Somatostatinoma. **A** CT of a large tumour in the pancreatic head. **B** Gross appearance of a large tumour with yellow to tan parenchyma and a multinodular growth pattern.

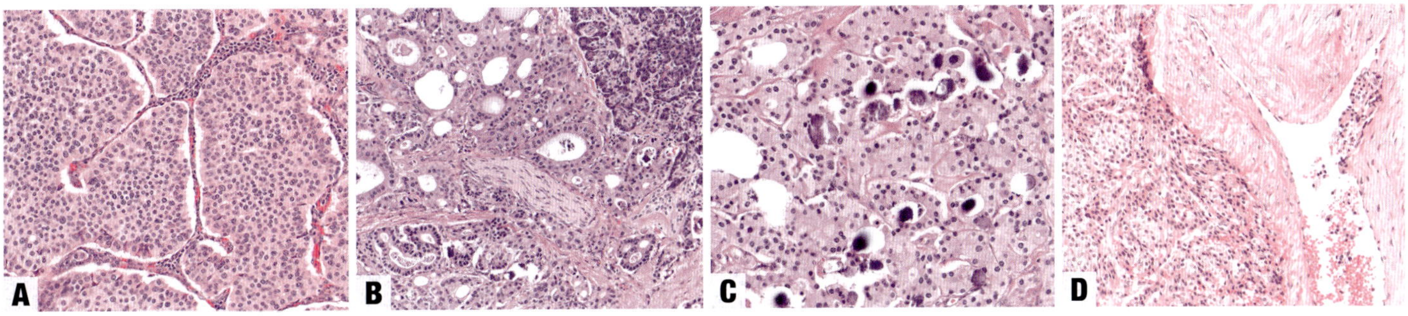

Fig. 7.18 Somatostatinoma. **A** Most pancreatic tumours have the typical appearance of other pancreatic neuroendocrine tumours (PanNETs), with trabecular, solid, and/or acinar architecture. **B** Perineural invasion is frequent. **C** A subset of pancreatic tumours show histological features similar to those of their ampullary/duodenal analogues, with tubular and glandular architecture and intraglandular psammomatous calcification. **D** Vascular invasion is frequent.

but pancreatic somatostatinomas are rarely found in neurofibromatosis {2833}. Patients with other predisposing genetic syndromes for PanNETs, such as multiple endocrine neoplasia type 1 and von Hippel–Lindau syndrome, infrequently develop somatostatinomas {2806,4211,1761,2621}.

Pathogenesis

Unknown

Macroscopic appearance

Pancreatic somatostatinomas are grossly indistinguishable from other PanNETs. These neoplasms are solitary, well circumscribed, and large (average diameter: 50–60 mm) {4211}. On cross-section, pancreatic somatostatinomas are unencapsulated and composed of yellow to tan parenchyma. They are usually multinodular and demonstrate invasive growth into adjacent structures, such as the duodenum and spleen. Because ampullary and duodenal somatostatinomas are considerably more common than pancreatic somatostatinomas, careful inspection of the central location of the tumour and correlation with the microscopic findings are critical.

Histopathology

Most somatostatinomas have the typical appearance of other PanNETs. The neoplastic cells are cuboidal to round, with eosinophilic cytoplasm and uniform nuclei. They are often characterized by a trabecular, solid, and/or acinar architecture. PanNETs with a striking nested pattern, resembling paragangliomas, often immunolabel for somatostatin {2390}. Vascular invasion and perineural invasion are frequent, but extensive necrosis is typically absent. A few pancreatic somatostatinomas exhibit histological features similar to those of ampullary/duodenal somatostatinomas, with a tubular and glandular architectural pattern and intraglandular psammomatous calcifications.

Grading

A systematic analysis of mitotic count and Ki-67 proliferation index has not been documented for pancreatic somatostatinomas, but most cases are intermediate-grade (G2) {2760}.

Immunohistochemistry

The tumour shows diffuse positivity for keratins, INSM1, synaptophysin, and somatostatin and is less consistently positive or negative for chromogranin A. Scattered positivity for PP, calcitonin, gastrin, ACTH, glucagon, and insulin can also occur. Tumours that demonstrate D-cell differentiation based on immunohistochemical labelling with somatostatin but lack symptoms of somatostatinoma syndrome are designated as somatostatin-producing well-differentiated NETs rather than somatostatinomas.

Cytology

The cytology is similar to that of other PanNETs {1119}.

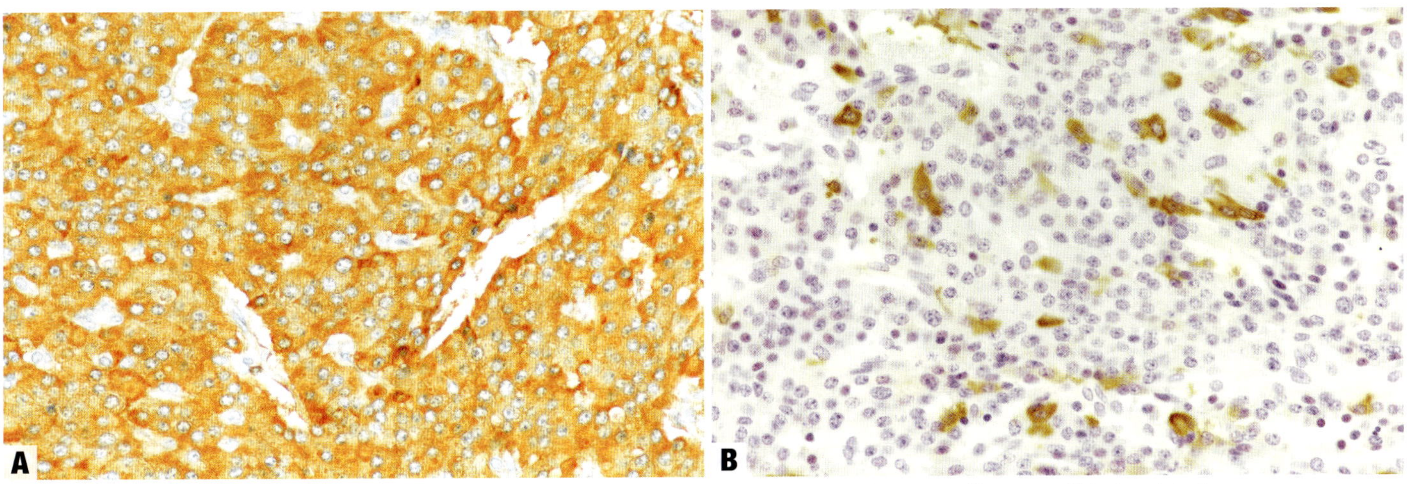

Fig. 7.19 Somatostatinoma. **A** Tumour showing diffuse immunopositivity for somatostatin. **B** Tumour showing scattered immunopositivity for calcitonin.

Diagnostic molecular pathology

The molecular pathology of sporadic pancreatic somatostatinomas is not well studied. There are no known genetic differences from non-functioning PanNETs.

Essential and desirable diagnostic criteria

Essential: a keratin-positive PanNEN (PanNET) with clinical and laboratory diagnosis confirming somatostatin excess (fasting plasma somatostatin level > 18.33 pmol/L or > 30 pg/mL); Ki-67 immunohistochemistry.

Desirable: immunoreactivity for somatostatin.

Staging

The staging of pancreatic somatostatinomas, like that of all pancreatic neuroendocrine neoplasms (PanNENs), follows the eighth editions (2017) of the Union for International Cancer Control (UICC) TNM classification {532} and the American Joint Committee on Cancer (AJCC) cancer staging manual {132, 850}, which rely on macroscopic assessment of site, tumour size, and metastases. This approach largely corresponds to that of the European Neuroendocrine Tumor Society (ENETS) classification {3747}.

Prognosis and prediction

There are insufficient survival data for patients with pancreatic somatostatinomas. However, the 5-year overall survival rate ranges from 60–100% in patients with localized disease to 15–60% in patients with distant metastases. Large tumour size (> 30 mm) and lymph node involvement are poor prognostic markers {4211}.

Gastrinoma

Basturk O
Brosens LAA
de Herder WW
Hong SM
La Rosa S
Mete O

Definition

Gastrinoma of the pancreas is a functioning well-differentiated pancreatic neuroendocrine tumour (PanNET) composed of gastrin-producing cells (G cells), with uncontrolled gastrin secretion causing Zollinger–Ellison syndrome.

ICD-O coding

8153/3 Neuroendocrine tumour, gastrin-producing (gastrinoma)

ICD-11 coding

2C10.1 & XH0GY2 Neuroendocrine neoplasms of pancreas & Gastrinoma, malignant

Related terminology

None

Subtype(s)

None

Localization

Although > 80% of gastrinomas are located within the gastrinoma triangle, in patients with multiple endocrine neoplasia type 1 (MEN1), 60–90% of the tumours are in the duodenum. These duodenal gastrinomas are usually very small and may not be visible on endoscopic ultrasound or preoperative imaging studies {4089}. Therefore, a gastrinoma that presents as a tumour adjacent to the pancreas or with predominantly peripancreatic lymph node involvement requires careful exclusion of metastatic disease from occult duodenal gastrinoma {154}. Pancreatic gastrinomas have no preferential localization within the pancreas {868,2099,2424}.

Clinical features

The typical clinical features of Zollinger–Ellison syndrome are advanced peptic ulcer disease, gastro-oesophageal reflux disease, diarrhoea, nausea, vomiting, and abdominal pain {1077}. Hypergastrinaemia may also lead to fundic enterochromaffin-like cell (ECL-cell) proliferations. MEN1-associated pancreatic gastrinomas may lead to type 2 ECL-cell fundic neuroendocrine tumours (NETs) {2534,4866}.

Biochemical investigations

Symptoms are caused by elevated circulating gastrin levels (> 150 pg/L) and gastric acid hypersecretion (gastric pH $\leq$ 2). Serum chromogranin A levels are also increased in about 90% of pancreatic gastrinoma cases {2099,2424}.

Imaging

The primary tumour site and its metastatic spread are determined using conventional imaging (CT, MRI, EUS) and functional imaging studies such as SSTR scintigraphy (111In-pentetreotide scan) and 68Ga-DOTATATE/DOTATOC PET-CT {2433, 1018,2099,2424}.

Epidemiology

Pancreatic gastrinomas account for 4–8% of all PanNETs {155, 2054}, with an estimated annual incidence of 0.5–2 cases per 1 million people. Zollinger–Ellison syndrome is the second most common hormonal syndrome associated with functioning PanNETs {2905,2054}. Patients with sporadic pancreatic gastrinomas, who usually are younger than those with nonfunctioning PanNETs, are often in their fifth or sixth decade of life, and the male and female distributions are equal {2099, 3747}. MEN1-associated pancreatic gastrinomas usually arise in patients who are about a decade younger {1567,1566,2099, 4008}.

Etiology

With the exception of MEN1, there are no known pancreatic gastrinoma-specific etiological factors {4866}.

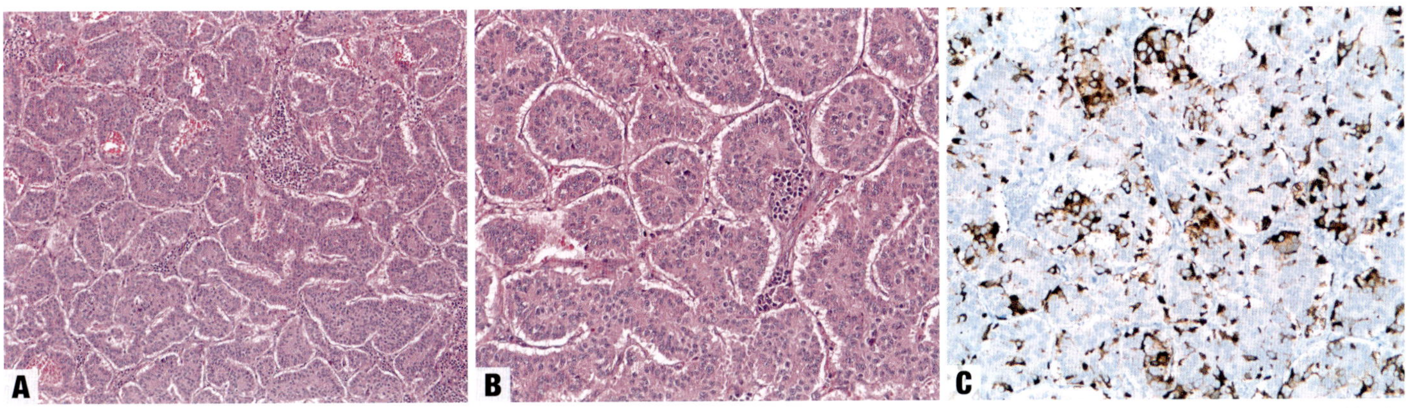

Fig. 7.20 Gastrinoma. An example with a typical tubuloacinar and pseudoglandular growth pattern (**A**) and low nuclear atypia (**B**). The tumour cells are immunopositive for gastrin (**C**).

Pathogenesis

The gastrin cell hyperplasia-to-neoplasia (gastrinoma) sequence has only been identified in MEN1-associated duodenal gastrinomas {156,1733}. The pathogenesis of pancreatic gastrinomas is largely unknown. They are often sporadic. Rare cases occur in the setting of familial predisposing conditions such as MEN1, neurofibromatosis type 1, neurofibromatosis type 2 {2589,2867}, or tuberous sclerosis {4034}.

Specific *MEN1* mutations have been reported to lead to abnormal menin interaction with FOXN3 (CHES1). This may be associated with a higher risk of aggressive behaviour {329}.

Macroscopic appearance

Pancreatic gastrinomas are usually large (mean: 38 mm) but do not have distinctive macroscopic features.

Histopathology

Pancreatic gastrinomas are often indistinguishable from other PanNETs but they tend to display trabecular and/or glandular structures. The margin of the tumour can be expansive or focally infiltrative. The stroma is normally delicate but may be prominent in large tumours.

Grading

Most are G1 or G2 tumours.

Immunohistochemistry

The tumour cells are positive for keratins (AE1/AE3, CAM5.2, CK8/18, CK19), neuroendocrine differentiation markers (chromogranin A, synaptophysin, INSM1), pancreas lineage–related transcription factors (insulin gene enhancer protein ISL1 and PDX1) {4259,1351,1865,28}, and SSTR2A {2444,2397}. Gastrin expression may be focal, but the proportion of gastrin-producing cells is irrelevant for the concurrent clinical syndrome. Additional hormones that may be expressed include insulin, glucagon, PP, and serotonin.

Cytology

The cytology is indistinguishable from that of other PanNETs.

Diagnostic molecular pathology

None

Essential and desirable diagnostic criteria

Essential: a keratin-positive well-differentiated NEN (PanNET) and elevated fasting plasma gastrin levels (> 150 pg/L); Ki-67 immunohistochemistry.

Desirable: gastrin immunoreactivity in a PanNET; gastric acid hypersecretion; duodenal ulcer.

Staging

The pathological staging of pancreatic gastrinomas, like that of all PanNETs, is based on the eighth edition (2017) of the Union for International Cancer Control (UICC) TNM classification {532} and the American Joint Committee on Cancer (AJCC) cancer staging manual {132}.

Prognosis and prediction

Tumour stage and grade are important prognostic factors. Approximately 60% of pancreatic gastrinomas metastasize to regional lymph nodes {1064,330}. Although regional lymph node metastases do not seem to influence the prognosis too much, survival does decrease once liver metastases occur {4212, 1350,330,5116}. Recently, initial fasting serum gastrin levels (≥ 20 times the upper limit of normal), PanNET size (≥ 20 mm), and multiple concurrent NETs have been also reported to be associated with overall survival in MEN1 patients with gastrinomas {4641}.

Pancreatic gastrinomas expressing SSTR2A, either by immunohistochemistry or by imaging procedures, usually qualify for treatment with somatostatin analogues {3753,639,2166,5116, 5115} and SSTR-targeted radiotherapy {509}.

VIPoma

Mete O
Basturk O
Brosens LAA
de Herder WW
Hong SM
La Rosa S

Definition

VIPoma is a vasoactive intestinal peptide (VIP)-producing pancreatic neuroendocrine neoplasm (PanNEN) that causes WDHA syndrome (watery diarrhoea, hypokalaemia, and achlorhydria; also known as Verner–Morrison syndrome).

ICD-O coding

8155/3 VIPoma

ICD-11 coding

2C10.1 & XH8LS0 Neuroendocrine neoplasms of pancreas & VIPoma, malignant

Related terminology

Acceptable: VIP-producing pancreatic neuroendocrine tumour.
Not recommended: diarrhoeagenic tumour; islet cell tumour with watery diarrhoea.

Subtype(s)

None

Localization

Most pancreatic VIPomas are located in the tail, with 70% in the body or tail and 30% in the head {4192,4213,1543,4135}.

Clinical features

About 75–90% of cases of WDHA syndrome originate from a VIP-secreting pancreatic neuroendocrine tumour (PanNET). Approximately 10–25% of WDHA syndrome cases originate from extrapancreatic sources {4213,1321} that are often linked to neurogenic (neuroblastoma, ganglioneuroblastoma, ganglioneuroma) and sympathetic paraganglial (phaeochromocytoma, composite phaeochromocytoma, paraganglioma) neoplasms of the retroperitoneum, adrenal medulla, and mediastinum {2432,4213,3355,2598,3138}. VIP production from medullary thyroid carcinoma and respiratory tract / lung neoplasms can also occur, but this often does not lead to WDHA syndrome {3890,3891,1768}.

The cardinal features of WDHA syndrome consist of profuse secretory-type watery diarrhoea (usually > 1 L of stool volume per day) that persists with fasting, weight loss, flushing, hypokalaemia, hypochlorhydria/achlorhydria, and metabolic acidosis due to bicarbonate and potassium loss via the stools together with hypovolaemia. Other (less common) manifestations are hypercalcaemia and glucose intolerance {2432,4192,4213}.

Biochemical investigations

An excess of various hormones and peptides, including but not limited to neurotensin and secretin, can simulate WDHA syndrome {812,4713}. The diagnosis requires documentation of elevated plasma VIP levels (often > 60 pmol/L or > 190 pg/mL).

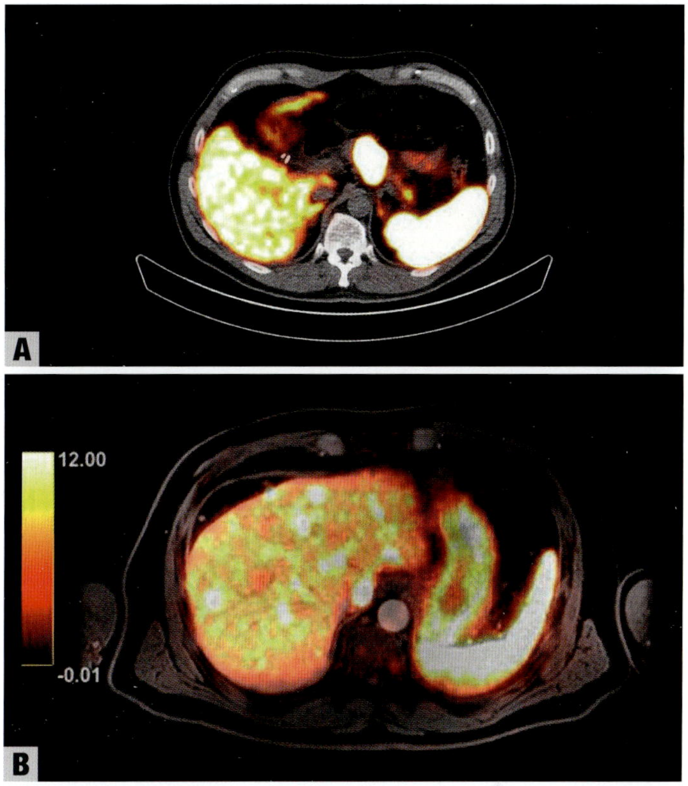

Fig. 7.21 VIPoma. **A** Functional imaging studies of a 54-year-old man with WDHA syndrome (watery diarrhoea, hypokalaemia, and achlorhydria) due to pancreatic VIPoma. 68Ga-DOTATATE PET-CT showing a 45 mm SSTR2-positive neuroendocrine tumour (NET) in the pancreatic body–tail area. **B** Functional imaging showing liver metastases of a pancreatic VIPoma. 68Ga-DOTATATE PET-MRI performed 1 year after surgery, showing multiple SSTR2-positive liver metastases.

Imaging

Primary tumour localization and the presence of metastatic spread are determined using conventional imaging (CT, MRI, EUS) and functional imaging studies (111In-pentetreotide [Octreoscan] SPECT-CT, 68Ga-DOTATATE/DOTATOC PET-CT) {4192,2445,150}. A series identified a T2 hyperintensity and T1 hypointensity on MRI studies of pancreatic VIPomas {150}. Functional imaging studies (111In-pentetreotide and/or 68Ga-DOTATATE PET-CT) yielded positivity in about 80% of pancreatic VIPomas {150}, and scan positivity is further required for peptide receptor radionuclide therapy (PRRT).

Epidemiology

Pancreatic VIPomas account for 0.6–1.5% of all PanNENs {2905,2054} and approximately 2–6% of functioning tumours {2054,2266}. The incidence is 0.05–0.2 cases per 1 million person-years {1321} and there is no sex predilection {4135,150}. Neurogenic tumours such as neuroblastomas and ganglioneuroblastomas are more common in the paediatric population

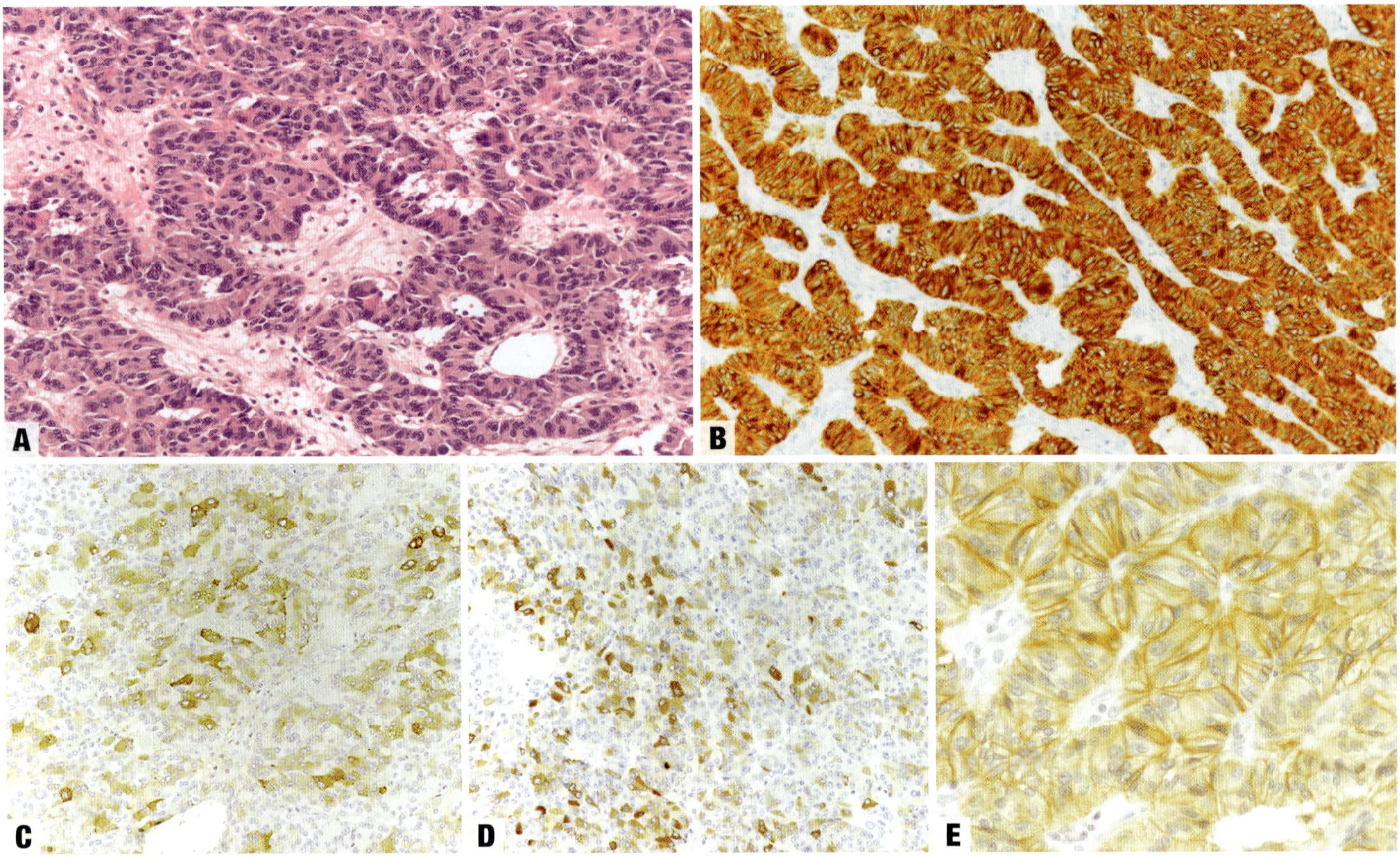

Fig. 7.22 VIPoma. **A** Well-differentiated VIPoma. This photomicrograph shows a tumour with predominant trabecular growth. **B** The tumour cells are diffusely and strongly positive for CK8/18. **C** The extent of VIP immunoreactivity in pancreatic VIPoma is often variable. **D** This photomicrograph shows a tumour that shows coexpression of PP. **E** Diffuse membranous SSTR2A expression.

(mean age: 7.3 years) than are pancreatic VIPomas (mean age: 50.5 years) {372,4213}.

Etiology

There are no established etiological factors. About 3–10% of pancreatic VIPomas occur in the context of multiple endocrine neoplasia type 1 {4213,4192,3947}.

Pathogenesis

Autonomous VIP secretion activates G protein–coupled receptors on the intestinal epithelial cells, which leads to watery diarrhoea and related findings {3761,1317}.

Somatic mutations in *MEN1*, *VHL*, *PTEN*, or *SMAD4* (*DPC4*) mutations have been reported {327,314}. Frequent aberrations of 11q, Xq, and the Y chromosome are detected {4246}. Allelic losses of 3p and 6q in the tumours, found by loss-of-heterozygosity analysis, may be involved in tumour progression {315, 314}.

Macroscopic appearance

Pancreatic VIPomas are usually solitary and well-delineated tumours (mean size: 45–53 mm) {4216,4213,1543,150} and can show solid and cystic components {150}.

Histopathology

These tumours are often indistinguishable from other well-differentiated PanNETs, but they tend to show solid, trabecular, or tubuloacinar patterns {4216}. Variable oncocytic or clear cell change can occur {4216}. Vascular and lymphatic invasion are common {4213}. Some functioning VIPomas can manifest as neuroendocrine microtumours (measuring < 5 mm) {2423}.

Grading

They are graded similarly to other PanNETs, and most are G1 or G2 {2905,150}, but G3 tumours also occur {150}.

Immunohistochemistry

Tumour cells express neuroendocrine differentiation markers (chromogranin A, synaptophysin, INSM1), keratins (AE1/AE3, CAM5.2, CK8/18, CK19), and functional markers (SSTR2A). Some tumours display paranuclear fibrous bodies on low-molecular-weight keratin immunohistochemistry. VIP immunolabelling is found in 90% of cases, but the extent of labelling is variable given the rapid turnover of protein biosynthesis. Although PP coexpression is frequent {4216}, synchronous calcitonin expression can also occur {2374}. Insulin coexpression was also reported at time of metastatic spread {2853}.

Cytology

The cytology is indistinguishable from that of other neuroendocrine neoplasms (NENs).

Diagnostic molecular pathology

None

Essential and desirable diagnostic criteria

Essential: a keratin-positive PanNEN with elevated plasma VIP levels; Ki-67 immunohistochemistry.

Desirable: VIP immunoreactivity; confirmation of pancreatic origin on imaging studies.

Staging

The eighth edition of the American Joint Committee on Cancer (AJCC) / Union for International Cancer Control (UICC) TNM staging system is currently applied to these tumours, which relies on the tumour size, extent of tumour spread, and metastases {532,132}. This approach largely corresponds to that of the European Neuroendocrine Tumor Society (ENETS) classification {3747}.

Prognosis and prediction

Approximately 50–80% of cases present with distant metastases at diagnosis, mostly in the liver {2432,4192,4213}. Ovarian metastases are also reported {2850}. Tumour stage and grade (based on the Ki-67 labelling index and mitotic count) are important prognostic factors. The management of VIP excess (using somatostatin analogues, PRRT, or cytoreductive therapies) is also a critical factor {150}. The 5-year survival rates are 60% and 94%, respectively, for patients with metastatic disease and those who underwent intended curative surgery {4213}.

Serotonin-producing tumours with and without carcinoid syndrome

La Rosa S
Basturk O
Brosens LAA
de Herder WW
Hong SM
Kasajima A
Mete O

Definition

Serotonin-producing pancreatic neuroendocrine tumours (PanNETs) are well-differentiated neuroendocrine neoplasms (NENs) composed of serotonin-producing cells. They are usually clinically non-functioning, but in rare cases they produce carcinoid syndrome (functioning PanNET).

ICD-O coding

8241/3 Serotonin-producing tumour

ICD-11 coding

2C10.1 & XH7NM1 Neuroendocrine neoplasms of pancreas & Enterochromaffin cell carcinoid (includes serotonin-producing carcinoid)

Related terminology

Not recommended: pancreatic carcinoid.

Subtype(s)

None

Localization

They are evenly distributed in the pancreas. Some cases show a ductocentric localization {2480,2906}.

Clinical features

Patients bearing non-functioning serotonin-producing PanNETs can be asymptomatic or can present with nonspecific symptoms due to local growth. Functioning tumours are rare and generally metastatic to the liver, and they present with carcinoid syndrome, including abdominal pain (in 66% of cases), diarrhoea (in 52%), and flushing (in 34%) {2895}. Carcinoid heart disease has been rarely reported {1542}. It is worth noting that not every patient with a metastatic tumour and increased circulating serotonin levels presents with symptoms of carcinoid syndrome {5117,1923}. Functioning tumours are larger than non-functioning ones {2480}.

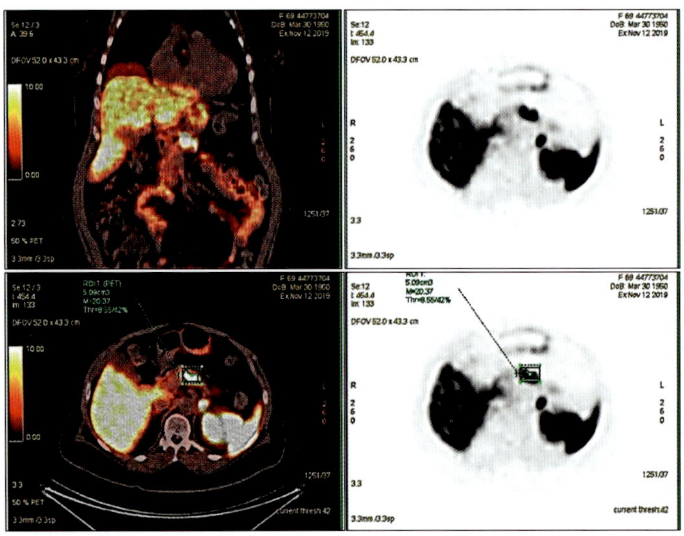

Fig. 7.23 Serotonin-producing pancreatic neuroendocrine tumour (PanNET). 68Ga PET-CT total body: high tracer uptake by a non-functioning neuroendocrine tumour (NET) of the pancreatic body.

Biochemical investigations

The breakdown metabolite of serotonin is 5-HIAA, which can be measured in the urine or plasma as a diagnostic test.

Imaging

Serotonin-producing PanNETs can be visualized using CT, ultrasound, EUS, MRI, 111In-pentetreotide (Octreoscan), or 68Ga-DOTATATE/DOTATOC PET-CT {1923,1924}.

Epidemiology

Serotonin-producing PanNETs represent 0.58–1.4% of digestive serotonin-producing tumours {3055,3056} and 1.4–4% of PanNETs {4207,2480,3000}. In a recently published large international cohort study, functioning serotonin-producing PanNETs represented 1.4% of all PanNETs {3747}. Serotonin-producing PanNETs have a slight female predilection, and patients with functioning tumours are younger (mean age: 41 years) than patients with non-functioning tumours (mean age: 54 years) {2487}.

Etiology

Unknown

Pathogenesis

Similarly to ileal enterochromaffin-cell (EC-cell) neuroendocrine tumours (NETs), serotonin-producing PanNETs show monosomy and rearrangement of chromosome 18 {2480}.

Macroscopic appearance

There are no specific macroscopic features. Tumour size ranges from 5 to 90 mm (mean: 34 mm) {4207,2480}. Some non-functioning tumours originate close to the main pancreatic duct, causing a dilatation of the upstream duct system, which can simulate an intraductal papillary mucinous neoplasm radiographically. These tumours tend to be smaller and more fibrotic than tumours not close to the pancreatic duct system {4768,2240,2906}.

Histopathology

Most cases are well-differentiated PanNETs, although rare serotonin-producing neuroendocrine carcinomas (NECs) have been described (see *Pancreatic neuroendocrine carcinoma*, p. 325) {2480}. Serotonin-producing PanNETs can show different architectural features, including trabecular (the most frequent), solid-nested, or acinar patterns of growths. Some cases can show marked stromal fibrosis and, when they are located close to the

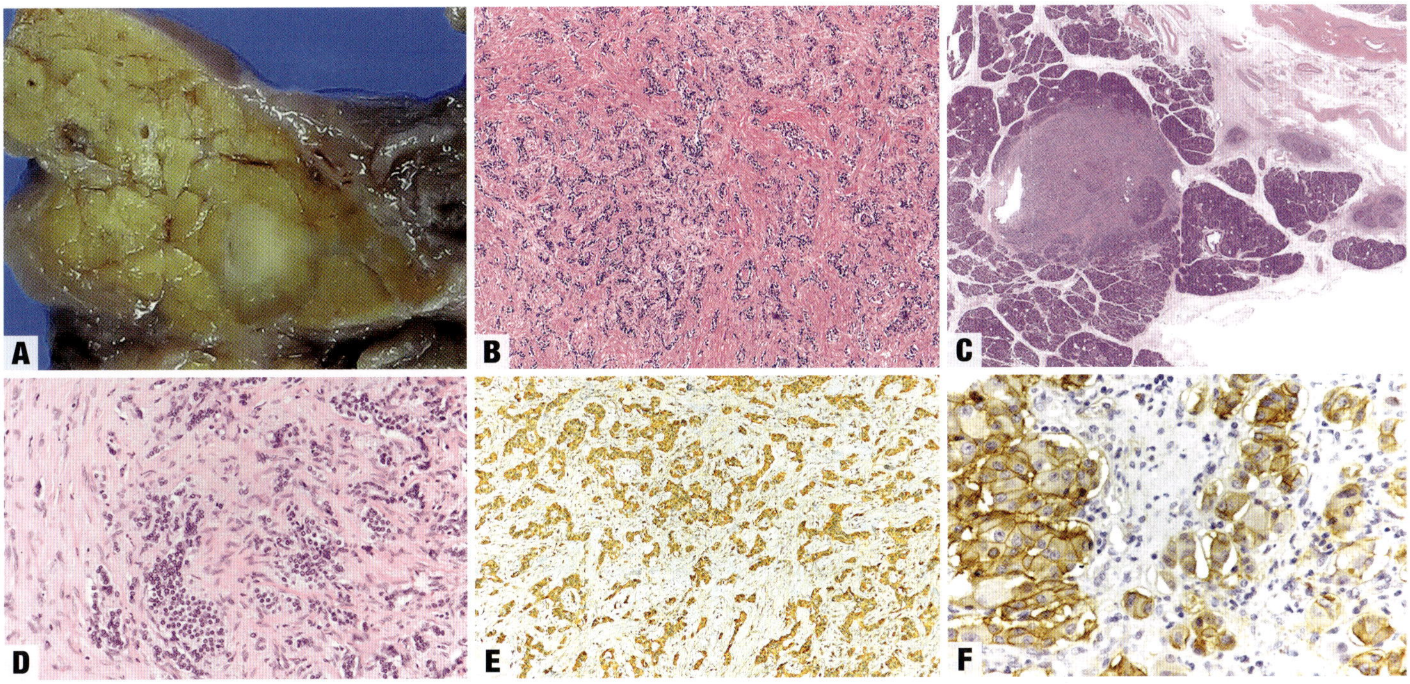

Fig. 7.24 Serotonin-producing pancreatic neuroendocrine tumour (PanNET). **A** Macroscopic appearance of a 7 mm tumour of the head of the pancreas, located close to the main pancreatic duct, causing obstruction. **B** Low-power magnification of a case showing trabecular architecture and marked stromal fibrosis. **C** Microscopic appearance of the tumour at low magnification. **D** The tumour cells show mild atypia. **E** The tumour cells express serotonin. **F** The tumour cells show membrane immunoreactivity for SSTR2A.

pancreatic duct system, may lead to pancreatic duct obstruction with consequent chronic obstructive pancreatitis {2240}. Vascular, lymphatic, and perineural invasion can be observed.

Grading

Most serotonin-producing PanNETs are G1 or G2.

Immunohistochemistry

Serotonin-producing PanNETs express keratins, neuroendocrine differentiation markers (synaptophysin, chromogranin A, and INSM1), serotonin, and SSTR2A, and they generally are negative for pancreatic hormones (insulin, glucagon, somatostatin, and PP) and gastrin {2906}. They may be positive for VMAT2, they are negative for substance P and FGF1 (aFGF), and they show low expression of CTGF and VMAT1 {2480, 2906}. In contrast to some gastrointestinal EC-cell NETs, PanNETs usually show negative or only focally positive SATB2 and CDX2 {3060}. The overall immunoprofile suggests that serotonin-producing PanNETs are different from their intestinal counterparts, as also demonstrated by ultrastructural investigations showing that the serotonin-producing PanNETs are composed of gastric-type and not intestinal-type EC cells {2480}.

Cytology

The cytology is the same as that of other PanNETs.

Diagnostic molecular pathology

Not clinically relevant

Essential and desirable diagnostic criteria

Essential: a keratin-positive PanNEN (PanNET) with serotonin immunoreactivity with or without carcinoid syndrome; Ki-67 immunohistochemistry.

Desirable: VMAT2 positivity; negativity or focal positivity for CDX2 and SATB2.

Staging

The staging of serotonin-producing PanNETs is the same of other PanNETs.

Prognosis and prediction

In a recent study including 7 serotonin-producing PanNETs (both functioning and non-functioning), disease-related survival rates at 1, 3, and 5 years were estimated to be 71%, 43%, and 43%, respectively {3000}. The prognosis of non-functioning serotonin-positive and serotonin-negative PanNETs does not differ and is related to tumour grade and stage {2480,2906}. However, functioning serotonin-producing PanNETs have a worse prognosis than non-functioning ones, presumably because of the more common presence of liver metastases in the functioning cases {2480}.

Other pancreatic neuroendocrine tumours with ectopic hormone production

Basturk O
Asa SL
Brosens LAA
Ezzat S
Hong SM
La Rosa S
Mete O

Definition

Other pancreatic neuroendocrine tumours (PanNETs) with ectopic hormone production are defined as well-differentiated PanNETs producing hormones that are not eutopic to the pancreas.

ICD-O coding

8158/3 ACTH-producing tumour
8158/3 Calcitonin-producing pancreatic neuroendocrine tumour
8158/3 CRH-producing pancreatic neuroendocrine tumour
8158/3 Cholecystokinin-producing pancreatic neuroendocrine tumour
8158/3 Erythropoietin-producing pancreatic neuroendocrine tumour
8272/3 GH-producing tumour
8158/3 GHRH-producing pancreatic neuroendocrine tumour
8158/3 Ghrelin-producing pancreatic neuroendocrine tumour
8272/3 Gonadotropin-producing tumour
8158/3 PTH/PTHrP-producing pancreatic neuroendocrine tumour
8158/3 Vasopressin-producing pancreatic neuroendocrine tumour

ICD-11 coding

2C10.1 & XH7AG8 Neuroendocrine neoplasms of pancreas & ACTH-producing tumour
(No ICD-11 codes for the other subtypes)

Related terminology

Acceptable: ectopic hormone–producing PanNET.

Subtype(s)

ACTH-producing tumour; calcitonin-producing PanNET; CRH-producing PanNET; CCK-producing PanNET; erythropoietin-producing PanNET; growth hormone–producing tumour; GHRH-producing PanNET; ghrelin-producing PanNET; gonadotropin-producing tumour; PTH/PTHrP-producing PanNET; vasopressin-producing PanNET

Localization

There is no site predilection.

Clinical features

Rare PanNETs with ectopic hormone secretion produce endocrine syndromes that are not expected from the pancreas. Patients may develop some or all of the symptoms of the syndrome. In the commonest scenario, PanNETs producing ACTH and/or CRH cause Cushing syndrome {3442, 2197,2836,1413}; approximately 40% of patients develop Zollinger–Ellison syndrome and 5% may develop inappropriate insulin secretion {4866,2883,871}. PanNETs expressing and secreting PTH or PTHrP may cause hypercalcaemia {187, 12,4643,2182,1545,2180}. PTH is ectopic, whereas PTHrP is not {1156}; however, clinical manifestation of hormone excess is unusual, because it requires gene de-repression to cause clinically relevant hypersecretion. PanNETs with growth hormone or GHRH production cause acromegaly {2933,1305, 3937,4842,3051,3901,4257}. Although calcitonin expression in PanNETs is common {4601}, it is often not associated with a well-defined endocrine syndrome; rare patients may present with diarrhoea and hypercalcaemia {1390,4015,3304,4718}, but the presentation may be complicated by plurihormonal ectopic secretion with other causes of diarrhoea such as carcinoid syndrome or Zollinger–Ellison syndrome, and it is often associated with Cushing syndrome {205,1390,4643, 4015,2374,3304}.

Even more rare endocrine syndromes attributed to PanNETs include only a few reported cases. These include persistent steatorrhoea, weight loss, and gallstones combined with peptic ulcer disease due to CCK excess in the absence of other

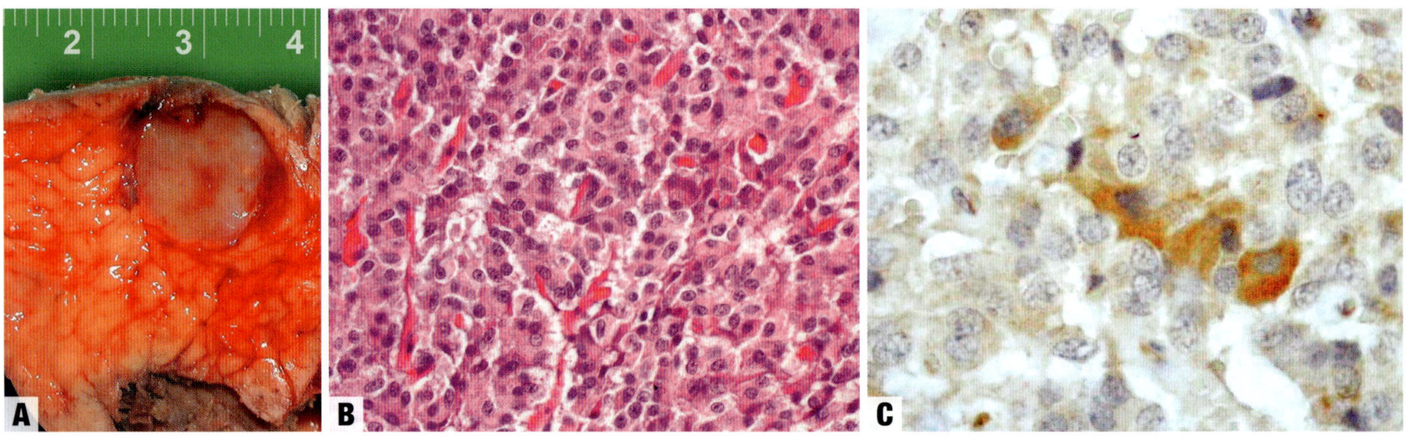

Fig. 7.25 Other pancreatic neuroendocrine tumours (PanNETs) with ectopic hormone production. **A** GHRH-producing PanNET. The tumour is well circumscribed. **B** Sections reveal trabecular architecture and bland cytology. **C** The tumour cells are positive for GHRH immunohistochemical stain.

elevated hormones (cholecystokininoma syndrome) {3709, 1054}; hyponatraemia due to vasopressin excess (syndrome of inappropriate antidiuresis [SIAD]) {114}; erythroblastosis due to erythropoietin secretion {3930}; ovarian hyperstimulation due to FSH excess {3026}; and masculinization due to LH excess {533,3545}. An exceptional case of a ghrelin-secreting PanNET manifesting with a 50-fold increase of circulating ghrelin levels and no associated growth hormone / IGF1 abnormality has also been reported {908}.

Ectopic hormone production may evolve during progression of the PanNET {3657,3442,114}; it may even be seen in recurrences or metastases after an initial diagnosis of non-functioning PanNET {4369,114}.

Epidemiology

The most common ectopic hormone–producing PanNET is the ACTH-secreting PanNET, and pancreatic primaries account for 10–15% of ectopic (i.e. non-pituitary, non-adrenal) Cushing syndrome cases {2377,2485,2836,1413}. The tumours occur most frequently in young or middle-aged female patients (M:F ratio: 0.5:1). They can also occur in children {2197}.

Etiology

Except for extremely rare cases related to genetically transmitted syndromes, including multiple endocrine neoplasia type 1 {4311,4337,3901} and von Hippel–Lindau syndrome {2836}, the etiology of these functioning PanNETs is unknown.

Pathogenesis

The pathogenesis is unknown. The factors involved in derepression with aberrant hormone expression and secretion remain to be determined.

Macroscopic appearance

The gross features of these ectopic hormone–producing PanNETs are not distinctive.

Histopathology

PanNETs with ectopic hormone production are often indistinguishable from other PanNETs.

Grading

They are well differentiated {2836}, and most are G2 tumours.

Immunohistochemistry

Immunolabelling for the neuroendocrine biomarkers and hormones can be focal or diffuse, and other related or diverse peptide hormones may also be detected. For example, all ACTH-producing PanNETs label for chromogranin A and synaptophysin, as well as for the ACTH precursor protein POMC and the various hormones that are cleaved from POMC, such as MSH (melanotropin), β-endorphin, and met-enkephalin {3347,93,2836,2929}. These tumours may also be positive for SSTR2A {715,1055,862,2374,5133}.

Differential diagnosis

PanNETs with ectopic hormone production should be distinguished from pancreatic paragangliomas with aberrant hormone expression and from metastatic neuroendocrine tumours (NETs). A lack of reactivity for keratins (AE1/AE3, CAM5.2) and reactivity for GATA3 and tyrosine hydroxylase can help distinguish paragangliomas. Metastatic NETs are distinguished using anatomical site and/or cell lineage–specific transcription factors and hormones, like in other organs.

Cytology

The cytology is the same as that of other PanNETs.

Diagnostic molecular pathology

Not clinically relevant

Essential and desirable diagnostic criteria

Essential: a keratin-positive PanNEN (PanNET); immunohistochemical expression of keratin, neuroendocrine markers, and ectopic hormones; Ki-67 immunohistochemistry.

Desirable: elevated circulating levels of the ectopic hormone and symptoms of the related endocrine syndrome.

Staging

The pathological staging of PanNETs with ectopic hormone production, like that of all PanNETs, is based on the eighth edition

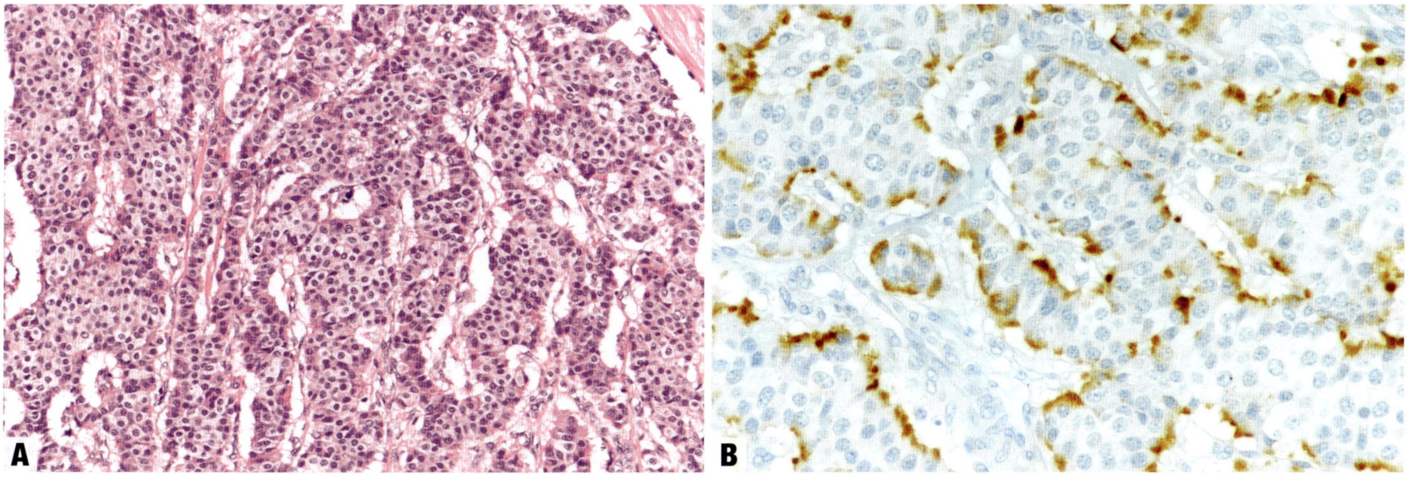

Fig. 7.26 Other pancreatic neuroendocrine tumours (PanNETs) with ectopic hormone production. **A** An ACTH-producing PanNET with a trabecular growth pattern. **B** The tumour cells are positive for ACTH immunohistochemical stain.

(2017) of the Union for International Cancer Control (UICC) and American Joint Committee on Cancer (AJCC) TNM classification.

Prognosis and prediction

The prognosis of PanNETs with ectopic hormone production depends on the grading and staging of the tumour. However, most patients present with metastases at the time of diagnosis or develop distant metastases during follow-up, and their prognosis is poor {5128}. For example, the 5- and 10-year survival rates of ectopic ACTH-producing PanNETs are 35% and 16%, respectively {2836}. Cases positive for SSTR2 may respond to somatostatin analogue therapy and peptide receptor radionuclide therapy (PRRT) {1131,2377,2374,2056,5133}.

(Poly)functioning PanNETs with multiple clinical endocrine syndromes can be particularly aggressive {93,2836,114}. The mean survival time after the appearance of the second endocrine syndrome is only 5–7 months.

Pancreatic neuroendocrine carcinoma

Basturk O
Brosens LAA
Hong SM
Klöppel G
La Rosa S
Mete O
Ohike N
Tang LH
Volante M

Definition

Pancreatic neuroendocrine carcinoma (PanNEC) is a poorly differentiated, high-grade malignant epithelial neoplasm with diffuse neuroendocrine differentiation. Small cell and large cell subtypes occur.

ICD-O coding

8246/3 Neuroendocrine carcinoma, NOS
8041/3 Small cell neuroendocrine carcinoma
8013/3 Large cell neuroendocrine carcinoma

ICD-11 coding

2C10.1 & XH0U20 Neuroendocrine neoplasms of pancreas & Neuroendocrine carcinoma, NOS
2C10.1 & XH9SY0 Neuroendocrine neoplasms of pancreas & Small cell neuroendocrine carcinoma
2C10.1 & XH0NL5 Neuroendocrine neoplasms of pancreas & Large cell neuroendocrine carcinoma

Related terminology

Acceptable: high-grade (poorly differentiated) neuroendocrine carcinoma (NEC); large cell neuroendocrine carcinoma (LCNEC); small cell neuroendocrine carcinoma (SCNEC); small cell carcinoma.
Not recommended: high-grade neuroendocrine tumour.

Subtype(s)

Large cell PanNEC; small cell PanNEC

Localization

The majority of PanNECs occur in the head of the pancreas {339}.

Clinical features

The presentation of PanNECs is similar to that of pancreatic ductal adenocarcinomas {2319,339,340,1850} and includes back pain, jaundice, and/or nonspecific abdominal symptoms {2611,4235}. In contrast to well-differentiated pancreatic neuroendocrine tumours (PanNETs), PanNECs are usually clinically non-functioning {919}. Serum calcitonin level may be elevated in some patients {4601}. SSTRs (in particular SSTR2) usually are not expressed {2389}, which may be helpful in distinguishing PanNECs from PanNETs, because functional imaging studies such as SSTR scintigraphy (111In-pentetreotide [Octreoscan]) and 68Ga-DOTATATE PET-CT {4256,4603,207} are often negative in PanNECs. However, FDG PET-CT is usually positive {4256}.

Epidemiology

PanNECs are uncommon and represent < 1% of all pancreatic neoplasms and no more than 2–3% of all pancreatic neuroendocrine neoplasms (PanNENs) {3731,1752,3237,340}. Most of the patients are in their late fifties, and there is a slight male predilection (M:F ratio: 1.4:1) {4235,339,340,1850}.

Etiology

The genetic syndromes associated with PanNETs (multiple endocrine neoplasia type 1, von Hippel–Lindau syndrome, neurofibromatosis type 1, etc.) are not associated with PanNECs.

Pathogenesis

The most frequently mutated gene in PanNECs is *TP53*, followed by *RB1* and, to a lesser extent, *KRAS*, *BRAF*, *APC*, and others {4992,1609,4704,2389,2388,4603}. *KRAS* mutations, which are very common in pancreatic ductal adenocarcinoma, have

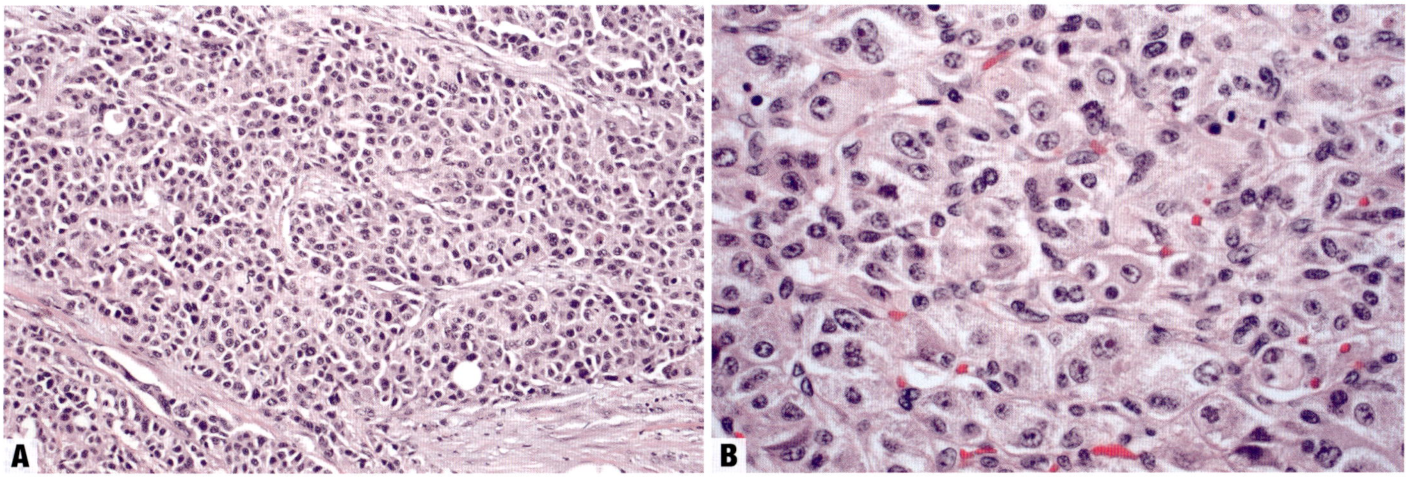

Fig. 7.27 Pancreatic neuroendocrine carcinoma (poorly differentiated neuroendocrine neoplasm), large cell type. **A** Diffuse growth of relatively monotonous cells with a nested/organoid pattern indicating neuroendocrine differentiation, which was confirmed by synaptophysin staining. Cytological atypia and prominent mitotic activity indicate the high-grade nature of this carcinoma. **B** The cells have moderate cytoplasm and large nuclei with prominent nucleoli.

Chapter 7

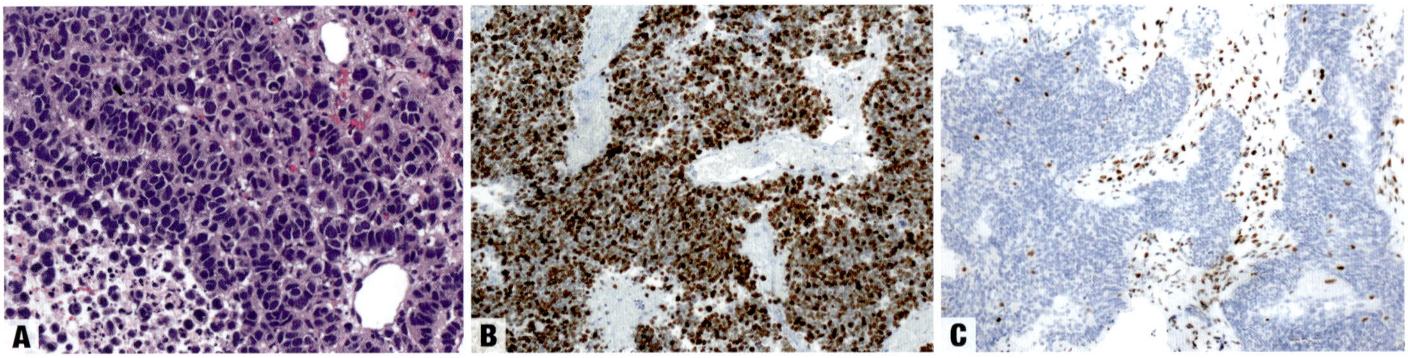

Fig. 7.28 Pancreatic neuroendocrine carcinoma (poorly differentiated neuroendocrine neoplasm). **A** The cells have high-grade cytology, with minimal cytoplasm and a high N:C ratio. Mitotic activity is brisk, and necrosis is readily evident. **B** Ki-67 immunostaining shows diffuse nuclear labelling, with a Ki-67 proliferation index > 90%. **C** Loss of RB1 protein expression.

been observed in about 40% of PanNECs, and their presence supports the pathogenetic relationship between PanNECs and non-neuroendocrine pancreatic carcinoma (pancreatic ductal adenocarcinoma) {2309,2388}. The potential for well-differentiated PanNETs to transform to poorly differentiated PanNECs could be considered, and anecdotal cases exist.

The following specific genetic alterations common in PanNETs are not features of PanNECs: alterations in *MEN1*, as well as in DNA damage repair (*MUTYH*, *CHEK2*, *BRCA2*), chromatin remodelling (*ARID1A*, *SMARCA4*), telomere alteration (*DAXX/ATRX*), and PI3K/mTOR signalling (*EWSR1* fusions, *PTEN*, *HIF1A/EPAS2*) pathways (see *Pancreatic neuroendocrine neoplasms: Introduction*, p. 296) {4992,3977,207}.

Macroscopic appearance

PanNECs present as large (mean size: 40 mm, range: 20–180 mm), relatively circumscribed, solid tumours that are typically fleshier than pancreatic ductal adenocarcinomas. They tend to be white-grey or yellow, and often reveal vague nodularity. Haemorrhage is common, and necrosis may be seen {339}.

Histopathology

The histology of PanNECs is similar to that of their counterparts in other organs, particularly their counterparts in the lung {4308, 3714,339,340}. These poorly differentiated carcinomas are subdivided on the basis of cell size into large cell and small cell subtypes.

The large cell PanNEC (LCNEC) is more common (60%) and is characterized by relatively uniform round to polygonal cells with amphophilic cytoplasm, large nuclei, vesicular chromatin, and (in some cases) prominent nucleoli. Diffuse large irregular nests, and trabecular and peripheral palisading growth patterns, often intermingled in various proportions, are seen in most of these carcinomas {339,340,4412,2716}.

The small cell PanNEC reveals diffuse sheets of small to intermediate cells with finely granular chromatin, high N:C ratios, inconspicuous nucleoli, prominent nuclear moulding, and crush artefact {2716}.

In both subtypes, mitotic activity is brisk (often > 20 mitoses/2 mm^2) and there is extensive tumour necrosis. The Ki-67 proliferation index is by definition > 20%, and commonly 60–80%, particularly in the small cell subtype {4235,339,340}. The Ki-67 index tends to be lower in the large cell subtype.

PanNECs can be associated with non-NEC components, in particular ductal adenocarcinoma or very rarely acinar cell carcinoma. When each component accounts for ≥ 30% of the tumour, the term "mixed ductal–neuroendocrine carcinoma", a type of mixed neuroendocrine–non-neuroendocrine neoplasm (MiNEN), is applied {339} (see *Mixed ductal adenocarcinoma–neuroendocrine neoplasms*, p. 328, and *Mixed acinar–neuroendocrine carcinoma*, p. 330).

Immunohistochemistry

Demonstration of neuroendocrine differentiation is required to confirm the diagnosis of PanNEC {339,340,4308,3714,1170, 3749,2091,2716}. Synaptophysin is the most sensitive marker. In contrast, chromogranin A is a highly specific marker, but its sensitivity is relatively low, and its expression can be limited in the small cell subtype, where the cytoplasm contains fewer secretory granules {4105}. Moreover, the expression of these neuroendocrine markers may be focal or show a dot-like staining pattern {339,1170}. INSM1 may be expressed in neoplasms with variable synaptophysin or focal/negative chromogranin A expression {4418,376,378,2154,2532}. The use of nonspecific biomarkers alone (e.g. CD56, CD57, and NSE) is discouraged.

Differential diagnosis

An important mimic of PanNEC, especially of the large cell subtype, is acinar cell carcinoma, because of its monotonous appearance, high proliferative rate, and common expression of neuroendocrine markers (at least focally). In fact, the diagnosis of large cell PanNEC should not be established without immunohistochemical evaluation for acinar differentiation markers (e.g. trypsin, chymotrypsin, BCL10) {2532}. In one study, 15% of cases originally classified as PanNEC proved to be mixed acinar–neuroendocrine carcinomas on further analysis {339}.

Metastatic carcinoma to the pancreas should also be excluded and requires clinical correlation {26}. Immunohistochemical analysis may not be helpful in this regard, given the common expression in PanNECs of otherwise organ-specific transcription factors, such as thyroid transcription factor 1 (TTF1), CDX2, and insulin gene enhancer protein ISL1 or PDX1{4693,28}.

The crushed and moulded tumour cells of the small cell subtype may resemble lymphoma. Immunohistochemistry is helpful for the diagnosis. Other small round cell tumours, such as the Ewing family of tumours, may also involve the pancreas and need to be distinguished. Immunolabelling for CD99 can be helpful because most Ewing-family tumours show staining {3117,437}.

Cytology

The features of PanNEC are similar to those of other organs {3712}. Smears are hypercellular and show sheets of small cells with very high N:C ratios, poorly defined cytoplasm, hyperchromatic angulated and elongated nuclei with uniformly distributed fine salt-and-pepper chromatin, inconspicuous nucleoli, nuclear moulding, numerous mitotic figures, and apoptotic bodies. Nuclear crush artefact and necrotic debris in the background are prominent, along with stripped nuclei and a variable number of intact single tumour cells. The carcinomas should be differentiated from other malignancies, including other carcinomas, melanomas, and lymphomas; immunohistochemical studies on cell blocks may be helpful {4139,1170,4140}. Their distinction from well-differentiated neuroendocrine tumours (NETs) can be also be challenging. Proliferation index analysis may serve as an adjunct {1462,4140}.

Diagnostic molecular pathology

PanNECs show abnormal p53 expression and/or complete loss of RB1 expression in 95% and 74% of cases, respectively, which correspond to intragenic mutated *TP53* and *RB1* genes; PanNECs lack mutations in *DAXX*, *ATRX*, and *MEN1* {4992,2388}. Therefore, genomic profiling can be useful in the distinction of PanNECs from PanNETs in selected cases.

Essential and desirable diagnostic criteria

Essential: a keratin-positive poorly differentiated epithelial neoplasm of small to intermediate or large cells; neuroendocrine morphology; a mitotic count of > 20 mitoses/2 mm^2; Ki-67 proliferation index > 20%; expression of neuroendocrine markers.
Desirable: abnormal p53 expression; loss of RB1 expression.

Staging

The pathological staging of PanNECs is based on the eighth edition (2017) of the Union for International Cancer Control (UICC) TNM classification {532} for carcinomas of the exocrine pancreas.

Prognosis and prediction

PanNECs are highly aggressive malignant neoplasms {4235, 4020,339,340}. Advanced stage at presentation is common {2611,4235,1850}; therefore, chemotherapy is often the primary therapeutic approach {4308,3664,2091}. The aggressive behaviour of PanNECs warrants consideration of adjuvant therapy after surgery, even for locoregional disease, and although definite data are lacking, platinum and etoposide are recommended {4235,340,2091}. However, even with resection and platinum-based therapy, the median survival time is very short (< 1 year), and < 25% of patients survive beyond 2 years {4235, 339,3633,2091}. In addition, PanNECs with other carcinoma components (e.g. ductal adenocarcinoma) appear to be similarly aggressive, emphasizing the importance of recognizing the PanNEC component in such cases.

There are no data to support the use of somatostatin analogue therapy in PanNECs. Immunotherapy with checkpoint inhibitors is currently under investigation in extrapulmonary NECs {2091}.

Mixed ductal adenocarcinoma–neuroendocrine neoplasms

La Rosa S
Basturk O
Brosens LAA
Hong SM
Mete O

Definition

Mixed ductal adenocarcinoma–neuroendocrine neoplasms are pancreatic mixed neuroendocrine–non-neuroendocrine neoplasm (MiNEN) subtypes composed of morphologically and immunohistochemically recognizable ductal adenocarcinoma associated with a neuroendocrine component, represented by poorly differentiated neuroendocrine carcinoma (NEC) or, very rarely, by well-differentiated neuroendocrine tumour (NET). Both components constitute ≥ 30% of the tumour volume, and they are presumed to be clonally related.

ICD-O coding

8154/3 Mixed ductal adenocarcinoma–neuroendocrine carcinoma

8244/3 Mixed ductal adenocarcinoma–neuroendocrine tumour

ICD-11 coding

2C10.1 & XH6H10 Neuroendocrine neoplasms of pancreas & Mixed adenoneuroendocrine carcinoma

Related terminology

Acceptable: mixed adenoneuroendocrine carcinoma (MANEC); mixed ductal–neuroendocrine carcinoma.

Subtype(s)

Mixed ductal adenocarcinoma–NEC; mixed ductal adenocarcinoma–NET (very rare)

Localization

Mixed ductal adenocarcinoma–neuroendocrine neoplasms are most frequently located in the pancreatic head.

Clinical features

The symptoms are usually nonspecific and related to tumour growth and/or metastatic dissemination. One patient with mixed ductal adenocarcinoma–NET presenting with Zollinger–Ellison syndrome has been reported {4436}.

Epidemiology

Mixed ductal adenocarcinoma–NECs account for about 0.5–2% of all ductal adenocarcinomas {2340,3328}. About 18% of pancreatic NECs (PanNECs) have components of adenocarcinoma {339}. There is no sex predilection. The average patient age at presentation is 68 years (range: 21–84 years).

Etiology

Unknown

Pathogenesis

No association with genetic syndromes has been documented. No definitive molecular pathogenetic data are yet available. Data from gastrointestinal MiNENs suggest a monoclonal origin of the two components, but this has not been well tested in pancreatic mixed ductal adenocarcinoma–NECs {1599}. Considering the molecular information of conventional ductal adenocarcinomas (*KRAS*, *CDKN2A*, *TP53*, and *SMAD4* somatic mutations) and of NECs (*TP53* and *RB1* somatic mutations), mixed ductal adenocarcinoma–NECs are expected to show the same molecular profile.

Macroscopic appearance

Mixed ductal adenocarcinoma–NEC and mixed ductal adenocarcinoma–NET are solid tumours measuring 20–100 mm in diameter.

Histopathology

In some mixed ductal adenocarcinoma–NECs, the two morphologically recognizable components are intermingled and characterized by neoplastic ductal and neuroendocrine cells forming glandular, cribriform, solid, and/or trabecular structures. In other cases, the two components are distinct and consist of a ductal adenocarcinoma usually combined with a NEC, either small cell or large cell subtype. In very rare cases, the neuroendocrine component is well-differentiated NET {3243}.

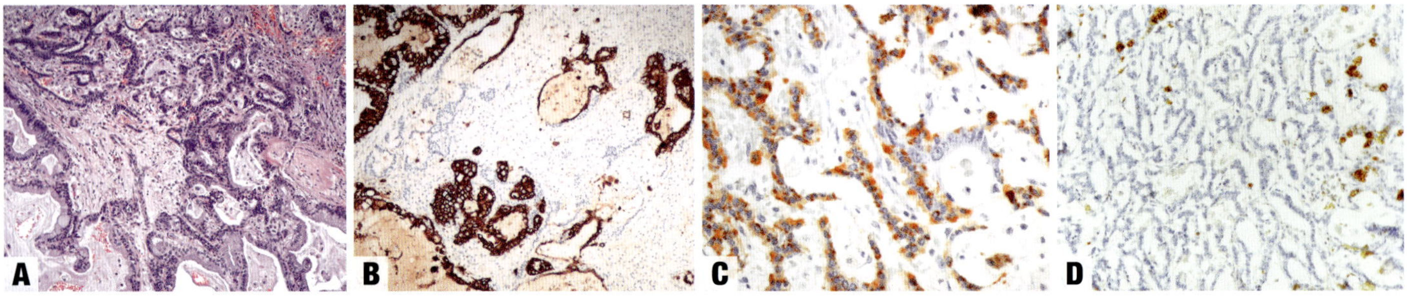

Fig. 7.29 Mixed ductal adenocarcinoma–neuroendocrine tumour (NET). **A** The tumour is composed of ductal adenocarcinoma (bottom of image) associated with a well-differentiated NET showing a trabecular pattern of growth. **B** The adenocarcinoma component is positive for CK7, which is negative in the trabecular NET component. **C** The NET component is positive for chromogranin A. A glandular structure is chromogranin A–negative. **D** The Ki-67 proliferation index of the trabecular NET component is low.

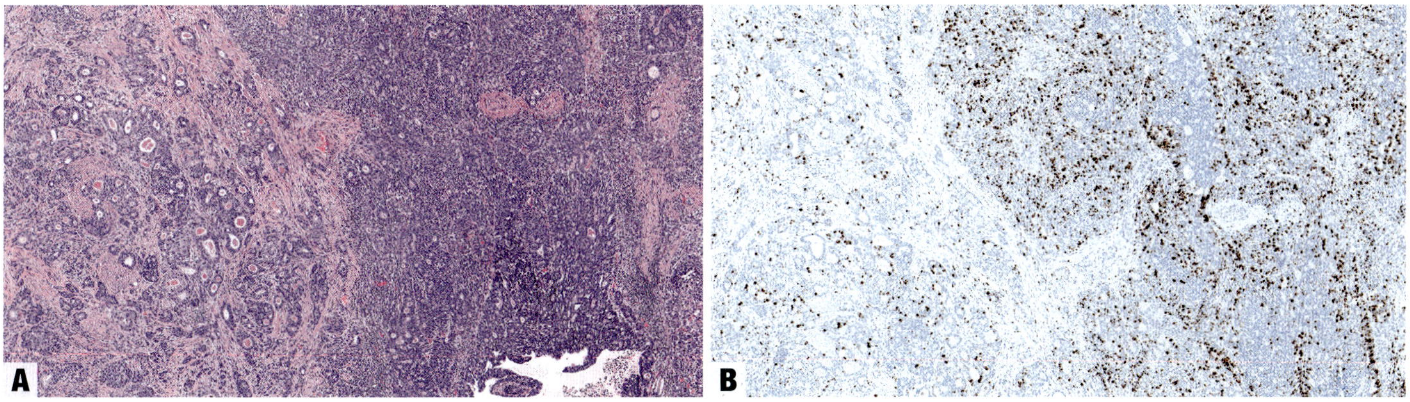

Fig. 7.30 Mixed ductal adenocarcinoma–neuroendocrine carcinoma (NEC). **A** This tumour is composed of ductal adenocarcinoma (left) and large cell neuroendocrine carcinoma (LCNEC; right). The two components are morphologically recognizable. **B** The Ki-67 proliferation index of the NEC component is > 20%.

Immunohistochemistry

The ductal adenocarcinoma component is positive for CEA, EMA (MUC1), and/or MUC2, whereas the neuroendocrine component is positive for synaptophysin, chromogranin A, and INSM1.

Differential diagnosis

The most important differential diagnoses include ductal adenocarcinoma with entrapped islets, which can be intimately attached to well-differentiated neoplastic glands, and pancreatic NETs (PanNETs) with entrapped ductules {4605}. Another consideration in the case of mixed ductal adenocarcinoma–NET is the coincidental occurrence of a clonally distinct PanNET within the same pancreas as a ductal adenocarcinoma (collision tumour), which must be excluded before establishing the diagnosis of mixed ductal adenocarcinoma–NET. The neuroendocrine component of mixed ductal adenocarcinoma–NEC shows a high Ki-67 index (> 20%); the NET component of mixed ductal adenocarcinoma–NET has a Ki-67 index < 20%.

Cytology

Cytology is not clinically relevant, because the diagnosis is made on resected specimen.

Diagnostic molecular pathology

Not clinically relevant

Essential and desirable diagnostic criteria

Essential: a mixed tumour composed of two morphologically recognizable components; ≥ 30% of the neoplasm composed of each type; neuroendocrine marker expression in the neuroendocrine component.

Staging

Pancreatic MiNENs are staged using the Union for International Cancer Control (UICC) or American Joint Committee on Cancer (AJCC) staging system for pancreatic carcinoma.

Prognosis and prediction

Mixed ductal adenocarcinoma–NECs usually metastasize to lymph nodes and liver. Resectability is the most important prognostic factor. Patients rarely survive > 3 years. The 2-year and 5-year survival rates are 25% and 0%, respectively. However, the few prognostic data available seem to suggest that mixed ductal adenocarcinoma–NECs have a slightly longer median survival time than pure NECs (20 months vs 12 months) {339}. Mixed ductal adenocarcinoma–NETs seem to show a better survival than mixed ductal adenocarcinoma–NECs {3243}.

Mixed acinar–neuroendocrine carcinoma

Basturk O
Brosens LAA
Hong SM
La Rosa S
Mete O
Ohike N

Definition

Mixed acinar–neuroendocrine carcinoma is a pancreatic mixed neuroendocrine–non-neuroendocrine neoplasm (MiNEN) composed of morphologically and immunohistochemically recognizable acinar cell carcinoma associated with a neuroendocrine component, usually neuroendocrine carcinoma (NEC), each of which constitutes ≥ 30% of the tumour volume.

ICD-O coding

8154/3 Mixed acinar-neuroendocrine carcinoma

ICD-11 coding

2D12.Y & XH8E54 Other specified malignant neoplasms of other endocrine glands or related structures & Mixed neuroendocrine non-neuroendocrine neoplasm

Related terminology

Acceptable: mixed acinar–endocrine carcinoma.

Not recommended: acinar cell carcinoma–neuroendocrine carcinoma.

Subtype(s)

None

Localization

These carcinomas are located throughout the pancreas {4866, 3329,2477,2291}.

Clinical features

Patients usually present with nonspecific symptoms like abdominal pain and weight loss {2477}. However, mixed acinar–neuroendocrine carcinomas causing jaundice or lipase hypersecretion syndrome have been reported {338}.

Epidemiology

Mixed acinar–neuroendocrine carcinomas account for 15–20% of all acinar cell carcinomas {2338,2477,2337}. Most of the patients are in their sixties (age range: 37–88 years), and there is no sex predilection {2338,3329,2477,4469}.

Etiology

Unknown

Pathogenesis

No association with genetic syndromes has been documented. Mixed acinar–neuroendocrine carcinomas are reported to have the same genetic changes as those seen in pure acinar cell carcinomas, including APC/β-catenin pathway alterations, *BRAF* rearrangements, and DNA repair defects such as mismatch repair deficiency and BRCA pathway defects {1465,822,4932, 4469,3604}. A recent molecular study suggested that *MYC* amplification may be a mechanism involved in the neuroendocrine differentiation of acinar cell carcinomas {2478}.

Macroscopic appearance

These carcinomas typically present as large (range: 15–300 mm), poorly defined, multilobulated tumours with a fleshy cut surface. Haemorrhage and necrosis are common. Intraductal spread may be seen {3330,2337,4605}.

Histopathology

Most acinar–neuroendocrine carcinomas resemble acinar cell carcinomas and display neuroendocrine differentiation but have a homogeneous morphology. Such cases do not fit the definition of a MiNEN and are best regarded as acinar cell carcinomas with extensive neuroendocrine differentiation, which does not affect their clinical behaviour {822,4866}. Acinar cell carcinomas with scattered neuroendocrine cells (< 30% of the

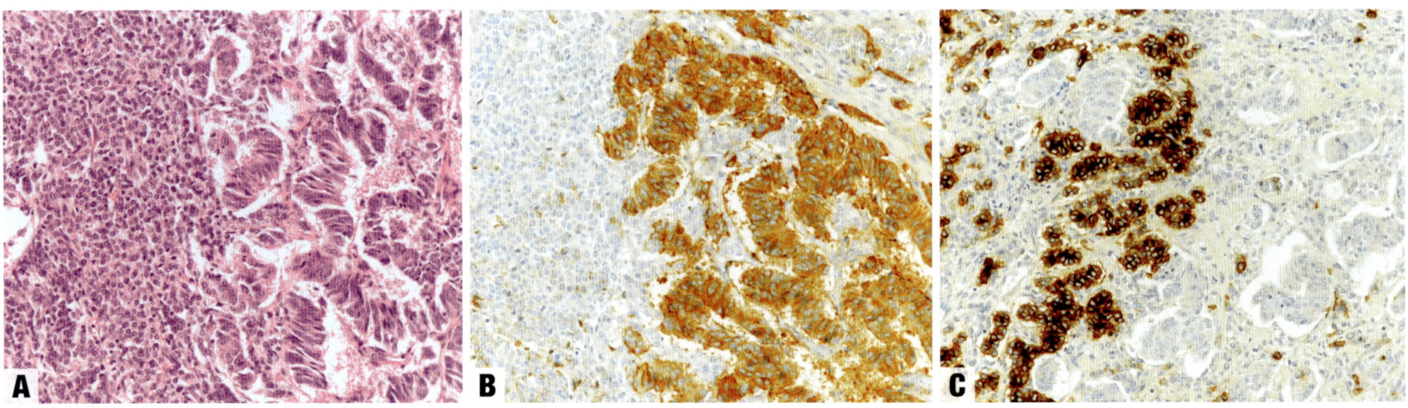

Fig. 7.31 Mixed acinar–neuroendocrine carcinoma. **A** The tumour is showing morphologically distinguishable solid acinar (left) and trabecular neuroendocrine (right) components. **B** The neuroendocrine component is strongly positive for chromogranin A. **C** The neuroendocrine component is negative for trypsin, which is positive in the acinar component.

tumour cells) do not qualify as mixed carcinomas and should be diagnosed as acinar cell carcinoma {4866}.

A few cases show morphologically and immunohistochemically discernible acinar and neuroendocrine components, which form closely connected sheets and nests {2337}, and these cases fit the definition of a MiNEN.

Immunohistochemistry

In cases fitting the definition of a MiNEN, immunoexpression of both acinar (e.g. trypsin, chymotrypsin, and BCL10) and neuroendocrine (e.g. chromogranin A, synaptophysin, and INSM1) markers, each in ≥ 30% of the tumour cell population, can help recognize the mixed nature of these neoplasms {2338,2481}.

Differential diagnosis

The distinction of mixed acinar–neuroendocrine carcinoma from pancreatic NEC (PanNEC) and even well-differentiated pancreatic neuroendocrine tumour (PanNET) can be problematic. In fact, in one study, 15% of cases originally classified as PanNEC proved to be mixed acinar–neuroendocrine carcinomas on further analysis {339,2337,2532}.

Cytology

Smears from mixed acinar–neuroendocrine carcinomas are often cellular and reveal a monotonous population of predominantly single, atypical tumour cells; some loosely cohesive clusters; and rare pseudoacinar formations. The tumour cells are round to oval with small to moderate amounts of delicate to granular cytoplasm. The nuclei have mild to moderate anisonucleosis and granular chromatin with small nucleoli {4138, 4294,3246,4863}. However, these features significantly overlap with those of well-differentiated PanNET, PanNEC, and acinar cell carcinoma. Therefore, demonstration of both acinar and neuroendocrine differentiation by immunohistochemistry is required to suggest the possibility of mixed acinar–neuroendocrine carcinoma.

Diagnostic molecular pathology

Diagnostic molecular pathology is not yet required for diagnosis. However, molecular investigation may be helpful in distinguishing the components of these tumours in small biopsies.

Essential and desirable diagnostic criteria

Essential: a mixed tumour composed of two components; ≥ 30% of the neoplasm should be composed of each type; immunohistochemical evidence of acinar and neuroendocrine differentiation.

Desirable: Ki-67 immunohistochemistry.

Staging

The pathological staging of mixed acinar–neuroendocrine carcinomas is based on the eighth edition (2017) of the Union for International Cancer Control (UICC) TNM classification {532} for carcinomas of the exocrine pancreas.

Prognosis and prediction

Mixed acinar–neuroendocrine carcinomas mainly behave like acinar cell carcinomas {2338,3329,2477} and are more aggressive than PanNETs {2291}. Most patients have nodal and/or distant metastases at presentation {2291}. After resection, the reported 5-year survival rate for patients who undergo surgery is 30–50%, similar to the rate associated with acinar cell carcinomas {2745,2477,2291,3243,4605}. There is no evidence that the presence of a neuroendocrine component should affect the oncological treatment of mixed acinar–neuroendocrine carcinomas.

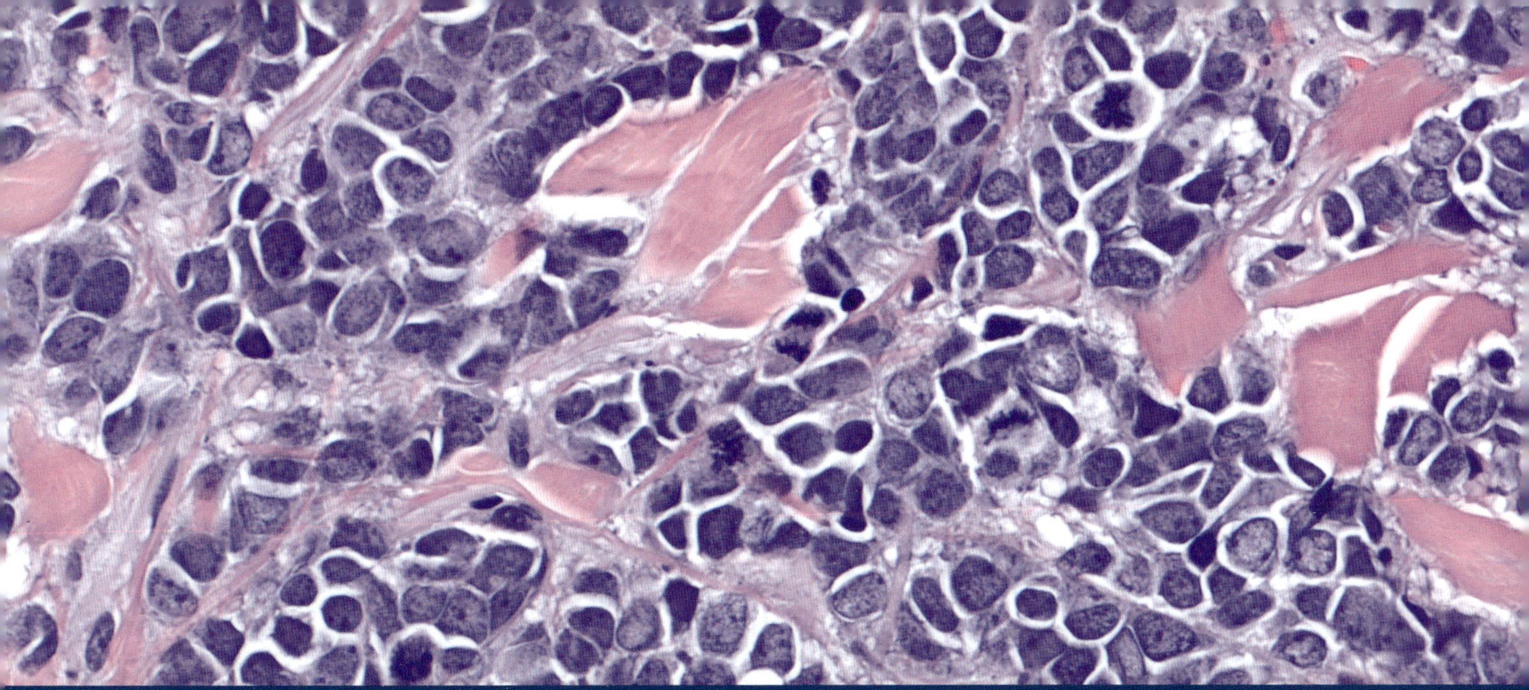

8

Neuroendocrine neoplasms in non-endocrine organs

Edited by: Asa SL, Klimstra DS, Mete O, Osamura RY, Rindi G, Thompson LDR, Washington MK

- Neuroendocrine neoplasms
  - Neuroendocrine tumours
    - Neuroendocrine tumours
  - Neuroendocrine carcinomas
    - Small cell neuroendocrine carcinoma
    - Large cell neuroendocrine carcinoma
    - Merkel cell carcinoma
  - Mixed neuroendocrine neoplasms
    - Mixed neuroendocrine–non-neuroendocrine neoplasms
  - Paraganglioma-like neuroendocrine neoplasms
    - Composite gangliocytoma/neuroma and neuroendocrine tumour
    - Cauda equina neuroendocrine tumour (previously paraganglioma)

Neuroendocrine neoplasms in non-endocrine organs: Introduction

Rindi G
Asa SL
Klimstra DS
Papotti M

Neuroendocrine cells exist in almost every organ and tissue. Neuroendocrine neoplasms (NENs) encompass all tumour types expressing markers of neuroendocrine differentiation. Neuroendocrine biomarkers comprise antigens specific to neuroendocrine cells and neurons. In contrast to neurons usually secreting neurotransmitters to affect an adjacent cell at a synapse, neuroendocrine cells produce peptides for distant (endocrine) and/or local (paracrine and autocrine) function(s). Neuroendocrine markers are constituents of peptide hormone or bioamine synthesis and secretion machinery {209,3751}. They include (1) transcription factors driving neuroendocrine differentiation, like INSM1 and insulin gene enhancer protein ISL1; (2) components of dense-core vesicles that store peptide hormones like chromogranins/secretogranins; (3) components of small synaptic-like vesicles that store small mediators (taurine, choline, GABA, etc.) like synaptophysin; and (4) receptors involved in neuroendocrine cell control, like SSTR1–5. In addition, neuroendocrine cells express transcription factors specific to their location (e.g. thyroid transcription factor 1 [TTF1], CDX2, SATB2), hormones, and enzymes associated with hormone processing {3752}. Two main groups of neuroendocrine cells exist: epithelial and neuronal or paraneuronal, distinguished by the expression of keratins in the former.

Neuroendocrine biomarkers display different degrees of specificity and sensitivity when used for diagnostic purposes (see Table 8.01). INSM1 and synaptophysin are expressed in almost all neoplastic cells with neuroendocrine differentiation {376}. Both, however, have limitations: INSM1 is expressed in a fraction of non-neuroendocrine thoracic carcinomas and in sarcomas {4568}, and synaptophysin is expressed in adrenal cortex and pancreatic exocrine neoplasms like solid pseudopapillary neoplasms {3324,2191}. In contrast, expression of chromogranin A and SSTRs is usually strong in well-differentiated epithelial NENs and weak to absent in many/most poorly differentiated epithelial NENs {3749,3751}.

Epithelial neuroendocrine cells are encountered in the anterior pituitary, parathyroids, and pancreatic islets. Widespread neuroendocrine cells constitute the diffuse neuroendocrine system of several body sites, including the lungs, gut, thyroid, thymus, kidneys, urinary tract, liver, reproductive organs, breast, and skin {3749}. Non-epithelial neuroendocrine tissues include the sympathetic and parasympathetic paraganglia found in every organ and in the soft tissue of the torso {203}, and the hypothalamus and posterior pituitary neurons {4731}.

A rational and coherent classification system has been proposed for NENs for a unified approach to these lesions {3749}, while recognizing that important organ-specific differences exist, as follows.

Epithelial well-differentiated NEN: Neuroendocrine tumour

Well-differentiated epithelial NENs (neuroendocrine tumours, NETs) are malignant tumours whose cells retain the structural

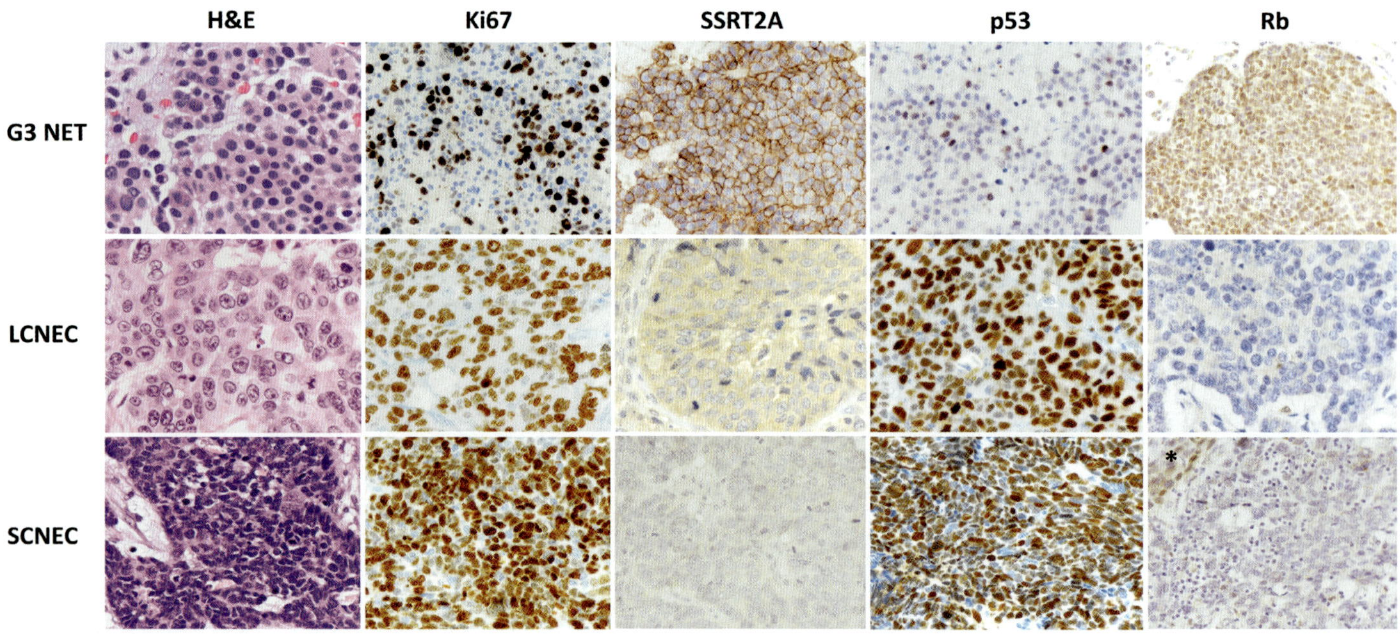

Fig. 8.01 Morphology and immunophenotype of high-grade neuroendocrine neoplasms (NENs). **Top row:** High-grade, well-differentiated neuroendocrine tumour (G3 NET). **Middle row:** Poorly differentiated neuroendocrine carcinoma (NEC), large cell type (LCNEC). **Bottom row:** Poorly differentiated NEC, small cell type (SCNEC). Along the NET–NEC spectrum there is an increase in the proliferation index (Ki-67, MIB1), loss of SSTR2A, accumulation of p53, and loss of RB1.

features of hormone synthesis and secretion of normal neuroendocrine cells. The terminology for well-differentiated NENs remains somewhat organ-specific. Based on recommendations from an expert consensus group assembled by WHO in 2017, "neuroendocrine tumour" is the preferred term in most organs, and "carcinoid tumour" is not recommended {3749}. However, in the lung, "carcinoid tumour" and "atypical carcinoid tumour" remain in widespread use and are considered to be acceptable {4871}.

Table 8.01 Biomarkers of neuroendocrine cells and tumours

Location	Cell type	Transcription factor(s)	Hormones	Other
Hypothalamus	Neurons	NeuN, TTF1	GRH, TRH, CRH, GnRH, dopamine, somatostatin, vasopressin, oxytocin	Neurofilaments
Pituitary	Corticotroph	TPIT, NeuroD1	ACTH, other POMC derivatives	Keratins (+++)
	Somatotroph	PIT1	GH, α-subunit	Keratins[a]
	Lactotroph	PIT1, ER	Prolactin	Keratins[b]
	Mammosomatotroph	PIT1, ER	GH, prolactin, α-subunit	Keratins
	Thyrotroph	PIT1, GATA2/3	TSH	Keratins[b]
	Gonadotroph	SF1, ER, GATA2/3	FSH, LH	Keratins[b]
Thyroid	C cell	PAX8, TTF1	Calcitonin, CGRP	Keratins, CEA[c]
Parathyroid	Chief cell + subtypes	GATA3, GCM2	PTH	Keratins
Thymus	Unclassified neuroendocrine cells	TTF1[b], PAX8[b,d]	Calcitonin, CGRP	
Lung	P1, P2, P3	TTF1	Bombesin (GRP), serotonin, calcitonin, CGRP	Keratins, CEA[b,c]
Stomach	ECL	CDX2[b]	Histamine	VMAT2, keratins
	EC		Serotonin	Keratins
	D		Somatostatin	Keratins
	G		Gastrin	Keratins
	XP, D		Xenin, ghrelin	Keratins
Pancreas	A	ARX, PDX1, ISL1, CDX2, PAX6	Glucagon	Keratins
	B		Insulin	Keratins
	D		Somatostatin	Keratins
	PP		PP	Keratins
Bowel	G	Duodenum: ISL1, PDX1, CDX2 Jejunum and ileum: CDX2 Colon and appendix: CDX2[b]	Gastrin	Keratins Colon: PAP
	D		Somatostatin	
	I		CCK	
	K		GIP	
	S		Secretin	
	MO		Motilin	
	N		Neurotensin	
	L		GLI, PYY, PP	
	EC		Serotonin	
Prostate, kidney, bladder, gonads, breast	Unclassified neuroendocrine cells	Variable	Variable	Keratins, PAP[b]
Skin	Merkel cell	PAX5, SATB2	Unknown	Dot-like CK20, TdT, Merkel cell polyomavirus
Paragangliomas	Neuroendocrine or chief cells	GATA3, PHOX2B, HAND2	Dopamine. epinephrine (adrenaline), norepinephrine (noradrenaline)	Tyrosine hydroxylase, L-DOPA decarboxylase, PNMT

EC, enterochromaffin; ECL, enterochromaffin-like; GH, growth hormone; ISL1, insulin gene enhancer protein ISL1; TTF1, thyroid transcription factor 1.
[a]Pattern of keratin positivity distinguishes tumour types. [b]Not a consistent finding in normal cells; tumours may have significant variability. [c]Using a monoclonal antibody. [d]PAX8 in thymic lesions is controversial and likely due to cross-reactivity of polyclonal antisera.

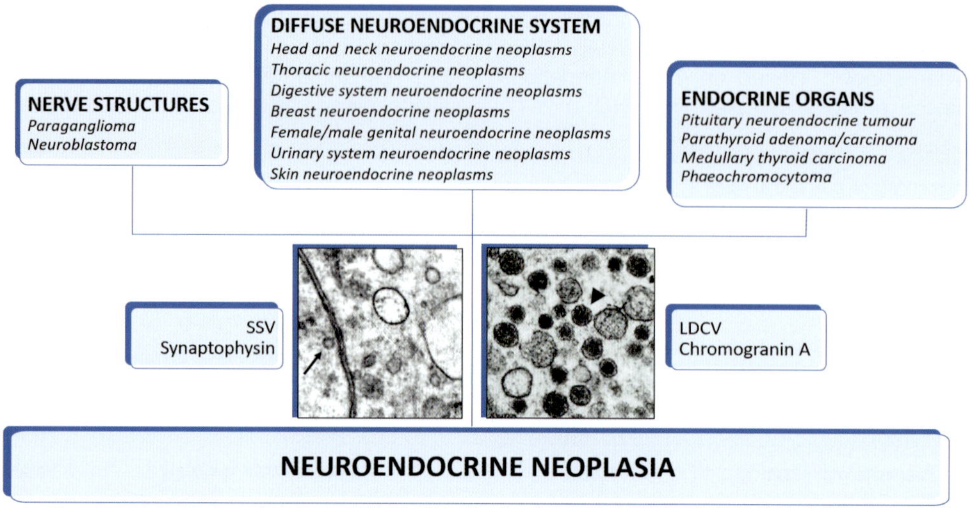

Fig. 8.02 The neuroendocrine neoplasm (NEN) family. NEN cells display small synaptic-like vesicles (SSV, centre left, arrow; pulmonary carcinoid) and large dense-core vesicles (LDCV, centre right, arrowhead; pulmonary carcinoid); the main markers are synaptophysin for SSV and chromogranin A for LDCV {3200;556}. NEN comprises non-epithelial neoplasms of nerve structures and epithelial neoplasms of endocrine organs and of multiple organs within the diffuse neuroendocrine system.

In sites where specific grading systems have been established, three grades are usually defined: grade 1 (G1), grade 2 (G2), and grade 3 (G3). Most NETs are G1 or G2 and relatively indolent, but high-grade malignancy can also occur, with proliferation in the G3 range. NETs have unique molecular alterations that are distinct from the usual cancer drivers, with prominent epigenetic changes at all sites and different expression profiles {740,2143,214,207,4731,2532,4149,1732}. Differences occur, based on anatomical site. In about one third of NETs there is a familial predisposition (see Chapter 13: *Genetic tumour syndromes associated with endocrine lesions and tumours*).

Epithelial poorly differentiated NEN: Neuroendocrine carcinoma

Poorly differentiated epithelial NENs (neuroendocrine carcinomas [NECs]) are high-grade malignant neoplasms whose cells often express little or no chromogranin A, SSTRs, or hormones, but retain a high expression of INSM1 and synaptophysin (as well as the less specific CD56, NSE, and PGP9.5, which are no longer recommended diagnostically). NECs are high-grade by definition, with high proliferative activity and small cell or large cell morphology; they have limited or no site-specific features {3749}. The molecular profile of NEC is strikingly different from that of NETs and is characterized by *TP53* and *RB1* gene alterations at most anatomical sites {3749,4603}, with additional site-specific genomic alterations. Poorly differentiated NECs may also contain a minor component of non-neuroendocrine differentiation; especially uncommon is a component of well-differentiated NET.

Epithelial mixed neuroendocrine–non-neuroendocrine neoplasm

Mixed neuroendocrine–non-neuroendocrine neoplasms (MiNENs; defined as "combined" in the lung and other sites) are epithelial cancers whose cells express neuroendocrine and non-neuroendocrine features in separate morphologically and immunohistochemically recognizable populations {3751,2869,3010,4727,2532}. Equally significant components express neuroendocrine differentiation and a squamous, glandular, or other non-neuroendocrine phenotype. Although the two cell subsets of MiNEN are usually morphologically distinct, transitional areas may be seen. The presence of only minor cancer subpopulations of either phenotype do not qualify for a MiNEN diagnosis. In the digestive system, cut-off points are defined {4866}. Both MiNEN cancer components are graded according to current grading systems. The neuroendocrine component is usually a NEC, but NETs can be rarely seen.

Non-epithelial NEN: Paraganglioma

Non-epithelial NENs are represented by paragangliomas, both intra-adrenal (known as phaeochromocytoma) and extra-adrenal {203}. Although they also show a spectrum of differentiation, they express INSM1, GATA3, synaptophysin, and chromogranin A. Unlike epithelial NENs, paragangliomas express vimentin and are negative for keratins. Most paragangliomas also express tyrosine hydroxylase, a key enzyme in the catecholamine biosynthetic pathway. They all have malignant potential, but metastasis is uncommon. Paragangliomas very commonly have a genetic predisposition, and some of the familial syndromes overlap with those associated with NETs {3415}.

Other NEN types

NEN types that bridge epithelial and neuronal NENs may be observed but are extremely rare. These epithelial-neuronal NENs are characterized by two neuroendocrine cell components, one expressing markers of neural differentiation (usually ganglion cells, with or without Schwannian stroma, but occasionally neurocytic) and one epithelial. Both epithelial and neuronal components are well differentiated and produce peptide hormones. Epithelial-neuronal NENs, termed composite gangliocytoma/neuroma and neuroendocrine tumours (CoG-NETs), occur in the pituitary, gut, and cauda equina region of the spine.

NENs belonging to endocrine organs, including the pituitary, thyroid, parathyroid, and endocrine pancreas, as well as paragangliomas, are discussed in dedicated chapters elsewhere in this volume. This chapter provides an overview of epithelial NENs in non-endocrine organs.

Neuroendocrine tumours

Rindi G
de Herder WW
McCluggage WG
Moch H
Osamura RY
Papotti M
Travis WD

Definition

Neuroendocrine tumours (NETs) are malignant, well-differentiated epithelial neuroendocrine neoplasms (NENs).

ICD-O coding

8240/3 Neuroendocrine tumour, NOS
8240/3 Neuroendocrine tumour, grade 1
8249/3 Neuroendocrine tumour, grade 2
8249/3 Neuroendocrine tumour, grade 3
8242/3 ECL-cell neuroendocrine tumour
8156/3 D-cell neuroendocrine tumour
8153/3 G-cell neuroendocrine tumour
8241/3 EC-cell neuroendocrine tumour
8152/3 L-cell neuroendocrine tumour
9091/1 Ovarian neuroendocrine tumour

ICD-11 coding

2C6Y & XH9LV8 Other specified malignant neoplasms of breast & Neuroendocrine tumour, grade 1
2C7Y & XH9LV8 Other specified malignant neoplasms of female genital organs & Neuroendocrine tumour, grade 1
2C25.4 & XH9LV8 Carcinoid or other malignant neuroendocrine neoplasms of bronchus or lung & Neuroendocrine tumour, grade 1
2C25.4 & XH51K1 Carcinoid or other malignant neuroendocrine neoplasms of bronchus or lung & Neuroendocrine tumour, grade 2

Related terminology

Acceptable: well-differentiated NET; carcinoid; typical carcinoid; atypical carcinoid (see *Neuroendocrine neoplasms in non-endocrine organs: Introduction*, p. 334).
Not recommended: well-differentiated neuroendocrine carcinoma (NEC).

Subtype(s)

There are no subtypes at most anatomical sites except for the digestive tract (see Table S8.1, available as supplementary material at https://publications.iarc.who.int/645).

Localization

NETs may occur in the upper and lower airways {3518}, the digestive and urological tracts, the male and female genital tracts, the breast, and the skin {2279,2410,1643,134}. The most common sites are the digestive tract and the lung {995,119,988}. Preferential localizations are the larynx for the head and neck {3518}; for the thorax, the lung; for the digestive tract, the colorectum, small intestine, and pancreas; for the urogenital tract, the kidney {3227}; and for the gynaecological tract, the ovary. See Table S8.1 (available at https://publications.iarc.who.int/645).

Clinical features

The majority of NETs do not manifest with signs and symptoms of active hormone secretion; typically, patients present with nonspecific, site-dependent, mass-related symptoms. They may also be discovered during screening or investigation for unrelated clinical reasons. Fewer than one third are associated with hormonal manifestations that include carcinoid syndrome, gastrinoma-associated Zollinger–Ellison syndrome, insulinoma syndrome, and other (rarer) syndromes {3751}. Ovarian tumours are usually incidental findings in mature teratomas. See Table S8.1 for details (available at https://publications.iarc.who.int/645).

Epidemiology

The incidence is approximately 7 new cases per 100 000 person-years and has been steadily increasing over the last 20 years {995,119,988,2871}. Both sexes are equally affected, with a slight male prevalence in the digestive tract {988,2871}. Most patients are in their sixth to eighth decade of life, but younger patients can be affected in conjunction with hereditary conditions and in ovarian neoplasms (given the association with mature teratomas). NETs rarely occur in infancy and childhood {1335,4191}. See Table S8.1 (available at https://publications.iarc.who.int/645).

Etiology

The etiology is unknown. Hereditary genetic defects including multiple endocrine neoplasia type 1, von Hippel–Lindau syndrome, and neurofibromatosis type 1 are associated with NETs in the thorax and upper digestive tract {4871,4866}. Known risk factors are a family history of cancer; old age; a high body mass index; and site-specific risk factors shared with non-neuroendocrine cancer, including smoking and alcohol consumption {10,2506,1598}. See Table S8.1 (available at https://publications.iarc.who.int/645).

Pathogenesis

The pathogenesis is unknown, except for enterochromaffin-like cell (ECL-cell) NET of the stomach, for which hypergastrinaemia is the obligate promoting factor. The related settings include chronic atrophic gastritis (autoimmune or *Helicobacter pylori* infection–related), and multiple endocrine neoplasia type 1 (Zollinger–Ellison syndrome) may be involved. See Table S8.1 (available at https://publications.iarc.who.int/645).

Macroscopic appearance

In tubular structures (airways, digestive and urinary tracts), NETs are often polypoid lesions a few millimetres in size, projecting into the lumen, sometimes with an ulcerated surface. In clinically silent organs (lung, thymus, kidney, female genital organs, and the right colon), NETs may be much larger {2279,409}. NETs are usually expansive, highly vascularized, reddish nodules. See Table S8.2 (available at https://publications.iarc.who.int/645).

Histopathology

Classic patterns include islets and nests (solid islet structure); anastomosing trabeculae and ribbons (trabecular structure); and tubules, acini, and rosette-like structures (glandular structure) {4209}. Patterns may be site-specific {2213}. Mixed patterns are often observed. Necrosis is usually absent, and when present it is spotty and may be associated with atypia. Cells are monomorphic, polygonal, and of medium size, with abundant eosinophilic, sometimes granular cytoplasm and round, regular nuclei with dispersed granular salt-and-pepper chromatin, usually with inconspicuous nucleoli. Mitoses are uncommon and when increased indicate a higher-grade NET. Minor mucin production may be observed in NETs of the digestive tract {4209} and middle ear. See Table S8.2 (available at https://publications.iarc.who.int/645).

Immunohistochemistry

The majority of NETs are diffusely and intensely positive for cytokeratin(s) (e.g. AE1/AE3 cocktail) and for neuroendocrine markers including chromogranin A, synaptophysin, and INSM1. Expression of SSTR2 or SSTR5 is often observed. Ki-67 staining (MIB1 clone) is recommended for grading when required and for clinical decision-making. Immunohistochemistry for hormones and transcription factors is often site-specific and recommended in metastatic settings and in the presence of hormonal syndromes. See Table S8.2 (available at https://publications.iarc.who.int/645).

Differential diagnosis

Paraganglioma is usually negative for cytokeratin(s) and positive for GATA3 and tyrosine hydroxylase {2817}. Other than in the lung and liver, metastases of NET from other sites including the thyroid (calcitonin-positive) are, rarely, also seen in the breast {4209} and skin {1109} and should be considered. Different anatomical sites may call for site-specific differential diagnoses (e.g. low-grade adenocarcinoma in the lung and breast, sex cord tumours in the ovary).

Grading

Grading is recommended in some sites and performed by measuring proliferation either by mitotic count and/or Ki-67 index assessment. The presence of necrosis is also a marker of aggressive behaviour and is included in grading definitions at some sites. The vast majority of NETs are low-grade (G1–G2). High-grade (G3) NETs are uncommon (< 10%) and occur mainly in the thymus, stomach, and colon. In the lung and thymus, high-grade NETs are recognized, although they are still classified with large cell neuroendocrine carcinoma (LCNEC). See Table S8.2 (available at https://publications.iarc.who.int/645).

Cytology

FNA smears usually display a clean background and small to medium-sized round to oval cells (either isolated or in groups) with evident cytoplasm, regular nuclei, and granular chromatin. A cytological diagnosis of NET requires immunohistochemistry and, when possible, histological confirmation is advised. See Table S8.2 (available at https://publications.iarc.who.int/645).

Diagnostic molecular pathology

There is no diagnostic molecular pathology.

Essential and desirable diagnostic criteria

Essential: neuroendocrine morphology; diffuse and intense expression of cytokeratin(s) and chromogranin A or two other neuroendocrine markers; Ki-67.

Desirable: SSTR2; see Table S8.2 for details (available at https://publications.iarc.who.int/645).

Staging

Staging is performed using a NET-specific system for the digestive tract only {4866}. The other sites adopt the staging systems of non-neuroendocrine cancer. See Table S8.2 (available at https://publications.iarc.who.int/645).

Prognosis and prediction

The prognosis depends on the tumour site, grade, and stage. Low-grade (G1–G2) NETs typically have an indolent course, with 5-year survival rates as high as 90%, depending on the site. High-grade (G3) NETs display aggressive behaviour, similar to that of non-neuroendocrine carcinomas in the digestive tract. See Table S8.2 (available at https://publications.iarc.who.int/645).

Small cell neuroendocrine carcinoma

Volante M
Beasley MB
Busam KJ
Inzani F
Osamura RY
Rekhtman N
Scoazec JY
Shia J
Ströbel P

Definition

Small cell neuroendocrine carcinoma (SCNEC) is a malignant epithelial neoplasm composed of small cells with high mitotic and proliferation indexes. Most SCNECs express neuroendocrine differentiation markers. SCNEC may occur either in pure form or combined (mixed) with any other carcinoma histotype, demonstrating different site-specific prevalence for the various combinations.

ICD-O coding

8041/3 Small cell neuroendocrine carcinoma
8045/3 Combined small cell neuroendocrine carcinoma

ICD-11 coding

2C25.1 Small cell carcinoma of bronchus or lung
2C27.Y & XH0YB0 Other specified malignant neoplasms of thymus & Small cell carcinoma, NOS
2C7Z & XH0YB0 Malignant neoplasms of female genital organs, unspecified & Small cell carcinoma, NOS

Related terminology

Acceptable: neuroendocrine carcinoma (NEC), small cell type.
Not recommended: oat cell carcinoma; intermediate cell type small cell carcinoma; microcytoma.

Subtype(s)

None

Localization

SCNEC may arise in every epithelial organ/tissue. Site-specific main features are detailed in Table S8.3 and Table S8.4 (both available as supplementary material at https://publications.iarc.who.int/645). SCNECs most frequently arise in the lung, outnumbering the extrapulmonary locations 10:1 {994}. The most frequent sites of extrapulmonary SCNEC include the female genital (26%), gastrointestinal (23%), and genitourinary (19%) tracts, and the head and neck (16%); in 13% of cases, the primary site is unknown {524}.

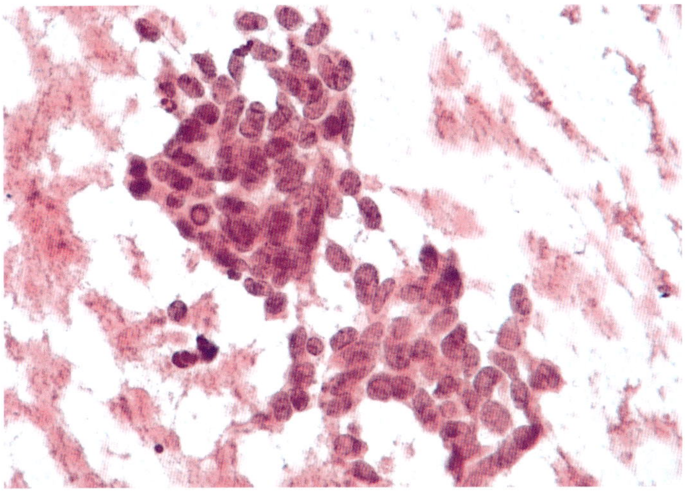

Fig. 8.03 Small cell carcinoma of the lung. FNAC. A dirty background containing clusters of cells with scant cytoplasm and overlapping nuclei with moulding and dispersed chromatin. Nucleoli are inconspicuous.

Clinical features

SCNEC is a rapidly growing neoplasm with signs and symptoms related to the obstruction/infiltration of surrounding structures,

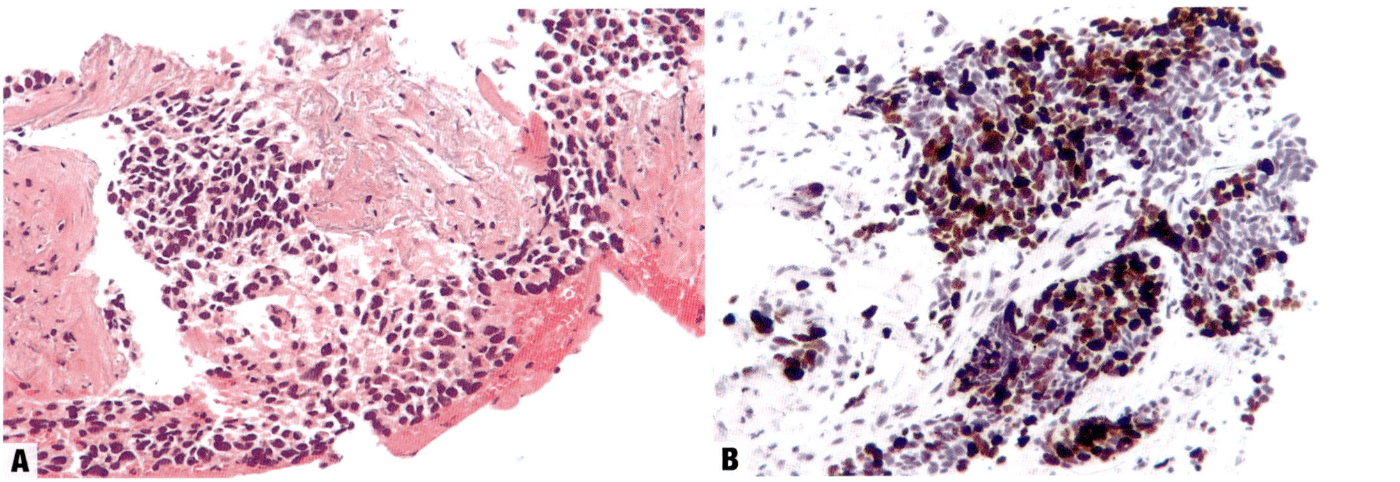

Fig. 8.04 Small cell carcinoma of the lung. **A** Core biopsy. Sheets of small cells showing discohesive pattern in a fibrotic stromal background. Nuclei are irregular, with finely granular chromatin and no evident nucleoli. **B** Ki-67 (MIB1) immunohistochemistry on a core biopsy. Necrosis may be absent and mitotic figures may be difficult to evaluate in biopsy samples. Ki-67 (MIB1) staining may be very helpful to sustain a diagnosis of small cell carcinoma in this setting, such as in the present case with a high (albeit heterogeneous) proliferation rate (exceeding 70%).

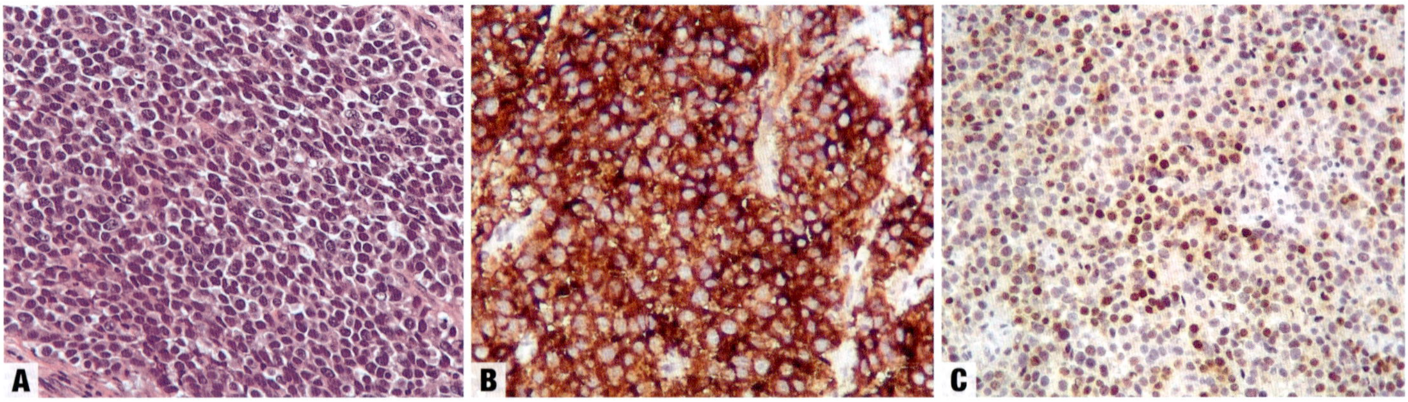

Fig. 8.05 Gastric small cell carcinoma. **A** Tumour cells are densely packed in a discohesive pattern with a poor stroma component. Nuclear chromatin is finely dispersed or has a salt-and-pepper appearance. Small nucleoli are present in only very few cells. **B** Neoplastic cells show diffuse and intense cytoplasmic positivity for synaptophysin. **C** Neoplastic cells show diffuse nuclear positivity for INSM1, although with heterogeneous intensity.

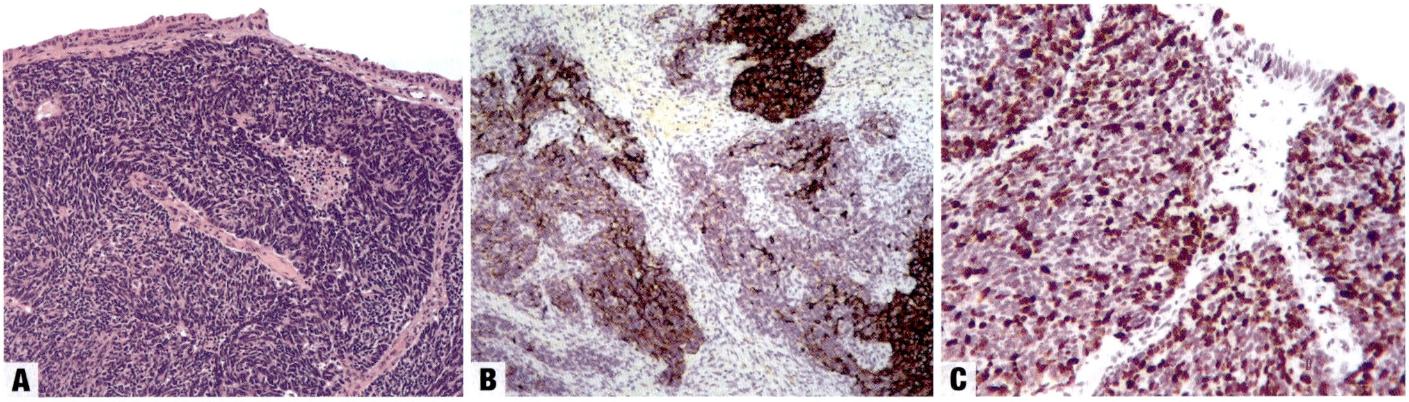

Fig. 8.06 Bladder small cell carcinoma. **A** A malignant neoplasm infiltrating the bladder wall made of spindling small cells in a solid growth pattern intersected by rare fibrotic bands. **B** Neoplastic cells show a heterogeneous pattern of cytoplasmic positivity for synaptophysin. **C** The Ki-67 index in neoplastic cells is homogeneously high (> 70% in this example).

or (often) to the presence of distant metastases. Paraneoplastic syndromes occur in approximately 10% of lung cases, with hyponatraemia, Cushing syndrome, and Lambert–Eaton myasthenic syndrome {2181,3027}. In extrapulmonary SCNECs, inappropriate vasopressin (antidiuretic hormone) secretion in bladder and cervical SCNEC {4290,5153} and Lambert–Eaton myasthenic syndrome in thymic SCNEC are described {1807}.

Epidemiology

Pulmonary SCNEC age-adjusted incidence rates show a decline from 8.6 cases per 100 000 person-years in 1988 to 5.3 cases per 100 000 person-years in 2015, an inverse trend to that of all other pulmonary neuroendocrine neoplasms (NENs) {4081}. The incidence of extrapulmonary SCNECs is difficult to estimate; in the United Kingdom it has been calculated as 0.45 cases per 100 000 person-years in males and 0.37 cases per 100 000 person-years in females in 2000–2004 {4925}.

Etiology

Heavy smoking is the main risk factor for pulmonary SCNEC and is suggested to play a role at other locations too. SCNEC may also arise as the result of histological transformation after therapy with various agents such as tyrosine kinase inhibitors in oncogene-addicted non-small cell lung cancers {4807} or androgen deprivation in prostate cancer {4738}. HPV infection has been associated with SCNEC in the uterine cervix.

Pathogenesis

Biallelic inactivation of *TP53* and/or *RB1* is by far the most common genomic alteration in SCNEC, irrespective of the primary site. Associated alterations vary depending on the site of origin. At the transcriptional level, pulmonary SCNECs have been classified into four major classes, each with a different prominence of neuroendocrine marker expression and potential clinical implications for therapy {270,2525}. In other systems, SCNEC of the urinary tract {1401} was classified into a specific molecular group with potential but unvalidated clinical impact. Even without prior therapy, SCNEC can arise as a component of a non-neuroendocrine carcinoma, presumably reflecting clonal genomic evolution.

Macroscopic appearance

Irrespective of the site, SCNEC presents as a poorly circumscribed necrotic mass, with a soft or firm consistency depending on the amount of stroma, and with infiltration of the surrounding tissues.

Histopathology

Small cell size is usually defined as smaller than three resting lymphocytes and should be predominant (> 90% of the tumour); a minor component of larger or giant cells does not preclude an SCNEC diagnosis. Definitional cytological characteristics are the presence of scant cytoplasm with poorly defined borders and finely granular nuclear chromatin with no evident nucleoli. Nuclei are often fusiform. The architecture is sheet-like or diffuse. However, in surgically resected samples, SCNEC may show more overt neuroendocrine growth patterns such as nests or trabeculae {3233}. Necrosis is frequent and often extensive. Apoptotic bodies are usually conspicuous. The mitotic count is high, averaging > 50 mitoses/2 mm^2, with definitional cut-off points of > 10 mitoses/2 mm^2 in the lung and thymus and > 20 mitoses/2 mm^2 in the digestive system.

Immunophenotype

Cytokeratin (pancytokeratin and/or low-molecular-weight cytokeratin) expression may be diffuse or focal in a dot-like paranuclear pattern. Neuroendocrine differentiation by at least one positive neuroendocrine marker (in a panel including chromogranin A, synaptophysin, and INSM1) is present in the majority of cases. Despite INSM1 proving the most sensitive in different locations, a small proportion of SCNECs, more frequently in the lung, urinary tract, and head and neck, may be completely negative for neuroendocrine markers {3810,2283,3808}. Thyroid transcription factor 1 (TTF1) is not a lung primary–specific marker. CDX2 expression may indicate a gastrointestinal origin but should be interpreted in an appropriate clinical context. SCNECs in the urinary tract and prostate have variable (most frequently negative) expression of GATA3 and NKX3-1, respectively. Aberrant immunolabelling for p53 is very common, as is loss of RB1 immunoexpression, reflecting the most common molecular alterations in this neoplasm. The Ki-67 labelling index is very high, > 75% in most cases, and by definition > 20% in gastroenteropancreatic SCNECs. After therapy, however, the Ki-67 index may be reduced, even into the range typical for G2 (3–20%) or G1 (< 3%) neuroendocrine tumours (NETs) {4754}.

Differential diagnosis

The diagnosis of SCNEC in the appropriate pathological and clinical context is usually easily established on surgical material but may be challenging in the preoperative setting. On small, crushed biopsies or cytological samples, SCNEC may be difficult to distinguish from other NENs, including carcinoids/NETs. A low Ki-67 index and intense diffuse expression of chromogranin A suggest a NET. The distinction between SCNEC and large cell neuroendocrine carcinoma (LCNEC) is based on cytological features (see *Large cell neuroendocrine carcinoma*, p. 342) and can be very challenging, especially in extrapulmonary locations {4111}. Merkel cell carcinoma may be distinguished on the basis of CK20 expression and its peculiar immunoprofile (see *Merkel cell carcinoma*, p. 346) {3457, 2263,377}. SCNEC should be distinguished from other small cell neoplasms, including lymphomas, melanomas, small cell sarcomas (i.e. osteosarcoma), or basaloid squamous cell carcinomas. A panel of pertinent immunohistochemical markers is conclusive in most cases. A more problematic issue are small cell neoplasms that can express epithelial and neuronal/neuroendocrine markers, such as the ubiquitous Ewing sarcoma family of tumours, which is characterized by the coexpression of FLI1 and CD99, retained RB1 expression, and the presence of *EWSR1* (or, more rarely, *CIC* or *BCOR*) fusions. In specific subsites, the range of differential diagnoses may include other entities, such as olfactory neuroblastoma in the sinonasal tract, *YWHAE::NUTM2A* or *NUTM2B*-translocated high-grade endometrial stromal sarcoma in the uterus, and hypercalcaemic-type small cell carcinoma in the ovary, this last entity representing a non-neuroendocrine *SMARCA4*-mutated cancer. In metastatic diseases, the primary origin is nearly always impossible to determine from pathological criteria alone. At variance with well-differentiated NETs, the expression of lineage-specific transcription factors in SCNEC is not organ-specific {2232}.

Cytology

Neoplastic cells are present, with scant cytoplasm, oval or spindle shape, and speckled fine and coarse chromatin with absent or inconspicuous nucleoli, arranged in a loosely cohesive pattern or small tissue fragments. The presence of necrotic debris and apoptotic bodies is also frequent. Mitotic figures may be difficult to assess on smears. Nuclear moulding and chromatin streaking are typical. Cytological features may differ according to different sampling methods (e.g. FNAB for breast, brushings for lung central lesions, or urines for the urinary tract), therefore standardization of preanalytical conditions is essential.

Diagnostic molecular pathology

No molecular tests are essential for the diagnosis.

Essential and desirable diagnostic criteria

Essential: small cell epithelial neoplasm with high-grade features (definitional mitotic counts in lung and thymus and digestive system); finely granular nuclear chromatin with no prominent nucleoli.

Desirable: neuroendocrine differentiation, defined by positive neuroendocrine markers; a high proliferation index (Ki-67 index > 30%, most frequently > 75%; by definition > 20% in tumours of the digestive system); p53 immunohistochemical overexpression and/or RB1 protein loss; negative immunolabelling for SSTR2.

Staging

Site-specific TNM staging follows the rules for non-neuroendocrine carcinomas.

Prognosis and prediction

SCNEC is a highly aggressive and lethal neoplasm irrespective of the site of origin, with a high predisposition for distant metastases, mainly in the liver, bone, brain, lung, and adrenal gland. Pulmonary SCNECs are diagnosed at stage IV in the majority of cases and have a 5-year survival rate of 2%. The prognosis of extrapulmonary SCNECs is generally slightly better than that of SCNECs in the lung, although it varies depending on site. The 1-, 3-, and 5-year overall survival rates for extrapulmonary SCNEC are 41.3%, 17.7%, and 12.8%, respectively {4989}. Favourable prognostic factors include an origin in the breast or the head and neck, younger age, female sex, localized stage, and treatment by surgery or combinatory radiochemotherapy as compared with chemotherapy alone {4989,2819}.

Large cell neuroendocrine carcinoma

Uccella S
Busam KJ
Inzani F
Osamura RY
Papotti M
Rekhtman N
Shia J

Definition

Large cell neuroendocrine carcinoma (LCNEC) is a poorly differentiated neuroendocrine neoplasm (NEN) composed of non-small cells.

ICD-O coding

8013/3 Large cell neuroendocrine carcinoma

ICD-11 coding

2C25.4 & XH0NL5 Carcinoid or other malignant neuroendocrine neoplasms of bronchus or lung & Large cell neuroendocrine carcinoma
2C27.Y & XH0NL5 Other specified malignant neoplasms of thymus & Large cell neuroendocrine carcinoma
2C7Z & XH0U20 Malignant neoplasms of female genital organs, unspecified & Neuroendocrine carcinoma, NOS
2C7Z & XH0NL5 Malignant neoplasms of female genital organs, unspecified & Large cell neuroendocrine carcinoma

Related terminology

Acceptable: neuroendocrine carcinoma (NEC), large cell type.

Subtype(s)

None

Localization

LCNEC can arise in any epithelium-containing organ (see Table S8.5, available as supplementary material at https://publications.iarc.who.int/645). In absolute numbers, the main site of LCNEC is the lung, where it represents 15% of all NENs {1337}, although in other sites it may represent a higher relative proportion of NENs {4111,3718,1120,4262}.

Clinical features

The clinical presentation of LCNEC overlaps with that of any non-neuroendocrine cancer occurring at various sites and is dominated by mass compressive symptoms, lumen occlusion, ulceration, and bleeding. The disease often presents at an advanced stage, with early metastatic dissemination. Circulating neuroendocrine markers (e.g. chromogranin A, NSE) do not directly correlate with tumour grade {3310}, and their levels may be lower than in neuroendocrine tumour (NET) {4414}. 68Ga-DOTATOC/DOTANOC PET-CT and FDOPA PET-CT are

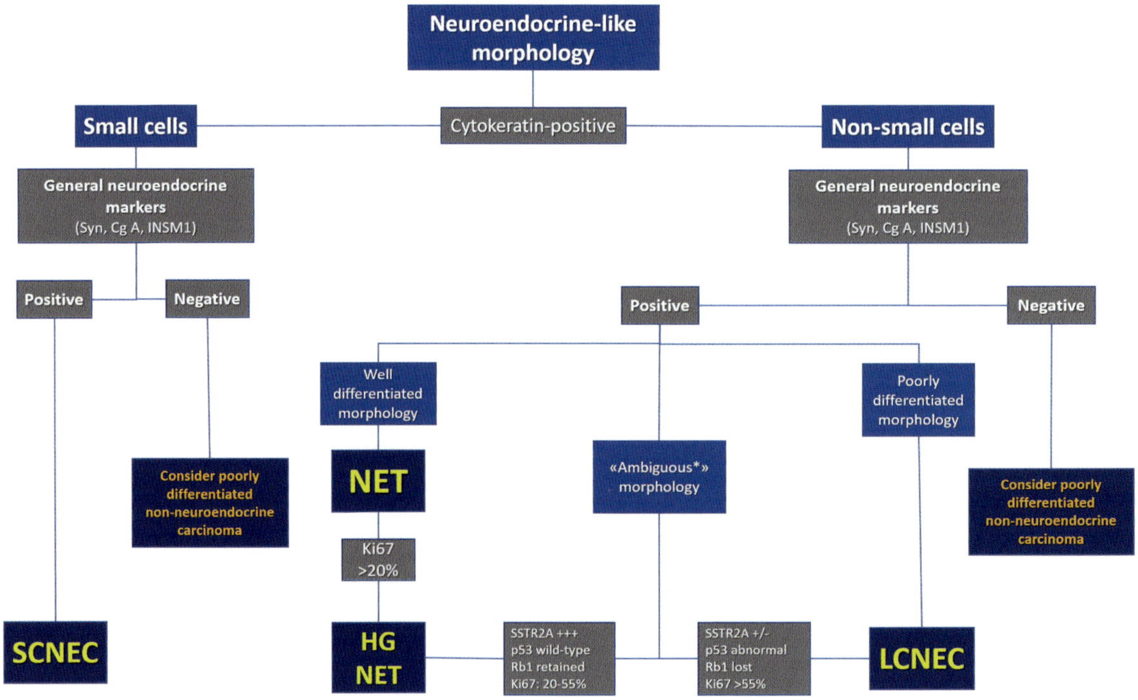

Fig. 8.07 Differential diagnostic algorithm for high-grade neuroendocrine neoplasms (NENs). Cases with ambiguous morphology (asterisk) are those that cannot be assigned to a definite histotype from morphology alone. Cg A, chromogranin A; HG NET, high-grade neuroendocrine tumour (G3 NET in the digestive tract, NET with elevated mitotic count and/or Ki-67 proliferation index in thoracic organs); LCNEC, large cell neuroendocrine carcinoma; NET, neuroendocrine tumour; SCNEC, small cell neuroendocrine carcinoma; Syn, synaptophysin.

Table 8.02 Histological diagnostic features of large cell neuroendocrine carcinoma (LCNEC) and other high-grade NENs

Feature	LCNEC	SCNEC	HG-NET
Growth pattern[a]	Organoid > diffuse	Diffuse > organoid	Organoid
Cell size	Large (> 3 resting lymphocytes)	Small/intermediate (≤ 3 resting lymphocytes)	Intermediate
N:C ratio	Low	High	Low
Nuclear moulding	Absent	Present	Absent
Nuclear form	Round to oval	Round, oval, spindle	Round to oval
Chromatin pattern	Coarse (clear, vesicular nucleus)	Homogeneously dispersed (blue nucleus)	Finely dispersed, granular (salt-and-pepper nucleus)
Nucleolus	Evident, sometimes large and eosinophilic	Absent or inconspicuous	Evident
Cell borders	Distinct	Indistinct	Distinct
Cytoplasm	Moderately abundant, amphophilic or eosinophilic, may be granular	Scant, barely visible	Moderately abundant or abundant, eosinophilic, granular
Necrosis	Abundant, may be focal	Usually abundant	Focal or punctate
Mitoses/2 mm^2	Lung: > 10 (median: 70) Digestive: > 20	Lung: > 10 (median: 80) Digestive: > 20	Lung: > 10 (but lower than NEC) Digestive: rarely > 20

HG-NET, high-grade neuroendocrine tumour (NET/carcinoid with proliferative activity; G3 NET); NEC, neuroendocrine carcinoma; SCNEC, small cell neuroendocrine carcinoma.
[a]Organoid pattern: solid nests, trabeculae, pseudoglands, or rosettes.

not typically positive in LCNEC, which instead shows high FDG avidity {1820,2245}.

Epidemiology

LCNEC is rare, accounting for about 2% of all primary malignancies outside the lung {4723}. In extragenital organs, LCNEC preferentially affects male patients, except in the biliary tree, where the M:F ratio is 1:2.1 {2584}. The mean age at diagnosis is in the sixth to seventh decade of life, but it varies with site: LCNEC of the uterine cervix affects premenopausal women in their fourth or fifth decade of life {3718,2038}.

Etiology

Although etiological factors have not been defined, specific causative agents have been identified in selected locations (see Table S8.5, available at https://publications.iarc.who.int/645).

Pathogenesis

Although many LCNECs share genomic alterations with small cell neuroendocrine carcinoma (SCNEC), LCNECs also share the genetic landscape of non-neuroendocrine carcinomas {4603}. Specific data on lung LCNECs demonstrate distinct pathogenetic pathways, including mutations of *TP53* and *RB1* (78% and 38%, respectively) {3720}. Three alternative or only partially overlapping molecular profiles have been demonstrated: (1) LCNEC with pulmonary SCNEC-like features, characterized by *TP53* and *RB1* mutations and, to a lesser extent, *MYC* amplifications and *PTEN* mutations; (2) LCNEC with non-small cell lung carcinoma–like features, which lacks *TP53* and *RB1* alterations and is characterized by *STK11*, *KRAS*, *KEAP1*, *PIK3CA*, and NOTCH-family gene alterations; and (3) LCNEC with NET (carcinoid)-like features, with a low mutation burden and *MEN1* alterations {3720,1535, 1091}. Some cases classified as LCNEC in the lung or thymus would be regarded as well-differentiated G3 NET in the gastroenteropancreatic system. In analogy to the lung, *TP53* mutations represent the most common molecular alteration in LCNEC of extrapulmonary sites, with the exception of LCNEC of the cervix, the pathogenesis of which is HPV-related {1888}. LCNEC of colorectal and sinonasal sites lacks frequent *RB1* mutations, which are found at nearly all other sites {4603}.

Macroscopic appearance

The macroscopic appearance of LCNEC does not differ from that of non-neuroendocrine cancer at various sites (see Table S8.6, available at https://publications.iarc.who.int/645). LCNECs are often large and infiltrative lesions, with areas of necrosis and haemorrhage.

Histopathology

LCNEC shows organoid (solid nests, trabeculae, rosettes, and glandular structures) or diffuse growth. Necrosis is frequent, either extensive (geographical-chart necrosis) or focal. The cells are large, with irregular nuclei, prominent nucleoli, and distinct cell borders (see Table 8.02) {4541,4538}. Merkel cell carcinoma may show a spectrum of cytological features from small cells to intermediate and large cells. In the small and intermediate cell subtypes, a fine granular salt-and-pepper chromatin pattern is observed, nuclear moulding is uncommon, and nucleoli are small but distinct {4767}. A high mitotic count is present, > 10 mitoses/2 mm^2 by definition in the lung and > 20 mitoses/2 mm^2 in digestive organs, and the Ki-67 (MIB1) proliferation index is usually > 55% {4542,4541,4111,4538}. In a significant subset of cases, LCNEC associates with a clonally related non-neuroendocrine carcinoma (see the sections on mixed neuroendocrine–non-neuroendocrine neoplasms, p. 328) {2533}.

Immunohistochemistry

Expression of general neuroendocrine markers (synaptophysin, chromogranin A, INSM1) is mandatory to confirm the diagnosis.

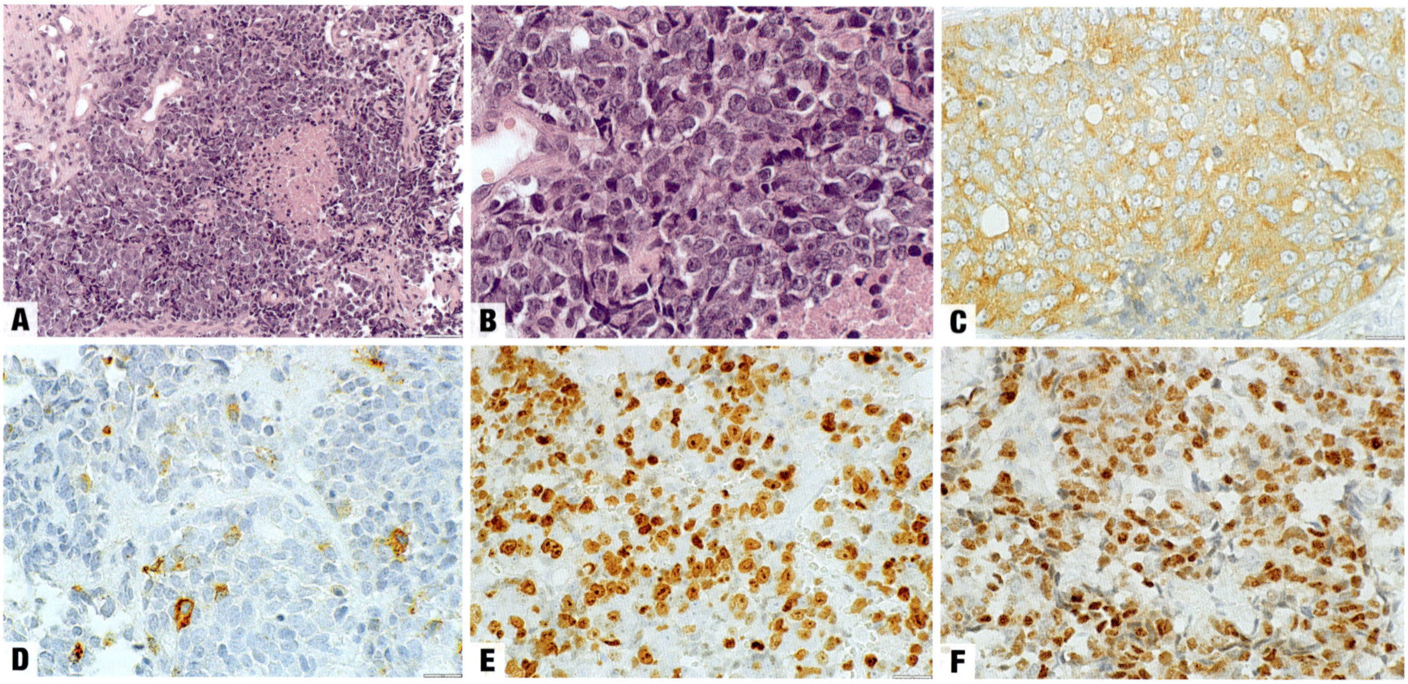

Fig. 8.08 Large cell neuroendocrine carcinoma (LCNEC) of the nasal cavity. **A** Sheets and irregular cords of large atypical cells with zonal necrosis. **B** Neoplastic cells have moderately abundant eosinophilic and granular cytoplasm, large nuclei with evident nuclear membranes, and eosinophilic macronucleoli. **C** Neoplastic cells display diffuse immunoreactivity for synaptophysin. **D** Chromogranin A is expressed in scattered cells, with a punctate pattern. **E** The Ki-67 proliferation index is very high. **F** INSM1 is strongly and diffusely positive.

Synaptophysin is considered the most sensitive marker and often is diffusely expressed in the neoplastic cells, whereas chromogranin A may be focal {4604}. INSM1 has been reported to have a high sensitivity and specificity in NEC {376}. Low-molecular-weight cytokeratins are always expressed {4604}. Site-specific transcription factors are not useful in identifying the site of origin of a metastatic LCNEC, with thyroid transcription factor 1 (TTF1) being expressed in as many as 50% of cases, independently of the primary location; Merkel cell carcinoma displays a characteristic immunoprofile (see Table S8.6, available at https://publications.iarc.who.int/645) {4604,376,3457, 2263,377}. SSTR2 may be expressed in a subset of LCNECs, usually with a weaker intensity than in NETs {4604,376}. Abnormal expression (hyperexpression or complete absence) of p53 and, to a lesser extent, a lack of RB1 are frequently observed {4992,4413,2104}. The Ki-67 proliferation index is generally elevated. In the digestive system the Ki-67 proliferation index is > 20% by definition and averages 50–80%, which is generally lower than in SCNEC {1353}. In a series of 77 lung LCNECs, a wide range of Ki-67 proliferation indexes (1–64%) was observed {4771}, generally lower than in SCNEC {1353}. The Ki-67 index may be focally or diffusely reduced after treatment {4754}.

Differential diagnosis

This includes SCNEC, high-grade (proliferating) NET (G3 NET in the digestive system), and poorly differentiated non-neuroendocrine carcinomas with neuroendocrine-like morphology or with classic morphology and (focal) immunohistochemical expression of neuroendocrine markers. A diagnostic algorithm, including morphological and immunohistochemical analysis, is helpful in discriminating among the various entities. The diagnosis of LCNEC should rely on morphology, proliferation index, and the expression of general neuroendocrine markers {4604, 1090}. Merkel cell carcinoma may be distinguished on the basis of CK20 expression and its peculiar immunoprofile (see *Merkel cell carcinoma*, p. 346) {3457,2263,377}.

Cytology

In smears, LCNEC exhibits intermediate to large cells containing variably prominent nucleoli, frequently in a necrotic background; single-cell component and crush artefact with nuclear streaming are frequent features {4873,5038,2851,2112,1980, 2034}. The application of pertinent immunostains, most feasible on cell blocks, is mandatory for a definitive diagnosis.

Diagnostic molecular pathology

Not clinically relevant

Essential and desirable diagnostic criteria

Essential: poorly differentiated neuroendocrine morphology; large cell (non-small cell) cytology; a high proliferation rate; immunohistochemical evidence of neuroendocrine differentiation (e.g. chromogranin A, synaptophysin, and/or INSM1).

Desirable: a high Ki-67 proliferation index (often > 55%); negative immunohistochemistry for SSTR2 and SSTR5.

Staging

Staging is the same as for non-neuroendocrine carcinoma of each primary site.

Prognosis and prediction

LCNEC has an ominous prognosis, with shorter survival times and higher recurrence rates than stage-adjusted non-neuroendocrine carcinoma at each site {3834,1360,2070,3952,4077,

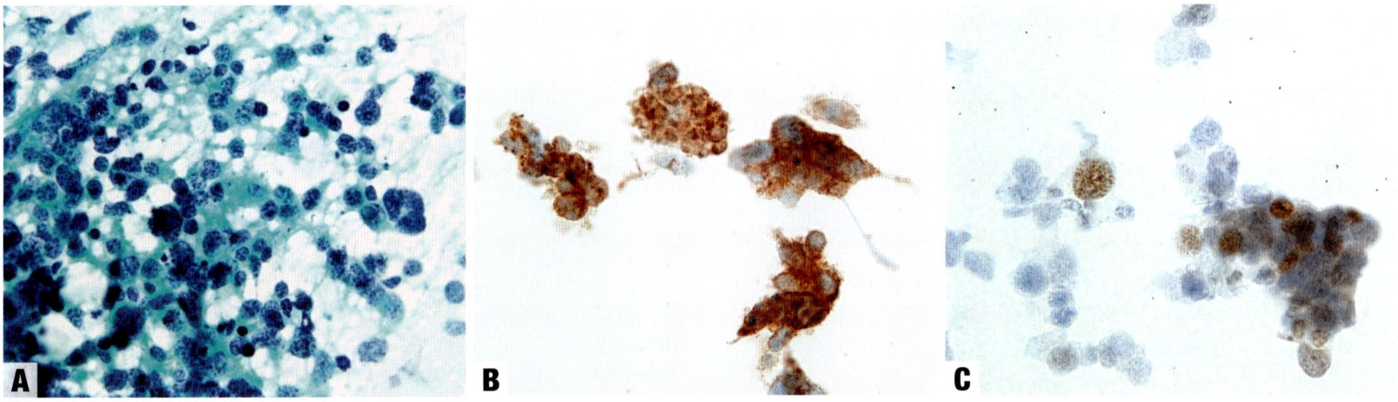

Fig. 8.09 Large cell neuroendocrine carcinoma (LCNEC). **A** Many large and loosely cohesive tumour cells contain abundant cytoplasm and vesicular nuclei. **B** Most tumour cells are immunohistochemically positive for synaptophysin in the cytoplasm. **C** Some tumour cell nuclei are immunohistochemically positive for thyroid transcription factor 1 (TTF1).

1382}. Compared with SCNEC, LCNEC presents at a lower stage and is more likely to be surgically treated and to have a better outcome (e.g. colonic LCNEC has a 5-year survival rate of ~20%, vs ~10% for SCNEC) {2402,4077}. In a non-surgical metastatic setting, median survival times are similar to those for SCNEC (~10 months) for chemotherapy-treated pulmonary and extrapulmonary LCNECs {4235,3156,4666,89,4787,2317}. Adjuvant or neoadjuvant chemotherapy regimens are largely based on those employed in both SCNEC and LCNEC of the lung {3156,89}. Although controlled clinical studies are lacking, isolated cases of LCNEC responsive to PD1/PDL1 checkpoint inhibitors have been reported {4805,2894,4387}. PDL1 is expressed in a fraction of tumour cells in 10–20% of LCNECs at various sites {4578,3768,1206,1866,186} and in the inflammatory cells in the majority of cases {186}. Systematic studies on the predictive value of PDL1 expression in LCNEC are lacking.

Chapter 8

Merkel cell carcinoma

Tetzlaff M
Messina JL
Tsai KY

Definition
Merkel cell carcinoma (MCC) is a high-grade primary cutaneous neuroendocrine carcinoma (NEC).

ICD-O coding
8247/3 Merkel cell carcinoma

ICD-11 coding
2C34 & XH81N8 Cutaneous neuroendocrine carcinoma & Merkel cell carcinoma

Related terminology
Not recommended: primary neuroendocrine carcinoma of skin.

Subtype(s)
None

Localization
MCC most commonly arises on sun-exposed sites. A review of 14 414 patients with MCC demonstrated that 43% of cases developed on the head or neck {1790}.

Clinical features
MCC presents as a rapidly growing, often violaceous papule or nodule. The broad clinical differential diagnosis includes basal cell and squamous cell carcinomas, lymphoma, atypical fibroxanthoma, and melanoma. The majority (65%) of patients present with disease localized to the skin, 26% with regional lymph node metastases, and 8% with distant metastases {1790}.

Epidemiology
MCC most commonly affects older White, non-Hispanic males. A population-based survey of 11 028 cases from 21 countries showed the highest rates in Australia, New Zealand, and the USA {4268}. MCC incidence per 1 million person-years has increased significantly in the USA from 1.5 cases in 1986, to 4.4 cases in 2001, to 7.9 cases in 2011 {1919,1388,3471}.

Etiology
Risk factors for MCC development include male sex, old age, chronic sun exposure, and immunosuppression. Merkel cell polyomavirus (MCPyV) infection and ultraviolet (UV) radiation–induced mutagenesis reflect two distinct pathways for MCC development. Asymptomatic MCPyV infection occurs early in life, with seropositivity rates of 60–70% {1046}.

Pathogenesis
Clonally integrated MCPyV expresses the viral oncoproteins large T-antigen (LT) and small T-antigen {4850,1792,360,1323} and is responsible for 60–80% of cases {1352,3102}. Truncated LT binds and inactivates RB1 protein, allowing cell-cycle progression. Virus-negative MCC possesses a significantly higher genomic instability and somatic mutation burden than MCPyV-positive MCC – predominantly UV radiation signature mutations affecting *TP53*, *RB1*, and NOTCH family members {1388, 1793,1619,4924,2350}. MCPyV-positive MCCs predominate in areas with high ambient UV radiation, whereas MCPyV-negative MCCs predominate in low-exposure areas {1323}.

Macroscopic appearance
See *Clinical features*.

Histopathology
Scanning magnification shows a densely cellular dermal malignancy with frequent extension into the subcutis, infiltrative or pushing borders, and variably dense lymphohistiocytic inflammatory infiltrate. Intraepidermal MCC is rare {1790,1792}. Tumour cells with scant cytoplasm, round to oval nuclei, and finely granular chromatin are arranged as sheets, cords, and trabeculae. Mitotic figures and apoptotic bodies are common. Tumour cells are usually intermediate in size, but large cell and small cell

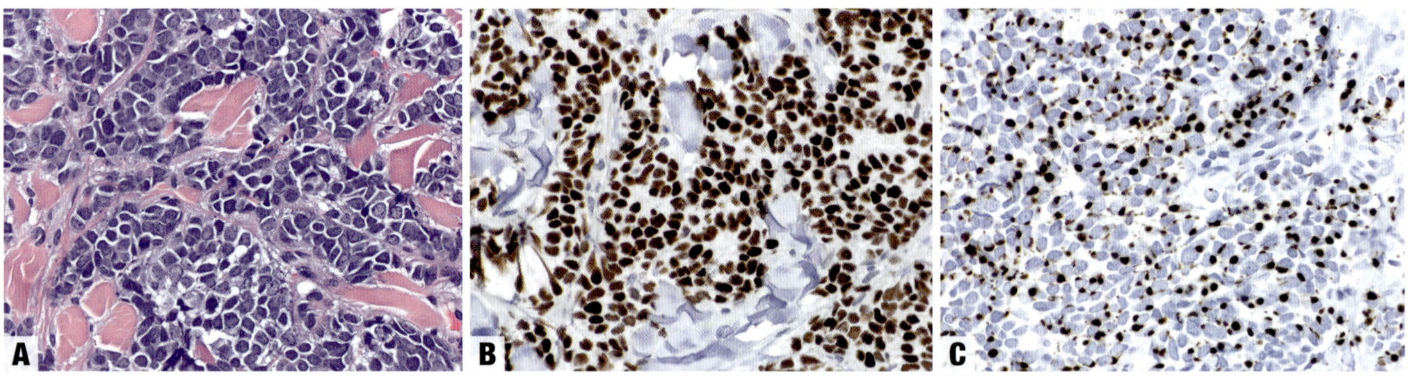

Fig. 8.10 Merkel cell carcinoma. **A** Histopathology. Tumour cells are arranged as syncytia and trabeculae, with large irregular nuclei and slight cytoplasm. The nuclei have finely granular chromatin, and mitotic figures are numerous. **B** Merkel cell polyomavirus T-antigen shows nuclear positivity. **C** CK20 stains Merkel cell carcinoma with a characteristic perinuclear dot-like positivity.

morphologies may occur {1792,4440}. MCC may show divergent differentiation, most commonly glandular {4046,2857,2357} or squamous {2013,576,4171,3387,2068,2857,2355}, and less commonly sarcomatoid or neuroblastic {1792}. Distinct foci of invasive squamous cell carcinoma or squamous cell carcinoma in situ are found in as many as 15% of cases, and there may be a relationship between them {1323,1794,2262}.

Immunohistochemistry

Immunohistochemical studies are essential for confirming the diagnosis of MCC. The most specific marker is CK20, which highlights most MCCs (~88%) {745,4042,804,2097,446,3457,2264} with characteristic perinuclear dots. MCCs show neuroendocrine differentiation, including synaptophysin (92%) and chromogranin A (84%). Neurofilament is expressed in ~80% of MCCs. Immunohistochemical detection of MCPyV LT (CM2B4) is sensitive (88%) and specific (94%) {3102}. A subset of MCPyV-negative MCCs demonstrate divergent immunophenotypic findings (thyroid transcription factor 1 [TTF1] positivity, or negativity for neurofilament and/or CK20) {3457,2264}. CK20-negative MCCs may be diagnosed by neurofilament positivity and TTF1 negativity; MCPyV staining has limited sensitivity for CK20-negative tumours {3021}. A meta-analysis identified frequent PAX5 (~90%), TdT (~65%), and KIT (CD117) (63%) in MCC {3971}. SATB2 is also expressed in MCCs {2263,377}. Expression of B-cell markers is associated with MCPyV {1911}. These are all important pitfalls, because detection of these biomarkers and MCPyV can assist the distinction of MCCs from other NECs {2263}.

Cytology

Smears are highly cellular and have a predominantly dispersed pattern, with scattered irregular tissue fragments consisting of crowded cells that have tightly packed, moulded nuclei with minimal cytoplasm, although in some cases delicate cytoplasm can be seen. Single dispersed tumour cells have high N:C ratios, scant pale blue (Giemsa) cytoplasm, variable nuclear size and shape, finely stippled chromatin, and indistinct nucleoli. Stripped nuclei are plentiful, and apoptotic debris is often prominent, but necrosis is not usually seen {4115}.

Diagnostic molecular pathology

Molecular studies are not typically used in the diagnosis of MCC, although viral gene expression and UV radiation signature mutation detection have enabled distinction from histological mimickers {4333,2548}. Immunohistochemical detection of MCPyV LT (CM2B4) is sensitive (88%) and specific (94%) {3102}.

Essential and desirable diagnostic criteria

Essential: a rapidly growing skin lesion; a highly cellular dermal malignancy composed of cells with round to oval nuclei and finely granular chromatin; immunopositive for cytokeratin (e.g. CK20) with dot-like perinuclear staining and for markers of neuroendocrine differentiation.

Desirable: expression of B-cell markers and/or MCPyV may be helpful in the distinction from other NECs.

Staging

The eighth edition of the American Joint Committee on Cancer (AJCC) TNM system forms the basis for MCC staging {1790}.

Prognosis and prediction

Five-year overall survival rates are about 51% for those with localized disease, 35% for patients with regional lymph node metastases, and 14% when distant metastases are present. In node-negative patients, T stage robustly predicts 5-year overall survival: 55.8% for pT1 disease, 41.1% for pT2/pT3, and 31.8% for pT4 {1790}, although recent data suggest that survival rates are substantially higher {1334}. Cases with clinically evident lymph node metastases have a worse prognosis than cases with clinically occult lymph node involvement {1790}, and the pattern and extent of sentinel lymph node involvement are additional prognostic factors {1347,1279}. Patients with clinically evident regional lymph node disease without a known primary MCC are distinguished from patients with a known primary MCC (stage IIIA vs stage IIIB) and have a better prognosis {1406,4421,780}.

Additional prognostic features of the primary tumour include tumour thickness, pattern of growth, lymphovascular invasion, and tumour-infiltrating lymphocytes, all of which are independently associated with patient survival {139,3470,4141,1347}. The pattern of sentinel lymph node involvement and the extent of disease burden in the sentinel lymph node are additional prognostic factors in MCC {1347,1279}.

MCPyV-positive MCCs may have better survival rates than MCPyV-negative MCCs {4142,4143,3189,1885,3102,1833}, although this is controversial {3470,1753} and MCPyV status does not predict survival independently of stage {3102}. Expression of p63 correlates with shorter survival times in MCC {234,232,1885,1389}, but not independently of stage {4282}. Ki-67 labelling index ≥ 55% {2479} and TERT methylation {3734} were associated with a bad prognosis.

Integrity of the host immune system is both a risk factor and a prognostic factor in MCC {3508,1251,1846,1858}. Immunocompromised patients have worse survival rates than immunocompetent patients {3469}. Increased expression of immune-related genes (e.g. *CD8A* and granzyme genes) and higher levels of tumour-infiltrative CD8+ T cells independently correlate with longer survival {3470,4141,1347}. Furthermore, in MCPyV-positive MCCs, decreased expression of immune markers including granzyme and IDO1 correlated with shorter survival, whereas in MCPyV-negative MCCs, expression of several genes, including *UBE2C*, correlated with shorter survival {1791}.

Mixed neuroendocrine–non-neuroendocrine neoplasms

La Rosa S
Milione M
Osamura RY
Rekhtman N
Tang LH
Uccella S

Definition

Mixed neuroendocrine–non-neuroendocrine neoplasms (MiNENs) are mixed epithelial neoplasms in which a neuroendocrine component is combined with a non-neuroendocrine one, each of which is morphologically and immunohistochemically recognizable. The term "MiNEN" is a descriptive category for these mixed neoplasms; site-specific terms that reflect the different components should be used as diagnoses.

ICD-O coding

8154/3 Mixed neuroendocrine–non-neuroendocrine neoplasm
8013/3 Combined large cell neuroendocrine carcinoma
8045/3 Combined small cell neuroendocrine carcinoma

ICD-11 coding

Code according to site of origin and tumours
2C10.1 & XH6H10 Neuroendocrine neoplasms of pancreas & Mixed adenoneuroendocrine carcinoma

Related terminology

Acceptable: combined neuroendocrine carcinoma (NEC) and non-neuroendocrine carcinoma (i.e. squamous cell carcinoma or adenocarcinoma).

Subtype(s)

The various combinations of neuroendocrine and non-neuroendocrine components give rise, in different anatomical sites, to several different MiNEN subtypes. The neuroendocrine component can be poorly differentiated (NEC) and of small cell or large cell type or, rarely, well differentiated (neuroendocrine tumour [NET]). The non-neuroendocrine component usually has the morphological features of autochthonous carcinomas of each primary site {2533} (see Box 8.01).

Localization

All organs in which a neuroendocrine neoplasm (NEN) can arise can give rise to MiNENs (see Table S8.7, available as supplementary material at https://publications.iarc.who.int/645).

Clinical features

Clinical presentation and symptoms depend on the site of origin and are related to tumour growth and/or metastatic dissemination (see Table S8.7, available at https://publications.iarc.who.int/645). Specific endocrine syndromes have not been described in MiNENs in which the neuroendocrine component is represented by a NET. In rare cases of MiNENs in which the neuroendocrine component is a NEC, paraneoplastic syndromes (e.g. syndrome of inappropriate antidiuresis [SIAD]) have been reported {2244,2533,4605}.

Epidemiology

MiNENs account for 2–30% of all NENs, with a variable site-specific incidence. Men are more frequently affected than women, and the age at diagnosis is generally in the sixth or seventh decade of life {4606,4595,4605}.

Etiology

The etiological factors are not known, and an association with specific hereditary genetic syndromes has not been demonstrated. However, in some organs, associations with possible etiological factors have been observed, such as high-grade HPV infection in oropharyngeal and cervical MiNENs {2044,433} and cigarette smoking in lung MiNENs {1662}. For sinonasal MiNENs, no occupational exposure to carcinogens has been demonstrated. Skin MiNENs are not apparently associated with Merkel cell polyomavirus {2533}.

Pathogenesis

Several molecular studies demonstrated that the two components are clonally related and therefore derive from a common

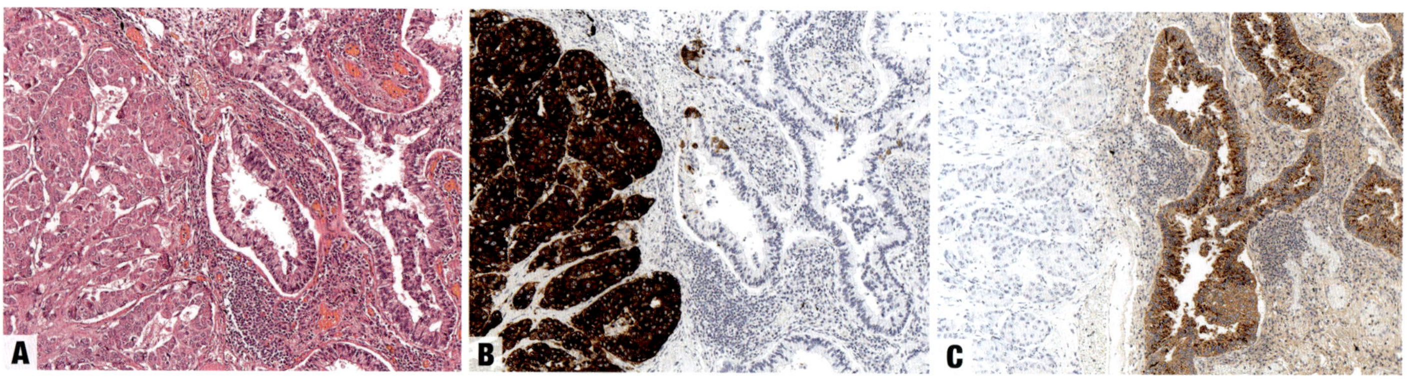

Fig. 8.11 Mixed neuroendocrine–non-neuroendocrine neoplasm (MiNEN) of the lung (combined neoplasm). **A** This MiNEN is composed of large cell neuroendocrine carcinoma (LCNEC; left) and adenocarcinoma (right). **B** The LCNEC component is positive for synaptophysin. **C** The adenocarcinoma component is positive for napsin A.

Box 8.01 Specific types of mixed neuroendocrine–non-neuroendocrine neoplasms (MiNENs) by organ

Head and neck
- **Middle ear**
  - Glandular adenoma–NET
- **Sinonasal tract**
  - Mixed inverted papilloma–SCNEC
  - Mixed intestinal-type adenocarcinoma–SCNEC
  - Mixed intestinal-type adenocarcinoma–LCNEC
  - Mixed squamous cell carcinoma–SCNEC
  - Mixed squamous cell carcinoma–LCNEC
  - Mixed adenosquamous carcinoma–SCNEC
- **Oropharynx**
  - Mixed squamous cell carcinoma–SCNEC
- **Larynx**
  - Mixed squamous cell carcinoma–SCNEC
  - Mixed squamous cell carcinoma–NET

Thorax
- **Lung**
  - Mixed adenocarcinoma–NEC (SCNEC or LCNEC)
  - Mixed squamous cell carcinoma–NEC (SCNEC or LCNEC)
  - Mixed large cell carcinoma–NEC (SCNEC or LCNEC)
  - Mixed spindle/giant cell carcinoma–NEC (SCNEC or LCNEC)
  - Mixed adenocarcinoma–NET
  - Mixed squamous cell carcinoma–NET
- **Thymus**
  - Mixed thymoma–NEC (SCNEC or LCNEC)
  - Mixed thymic carcinoma–NEC (SCNEC or LCNEC)
  - Mixed thymoma–NET
  - Mixed thymic carcinoma–NET

Digestive system
- **Oesophagus**
  - Mixed adenocarcinoma–NEC (SCNEC or LCNEC)
  - Mixed squamous cell carcinoma–NEC (SCNEC or LCNEC)
  - Mixed adenocarcinoma–NET
- **Stomach**
  - Mixed adenocarcinoma–NEC (SCNEC or LCNEC)
  - Mixed adenocarcinoma–NET
- **Small intestine and ampulla**
  - Mixed adenocarcinoma–NEC (SCNEC or LCNEC)
  - Mixed adenocarcinoma–NET (G1, G2, G3)
- **Appendix (goblet cell adenocarcinoma excluded)**
  - Mixed adenocarcinoma–NEC (SCNEC or LCNEC)
- **Colorectum**
  - Mixed adenocarcinoma–NEC (SCNEC or LCNEC)
  - Mixed adenocarcinoma–NET
- **Liver**
  - Mixed hepatocellular carcinoma–NEC (SCNEC or LCNEC)
  - Mixed hepatocellular carcinoma–NET
  - Mixed cholangiocarcinoma–NEC
- **Gallbladder and bile ducts**
  - Mixed adenocarcinoma–NEC (SCNEC or LCNEC)
  - Mixed adenocarcinoma–intracholecystic papillary neoplasm–NEC (SCNEC or LCNEC)

Female genital tract
- **Vulva**
  - Mixed adenocarcinoma–LCNEC
- **Cervix and vagina**
  - Mixed adenocarcinoma–SCNEC
  - Mixed adenocarcinoma–LCNEC
  - Mixed squamous cell carcinoma–SCNEC
  - Mixed squamous cell carcinoma–LCNEC
  - Mixed adenosquamous carcinoma–SCNEC
  - Mixed carcinosarcoma–SCNEC
  - Mixed mesonephric adenocarcinoma–LCNEC
  - Mixed adenoid-cystic adenocarcinoma–SCNEC
- **Endometrium**
  - Endometrioid carcinoma–LCNEC
  - Endometrioid carcinoma–SCNEC
  - High-grade serous carcinoma–LCNEC
  - Carcinosarcoma–SCNEC
- **Ovary**
  - Mixed mucinous carcinoma–LCNEC
  - Mixed endometrioid carcinoma–LCNEC
  - Mixed endometrioid carcinoma–SCNEC
  - Mixed high-grade serous carcinoma–LCNEC
  - Mixed undifferentiated carcinoma–LCNEC

Urinary and male genital tracts
- **Kidney**
  - Mixed urothelial carcinoma–SCNEC
  - Mixed urothelial carcinoma–LCNEC
  - Mixed squamous cell carcinoma–SCNEC
  - Mixed papillary renal cell carcinoma–SCNEC
  - Mixed clear cell renal carcinoma–NET
- **Urinary tract**
  - Mixed urothelial carcinoma (including subtypes)–SCNEC
  - Mixed adenocarcinoma–SCNEC
  - Mixed adenocarcinoma–LCNEC
- **Prostate**
  - Mixed acinar adenocarcinoma–LCNEC
  - Mixed acinar adenocarcinoma–SCNEC

Skin
  - Mixed squamous cell carcinoma–MCC
  - Mixed basal cell carcinoma–MCC
  - Mixed trichoblastoma–MCC
  - Mixed sebaceous carcinoma–MCC

LCNEC, large cell neuroendocrine carcinoma; MCC, Merkel cell carcinoma; NEC, neuroendocrine carcinoma; NET, neuroendocrine tumour; SCNEC, small cell neuroendocrine carcinoma.

progenitor cell. Pathogenetic mechanisms involved in MiNENs with a NEC component are similar to those observed in non-neuroendocrine carcinomas of each anatomical site. Although there are some site-specific characteristics, mutations in *TP53*, *RB1*, *KRAS*, *STK11*, and *KEAP1* are the most common molecular alterations, independently of the site of origin {2664, 3143,1456,2484,4907,2104,3976,4732,2482,3190,4605}. In lung MiNENs composed of adenocarcinoma and small cell neuroendocrine carcinoma (SCNEC), *EGFR* mutations have been described {1456}.

Macroscopic appearance

The macroscopic appearance resembles that of non-neuroendocrine carcinoma of the same site (e.g. adenocarcinoma, squamous cell carcinoma, ovarian serous carcinoma, renal cell carcinoma).

Histopathology

The diagnosis of MiNEN subtypes requires that both components are morphologically recognizable. Some neoplasms in various organs exhibit mixed differentiation, including neuroendocrine

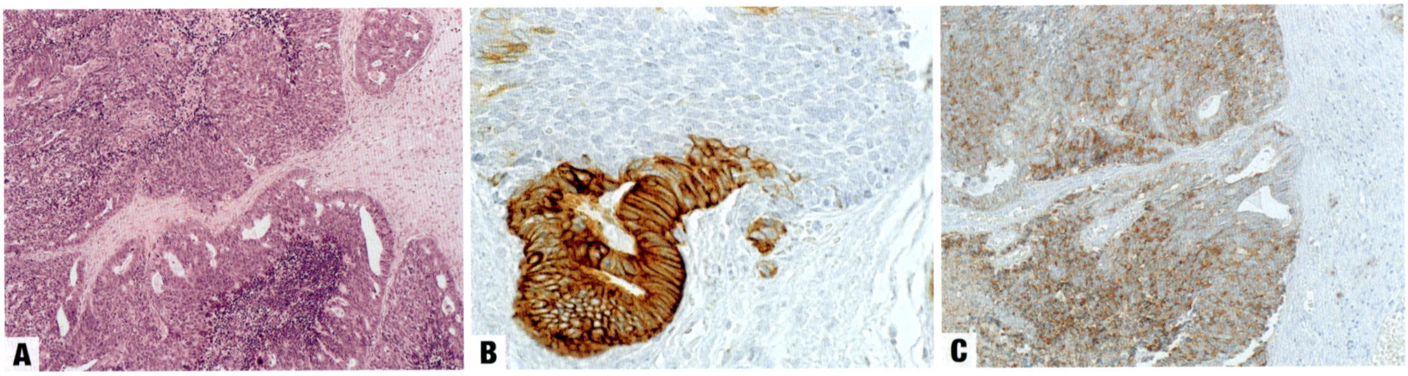

Fig. 8.12 Nasal mixed neuroendocrine–non-neuroendocrine neoplasm (MiNEN) composed of intestinal-type nasal adenocarcinoma and large cell neuroendocrine carcinoma (LCNEC). **A** Intermingled glandular structures and solid sheets of poorly differentiated large cells with central necrosis. **B** The glandular component is positive for CK20. **C** The solid component is positive for synaptophysin.

and non-neuroendocrine lineages, which can be demonstrated using immunolabelling, but the components are so intimately admixed that they cannot be recognized histologically; these neoplasms do not fit the definition of MiNEN, although they may be diagnosed as mixed neoplasms nonetheless. The clinical significance of mixed differentiation in such cases is not clear. The histological features of the neuroendocrine and non-neuroendocrine components are similar to those of their pure counterparts. The neuroendocrine component is usually represented by a NEC of either the small cell (SCNEC) or large cell (LCNEC) subtype. Their morphological features are described in *Small cell neuroendocrine carcinoma* (p. 339) and *Large cell neuroendocrine carcinoma* (p. 342). More rarely, the neuroendocrine component is represented by a NET showing the morphological features described in *Neuroendocrine tumours* (p. 337). The Ki-67 proliferation index is necessary to grade the NET component. In addition, in the digestive system the Ki-67 index of the NEC component (≤ 55% vs > 55%) is also useful for stratifying MiNENs into two prognostic groups {3008}. However, in other sites, like the uterine cervix, the Ki-67 proliferation index does not seem to have a prognostic impact {1940}. The non-neuroendocrine component can be represented by different non-neuroendocrine carcinoma types. Adenocarcinoma and squamous cell carcinoma, including their respective organ-specific subtypes, are the most common components. In addition, depending on the site of origin, other specific carcinomas can be observed, such as ovarian mucinous carcinoma, basal cell carcinoma, thymoma, urothelial carcinoma, renal papillary carcinoma, etc.

Immunohistochemistry is mandatory for confirming the neuroendocrine nature of the neuroendocrine component. Synaptophysin, chromogranin A, and INSM1 are the most sensitive and specific markers. However, it is worth noting that chromogranin A in NECs, especially in the SCNEC subtype, can be negative or focally expressed with a paranuclear dot-like pattern of positivity. The immunohistochemical profile of the non-neuroendocrine component depends on the type of cancer and on the site.

In the digestive tract, rare cases of mixed neoplasms including a non-malignant non-neuroendocrine component such as adenoma {2494} or intracholecystic papillary neoplasm {1416} have been described, but these should not be considered MiNENs, because the non-neuroendocrine component is not an invasive carcinoma. These cases rather represent a NEC arising from a non-neuroendocrine preinvasive (precursor) neoplasm.

Cytology

FNA cytopathology will demonstrate the features of neuroendocrine carcinoma with a second component such as adenocarcinoma.

Diagnostic molecular pathology

Not clinically relevant

Essential and desirable diagnostic criteria

See Table S8.8 (available at https://publications.iarc.who.int/645).

Essential: mixed tumour morphology with the two components morphologically recognizable, with pertinent immunohistochemistry to confirm the neuroendocrine component; in digestive system MiNENs, each component must be malignant and represent ≥ 30% of the tumour mass.

Desirable: Ki-67 proliferation index to grade the NET component and to prognostically stratify the NEC component.

Staging

MiNENs are staged using the Union for International Cancer Control (UICC) or American Joint Committee on Cancer (AJCC) staging system for primary cancers arising in the involved organ.

Prognosis and prediction

The careful typing, grading, and quantification of both components is crucial to patient outcome and case management. Although specific organ-related characteristics influence clinical behaviour, MiNENs in which the neuroendocrine component is represented by a NEC (either SCNEC or LCNEC) are generally very aggressive neoplasms with an ominous prognosis similar to that of pure NECs {3009,3007}, showing a median overall survival time of 8–61 months. For digestive MiNENs, the Ki-67 proliferation index plays a prognostic role, with a Ki-67 index > 55% representing a poor prognostic marker {3008}. MiNENs in which the neuroendocrine component is represented by a NET seem to have a better prognosis, probably driven by the non-neuroendocrine (adenocarcinoma or squamous cell carcinoma) component {2533,4605}.

Composite gangliocytoma/neuroma and neuroendocrine tumour

Gill AJ
Fuchs TL
Okubo Y
Uccella S

Definition

Composite gangliocytoma/neuroma and neuroendocrine tumour (CoGNET), previously known as gangliocytic paraganglioma, is a triphasic tumour composed of neuroendocrine epithelial cells, Schwannian spindle cells, and ganglion cells.

ICD-O coding

8683/3 Composite gangliocytoma/neuroma and neuroendocrine tumour

ICD-11 coding

2B80.01 & XH3JF3 Neuroendocrine neoplasm of duodenum & Composite paraganglioma

Related terminology

Acceptable: mixed ganglioneuroma–neuroendocrine neoplasm (MiGNEN); gangliocytic neuroendocrine tumour.

Not recommended: duodenal ganglioneuroma; duodenal paraganglioma; gangliocytic paraganglioma.

Subtype(s)

None

Localization

CoGNET almost exclusively arises in the second part of the duodenum (periampullary region) {3339,2817}. Extremely rare cases have been reported in the jejunum, pylorus, oesophagus, pancreas, appendix, lung, and thymus {4338,4903,5028,3343, 3287,2177}.

Clinical features

Patients with CoGNET usually present with gastrointestinal bleeding due to mucosal ulceration or nonspecific epigastric pain {817}. Biliary and intestinal obstruction have been reported {2824}. Most CoGNETs are clinically non-functioning, although high serum levels of somatostatin and PP have been reported {4516,133}.

Epidemiology

Most frequent in the sixth decade of life {2774,3339}, CoGNETs occur across a broad age range (15–92 years) {2774,817}. A slight male predominance (M:F ratio: ~3:2) {3339} was reported in some series but not in others {817}.

Etiology

Although a few cases were reported in the setting of neurofibromatosis type 1 {702,4279}, the majority of CoGNETs are sporadic, with no known risk factors or syndromic associations.

Pathogenesis

CoGNET is thought to derive from a defective sheet of intraembryonic endodermal progenitor cells, progenitor neuroectodermal cell rests, and smooth muscle {1688,3528,4905,569}. About 20% of CoGNETs harbour somatic gain-of-function mutations in *EPAS1* (*HIF2A*) {5184}.

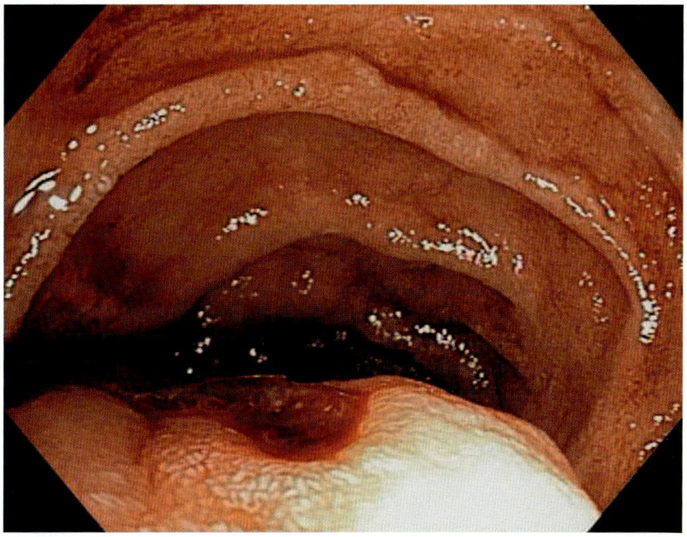

Fig. 8.13 Composite gangliocytoma/neuroma and neuroendocrine tumour (CoGNET). Endoscopic image of a CoGNET presenting as a 20 mm submucosal mass with mucosal ulceration in the second part of the duodenum.

Macroscopic appearance

CoGNETs are solitary, polypoid, pedunculated or sessile lesions {3994}, 20–30 mm in median size (range: 7–190 mm) depending on site {817,3339}. In the pancreatic head, CoGNETs are larger (median size: 40 mm) {817}. Tumours are typically centred in the submucosa and are well demarcated but unencapsulated, with borders infiltrating the mucosa and/or muscularis propria in more than half of the cases {3342}. The cut surface varies from tan-grey to yellow-white. The overlying mucosa is often ulcerated, even in the absence of mucosal invasion.

Histopathology

CoGNETs display three morphologically distinct cell components: (1) an epithelial cell component, arranged in nests and gland-like structures with granular eosinophilic cytoplasm, round to oval nuclei, speckled chromatin, and inconspicuous nucleoli; (2) a spindle cell Schwannian component, in slender fascicles with elongated plump nuclei and attenuated eosinophilic cytoplasm, wrapping around nests of epithelial cells; and (3) a ganglion cell component, scattered or in clusters, intermixed with the epithelial and spindle cell components. The proportions of the three components vary widely; ganglion cells may be difficult to identify. Mitoses are rare. Cytological atypia is minimal, and necrosis is absent. Any one or all three components may be present in metastases.

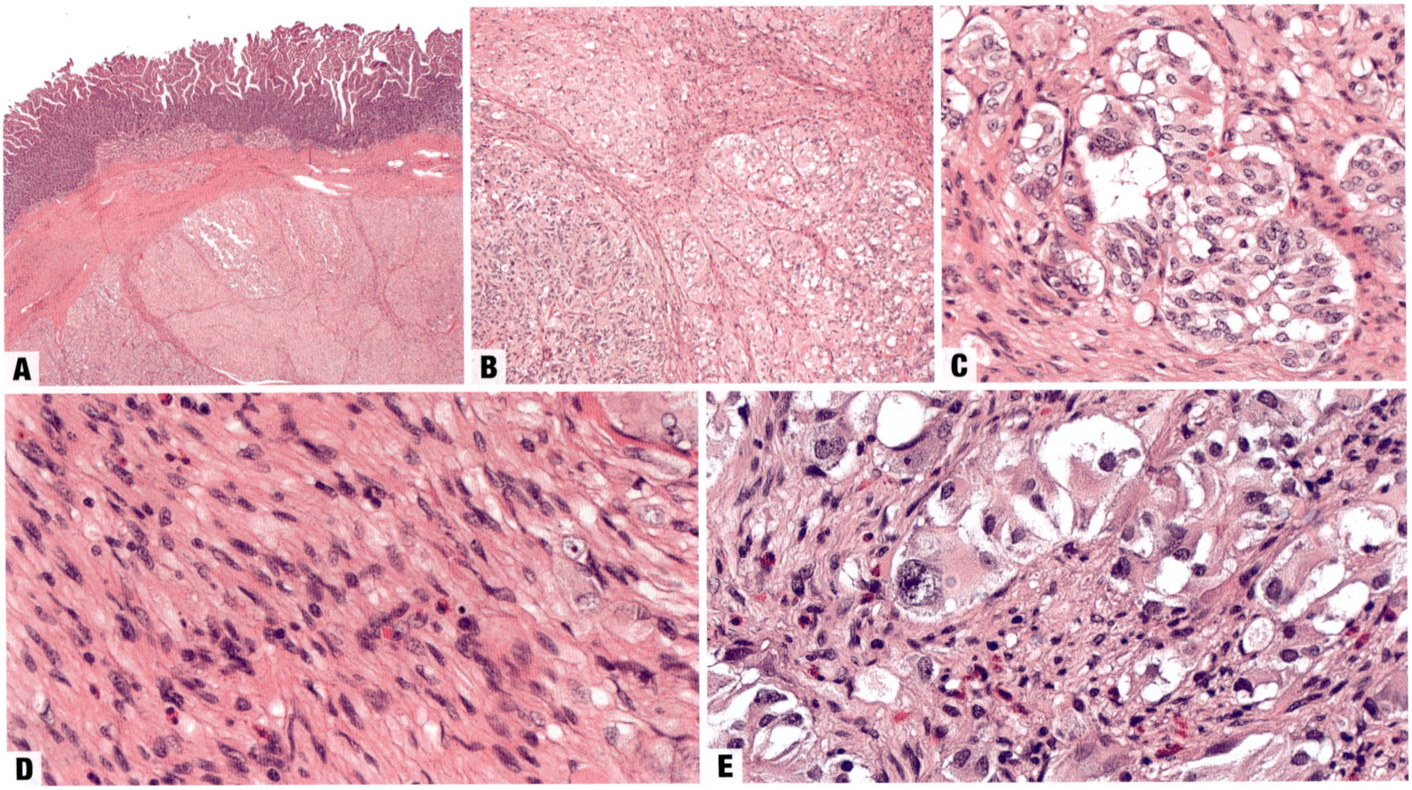

Fig. 8.14 Composite gangliocytoma/neuroma and neuroendocrine tumour (CoGNET). **A** CoGNET typically presents as a polypoid submucosal mass in the duodenum. **B** Characteristic triphasic appearance including epithelioid neuroendocrine cells, ganglion cells, and spindle cells with Schwann cell differentiation. **C** Epithelioid cells with neuroendocrine features. **D** Spindle cells with Schwann cell differentiation. **E** Ganglion cells intermixed with the spindle cell component.

Immunohistochemistry

Almost all epithelial cells express cytokeratins {2817}, chromogranin A, synaptophysin, NSE, and PR. PP and somatostatin may also be expressed. Spindle cells express SOX10, S100, and NSE. Ganglion cells express NSE and synaptophysin but are negative for SOX10 {2817}. CoGNETs are usually negative for or show only very focal, weak expression of GATA3 and tyrosine hydroxylase {2817}.

Differential diagnosis

Exclusion of gastrointestinal stromal tumour, leiomyoma, schwannoma, neuroendocrine tumour (NET), adenocarcinoma, ganglioneuroma, and paraganglioma is based on specific markers (KIT [c-KIT] and DOG1 for gastrointestinal stromal tumour, desmin for leiomyoma) and adequate sampling. Ganglioneuroma lacks the epithelial component of CoGNET, whereas conventional paraganglioma lacks the ganglion and Schwannian components and is usually cytokeratin-negative {5184,5183,3344,2817}. CoGNET is often misdiagnosed as conventional well-differentiated NET (G1). Increasing evidence indicates that CoGNET is more closely related to NET than to conventional paraganglioma {2817,5184}. Immunohistochemistry for PR and PP, although not specific, may be useful {3340}.

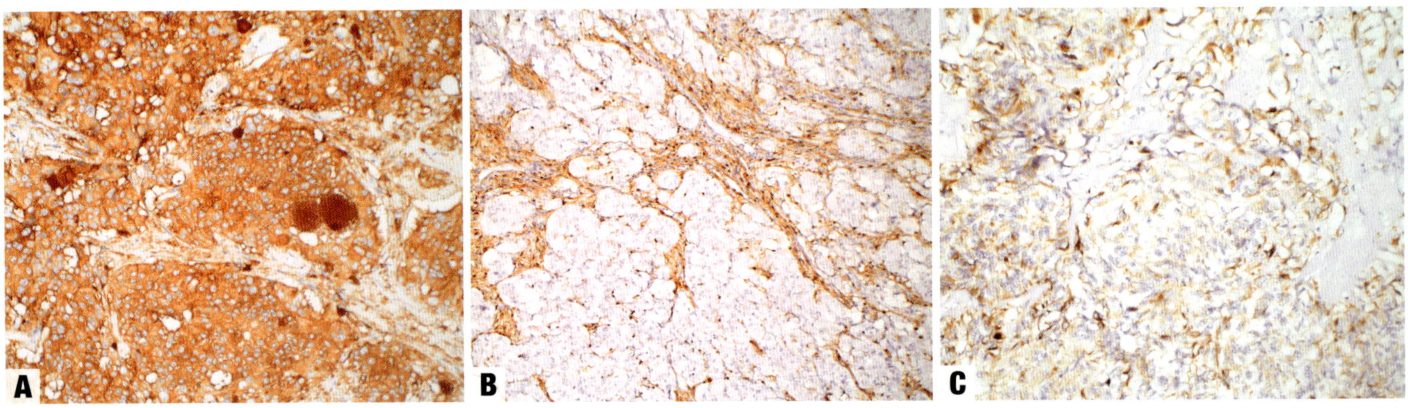

Fig. 8.15 Composite gangliocytoma/neuroma and neuroendocrine tumour (CoGNET). **A** Synaptophysin is positive in the epithelioid cells and the ganglion cells. **B** S100 is positive in the spindle cells with Schwann cell differentiation. **C** CK8/18 may show limited positivity in the epithelioid cells.

Cytology

Aspirates are often hypercellular and predominantly composed of epithelial cells, with a minor component of spindle and ganglion cells {1192,2408}. Rare cases with predominant spindle cells have been described {345}.

Diagnostic molecular pathology

None

Essential and desirable diagnostic criteria

Essential: triphasic differentiation with variable neuroendocrine epithelial cells, spindle cells with Schwannian differentiation, and ganglion cells.

Desirable: location in the periampullary region of the duodenum.

Staging

Staging utilizes a NET-specific system for the digestive tract only {4866}. The other (exceedingly rare) sites adopt the staging systems of non-neuroendocrine cancer.

Prognosis and prediction

Most CoGNETs are indolent and do not recur after complete removal. However, lymph node metastases were reported in 10–14.5% of cases and liver metastases in 1.8% of cases {4665, 3344,817}. In a recent study, the 1-year, 3-year, and 5-year survival rates for periampullary CoGNETs were 100%, 83.3%, and 55.6%, respectively {817}. No known histopathological factors are predictive of metastasis. Tumour size > 20 mm, young age, and submucosal invasion could be risk factors for lymph node metastasis {3342,3434,4665,1696,3343,3407}. Pancreatic CoGNETs are thought to have a greater potential for malignant behaviour {3287}. Because of the lack of validated predictive malignancy markers, all CoGNETs should be regarded as potentially malignant; long-term follow-up is recommended.

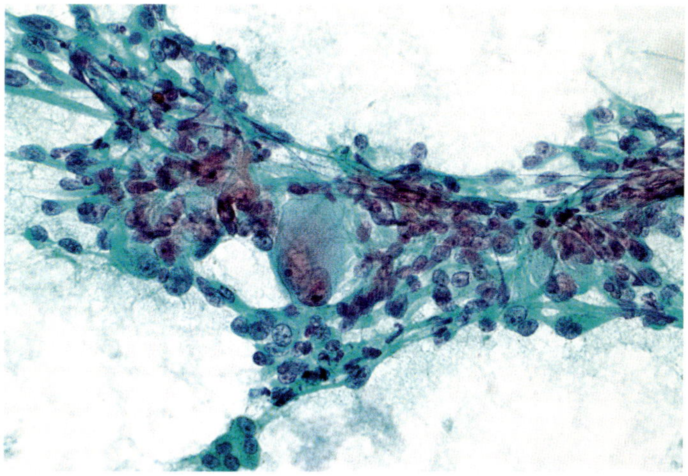

Fig. 8.16 Composite gangliocytoma/neuroma and neuroendocrine tumour (CoGNET). FNAB demonstrating epithelioid neuroendocrine cells and a large binucleated ganglion cell. The specimen was diagnosed as CoGNET after excision (Pap).

Cauda equina neuroendocrine tumour (previously paraganglioma)

Brandner S
Kleinschmidt-DeMasters BK
Perry A
Sarkar C

Definition

Cauda equina neuroendocrine tumour (NET), previously called paraganglioma, is a neuroendocrine neoplasm (NEN) arising from specialized neural crest cells in the cauda equina / filum terminale region.

ICD-O coding

8693/3 Cauda equina neuroendocrine tumour

ICD-11 coding

XH1X68 Paraganglioma, benign
XH0EW6 Paraganglioma, NOS

Related terminology

Not recommended: paraganglioma of the cauda equina; cauda equina paraganglioma.

Subtype(s)

None

Localization

Cauda equina / filum terminale region (intradural)

Clinical features

Cauda equina NETs exhibit no clinical features that allow their distinction from other intradural lumbosacral tumours (see Table 8.03). The most common presenting symptoms include a history of low back pain and sciatica. Less common manifestations are numbness, paraparesis, and incontinence {1525}. Fully developed cauda equina syndrome is uncommon. Signs of increased intracranial pressure and papilloedema are unusual at presentation {3936,1525,307,25,577}. Cerebrospinal fluid protein is usually markedly increased {4229,4205}.

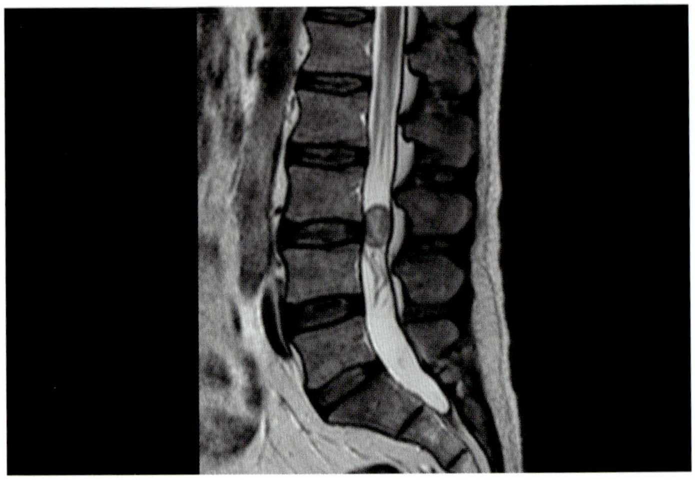

Fig. 8.17 Cauda equina neuroendocrine tumour (NET). Hyperintense T2-weighted image showing the well-demarcated tumour in the cauda equina region.

Imaging

MRI appearances of cauda equina NETs are indistinguishable from those of schwannoma or (myxopapillary) ependymoma

Table 8.03 The immunohistochemistry, chromosomal copy number, DNA methylation, and clinical profiles of cauda equina neuroendocrine tumours (NETs) are distinct from those of other paragangliomas

Features	Extraspinal paragangliomas	Cauda equina NET
Immunohistochemical		
Cytokeratin expression	Generally negative	Positive with variable staining patterns
Cytoplasmic SDHB expression	Loss of expression in most hereditary cases	Retained expression
GATA3 nuclear expression	Positive	Negative
HOXB13 expression	Negative	Positive
Molecular		
Germline mutations	Present in as many as 40% of cases (most commonly of SDH genes)	Not present
Chromosomal copy-number profile	Mostly aneuploid with recurrent trisomy 1q and monosomies of 1p, 3, and 11	Generally a diploid genome Chromosomal losses, gains, focal amplifications, or deletions are extremely rare
Fusion genes	Present, e.g. *MAML3* fusion associated with poor prognosis	Not observed
Genome-wide methylation profiling	Cauda equina NETs are epigenetically distinct from extraspinal paragangliomas	
Clinical	Can be hormonally active and can show a clinically aggressive behaviour with metastasis	Hormonally silent and clinically indolent with no reports of metastasis outside CNS

{25,3032}. Tumours are sharply circumscribed and occasionally partly cystic, and they can be hypointense, isointense, or hyperintense on T1- and T2-weighted images; contrast enhancement may be present or absent. A low-signal-intensity rim (cap sign) on T2-weighted images can be caused by subcapsular haemosiderin {2620,5033,5014}. The hypervascular architecture can give a salt-and-pepper appearance on T2-weighted images. Serpentine flow voids along the tumour surface or spinal cord margin may also be seen on MRI {1085,2938}.

Epidemiology

A meta-analysis of 297 cases {1934} identified a peak in incidence between the ages of 40 and 49 years, with a mean age at presentation of 47.0 years (range: 9–77 years). The M:F ratio was 1.5:1.

Etiology

These are sporadic NETs. The etiology is unknown.

Pathogenesis

Cauda equina NETs are histogenetically and molecularly distinct from paragangliomas and phaeochromocytomas outside the CNS. They overexpress the transcription factor HOXB13 {449}, which is developmentally expressed in the caudal extent of the spinal cord and in the urogenital sinus. This coincides with dynamic changes associated with the formation of the secondary neural tube {5123,1201}, providing circumstantial evidence of a cell of origin. To date, these tumours have not been seen in patients with familial paraganglioma phaeochromocytoma syndrome due to mutations in SDH genes {1667}.

Macroscopic appearance

Tumours are oval to sausage-shaped, delicately encapsulated, soft, red-brown masses that bleed freely and may cause superficial siderosis of the CNS {4090,2313,2726,3606}. In five series of 59 spinal tumours, sizes ranged from 10 to 112 mm in greatest dimension {2877,3032,5014}. Capsular calcification and cystic components may be found. Occasional tumours penetrate the dura to invade bone. A macroscopically identifiable attachment may be found, either to the filum terminale or (less often) to a caudal nerve root {4229}.

Histopathology

These well-differentiated NETs are composed of neuroendocrine cells arranged in nests or lobules surrounded by an inconspicuous single layer of sustentacular cells. The nests are surrounded by a delicate capillary network and a delicate supporting reticulin fibre network that may undergo sclerosis. The uniform round or polygonal neuroendocrine cells possess central round to oval nuclei with finely stippled chromatin and inconspicuous nucleoli. Degenerative nuclear pleomorphism (endocrine anaplasia) is generally mild. Cytoplasm is usually eosinophilic and finely granular. In some instances, it is amphophilic or clear. Sustentacular cells are thin and spindle-shaped. Encompassing the lobules, their long processes are often so attenuated as to be undetectable by routine light microscopy and are visible only on immunostaining for S100. Approximately 25% of cauda equina NETs contain mature ganglion cells and/or Schwann cell components (gangliocytic or ganglioneuromatous tumours). Ependymoma-like perivascular formations are common. Some tumours show angiomatous, adenomatous, and pseudorosette patterns {4229}. Tumours with spindled cytology {3086}, melanin-containing cells {1477,3086}, and oncocytic change {3433} have been described. Foci of haemorrhagic necrosis may occur, and scattered mitotic figures can be seen. Neither these features nor nuclear pleomorphism are of prognostic significance {4229}.

The neuroendocrine cells are immunoreactive for chromogranin A and synaptophysin {2977,2335,4229} and show

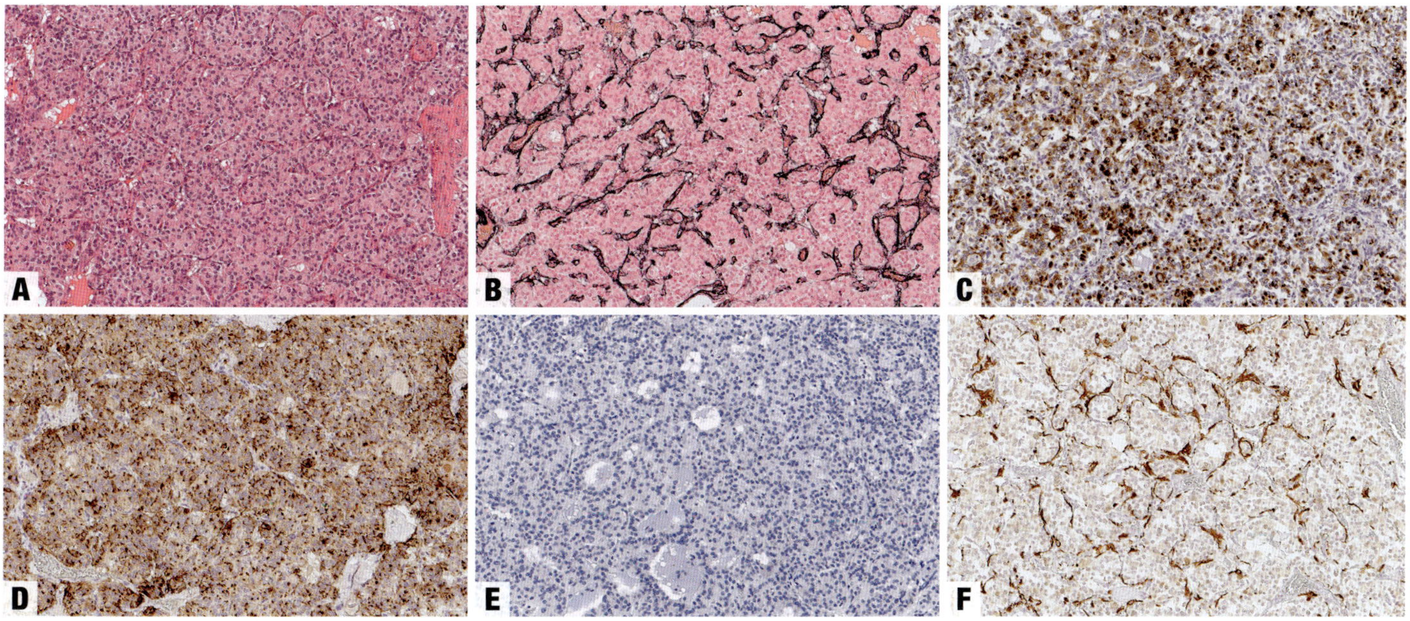

Fig. 8.18 Cauda equina neuroendocrine tumour (NET). **A** Nests of uniform round or polygonal chief cells surrounded by a capillary and fibre network. **B** The nests of tumour cells are surrounded by a delicate supporting reticulin fibre network (reticulin silver stain). **C** Cytokeratin is expressed in most tumours (MNF116). **D** Chromogranin A immunostaining labels the neuroendocrine (chief) cells. **E** These tumours do not express GATA3. **F** S100 immunohistochemistry labels the sustentacular cells, encompassing the lobules.

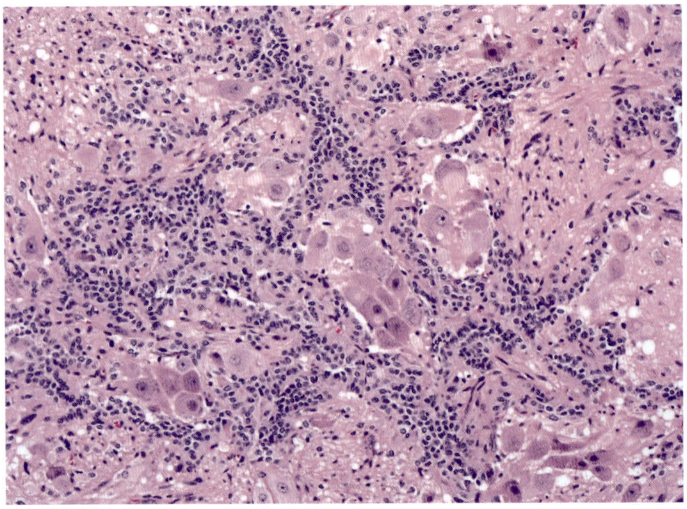

Fig. 8.19 Gangliocytic cauda equina neuroectodermal tumour. This example featured extensive ganglion cell differentiation with associated neuropil-rich stroma, interspersed with nests and ribbons of small round to polygonal neuroendocrine cells.

variable S100 immunoreactivity. Immunoreactivity for cytokeratins (especially CAM5.2, AE1/AE3, and MNF116) has been described in a majority of these lesions {4306,3361,796,1693, 2977,1092,3670}. Furthermore, gangliocytic tumours containing a variable mixture of epithelioid neuroendocrine cells, Schwann-like cells, and scattered ganglion-like cells can show cytokeratin positivity in the epithelioid cells {3638,4085}. Expression of serotonin (5-HT) and of various neuropeptides (somatostatin, gastrin, calcitonin, PP, PYY, leu-enkephalin, and met-enkephalin) has been demonstrated {4229,3086}.

Sustentacular cells show inconsistent S100 reactivity {4199, 4587} and occasionally express GFAP {4240}; the latter may also highlight a thin rim of peripheral non-neoplastic tissue. They often express the neural crest transcription factor SOX10 {3284}. The value of proliferation markers has not been established.

Although previously considered to be paragangliomas, unlike paragangliomas of the autonomic nervous system, these tumours do not express the zinc finger transcription factor GATA3 {4199,215}. They express HOXB13 (a transcription factor that is developmentally expressed in progenitor cells of the caudal spinal cord {449,215}), a feature they share with myxopapillary ependymoma {449}. A minority express SATB2 {215}.

Cytology

Not reported

Diagnostic molecular pathology

DNA methylation and chromosomal copy-number profiles of cauda equina NETs are distinct from paragangliomas {3670, 4037}.

Essential and desirable diagnostic criteria

Essential: a well-demarcated tumour with nested architecture; synaptophysin and chromogranin immunoreactivity; cauda equina / filum terminale location; methylation profile (in selected cases).

Staging

Not relevant

Prognosis and prediction

The vast majority of cauda equina NETs are slow-growing and curable by total excision; only 4% recur after gross total removal {4306}. Cerebrospinal fluid seeding has occasionally been documented {4306,3775,4464,4491}.

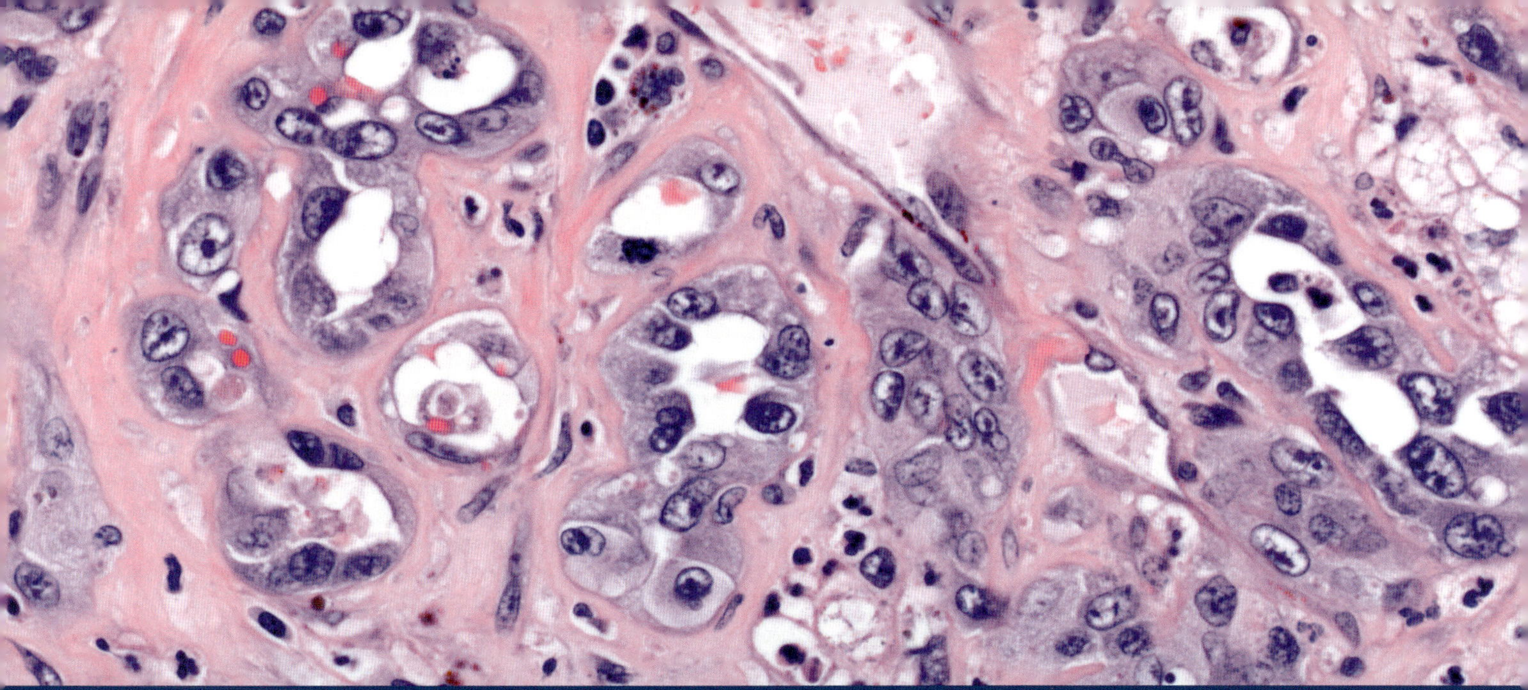

9

Mesenchymal and stromal tumours

Edited by: Hyrcza MD, Lazar AJ, Tallini G

Mesenchymal and stromal tumours: Introduction

Hyrcza MD

Although most tumours of the endocrine organs are of epithelial origin, a wide variety of mesenchymal tumours can also occur. Only the most commonly encountered tumours are discussed in this chapter. For entities not found, please refer to the fifth-edition *Soft tissue and bone tumours* volume of this series. For the more detailed classification and descriptions of fibromas and haemangiomas, please refer to the *Skin tumours* volume. Radiographic and cytological characteristics of the mesenchymal lesions may mimic epithelial tumours and therefore they should always be considered in the differential diagnosis. As seen in Table 9.01, the thyroid is the organ with the greatest variety of mesenchymal tumour types reported. Many such tumours have also been reported in the adrenal, pituitary, and pancreas, whereas few have been detected in the parathyroid glands.

Table 9.01 The mesenchymal lesions listed in this chapter and the endocrine organs in which they have been reported

Lesion	Pituitary	Thyroid	Parathyroid	Adrenal
Lipoma	×	✓ (thyrolipoma)	✓ (lipoadenoma)	✓ {2508}
Solitary fibrous tumour	✓ {1467}	✓ {4488}	×	✓ {3612}
PEComa	✓ {2007}	× {4859}	×	✓ {5120}
Glomangioma and glomus tumour	✓ {3647}	✓ {853}	×	×
Angiosarcoma	✓ {531}	✓ {2249}	×	✓ {1265}
Leiomyoma	×	✓ {1274}	×	✓ {3896}
Leiomyosarcoma	✓ {1699}	✓ {3416}	×	✓ {3896}
Rhabdomyosarcoma	✓ {1699}	✓ {1345}	×	✓ {4775}
Schwannoma	✓ {3089}	✓ {3416}	×	✓ {5170}
Neurofibroma	×	✓ {137}	×	✓ {1712}
Granular cell tumour	✓ {2973}	✓ {3005}	×	×
MPNST	✓ {1708}	✓ {3416}	×	✓ {3893}

✓, reported; ×, not reported; MPNST malignant peripheral nerve sheath tumour; PEComa, perivascular epithelioid cell tumour.

Lipoma

Fritchie KJ
Rossi S

Definition
Lipoma is a benign neoplasm of mature adipocytes.

ICD-O coding
8850/0 Lipoma, NOS

ICD-11 coding
2E80.0Z Lipoma

Related terminology
None

Subtype(s)
None

Localization
Lipomas may arise in the adrenal gland and pancreas {5154, 2512,2508,4961,2586,421}. Pancreatic lipomas most commonly arise in the head, followed by the body and tail {581,4961}. Lipomas have not been described in the thyroid. The term "thyroid lipoadenoma" (thyrolipoma; adenolipoma) indicates a subtype of follicular adenoma containing a variable amount of mature adipose tissue (see *Follicular thyroid adenoma*, p. 122). Rare cases of diffuse fat infiltration throughout the thyroid parenchyma, i.e. thyrolipomatosis, have been also reported {1523, 2045}. For parathyroid lipoadenomas, see *Parathyroid lipoadenoma* (p. 213).

Clinical features
Most lipomas of the pancreas and adrenal gland are usually asymptomatic and incidentally discovered; a small subset of patients may report abdominal pain {2512,581}. Rare cases of pancreatic lipoma result in pancreatitis. CT shows a well-circumscribed, lobulated, purely fat-density mass.

Epidemiology
Adrenal lipomas are rare, accounting for < 1% of primary adrenal neoplasms {2512}. The proportion of pancreatic lipomas is even rarer (~0.01%) {581}. Both sexes are affected equally, and these tumours typically present in the sixth and seventh decades of life.

Etiology
Unknown

Pathogenesis
Most lipomas harbour translocations involving 12q13-q15, resulting in the fusion of *HMGA2* with a variety of gene partners, driving the pathogenesis of these tumours {4881}.

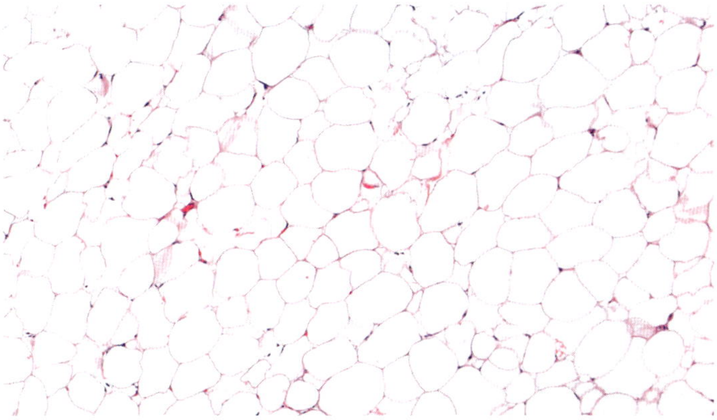

Fig. 9.01 Lipoma. Lipomas consist of mature adipocytes without fibrous septa or atypical hyperchromatic stromal cells.

Macroscopic appearance
Gross examination reveals a circumscribed mass with a homogeneous yellow cut surface. Most adrenal lipomas measure 50–100 mm but may reach sizes as large as 200 mm, whereas the average size of pancreatic lipomas is approximately 20 mm {2508,581}.

Histopathology
Histological review shows a sheet-like proliferation of mature adipocytes without atypical hyperchromatic stromal cells. Fat necrosis and dystrophic calcification may be present.

Cytology
Aspiration specimens show adipocytes containing a single large lipid droplet with a compressed rim of cytoplasm and a flattened, inconspicuous nucleus.

Diagnostic molecular pathology
FISH studies for *MDM2* amplification may be helpful in excluding well-differentiated liposarcoma {4172,4831,876}.

Essential and desirable diagnostic criteria
Essential: a circumscribed yellow mass; a uniform proliferation of mature adipose tissue; no atypical hyperchromatic stromal cells.
Desirable: an absence of *MDM2* amplification by FISH (in selected cases).

Staging
Not clinically relevant

Prognosis and prediction
Lipomas are benign. Surgical excision is generally reserved for symptomatic lesions.

Solitary fibrous tumour

Demicco EG
Thompson LDR
Wenig BM

Definition

Solitary fibrous tumour (SFT) is a fibroblastic mesenchymal tumour characterized by *NAB2::STAT6* gene rearrangement.

ICD-O coding

8815/0 Solitary fibrous tumour, benign
8815/1 Solitary fibrous tumour, NOS
8815/1 Fat-forming (lipomatous) solitary fibrous tumour
8815/1 Giant cell–rich solitary fibrous tumour
8815/3 Solitary fibrous tumour, malignant

ICD-11 coding

2F7C & XH7E62 Neoplasms of uncertain behaviour of connective or other soft tissue & Solitary fibrous tumour, NOS
2B5Y & XH1HP3 Other specified malignant mesenchymal neoplasms & Solitary fibrous tumour, malignant

Related terminology

Acceptable: extrapleural solitary fibrous tumour.
Not recommended: haemangiopericytoma; giant cell angiofibroma; benign solitary fibrous tumour.

Subtype(s)

Fat-forming (lipomatous) solitary fibrous tumour; giant cell–rich solitary fibrous tumour

Localization

SFTs can develop at any anatomical site, but within endocrine organs (a rare location) they most commonly involve the thyroid gland {2371,4488,4326} or pituitary fossa {694,2282,1467}, with only rare reports in other endocrine organs {1909,2825,1524, 1529,2631}.

Clinical features

Symptoms are nonspecific, and SFTs usually present as slow-growing, painless masses {4488}. Large tumours may cause mass effect or obstructive symptoms. Paraneoplastic syndromes have been reported, such as Doege–Potter syndrome, with the induction of severe hypoglycaemia or (more rarely) acromegaloid changes due to tumour production of IGF2 {783,1027}.

Imaging

Radiographic features are nonspecific, with CT showing heterogeneous contrast enhancement {2260,5069}, whereas MRI shows intermediate T1 intensity and variable T2 intensity corresponding to fibrous and cellular or myxoid tumour components {2260,1358}.

Epidemiology

There is an equal sex distribution, with a peak incidence between 50 and 60 years of age {1081,4032,3904,1082,1548, 1441,4488,1728}.

Etiology

Unknown

Pathogenesis

Paracentric inversion involving chromosome 12q, resulting in the fusion of *NAB2* and *STAT6* {821,3057,3771}, is pathognomonic of SFT.

Macroscopic appearance

SFTs are well circumscribed and usually measure 50–100 mm, but they may be larger.

Histopathology

SFTs are unencapsulated and variably cellular, with a patternless architecture interspersed with loosely to densely collagenized or myxoid stroma. Tumours are highly vascular, with dilated round to angulated branching blood vessels, which may be hyalinized. Cells are ovoid to spindled and typically monotonous, with bland nuclear features and few mitotic figures. Features suggestive of aggressive clinical behaviour include increased

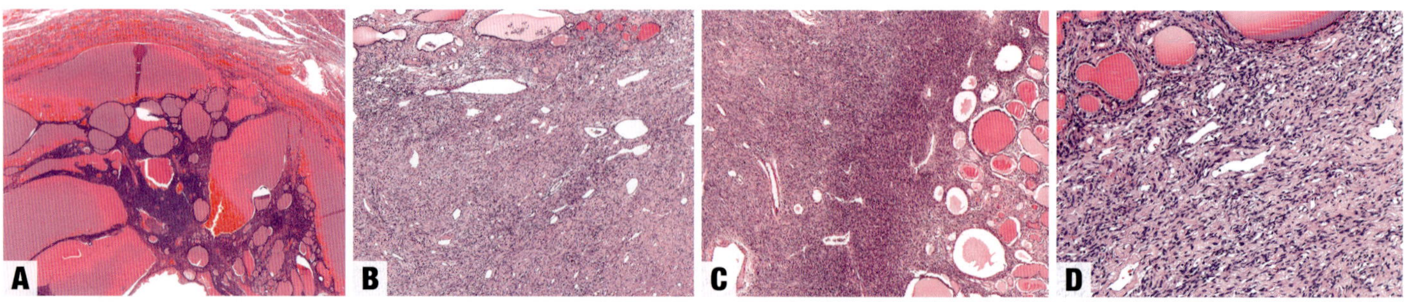

Fig. 9.02 Solitary fibrous tumour. **A** A well-defined mass is identified within the thyroid gland parenchyma. There is a spindled cell proliferation set within thyroid gland follicles. **B** Entrapped thyroid follicles are noted at the periphery, whereas patulous, open vessels are identified in the spindled cell neoplastic proliferation. Collagenized stroma is present. **C** There is a hypercellular spindled cell proliferation, showing tight, short bundles, meandering between the thyroid follicles, with open, patulous vessels easily identified. **D** Entrapped thyroid follicles are seen at the periphery of the spindled cell proliferation. There is a background collagenized stroma.

mitotic activity and necrosis. Metastatic presentations of SFT in endocrine organs have been reported {3464,3371,2371}.

Subtypes

Lipomatous (fat-forming) SFT harbours a component of mature adipose tissue {1395,1701,3239,788}. Giant cell–rich SFT has multinucleated giant cells within the stroma and lining pseudovascular spaces {1058,1702}. Dedifferentiated (anaplastic) SFT, although not yet reported in endocrine organs, shows transition to high-grade sarcoma with or without heterologous elements {2790,3106,4314,892,4493,2870,55,4422}.

Immunohistochemistry

By immunohistochemistry, SFT typically shows strong and diffuse cytoplasmic expression with CD34 and nuclear STAT6 {4036,1151,1080}, but expression may be lost in dedifferentiated SFT or embolized tumours {3106,892,963,4013}.

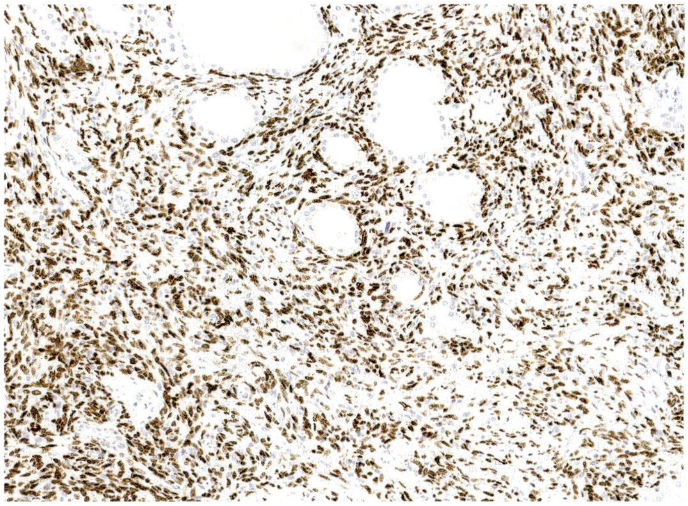

Fig. 9.03 Solitary fibrous tumour. The neoplastic cells show strong and diffuse nuclear immunoreactivity for STAT6, whereas the nuclei of the native thyroid follicles are negative.

Cytology

Smears are cellular, with loosely cohesive clusters around blood vessels or dispersed cells with bare nuclei. The cells are oval, elongated, or rounded, with wispy cytoplasm and eosinophilic collagenous stroma {3452,3050,4417,3830}.

Diagnostic molecular pathology

Molecular assays may be insensitive for the diverse *NAB2*::*STAT6* fusion types. Conventional cytogenetic methods are not recommended, because of the small size of the inversion, but STAT6 immunohistochemistry is a sensitive and specific surrogate for all fusion types {4036,1151,2364}.

Essential and desirable diagnostic criteria

Essential: spindled to ovoid cells arranged around a branching vasculature; variable stromal collagen deposition; demonstration of CD34 and/or STAT6 expression by immunohistochemistry.

Desirable: NAB2::*STAT6* fusion (in selected cases).

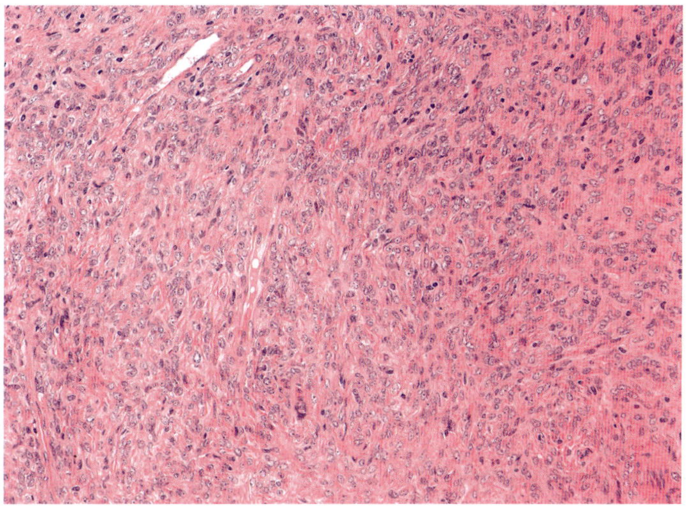

Fig. 9.04 Solitary fibrous tumour. Tumour involving the pituitary.

Staging

Multivariable risk-stratification models are preferred over staging.

Prognosis and prediction

Recurrence (distant or local) occurs in 10–30% of SFTs, often after a long latency (> 5 years) {1081,1548,3904,3456,1441, 2922,4640,1538}. Risk stratification based on multivariable models may be applied in order to aid management {1538, 1081,4652,3456,3904,1548}; most are site-agnostic. The most widely used multivariate model for metastatic risk incorporates mitotic count (> 2 mitoses/mm^2, equating to ≥ 4 mitoses/10 HPF of 0.55 mm in diameter and 0.24 mm^2 in area), patient age (≥ 55 years), and tumour size stratified by 50 mm tiers, with or without the additional variable of necrosis, to classify tumours into low-risk, intermediate-risk, and high-risk groups {1081, 1082,3717,1079}. Secondary *TERT* promoter mutations {55,263, 2669,1083} and *TP53* loss {4314,2456,55,963} may be associated with disease progression.

Benign vascular tumours

Hyrcza MD
Calonje JE

Definition

Benign vascular tumours encompass a variety of haemangiomas, lymphangiomas, and vascular malformations. These tumours are characterized by proliferation of mature blood vessels or lymphatics.

ICD-O coding

9120/0 Haemangioma, NOS
9131/0 Capillary haemangioma
9131/0 Lobular capillary haemangioma
9121/0 Cavernous haemangioma
9131/0 Infantile haemangioma
9122/0 Venous haemangioma
9123/0 Arteriovenous haemangioma
9125/0 Epithelioid haemangioma
9170/0 Lymphangioma, NOS

ICD-11 coding

2F37.Y & XH5AW4 Other specified benign neoplasm of endocrine glands & Haemangioma, NOS
2F37.Y & XH3U29 Other specified benign neoplasm of endocrine glands & Capillary haemangioma
2F37.Y & XH1GU2 Other specified benign neoplasm of endocrine glands & Cavernous haemangioma
2F37.Y & XH4NS3 Other specified benign neoplasm of endocrine glands & Venous haemangioma
2F37.Y & XH9MR8 Other specified benign neoplasm of endocrine glands & Lymphangioma, NOS

Related terminology

None

Subtype(s)

Haemangiomas

Capillary haemangioma; lobular capillary haemangioma; cavernous haemangioma; infantile haemangioma; venous haemangioma; arteriovenous haemangioma; epithelioid haemangioma

Arteriovenous malformations

Lymphangioma; lymphangiomatosis; papillary endothelial hyperplasia

Localization

Benign vascular lesions have been described in the thyroid {3550,3754,2585,1508}, parathyroid {2945,4351,3230,4198}, adrenal glands {5161}, and pituitary {3941,1650,993,2517}.

Clinical features

Adrenal vascular tumours are unilateral, and patients present most commonly with abdominal, flank, or back pain (in about half of cases) and non-refractory hypertension (in about a quarter of cases) {5161}. Sellar haemangiomas often mimic a non-functioning pituitary neuroendocrine tumour (PitNET) and present with headache, hypopituitarism, and (rarely) pituitary apoplexy {993}. Cranial nerve palsies can be seen when lesions involve the cavernous sinus {993}. Thyroid haemangiomas tend to present as an asymptomatic thyroid nodule {996,2986}. Occasionally, fast growth and calcification may mimic thyroid carcinoma {2986}. Of the 5 reported parathyroid haemangiomas, 3 have been found incidentally during surgery for parathyroid adenoma causing hyperparathyroidism, 1 case presented with acute unilateral neck swelling and pain with swallowing {3230}, and 1 case was a retropharyngeal tumour found incidentally on MRI {4198}.

Epidemiology

Benign vascular tumours of endocrine organs are rare, with most cases reported in the adrenal {5161,4572}, followed by the thyroid, pituitary, and parathyroid glands. Patients of any age can be affected, with congenital cases described {2076}. In one series of 17 adrenal haemangiomas, the mean age at diagnosis was 65 years (range: 48–87 years) {5161}. In a series of adrenal lymphangiomas, the mean age at presentation was 42 years (range: 28–56 years) {1225}.

Etiology

Many haemangiomas and lymphangiomas are probably non-neoplastic vascular malformations. Most are solitary and sporadic. Congenital vascular lesions of the thyroid have been documented, including arteriovenous malformations and infantile haemangiomas {2076}.

Pathogenesis

Lymphangioma / lymphatic malformations have been linked to mutations in *FLT4* (*VEGFR3*) {1373,1374} and *FOXC2* {1328}.

Macroscopic appearance

Haemangiomas tend to present grossly as red or dark-brown spongy tumours. Phleboliths may be seen. Adrenal lymphangiomas show multiloculated cysts without papillary excrescences, filled with non-viscous, clear, yellow to brown fluid {1225}.

Histopathology

Haemangiomas of endocrine organs tend to be of cavernous, venous, and capillary types {2986}, with other subtypes reported rarely. All haemangiomas show multiple vascular channels but differ in their calibre, wall thickness, and size. Cavernous haemangiomas are composed of multiple thin-walled, large-diameter, blood-filled channels lined by endothelial cells lacking atypia and multilayering, and separated by scant connective tissue stroma. Venous haemangiomas consist of veins of various sizes, often with thick muscular walls, frequently containing thrombi and occasionally phleboliths. Venous haemangiomas with widely dilated vessels can mimic cavernous

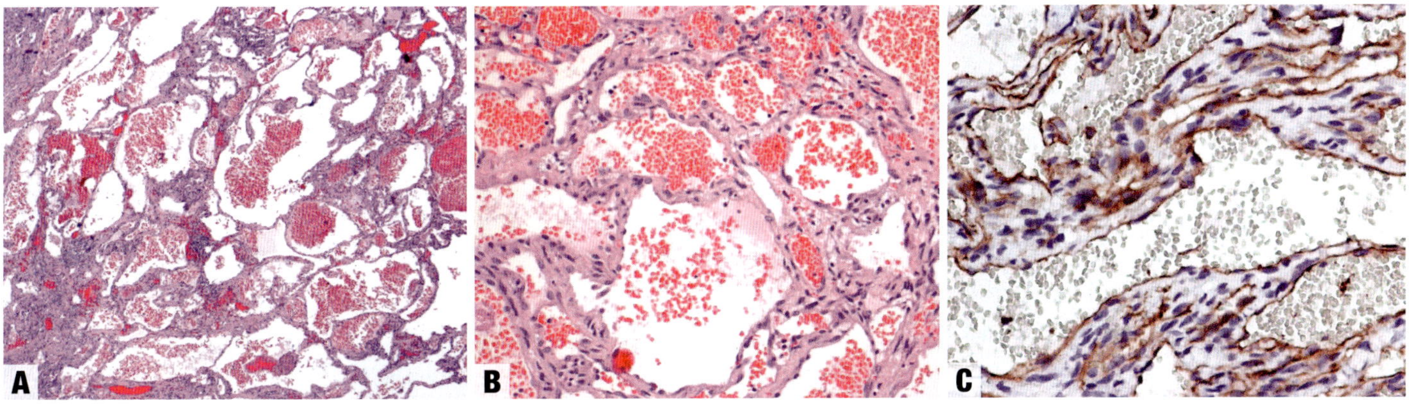

Fig. 9.05 Thyroid haemangioma. **A** In some cases, cavernous vascular spaces predominate. **B** At higher magnification, the endothelial cells lack cytological atypia. **C** There is strong and diffuse CD31 immunoreactivity in endothelial cells.

haemangioma. Arteriovenous malformations show a variety of vessels of different sizes, including veins and arteries, and occasionally lymphatics. Veins typically predominate. Thrombosis and calcification can be seen. Lymphangiomas show dilated thin-walled vascular channels with empty-appearing lumina and occasional small, delicate valves. Adrenal haemangiomas and lymphangiomas may contain fat tissue {4437} and in rare cases may coexist with other adrenal tumours such as cortical adenomas {1408}. In the thyroid gland, vascular tumours must be distinguished from papillary endothelial hyperplasia secondary to FNA {246}, which can occasionally resemble cavernous haemangioma {4572}, and from papillary endothelial hyperplasia within or around the capsule of thyroid nodules {3419}. The latter has been associated with the production of lymphangiogenic factors by proliferating follicular cells {4011}.

Histochemistry

Elastin stains may help to distinguish between arteries, which contain elastic lamina, and veins, which usually do not.

Immunohistochemistry

Endothelial cells in haemangiomas and vascular malformations show immunoreactivity for CD34, CD31, FLI1, and ERG. They are negative for D2-40, keratin, and KSHV/HHV8. Infantile haemangiomas are positive for GLUT1, which distinguishes this subtype from other haemangiomas, although positive staining can also be seen in arteriovenous malformations {4550}. Lymphatic endothelial cells show characteristic podoplanin immunoreactivity recognized by D2-40.

Cytology

Not relevant

Diagnostic molecular pathology

None

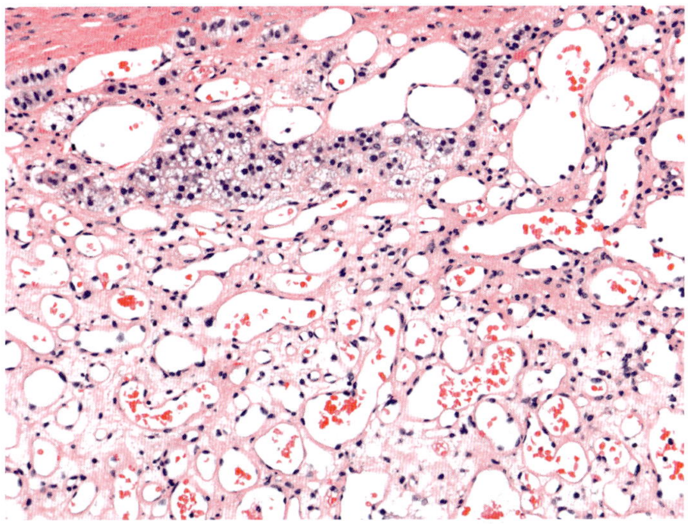

Fig. 9.06 Haemangioma of the adrenal cortex. Well-developed vascular channels are intermixed with adrenal cortical cells.

Essential and desirable diagnostic criteria

Essential: a tumour-forming proliferation of vascular channels lined by endothelial cells lacking atypia.

Staging

Not applicable

Prognosis and prediction

Benign vascular lesions are cured with complete surgical resection, but completeness of removal may not be achievable in certain locations such as the pituitary or with extensive tumours. Recurrences are common in incompletely resected cases {476}.

PEComa

Doyle LA
Argani P
Hyrcza MD

Definition

Perivascular epithelioid cell tumour (PEComa) is a mesenchymal neoplasm composed of perivascular epithelioid cells (PECs) – distinctive epithelioid cells that are often closely associated with blood vessel walls and express both melanocytic and smooth muscle markers.

ICD-O coding

8714/0 Perivascular epithelioid tumour, benign
8714/3 Perivascular epithelioid tumour, malignant
8860/0 Angiomyolipoma
8860/1 Angiomyolipoma, epithelioid

ICD-11 coding

2F7C & XH4CC6 Neoplasms of uncertain behaviour of connective or other soft tissue & Perivascular epithelioid tumour, benign
2B5F.2 & XH9WD1 Sarcoma, not elsewhere classified, of other specified sites & Perivascular epithelioid tumour, malignant

Related terminology

Acceptable: angiomyolipoma; epithelioid angiomyolipoma; lymphangioleiomyomatosis.
Not recommended: clear cell myomelanocytic tumour.

Subtype(s)

Perivascular epithelioid tumour, benign; perivascular epithelioid tumour, malignant; angiomyolipoma; angiomyolipoma, epithelioid

Localization

PEComas show a wide anatomical distribution but are extremely rare in the thyroid, pituitary, pancreas, and adrenal glands {2512,2944,1400,2653,5007,2542,1150,2007,387,4618}.

Clinical features

Clinical presentation is site-dependent; many PEComas of endocrine organs are incidentally detected radiologically, but some present as a mass or with endocrine dysfunction, depending on the site of involvement {2403,1436}.

Epidemiology

PEComas are rare and show a female predilection (M:F ratio: ~0.2:1), with a wide age range and a peak in young to middle-aged adults (mean age: 45 years) {1397,1400,1941,1150}.

Etiology

Most PEComas are sporadic; a small subset are associated with tuberous sclerosis {462,1400,1941}.

Pathogenesis

Loss of heterozygosity involving the *TSC2* locus has been found {3396}. Deletion of 16p, the location of the *TSC2* gene, indicates the oncogenetic relationship of PEComas and angiomyolipomas as *TSC2*-linked neoplasms. *TP53* mutations have been identified in 63% of *TSC2*-mutated PEComas {34}. A small subset of PEComas harbour *TFE3* gene fusions, correlating with strong nuclear immunoreactivity for TFE3 {174}. The most common fusion partner of *TFE3* is *SFPQ* (*PSF*) {4409, 34,3678}. *DVL2::TFE3* and *NONO::TFE3* gene fusions have also been identified in PEComas arising in soft tissues {175}. *TFE3*-rearranged PEComa lacks *TSC2* mutations / loss of heterozygosity and thus appears to be pathogenetically distinct {2816,34}. The molecular alterations found in PEComas are associated with an aberrant increase in mTOR pathway signalling {3504}.

Macroscopic appearance

PEComas are grossly well circumscribed, with a firm and fibrous or fleshy cut surface. Tumours show a wide size range (mean: 50–80 mm) {1400,1150,387}.

Histopathology

PEComas typically show a nested architecture and are composed of epithelioid cells with abundant granular eosinophilic or clear cytoplasm and round nuclei with small nucleoli. The

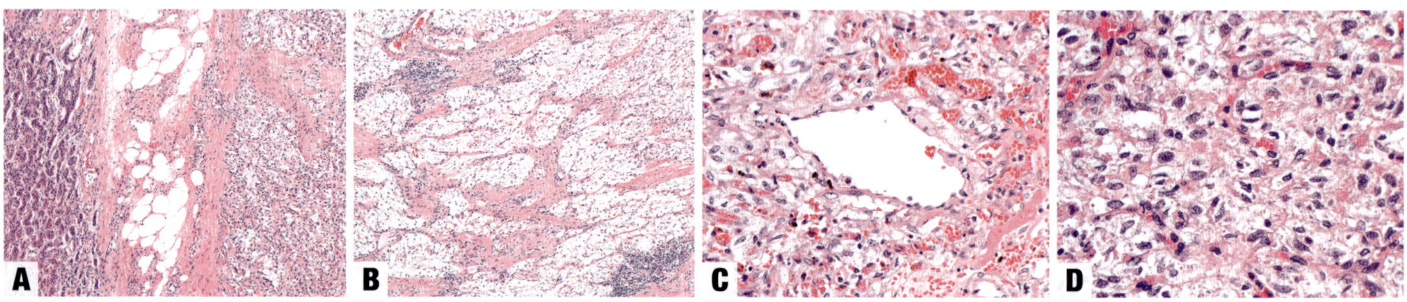

Fig. 9.07 PEComa of the adrenal gland. **A** The neoplasm is well circumscribed, and adrenal cortex can be seen to the left. **B** A nested growth pattern is characteristic of PEComa. The stroma may be collagenous or hyalinized. **C** The tumour cells are characteristically arranged around blood vessels, often approximating the endothelium. **D** The cells may be spindled or epithelioid, are typically bland, and have variable amounts of clear or granular eosinophilic cytoplasm.

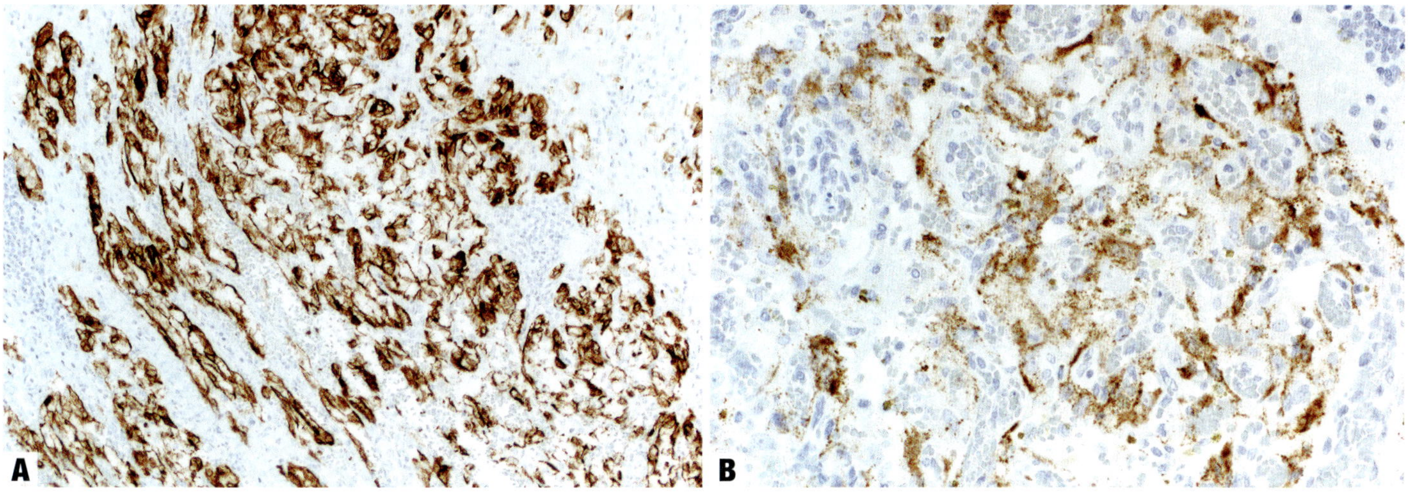

Fig. 9.08 PEComa of the adrenal gland. **A** Strong diffuse desmin expression in neoplastic cells. **B** Focal expression of HMB45 in neoplastic cells.

nests or trabeculae are typically surrounded by thin-walled capillary vessels. A small subset of tumours have predominantly spindle cell morphology {1400,1150}. PEComa usually shows a distinctive perivascular pattern of growth, with tumour cells radially arranged around vessels, replacing the vessel wall and approaching the endothelium. Epithelioid angiomyolipoma is synonymous with PEComa {247,534}. Typical PEComa may contain occasional multinucleated cells and show limited pleomorphism (symplastic change), but mitotic figures are usually scarce or absent.

Within the adrenal gland, angiomyolipoma is the most common subtype of PEComa and is composed of variable amounts of mature fat, bland spindle cells with granular eosinophilic cytoplasm, and branching thin- and thick-walled vessels.

Malignant PEComas are characterized by a variable combination of mitotic activity, necrosis, and pleomorphism {462,1400, 1150,387}.

Immunohistochemistry

PEComas characteristically express both melanocytic markers (e.g. HMB45, the most sensitive immunomarker; melan-A; and MITF) and muscle markers (e.g. SMA, desmin, and caldesmon {2805,1941,1398,1150,387}. Expression of melanocytic markers is more common in epithelioid cells than spindled tumour cells. Desmin and h-caldesmon are often less extensively positive than SMA {1941}. Some tumours lack expression of muscle markers {1398}. Nuclear expression of S100 is generally not observed in PEComas. Approximately 15% of cases show strong nuclear staining for TFE3 {1400,174,1150,175}. PEComas with *TFE3* rearrangement tend to occur in younger patients, have a prominent alveolar growth pattern and epithelioid morphology, and often lack expression of smooth muscle markers {2816,34,3678,175}.

Cytology

Not clinically relevant

Diagnostic molecular pathology

For cases with strong TFE3 protein expression, identification of *TFE3* gene rearrangement or a corresponding fusion gene can help confirm the diagnosis.

Essential and desirable diagnostic criteria

Essential: epithelioid and/or spindle cells with granular eosinophilic to clear cytoplasm; nested, trabecular, or sheet-like architecture with frequent perivascular orientation; variable coexpression of melanocytic and smooth muscle markers.

Desirable: TFE3 expression if smooth muscle markers are negative.

Staging

Not clinically relevant

Prognosis and prediction

Typically, malignant tumours are large; show marked nuclear atypia and pleomorphism, conspicuous mitoses, necrosis, and infiltrative margins; and tend to pursue an aggressive clinical course {1400,387}. Tumour size > 50 mm has been significantly associated with recurrence {443}. The most common metastatic sites are the liver, lymph nodes, lungs, and bone {1400,1150, 387}. Patients with unresectable/advanced malignant PEComas may respond to mTOR inhibitors {3504}.

Glomangioma and glomus tumour

Hyrcza MD

Definition

Glomangioma and glomus tumour are mesenchymal neoplasms composed of cells with features of the modified smooth muscle cells of the normal glomus body.

ICD-O coding

8711/0 Glomus tumour, benign
8711/1 Glomangiomatosis
8711/1 Glomus tumour of uncertain malignant potential
8711/3 Glomus tumour, malignant

ICD-11 coding

2E81.0Y Glomangioma

Related terminology

Glomus tumour
Acceptable: glomangioma; glomangiomyoma.

Malignant glomus tumour
Acceptable: glomangiosarcoma.

Subtype(s)

Oncocytic glomus tumour {4182}; epithelioid glomus tumour {3630}; myxoid glomus tumour {2648}; signet ring glomus tumour {1775}; hyalinized glomus tumour {4703}; symplastic glomus tumour {1396}; glomangiomatosis {1396}; glomus tumour of uncertain malignant potential {1396}; benign glomus tumour; malignant glomus tumour {1396}; glomuvenous malformation

Localization

Glomus tumours arise most commonly in the skin and soft tissues, especially in the distal extremities {1396,4134,4285}; however, they can also rarely occur in visceral locations, including endocrine organs. Cases have been reported in the pituitary {204,1766,1200,4571,3647}, thyroid {853,2697}, and pancreas {3006,4396}, but not in the adrenal or the parathyroid.

Clinical features

Cutaneous glomus tumours typically present as solitary, painful, pink to blue nodules, whereas glomuvenous malformations are typically larger and more common in patients with multiple or familial lesions {543}. The 6 cases reported in the pituitary presented with headache, decreased visual acuity, intermittent diplopia, bitemporal hemianopia, and panhypopituitarism {204,3647,1766,1200,4571}. All had suprasellar extension, with 4 cases also involving the cavernous sinus {3647}. The 2 reported thyroid cases presented initially as painless nodules, with 1 case progressing to a painful tumour {853,2697}. The pancreatic cases presented with postprandial epigastric and back pain, weight loss, episodic precordial pain, and vomiting {3006,4396}.

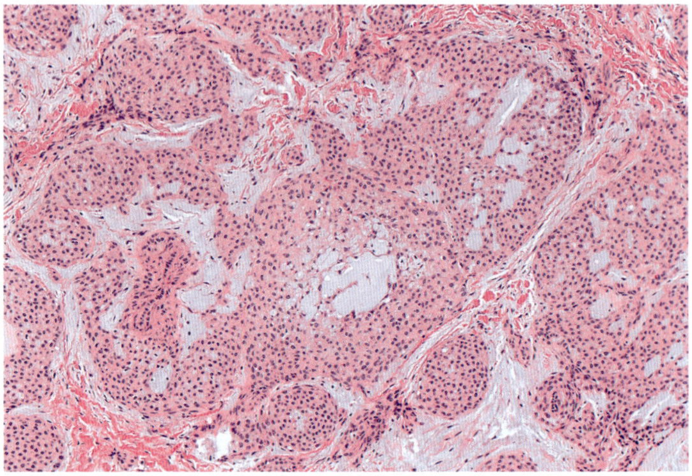

Fig. 9.09 Glomus tumour. Tumour composed of nests of cells surrounding capillaries and small vessels in a myxoid to hyalinized stroma.

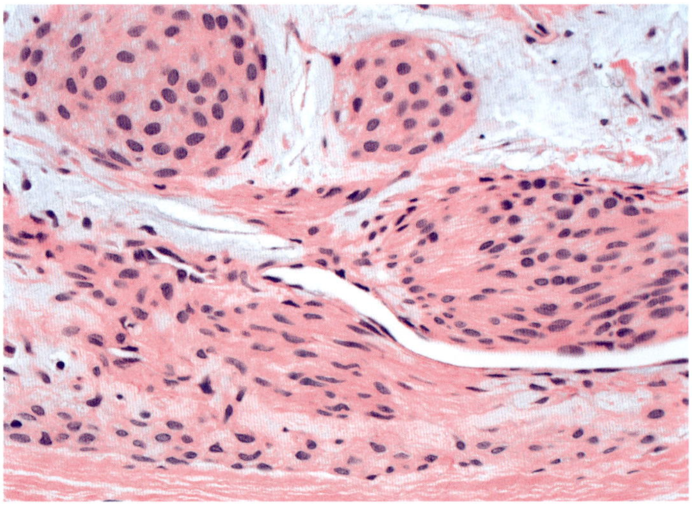

Fig. 9.10 Glomus tumour. Tumours are composed of small, uniform, round or polygonal cells with a central nucleus and amphophilic or eosinophilic cytoplasm.

Epidemiology

The pituitary cases occurred in patients aged 8–72 years; 3 patients were male and 3 were female {204,3647,1766,1200, 4571}. The 2 reported thyroid cases occurred in men aged 55 and 68 years {853,2697}. The pancreatic cases occurred in a 17-year-old girl and a 46-year-old woman {3006,4396}.

Etiology

Multiple familial glomus tumours are caused by inactivating mutations in *GLMN* (encoding glomulin), inherited in an autosomal dominant pattern {543}.

Pathogenesis

Inactivating mutations in *GLMN* (1p22.1) are associated with familial glomus tumours inherited in an autosomal dominant pattern {543}. Multiple digital glomus tumours have also been linked to neurofibromatosis type 1 {523,1799,1800}. NOTCH gene fusions were identified in about half of the cases, with *NOTCH2* rearranged in most (88%) and *NOTCH3* and *NOTCH1* in a minority {3107,35}. In about three quarters of these fusion tumours, the gene partner was the microRNA gene *MIR143* {35}. NOTCH fusions were seen in both benign and malignant glomus tumours and in both superficial and visceral cases {3107,35}. *BRAF* p.V600E mutations have been detected in 6% of glomus tumours, including 3 (12%) of 24 malignant tumours {2201}.

Macroscopic appearance

Glomus tumours tend to be grossly well circumscribed, even in malignant cases {4396}. Reported sellar cases were described as firm and rubbery {3647}.

Histopathology

Tumours are composed of small, uniform, round or polygonal cells with a central nucleus and amphophilic or eosinophilic cytoplasm. Cell borders may be well delineated or indistinct. Predominantly oncocytic {4182}, epithelioid (large cell) {3630}, and signet-ring cell {1775} subtypes have been described. The cells are typically arranged in nests surrounding capillaries and small vessels. Myxoid or hyalinized stroma may be seen in some cases {2648,4703}. Most tumours are solid, but a vascular component predominates in glomangiomas, glomangiomatosis, and glomuvenous malformations, with small nests of glomus cells present in vessel walls {5173}. Haemangiopericytoma-like vessels may also be seen {1665}. Spindle cells resembling smooth muscle are seen in a minority of cases (glomangiomyomas). The symplastic subtype displays degenerative nuclear atypia lacking mitotic activity and necrosis {1396,2168, 3933}. Malignant glomus tumours show atypical mitotic figures and/or a combination of high nuclear grade and mitotic activity (≥ 5 mitoses/10–11 mm^2) {1396,2519,5072}. They can arise from a benign precursor and may show leiomyosarcoma- or fibrosarcoma-like components.

Immunohistochemistry

A typical glomus tumour shows diffuse reactivity for SMA, with the majority of cases also showing MSA (recognized by HHF35), vimentin, pericellular collagen IV, caldesmon, SIRT1, and laminin staining. TLE1 expression has been reported in one study {508}. Synaptophysin expression may be present, a confounding factor in the differential diagnosis with neuroendocrine tumours (NETs) {4571,2993}. Tumours are negative for keratins, chromogranin A, CD56, S100, and KIT (CD117). CD34 highlights the endothelial cells but may be focally positive in the neoplastic glomus cells {1396,3121}. The Ki-67 labelling index in the pituitary cases ranged between 10% and 30% {3647}.

Cytology

Cytological reports of glomus tumours are infrequent and mostly describe cutaneous and superficial lesions. One report of a visceral glomus tumour described groups of cohesive, uniform, small, round to polygonal cells with scant cytoplasm, indistinct cell borders, and round, hyperchromatic nuclei with homogeneous chromatin {1045}.

Diagnostic molecular pathology

About half of glomus tumours harbour NOTCH gene fusions, with *NOTCH2* being involved most commonly (88%) and *MIR143* being the most common fusion partner (76%) {35}; however, these fusions are not entirely specific for glomus tumours because they have also been demonstrated in myopericytoma and angioleiomyoma {35}.

Essential and desirable diagnostic criteria

Essential: small, round to polygonal glomoid cells with central nuclei and diffuse SMA expression.
Desirable: pericellular collagen IV expression.

Staging

Malignant cases are staged by the staging criteria appropriate to the site in which they arise.

Prognosis and prediction

Most glomus tumours are benign and are cured by complete resection. Malignant glomus tumours are highly aggressive, with frequent metastases, often resulting in the death of the patient {1396}. Deep or visceral location is one of the proposed criteria for the diagnosis of glomus tumour of uncertain malignant potential {1396}, which would indicate that all endocrine organ glomus tumours have uncertain malignant potential. In line with this, among the 5 pituitary cases with available follow-up, all 5 recurred and 2 patients died of the disease {3647}. The 2 reported glomus tumours of the thyroid also behaved in a malignant fashion, with the patients developing metastases and dying from their disease, one at 30 months and one at 6 months after their initial diagnosis {853,2697}.

Angiosarcoma

Erickson LA
Bongiovanni M
Folpe AL
Piana S

Definition

Angiosarcoma is a highly malignant tumour showing endothelial differentiation.

ICD-O coding

9120/3 Angiosarcoma

ICD-11 coding

2B56.Y & XH6264 Angiosarcoma, other specified primary site & Haemangiosarcoma

Related terminology

Not recommended: malignant haemangioendothelioma; haemangiosarcoma.

Subtype(s)

None

Localization

Tumours primary to endocrine organs are often centred in the organ rather than involving the periphery of the organ secondarily.

Clinical features

Angiosarcoma of endocrine organs predominantly affects older patients, often those in their sixth or seventh decade of life {4851,531,1016}. Patients with thyroid angiosarcoma are more commonly female, whereas adrenal angiosarcoma affects both sexes similarly {4851}. Primary thyroid angiosarcoma may present as painless thyroid enlargement, or as a rapidly enlarging neck mass with compressive symptoms of dysphagia or dyspnoea. Paraneoplastic hypercalcaemia, transient increase of blood sugar, and leukocytosis are not uncommon {4342, 1016}. Patients with primary thyroid angiosarcoma often have a history of goitre {1016}. Primary adrenal angiosarcoma presents as an abdominal mass with or without pain, fever, weight loss, and weakness {4851}. Angiosarcoma involving the pituitary gland can be associated with panhypopituitarism and intracranial hypertension {531}. Primary angiosarcoma of the pancreas may present with nonspecific symptoms, abdominal epigastric pain, and nausea, and it can mimic acute pancreatitis {953,1332}. Pancreatic angiosarcoma has been reported as an incidental finding in an individual undergoing imaging for metastatic breast cancer {4938}.

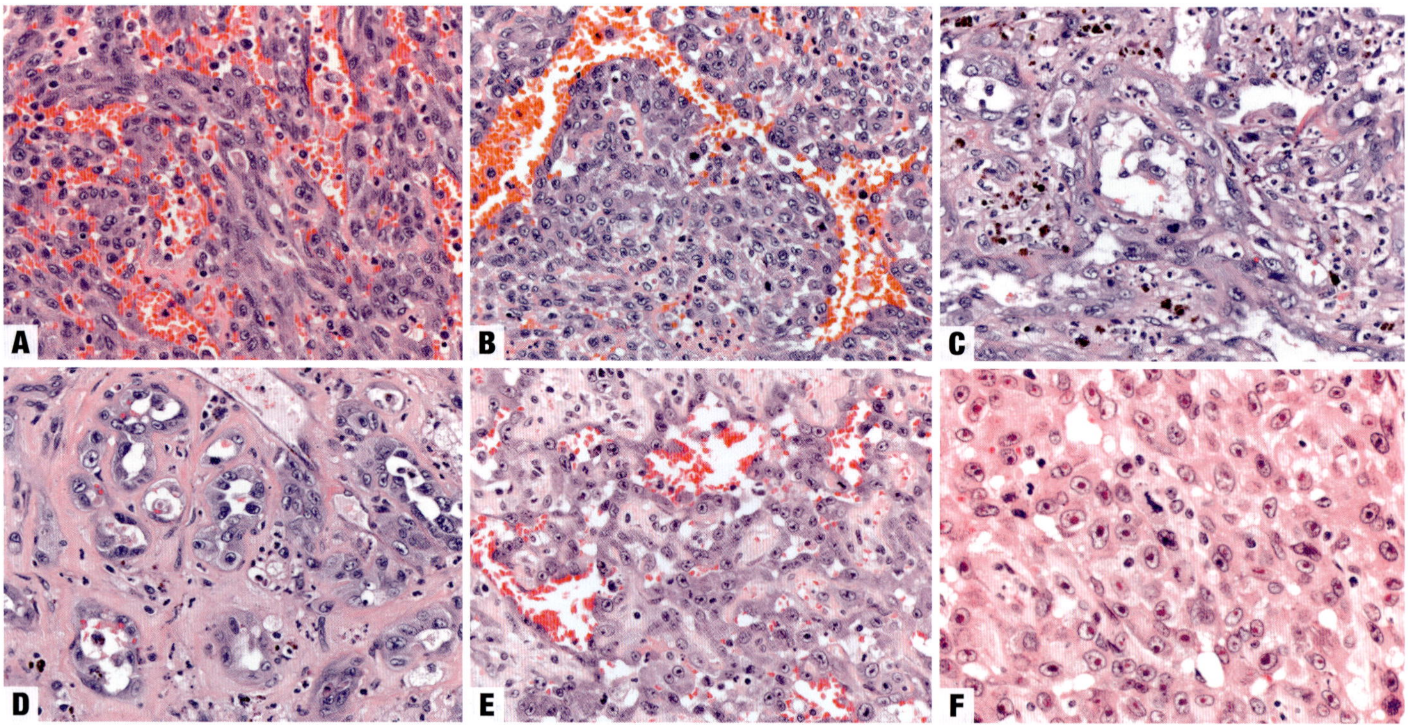

Fig. 9.11 Angiosarcoma. **A** This thyroid angiosarcoma is highly cellular, with a spindled growth pattern. **B** This angiosarcoma has areas of sheet-like growth and marked haemorrhage. **C** Prominent vasoformative features are present in this angiosarcoma in the thyroid. **D** Markedly epithelioid cells are seen lining vascular-like spaces in this angiosarcoma. **E** This primary adrenal angiosarcoma has prominent vasoformative features, helpful in recognizing the tumour as an angiosarcoma rather than an adrenal cortical carcinoma. **F** Primary angiosarcomas of endocrine organs usually have an epithelioid morphology, with epithelioid cells exhibiting large pleomorphic nuclei and prominent eosinophilic nucleoli.

Epidemiology

Angiosarcoma, the most common primary thyroid sarcoma, is a rare tumour {4342}. Older series have reported a relative high incidence in Alpine regions of Switzerland, Italy, and Austria, in association with endemic goitre {1016}. Adrenal angiosarcomas are very rare, without well-defined epidemiological characteristics. Sarcomas account for < 0.1% of all pancreatic malignancies, and fewer than 10 primary pancreatic angiosarcomas have been reported {4070,953,2925,989,4938,1332}. An exceptional example of pituitary angiosarcoma has also been reported {531}. With so few angiosarcomas reported in endocrine organs other than the thyroid, well-defined epidemiological characteristics for angiosarcomas at these sites have yet to be established.

Etiology

Iodine deficiency is a likely etiological factor for primary thyroid angiosarcoma, at least for cases that arise in longstanding goitres in areas where the goitre is endemic {1016}.

Pathogenesis

Primary thyroid angiosarcoma is a distinct entity. Although historically it was debated whether primary thyroid angiosarcoma was an angiomatoid subtype of anaplastic thyroid carcinoma rather than a true sarcoma with endothelial differentiation, thyroid angiosarcoma and anaplastic thyroid carcinoma are now regarded as two distinct and unrelated entities. Unlike anaplastic thyroid carcinoma, angiosarcomas of the thyroid harbour few mutations, and in particular they lack mutations of *TP53* and/or *TERT* {2442}. Because of the rarity of primary angiosarcomas of other endocrine organs, little is known about their pathogenesis and underlying genetic abnormalities.

Macroscopic appearance

Thyroid angiosarcomas may appear deceptively circumscribed, but they are invariably infiltrative lesions. Extension into adjacent structures is common {1291}. The cut surface is haemorrhagic and variegated, with cystic and solid areas which may be necrotic. Thyroid angiosarcomas range in size from 30 to 120 mm {2798,2442}. Adrenal angiosarcomas range from relatively small to massive, haemorrhagic masses {4851}. Angiosarcomas of the pancreas are variably sized and may involve any part of the gland {4070,953,2925,989,4938,1332}.

Histopathology

Angiosarcomas primary to endocrine organs have the same general features as angiosarcomas at any other anatomical site. They may be well-differentiated and vasoformative, or poorly differentiated, with chiefly epithelioid or spindled morphology. Diffusely infiltrative growth into surrounding non-neoplastic tissues is the rule. Although some cases have relatively subtle degrees of nuclear atypia, most are obviously malignant, with high nuclear grade and easily identified mitotic figures. Tumours with epithelioid differentiation display cells with abundant eosinophilic or amphophilic cytoplasm, large nuclei with well-defined nuclear membranes, and prominent nucleoli. They are common, and particularly well characterized in the thyroid gland {1291,1016,3419}. Predominantly epithelioid angiosarcomas may be easily confused with primary epithelial malignancies at all endocrine locations {531,1992}. Angiosarcoma of the thyroid may have surrounding areas of multinodular goitre and must be

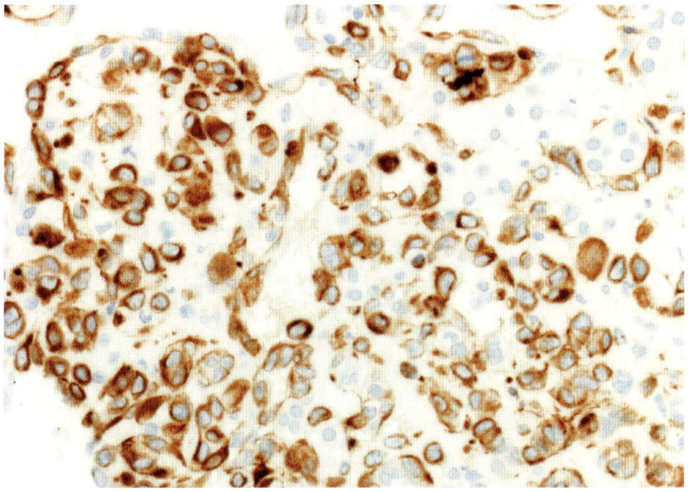

Fig. 9.12 Angiosarcoma, CAM5.2 immunostain. Angiosarcomas of endocrine organs are often epithelioid and frequently show immunopositivity for low-molecular-weight keratins such as CAM5.2.

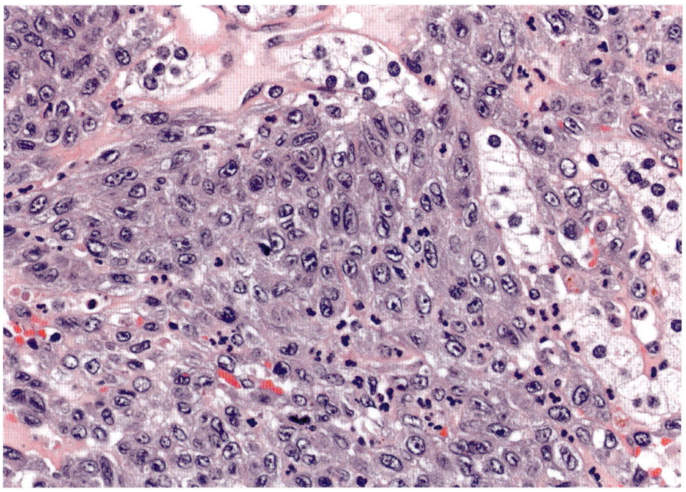

Fig. 9.13 Angiosarcoma. Focal residual adrenal cortical cells are identified in the background of this primary adrenal angiosarcoma that shows a sheet-like growth pattern.

distinguished from reactive vascular proliferation and anaplastic carcinoma {3419,2442}. Adrenal angiosarcomas have been misdiagnosed as adrenal cortical carcinomas and must also be distinguished from metastatic tumours {1186}.

Immunohistochemistry

Angiosarcomas express the panendothelial markers CD31, CD34, FLI1, von Willebrand factor (factor VIII–related antigen), and ERG, and they may be positive for the lymphatic marker podoplanin (D2-40). Expression of low-molecular-weight keratins is seen in approximately 50% of angiosarcomas, typically those with epithelioid features {1291,4851,953,531,1992,2442}. Angiosarcomas of the thyroid lack expression of thyroid-related markers (thyroglobulin, thyroid transcription factor 1 [TTF1], PAX8). Expression of MYC (c-myc) may occasionally be present but is not helpful in the distinction of angiosarcoma from non-vascular malignancies at endocrine sites {2442}. For the differential diagnosis, a panel of immunohistochemical markers including those of endothelial lineage, organ-specific markers (e.g. TTF1, pituitary hormones, pancreatic hormones), and endocrine/neuroendocrine markers (e.g. SF1, synaptophysin, chromogranin A) is essential.

Cytology

FNAB of angiosarcoma may be highly cellular, and there is often a bloody and variably necrotic background. Cells are arranged in loosely cohesive groups and can be spindled, plasmacytoid, or epithelioid with abundant cytoplasm; scattered binucleated cells with prominent nucleoli may be seen. Mitotic figures may be present. The diagnosis of angiosarcoma should be made with great caution in patients who have undergone prior FNAB, because biopsy-related reactive stromal changes can closely mimic a malignant vascular tumour {3419,1959}.

Diagnostic molecular pathology

Not clinically relevant

Essential and desirable diagnostic criteria

Essential: a malignant vascular neoplasm showing histological and/or immunohistochemical evidence of endothelial differentiation.

Staging

The Union for International Cancer Control (UICC) TNM staging system is used.

Prognosis and prediction

Primary angiosarcomas of endocrine organs are highly aggressive tumours, with rapid growth, extensive local invasion and infiltration of adjacent organs, regional and distant metastasis, and a poor outcome with death often within 6 months, although cases with long survival have been reported {3419,4342,1016}.

Leiomyoma

Wenig BM
Thompson LDR

Definition
Leiomyoma is a benign neoplasm with smooth muscle differentiation.

ICD-O coding
8890/0 Leiomyoma, NOS

ICD-11 coding
2E86.1 Leiomyoma of other or unspecified sites

Related terminology
None

Subtype(s)
None

Localization
The most common endocrine organ site for leiomyoma is the adrenal gland {3896}, followed by the thyroid gland {5150}.

Clinical features
Adrenal leiomyomas most often present with abdominal or flank pain/discomfort, and less often with weight loss, anorexia, and malaise {3896}. Symptom duration may be from 2 weeks to months or years {3896}. In general, adrenal leiomyomas manifest as hormonally non-functioning masses and are not associated with signs or symptoms of hormonal secretion. In some patients, the tumour was found incidentally during workup (e.g. imaging studies) for other unrelated symptoms or other conditions {964,2662,3077,1986}. The lack of specific imaging characteristics of these tumours makes them indistinguishable from other adrenal lesions, such as adrenal cortical adenoma, adrenal cortical carcinoma, or phaeochromocytoma, so often a diagnosis is established only after surgical excision {3896}. Thyroid leiomyoma presents as a painless, slow-growing mass that on thyroid scan appears as a cold nodule {4478,143,419,1860, 1274,3058,5150}. Thyroid function testing is normal.

Epidemiology
Primary leiomyomas of endocrine organs including the adrenal and thyroid are rare. Almost 50% of adrenal leiomyomas occur in HIV-positive patients {3896}. Adrenal leiomyomas occur over a wide age range, from the first {2111} to the eighth decade of life (median age: 34.5 years) {1986,3896}, and are more common in women than in men {3896}.

Thyroid leiomyomas are rare {4478,143,419,1860,1274,3058, 5150}. They occur over a wide age range, from the first to the seventh decade of life (median age: 45 years), and tend to be more common in women than in men {5150}.

Etiology
Unknown

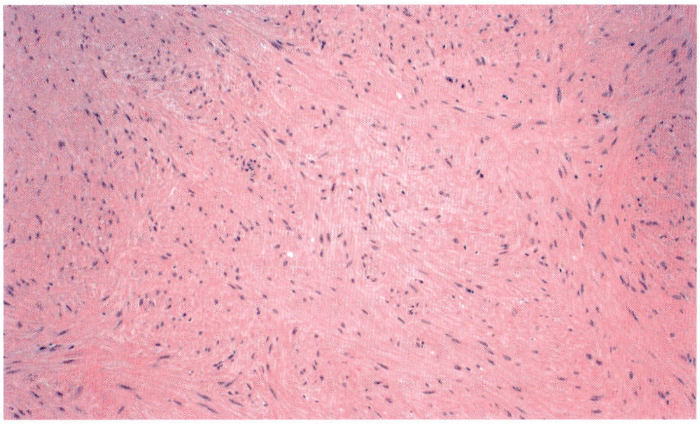

Fig. 9.14 Leiomyoma. This thyroid gland leiomyoma demonstrates hypocellular fascicles of spindled smooth muscle cells.

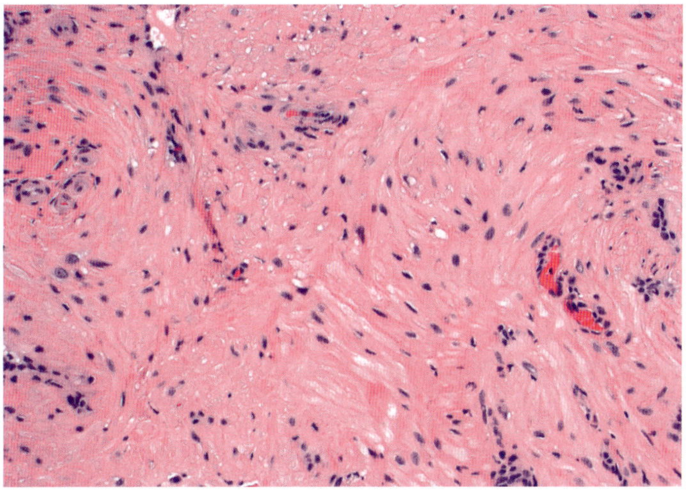

Fig. 9.15 Leiomyoma. High-power view of a thyroid gland leiomyoma showing spindled cells without pleomorphism, necrosis, or increased mitoses.

Pathogenesis
For adrenal leiomyomas, risk factors include immunodeficiency (acquired or congenital, including HIV/AIDS), reported in almost 50% of patients {964,2662,1986,3896}. In some of these cases, EBV was identified by in situ hybridization {2907,3896}. The pathogenetic reason for the association between (adrenal) leiomyoma and HIV or EBV infections is unclear and needs further investigation. EBV-associated smooth muscle tumours were initially reported as a complication of renal transplantation and immunosuppression and were subsequently identified in patients with HIV/AIDS as well as in patients who had undergone cardiac or liver transplantation. The cause of thyroid gland smooth muscle tumours is not known, and there is no viral or organ-transplant association with thyroid gland–related smooth muscle tumours.

Macroscopic appearance

Adrenal leiomyomas are solid, white, tan-white, and cream-coloured masses that are encapsulated or well circumscribed but may appear unencapsulated and multilobulated {4255}. The tumours vary in size, with a median size at diagnosis of 80 mm {3896}. Most tumours are unilateral, but bilateral occurrence has been reported {3896}. Thyroid leiomyomas are polypoid, nodular, and usually well demarcated, with a white to tan trabecular cut surface, and they measure 15–90 mm {4478,5150}.

Histopathology

Regardless of the site of origin, the histology of leiomyomas is similar and includes well-circumscribed to encapsulated nodules composed of intersecting fascicles of spindle-shaped to slightly epithelioid cells with eosinophilic cytoplasm and blunt-ended, cigar-shaped nuclei. Perinuclear cytoplasmic vacuoles may be identified. There is no significant nuclear atypia, increased mitotic activity, or tumour necrosis. Neoplastic cells show immunoreactivity for SMA, MSA, desmin, and caldesmon but are negative for S100, KIT, CD34, STAT6, myogenin, and myoglobin {3896}. In situ hybridization for EBV-encoded small RNA (EBER) may be positive {3966,3428}.

Smooth muscle cell tumours of the adrenal gland are thought to derive from the adrenal vein or its branches, considering its smooth muscle differentiation. However, it is not clear if all tumours originate from the adrenal vein or other smaller intra-adrenal vasculature {2074,3896}. In reported cases of adrenal gland leiomyomas, adrenal gland parenchyma was reported to be present in association with the tumours in some but not all cases, raising the possibility of an extra-adrenal origin (e.g. retroperitoneum) {3896}. Thyroid leiomyomas are thought to arise from vascular smooth muscle {4478}, and thyroid gland parenchyma can be seen entrapped by or separate from the tumour.

Immunohistochemistry

In adrenal tumours, the tumour cells are negative for markers associated with adrenal cortical adenoma/carcinoma (e.g. SF1, synaptophysin, inhibin, calretinin, and melan-A) and phaeochromocytoma (e.g. tyrosine hydroxylase, DBH {2303}, synaptophysin, chromogranin, INSM1). In thyroid tumours, the tumour cells are negative for cytokeratins, thyroglobulin, thyroid transcription factor 1 (TTF1), PAX8, calcitonin, CEA, and neuroendocrine markers (synaptophysin, chromogranin, INSM1). Proliferation rates by Ki-67 or MIB1 staining are low, typically < 5% {3896}.

Differential diagnosis

The clinical and/or imaging differential diagnosis for adrenal gland–based leiomyomas includes adrenal cortical neoplasms (adenoma, carcinoma) and phaeochromocytoma. The histological differential diagnosis includes peripheral nerve sheath tumours, solitary fibrous tumour, gastrointestinal stromal tumour, and leiomyosarcoma.

The differential diagnosis for thyroid leiomyoma includes other spindle cell lesions of the thyroid gland, including solitary fibrous tumour, invasive fibrous thyroiditis (Riedel disease), post-FNA spindle cell nodules, follicular adenoma with prominent spindle cells, papillary thyroid carcinoma with nodular fasciitis–like stroma, medullary thyroid carcinoma with a spindle cell pattern, anaplastic thyroid carcinoma, peripheral nerve sheath tumours, leiomyosarcoma, spindle epithelial tumour with thymus-like elements, and intrathyroidal thymic carcinoma {3423,3416,29,1588,5150}. Psammoma bodies were reported in a thyroid leiomyoma {3058}, but thyroglobulin, TTF1, and PAX8 were not performed, engendering doubt about the validity of the diagnosis as opposed to a possible diagnosis of papillary thyroid carcinoma with nodular fasciitis–like stroma.

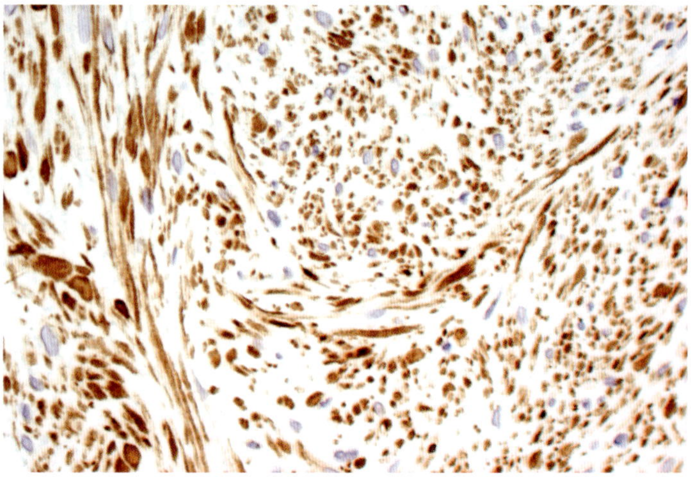

Fig. 9.16 Leiomyoma. The neoplastic cells of a thyroid gland leiomyoma show strong and diffuse desmin immunoreactivity.

The characteristic and reproducible histology and immunohistochemical findings in leiomyoma allow for its differentiation from these other adrenal and thyroid lesion/tumour types.

Cytology

Not clinically relevant

Diagnostic molecular pathology

There are no known markers of genetic relevance.

Essential and desirable diagnostic criteria

Essential: intersecting fascicles of bland spindled cells with blunt-ended, cigar-shaped nuclei; immunoreactivity for actins, desmin, and caldesmon.

Desirable: a well-circumscribed or encapsulated mass with a white trabecular cut surface; presence of adrenal or thyroid parenchyma.

Staging

None

Prognosis and prediction

Endocrine leiomyomas have an excellent prognosis. Surgical excision is curative {4478,143,419,1860,1274,3058,5150,3896}.

Leiomyosarcoma

Wenig BM
Thompson LDR

Definition

Leiomyosarcoma (LMS) is a sarcoma composed of cells showing smooth muscle differentiation.

ICD-O coding

8890/3 Leiomyosarcoma, NOS

ICD-11 coding

2D12.Y & XH7ED4 Other specified malignant neoplasms of other endocrine glands or related structures & Leiomyosarcoma, NOS

Related terminology

None

Subtype(s)

None

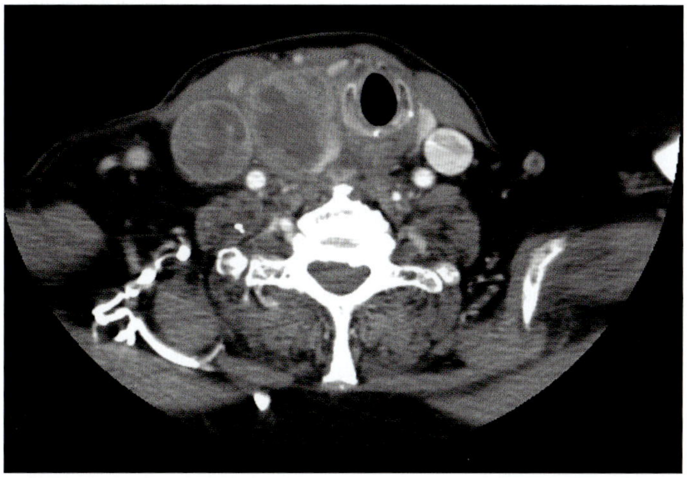

Fig. 9.17 Leiomyosarcoma. There is a large destructive mass within the thyroid gland, with cystic metastasis in a neck lymph node (CT).

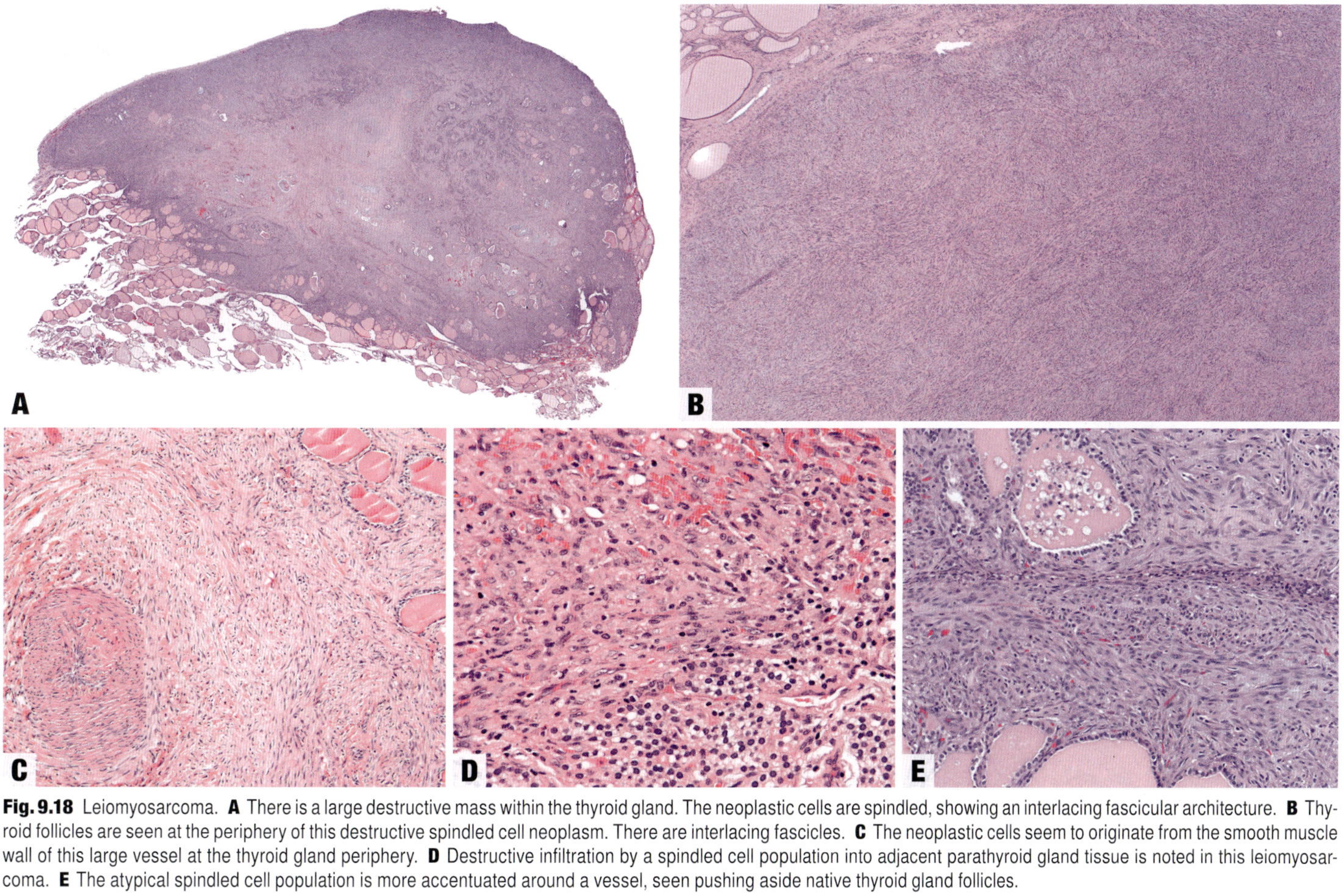

Fig. 9.18 Leiomyosarcoma. **A** There is a large destructive mass within the thyroid gland. The neoplastic cells are spindled, showing an interlacing fascicular architecture. **B** Thyroid follicles are seen at the periphery of this destructive spindled cell neoplasm. There are interlacing fascicles. **C** The neoplastic cells seem to originate from the smooth muscle wall of this large vessel at the thyroid gland periphery. **D** Destructive infiltration by a spindled cell population into adjacent parathyroid gland tissue is noted in this leiomyosarcoma. **E** The atypical spindled cell population is more accentuated around a vessel, seen pushing aside native thyroid gland follicles.

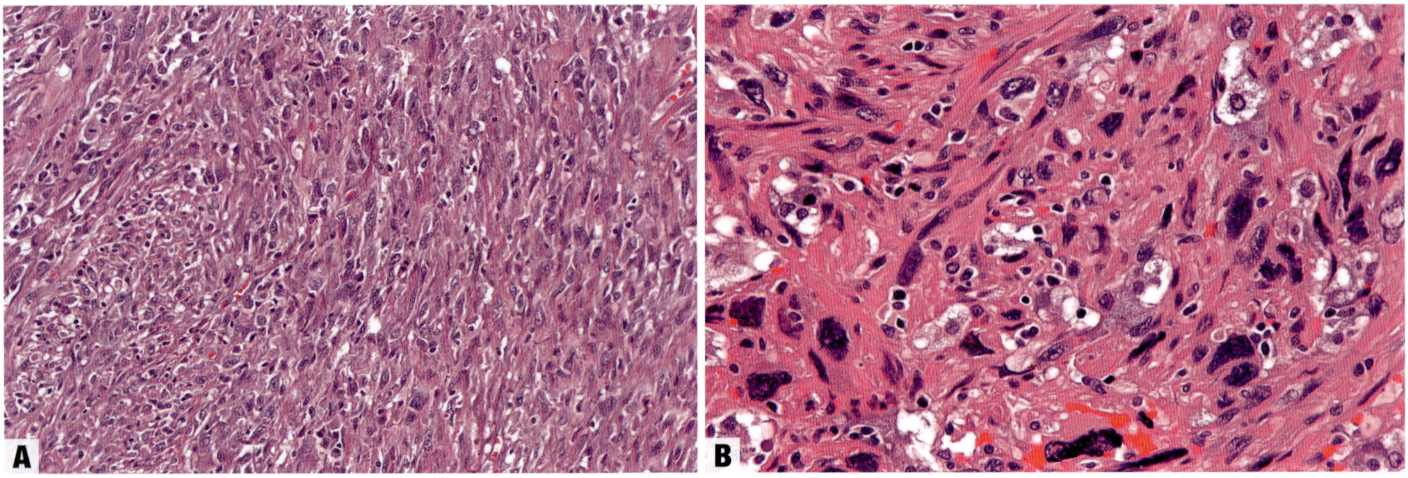

Fig. 9.19 Leiomyosarcoma. **A** The spindled neoplastic cells have a vaguely epithelioid quality. Numerous mitotic figures are seen. **B** Leiomyosarcomas of the adrenal gland usually arise around the central vessels. Note the destroyed adrenal cortical cells.

Localization

The most common endocrine organ site for LMS is the adrenal gland {3896}, followed by the thyroid gland {4478}.

Clinical features

Adrenal LMSs most often present with abdominal or flank pain/discomfort, and less often with weight loss, anorexia, and an enlarging abdominal mass {3896}. Symptom duration varies from sudden onset to days to several months and years {3896}. Adrenal LMSs are non-functioning and are not associated with signs/symptoms of hormonal secretion. However, elevated levels of serum NSE may occur (normalizing after excision) {1642}, and elevated serum CA125 {4802} may rarely occur. On imaging, adrenal LMSs are heterogeneous-appearing; they may be well-defined, lobulated, or with irregular borders; and they may have necrosis {3896}. Some tumours show infiltrative growth (including into the inferior vena cava through tumour thrombus), infiltration of adjacent organs (e.g. kidney, liver, pancreas), or lymph node or visceral metastases (liver, lung, bone) {3896}. Tumours are unilateral, with no side predilection {3896}.

Thyroid LMS typically presents as a painless, rapidly growing neck mass {4478,5195}. Additional symptoms may include hoarseness, dysphagia, dyspnoea, weight loss, and arm pain {5195}. The majority of patients with LMS are euthyroid with no prior history of radiation exposure {5195}. Tumours are typically solitary and limited to a single lobe {4478,5195}, although large tumours may involve both lobes and the isthmus {5195}. Thyroid nuclear scans may identify a cold nodule or an enlarged gland with areas of increased or decreased uptake of radioactive iodine {5195}. Ultrasound may reveal a poorly defined or well-defined hypoechoic mass, a solid or partially cystic nodule, or a calcified nodule {5195}. CT may show a low-density mass with dense calcification and necrosis, a well-demarcated mass, a soft tissue mass with calcification, or (in select cases) direct tumorous invasion of the adjacent structures {5195}. MRI may reveal a mass of intermediate signal on T2-weighted images and an isointense mass on T1-weighted images with a fair gadolinium enhancement {4382}.

Epidemiology

Primary LMSs of endocrine organs, including the adrenal and thyroid, are rare. Adrenal LMS may occur over a wide age range, from the second to the ninth decade of life (median: 60 years) {3896}. There is no sex preference {3896}.

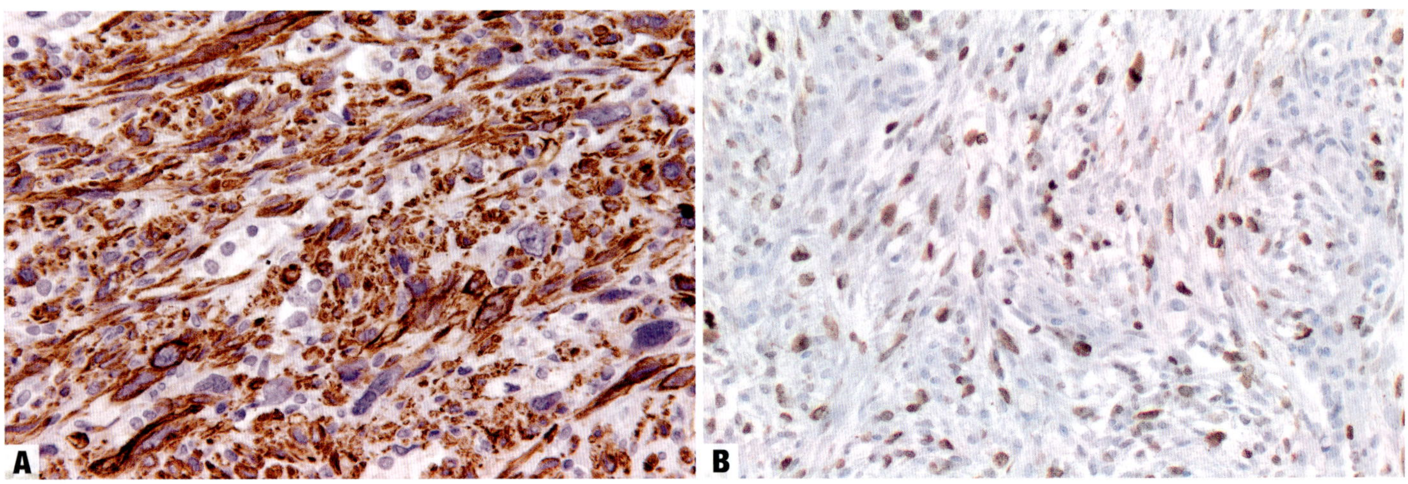

Fig. 9.20 Leiomyosarcoma. **A** The neoplastic cells this adrenal gland leiomyosarcoma are strongly reactive for desmin, whereas the native cortical cells are negative. **B** There is usually a high proliferation index in leiomyosarcoma, as detected by Ki-67 labelling.

Thyroid LMS is rare: about 0.014% of all LMSs develop in the thyroid gland {5195}. Primary thyroid gland LMS may occur over a wide age range, from the fourth to the tenth decade of life (median: 65 years). There is a slight female predilection (M:F ratio: 1:1.3) {5195}.

Etiology

Unknown

Pathogenesis

Smooth muscle cell tumours of the adrenal gland are thought to derive from the adrenal vein or its branches, considering its smooth muscle differentiation. However, it is not clear if all tumours originate from the adrenal vein or from other, smaller, intra-adrenal vasculature {2074,3896}. Thyroid gland LMSs are thought to arise from perithyroidal vascular smooth muscle cells {4478}.

A subset of patients with adrenal LMS have AIDS {5126,457, 2673}, which in turn may be associated with EBV {5126}. Thyroid LMS may occur in children in the setting of congenital immunodeficiency {4584}.

Macroscopic appearance

Adrenal LMS appears as a lobulated/multinodular, greyish to white-tan, well-defined, roundish tumour that may have areas of cystic degeneration, haemorrhage, myxoid-appearing change and/or necrosis. These tumours may be encapsulated or unencapsulated and extra-adrenal invasion may be identified, including into the inferior vena cava or tumour thrombus in the adrenal vein {3896}. Tumour size ranges from 8 to 270 mm (median: 90 mm).

Thyroid LMS is circumscribed to widely infiltrative, and on cut section it is white or tan-grey with a whorled appearance and may have areas of haemorrhage, cystic degeneration, and/or necrosis. The tumour size ranges from 11 to 160 mm (mean diameter: 66 mm) {4478,5195}.

Histopathology

Regardless of site, the histology of LMS shows spindle cells arranged in compact interlacing fascicles. Tumour cells include oval to elongated (cigar-shaped) and frequently blunt-ended hyperchromatic nuclei with a perinuclear vacuole and eosinophilic to clear cytoplasm. The cellularity, nuclear pleomorphism, mitotic activity, and tumour necrosis vary, but typically these tumours are hypercellular with moderate to marked nuclear pleomorphism, increased mitotic activity (with or without atypical forms), and tumour necrosis {4478}. Tumour giant cells may be present. Entrapped adrenal or thyroid parenchyma may be seen.

Immunohistochemistry

Neoplastic cells show immunoreactivity for SMA, MSA, desmin, and caldesmon {4478,3887,625,3703,3896} but are negative for cytokeratins, S100, SOX10, KIT (CD117), CD34, STAT6, myogenin, and myoglobin. In situ hybridization for EBV-encoded small RNA (EBER) may be positive {4584}.

In adrenal tumours, the tumour cells are negative for markers associated with adrenal cortical neoplasms (e.g. SF1, synaptophysin, inhibin, and melan-A) and for phaeochromocytoma (e.g. tyrosine hydroxylase, dopamine hydroxylase {2303}, synaptophysin, chromogranin, INSM1, and sustentacular S100/ SOX10). In thyroid tumours, the tumour cells are negative for cytokeratins, thyroglobulin, thyroid transcription factor 1 (TTF1), PAX8, calcitonin, CEA, and neuroendocrine markers (synaptophysin, chromogranin, and INSM1). Proliferation rates by Ki-67 staining vary but typically are increased and may be as high as 60% {3703}.

Differential diagnosis

The differential diagnosis for adrenal LMS includes leiomyoma, peripheral nerve sheath tumours, solitary fibrous tumour, and sarcomas of the retroperitoneum secondarily invading the adrenal gland.

The differential diagnosis for thyroid LMS primarily includes anaplastic thyroid carcinoma; secondary invasion of the thyroid from a neoplasm in the neck; and metastasis to the thyroid gland from LMS originating in other organs including the uterus {1234,2042,1521,1562,2555,2990,326}, vagina {1624}, lung {4928}, soft tissues of the lower extremity {3206,4804}, and the pulmonary artery {980}.

Cytology

FNA preoperative diagnosis of thyroid LMS may be useful in demonstrating malignant spindle-shaped cells with nuclear pleomorphism and increased mitotic activity {3206,2233,3112}.

Diagnostic molecular pathology

Not clinically relevant

Essential and desirable diagnostic criteria

Essential: a sarcoma arranged in fascicles composed of spindled cells with blunt-ended hyperchromatic nuclei, nuclear pleomorphism, and increased mitoses.

Desirable: tumour necrosis; atypical mitoses; immunoreactivity for SMA, desmin, and/or caldesmon; presence of adrenal or thyroid parenchyma.

Staging

Union for International Cancer Control (UICC) TNM eighth edition

Prognosis and prediction

Surgery is the treatment of choice. For adrenal LMS, the 1-year survival rate is reported to be 60%, and the 2-year survival rate is 15.3% {3896}. For thyroid LMS the prognosis is poor, with an estimated 1-year survival rate of 5–10% {2830}.

Rhabdomyosarcomas

Kohashi K
Rudzinski ER
Thompson LDR

Definition

Rhabdomyosarcomas are a group of malignant mesenchymal tumours with skeletal muscle differentiation.

ICD-O coding

8900/3 Rhabdomyosarcoma, NOS
8910/3 Embryonal rhabdomyosarcoma
8920/3 Alveolar rhabdomyosarcoma
8901/3 Pleomorphic rhabdomyosarcoma
8912/3 Spindle cell / sclerosing rhabdomyosarcoma

ICD-11 coding

2D12.Y & XH0GA1 Other specified malignant neoplasms of other endocrine glands or related structures & Rhabdomyosarcoma, NOS
2B55.Z & XH83G1 Rhabdomyosarcoma, unspecified primary site & Embryonal rhabdomyosarcoma, NOS
2B55.Z & XH7099 Rhabdomyosarcoma, unspecified primary site & Alveolar rhabdomyosarcoma
2B55.Z & XH5SX9 Rhabdomyosarcoma, unspecified primary site & Pleomorphic rhabdomyosarcoma, NOS
2B55.Z & XH7NM2 Rhabdomyosarcoma, unspecified primary site & Spindle cell rhabdomyosarcoma

Related terminology

Not recommended: myosarcoma; malignant rhabdomyoma.

Subtype(s)

Embryonal rhabdomyosarcoma (ERMS); alveolar rhabdomyosarcoma (ARMS); pleomorphic rhabdomyosarcoma; spindle cell / sclerosing rhabdomyosarcoma (SCSRMS)

Localization

Rhabdomyosarcoma has been reported arising as a primary tumour in the pituitary {1394,5163,1037,1180}, adrenal {2224, 5068,4775} and thyroid glands {2725,1469,1738,1193,1345}, and (rarely) in the pancreas {5049,3516,4129}.

Clinical features

Rhabdomyosarcoma arising at endocrine sites is reported in both adult and paediatric populations. Patients with tumours may present with palpable masses (e.g. anterior neck / thyroid) or mass effect symptoms (e.g. visual disorders or headache from pituitary primary tumours, hypertension from adrenal tumours, or epigastric pain from pancreatic tumours) {5049, 5068,1699}. Rhabdomyosarcomas at endocrine sites are infrequently associated with prior irradiation {1394}.

Epidemiology

Rhabdomyosarcoma is extremely rare within endocrine organ sites. In several reports, rhabdomyosarcoma coexisted with another endocrine tumour (e.g. pituitary neuroendocrine tumour [PitNET]) {4494,1037,1180}. More commonly, however, rhabdomyosarcoma may present synchronously or metachronously with other endocrine tumours in some cancer predisposition syndromes. For instance, Li–Fraumeni syndrome (*TP53* mutations) is associated with rhabdomyosarcoma and adrenal cortical carcinoma, and *DICER1* syndrome is associated with rhabdomyosarcoma of the uterine cervix in addition to thyroid nodules or pituitary blastoma {3063,63,5140}.

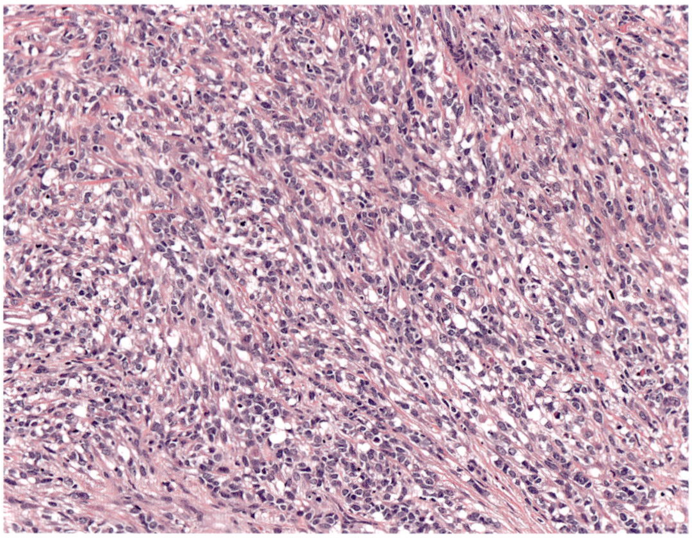

Fig. 9.21 Spindle rhabdomyosarcoma of thyroid. Slightly spindled, primitive rhabdoid cells are present in this rhabdomyosarcoma.

Etiology

ERMS is associated with radiation and several tumour predisposition syndromes, including Li–Fraumeni syndrome (associated with an inactivating mutation of *TP53*), Costello syndrome (also called faciocutaneoskeletal syndrome; *HRAS* mutation), neurofibromatosis type 1 (inactivating mutation of one allele of *NF1*), and Beckwith–Wiedemann syndrome (mutation or deletion of the 11p15.5 chromosomal region) {1141,3552,917,1511, 2629}. Such associations are not reported for other rhabdomyosarcoma subtypes.

Pathogenesis

ARMS harbours a *PAX3/7::FOXO1* fusion in most tumours {320,1007,1481}. PAX3 and PAX7 are transcription factors with essential roles in myogenesis {554}, with fusion proteins activating many downstream target genes, including *MET*, *ALK*, *MYCN*, and *MYOD1*, among others {389,369,628,1683,4179}. Less common fusions include *PAX3* with *FOXO4*, *NCOA1*, and *FGFR1* {321,4331,2684,4103}. SCSRMS separates into three genetic groups: *NCOA2::VGLL2* rearrangement; *MYOD1* mutation; and no identifiable genetic alteration {3108,33}. Skull/ mandibular intraosseous SCSRMS shows *EWSR1::FUS-TFCP2*

{4983}. As many as 50% of ERMS cases have RAS pathway mutations {4179}.

Macroscopic appearance

Rhabdomyosarcoma is soft, fleshy, and grey, with variable amounts of fibrous tissue and occasional necrotic areas and haemorrhage. Deep-seated tumours commonly infiltrate surrounding tissues.

Histopathology

ERMS consists of primitive round to spindle cells, with scant cytoplasm and hyperchromatic nuclei. There may be scattered rhabdomyoblasts. Botryoid ERMS typically shows linear aggregates of tumour cells close to the mucosa (cambium layer), with a cellularity gradient {1056,3649,1955,3648,1954}.

ARMS typically shows fibrovascular septa separating cellular nests of small monomorphic round cells with scant cytoplasm, which tend to coalesce in the centre and are dyscohesive at the periphery. The solid pattern lacks fibrovascular septa and forms sheets of tumour cells {3192,3432,4359,3855,4485}.

SCSRMS consists of a fasciculated proliferation of spindle cells with elongated nuclei and pale, indistinct cytoplasm, with interspersed spindled or polygonal rhabdomyoblasts with abundant, brightly eosinophilic cytoplasm {2368}.

Immunohistochemistry

The skeletal muscle–specific proteins myogenin (MYF4) and MYOD1 are variably expressed both within and between tumours, the proportion of positive cells reflecting the degree of differentiation {3097}. Occasional expression of keratin, neuroendocrine markers, S100, and ALK may also be observed {885,3192,5050,5080,4485,4983}, informing a panel approach to avoid misdiagnosis.

Differential diagnosis

The major differential diagnoses depend on the pattern of tumour, and metastatic tumours must be excluded {2205}. Fetal rhabdomyoma, dedifferentiated liposarcoma, malignant peripheral nerve sheath tumour with rhabdomyoblastic differentiation (formerly malignant triton tumour), Ewing sarcoma, haematolymphoid tumours, melanoma, carcinoma, and neuroendocrine tumours (NETs) must be actively excluded.

Cytology

Smears are highly cellular, with primitive uniform round, spindled, and stellate cells with scattered rhabdomyoblasts, sometimes in a tigroid background {999,2336,3306}.

Diagnostic molecular pathology

PAX3::FOXO1, *PAX7::FOXO1*, or *NCOA2::VGLL2* rearrangement or *MYOD1* mutation can aid diagnosis.

Essential and desirable diagnostic criteria

Essential: for all rhabdomyosarcoma subtypes, a malignant skeletal muscle tumour showing:

- ERMS: primitive round to spindle cell morphology
- ARMS: monomorphic, primitive-appearing round cells, usually dyscohesively arranged in a nested to solid pattern
- SCSRMS: spindled morphology with/without sclerotic collagenous matrix

Desirable (in selected cases): rhabdomyoblasts; myogenin/MYOD1 immunohistochemistry; detection of supporting genetic alterations.

Staging

Rhabdomyosarcoma may be staged according to the site of origin, using the Union for International Cancer Control (UICC) system for soft tissue sarcomas, with the exception of head and neck tumours, which are excluded. In paediatric rhabdomyosarcoma, modified TNM staging (the Intergroup Rhabdomyosarcoma Study Group [IRSG] grouping system) is used. This system relies on the site of origin, with risk stratification based on favourable site (e.g. bile ducts, orbit, head and neck, or genitourinary tract [excluding bladder, prostate, or parameningeal]) or unfavourable (other) site. The IRSG grouping system is used

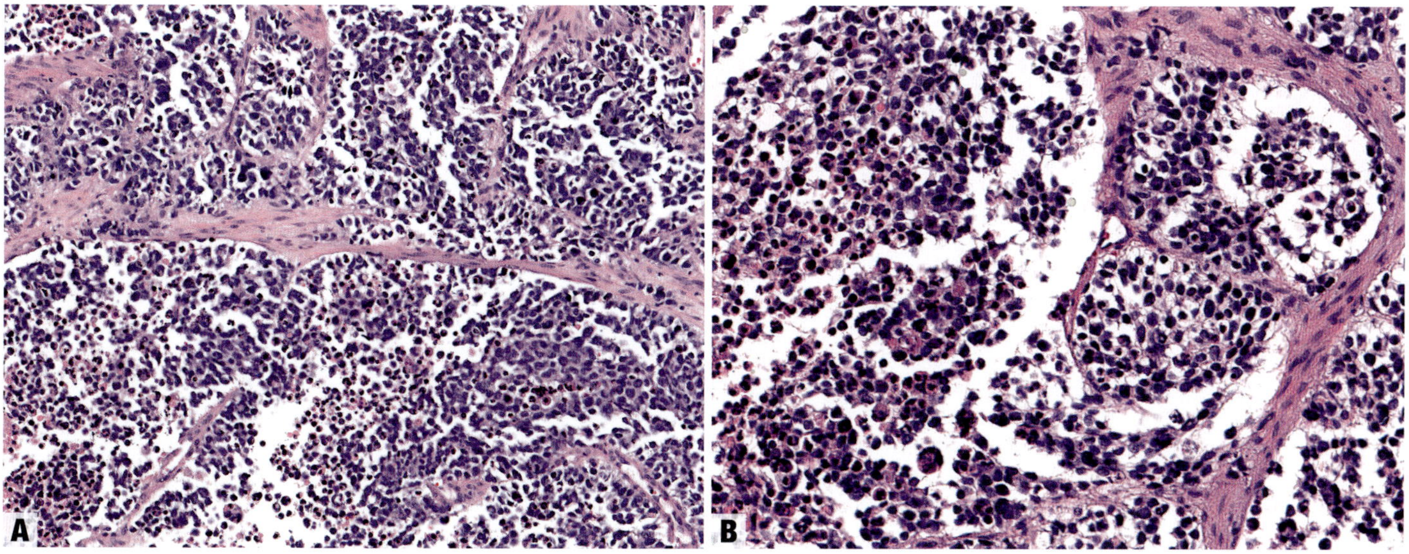

Fig. 9.22 Alveolar rhabdomyosarcoma of the thyroid. **A** There are nests with a dilapidated periphery, showing small blue round cells within the alveolar spaces. Tumour necrosis is present. **B** Nests with degenerative changes in the centre are noted, composed of small neoplastic cells with eccentric, eosinophilic cytoplasm.

for surgicopathological evaluation, including assessment of margins and residual disease {2813}.

Prognosis and prediction

Risk stratification predictive of outcome has been addressed with surgicopathological staging and fusion-based classification (IRSG grouping system) {1826,3231,4179}. Overall, rhabdomyosarcomas are considered systemic diseases, with specific sites showing a relatively poor prognosis (5-year survival rate: 40–45%) {4950,4941,4359,4485}. Age and tumour stage (most adult patients have stage IV disease at presentation) are the most important risk factors, with children and female patients having a better outcome than adults or male patients {4467,3934,1880}. Patients with fusion-positive ARMS have a worse outcome than those with fusion-negative ARMS and ERMS, with a worse prognosis for *PAX3::FOXO1* versus *PAX7::FOXO1* fusions {4890,1162,3034,4178,1826,4059,3231,4179,1880}. SCSRMS with *MYOD1* mutations has a poor prognosis, whereas infants with *VGLL2::NCOA2*-positive SCSRMS have an excellent outcome {72,33}.

Schwannoma

Perry A
Thompson LDR

Definition

Schwannoma is a benign peripheral nerve sheath tumour composed entirely or nearly entirely of differentiated neoplastic Schwann cells.

ICD-O coding

9560/0 Schwannoma, NOS
9560/0 Ancient schwannoma
9560/0 Cellular schwannoma
9560/0 Plexiform schwannoma
9560/0 Epithelioid schwannoma
9560/0 Microcystic/reticular schwannoma

ICD-11 coding

2F37.Y & XH98Z3 Other specified benign neoplasm of endocrine glands & Schwannoma, NOS

Related terminology

Not recommended: neurilemoma, neurinoma.

Subtype(s)

Ancient schwannoma; cellular schwannoma; plexiform schwannoma; epithelioid schwannoma; microcystic/reticular schwannoma

Localization

Rare examples have been reported within the pituitary, thyroid, and adrenal glands, as well as the pancreas {4477,2186,1656, 773,5134,4828,5170,103}, and are considered to arise from sympathetic or parasympathetic plexus or sensory nerves.

Clinical features

Schwannomas are slowly growing tumours and are often asymptomatic or incidental. They are usually mistaken for hormonally non-functioning primaries at these endocrine organ locations {4477,2186,1656,773,5134,4828,5170,103}.

Epidemiology

Tumours in endocrine organs are extremely rare, representing < 0.02% of all thyroid gland tumours {4477}. More than 90% of schwannomas are solitary and sporadic, affecting all ages but peaking in the fourth to sixth decade of life, without a sex predilection. Syndrome-associated tumours develop at a younger age {2615,137} and may show malignant transformation.

Etiology

The etiology of most sporadic schwannomas is not known, although prior irradiation is associated with an increased incidence {3802,3610}.

Pathogenesis

A causal relationship exists between schwannoma tumorigenesis and loss of expression of merlin (NF2; also known as schwannomin), the protein product of the gene *NF2* located at 22q12 {4275}. Inactivating mutations have been detected in 50–75% of sporadic cases {2077,2540,3321,1824}. Multiple schwannomas are a feature of neurofibromatosis type 2 and schwannomatosis, although they have not specifically been reported in endocrine organs {441,2250}.

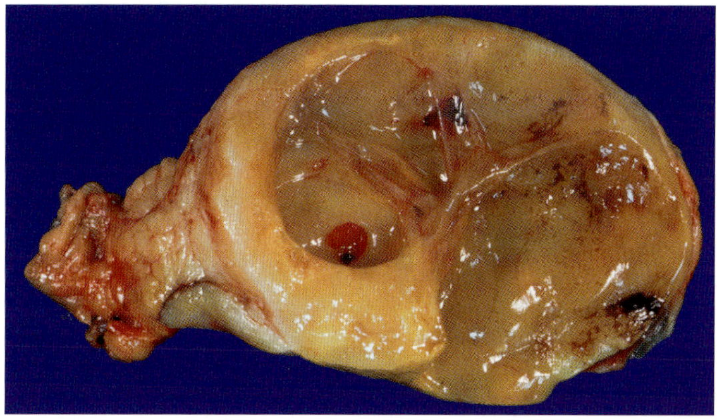

Fig. 9.23 Schwannoma. There is a well-defined, gelatinous to myxoid neoplasm within the adrenal gland, identified as a schwannoma histologically.

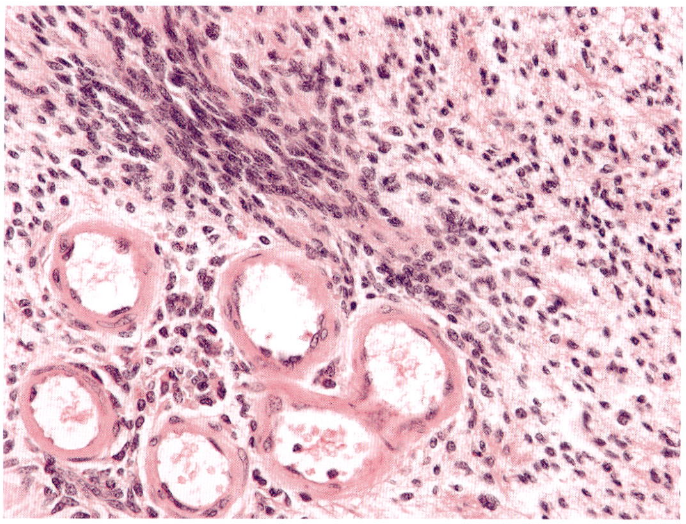

Fig. 9.24 Schwannoma. This thyroid gland schwannoma demonstrates perivascular hyalinization. The neoplastic cells are spindled and have a vaguely palisaded appearance.

Macroscopic appearance

These tumours are mainly solitary, variably encapsulated, and smooth-surfaced, growing to a considerable size (with adrenal tumours reaching even larger sizes than thyroid tumours). Endocrine organ tumours often lack an attached nerve. Sectioned tumours reveal firm, light-tan, glistening tissue; cystic spaces; white/yellow areas; and/or patchy haemorrhage.

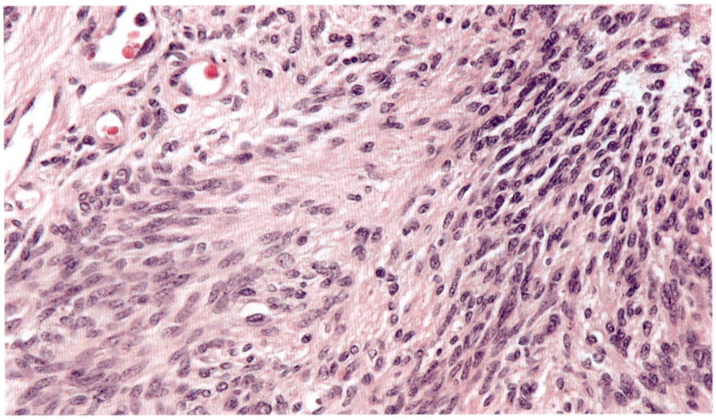

Fig. 9.25 Schwannoma. The spindled cells are bland and show bent to wavy nuclei within a syncytial-appearing cytoplasm.

Histopathology

Schwannoma is a well-circumscribed to partially encapsulated spindle cell tumour composed nearly entirely of well-differentiated Schwann cells. Most are biphasic tumours with compact hypercellular areas (Antoni A) showing variable nuclear palisading, alternating with loosely arranged foci (Antoni B). Cells within Antoni A zones possess modest eosinophilic cytoplasm; no discernible cell borders; and normochromatic, elongated, tapered to buckled nuclei. Intranuclear cytoplasmic inclusions, nuclear pleomorphism, and mitoses may be seen. Palisading (Verocay bodies) takes the form of parallel rows of nuclei separated by their aligned cell processes. Antoni B zones contain a cobweb-like network of cell processes with collections of lipid-laden histiocytes and thick-walled, hyalinized blood vessels. Lymphoid aggregates are often at the periphery.

Immunohistochemistry

Immunoreactivity for S100 and SOX10 is usually extensive {4477,3284,2200}. In contrast to the lattice-like staining pattern in neurofibromas, CD34 is usually positive only in subcapsular and septal areas. EMA also highlights perineurial cells in the capsule. In the differential with thyroid gland lesions, thyroid transcription factor 1 (TTF1; clone-specific) is aberrantly expressed in schwannoma {4777}.

Differential diagnosis

The differential diagnosis is with leiomyoma, solitary fibrous tumour, neurofibroma, meningioma (when tumours are within the pituitary gland), and spindle cell follicular adenoma (in the thyroid gland).

Cytology

Aspirate smears are typically cellular, with cohesive syncytial fragments of spindle cells. Within the fragments, variably wavy and bent tumour cell nuclei with tapered edges and fibrillary cytoplasm are seen. Organ-specific features (i.e. thyroid follicles, adrenal cortex) are inconspicuous. S100/SOX10 aids in confirming a neural tumour {767,4677,53}.

Diagnostic molecular pathology

Not routinely performed

Essential and desirable diagnostic criteria

Essential: densely packed spindled cell areas with loosely arranged hypocellular myxoid areas; spindled cells with buckled, elongated, fusiform nuclei.

Desirable: hyalinized blood vessel walls; Verocay bodies; extensive S100 and SOX10 immunoreactivity.

Staging

Not applicable

Prognosis and prediction

Schwannomas are benign. Multifocality may mimic recurrence or malignancy.

Neurofibroma

Perry A

Definition

Neurofibroma is a benign peripheral nerve sheath tumour consisting of mature neoplastic Schwann cells intermixed with non-neoplastic cell types.

ICD-O coding

9540/0 Neurofibroma, NOS
9540/0 Ancient neurofibroma
9540/0 Cellular neurofibroma
9540/1 Atypical neurofibroma
9540/0 Plexiform neurofibroma

ICD-11 coding

2F37.Y & XH87J5 Other specified benign neoplasm of endocrine glands & Neurofibroma, NOS

Related terminology

None

Subtype(s)

Ancient neurofibroma; cellular neurofibroma; atypical neurofibroma; plexiform neurofibroma (see the *Soft tissue and bone tumours* or *Central nervous system tumours* volumes of this series)

Localization

Neurofibromas arising within endocrine organs are extremely rare, with only a few reported cases in the thyroid gland, adrenal gland, and pancreas {137,4569,1148,1070,1712}.

Clinical features

Sporadic and neurofibromatosis type 1–associated neurofibromas of endocrine organs typically mimic more common primary tumours in those locations {137,4569,1148,1070,1712}.

Epidemiology

Epidemiological studies of neurofibromas in endocrine organs do not exist, because of their rarity, although these tumours have been reported in both paediatric and adult patients.

Etiology

Unknown

Pathogenesis

Only the subpopulation of Schwann cells is considered neoplastic within neurofibromas {3531}, and biallelic genetic inactivation of the tumour suppressor gene *NF1* in this Schwann cell population is generally the only recurrent somatic event detectable {1245,3502}. Therefore, complete loss of function of the *NF1* gene product, neurofibromin (NF1), is considered a prerequisite for tumour development. Neurofibromin (NF1) is a negative regulator of RAS oncogenes {4148}.

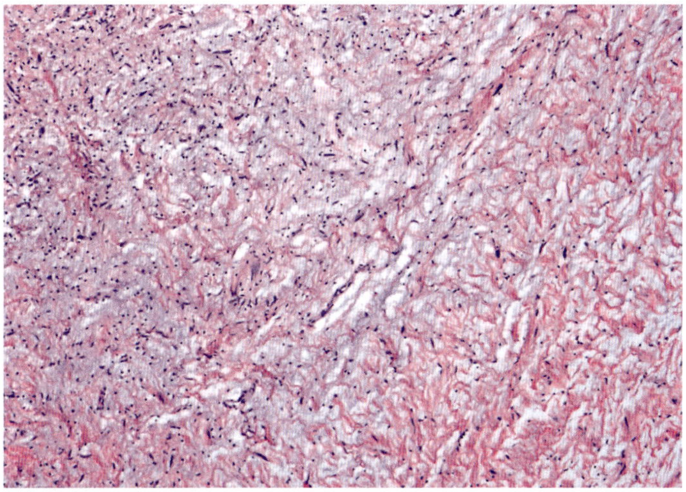

Fig. 9.26 Neurofibroma. This tumour is predominantly composed of small tumour cells with slender, spindled nuclei and thin, wavy, eosinophilic cytoplasm, embedded within a variably myxoid to collagenous stroma.

Macroscopic appearance

Neurofibromas are usually unencapsulated nodular or polypoid lesions. Cut surfaces are most often uniformly tan or grey, glistening, mucoid, semitranslucent, and firm.

Histopathology

Neurofibromas are unencapsulated tumours characterized by bland spindle cells with thin, wavy nuclei, representing the neoplastic Schwann cell, immersed in a variably loose myxoid stroma. The tumour cells are typically smaller than those of schwannoma. Stromal collagen is characteristic, often likened in classic pathology descriptions to shredded carrots. A variety of other cell components are also identifiable in neurofibroma, including perineurial and perineurial-like cells, fibroblasts, and mast cells. Nerve fibres are variably identifiable in intraneural subtypes, which are characterized by the expansion of single or multiple nerve fascicles; plexiform neurofibroma is associated with neurofibromatosis type 1.

Immunohistochemistry

Individual nerve fascicles are recognized by a peripheral EMA-positive perineurial layer. The neoplastic Schwann cells are positive for S100, SOX10, and collagen IV, albeit in smaller proportions than in schwannomas. Non-neoplastic cellular components include a limited number of EMA-positive and GLUT1-positive perineurial cells, as well as CD34-positive fibroblastic cells, this last component often forming a lattice-like network that is not seen in schwannomas.

Cytology

Intraoperative smears and FNA specimens of neurofibroma are often paucicellular, owing to the increased collagen matrix.

Nevertheless, the presence of a mucin-rich background and small spindled cells with thin, wavy nuclei can provide diagnostic clues.

Diagnostic molecular pathology

Molecular analyses do not have an established role in the diagnosis of neurofibroma.

Essential and desirable diagnostic criteria

Essential: an infiltrative, low-cellularity spindle cell neoplasm associated with a variably myxoid to collagenous stroma.

Desirable: S100 positivity in the Schwann cell population, with CD34 highlighting a lattice-like stromal component.

Staging

Not applicable

Prognosis and prediction

Neurofibromas are benign, although plexiform neurofibromas in patients with neurofibromatosis type 1 are at increased risk of transformation to malignant peripheral nerve sheath tumour.

Granular cell tumour

Perry A

Definition

Granular cell tumour is most probably of Schwannian origin and is composed of epithelioid to polygonal cells with abundant granular cytoplasm due to lysosomal accumulation.

ICD-O coding

9580/0 Granular cell tumour, NOS
9580/3 Granular cell tumour, malignant

ICD-11 coding

2F37.Y & XH09A9 Other specified benign neoplasm of endocrine glands & Granular cell tumour, NOS
2D12.Y & XH90D3 Other specified malignant neoplasms of other endocrine glands or related structures & Granular cell tumour, malignant

Related terminology

Not recommended: granular cell schwannoma; granular cell nerve sheath tumour; granular cell myoblastoma; Abrikossoff tumour.

Subtype(s)

Malignant granular cell tumour (see the *Soft tissue and bone tumours* volume of this series {4870})

Localization

Granular cell tumours within endocrine organs are extremely rare. Roughly a dozen cases have been reported in the thyroid gland {1842}, with even fewer cases in the pancreas {1505}. For granular cell tumour of the sellar region, which arises from pituicytes, please refer to *Pituicytomas* (p. 92).

Clinical features

Although usually asymptomatic, clinically and on imaging they may mimic malignancies within the thyroid and pancreas, including neuroendocrine tumours (NETs). A single thyroid case has recurred {1842}, and 1 pancreatic example was multicentric, with a second tumour found in the caecum {1505}.

Epidemiology

Nearly all reported cases of granular cell tumour of the thyroid have occurred in young women {1842}. Pancreatic examples show a similar female predominance {4379}.

Etiology

Multiple granular cell tumours have been reported in association with various RASopathy syndromes, such as neurofibromatosis type 1, Noonan syndrome, and LEOPARD syndrome (multiple lentigines, electrocardiographic conduction abnormalities, ocular hypertelorism, pulmonic stenosis, abnormal genitalia, retardation of growth, and sensorineural deafness) {2722,4021, 3671,4136}.

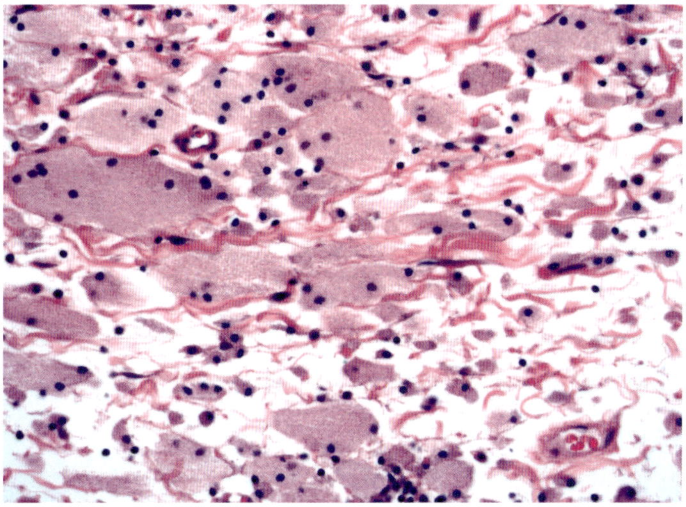

Fig. 9.27 Granular cell tumour. A loose collection of large tumour cells with small, cytologically bland nuclei and abundant granular cytoplasm.

Pathogenesis

Pathognomonic loss-of-function mutations affecting the V-ATPase accessory genes, *ATP6AP1* (61%) and *ATP6AP2* (11%), are found in 72% of granular cell tumours collectively {3427,4057}. These genes play pivotal roles in endosomal pH regulation {3427}. Granular cell tumours lacking mutations in these genes have been reported to harbour mutations affecting other V-ATPase–related genes {4057}. Inactivation of either *ATP6AP1* or *ATP6AP2* in Schwann cells leads to the accumulation of intracytoplasmic granules that are characteristic of granular cell tumour.

Macroscopic appearance

Granular cell tumours are unencapsulated, uninodular, firm masses with a yellowish, finely granular texture on cut surface.

Histopathology

Granular cell tumour has poorly defined borders with sheets, nests, and trabeculae of large, monotonous epithelioid to polygonal cells with intensely eosinophilic, granular cytoplasm due to massive lysosomal accumulation. They often infiltrate retained normal structures, including those of the thyroid and pancreas. A syncytial appearance may be seen, due to indistinct cell borders. Nuclei are usually centrally situated and range from uniformly small and mildly hyperchromatic to larger and vesicular with distinct nucleoli. Mitoses are typically inconspicuous.

Histological features associated with malignancy include increased cellularity, prominent spindling, high N:C ratios, vesicular nuclei with prominent nucleoli, marked pleomorphism, increased mitotic activity (> 2 mitoses/2 mm^2), and geographical necrosis {1327,2002,4788}.

Immunohistochemistry

Granular cell tumours are generally immunoreactive for S100, SOX10, nestin, inhibin, and calretinin {3431,736}. Tumours are also positive for CD68, CD63 (NKI/C3 clone), and NSE {1381}.

Cytology

In FNA samples, the characteristic granular cytoplasm and bland nuclei are useful, although carcinomas and histiocytic processes remain in the differential.

Diagnostic molecular pathology

Not applicable

Essential and desirable diagnostic criteria

Essential: nests and sheets of epithelioid to polygonal cells with abundant, intensely eosinophilic, granular cytoplasm; positivity for S100 and SOX10 by immunohistochemistry.

Staging

Not applicable

Prognosis and prediction

All of the reported granular cell tumours of the thyroid and pancreas have been both pathologically and clinically benign. Recurrences are exceedingly rare {1842}.

Malignant peripheral nerve sheath tumour

Perry A
Thompson LDR

Definition

Malignant peripheral nerve sheath tumour (MPNST) is a malignant spindle cell tumour with limited Schwannian differentiation. Molecular hallmarks are the combined genetic inactivation of *NF1*, *CDKN2A* and/or *CDKN2B*, and *SUZ12* or *EED*, as well as complex genomic rearrangements.

ICD-O coding

9540/3 Malignant peripheral nerve sheath tumour, NOS
9542/3 Epithelioid malignant peripheral nerve sheath tumour

ICD-11 coding

2D12.Y & XH2XP8 Other specified malignant neoplasms of other endocrine glands or related structures & Malignant peripheral nerve sheath tumour

Related terminology

Not recommended: malignant schwannoma; neurofibrosarcoma; neurogenic sarcoma.

Subtype(s)

Epithelioid MPNST

Localization

Rare MPNSTs have been reported in the pituitary {1708,16, 4442}, thyroid {3393,984}, pancreas {3393,5042,283}, and adrenal glands {3018,1014,1713,271,4926,3177}, with tumours in the adrenal glands often arising in association with phaeochromocytoma or ganglioneuroma. A rare case of epithelioid MPNST has been reported in the thyroid {5070}.

Clinical features

MPNSTs have a slight male sex predilection and typically present in patients aged 20–50 years, with most paediatric and young adult cases arising in patients with neurofibromatosis type 1 (NF1). Symptoms are nonspecific. Tumours are identified during imaging studies or as an enlarging mass; pain and anorexia may be reported. Organ-specific findings include dyspnoea (thyroid) or dyspepsia and other bowel/biliary disturbances (pancreas) {984,283}.

Epidemiology

MPNST is extremely rare within endocrine organ sites.

Etiology

MPNST may be associated with NF1 or prior irradiation.

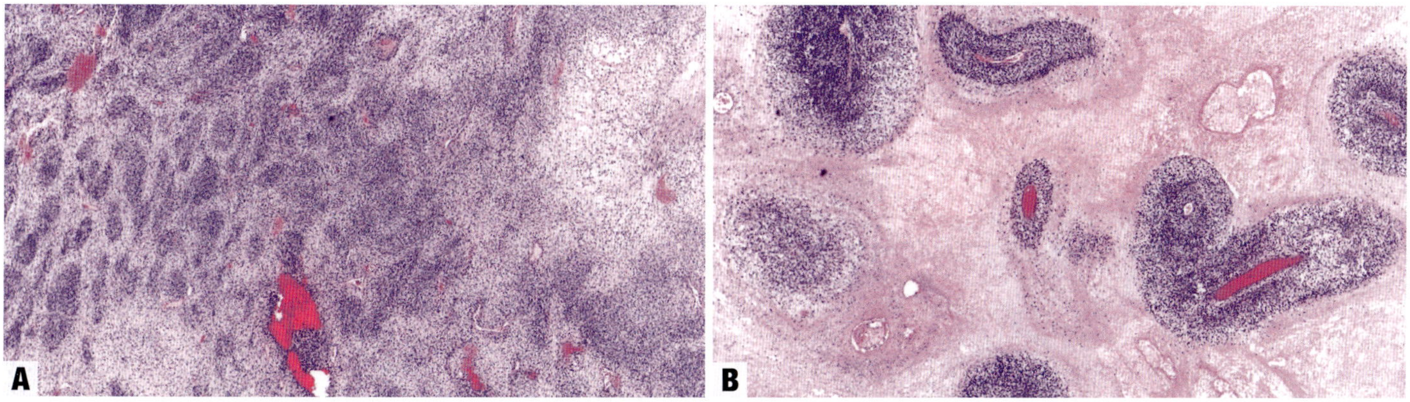

Fig. 9.28 Malignant peripheral nerve sheath tumour. **A** Marbled appearance at low magnification, with alternating dark and pale zones. **B** Extensive geographical necrosis.

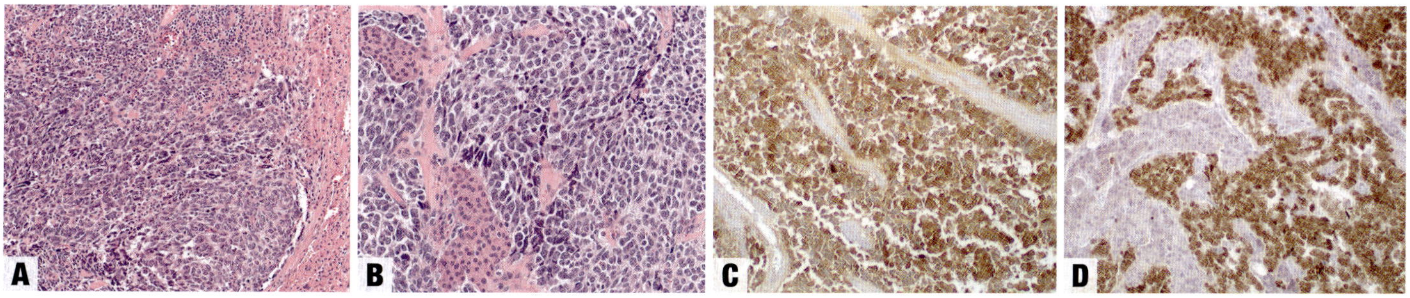

Fig. 9.29 Epithelioid malignant peripheral nerve sheath tumour. **A** An adrenal gland tumour with destruction of the adjacent adrenal cortex. **B** The native adrenal cortex is captured by the pleomorphic, epithelioid to spindled cell population. **C** Extensive nuclear and cytoplasmic reactivity for S100. **D** Extensive nuclear reactivity for SOX10.

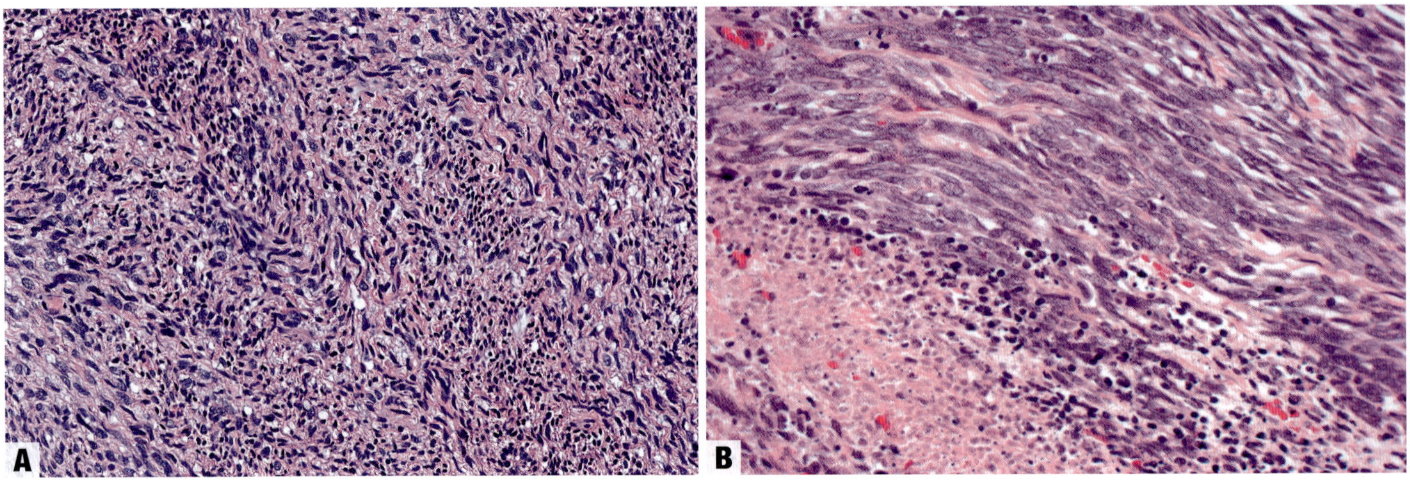

Fig. 9.30 Malignant peripheral nerve sheath tumour. **A** The atypical spindled cells of this malignant peripheral nerve sheath tumour demonstrate a fascicular architecture, with wavy, buckled, pointed nuclei. **B** There is comedonecrosis adjacent to the atypical spindled cells of this thyroid gland malignant peripheral nerve sheath tumour.

Pathogenesis

Conventional MPNSTs have complex karyotypes and frequent concurrent inactivating mutations involving three pathways: *NF1*, *CDKN2A* and/or *CDKN2B*, and PRC2 core components (*EED* or *SUZ12*) {2588,1034,5141,3501}. About 80% of all high-grade MPNSTs exhibit complete loss of PRC2 activity through loss of the PRC2 core component (*EED* or *SUZ12*) and complete loss of H3 p.K27me3 expression {2588,3982,3619}. In contrast to the conventional subtype, epithelioid MPNST is not NF1-associated, often arises from schwannoma rather than neurofibroma, and is associated with *SMARCB1* inactivation {2588,2117,3981}.

Macroscopic appearance

MPNSTs are usually large and have a tan-white, fleshy cut surface, often with areas of haemorrhage and necrosis. They are destructively infiltrative into the native organ, but may appear pseudoencapsulated.

Histopathology

MPNST is a destructively infiltrative malignancy composed of fascicles of spindle-shaped cells, a variably haemangiopericytoma-like vascular pattern, and alternating hypercellular and hypocellular areas (marbled appearance). A peritheliomatous concentration of tumour cells may be seen. There are often areas of geographical necrosis and high mitotic activity. The cells have pale cytoplasm and hyperchromatic, wavy, buckled, and tapered nuclei. Occasional MPNSTs (especially radiation-induced ones) feature highly atypical nuclei, simulating an undifferentiated pleomorphic sarcoma. Heterologous skeletal muscle (malignant triton tumour), bone, cartilage, or vascular differentiation is seen in about 15% of tumours {1713}.

Epithelioid MPNST consists of lobules of large epithelioid, melanoma-like cells with vesicular nuclei, prominent nucleoli, and abundant eosinophilic cytoplasm.

Immunohistochemistry

MPNSTs may be positive for S100 (< 50% of tumours), SOX10 (< 70%), and GFAP (20–30%) {2190}, although staining is patchy, focal, and weak; in fact, diffuse staining for S100 or SOX10 is not usually compatible with conventional MPNST. Complete loss of immunostaining for H3 p.K27me3 can be diagnostically useful, with high-grade sporadic and radiation-induced MPNST tumours showing the most frequent loss {3619, 3982,3490,3373}. Epithelioid MPNST is typically strongly and extensively positive for S100 and SOX10, is negative for more specific melanoma markers, retains H3 p.K27me3, and shows loss of SMARCB1 (INI1) expression {3981}.

Cytology

Fine-needle aspirates of MPNST are similar in endocrine and soft tissue sites, but they are often not sufficiently specific to obviate the need for biopsy or resection confirmation.

Diagnostic molecular pathology

In diagnostically challenging cases, DNA methylation profiling can identify a specific tumour signature of MPNST {2363}. Other molecular data providing support for an MPNST diagnosis include mutations in *NF1* and *SUZ12* or *EED*.

Essential and desirable diagnostic criteria

Essential: alternating light and dark zones with pleomorphic spindled cells showing tapered, buckled nuclei; epithelioid cytology and loss of SMARCB1 (INI1) expression (epithelioid MPNST).

Desirable: a haemangiopericytoma-like vascular pattern; variable S100 and/or SOX10 reactivity; loss of H3 p.K27me3 expression; association with a large nerve, NF1, pre-existing neurofibroma, and/or prior irradiation; association with pre-existing schwannoma and extensive expression of S100 and SOX10 (epithelioid MPNST).

Staging

Not clinically relevant

Prognosis and prediction

The reported 5-year overall survival rate for NF1-associated MPNST (35%) is lower than that for sporadic tumours (65%); deep location, positive surgical margins, and high-grade histology were additionally associated with worse outcomes {2553}. Radiation-associated MPNSTs have a reported 5-year overall survival rate of 23.5% {2987}. Specific prognostic factors for endocrine organs have not been reported.

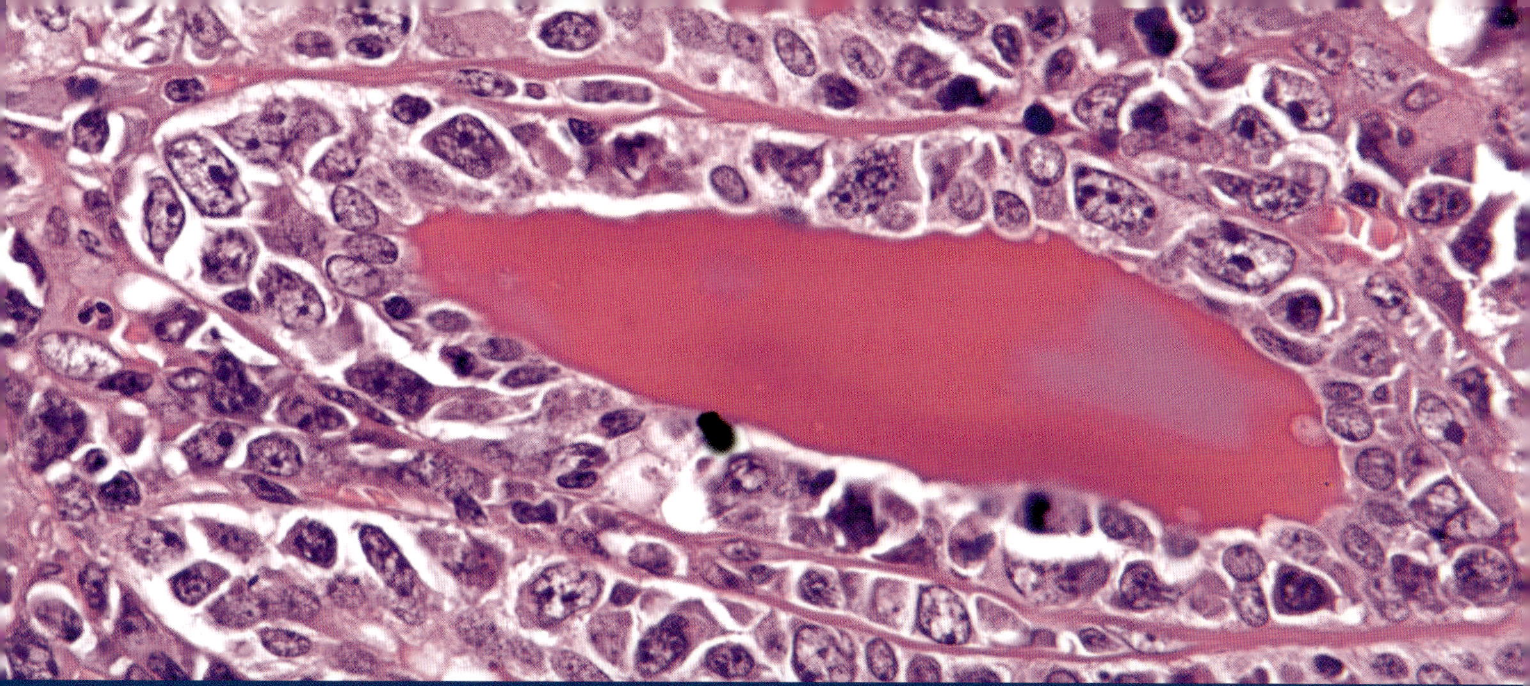

10

Haematolymphoid tumours

Edited by: Erickson LA, Khoury JD

IgG4-related disease
Extranodal marginal zone lymphoma of mucosa-associated lymphoid tissue
Diffuse large B-cell lymphoma NOS
Langerhans cell histiocytosis
Rosai–Dorfman disease
Erdheim–Chester disease
Follicular dendritic cell sarcoma

Haematolymphoid tumours: Introduction

Erickson LA
Hyrcza MD

This chapter begins with a disease that mimics haematolymphoid neoplasms, IgG4-related disease, then describes lymphomas and histiocytic proliferations that occasionally involve endocrine organs, and concludes with follicular dendritic cell sarcoma, a mesenchymal dendritic cell neoplasm.

IgG4-related disease is new to this edition of the WHO classification of endocrine and neuroendocrine tumours. IgG4-related disease is a chronic fibroinflammatory condition characterized by a lymphoplasmacytic infiltrate enriched in IgG4-positive plasma cells, often with storiform fibrosis, obliterative phlebitis, and elevated serum IgG4. The pancreas is the most commonly involved endocrine organ. In the thyroid gland, IgG4-related disease can present as Riedel-like thyroiditis or the fibrotic subtype of Hashimoto thyroiditis. IgG4-related disease also affects the pituitary.

Primary lymphomas of the thyroid account for 1–5% of all thyroid malignancies {160,4460}. Diffuse large B-cell lymphoma accounts for > 65% of all thyroid lymphomas {4446,120,5066}. Approximately 1–5% of extranodal marginal zone lymphomas of mucosa-associated lymphoid tissue, the second most frequent type of primary thyroid lymphoma, are located in the thyroid {5190,1093,719}. Primary lymphoma of the adrenal gland is rare; > 85% of cases are diffuse large B-cell lymphomas {5100,4813, 781}. Primary pituitary lymphomas account for up to 0.2% of pituitary lesions; 55% of cases are diffuse large B-cell lymphomas {4636,1325,645}.

Histiocytic proliferations affecting endocrine organs include Langerhans cell histiocytosis, Rosai–Dorfman disease, and Erdheim–Chester disease. In endocrine organs, Langerhans cell histiocytosis most often affects the pituitary and thyroid {3884}. Fewer than 10 cases of thyroid Rosai–Dorfman disease have been described, and only rare cases affect the posterior pituitary or adrenal glands {4746,1559,4551,1393}. Erdheim–Chester disease is rare, but endocrine involvement is frequent in this disorder {933}. Mutations (particularly *BRAF* p.V600E and *MAP2K1* mutations) leading to the activation of the RAS/RAF/MAPK pathway are a common feature of Langerhans cell histiocytosis {3777,548,735} and Erdheim–Chester disease {1114, 3418,1652}. Recent evidence of similar gain-of-function mutations raises the possibility of a clonal origin in some cases of Rosai–Dorfman disease {8,1503}. Follicular dendritic cell sarcoma is rare in endocrine organs, with cases showing recurrent alterations in NF-κB pathway genes and an absence of MAPK pathway abnormalities {1670,2868}.

IgG4-related disease

Hyrcza MD

Definition

IgG4-related disease is a chronic fibroinflammatory condition characterized by a lymphoplasmacytic infiltrate enriched in IgG4-positive plasma cells, often with storiform fibrosis, obliterative phlebitis, and elevated serum IgG4.

ICD-O coding

9760/1 IgG4-related disease

ICD-11 coding

4A43.0 IgG4-related disease

Related terminology

Not recommended: IgG4-related autoimmune disease; IgG4-related systemic disease; IgG4-related sclerosing disease.

Subtype(s)

None

Localization

IgG4-related disease can affect a single organ or multiple sites. Among endocrine organs, the pancreas is most commonly involved {4765,1199}. The thyroid was involved in 5.6% of patients with IgG4-related disease in one series {4765}, and the pituitary was involved in 8% of cases in another study {1199}. Rare cases of adrenal involvement by IgG4-related disease have been reported {3875,2769}.

Clinical features

The clinical presentation varies with the site of involvement. In the thyroid, IgG4-related disease can present with hypothyroidism, or painless thyroid enlargement in IgG4-related Riedel-like thyroiditis {3865,3847}. IgG4-related disease involving the pituitary may be associated with clinical symptoms of hypophysitis, such as nausea, headache, sexual dysfunction, fatigue, weight loss, polydipsia, generalized weakness, or blurred vision {2612,135}.

Imaging

Radiographic features of IgG4-related disease in the pancreas include a focal mass-like lesion mimicking pancreatic carcinoma and diffuse or segmental pancreatic enlargement {1849}. IgG4-related thyroiditis may show hypoechoic lesions by ultrasound. IgG4-related hypophysitis may cause pituitary gland and stalk mass-like thickening {148}.

Epidemiology

The incidence of IgG4-related disease is 0.28–1.08 cases per 100 000 person-years, and the prevalence was 62 per million in a Japanese cohort {4607}. There is a male predominance (M:F ratio: 1:0.8), and the average age of onset is 59 years {4607}. The disease can occur at any age, including childhood {2203}. The incidence of IgG4- related Riedel-like thyroiditis is 1.06 cases per 100 000 person-years, whereas the reported prevalence of IgG4-related Hashimoto thyroiditis ranges from 5% to 34% {3847}. IgG4-related hypophysitis constituted 30% of hypophysitis cases and 4% of hypopituitarism cases in one study {303}.

Etiology

The etiology of IgG4-related disease is not well understood. Environmental exposures, immune dysfunction, infections, and genetic predispositions linked to a variety of genes have

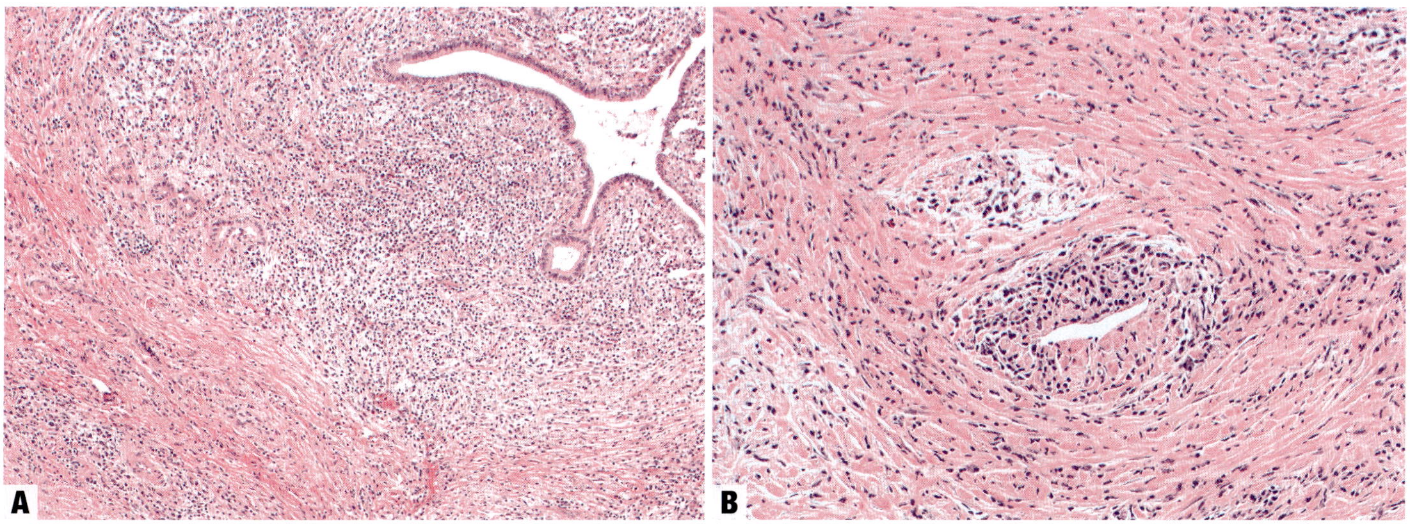

Fig. 10.01 IgG4-related disease. **A** IgG4-related pancreatitis shows a lymphoplasmacytic infiltrate associated with fibrosis, often in a storiform pattern. **B** This example shows obliterative phlebitis.

Table 10.01 Common endocrine organs involved by IgG4-related disease, and clinical features

Site	Clinical presentation	IgG4+/mm^2	IgG4:IgG
Pancreas	Parenchymal mass lesion mimicking pancreatic carcinoma (painless obstructive jaundice, pancreatic mass, abdominal pain) and/or pancreatic insufficiency (new-onset diabetes mellitus, steatorrhoea)	> 40 (biopsy) > 200 (excision)	> 40%
Pituitary	Headache, visual field defect, hyperprolactinaemia (galactorrhoea), hypopituitarism (diabetes insipidus, fatigue, amenorrhoea) {2640}	> 40	> 40%
Thyroid	Goitre and/or hypothyroidism {4386}	> 80	> 40%

all been proposed to contribute to the development of IgG4-related disease {1391}.

Pathogenesis

The pathogenetic mechanisms leading to IgG4-related disease are unclear. TGF-β and IL-10 are elevated and the TGF-β pathway is activated, stimulating fibrogenesis {1391}. Whether the increased number of IgG4-producing plasma cells is part of the pathogenesis or a downstream effect is unknown.

Macroscopic appearance

There are no macroscopic findings specific for IgG4-related disease, because the features can be highly variable in different organs.

Histopathology

The characteristic histological features of IgG4-related disease in various organs are quite similar to those of IgG4-related pancreatitis (type 1 autoimmune pancreatitis), which is the prototype of endocrine IgG4-related disease. A dense lymphoplasmacytic infiltrate is associated with fibrosis, which often shows a storiform pattern. Obliterative phlebitis is seen in a subset of cases and is considered almost pathognomonic of IgG4-related disease in some organs. Eosinophils are often present. A prominent neutrophilic infiltrate, tissue necrosis, and epithelioid granulomas are generally not seen {5124}. Depending on the specimen type and particular endocrine organ, different densities of IgG4-positive plasma cells define IgG4-related disease {2642,5136,2242,3659,2131,3847}. See Table 10.01 for specific thresholds of IgG4-positive plasma cells per mm^2 for the diagnosis of IgG4-related disease in various endocrine organs {1103}. IgG4-related thyroid disease exhibits features of Riedel-like thyroiditis or the fibrotic subtype of Hashimoto thyroiditis; for other types of thyroid disease that do not fulfil all the main criteria for IgG4-related disease, terms such as "thyroid disease with an elevation of IgG4" have been suggested, particularly in cases without histological confirmation {3847}. IgG4-related hypophysitis shows lymphoplasmacytic infiltration of the pituitary gland and IgG4 serum levels exceeding 140 mg/dL {148}. When the pituitary gland is involved by IgG4-related disease, fibrosis and phlebitis are rarely seen. IgG4-related pancreatitis has been studied more extensively than IgG4-related disease affecting other endocrine organs {1103}. Depending on the specimen cellularity, a ratio of IgG4-positive to IgG-positive plasma cells of > 40% is a general cut-off point for possible involvement by IgG4-related disease. Of note, IgG4-related disease cannot be diagnosed solely on the basis of IgG4-positive plasma cell count or the IgG4+:IgG+ plasma cell ratio.

Differential diagnosis

Many conditions can be associated with increased numbers of IgG4-positive plasma cells that are not considered IgG4-related disease, including inflammatory diseases, antineutrophil cytoplasmic antibody (ANCA)-associated inflammatory diseases, infections, low-grade B-cell lymphoproliferative disorders, carcinomas with prominent intratumoural or peritumoural IgG4-positive plasma cells, among others.

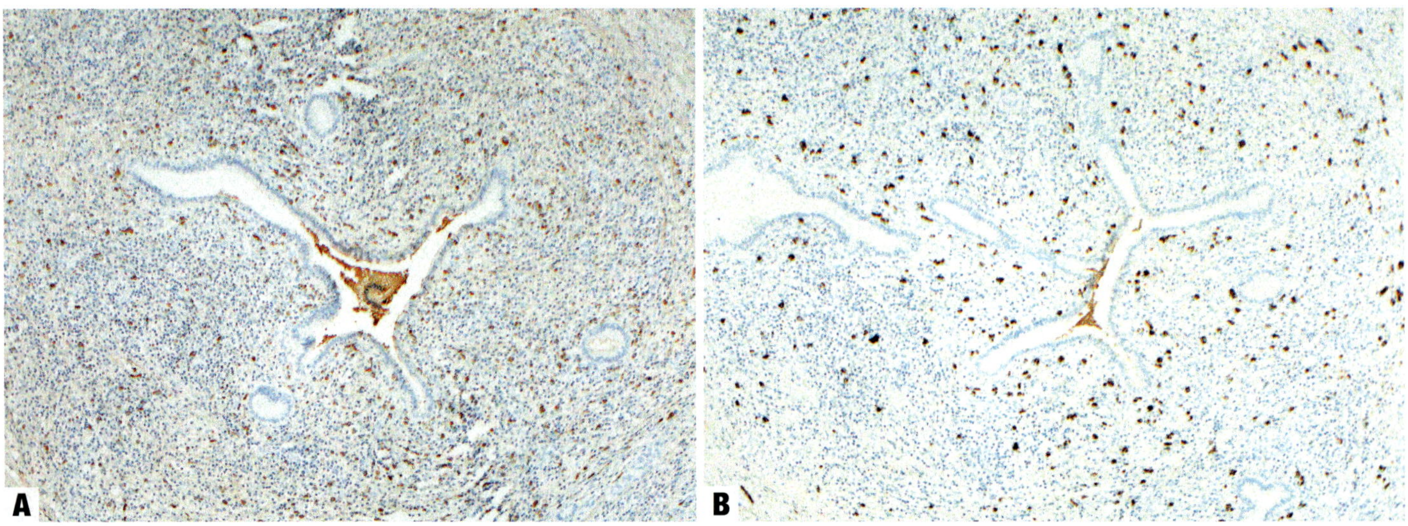

Fig. 10.02 IgG4-related disease. IgG (**A**) and IgG4 (**B**) immunostaining in a case of IgG4-related pancreatitis.

Cytology

There are no specific features of IgG4-related disease in cytology specimens. Aspirates show low cellularity; an inflammatory background of lymphocytes, plasma cells, and eosinophils; and spindle cells {2236}. Cases diagnosed on cytology have relied on the integration of clinical, radiographic, and serological parameters {2236,2157}.

Diagnostic molecular pathology

None

Essential and desirable diagnostic criteria

Essential: characteristic histological features (lymphoplasmacytic infiltrate; storiform fibrosis; obliterative fibrosis) and plasma cell density depending on specimen type and individual organ in the appropriate clinical and radiographic settings; an IgG4+:IgG+ plasma cell ratio of > 40%.

Desirable: elevated serum IgG4 (> 140 mg/dL); evidence of other organ involvement; response to glucocorticoid therapy.

Staging

None

Prognosis and prediction

IgG4-related disease is a chronic condition with a relapsing and remitting course. Glucocorticoids and B-cell depletion treatments generally effect a good response {2273}.

Extranodal marginal zone lymphoma of mucosa-associated lymphoid tissue

Tallini G
Kakkar A

Definition

Extranodal marginal zone lymphoma (EMZL) of mucosa-associated lymphoid tissue (MALT) is an indolent primary extranodal B-cell lymphoma with cytological and architectural features reminiscent of Peyer patch lymphoid tissue, the prototypical MALT. EMZL typically arises from marginal zone B cells of acquired MALT and is often associated with an underlying chronic inflammatory disorder.

ICD-O coding

9699/3 Extranodal marginal zone lymphoma of mucosa-associated lymphoid tissue

ICD-11 coding

2A85.3 Extranodal marginal zone B-cell lymphoma, primary site excluding stomach or skin

Related terminology

Acceptable: extranodal marginal zone lymphoma; mucosa-associated lymphoid tissue (MALT) lymphoma.

Subtype(s)

None

Localization

About 5% of EMZLs occur in the thyroid, and EMZLs account for about 2% of all malignant thyroid tumours {4458,5190,1093}. EMZLs of the adrenal and pituitary glands are very rare (< 0.5% of all pituitary or adrenal tumours), and those of the parathyroid gland are even rarer {1603,3877,3119,3682,2217}.

Clinical features

The typical presentation in the thyroid is an enlarging mass that is markedly hypoechoic on ultrasound and cold on scintigraphy

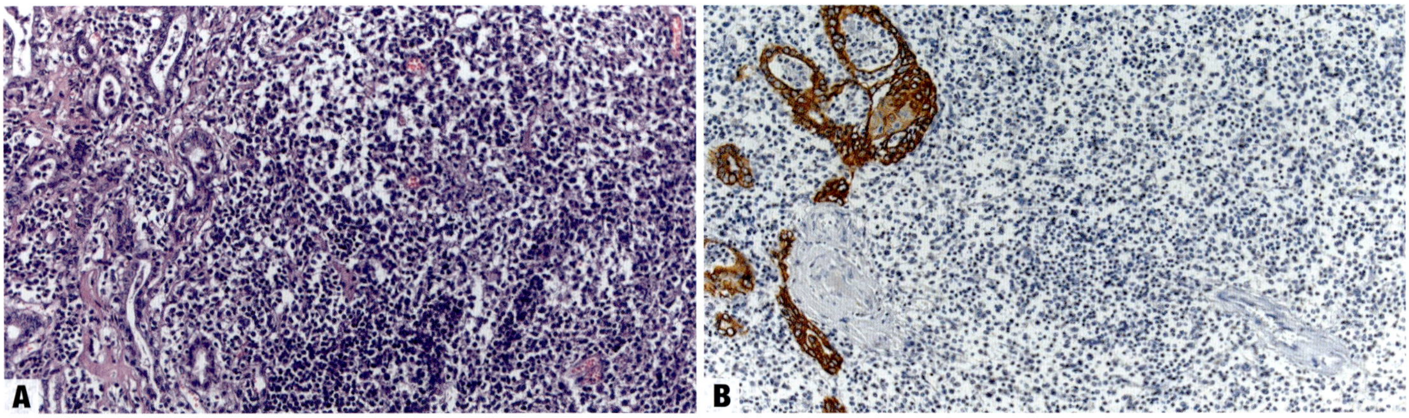

Fig. 10.03 Extranodal marginal zone lymphoma of the thyroid. **A** Thyroid parenchyma replaced by lymphoma. **B** Cytokeratin highlights destructive infiltration of the thyroid follicular epithelium by lymphoma cells (lymphoepithelial lesions).

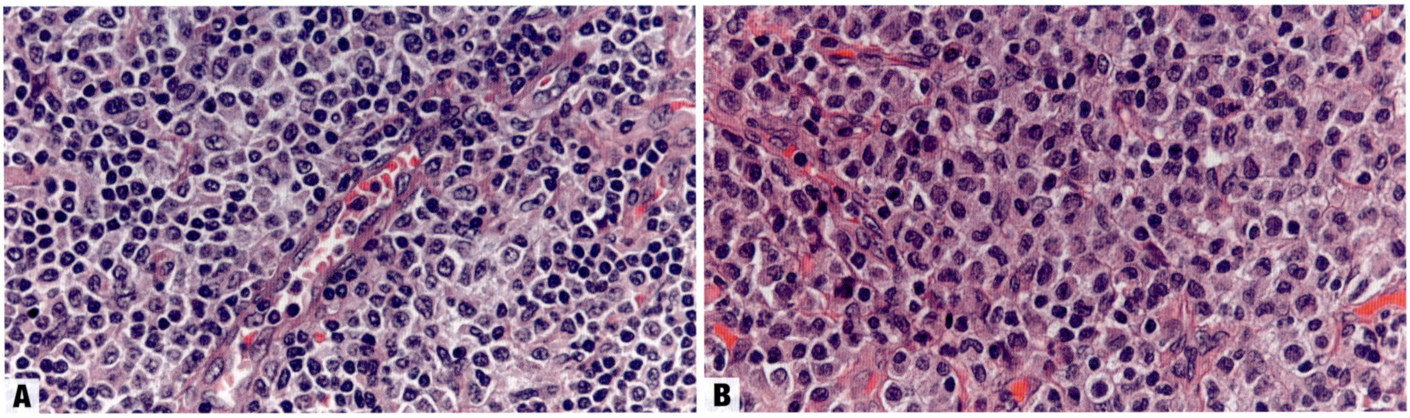

Fig. 10.04 Extranodal marginal zone lymphoma of the thyroid. **A** Heterogeneous infiltrate with small lymphocytes intermixed with scattered cells showing plasmacytic differentiation and a few large cells. **B** Tumour cells with pale cytoplasm, slightly irregular or indented nuclei, dispersed chromatin, and inconspicuous nucleoli, intermixed with monocyte-like cells with abundant pale cytoplasm.

{5030}. EMZL in the pituitary usually manifests as a sellar mass {679}. With EMZL in the adrenal there may be endocrine insufficiency {3682}.

Epidemiology

The median age is 60–70 years, and the M:F ratio is 1:4–5 {4827}. Concomitant thyroid EMZL and papillary thyroid carcinoma may rarely occur in the setting of Hashimoto thyroiditis {791}.

Etiology

EMZL usually occurs in the setting of autoimmune disorders or other causes of longstanding chronic inflammation {4184,1603}. Patients with Hashimoto thyroiditis have a 9- to 17-fold increased risk of developing lymphoma, particularly EMZL {2646,3272, 3730,2225}. The role of Hashimoto thyroiditis is supported by a clonal relationship between the lymphoma and the associated thyroiditis as demonstrated by identical IGH gene rearrangements {3103,4945,3082}.

Pathogenesis

An accumulation of extranodal lymphoid tissue (acquired MALT) due to chronic inflammation such as in autoimmune disorders results in clonal B-cell proliferation and acquisition of successive genetic alterations {4184,1603}.

The t(3;14)(p14;q32) translocation with the *FOXP1*::IGH gene fusion has been described in thyroid EMZL {3958}. It may also be seen in diffuse large B-cell lymphomas that have an EMZL component {3958}. FOXP1 is a repressor of proapoptotic genes, and its overexpression caused by the *FOXP1*::IGH fusion promotes B-cell survival by inhibiting caspase-dependent apoptosis, in cooperation with the NF-κB pathway, the latter having been implicated in the pathogenesis of EMZL at various locations {4653}. Thyroid EMZL commonly shows trisomy 3 (~20% of cases) and mutations in *TET2* (62%), *TNFRSF14* (46%), and *PIK3CD* (23%), whereas *TNFAIP3* and *MYD88* mutations are rare {4303,3722,4304,3082}.

Macroscopic appearance

EMZL is a solid infiltrative mass with a bulging white cut surface.

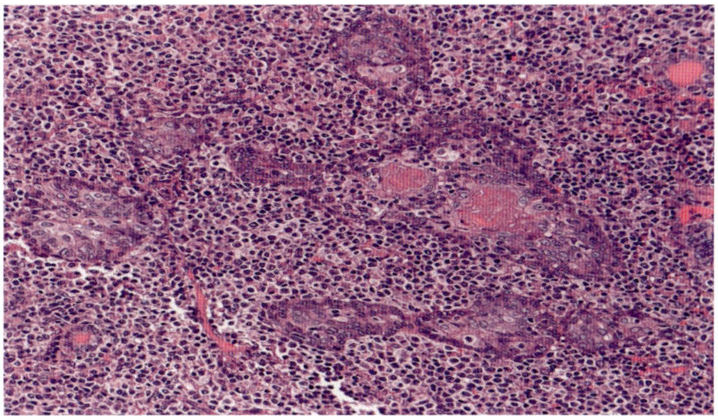

Fig. 10.05 Extranodal marginal zone lymphoma of the thyroid. Lymphoepithelial lesions with squamous metaplasia of thyroid follicular cells.

Histopathology

The histopathology shows a heterogeneous infiltrate predominantly composed of small B cells including marginal zone–like cells and small lymphocytes, with scattered plasma cells, immunoblasts, and centroblast-like cells replacing the glandular parenchyma. The marginal zone–like cells (also called centrocyte-like cells) are small to medium-sized, with pale cytoplasm, slightly irregular or indented nuclei, dispersed chromatin, and inconspicuous nucleoli. The presence of sheets of large cells unassociated with follicular dendritic cell meshworks is indicative of transformation to diffuse large B-cell lymphoma {2160}.

In the thyroid, EMZL accounts for 30–45% of all lymphomas. Thyroid follicles are commonly expanded by neoplastic lymphoid cells, forming lymphoepithelial lesions. Lymphoma cells may form expansile nodular aggregates within the thyroid follicular lumina, forming MALT balls. Hashimoto thyroiditis is identified in the background in virtually all cases {3482,4176,1093, 4827}.

Immunophenotype

The neoplastic cells are immunopositive for the B-lineage markers CD20, CD79a, and PAX5. They often express IgM, and less frequently, IgA or IgG. BCL2 is often positive, and the marginal

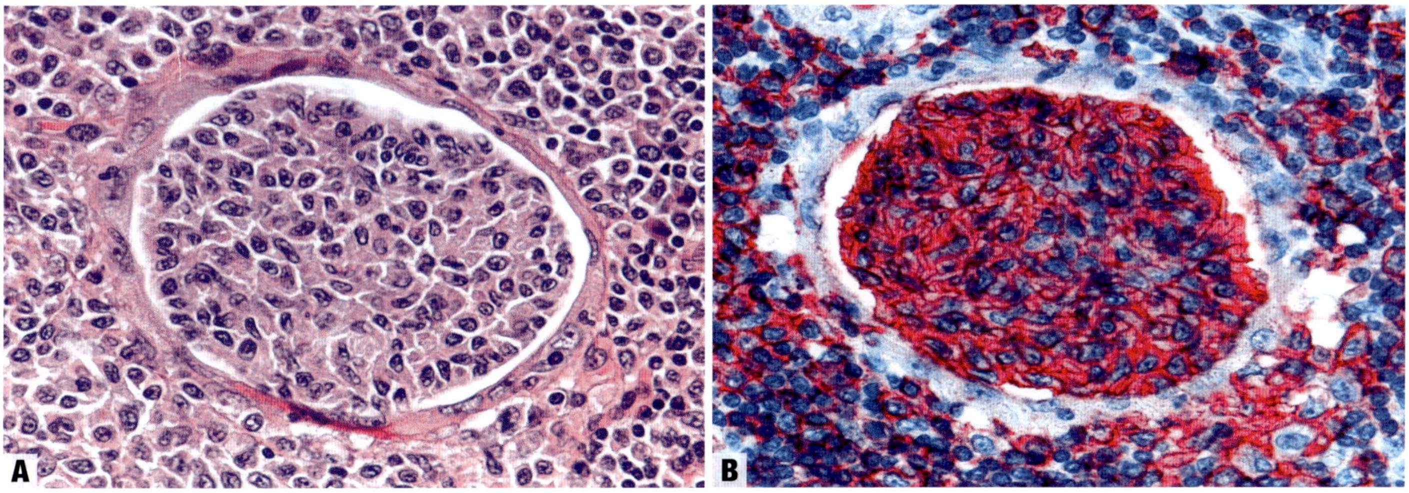

Fig. 10.06 Extranodal marginal zone lymphoma of the thyroid. **A** Expansile, ball-like collections of lymphoma cells within thyroid follicles (MALT balls) are distinctive lymphoepithelial lesions. **B** Lymphoma cells are positive for CD20.

zone marker IRTA1 is variably expressed. CD5, CD23, CD10, BCL6, cyclin D1, and SOX11 are usually negative, helping to distinguish from small lymphocytic lymphoma, follicular lymphoma, and mantle cell lymphoma.

Differential diagnosis

The differential diagnosis includes Hashimoto thyroiditis and chronic lymphocytic thyroiditis, which typically do not obliterate the thyroid parenchyma but may show destruction of the parenchyma, reminiscent of lymphoepithelial lesions. In difficult cases, immunohistochemical markers may be helpful, and keratin may be useful in highlighting destroyed follicles.

Cytology

Cytological specimens of EMZL often comprise a polymorphous proliferation of intermediate-sized lymphoid cells with centrocyte-like or monocytoid features and variable plasma cells.

Diagnostic molecular pathology

Molecular studies are usually not required for diagnosis.

Essential and desirable diagnostic criteria

Essential: lymphoma composed predominantly of small to medium-sized centrocyte-like cells and monocytoid cells; effacement or distortion of organ tissue architecture; B-cell immunophenotype compatible with EMZL; absence of sheets of large cells unassociated with follicular dendritic cell meshworks.

Desirable: monotypic lymphoid and/or plasma cells, or clonal IG gene rearrangement.

Staging

Lugano modification of the Ann Arbor staging system {795}

Prognosis and prediction

The prognosis is excellent {4458,5190}. For cases in the thyroid, the median survival time is about 15 years {4960}, with a 5-year survival rate of about 90% {1093,4827,4960}. Poor prognostic factors include age > 70 years, high stage, elevated LDH as also incorporated into the MALT Lymphoma International Prognostic Index (MALT-IPI) {4459}.

Diffuse large B-cell lymphoma NOS

Chan JKC
Gujral S

Definition

Diffuse large B-cell lymphoma NOS (DLBCL-NOS) is a neoplastic proliferation of medium-sized to large B cells with a diffuse growth pattern, not meeting the diagnostic criteria for specific large B-cell lymphoma neoplasms.

ICD-O coding

9680/3 Diffuse large B-cell lymphoma, NOS

ICD-11 coding

2A81.Z Diffuse large B-cell lymphoma, NOS

Related terminology

None

Subtype(s)

Centroblastic subtype; immunoblastic subtype; anaplastic subtype; germinal-centre B-cell–like subtype; activated B-cell–like subtype; diffuse large B-cell lymphoma with *MYC* and *BCL6* rearrangements

Localization

In the endocrine organs, primary DLBCL-NOS can occur in the thyroid, adrenal, and pituitary, but it has not been described in the parathyroid.

Clinical features

Patients with thyroid DLBCL-NOS usually present with a mass in the thyroid, with or without cervical lymphadenopathy {120,4827, 1798,1093,4176}. Rapid enlargement of the mass, hoarseness, dyspnoea, and increased serum LDH are common {120,4827, 1798,1093,4176,827}. Most patients (84–100%) have stage I/II disease {5066,927}.

Primary adrenal DLBCL-NOS is defined as lymphoma involving one or both adrenals, lacking a history of lymphoma, and with or without involvement of lymph nodes or other organs but always with the adrenal lesions being unequivocally dominant {3682}. About 70% of cases are bilateral {781}. Patients usually present with abdominal pain and constitutional symptoms, although some patients are asymptomatic. Clinical and biochemical features of adrenal insufficiency are common {4813, 5035,2204,2022,5100}.

Patients with primary pituitary lymphoma usually present with a mass lesion manifesting as cranial nerve palsy, headache, and visual field defects, as well as impaired hormonal status such as anterior pituitary failure, panhypopituitarism, diabetes insipidus, and hyperprolactinaemia {645,4420,2874}.

Epidemiology

Primary lymphomas of the thyroid are uncommon, accounting for 1–5% of all thyroid malignancies and approximately 1–2% of extranodal lymphomas {160,3482,4460}. DLBCL-NOS accounts for > 65% of cases {1658}. Thyroid DLBCLs are about 2.5 times as prevalent in women as in men, with a median age of 65 years {4446,120,4827,4460,927,5066}.

Primary lymphomas of the adrenal gland are very rare, accounting for < 1% of all lymphomas, and with < 300 cases reported in the literature {2022,5100}. DLBCL-NOS accounts for > 85% of cases {4813}. The mean age is 70 years, and the M:F ratio is 7:1 {781}.

Primary lymphomas of the pituitary are even rarer, accounting for 0–0.2% of all pituitary lesions according to retrospective large surgical or radiological series {1432,3877,4636,1325}. DLBCL-NOS accounts for 55% of all cases {645,4420}. In a literature review published in 2020, 23 of the 44 reported cases represented DLBCL {645}, with a median age of 65 years and with no sex predilection.

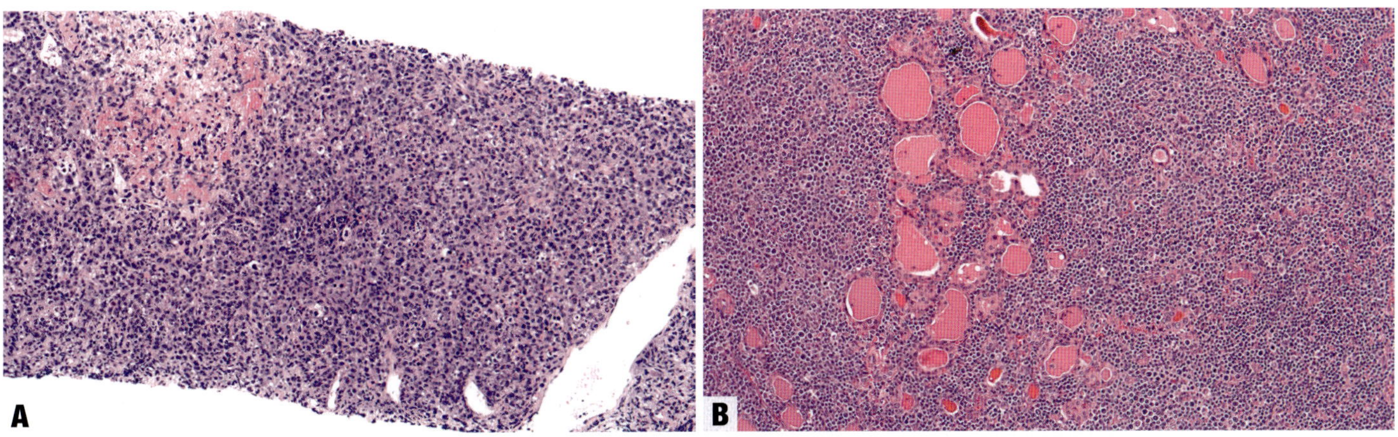

Fig. 10.07 Diffuse large B-cell lymphoma NOS (DLBCL-NOS). **A** Needle biopsy of an adrenal mass shows primary DLBCL-NOS with replacement of the normal parenchyma by a diffuse infiltrate of abnormal lymphoid cells. Focal necrosis is present. The interspersed sinusoidal blood vessels probably represent residual pre-existing vasculature of the adrenal cortex. **B** Primary thyroid DLBCL-NOS shows a diffuse, dense lymphomatous infiltrate replacing the thyroid parenchyma. The residual thyroid follicles show oncocytic changes.

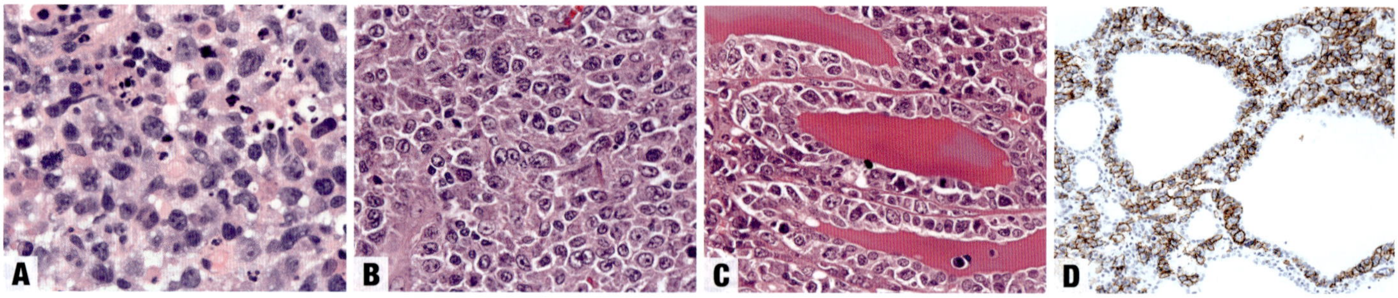

Fig. 10.08 Diffuse large B-cell lymphoma NOS (DLBCL-NOS). **A** Primary DLBCL-NOS involving the adrenal gland. The infiltrate comprises abnormal large lymphoid cells with irregularly folded nuclei and prominent nucleoli. Mitotic figures are seen. **B** Primary DLBCL-NOS involving the thyroid. The infiltrate comprises atypical large lymphoid cells with small distinct nucleoli. **C** Sometimes there can be striking infiltration of lymphoma cells into the thyroid follicular epithelium. **D** Primary DLBCL-NOS involving the thyroid. The lymphoma cells are immunoreactive for CD20. The infiltration into the thyroid follicular epithelium is highlighted.

Etiology

Thyroid lymphomas are strongly associated with chronic lymphocytic or Hashimoto thyroiditis {1093,3482,1009,2003,827}. The odds of developing thyroid lymphoma are significantly increased for patients with chronic lymphocytic thyroiditis {1929,2225, 4827}. Sequence similarity is reported in the clonal populations in Hashimoto thyroiditis and the ensuing thyroid lymphoma {3103}. Thyroid lymphomas often exhibit common homologous germline IGHV genes used by antithyroid antibodies, further implicating derivation from Hashimoto thyroiditis {3970,3826}.

Pathogenesis

The genomic profile of DLBCL-NOS has been characterized, with different genetic subtypes being recognized {1797,761, 4012,2500}. However, specific information on primary DLBCLs of endocrine organs is limited or lacking. In primary thyroid DLBCLs, *MYD88* mutation has not been detected, whereas *BCL2* or *MYC* translocation is found in a small proportion of cases {2351}. In primary adrenal DLBCL-NOS, *MYD88* p.L265P mutation and *CD79B* mutation are found in 24% and 48% of cases respectively, with the frequency being broadly comparable to that in various other extranodal large B-cell lymphomas.

Macroscopic appearance

The lymphoma forms a poorly defined, solid, fleshy tumour mass, which may exhibit necrotic or haemorrhagic foci {1093}.

Histopathology

DLBCL-NOS shows replacement of the normal parenchyma by a diffuse, dense infiltrate of large lymphoid cells with round or irregularly folded nuclei, distinct nucleoli, and amphophilic cytoplasm. Mitotic figures are readily identified.

In the thyroid, the lymphoma cells can infiltrate into the thyroid follicular epithelium and follicular lumina. In a proportion of cases, a component of extranodal marginal zone lymphoma or follicular lymphoma is present, suggesting transformation from these underlying indolent lymphomas {120,4827,1093,4176,2351}.

Immunohistochemistry

The neoplastic cells express pan–B cell markers, such as CD20, PAX5, and CD79a. They show variable expression of CD10, BCL6, IRF4 (MUM1), BCL2, and MYC. Subclassification into germinal-centre B-cell (GCB) and non-GCB subtypes can be achieved by immunohistochemical algorithms {4041, 2980}. For primary thyroid DLBCL-NOS, some studies report a predominance of the GCB subtype {4827,3245,2351}, whereas others report a predominance of the non-GCB subtype {5066}. In primary adrenal DLBCL-NOS, the non-GCB subtype markedly predominates {4813,5100}.

Cytology

The aspirates show non-cohesive large lymphoid cells with variable degrees of nuclear pleomorphism. The diagnostic sensitivity of FNA is increased when supplemented with cell-block production and immunohistochemistry {5139,1981,3578}.

Diagnostic molecular pathology

Usually not required for diagnosis

Essential and desirable diagnostic criteria

Essential: a destructive infiltrate of large lymphoid cells; mature B-cell phenotype; exclusion of other specific entities of large B-cell lymphoma.

Desirable: immunophenotype or gene expression profiling to determine GCB or activated B cell–like / non-GCB subtype; reporting of isolated *MYC* or dual *MYC* and *BCL6* rearrangements; genetic testing, if relevant for clinical decision-making.

Staging

Staging is by the Lugano classification, a modification of the Ann Arbor staging system {795}.

Prognosis and prediction

Patients with localized thyroid DLBCL have a favourable prognosis, with a median overall survival time of 9.3 years and a 5-year disease-specific survival rate of 75% {4460,1658}. Poor prognostic factors include high stage, poor performance status, bulky tumour, advanced age, non-GCB subtype, MYC/BCL2 dual expression, and a lack of administration of rituximab {1093, 2985,5066,927}.

For primary adrenal DLBCL, the 2-year overall survival rate is reported to be 68.3–72.5% {2301,4813}. Treatment with chemotherapy and early-stage disease are associated with longer survival.

Information on the outcome of patients with primary pituitary DLBCL is limited. Among 17 patients, 10 were alive with no or stable disease at 2–52 months, 5 died of disease at 1–24 months, and 2 died of unrelated causes {645}.

Langerhans cell histiocytosis

Rossi ED
Bychkov A
Chan JKC
Thompson LDR
Touraine PA

Definition

Langerhans cell histiocytosis (LCH) is a clonal neoplasm of myeloid dendritic cells that have a Langerhans cell phenotype (CD1a and CD207 expression) and lack high-grade cytological features.

ICD-O coding

9751/1 Langerhans cell histiocytosis, NOS
9751/3 Langerhans cell histiocytosis, disseminated

ICD-11 coding

2B31.2 Langerhans cell histiocytosis

Related terminology

Not recommended: eosinophilic granuloma; histiocytosis X (obsolete).

Subtype(s)

None

Localization

LCH can be localized to a single site (single-system LCH [SS-LCH]), occur in multiple sites within a single system (usually bone), or affect multiple systems (multisystem LCH [MS-LCH]) {3022,4511}. The most commonly affected endocrine organs are the pituitary and thyroid {3884}, usually as a single affected site {4476,5047}. Involvement of the parathyroid and adrenal glands is rare.

Clinical features

Involvement of the hypothalamic–pituitary–adrenal axis often leads to diabetes insipidus and growth hormone deficiency {3744,3884}, but there can also be a deficiency of gonadotropins (LH, FSH), TSH, and ACTH, as well as hyperprolactinaemia {3884}. Thyroid LCH typically presents as a diffuse goitre or a single nodule {2724,4688}.

Endocrine system involvement in LCH is evaluated using hormone assays and imaging {3079}. Increased uptake by FDG PET can be used for staging in hypothalamopituitary lesions {1596}. Neck sonography may reveal isolated or multiple hypoechoic and heterogeneous nodules in the thyroid {772}, which is a nonspecific finding.

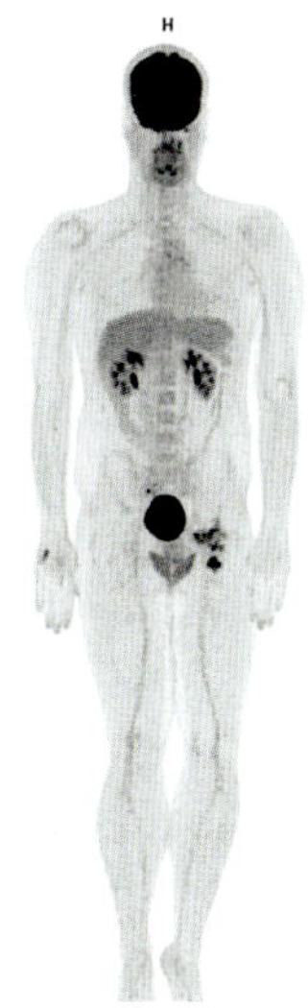

Fig. 10.09 Langerhans cell histiocytosis. FDG PET of a patient with Langerhans cell histiocytosis, showing widespread disease.

Epidemiology

LCH is a rare disease, with an annual incidence of 5–9 cases per 1 million children and 1–2 cases per 1 million adults {3783}. There is a slight male predilection {3744}. Endocrine manifestations are reported in 15–35% and are more prevalent in childhood-onset LCH than in adult-onset LCH {3744,3884}. Cases limited to the thyroid are extremely rare, and most cases with thyroid involvement occur in patients with multifocal disease {4957,3468}.

Etiology

The presence of frequent *BRAF* and *MAP2K1* mutations in LCH suggests it is a neoplastic process of myeloid origin {258,

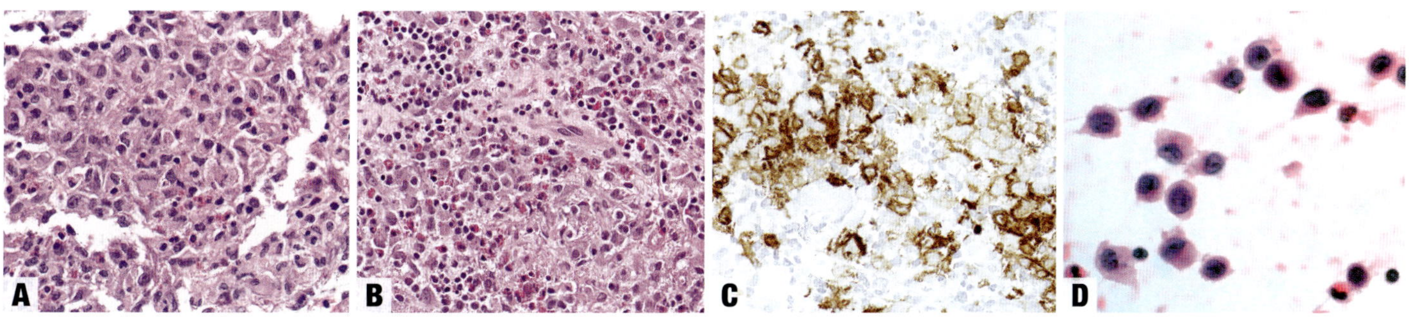

Fig. 10.10 Pituitary Langerhans cell histiocytosis. **A** Langerhans cell histiocytosis cells with contorted nuclei. **B** Eosinophils are prominent, in addition to the neoplastic Langerhans cells. **C** The histiocytes (Langerhans cells) are CD1a-positive. **D** Histiocytes with grooved nuclei admixed with eosinophils (intraoperative cytology).

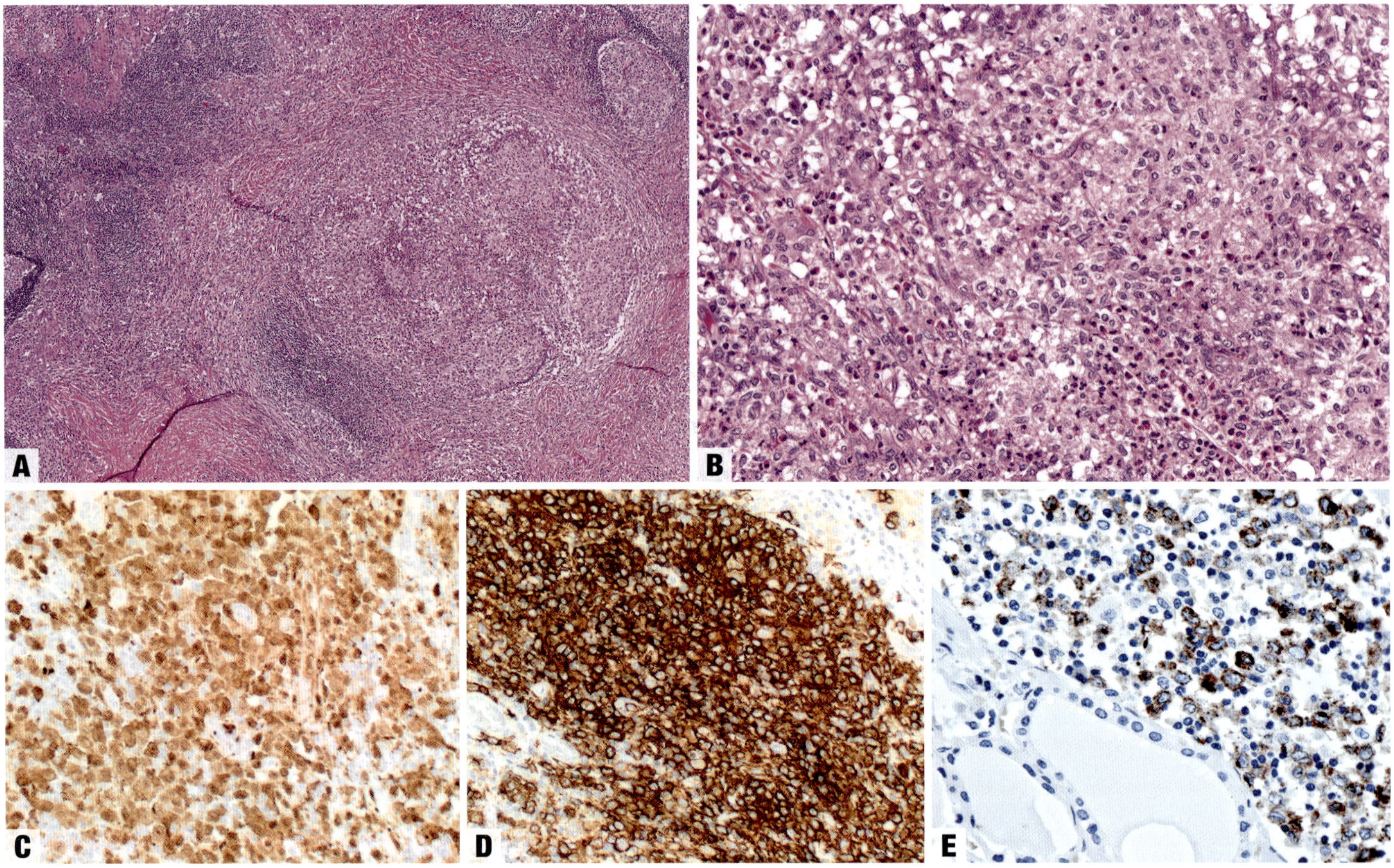

Fig. 10.11 Thyroid Langerhans cell histiocytosis. **A** The thyroid parenchyma is affected by chronic lymphocytic thyroiditis, in addition to showing a well-defined nodule of Langerhans cell histiocytosis. **B** Epithelioid histiocytes with curved, bean-shaped nuclei are associated with numerous eosinophils. **C,D** The neoplastic cells are strongly and diffusely immunoreactive for S100 in the nucleus and cytoplasm (**C**), and strongly and diffusely immunoreactive for CD1a (**D**). **E** There is CD207 (langerin) immunoexpression in the neoplastic cells adjacent to the thyroid follicles.

548,735,1078}. A subset of cases show antigen receptor gene rearrangements {785}. Cases of synchronous LCH and acute leukaemia of ambiguous or myeloid lineage suggest a possible clonal relationship {5073}. Nevertheless, the disorder shares features with other IL-17A–related inflammatory diseases {1078}.

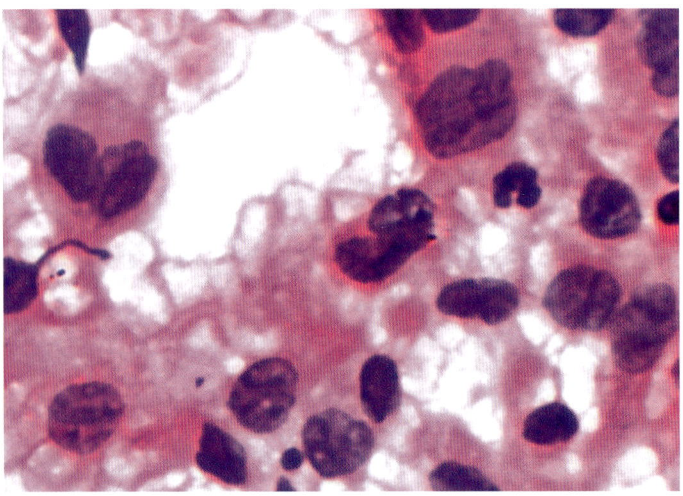

Fig. 10.12 Thyroid Langerhans cell histiocytosis. FNA. Large histiocytoid cells with convoluted nuclear membranes.

An IL-1 activation loop has been proposed, based on elevated levels of Merkel cell polyomavirus DNA sequences, high levels of the tyrosine phosphatase SHP-1 in lesional tissues, and increased IL-17A in peripheral blood and lesional tissues, particularly in multiorgan disease {3140,3139}.

Pathogenesis

About 50% of cases of LCH have *BRAF* p.V600E mutations {3777}. Mutations in *MAP2K1* are identified in one third to half of the *BRAF*-wildtype cases {548,735}. Mutations in other genes in the *MAPK* pathway (*ARAF* and *MAP3K1*) or other signalling pathways (*PIK3CA*) have also been described {1864,3204, 3205,1789}.

Macroscopic appearance

None

Histopathology

LCH is characterized by histiocytoid cells with grooved, convoluted, indented, or lobed nuclei {1789,4476} and moderately abundant, lightly eosinophilic cytoplasm. The background often includes eosinophils with a variable admixture of neutrophils and lymphocytes.

In the thyroid, the LCH cells show interstitial infiltration and destruction of thyroid follicles. A background of chronic lymphocytic thyroiditis is common. Sometimes, thyroid LCH can spread to cervical lymph nodes {728}.

The ultrastructural hallmark is the cytoplasmic Birbeck granules, which have a tennis-racket shape (200–400 nm long and 33 nm wide) and a zipper-like appearance.

LCH cells are positive for CD1a, S100, and CD207 (langerin) {1789}. VE1 immunostaining (anti–BRAF p.V600E) is positive in half of the cases and correlates with *BRAF* mutations by sequencing or PCR {3777}.

Cytology

Cytological preparations show cellular smears with large mononuclear or multinucleated histiocytoid cells with irregular nuclear contours, nuclear grooves, and foamy granular cytoplasm {1789,3830,296}. The inflammatory background contains eosinophils, occasional Charcot–Leyden crystals, and scattered lymphocytes {3830,3637,3949,1765}.

Diagnostic molecular pathology

Not applicable

Essential and desirable diagnostic criteria

Essential: clusters/sheets of histiocytoid cells with grooved to contorted nuclei positive for immunohistochemical markers of Langerhans cells (CD1a+, CD207+) in the correct histological/anatomical context.

Desirable: mutation analysis in the MAPK pathway, with sensitive testing for low-frequency allele detection.

Staging

None

Prognosis and prediction

In reports before targeted therapy was available, the clinical outcome depended largely on the extent of the disease (SS-LCH vs MS-LCH), with ≥ 99% survival for SS-LCH with unifocal disease. MS-LCH with risk-organ involvement has a variable course, with only ~60% of patients achieving no evidence of disease after 1 year on standard therapy. In MS-LCH without high-risk organ involvement, there is still about a 37% relapse/reactivation rate after 1 year of standard therapy with vinblastine and prednisone {1473,3022,1474,4511,99}. There are promising clinical responses in patients with relapsed and refractory LCH treated with BRAF or MEK inhibitors {3695}.

Rosai–Dorfman disease

Facchetti F
Chan JKC
Rossi S

Definition
Rosai–Dorfman disease (RDD) is a histiocytosis characterized by an accumulation of large S100-positive histiocytes commonly exhibiting emperipolesis.

ICD-O coding
9749/3 Rosai–Dorfman disease

ICD-11 coding
EK92 Histiocytoses of uncertain malignant potential

Related terminology
Acceptable: Rosai–Dorfman–Destombes disease.
Not recommended: sinus histiocytosis with massive lymphadenopathy.

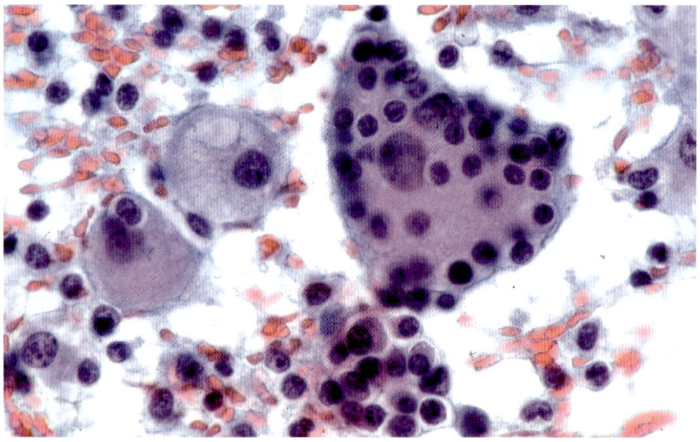

Fig. 10.13 Rosai–Dorfman disease of the thyroid. FNA. Large histiocytes with abundant pale cytoplasm showing pronounced emperipolesis.

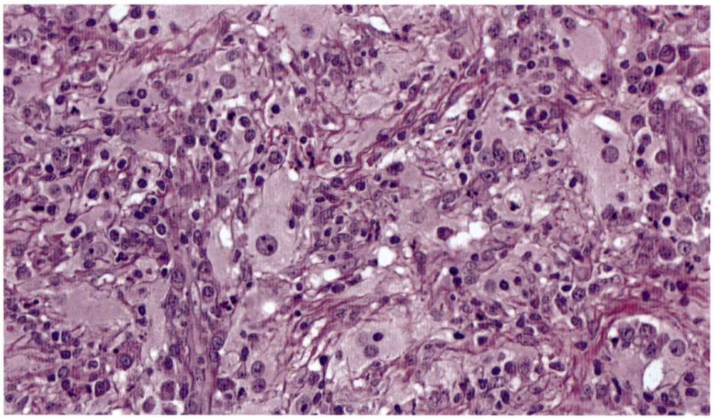

Fig. 10.14 Rosai–Dorfman disease involving the thyroid. The distinctive histiocytes are very large. They have round nuclei with distinct nucleoli and abundant pale-staining cytoplasm. Some contain lymphocytes or plasma cells in the cytoplasm. Abundant intermingled plasma cells are noticeable.

Subtype(s)
None

Localization
RDD typically involves cervical lymph nodes. In as many as 43% of cases, RDD develops in extranodal locations, most frequently the head and neck, skin and soft tissues, and CNS {8, 1243}. The thyroid is rarely affected, with < 10 cases published to date {4399,2567,3598,3120,4746,813,1559}. Isolated cases of RDD have been described in the posterior pituitary {3221, 2254,3848} and adrenal glands {1393}.

Clinical features
RDD of the thyroid is usually accompanied by involvement of cervical lymph nodes and other extranodal sites {3598,4746, 4399,813,2529,3120,2567}. Patients usually present with a cold thyroid nodule, which is typically tender on palpation. Systemic symptoms and abnormal laboratory findings (i.e. anaemia, leukocytosis, and hypergammaglobulinaemia) are common. RDD affecting the posterior pituitary presents as a suprasellar lesion and diabetes insipidus.

Epidemiology
In contrast to classic nodal RDD, which typically affects young men, most cases affecting endocrine organs arise in women between the fourth and sixth decades of life {4399,2567,3120, 3598,4746,1559,2254,3848}.

Etiology
The etiology is unknown. RDD may occur in a thyroid involved by autoimmune thyroid disease, for which a possible link has been postulated {3598}. A proportion of cases of RDD show an increased number of IgG4-positive plasma cells, but it is doubtful whether there is a relationship with IgG4-related disease {2942,2689}.

Pathogenesis
The pathogenesis is incompletely understood. Approximately 50% of cases carry gain-of-function mutations in MAPK/ERK pathway genes, including *KRAS*, *NRAS*, *MAP2K1*, *ARAF*, *CSF1R*, and (rarely) *BRAF* p.V600E, suggesting that at least a proportion of cases of RDD represent a neoplastic disorder {1114,4087,2891,1503,2075,734}.

Macroscopic appearance
RDD is usually well defined and tan-grey, with a soft or gritty texture.

Histopathology
The affected tissue shows infiltration by loose aggregates of large histiocytes with round vesicular nuclei, distinct nucleoli, and voluminous pale-staining cytoplasm, which typically exhibit

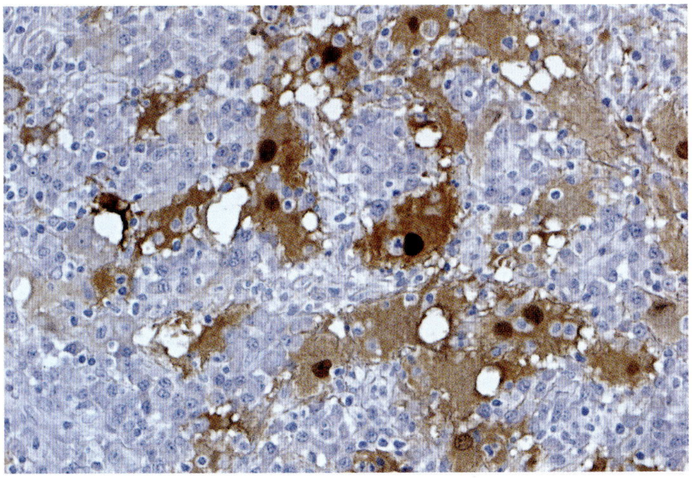

Fig. 10.15 Rosai–Dorfman disease involving the thyroid. The large histiocytes express S100. Emperipolesis is also obvious.

emperipolesis of lymphocytes, neutrophils, and plasma cells. There are usually many admixed plasma cells. The histiocytes are immunoreactive for S100, CD68, fascin, and OCT2 {3695} and variably immunoreactive for CD163 and CD14, but negative for CD1a and CD207. The background thyroid gland parenchyma often shows chronic lymphocytic thyroiditis. The differential diagnosis includes Erdheim–Chester disease, juvenile xanthogranuloma, and ALK-positive histiocytosis, all of which may express S100 and show focal emperipolesis {1243,4386,754}. The clinical, laboratory, and radiological context, as well as histopathological, immunohistochemical, and molecular features, will aid in their distinction.

Cytology

FNAC shows large histiocytes with emperipolesis in a background of mature lymphocytes, plasma cells, and neutrophils. Immunoreactivity for S100 is helpful for confirming the diagnosis {4746,813}.

Diagnostic molecular pathology

Not applicable

Essential and desirable diagnostic criteria

Essential: accumulation of large histiocytes with round vesicular nuclei, distinct nucleoli, and abundant pale cytoplasm; emperipolesis; expression of S100.

Desirable: in diagnostically challenging cases, expression of OCT2 and cyclin D1 in the absence of CD1a, CD207 (langerin), and ALK.

Staging

Not applicable

Prognosis and prediction

Individuals with thyroid RDD have remained well after treatment. Thyroid involvement is not known to change the generally good prognosis of RDD {3598}.

Erdheim–Chester disease

Paulus W
Chan JKC
Sahm F

Definition

Erdheim–Chester disease (ECD) is a clonal histiocytosis characterized by infiltration of foamy histiocytes and occasional Touton giant cells, chronic inflammation, and variable fibrosis, driven by alteration of a MAPK pathway gene.

ICD-O coding

9749/3 Erdheim–Chester disease

ICD-11 coding

2B31.Y & XH1VJ3 Other specified histiocytic or dendritic cell neoplasms & Erdheim–Chester disease

Related terminology

None

Subtype(s)

None

Localization

ECD is a multisystem disease where any organ may be involved. Long bones are affected in > 90% of cases. The most commonly involved endocrine organs are the pituitary and adrenal glands, whereas thyroid involvement has been described only occasionally {4108,933}.

Clinical features

Although ECD may be asymptomatic, most patients have general, inflammatory, or site-related symptoms. Endocrine involvement is frequent, and careful clinical, biological, and radiological evaluation reveals anterior pituitary dysfunction in 40–91% of patients, with diabetes insipidus in 25–50%, testicular insufficiency in as many as 53%, and adrenal infiltration/insufficiency in 6–39% of patients with ECD {933,1652}. Hypothyroidism is found in 20–28% of patients {1652,4098}. Among 64 patients with ECD, no patient was free of endocrine hormonal or structural involvement {933}.

Epidemiology

ECD is a rare but probably underdiagnosed disease. The median age at diagnosis is between 46 and 56 years, with an M:F ratio of 3:1 {1652}. Cases in children aged < 15 years are very rare and overlap with systemic juvenile xanthogranuloma.

Etiology

Unknown

Pathogenesis

ECD is a clonal neoplastic disorder driven by alteration of a MAPK pathway gene and ERK activation in nearly all cases {1114,1652}. Common alterations include *BRAF* p.V600E mutations (in as many as 60% of cases, depending on the study) {257,1795,1875,1244}, *MAP2K1* mutations (in as many as 30%), *KRAS* or *NRAS* mutations (in as many as 20%) {1244,1114,3418}, and other genetic alterations pertaining to the MAPK pathway, with single cases exhibiting *ARAF* mutations or *BRAF*, *NTRK1*, *ALK*, or *ETV3::NCOA2* fusions {1114,1189}. Single cases with *CSF1R* mutations or *RET* fusions have been reported {1189}. *PIK3CA* mutations can occur as single events or in combination with other alterations, mostly with *BRAF* p.V600E mutations (~11% of cases) {1244}. Activating mutations in *CSF1R* suggest that a subset of tumours may arise from extraembryonic macrophage progenitors {1189}, and mutant alleles in CD34-positive haematopoietic stem/progenitor cells have suggested several potential precursor pathways {1190}.

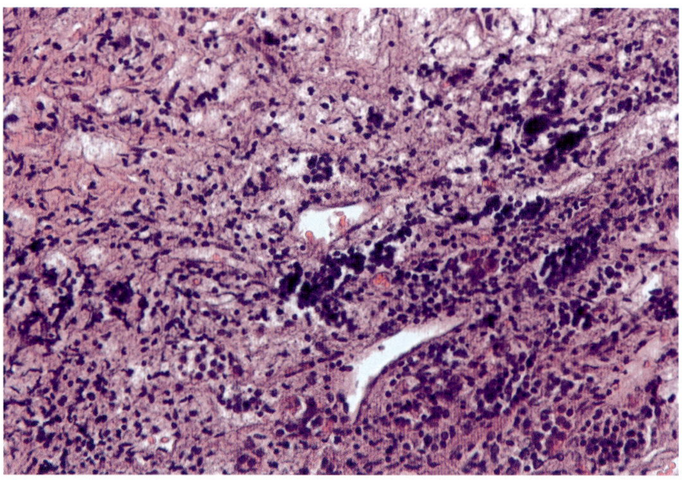

Fig. 10.16 Erdheim–Chester disease. An example from the sellar region showing histiocytic tumour cells (left) and anterior pituitary gland with atrophy and fibrosis (right).

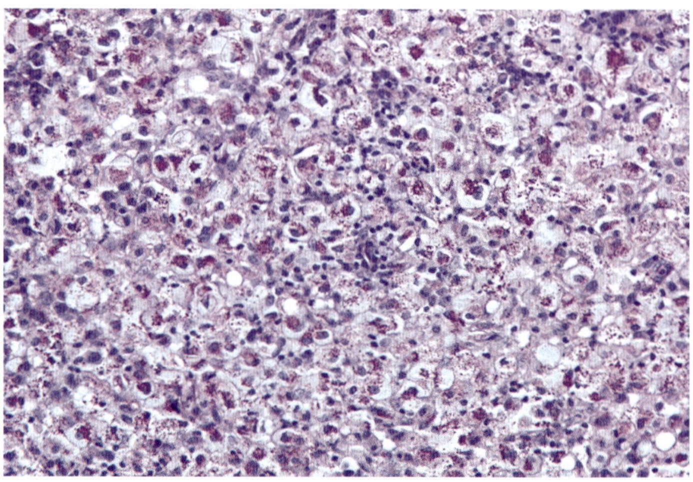

Fig. 10.17 Erdheim–Chester disease. An example from the sellar region showing histiocytic tumour cells and reactive lymphocytic cells (PAS).

Macroscopic appearance

The tissue samples in ECD often appear firm and sclerotic.

Histopathology

Like in juvenile xanthogranuloma, the affected tissue is infiltrated by foamy to epithelioid histiocytes with small nuclei, Touton-type multinucleated giant cells, scant lymphocytes and plasma cells, and rare neutrophils and eosinophils, accompanied by variable fibrosis.

The neoplastic histiocytes are positive for CD68, CD163, CD14, and factor XIIIa, variably positive for S100 (20–30% of cases), but negative for CD1a and CD207. About half express *BRAF* p.V600E mutations {3399}. Expression of phosphorylated ERK is frequent.

Cytology

Not clinically relevant

Diagnostic molecular pathology

Testing for potentially mutated genes (*BRAF*, in combination with *PIK3CA*, *MAP2K1*, and *KRAS*/*NRAS* in selected cases) should be performed with sensitive assays, because of the frequently low fraction of neoplastic cells. If this is negative, testing for fusions involving *NTRK1*, *ALK*, or *ETV3*::*NCOA2* may reveal rare variants of pathway activation.

Essential and desirable diagnostic criteria

Essential: infiltration of foamy cells positive for histiocytic antigens and negative for Langerhans cell markers; appropriate clinical and/or radiological context.

Desirable: exclusion of other lines of differentiation (epithelial, melanocytic, lymphocytic, etc.); exclusion of inflammatory lesions; mutation analysis of the MAPK pathway.

Staging

Not applicable

Prognosis and prediction

The prognosis depends on the site and extent of involvement. CNS involvement and multisystem disease are poor prognostic factors {180}. Therapeutic options include surgery, cladribine, immunomodulators, and molecular targeted therapies including BRAF inhibitors and MEK inhibitors {3353,1652}.

Follicular dendritic cell sarcoma

Chan JKC
Gujral S
Rossi ED

Definition

Follicular dendritic cell sarcoma (FDCS) is a malignant neoplasm showing morphological and phenotypic characteristics of follicular dendritic cells (FDCs), which are stromal-derived cells normally found in the germinal centres.

ICD-O coding

9758/3 Follicular dendritic cell sarcoma

ICD-11 coding

2B31.5 Follicular dendritic cell sarcoma

Related terminology

Acceptable: follicular dendritic cell tumour.

Subtype(s)

None

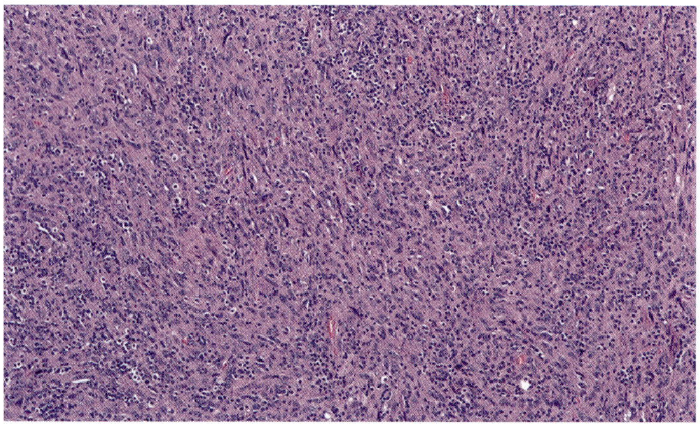

Fig. 10.18 Follicular dendritic cell sarcoma of the thyroid. Spindly cells show a storiform to whorled growth pattern. There are admixed small lymphocytes.

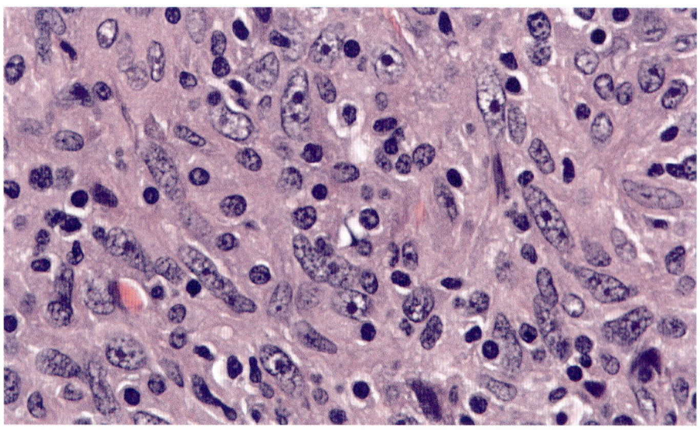

Fig. 10.19 Follicular dendritic cell sarcoma of the thyroid. The syncytial-appearing spindly tumour cells have elongated nuclei with pale chromatin and distinct nucleoli. There are intermingled small lymphocytes.

Localization

FDCS can occur in nodal sites or diverse extranodal sites. Cases occurring in endocrine organs include 7 cases reported in the thyroid and 1 case reported in the adrenal, with no cases reported so far in the parathyroid or pituitary {1480,5095,4271,5146,2748,2235}.

Clinical features

Patients with thyroid FDCS present with a slow-growing, painless thyroid mass, sometimes accompanied by cervical lymph node metastasis {1480,5095,4271,5146}. The patient with adrenal FDCS presented with paraneoplastic pemphigus {2748}.

Epidemiology

FDCS is extremely rare in endocrine organs {1312,3972}. Patients with thyroid FDCS are adults with a median age of 48 years, and there is a marked female predominance {1480,5095,4271,5146,2235}. The patient with adrenal FDCS was a boy aged 16 years {2748}.

Etiology

The etiology is generally unknown. FDCS shows no association with EBV.

Pathogenesis

Limited cytogenetic studies show a complex karyotype {3533}. Next-generation sequencing has revealed recurrent alterations in NF-κB pathway genes, *CDKN2A*, and *TP53* {1670,2868}. The frequent occurrence of NF-κB pathway gene mutations and the lack of MAPK pathway gene mutations contrast with the genomic profile of true histiocytic/dendritic cell neoplasms (including histiocytic sarcoma, interdigitating dendritic cell sarcoma, and Langerhans cell sarcoma) {2868}. Genomic analysis of a thyroid FDCS identified *CLTCL1*, *ATM*, *FLT1* (*VEGFR1*), and *TP53* mutations, as well as *HDGFRP3*::*SHC4* fusion {1005}.

Macroscopic appearance

FDCS has a fleshy appearance, with no distinctive features.

Histopathology

FDCS is composed of syncytial-appearing spindled to oval cells exhibiting a storiform, fascicular, whorled, or vague nodular pattern. The neoplastic cells have oval or elongated vesicular nuclei with a delicate nuclear membrane and distinct nucleoli. Nuclear pseudoinclusions and multinucleated tumour cells are common. The tumour is variably infiltrated by small lymphocytes. In some reported thyroid FDCS cases, the background thyroid shows features of chronic lymphocytic thyroiditis.

Immunohistochemistry

The neoplastic cells are positive for one or more of the FDC markers CD21, CD23, CD35, CXCL13, and podoplanin, and new FDC markers such as FDCSP and SRGN {5094,4692,970, 2734}. Expression of clusterin, desmoplakin, vimentin, fascin, EGFR, and HLA-DR is usually observed, whereas cytokeratin is usually negative {3559,4692,3332,970,1313}. The admixed small lymphocytes include B cells and T cells.

Cytology

FDCS is often difficult to diagnose on cytological materials alone. Spindled and epithelioid cells forming a fascicular, syncytial, and/or whorled pattern are often observed. The tumour cells have moderate amounts of cytoplasm, round to spindled nuclei, vesicular chromatin, and prominent nucleoli {3830}.

Diagnostic molecular pathology

Not required

Essential and desirable diagnostic criteria

Essential: a tumour with a storiform, fascicular, whorled, or nodular growth pattern; spindled or oval tumour cells with indistinct cell borders, vesicular nuclei, and distinct nucleoli; intermingled small lymphocytes; positivity for at least two FDC markers, such as CD21, CD23, CD35, and CXCL13; negative staining for lymphocyte-specific markers and generally negative staining for S100.

Staging

Not applicable

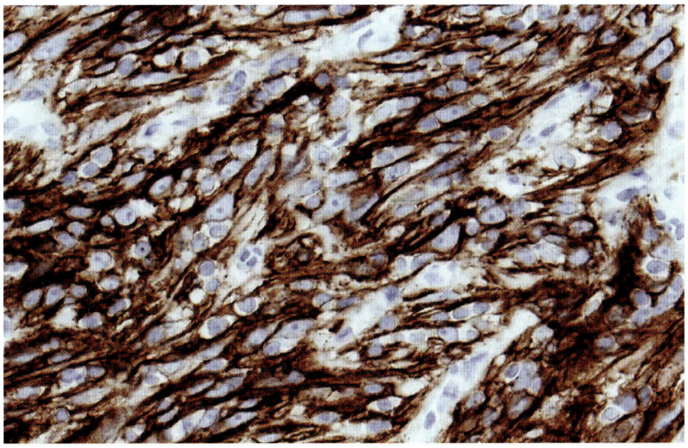

Fig. 10.20 Follicular dendritic cell sarcoma of the thyroid. Immunostaining for CD21 is positive. The long, interconnected cell processes are highlighted.

Prognosis and prediction

FDCS is a low- to intermediate-grade malignancy. A pooled analysis of the literature shows local recurrence and distant metastasis rates of 28% and 27%, respectively {3972}. Among the reported examples of thyroid FDCS, the patients were disease-free 6–36 months after diagnosis.

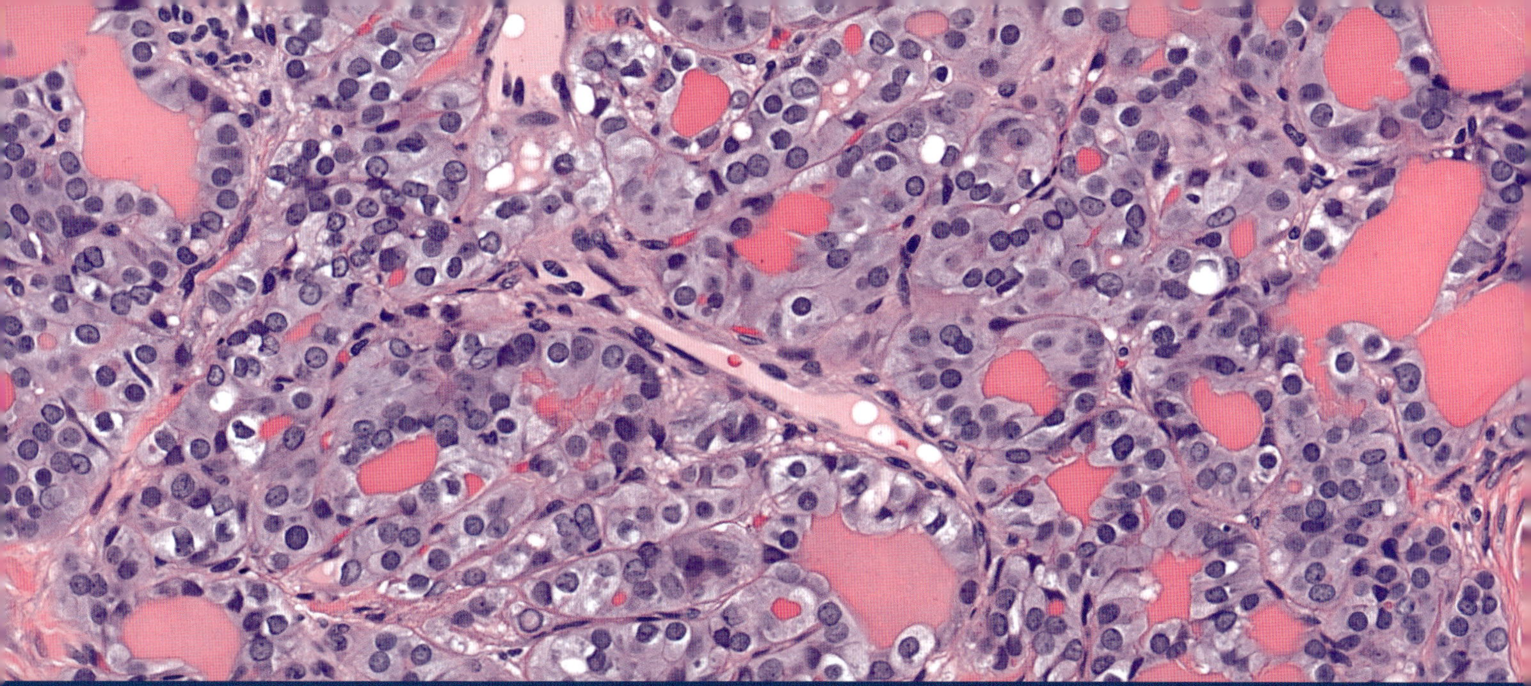

11

Germ cell tumours

Edited by: Erickson LA, Lax SF, Thompson LDR

Germ cell tumours: Introduction

Erickson LA
Papotti M
Tallini G

In this edition of the WHO classification of endocrine and neuroendocrine tumours, the classification of germ cell tumours in endocrine organs and teratomas with endocrine differentiation has been updated. The modifications and changes involve various organs and tumour entities. Germ cell tumours in endocrine organs include teratomas with mature or immature tissues derived from all three germ cell layers (endoderm, mesoderm, and ectoderm). Teratomas in endocrine organs are rare and found in the thyroid gland, the adrenal glands, and the pituitary gland. Most thyroid gland teratomas occur in neonates and young children, often as congenital tumours {4474,3743, 92}. Most adrenal gland teratomas are identified in adults {301}. Thyroid gland teratomas that are high-grade / highly malignant by histological criteria have been reclassified as thyroblastoma, supported by the recurrent finding of *DICER1* mutations, and are no longer regarded as true teratomas {3655,3809,32}. Thyroblastoma is discussed separately in the chapter on thyroid tumours, in the sections on embryonal thyroid neoplasms. Teratomas with endocrine differentiation that arise in non-endocrine organs include struma ovarii (teratomas with > 50% thyroid tissue or with functional or malignant thyroid tissue of any amount), thyroid carcinoma arising in struma ovarii, and ovarian neuroendocrine tumours (teratomas with unequivocal evidence of a neoplastic neuroendocrine component). Although endocrine differentiation is most often identified in ovarian teratomas, it can also arise in testicular or extragonadal teratomas {2685}.

Germ cell tumours in endocrine organs

Rooper LM
Barletta JA
Bell D
Looijenga LHJ
Thompson LDR

Definition

The most common germ cell tumours in endocrine organs are teratomas – germ cell tumours defined by the presence of mature or immature tissues derived from all three germ cell layers.

ICD-O coding

9080/0 Mature teratoma
9080/3 Immature teratoma
9084/3 Teratoma with somatic-type malignancy
9064/3 Germinoma
9070/3 Embryonal carcinoma
9071/3 Yolk sac tumour
9100/3 Choriocarcinoma
9085/3 Mixed germ cell tumour

ICD-11 coding

2D12.Y & XH1E13 Other specified malignant neoplasms of other endocrine glands or related structures & Germinoma
2D12.Y & XH8MB9 Other specified malignant neoplasms of other endocrine glands or related structures & Embryonal carcinoma, NOS
2D12.Y & XH09W7 Other specified malignant neoplasms of other endocrine glands or related structures & Yolk sac tumour
2D12.Y & XH83G5 Other specified malignant neoplasms of other endocrine glands or related structures & Teratoma, NOS
2D12.Y & XH8PK7 Other specified malignant neoplasms of other endocrine glands or related structures & Choriocarcinoma, NOS
2D12.Y & XH2PS1 Other specified malignant neoplasms of other endocrine glands or related structures & Mixed germ cell tumour

Related terminology

Acceptable: benign teratoma; immature teratoma.
Not recommended: malignant teratoma (now classified as thyroblastoma).

Subtype(s)

None

Localization

Endocrine organ teratomas are rare and found in the thyroid, adrenal, and pituitary glands. To be considered of endocrine organ origin, they should be centred in, be contiguous with, or completely replace the organ {4474,2451}.

Clinical features

Thyroid gland teratomas generally present as large neck masses that can cause airway compression and associated respiratory distress, particularly in the neonatal setting {4474, 92,3743}. Most adrenal gland teratomas are found incidentally on imaging {301}. In both sites, imaging demonstrates a heterogeneous cystic and solid mass with variable amounts of fat and calcifications {1834,769}.

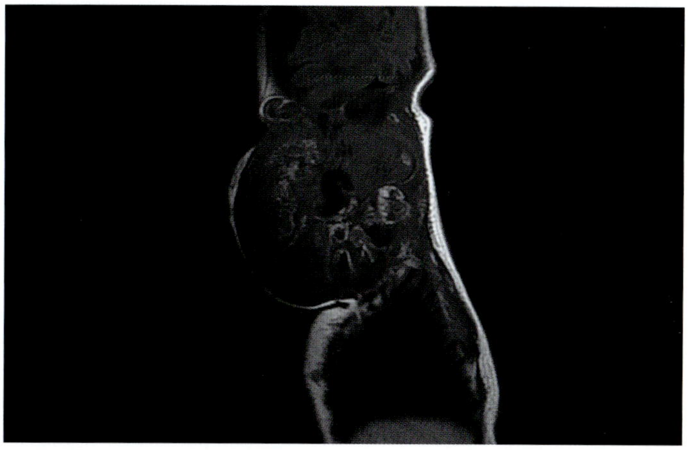

Fig. 11.01 Thyroid gland teratoma. Sagittal T1-weighted MRI showing a large mass in the neck of a neonate, resulting in compression of vital structures. Internal solid structures (calcifications) and cystic structures are seen.

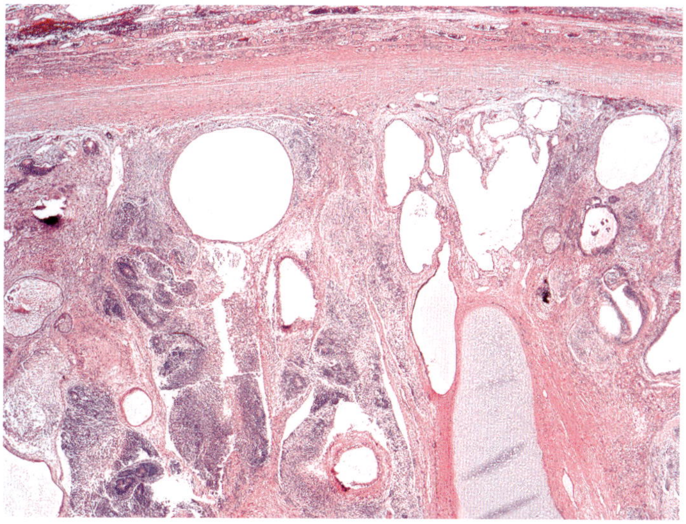

Fig. 11.02 Thyroid gland teratoma. Thyroid gland tissue is noted (top), and various elements of the germ cell layers are seen, including cartilage and glands. Immature neural elements are noted (immature teratoma).

Epidemiology

Teratomas account for < 0.1% of thyroid or adrenal gland tumours {1629,4474}. The majority of thyroid gland teratomas occur in neonates and young children, and most cases arise congenitally {4474,92,3743}. In contrast, the majority of adrenal gland teratomas are identified in adults {301,5165}.

Chapter 11

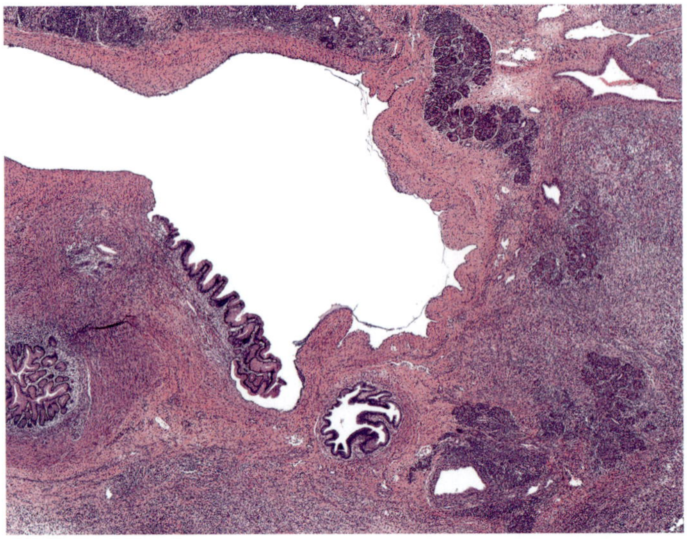

Fig. 11.03 Thyroid gland teratoma. A large cyst is lined by goblet-type epithelium, and more primitive stroma is seen around other glandular elements, in this mature teratoma.

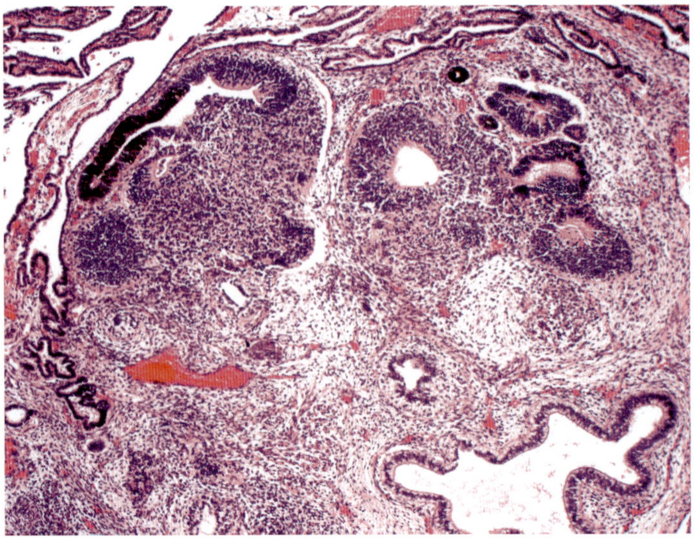

Fig. 11.04 Thyroid gland teratoma. Both mature and immature elements are noted in this teratoma. Pigmented retinal anlage epithelium is noted adjacent to glandular epithelium and immature skeletal muscle. Islands of immature neuroectodermal elements are seen.

Etiology

Unknown

Pathogenesis

Unknown

Macroscopic appearance

Tumours generally have a smooth but lobulated exterior and a heterogeneous, multiloculated, solid to cystic cut surface and contain variable amounts of serous, mucinous, or haemorrhagic fluid.

Histopathology

Teratomas are defined by the presence of mature or immature tissues from all embryonic germ cell layers (endoderm, mesoderm, and ectoderm). Tumours display multiple cystic spaces lined by a variety of epithelial types, including simple or stratified squamous epithelium, frequently in association with pilosebaceous units or other adnexal structures, pseudostratified and ciliated respiratory epithelium, mucin-producing intestinal epithelium, and transitional epithelium. Virtually all teratomas also contain a significant component of neural tissue, encompassing both mature glial elements, retinal anlage, or choroid plexus or immature neuroectodermal tissue composed of small to medium-sized cells with hyperchromatic nuclei and scant fibrillary cytoplasm arranged in sheets and rosettes. A variety of mesenchymal elements, including skeletal muscle, smooth muscle, cartilage, and bone, can be identified. Solid organ parenchyma, including pancreatic, liver, or lung tissue, is uncommonly seen.

Immunohistochemistry

Immunohistochemistry is usually unnecessary for diagnosis, with the various teratoma components displaying staining characteristics of their constituent tissues {4474,4744}.

Grading

Grading of endocrine organ teratomas is based on criteria for ovarian and sacrococcygeal teratoma, which rely on the quantity of immature neuroectodermal tissue {1632,4637,2391, 3290,3763,4474}. Grade 0 teratomas are considered benign, containing only mature elements. Grade 1 and grade 2 teratomas are classified as immature, with grade 1 having immature neuroectodermal tissue in only 1 low-power (4×) field and grade 2 having > 1 but < 4 low-power fields containing immature foci. Classically, tumours with > 4 low-power fields of immature neuroectodermal tissue, mitoses, and/or pleomorphism have been considered grade 3 or malignant teratomas {2557,4474,4502}. However, thyroid gland tumours that meet these criteria have been reclassified as thyroblastoma on the basis of recurrent *DICER1* mutations and should no longer be regarded as true teratomas {3655,3809,32}. Rarely, somatic-type malignancies have been reported to arise within otherwise benign or immature teratomas {3274}. Other germ cell tumours (e.g. yolk sac tumour, choriocarcinoma) are rarely reported in endocrine organs and are also malignant {4662, 5168,4537,1468}.

Differential diagnosis

Benign teratomas should be distinguished from other developmental cysts such as thyroglossal duct cyst, branchial cleft cyst, or duplication cysts on the basis of multiple tissue components. In limited sampling, immature teratomas can overlap with other primitive neoplasms such as Ewing sarcoma or neuroblastoma, but they can be correctly classified if mature elements are present.

Cytology

FNA is rarely performed but may reveal cystic acellular liquid {982,3308,1468}.

Diagnostic molecular pathology

An absence of *DICER1* hotspot mutations may help distinguish immature or benign tumours from malignant tumours (thyroblastoma), which typically harbour these mutations {3809}.

Essential and desirable diagnostic criteria

Essential: involvement or replacement of the thyroid or adrenal gland by a proliferation of tissue from all three germ layers; usually mature tissues, but small foci of immature neuroectodermal tissues may be seen.

Desirable: absence of the *DICER1* hotspot mutations seen in thyroblastoma (in selected cases).

Staging

Not applicable

Prognosis and prediction

Congenital thyroid gland teratomas can cause death due to airway compression and impaired development of other vital structures {344,4474,92,3743}. Among benign and immature teratomas in endocrine organs, the quantity of immature tissue does not appear to correlate with outcome, and patients have an excellent prognosis in the absence of an overtly malignant component {4474,92,3743}.

Teratomas with endocrine differentiation

Rooper LM
Asa SL
Baloch ZW
Bell D
Looijenga LHJ

Definition

Endocrine differentiation is frequently seen in teratomas that arise outside endocrine organs and ranges from benign endocrine tissue to malignant endocrine tumours.

ICD-O coding

9090/0 Struma ovarii, NOS
9090/3 Thyroid carcinoma arising in struma ovarii
9091/1 Ovarian neuroendocrine tumour

ICD-11 coding

2F76 & XH22M4 Neoplasms of uncertain behaviour of female genital organs & Struma ovarii, NOS

Related terminology

Acceptable: proliferative struma ovarii; ovarian carcinoid.
Not recommended: malignant struma ovarii; strumal carcinoid.

Subtype(s)

Struma ovarii; thyroid carcinoma arising in struma ovarii; ovarian neuroendocrine tumour

Localization

Endocrine differentiation is most commonly seen in ovarian teratomas but can also (rarely) arise in testicular or extragonadal teratomas {2685}. The most common manifestations include struma ovarii, a mature ovarian teratoma in which thyroid tissue is the predominant or sole component, and ovarian teratomas that either have components of well-differentiated neuroendocrine tumour (NET) or consist solely of well-differentiated NET. Struma ovarii can give rise to thyroid carcinomas.

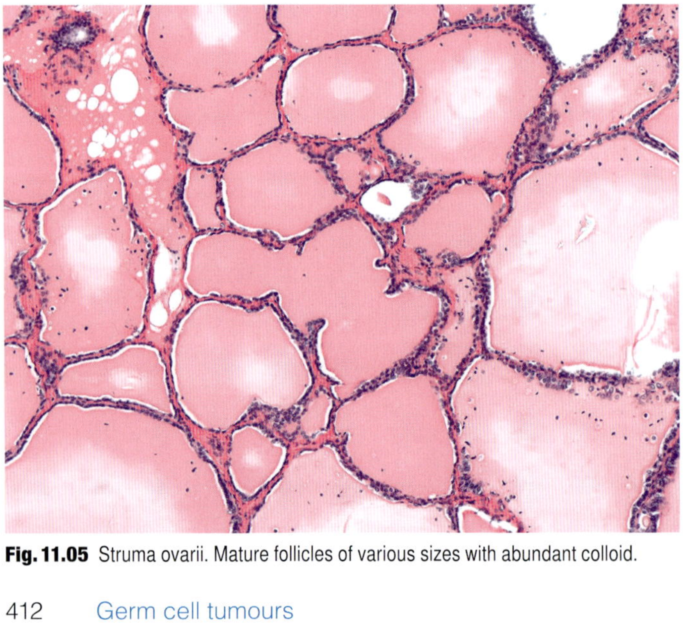

Fig. 11.05 Struma ovarii. Mature follicles of various sizes with abundant colloid.

In the retrorectal space (presacral region), embryonic hindgut remnants may give rise to retrorectal cystic hamartoma (tailgut cyst), which may demonstrate neuroendocrine neoplasms {2069,70,3085}.

Clinical features

Endocrine differentiation is usually an incidental finding in teratomas that otherwise present as a mass or with local mass effect. Among patients with struma ovarii, as many as one third have some degrees of ascites, and 5% show clinical evidence of hyperthyroidism {2256,1106}. As many as one third of patients with ovarian NET showing enterochromaffin-like cell (ECL-cell) differentiation can present with carcinoid syndrome, and rare patients with ovarian L-cell NET have chronic constipation due to PYY secretion {3762,3132,1260}. Although adrenal or pituitary tissue is quite rare, occasional functioning pituitary tumours arising in teratomas can manifest as hormone hypersecretion syndromes {3839,3118,623,1231,1917}.

Epidemiology

At least focal thyroid tissue can be seen in 15–20% of ovarian teratomas, but other endocrine tissues are only rarely seen {4935}. Struma ovarii accounts for 3% of ovarian teratomas, with thyroid carcinomas arising in just 3% of these cases {3766}. Ovarian NETs account for < 1% of ovarian teratomas {4935}. The peak incidence of struma ovarii and associated thyroid carcinomas is in the fifth decade of life {3839,3840}. Most patients with ovarian NET are postmenopausal {4389,3765}.

Etiology

Unknown

Pathogenesis

Ovarian teratomas are thought to derive from benign germ cells that develop into various mature tissues, including those of endocrine origin {4617}. It is not clear what drives the dominant thyroid differentiation in struma ovarii. Thyroid carcinomas arising in struma ovarii frequently demonstrate additional somatic mutations that are identical to those in their counterparts in the thyroid gland, including *BRAF*, *KRAS*, and *NRAS* mutations and *CCDC6*::*RET*, *NCOA4*::*RET*, and *PAX8*::*PPARG* rearrangements {2430,4005,4402,4577,956,3582}. Ovarian NETs are thought to arise from neuroendocrine cells within the constituent epithelia of mature teratoma {4389,3762}.

Macroscopic appearance

Struma ovarii is usually < 100 mm in size and has a red-tan, beefy cut surface with variable nodularity and cystic change that resembles normal or hyperplastic thyroid tissue {4367}. Thyroid-type carcinomas arising in struma ovarii may form more discrete masses {3766}. Ovarian NETs are generally small and form a homogeneous yellow to tan solid nodule {273}.

Histopathology

For classification as struma ovarii, teratomas should be composed of > 50% thyroid tissue, although tumours with functional or malignant thyroid tissue fall into this category regardless of proportion {3839}. The thyroid tissue generally consists of mature, colloid-filled follicles of various sizes. Cystic degeneration, a solid or microfollicular architecture, and oncocytic or clear cell features can confound recognition {4367}. The designation "proliferative struma ovarii" can be applied if the tumour demonstrates densely packed small follicles or pseudopapillary architecture but no specific features of malignancy {1106}. Struma ovarii expresses thyroglobulin, thyroid transcription factor 1 (TTF1), and PAX8 {2526,2913}.

Diagnosis of thyroid carcinoma arising in struma ovarii should be based on criteria for specific tumour types in the thyroid gland. The majority of these malignancies are classic papillary carcinoma, followed by the follicular subtype of papillary carcinoma, and follicular carcinoma {3766,1510,3838,493,4005,4075,3837,1106,2637,956,4833}; only rare cases of poorly differentiated or anaplastic carcinomas have been reported {2274,1457,2299}. A subset of cases can show minimal cytological atypia but still behave in a clinically malignant fashion {3766,1510,4075}.

Ovarian NETs can be subdivided into insular, trabecular, or mucinous types depending on architectural pattern {3762,4389,4390,273}. All of these histological patterns demonstrate uniform cuboidal to columnar cells with eosinophilic cytoplasm and centrally located nuclei with speckled chromatin and occasional cytoplasmic granules. The term "strumal carcinoid" has traditionally been used when other patterns are intimately mixed with thyroid follicles {3764}. Ovarian NETs demonstrate variable expression of chromogranin, synaptophysin, and CDX2, and most commonly are CK7-positive and CK20-negative {3653,1963}.

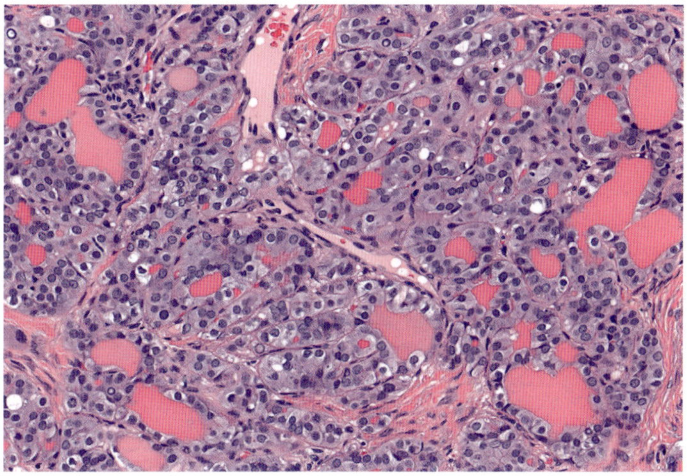

Fig. 11.06 Papillary thyroid carcinoma arising in struma ovarii. Diagnostic papillary nuclear features, including chromatin clearing, nuclear grooves, nuclear elongation, and intranuclear pseudoinclusions, are identified.

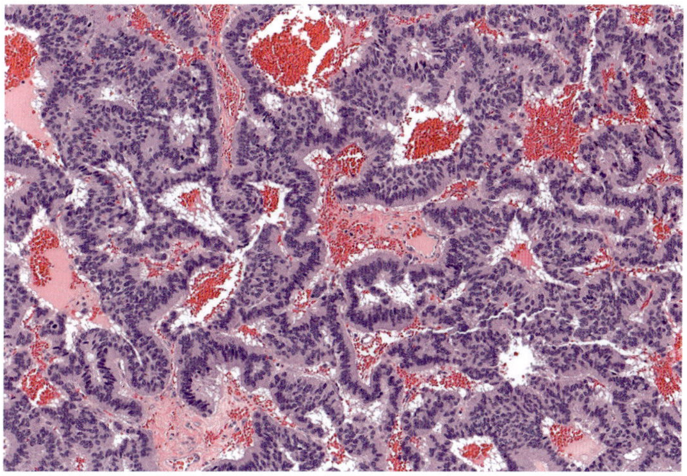

Fig. 11.07 Ovarian neuroendocrine tumour (NET). Ribbons and cords of uniform cells with pink cytoplasm and centrally located nuclei with salt-and-pepper chromatin.

Cytology

Not clinically relevant (aspiration of ovarian lesions is not performed)

Diagnostic molecular pathology

Not applicable

Essential and desirable diagnostic criteria

Essential:

- For struma ovarii: teratoma with thyroid tissue predominating
- For thyroid carcinoma arising in struma ovarii: meets diagnostic criteria for specific tumour type in the thyroid gland or demonstrates clinically malignant behaviour
- For ovarian NET: teratoma with unequivocal evidence of a neoplastic neuroendocrine component

Staging

Struma ovarii is not staged. Malignancies arising in teratoma are staged according to the American Joint Committee on Cancer (AJCC) / Union for International Cancer Control (UICC) TNM system.

Prognosis and prediction

The prognosis of struma ovarii is generally excellent {1106,4833}. The risk of recurrent disease for patients with thyroid carcinoma arising in struma ovarii is as high as 35% at 10 years, but these patients still have a 10-year survival rate of 90% {2637,1616,3766}. Risk factors for disease recurrence and progression are not well established, although carcinomas confined to the ovary at presentation have better outcomes {2637}. Ovarian NETs also have an excellent prognosis when confined to the ovary, with a 5-year survival rate of 95%, but can follow an aggressive course in advanced disease, with a 5-year survival rate of 53% {3194}.

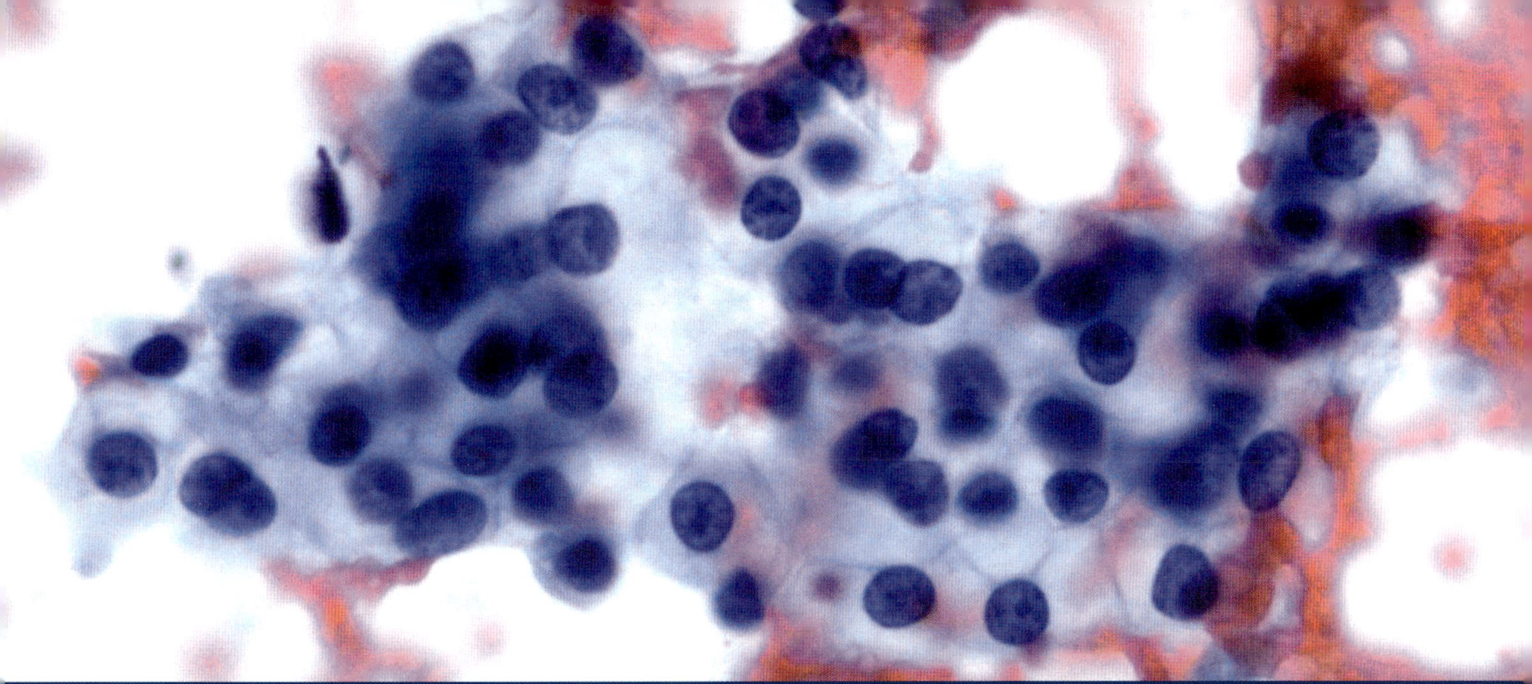

12

Metastasis

Edited by: Tallini G, Thompson LDR

Metastasis: Introduction

Tallini G
Thompson LDR

Endocrine glands are common targets of metastases from distant sites because their high vascularity promotes the homing of metastatic deposits. Interaction of the endocrine microenvironment recipient of the metastasis with the properties of specific tumour cell types is probably equally important for the successful implant and growth of these deposits {2072}, as shown by the spread of clear cell renal cell carcinoma to the thyroid gland {1549} or of lobular carcinoma of the breast to the pituitary gland or ovary {561}.

Metastases are frequently found in patients with a previous cancer diagnosis and disseminated disease (see Table 12.01). Intensive follow-up and prolonged patient survival have increased their identification in cytology or surgical pathology material {149}. An incidentally identified thyroid gland or adrenal gland nodule can be the first manifestation of metastases from occult neoplasms, typically clear cell renal cell carcinoma for the thyroid gland {1549} and lung carcinoma for the adrenal gland {3467}. By decision, metastases to the endocrine pancreas are not included here, because any metastatic deposit in the pancreas generally involves both the exocrine and endocrine pancreas. Metastases to the parathyroid glands are rare and not covered in a specific section in this volume, but they have been reported and analysed in a comprehensive literature review {348}.

Although endocrine organ dysfunction is rare, diabetes insipidus and adrenal insufficiency due to metastases to the pituitary or adrenal gland, respectively, are common manifestations {149}. Although they are excluded from the definition of metastatic disease, systemic haematolymphoid neoplasms also affect endocrine glands, and the testis is a well-known pharmacological sanctuary site in patients treated for acute lymphoblastic leukaemia.

Endocrine tumours are frequent recipients of tumour-to-tumour metastases (the uncommon phenomenon of metastatic dissemination of a primary donor tumour into a recipient tumour) reported in virtually every endocrine gland {2858, 2568,27,4407,1856}.

Table 12.01 Metastases to endocrine organs and origin of the primary tumour

Endocrine organ	Frequency of metastases	Reference	Primary tumours metastatic to endocrine organs	Reference
Pituitary	0.6–1.9%	Percentage of 3680 cancer patient autopsies {701}	Breast (37%), lung (24%), prostate (5%), kidney (5%)	{149}
Thyroid	0.1–2.1%	Percentage of all thyroid gland resections {1851,4931,859,3417,1549}	Kidney (48%), colorectum (10%), lung (8%), breast (8%), melanoma (4%), sarcoma (4%)	{149}
Parathyroid	Unknown[a]	{348}	Breast (67%), melanoma (12%), lung (6%)	{348}
Adrenal	2.2%	Percentage of metastases in adrenal incidentalomas {3467}	Melanoma (50%), breast and lung (30–40%), kidney and gastrointestinal tract (10–20%)	{149}
Ovary	7%	Percentage of metastases in lesions clinically presenting as primary ovarian tumours {2419}	Gastrointestinal tract (39%), breast (28%), endometrium (20%)	{1041}
Testis	0.02–2.5%	Percentage of secondary tumours in the testis[b] {2461}	Prostate (35%), lung (19%), colorectum (9%), melanoma (9%), kidney (7%)[b]	{149}

[a]A review of English-language publications between 1950 and 2017 identified 127 cases of metastasis to the parathyroid glands {348}. [b]Excluding involvement by systemic haematolymphoid malignancies.

Metastasis to the pituitary gland

Roncaroli FR
Erickson LA

Definition
Metastases to the pituitary gland are tumours involving the anterior and/or posterior pituitary secondarily by spread from primary sites in other organs.

ICD-O coding
Code according to histology of metastasis

ICD-11 coding
2E0Y & XA8J35 Malignant neoplasm metastasis in other specified sites & Pituitary gland

Related terminology
None

Subtype(s)
None

Localization
The posterior pituitary is more frequently involved than the anterior gland or the pituitary capsule {1839,1731}.

Clinical features
Pituitary metastases usually occur in patients with generalized metastatic disease {701,2674}. Although the pituitary can be the only site involved, pituitary metastases are rarely the first manifestation {1731,701}.

Headache, visual field defects, cranial nerve palsy, and ophthalmoplegia are presenting signs and symptoms {701}. Hypopituitarism and diabetes insipidus are common {701, 2674}. Apoplexy is rare {701}. Rapid growth of a sellar tumour with infiltration of adjacent structures should raise the suspicion of metastasis. Metastases can be asymptomatic and discovered when imaging is performed for other neurological deficits {2674}.

Epidemiology
Metastases represent about 0.6–1% of pituitary tumours {3877, 1731} and 0.14–28.1% of brain metastases at autopsy {1839}. The incidence is increasing because of patients' longer survival and more sensitive neuroimaging {1731}. Peak incidence is in the sixth or seventh decade of life; there is no sex predilection {1731,2095}. Metastases to pituitary neuroendocrine tumours (PitNETs)/adenomas have been reported {5015}.

Etiology
Unknown

Pathogenesis
Tumours can spread to the pituitary via direct blood supply to the posterior lobe, involve the infundibulum via the hypothalamic–hypophysial portal system, or disseminate from the suprasellar cistern {5192,2661,149,2674}.

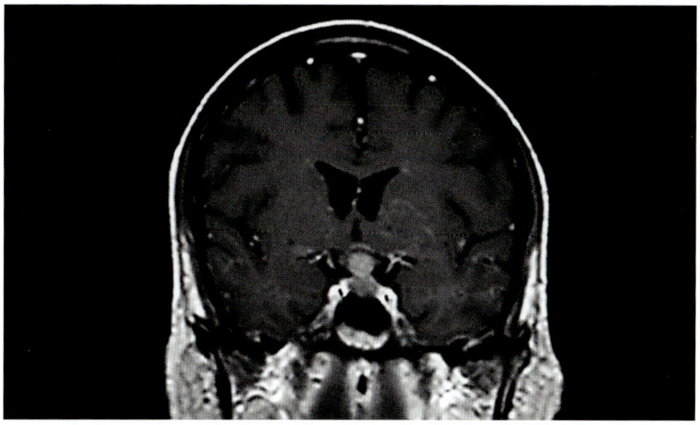

Fig. 12.01 MRI of breast carcinoma metastatic to the pituitary. Postcontrast axial T1-weighted sequence shows a dumbbell intrasuprasellar enhancing lesion.

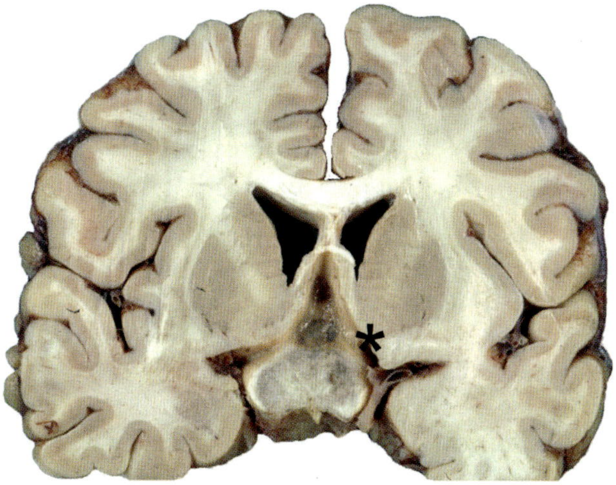

Fig. 12.02 Pancreatic adenocarcinoma metastatic to the pituitary, hypothalamus, and optic apparatus. Coronal brain section demonstrating a large tumour (adjacent to asterisk) replacing the pituitary gland and optic chiasm and invading the hypothalamus and third ventricle.

Macroscopic appearance
Metastases to the pituitary are intrasellar/suprasellar lesions, often with a dumbbell shape due to compression of the diaphragma sellae. Erosion of the sellar floor is common, and oedema of the optic apparatus can occur {1731}.

Histopathology
Any tumour can metastasize to the pituitary, with breast and lung the most common primary sites {1839,149}. Histological features are similar to those of the tumour of origin and may appear as a

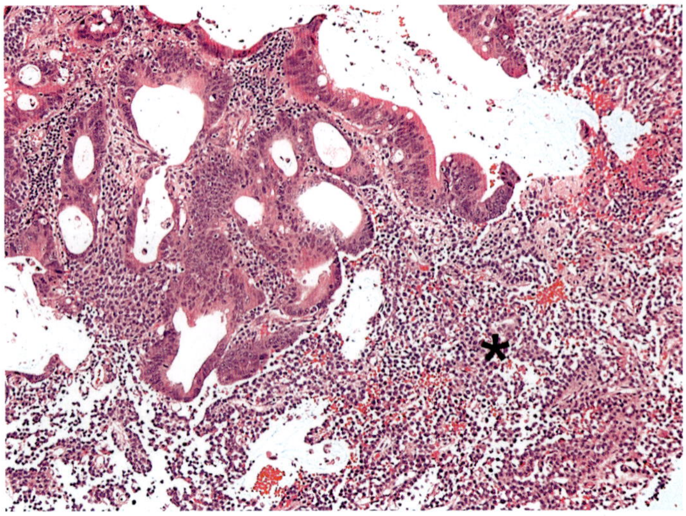

Fig. 12.03 Colon adenocarcinoma metastatic to gonadotroph pituitary neuroendocrine tumour (PitNET)/adenoma. Neoplastic glands composed of severely atypical columnar cells are admixed with acini of uniform tumour cells of the PitNET/adenoma (asterisk).

discrete mass, small aggregates, or single cells. Distinguishing metastatic low-grade neuroendocrine neoplasms (NENs) from a PitNET/adenoma is challenging. An absence of pituitary transcription factors favours metastasis.

Cytology

Squash and imprint preparations show atypical cells, at times admixed with normal adenohypophysial cells.

Diagnostic molecular pathology

Molecular testing may have a role in identifying the primary site of origin of the tumour or in guiding therapy, depending on the tumour type.

Essential and desirable diagnostic criteria

Essential: deposits of non-hypophysial malignant cells in the anterior and/or posterior pituitary.

Desirable: an absence of pituitary hormones and pituitary transcription factors in tumour cells (in selected cases).

Staging

Union for International Cancer Control (UICC) / American Joint Committee on Cancer (AJCC) staging system for the primary tumour metastatic to the pituitary gland

Prognosis and prediction

The prognosis is poor {1731}. Outcomes are improving with earlier diagnoses and better management of primary and systemic tumours {2661,2674}. Prognosis and treatment response depend on the primary tumour and extent of disease. A minority of patients die from progression of the pituitary lesion {1731}.

Metastasis to the thyroid gland

Ghossein RA
Baloch ZW
Rindi G

Definition

Metastases to the thyroid gland are tumours that involve the thyroid gland secondarily by haematogenous spread from primary sites in other organs.

ICD-O coding

Code according to histology of metastasis

ICD-11 coding

2E0Y & XA8RK3 Malignant neoplasm metastasis in other specified sites & Thyroid gland

Related terminology

None

Subtype(s)

None

Localization

Metastases to the thyroid gland arise in either or both thyroid gland lobes or the isthmus. They are most commonly a nodule but may be dispersed throughout the gland, and they are preferentially located at the periphery {3417,1549}.

Clinical features

Clinical symptoms are the most common mode of presentation {851}, often in the form of a palpable neck mass {4343, 3275}. Dysphonia and dysphagia may occur {3417}. Patients are typically euthyroid, with very rare cases of hyperthyroidism or hypothyroidism due to parenchymal destruction by the metastatic process {3040,5085,3417}. Twenty-five per cent of cases are found incidentally {851}. In clinical series, metastases most commonly originate from kidney tumours (40–50% of all metastases {1851}), followed by lung tumours, breast tumours, colorectal tumours, upper gastrointestinal tract

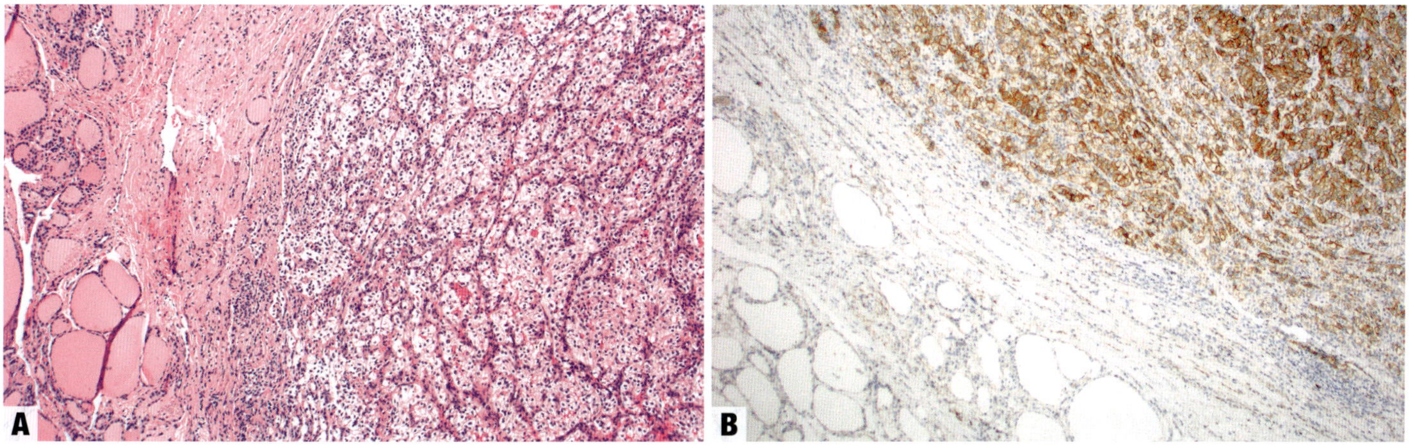

Fig. 12.04 Metastatic clear cell renal cell carcinoma (RCC) to the thyroid. **A** The clear cell RCC is separated from the thyroid by a fibrous capsule. Some lumina and solid nests are packed with blood in the RCC. **B** The cells of the RCC are immunopositive for CD10.

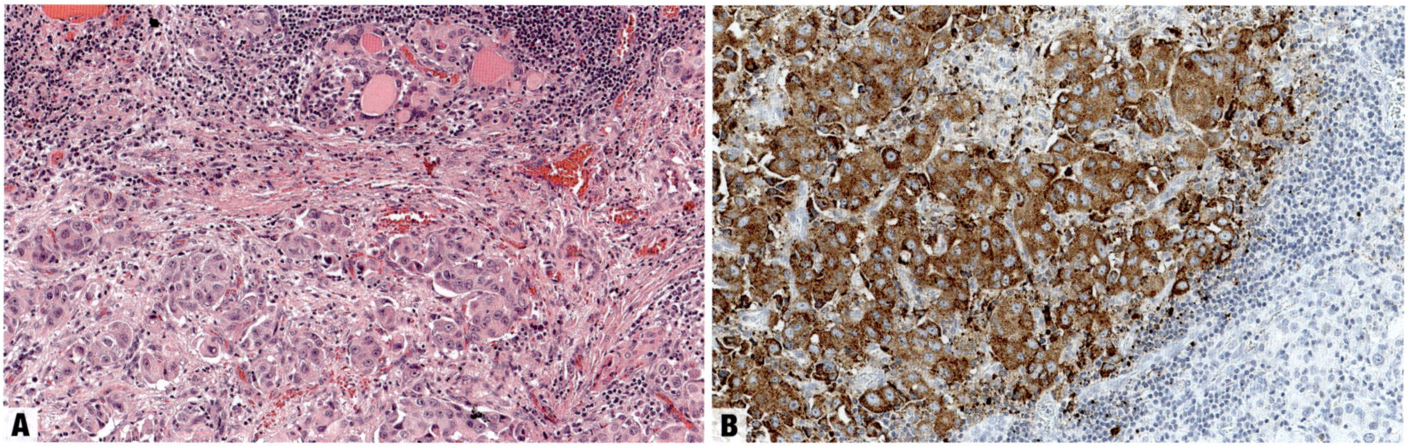

Fig. 12.05 Metastatic lung adenocarcinoma to the thyroid. **A** This metastasis has a solid pattern. **B** The metastatic tumour cells are immunopositive for napsin A.

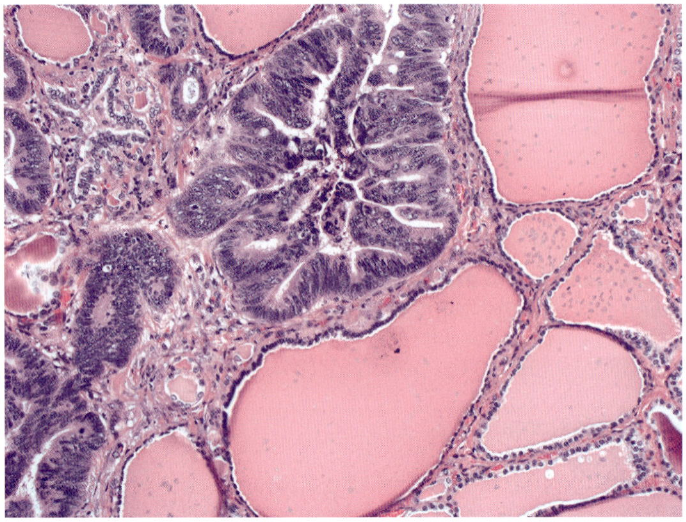

Fig. 12.06 Metastatic colorectal adenocarcinoma to the thyroid. The colorectal carcinoma infiltrates in between thyroid follicles.

tumours, melanoma, and sarcoma; the order of frequency of these other primary sites varies among different studies and when sex is taken into consideration {859,598,149,1549}. Rare primary sites include the uterus and bladder {3627,3584, 2042}.

Epidemiology

Metastases to the thyroid are identified in 1.9–25% of autopsy cases {851}, but their prevalence in surgical pathology practice is much lower (< 0.1%) {1851}. They occur in 0.36–2.1% of resected thyroid malignancies {4931,859,3417,1549}. There is a slight female preponderance (M:F ratio: 1:1.4) {851}. The mean and median ages at diagnosis are within the seventh decade of life {4931,859,3417,1549}. Metastases may be synchronous (20% of cases) but are usually metachronous, detected several years (median: 53 months) after the diagnosis of the primary tumour {851}.

Etiology

Unknown

Pathogenesis

The high vascularity of the thyroid gland predisposes to haematogenous dissemination. Interaction of the parenchymal microenvironment with the properties of specific tumour cell types is also important for the successful growth of tumour deposits, as demonstrated by the predominance of the thyroid gland as the recipient of clear cell renal cell carcinoma (RCC) {1851,2072, 1549}.

Macroscopic appearance

The metastases can be unifocal or multifocal {2762,1549}. Those of RCC are well circumscribed or encapsulated, are bright yellow on cross-section, and can be as large as 150 mm {1851}. Diffuse bilateral involvement of the gland may occur.

Histopathology

Clear cell RCC is the most frequent histotype {1851,859,1549}. Metastatic neoplastic cells can grow into the interstitium, form nodular masses, or develop within pre-existing thyroid nodules (tumour-to-tumour metastasis) {295}. Metastatic lung carcinoma can be mistaken for anaplastic thyroid carcinoma, and RCC for Hürthle cell or papillary thyroid carcinoma {1549}. Metastatic neuroendocrine neoplasms (NENs; including small cell neuroendocrine carcinomas [SCNECs] and large cell neuroendocrine carcinomas [LCNECs] from the lung and elsewhere, but also lung neuroendocrine tumours [NETs]) must be distinguished from medullary thyroid carcinoma {2881,3417, 1549}. Clinical history, histological clues (e.g. glandular lumina packed with red blood cells in RCC), and immunohistochemistry (e.g. absent calcitonin and CEA immunoreactivity in metastatic NENs, but positive reactions in medullary thyroid carcinoma) are important for the correct diagnosis. Importantly, direct extensions from other organs (i.e. larynx, oesophagus) should be excluded.

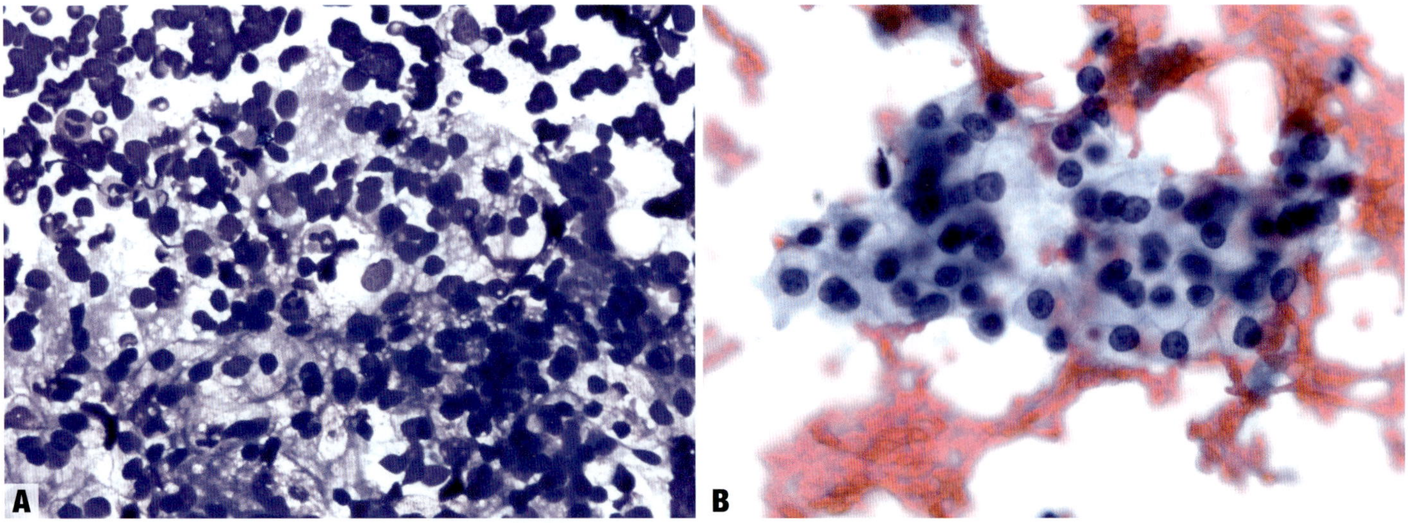

Fig. 12.07 FNA specimen of metastatic renal cell carcinoma to the thyroid gland. **A** Romanowsky-stained air-dried smear preparation showing a tissue fragment of tumour cells with clear cytoplasm and mild nuclear pleomorphism. **B** Pap-stained, alcohol-fixed smear preparation showing a tissue fragment of tumour cells with clear cytoplasm, distinct cell borders, and round to oval nuclei with even chromatin.

Cytology

FNA can accurately identify the metastasis in 74–81% of cases {851,3634}. High-grade nuclear atypia (often present) and tumour necrosis can help exclude common primary thyroid gland tumours {3634}. Immunohistochemistry is needed if nuclear atypia is mild and to exclude anaplastic thyroid carcinoma {3634}.

Diagnostic molecular pathology

Molecular testing may have a role in identifying the primary site of origin of the tumour or in guiding therapy, depending on the tumour type.

Essential and desirable diagnostic criteria

Essential: deposits of non-thyroidal malignant cells within the thyroid gland parenchyma.

Staging

Union for International Cancer Control (UICC) / American Joint Committee on Cancer (AJCC) staging system for the primary tumour metastatic to the thyroid

Prognosis and prediction

The 5-year overall survival rate ranges from 31% to 58% after thyroidectomy {2024,598,1549}, depending on the tumour type. Patients with unifocal thyroid involvement and oligometastatic disease have better outcomes {1851,598,3275,1549}.

Metastasis to the adrenal gland

Gill AJ
de Krijger RR

Definition
Metastases to the adrenal gland are tumours that involve the adrenal gland secondarily by haematogenous spread from primary sites in other organs.

ICD-O coding
Code according to histology of metastasis

ICD-11 coding
2E07 Malignant neoplasm metastasis in adrenal gland

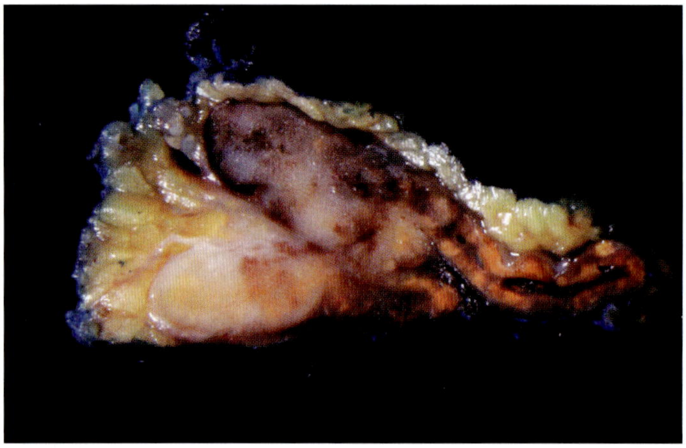

Fig. 12.08 Metastatic lung carcinoma to the adrenal. This example is from a 37-year-old woman with a history of lung carcinoma. The adrenal, 9 g, revealed a 12 mm homogeneous grey-white, firm, infiltrative lesion focally replacing the cortex and the medulla.

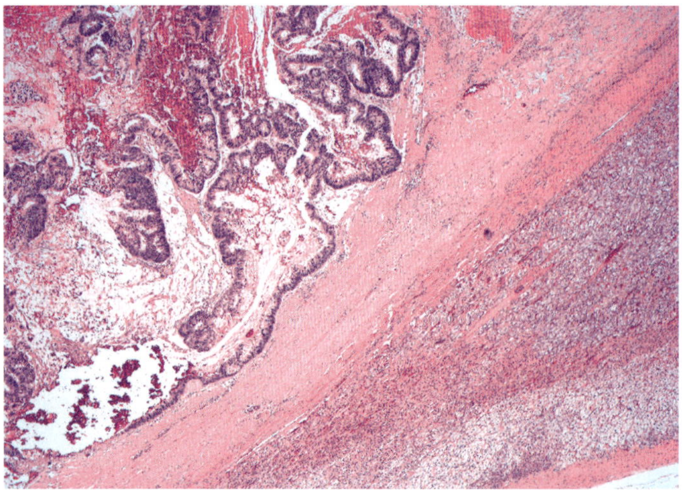

Fig. 12.09 Metastatic colorectal carcinoma to the adrenal gland. In this patient with known colorectal adenocarcinoma, the morphology of the metastatic deposit being composed of tall columnar cells with associated dirty necrosis allows definitive diagnosis without immunohistochemistry.

Related terminology
None

Subtype(s)
None

Localization
Adrenal cortex and/or medulla

Clinical features
Adrenal metastases are usually asymptomatic, but they may be associated with abdominal pain. Bilateral involvement is an important clue that a tumour is a metastasis. Adrenal insufficiency is unusual and requires bilateral involvement with destruction of > 90% of the cortex {2448,3706,1873}.

Epidemiology
Metastases are the second most common adrenal tumour after adrenal cortical adenomas. The adrenal glands are the fifth most common site for metastatic involvement, after the lymph nodes, lung, liver, and bone {1878}.

Etiology
None

Pathogenesis
The rich sinusoidal blood supply of the adrenal glands predisposes them as a site of haematogenous spread.

Macroscopic appearance
Metastatic tumours usually lack the typical yellow to orange colour of primary adrenocortical tumours, with the macroscopic appearance dependent on the primary tumour. Haemorrhage and cystic change are common.

Histopathology
Melanoma, as well as lung, breast, kidney, and gastrointestinal tract carcinomas, are among the most common primary tumours to spread to the adrenal, but virtually any tumour may do so {1878}. Definitive pathological diagnosis of metastasis is usually straightforward by morphology with or without immunohistochemistry when the primary site is known.

Differential diagnosis
Metastatic hepatocellular carcinoma, clear cell renal cell carcinoma, and melanoma may be particularly difficult to distinguish from primary adrenal cortical carcinomas because of morphological and immunohistochemical overlap, and a panel of immunohistochemical markers is usually necessary for the differential diagnosis. Nuclear expression of SF1 in tumour cells favours a primary adrenal cortical neoplasm.

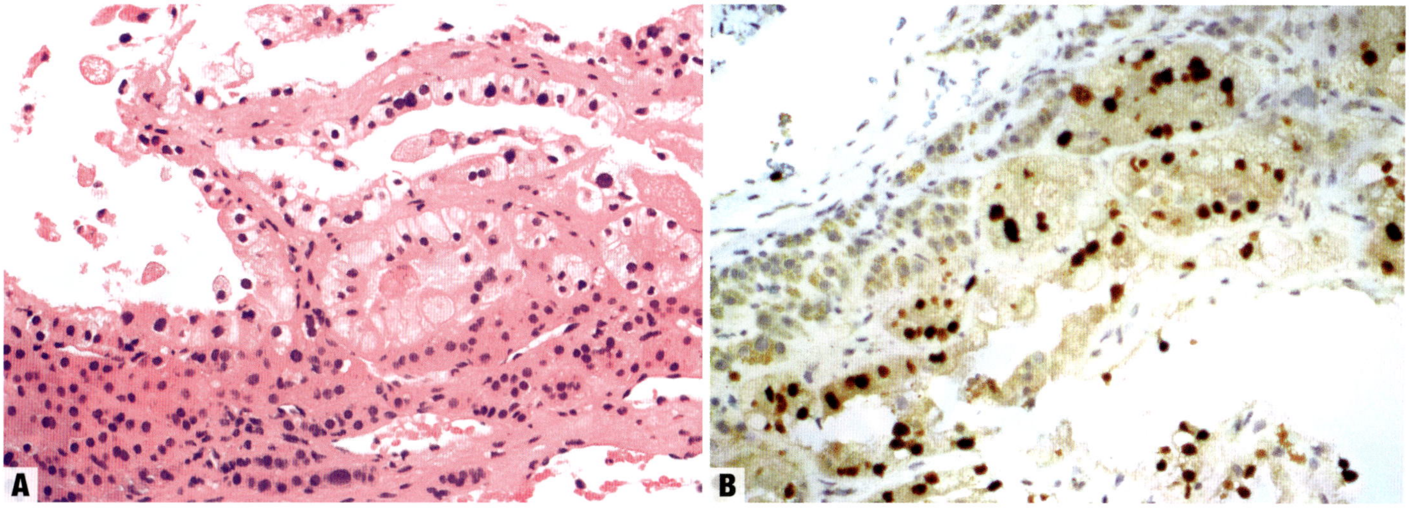

Fig. 12.10 Metastatic clear cell renal carcinoma in the adrenal gland. **A** Given the clear cytoplasm, the malignant cells are morphologically similar to zona fasciculata–type cells. The presence of cystic change is a clue, but immunohistochemistry would be required for a definitive diagnosis. **B** Diffuse strong nuclear expression of PAX8 in metastatic clear cell carcinoma in the adrenal gland allows ready distinction from zona glomerulosa–type adrenal cortical cells (PAX8 immunohistochemistry).

Cytology

Although rarely used for primary lesions, FNA may provide definitive diagnostic confirmation when used for metastases to the adrenal gland {3462}.

Diagnostic molecular pathology

Molecular testing may have a role in identifying the primary site of origin or in guiding therapy, depending on the tumour type.

Essential and desirable diagnostic criteria

Essential: deposits of non-adrenal malignant cells in the adrenal gland; appropriate pathological and/or clinical steps should be undertaken to exclude a primary adrenal tumour.

Staging

Union for International Cancer Control (UICC) / American Joint Committee on Cancer (AJCC) staging system for the primary tumour metastatic to the adrenal

Prognosis and prediction

Metastasectomy may be beneficial in carefully selected patients {3932,1498,1814,1649}. The prognosis of tumours that have metastasized to the adrenal gland is dependent on the underlying biology and extent of the primary tumour, but it is generally poor. In one study, the 2-year survival rate of patients with adrenal metastasis was 7% {3467}, which is considerably worse than the survival rate of patients with primary adrenal cortical carcinoma {1591}.

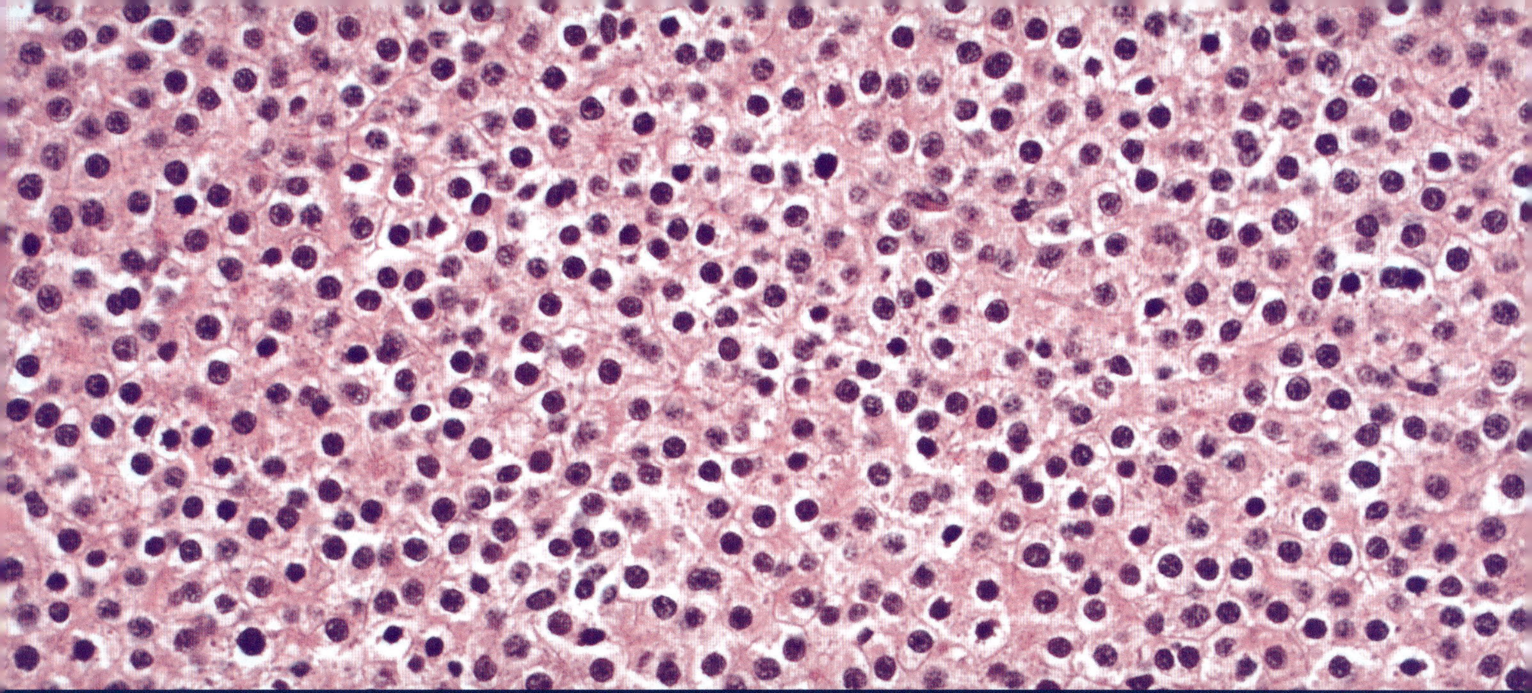

13

Genetic tumour syndromes associated with endocrine lesions and tumours

Edited by: Lax SF, Lazar AJ, Nosé V, Sobrinho-Simoes M

Genetic tumour syndromes associated with endocrine lesions and tumours: Introduction

Nosé V
de Krijger RR
Lax SF
Sobrinho-Simoes M

Since the first description of a patient with a combination of pituitary and parathyroid endocrine tumours in 1903, many tumours that were initially considered sporadic occurrences are now considered parts of well-defined syndromes. With the rapidly increasing use of molecular genetic techniques, including next-generation sequencing, in both diagnostic pathology and clinical genetics, numerous new constitutional gene mutations have been identified in tumours. These genetic alterations have other phenotypic consequences as well, resulting in clinically recognizable tumour-predisposing syndromes. It is increasingly challenging for pathology to keep pace with scientific discoveries by assimilating novel concepts in tumour classification, molecular genetics, and prognostication. Knowledge of underlying genetic variants can often have an important role in determining optimal therapy and surveillance guidelines.

Histopathology plays a critical role in the identification of hereditary disease, because it offers tools to complement molecular genetics, including morphological findings and immunohistochemistry. The latter can be a reliable and time-saving technique in the evaluation of some somatic mutations in tumours and/or of germline mutations in patients with familial cancer syndromes {966,317,3412,3411}.

The last edition of the WHO classification of tumours of endocrine organs, published in 2017, contained a chapter on inherited tumour syndromes, containing dedicated sections on 12 syndromes associated with endocrine tumours. Within the past few years, additional syndromes involving the endocrine organs have been identified. This current edition of the WHO classification of endocrine and neuroendocrine tumours now describes 15 syndromes associated with endocrine lesions

Table 13.01 Genetic syndromes with endocrine tumours (continued on next page)

Disease/phenotype	Syndrome MIM number	Inheritance	Locus	Gene(s)	Gene MIM number	Encoded protein(s)	Normal protein function
Multiple endocrine neoplasia type 1	131100	AD	11q13.1	*MEN1*	613733	Menin	DNA repair and regulation of apoptosis (tumour suppressor)
Multiple endocrine neoplasia type 2A	171400	AD	10q11.21	*RET*	164761	RET	Normal development of nerve cells
Multiple endocrine neoplasia type 2B	162300	AD	10q11.21	*RET*	164761	RET	Normal development of nerve cells
Multiple endocrine neoplasia type 4	610755	AD	12p13.1	*CDKN1B*	600778	p27	Prevention of aberrant cell division (tumour suppressor)
Multiple endocrine neoplasia type 5	171300	AD	14q23.3	*MAX*	154950	MAX	Essential component of the MYC/MAX/MXD1 network of transcription factors that regulate cell proliferation, differentiation, and apoptosis
Hyperparathyroidism–jaw tumour syndrome	145001	AD	1q25-q31	*CDC73*	607393	Parafibromin	Critical component of PAF1C that binds to RNA polymerase II and controls transcription
Von Hippel–Lindau syndrome	193300	AD	3p25.3	*VHL*	608537	VHL	Ubiquitination and degradation of HIF (tumour suppressor)
SDH-deficient tumour syndromes						SDH	Accumulation of succinate, which acts as an oncometabolite involved in tumorigenic pathways including hypoxic regulation and epigenetic reprogramming
PGL1	168000	AD;PT	11q23.1	*SDHD*	602690		
PGL2	601650	AD;PT	11q12.2	*SDHAF2*	613019		
PGL3	605373	AD	1q23.3	*SDHC*	602413		
PGL4	115310	AD	1p36.1-p35	*SDHB*	185470		
PGL5	614165	AD	5p15	*SDHA*	600857		

AD, autosomal dominant; AD;PT, autosomal dominant with paternal transmission (maternally imprinted, clinical disease is inherited only from paternal carrier); AR, autosomal recessive; PAF1C, polymerase-associated factor 1 complex; PGL1–5, paraganglioma syndrome types 1–5; SDH, succinate dehydrogenase; VHL, von Hippel–Lindau syndrome.

Table 13.01 Genetic syndromes with endocrine tumours (continued)

Disease/phenotype	Syndrome MIM number	Inheritance	Locus	Gene(s)	Gene MIM number	Encoded protein(s)	Normal protein function
Neurofibromatosis type 1	162200	AD	17q11.2	*NF1*	613113	Neurofibromin (NF1)	Negative regulation of RAS
Carney complex	160980	AD	17q24.2	*PRKAR1A*	188830	PRKAR1A	Regulatory subunit; *PRKAR1A* mutation results in overactive PKA
McCune–Albright syndrome	174800	Postzygotic	20q13	*GNAS*	139320	$G_s\alpha$	Signal transduction from seven-transmembrane receptors to the cAMP second messenger
***DICER1* syndrome**	606241	AD	14q32.13	*DICER1*	606241	DICER1	Processing microRNAs in the RNA interference pathway
Glucagon cell hyperplasia and neoplasia	619290	AR	17q25.3	*GCGR*	138033	GCGR	Glucagon signalling
Familial hyperinsulinism	147630	AD	8q24.3	*MAFA*	610303	MAFA	Transcription factor regulating Β-cell function and proliferation
Syndromic familial non-medullary thyroid carcinoma							
***PTEN* hamartoma tumour syndrome / Cowden syndrome**							
Cowden syndrome 1	158350	AD	10q23.31	*PTEN*	601728	PTEN	Phosphatase; regulation of cell division (tumour suppressor)
Cowden syndrome 4	615107	AD	10q23.31	*KLLN*	612105	Killin	Triggers apoptosis
Cowden syndrome 5	615108	AD	3q26.32	*PIK3CA*	171834	PIK3CA (p110α)	Catalytic subunit of PI3K
Cowden syndrome 6	615109	AD	14q32.33	*AKT1*	164730	AKT1	Modulation of the AKT/mTOR signalling pathway
Cowden syndrome 7	616858	AD	20p11.23	*SEC23B*	610512	SEC23B	ER-associated protein secretion
Familial adenomatous polyposis	175100	AD	5q22.2	*APC*	611731	APC	Negative regulation of β-catenin and WNT signalling
***DICER1* syndrome**	606241	AD	14q32.13	*DICER1*	606241	DICER1	Processing microRNAs in the RNA interference pathway
Carney complex	160980	AD	17q24.2	*PRKAR1A*	188830	PRKAR1A	Regulatory subunit; *PRKAR1A* mutation results in overactive PKA
Werner syndrome	277700	AR	8p12	*WRN*	604611	WRN	DNA helicase critical for DNA repair; universally expressed
Li–Fraumeni syndrome, *TP53*-associated	151623	AD	17p13.1	*TP53*	191170	p53	Regulation of cell division (tumour suppressor)
Li–Fraumeni syndrome, *CHEK2*-associated	609265	AD	22q12.1	*CHEK2*	604373	CHK2	Induction of cell-cycle arrest and apoptosis after DNA damage
Non-syndromic familial non-medullary thyroid carcinoma	See Table 13.09 (p. 489)						

AD, autosomal dominant; AD;PT, autosomal dominant with paternal transmission (maternally imprinted, clinical disease is inherited only from paternal carrier); AR, autosomal recessive; PAF1C, polymerase-associated factor 1 complex; PGL1–5, paraganglioma syndrome types 1–5; SDH, succinate dehydrogenase; VHL, von Hippel–Lindau syndrome.

and tumours. These hereditary syndromes are associated with a range of benign and malignant neoplasms involving multiple organ systems and are not limited to the endocrine system.

For the first time, germline mutation in *MAX* is discussed and classified as multiple endocrine neoplasia type 5 – a hereditary syndrome characterized by multiple endocrinopathies, including paraganglioma and/or phaeochromocytoma (PPGL) and pituitary and parathyroid disease, as well as tumours of neural crest origin, such as ganglioneuroma and neuroblastoma.

Knowledge of the molecular associations of the succinate dehydrogenase (SDH)-deficient tumour syndromes has recently expanded, necessitating clarification of the terminology for the family of SDH-deficient tumour syndromes {1573}. Although previously defined clinically, the term "Carney triad" is now defined by dual clinical and molecular criteria as a syndromic SDH-deficient tumour syndrome where no germline SDH mutation has been identified. Older terminology, such as "Carney–Stratakis dyad" (which was previously defined as the clinical association of familial SDH-deficient gastrointestinal stromal tumour and paraganglioma without consideration of the actual gene mutated) is now discouraged in favour of terminology based on the identification of the mutated gene {379}. Under this approach, the clinical association of SDH-deficient gastrointestinal stromal tumour, SDH-deficient paraganglioma, and pulmonary chondroma would now only be considered Carney triad if no pathogenic germline mutation is identified in any of the SDH genes. Similarly, the association of a personal and family history of SDH-deficient gastrointestinal stromal tumour and SDH-deficient paraganglioma, which would previously warrant clinical classification as Carney–Stratakis dyad, would now be classified on the basis of the underlying genetic abnormality – for example, germline *SDHA*, *SDHB*, *SDHC*, *SDHD*, or *SDHAF2* mutation syndrome {2085}.

Familial hyperinsulinism has also been added to the genetic tumour syndromes, with multifocal pancreatic B-cell proliferations and with the identification of *MAFA* mutation, which distinguishes this from sporadic insulinomatosis {2016}.

Besides the addition of a few newly discovered familial diseases, as a result of molecular tests and clinical and pathological correlation, it is now well recognized that the familial follicular cell–derived thyroid carcinoma (non-medullary thyroid carcinoma) is classified as either syndromic or non-syndromic familial follicular cell–derived thyroid carcinoma. This topic is well covered in two sections that highlight the important role the pathologist plays in recognizing some of these diseases. The distinct thyroid pathology in some of the syndromes should alert the pathologist to a possibility of a familial cancer syndrome {2545,615,507}. The genes involved in the non-syndromic subtypes have been better characterized more recently, and the thyroid tumours of the non-syndromic follicular cell–derived / non-medullary thyroid carcinoma subtypes are expanding rapidly {1703}.

These syndromes have been covered in detail because their clinical, histopathological, and genetic characteristics are well characterized in the endocrine system, and some may have associated neoplasms with unique features allowing distinction from their sporadic counterparts.

Not all of the syndromes described in this chapter on genetic tumour syndromes are linked to cancer; some are associated with benign (and premalignant) proliferations, the study of which has contributed to our understanding of the function of their causative genes in important biological processes such as development and tissue homeostasis.

The following sections provide detailed descriptions of selected syndromes, summarized in Table 13.01 (p. 426).

Multiple endocrine neoplasia type 1

Mete O
de Krijger RR
Gimenez-Roqueplo A-P
Osamura RY
Perren A
Valk GD

Definition

Multiple endocrine neoplasia type 1 (MEN1) is an autosomal dominant tumour syndrome caused by pathogenic germline *MEN1* variants.

MIM numbering

131100 Multiple endocrine neoplasia, type 1; MEN1

ICD-11 coding

2F7A.0 Multiple polyglandular tumours

Related terminology

Acceptable: MEN1 syndrome.

Not recommended: multiple endocrine adenomatosis type 1; familial Zollinger–Ellison syndrome; Wermer syndrome.

Subtype(s)

None

Localization

Patients with MEN1 present with multifocal endocrine neoplasms in the parathyroids (including ectopic or supernumerary parathyroid glands in the mediastinum), anterior pituitary, pancreas, and duodenum, and less commonly in the stomach, adrenal, thymus, and lungs. In addition, various non-endocrine lesions may occur in the skin, CNS, and soft tissues.

Clinical features

The cardinal components of MEN1 syndrome consist of primary hyperparathyroidism, pituitary adenomas / pituitary neuroendocrine tumours (PitNETs), and duodenopancreatic neuroendocrine tumours (NETs). Other endocrine tumours that can occur in patients with MEN1 include bronchopulmonary NETs, thymic NETs (TNETs), adrenocortical tumours, and phaeochromocytomas. Facial angiofibromas, collagenomas, lipomas, leiomyomas, and CNS tumours (e.g. meningiomas, ependymomas), as well as hibernomas and breast cancers, have also been described {4445,1153,110}. Lipomas, angiofibromas, and collagenomas occur in 30%, 85%, and 70% of patients, respectively, by the age of 4 years {516}.

Primary hyperparathyroidism is the most common manifestation and occurs in virtually all patients with MEN1. Hypercalcaemia should lead to the measurement of intact PTH {425}. Because multiglandular parathyroid involvement can be asymmetrical and asynchronous, most patients with MEN1 syndrome are not subjected to the more common restricted surgical procedure {4022,3554}. Prophylactic partial thymectomy is also considered by experienced surgeons, given that mediastinal recurrence due to ectopic or supernumerary parathyroid glands occurs in as many as 12% of cases {4022,969,3554}.

Duodenopancreatic NETs (functioning or non-functioning) are usually diagnosed from symptoms related to functioning NETs (e.g. gastrinoma, insulinoma, glucagonoma, VIPoma) or from imaging studies performed for digestive symptoms or during the screening of non-functioning NETs in *MEN1* variant carriers. Serum tumour markers are not useful for diagnosing non-functioning NET in patients with MEN1 {4657}. For diagnosing gastrinomas, which are often located in the duodenum, serum levels of gastrin (fasting) are assessed. For functioning pancreatic NETs (PanNETs), glucose (fasting), insulin, PP, glucagon, and VIP should be assessed. Conventional (e.g. CT, MRI, EUS) imaging studies are required for localizing small non-functioning NETs {4657}. Functional imaging studies (e.g. 111In-pentetreotide [Octreoscan] SPECT-CT, 68Ga-DOTATATE/DOTATOC

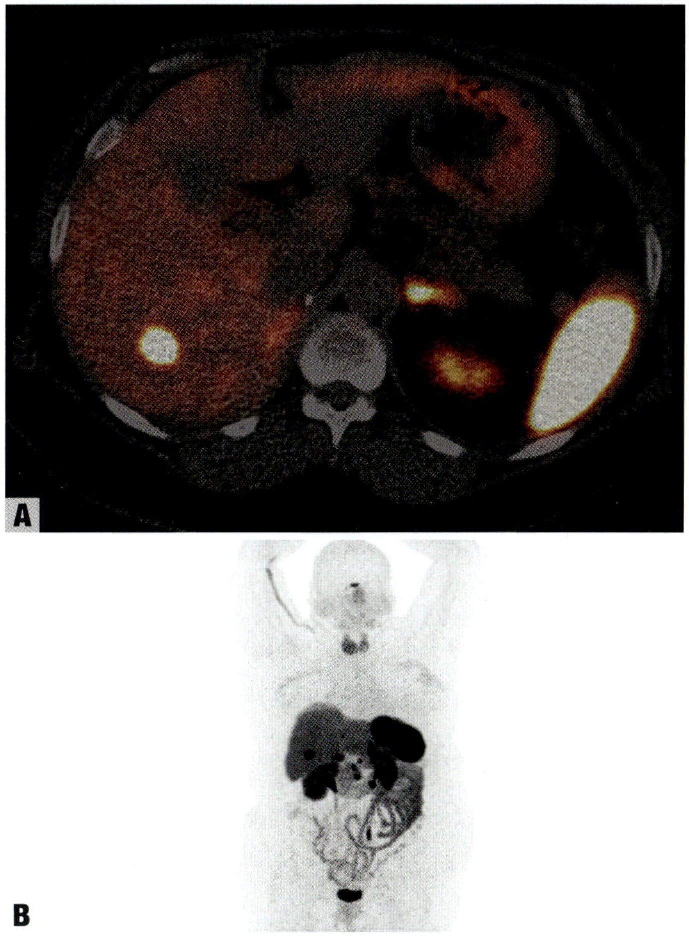

Fig. 13.01 68Ga-DOTA PET-CT in a patient with multiple endocrine neoplasia type 1. **A,B** These images show the diagnostic utility of 68Ga-DOTA PET-CT in a patient with multiple endocrine neoplasia type 1 with multiple small (< 10 mm) pancreatic neuroendocrine tumours (PanNETs) and metastatic spread to the liver. The functional imaging studies using 68Ga-DOTA PET-CT showed two hotspots corresponding to small PanNETs in the pancreatic head, another hotspot in the ventral pars ascendens of the duodenum (lymph node metastasis), and one larger and one small hotspot in the liver (metastases segment 6 and segments 3/4).

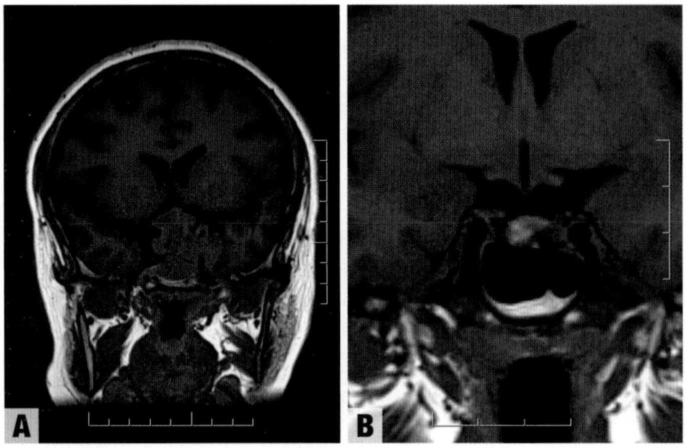

Fig. 13.02 MRI from a patient with multiple endocrine neoplasia type 1–related pituitary neuroendocrine tumour (PitNET) / pituitary adenoma, presenting with a macrotumour. **A** Coronal MRI reveals a large sellar mass with extensive suprasellar growth measuring approximately 40 mm. The lesion extends laterally into the left cavernous sinus surrounding most of the left internal carotid artery. The lesion extends through the floor of the sella into the sphenoidal sinus. The optic chiasm is draped over the superior aspect of the mass. **B** Coronal MRI shows an irregular 4–5 mm area of abnormal signal intensity without any mass effect.

PET-CT, FDG PET) can help determine the extent of various NETs in patients with MEN1 {2541,4552,2826,4657,3236}.

MEN1-associated PitNET/adenoma can be suspected when patients develop symptoms related to pituitary hormone excess (e.g. galactorrhoea and amenorrhoea, acromegaly, Cushing disease) or when a non-functioning macrotumour causes visual field defects or intracranial mass–related symptoms. Biochemical assessment (e.g. IGF1, prolactin, and dynamic endocrine tests) and MRI studies are typically performed {1023}. Screening protocols identified an increased frequency of pituitary microtumours (< 10 mm) on MRI studies {1023}; however, invasive pituitary macrotumours (> 10 mm) are overrepresented in some clinical series {4559}. When an ectopic source of GHRH is suspected as the cause of acromegaly {3938,1303,1544}, plasma GHRH over the threshold of 250–300 ng/L has been shown to have excellent specificity {1502,482}.

MEN1-associated adrenal lesions can be non-functioning {2523,4760}, or they can be seen in association with Cushing syndrome or primary aldosteronism {362,2523,5081,1517}. In general, adrenal cortical carcinomas are rare, but they are more common than sporadic manifestations {1517}.

Most paediatric-onset MEN1 manifestations are diagnosed after a positive predictive genetic test, and affected individuals are generally asymptomatic. In the absence of symptoms or hormone excess, biochemical screening is considered effective in patients aged 5–10 years, and imaging studies (e.g. brain, thoracic, and abdominal MRI) are performed in patients aged 10–15 years or older {4445,1647,4826,4664,3791}.

Epidemiology

The prevalence is estimated to be 3–20 cases per 100 000 population {515}. About 10% of patients have germline *MEN1* sequence variants arising de novo, with no family history {333, 4444}. The mean age at the time of diagnosis ranges between the fourth and fifth decade of life for various MEN1-associated manifestations {1602,3899,4687,1023,4949}. Age-related penetrance and variable expression can occur {4444,515}.

There is variable female prevalence recorded in MEN1 registries from Italy {1602}, Japan {3899}, and the Groupe d'Étude des Tumeurs Endocrines {1646}. No significant sex differences were identified in MEN1-related primary hyperparathyroidism {1646}. In addition, pulmonary NETs occurred equally in both sexes in large series {1024}. However, pancreatic neuroendocrine tumours (PanNETs) {1646} and TNETs {1646,1024,3899} were recorded more frequently in male patients. Unlike the exclusive male prevalence in some reported European databases {1646,1024}, the frequency of MEN1-associated TNET in female patients was significantly higher in Japan {3899}. Pituitary adenomas / PitNETs showed a female predilection {4687, 1646,1023,4949}.

The prevalence rates of primary hyperparathyroidism, gastroenteropancreatic NETs (GEP-NETs), and pituitary adenomas / PitNETs are 93–94%, 53–59%, and 38–50% in MEN1 registries, respectively {1602,3899,4687,1023}. The prevalence of insulinoma was higher in MEN1 patients in Japan than in patients of European descent {3899}. Gastric enterochromaffin-like cell (ECL-cell) NETs occur in 23–29% of such patients {477,399}. Depending on the diagnostic criteria applied (either histologically confirmed or radiologically identified), bronchopulmonary NETs can occur in about 5–23% of patients with MEN1 {3553, 1024,4160,328,2556,4642}. The estimated prevalence of TNETs is < 5% {1024}. Adrenal lesions have been reported in 20–70% of patients with MEN1 {3521,3979,3983,1517}.

Etiology

Pathogenic germline *MEN1* sequence variants, which are inherited as an autosomal dominant trait, are responsible for the development of MEN1 syndrome {4444,515}.

Pathogenesis

Pathogenic germline *MEN1* variants occur in the majority of patients with MEN1 and include a large variety of genetic abnormalities, including those leading to premature truncation, frameshift and nonsense mutations, or large deletions, including those in intronic areas leading to splice-site defects {2601, 901,515}. These are accompanied by loss of the wildtype allele in > 90% of *MEN1*-driven tumours. The 610-amino-acid protein product is called menin, for which the exact role in tumorigenesis remains to be established, although many roles have been proffered, including in the epigenetic regulation of gene transcription, cell division and proliferation, cell motility, cytoskeletal structure, DNA repair, genomic stability, cell signalling, and transcriptional regulation, through the potential interaction with about 50 proteins {750,2600,2601,4462,39,2882,1841,40,515}. Menin loss has shown correlations with various epigenetic aberrancies in MEN1-related tumours, such as loss of H3 p.K4me3 through inactivation of the KMT2 (MLL2) complex and gain of H3 p.K27me3 at specific genetic sites {2666}, DNA hypermethylation, and histone acetylation {515}. In the absence of loss of heterozygosity at the *MEN1* locus, epigenetic silencing via microRNAs may also contribute to the inactivation of the second allele {2766,515}.

Macroscopic appearance

Patients with MEN1 often present with multiglandular parathyroid disease. The individual parathyroid glands are variably involved, but all are grossly enlarged (> 6–8 mm) and increased in weight (> 40–60 mg). The cut section of parathyroid glands

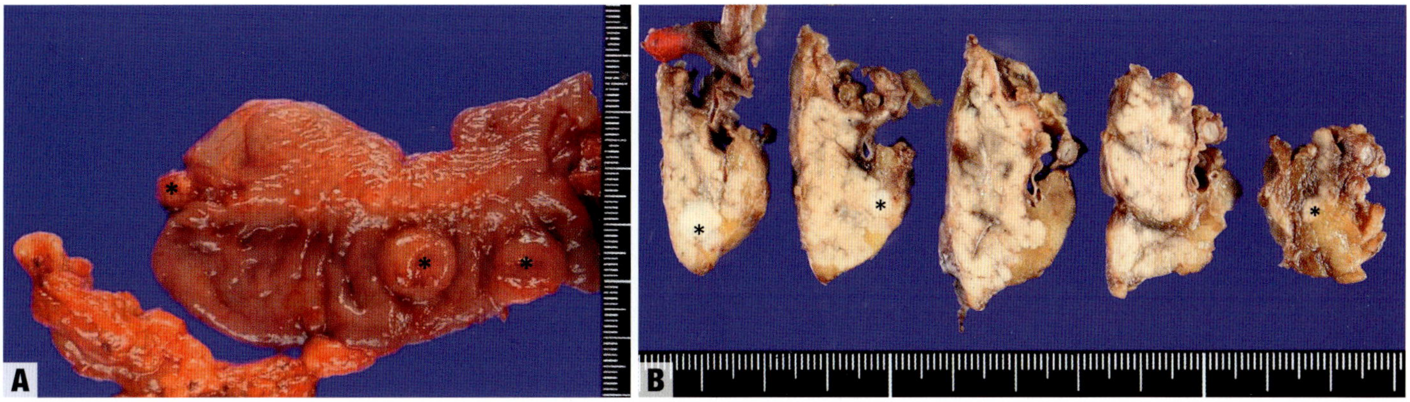

Fig. 13.03 Multiple endocrine neoplasia type 1–associated multiple neuroendocrine tumours (NETs). **A** Macroscopic appearance of multiple duodenal NETs (asterisks). **B** Macroscopic appearance of multiple NETs (asterisks) in the pancreatic tail of a patient with multiple endocrine neoplasia type 1.

may show nodularity. In patients with MEN1 syndrome, pituitary adenomas / PitNETs are grossly indistinguishable from their sporadic counterparts and are white to yellow soft tumours. Multiple contiguous adenomas/PitNETs cannot be distinguished with the naked eye. MEN1-associated pancreatic disease typically shows multiple tan to yellow parenchymal tumour nodules with a homogeneous cut surface. Cystic changes can occur in PanNETs with glucagon expression {2387}. Pancreatic neuroendocrine microtumours (0.5–5 mm) may be difficult to appreciate grossly. Duodenal NETs are often identified as multiple small nodules in the upper duodenum or at the margin of an ulcer. Duodenal NETs that measure less than 3–5 mm may be difficult to appreciate on gross examination. Multiple gastric nodules in the background of hypertrophic mucosa should raise the possibility of MEN1-associated gastric NETs (type 2 gastric ECL-cell neuroendocrine tumorigenesis). Individual lung NETs and TNETs are often indistinguishable from their sporadic counterparts. Multiple small pulmonary neuroendocrine microtumours (0.5–5 mm) can also be identified {328}. Adequate sampling of the non-tumorous duodenum, pancreas, stomach, and lung is often required because MEN1-associated tumours often show precursor lesions or associated microscopic tumours {2956,328}. Bilateral adrenal cortical nodules {1672,1517} and rare phaeochromocytomas {1517} can occur in patients with MEN1, but individual tumours are indistinguishable from their sporadic counterparts.

Histopathology

MEN1-related parathyroid disease

Multiglandular parathyroid disease is the hallmark of MEN1-related primary hyperparathyroidism {1130,4444,3996}. Because multiglandular parathyroid involvement can be asymmetrical and asynchronous, most patients with MEN1 syndrome are not subjected to the more common restricted surgical procedure {4022,3554}. As a consequence, surgical pathologists may be asked to evaluate multiple specimens during the full neck and mediastinal exploration of a patient with MEN1. The role of the diagnostician during the intraoperative consultation for MEN1-associated hyperparathyroidism typically involves the distinction of the parathyroid glands from other structures that could be mistaken for a parathyroid gland by the surgeon {1168}. Although the finding of multiple abnormal parathyroid glands generally results in a diagnosis of parathyroid hyperplasia, recent molecular data suggest that MEN1-related multiglandular parathyroid lesions are composed of multiple monoclonal proliferations, constituting multiple multiglandular microadenomas {1168,1438}. Histologically, they show multinodular proliferations composed primarily of chief cells, followed by oncocytic and/or clear cells {1168}. Unlike most sporadic parathyroid adenomas, MEN1-associated parathyroid proliferations lack the characteristic atrophic rim of non-lesional parathyroid tissue. Rim-like areas can occur in some glands; however, these regions are often cellular rather than being atrophic. Rarely, cystic changes can occur {4398}. Nuclear atypia, necrosis,

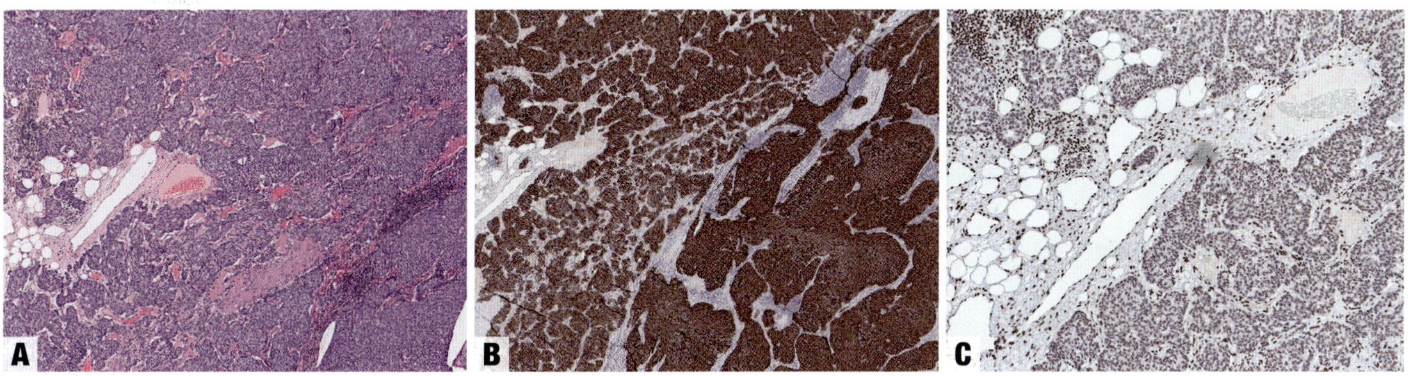

Fig. 13.04 Multiple endocrine neoplasia type 1–related thymic neuroendocrine tumour (TNET). A well-differentiated TNET in a patient with multiple endocrine neoplasia type 1. **A** At the histological level, this thymic NET is indistinguishable from its sporadic counterpart. **B** The tumour expresses chromogranin A. **C** There is global loss of nuclear menin expression in the tumour, supporting multiple endocrine neoplasia type 1–related pathogenesis. Note that the non-tumorous elements at the top of the image show a normal staining pattern for menin.

and prominent mitotic figures are uncommon. Glands may show stromal fibrosis and even irregular borders that can mimic the morphological features associated with parathyroid hyperplasia related to longstanding chronic renal failure or lithium exposure, atypical parathyroid tumour, and reactive changes associated with previous manipulations (e.g. FNABs, PTH washout, or therapeutic ethanol ablation) {118,1168,1172,1899}. Almost all MEN1-associated parathyroid neoplasms behave as benign tumours; carcinomas are extremely rare {1063,4159}, and their diagnosis requires the unequivocal demonstration of invasion into adjacent organs, vascular invasion, lymphatic invasion, or perineural invasion, and/or the presence of metastases {1065,1168,1172}. The parathyroid pathology of multiple endocrine neoplasia type 4 is histologically indistinguishable from that of MEN1. Patients presenting with MEN1-like parathyroid disease but lacking germline *MEN1* mutation should be tested for germline *CDKN1B* mutation {4444}.

MEN1-related pituitary disease

At the morphological level, individual tumours are indistinguishable from their sporadic counterparts {4559}. PIT1-lineage pituitary adenomas / PitNETs are common in MEN1-related pituitary disease {213}; however, other PitNETs, including those of TPIT lineage (e.g. densely granulated corticotroph tumour, sparsely granulated corticotroph tumour, Crooke cell tumour) and SF1 lineage (e.g. gonadotroph tumour) can also occur {2950,4559, 632,515}. Plurihormonal tumours have been reported frequently in a series {4559}; however, among functioning PIT1-lineage tumours, lactotroph tumours are the most frequent, followed by somatotroph and mammosomatotroph tumours {4949,1023, 4687}. Immature PIT1-lineage PitNETs (formerly known as poorly differentiated PIT1-lineage adenomas) can also occur in patients with MEN1 {2966}; this is not surprising given the increased frequency of immature PIT1-lineage PitNETs in young adults {2966,2961}. Multiple PitNETs of distinct cell lineages can also occur in patients with MEN1 {3686,3939,4559,2950}, significantly more frequently than in patients without MEN1 {4559}. Somatotroph or mammosomatotroph hyperplasia is an uncommon finding in MEN1 syndrome, but when it occurs in this setting, a GHRH-producing PanNET should be excluded {219, 4559}. MEN1-associated PitNETs show an increased number of S100-positive folliculostellate cells, as compared with their sporadic counterparts. The significance of this finding is unknown.

MEN1-related pancreatic disease

The hallmark of MEN1-related pancreatic disease is the presence of multifocal PanNETs (> 5 mm) or a unifocal PanNET arising in the background of neuroendocrine microtumours (each 0.5–5 mm; also known neuroendocrine microadenomatosis) {157,2342}. Monohormonal cell clusters inside normal islets, as well as neuroendocrine microtumours (microadenomas), have been shown to be clonal, with loss of the wildtype *MEN1* allele {3526}. Such microtumours are rarely found in ducts {3526}. At the morphological level, individual neoplasms are indistinguishable from their sporadic counterparts. Most are plurihormonal {2552,157}. Glucagon has been the most frequently identified hormone, followed by PP, insulin, and somatostatin {2342}. Glucagon-positive tumours may be cystic {2387}. Rarely, other hormones (e.g. calcitonin, PTHrP) may be expressed {346, 2999}. Gastrin is virtually never expressed. In cases of a MEN1-related hypoglycaemic syndrome, insulin-cell tumours can be the source of insulin excess. Very rarely, a PanNET may express a non-pancreatic hormone (e.g. GHRH causing ectopic acromegaly) {157}. Because *MEN1* inactivation can occur in about 40% of sporadic PanNETs {207}, loss of menin expression cannot be used to distinguish MEN1 syndrome in the absence of multifocal neuroendocrine microtumours (microadenomatosis). However, global loss of nuclear menin expression may help rationalize germline screening for MEN1-related pathogenesis, especially when global loss of nuclear menin expression occurs in multiple PanNETs and microtumours {2968}.

MEN1-related duodenal disease

Multifocal duodenal NETs that arise in the background of neuroendocrine cell hyperplasia is the hallmark of MEN1-related duodenal disease. Hyperplastic gastrin and somatostatin cells are typically identified in the crypts and in the Brunner glands {156,2342}. Multifocal gastrin-producing duodenal NETs are the most common cause of Zollinger–Ellison syndrome {1139,3567, 2956,2342}. In almost all MEN1 patients with Zollinger–Ellison syndrome, the source of gastrin excess is multicentric duodenal NETs {1139,2100,2341,3567}, typically in the mucosa and

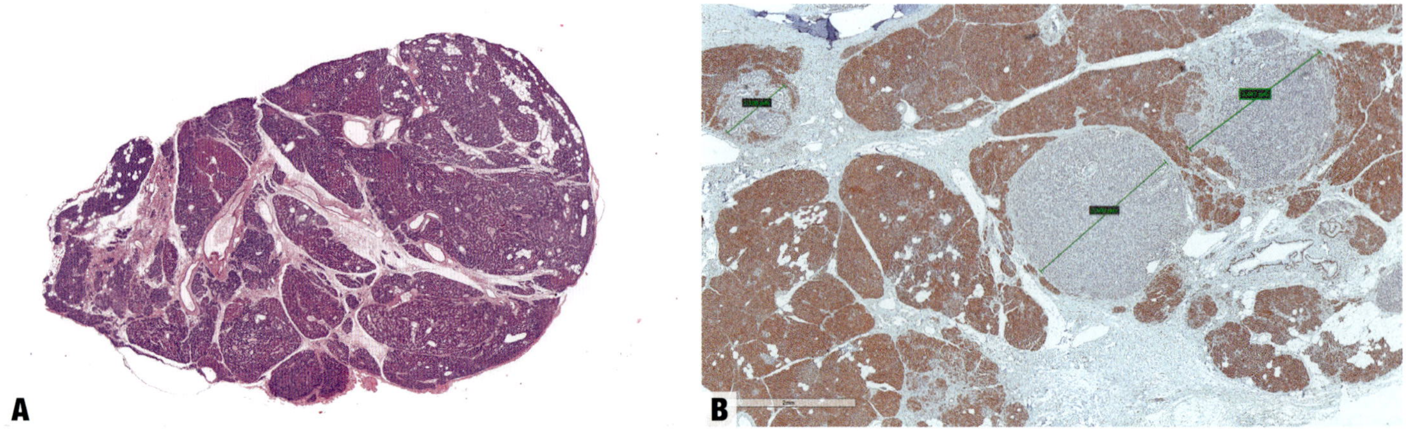

Fig. 13.05 Multiple endocrine neoplasia type 1. **A** Multiple endocrine neoplasia type 1–related parathyroid disease is characterized by multiglandular multiple adenomas. This photomicrograph shows one of the affected glands with multiple microscopic nodules/adenomas. **B** Global loss of nuclear menin expression (green bars) is illustrated in multiple pancreatic neuroendocrine microtumours, consistent with multiple endocrine neoplasia type 1 syndrome.

submucosa of the upper duodenum. The tumours are usually < 10 mm and may therefore be difficult to detect {154}. In as many as 80% of cases, the tumours give rise to large periduodenal and/or peripancreatic lymph node metastases, which were formerly interpreted as pancreatic gastrinoma primaries. Individual MEN1-related duodenal NETs look like sporadic ones. They show trabecular or pseudoglandular growth and are often associated with low-grade proliferative disease (grade 1). However, the multifocal nature of NETs and the presence of synchronous neuroendocrine cell hyperplasia often help distinguish MEN1-related disease from sporadic manifestations. Rare examples of MEN1-related duodenal NETs can be somatostatin-positive {156,2342,2956}.

MEN1-related gastric disease

The ECL-cell hyperplasia-to-neoplasia progression sequence due to autonomous gastrin secretion is the hallmark of MEN1-related gastric disease and defines type 2 ECL-cell NET pathogenesis {2956,2535,2536}. Affected patients show multifocal ECL-cell NETs arising in the background of ECL-cell hyperplasia in the oxyntic mucosa {2956,2535,2536}. Like in chronic atrophic gastritis (type 1 gastric ECL-cell neuroendocrine tumorigenesis), diffuse, linear, and micronodular ECL-cell hyperplasia can be seen in patients with MEN1; however, MEN1-related disease is distinguished by the presence of hyperplastic changes.

MEN1-related bronchopulmonary and thymic disease

Most MEN1 syndrome–associated bronchopulmonary neuroendocrine neoplasms (NENs) are well-differentiated NETs that show either low-grade (typical carcinoid) or intermediate-grade (atypical carcinoid) proliferative features; however, neuroendocrine carcinomas (small cell and large cell types) have been reported {2556}. At the morphological level, individual tumours are indistinguishable from their sporadic counterparts; evidence suggests that MEN1-related lung disease is enriched in multifocal neuroendocrine cell proliferations ranging from pulmonary neuroendocrine cell hyperplasia to neuroendocrine microtumours (formerly called tumourlets; each 0.5–5 mm) and NETs (> 5 mm) {328,4731}. Therefore, the identification of the multifocal pulmonary neuroendocrine cell hyperplasia-to-neoplasia sequence should alert the diagnostician to the possibility of an underlying genetic susceptibility. In an attempt to facilitate the genetic triaging in sporadic-looking presentations, global loss of nuclear menin expression has been suggested to be helpful in the setting of multifocal pulmonary NETs and microtumours {4731}. The distinction of MEN1-related TNET from sporadic tumours may be difficult in the absence of a relevant clinical history or synchronous manifestations of MEN1-related states. However, the application of menin immunohistochemistry may be helpful in young individuals. Ectopic ACTH-related Cushing syndrome can occur in MEN1-related TNETs {1546,2638}.

MEN1-related adrenal disease

Most MEN1-related adrenal lesions are benign cortical lesions that may be bilateral; they include adrenal cortical hyperplasia (e.g. paediatric-onset macronodular hyperplasia), cysts, and adrenal cortical adenomas. Adrenal cortical carcinomas may occur in just over 1% of patients with MEN1 {1517}. The histology of carcinomas or other adrenocortical tumours is comparable with that of sporadic cases, and both sarcomatoid and myxoid subtypes of adrenocortical carcinoma have been described {1784}. In addition to cortical lesions, phaeochromocytomas can occur in patients with MEN1, at a frequency of about 1% {2084,1088}.

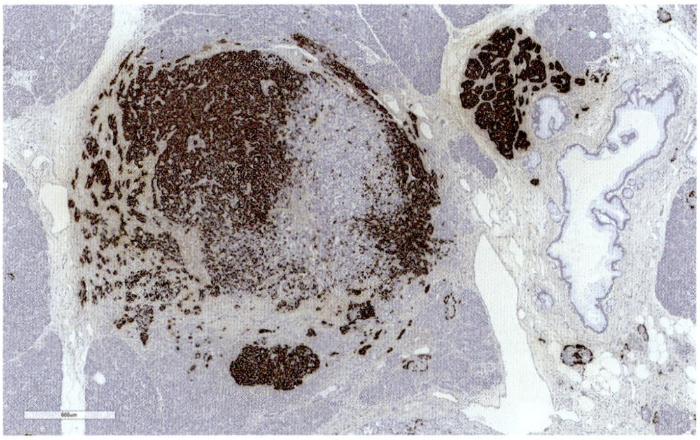

Fig. 13.06 Glucagon expression in multiple endocrine neoplasia type 1–related pancreatic neuroendocrine (micro)tumours. Plurihormonality is a common finding in multiple endocrine neoplasia type 1–related pancreatic neuroendocrine (micro)tumours. Glucagon is the most commonly expressed pancreatic hormone, as illustrated in this photomicrograph.

Other MEN1-related lesions

Many other entities have been reported to occur with increased frequency in patients with MEN1, although sufficient pathogenetic evidence has not been collected for all of these. This does not apply to cutaneous lesions, which have been firmly established as a component of MEN1 and include lipomas, angiofibromas, and collagenomas. These lesions are frequently multiple, and their combined occurrence may give a clue to the presence of MEN1 syndrome in such patients {226}. Another group of tumours that occur in MEN1 are CNS tumours, including meningiomas and spinal ependymomas {225,1459,954}, but again, their histopathology does not differ from that of their sporadic counterparts. Furthermore, the following soft tissue lesions have been reported to be associated with MEN1 syndrome: leiomyoma {2921,2030,830,3031}, gastrointestinal stromal tumour {2866}, deep-seated or visceral lipoma {4310}, and malignant peripheral nerve sheath tumour {3609}. Female patients with MEN1 are at increased risk for breast cancer; this subgroup of patients has been characterized by a loss of heterozygosity at the *MEN1* locus {1153}. So far, follicular nodular disease and thyroid neoplasms do not seem to be part of the MEN1 spectrum, and their occurrence has been attributed to chance {2717}.

Cytology

Cytologically, individual endocrine tumours are indistinguishable from their sporadic counterparts.

Diagnostic molecular pathology

Germline *MEN1* testing is offered to (1) an index patient with a clinical diagnosis of MEN1 syndrome (based on two or more MEN1 syndrome–related tumours), (2) asymptomatic first-degree relatives of a patient with a pathogenic *MEN1* variant (typically before the age of 5 years), (3) symptomatic first-degree relatives (with at least one MEN1-related tumour) of a proband with a pathogenic *MEN1* variant, (4) patients with primary hyperparathyroidism–related multiglandular parathyroid disease or parathyroid adenomas in young individuals (< 30 years), and (5) patients with gastrinoma or multifocal PanNETs at any age {515}. In general, DNA sequence analysis (exons and splice junction mutations) and multiplex ligation-dependent probe amplification for duplication/deletion analysis (screening for larger alterations) are usually used in most clinical laboratories {515}. About 10% of patients with MEN1-related clinical states may test negative for pathogenic *MEN1* variants {4444}. A fraction of *MEN1* mutation–negative patients may harbour pathogenic germline *CDKN1B* variants (multiple endocrine neoplasia type 4) or other CDKI gene variants {4444,1433}; however, the commonly used screening tools may also fail to capture some germline *MEN1* variants, as well as somatic mosaicism {515}. Therefore, whole-exome sequencing or whole-genome sequencing may help reduce the fraction of mutation-negative patients on first-line diagnostic molecular analyses {515}.

Essential and desirable diagnostic criteria

Essential:

- Clinical diagnostic criterion: at least two MEN1 syndrome–associated tumours; **or**
- Familial diagnostic criteria: at least one MEN1 syndrome–associated tumour and a first-degree relative with a confirmed diagnosis of MEN1 syndrome; **or**
- Genetic diagnostic criterion: germline *MEN1* mutation

Staging

Malignant tumours are staged using the American Joint Committee on Cancer (AJCC) / Union for International Cancer Control (UICC) TNM staging systems that are applied to sporadic manifestations.

Prognosis and prediction

Patients with MEN1 are at increased risk of death, usually related to the disease and its complications {1042,1648,2055, 515}. Mutation-negative patients with two out of three main MEN1 manifestations generally have a different phenotype and clinical course, with manifestations at an older age and a normal life expectancy {1025,3556}. Some studies suggest the existence of high-risk *MEN1* sequence variants. Mutation affecting the *JUND* interacting domain may be associated with an increased risk of death {4456}, and sequence variants affecting the *FOXN3* (*CHES1*) interacting domain may be associated with an increased risk of aggressive PanNETs {329}. However, further validation of these associations is required. Nevertheless, the well-established causes of high morbidity are TNETs, duodenal NETs, and PanNETs, along with rare cases of aggressive adrenal tumours {1042,1648,2055,1024,3553}. Female sex, family history of MEN1, and a more recently assessed diagnosis using improved criteria are associated with a lower risk of death {1648}. At the tumour level, the prognostic factors are the same as those for sporadic tumours; tumour stage, tumour size, and grade are important parameters {2055}. MEN1-associated lung NETs are slow-growing tumours with a good prognosis {4642}.

Multiple endocrine neoplasia type 2

Asa SL
de Krijger RR
Erickson LA
Gimenez-Roqueplo A-P
Osamura RY
Perren A
Valk GD

Definition

Multiple endocrine neoplasia type 2 (MEN2) is an autosomal dominant tumour syndrome caused by activating mutations in the *RET* proto-oncogene.

MIM numbering

171400 Multiple endocrine neoplasia, type 2A; MEN2A
162300 Multiple endocrine neoplasia, type 2B; MEN2B

ICD-11 coding

2F7A.0 Multiple polyglandular tumours

Related terminology

Acceptable: MEN2 syndrome.

Not recommended: Sipple syndrome; multiple endocrine neoplasia type 3; Gorlin syndrome; Wagenmann–Froboese syndrome; mucosal neuroma syndrome; Farndon syndrome.

Subtype(s)

Multiple endocrine neoplasia type 2A; multiple endocrine neoplasia type 2B (formerly called type 3)

Localization

Medullary thyroid carcinoma (MTC), which is the hallmark of this disorder, involves the thyroid gland and specifically arises most often at the junction of the upper third and lower two thirds of the lateral lobes of the gland. The disease begins as microscopic proliferations (classified as nodular C-cell hyperplasia) in this location, usually bilaterally, and progresses to multifocal invasive carcinoma.

Phaeochromocytoma arises in the adrenal medulla and again is often bilateral and multifocal. Extra-adrenal paragangliomas are not usually seen in this disorder.

Parathyroid proliferations arise in the parathyroid glands beside and below the thyroid in the neck. They are bilateral in 70% of patients.

Cutaneous lichen amyloidosis can be identified anywhere on the skin but most commonly involves the interscapular back.

Hirschsprung disease and oral-intestinal ganglioneuromas are manifestations of abnormal development of the myenteric and submucosal ganglionic plexus of the gastrointestinal tract. Loss of function leading to Hirschsprung disease most often affects the rectosigmoid colon. Ganglioneuromas can occur anywhere from the lips to the anus.

Clinical features

The disorder has several subtypes. MEN2A is the classic form, characterized by the development of MTC and often associated with phaeochromocytoma and/or parathyroid proliferations. MEN2B, originally called MEN3, is a rare subtype characterized by a highly aggressive early-onset MTC associated with a high risk of phaeochromocytoma, oral and intestinal ganglioneuromas, and a marfanoid body habitus.

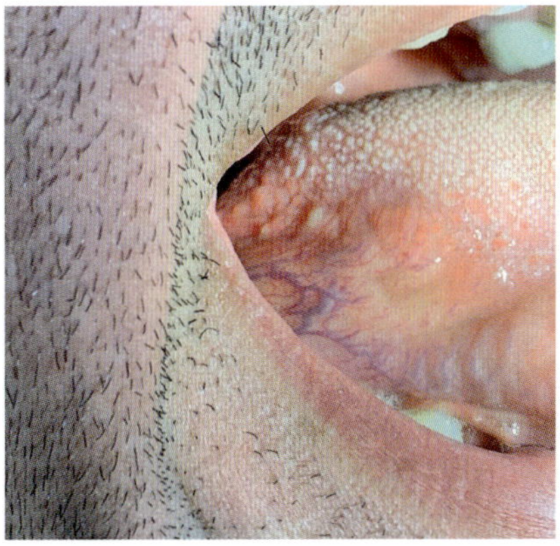

Fig. 13.07 Multiple endocrine neoplasia type 2. A 21-year-old man with multiple endocrine neoplasia type 2 with a mucosal neuroma of the tongue.

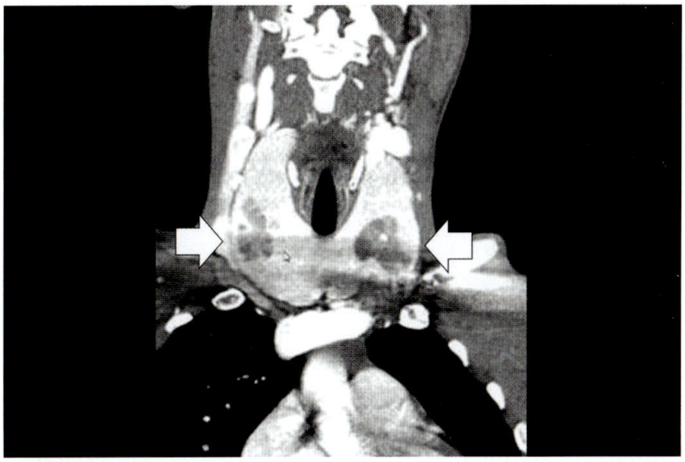

Fig. 13.08 Medullary thyroid carcinoma in multiple endocrine neoplasia type 2B. MRI shows bilateral medullary thyroid carcinomas (arrows) arising in the lateral thyroid lobes.

Isolated MTC can occur. Formerly known as familial MTC, it is recognized as a variant of MEN2A in the American Thyroid Association (ATA) guidelines on MTC published in 2015 {4848}. Other variants described include MEN2A with cutaneous lichen amyloidosis and MEN2A with Hirschsprung disease.

Patients with MEN2 usually present with signs and symptoms of MTC, including one or more neck masses sometimes causing pain, hoarseness, coughing, dysphagia, and dyspnoea. Occasional patients report diarrhoea and flushing caused by calcitonin excess. Rarer presentations are due to phaeochromocytoma that may cause hypertension, headache, tachycardia, sweating, tremors, and anxiety. Patients with Hirschsprung disease present in childhood with constipation, diarrhoea,

Table 13.02 *RET* mutations and associated risk of aggressive medullary thyroid carcinoma (MTC), phaeochromocytoma (Phaeo), and hyperparathyroidism (HPT) {4848}

RET mutation (protein change)	Aggressive MTC risk	Phaeo risk	HPT risk
M918T	Highest	High	Low
A883F	High	High	Low
C634S/R/G/Y/W/F/L	High	High	High
L790F	Moderate	Low	Low
S891A	Moderate	Low	Intermediate
V804M/L	Moderate	Low	Intermediate
D631Y	Moderate	High	Intermediate
C630R/Y/F	Moderate	Intermediate	Intermediate
C620F/R/S/G/Y/W	Moderate	Intermediate	Intermediate
C618F/R/S/G/Y/W	Moderate	Intermediate	Intermediate
C611F/G/S/Y/W	Moderate	Intermediate	Intermediate
C609F/G/R/S/Y	Moderate	Intermediate	Intermediate

vomiting, and abdominal distention. Patients with MEN2B have a marfanoid habitus, and ganglioneuromas may be seen on oral examination.

Increasingly, MEN2 is being diagnosed in younger patients, owing to genetic screening of known kindreds.

Epidemiology

The prevalence of MEN2 is estimated to be about 1 per 30 000 population {3688,4848}. The incidence of MEN2A is about 1 case per 1 973 500 person-years, and that of MEN2B is much lower, at 1 case per 38 750 000 person-years. The M:F ratio is about 1:1, but some studies have shown a slight female predominance. Geographical heterogeneity of *RET* variants has been documented {2781}, likely due to founder effects in different populations {2875}.

Etiology

Monoallelic gain-of-function germline mutations of *RET* induce constitutive activation of the RET receptor and are responsible for MEN2. In any given patient with one of the associated disorders, a negative family history does not exclude germline disease, because the disorder can skip generations or be misdiagnosed. MEN2B is more often due to a de novo germline mutation.

Pathogenesis

The proto-oncogene *RET*, on 10q11.2 was discovered in 1985, owing to its ability to transform NIH-3T3 cells {4380}. Activating *RET* proto-oncogene germline mutations were reported to cause MEN2A a few years later {3136}, followed by the detection of germline mutations in patients with MEN2B and familial MTC {3945,1927}.

The *RET* gene is a proto-oncogene that encodes a tyrosine kinase receptor. Physiologically, the RET receptor is activated by GDNF-family ligands bound to GFRαs and forms dimers, recruited to lipid rafts {2237}. Specific tyrosine residues within the tyrosine kinase domain (TKD) of RET are autophosphorylated after RET dimer formation, which in turn activates the MAPK, PI3K, JAK/STAT, PKA, and PKC pathways {2237}. Intracellular RET signalling is needed for the development of the enteric nervous system, kidney, and urinary tract {2237}.

There are clear correlations between genotype and phenotype. MEN2A mutations are mainly found in cysteines of codons 609, 611, 618, 620 (exon 10), or 634 (exon 11) of the extracellular domain, leading to bisulfide-bonded homodimers and constitutive activation {3135,1248,3068}. *RET* p.C634R is the most frequent mutation and is associated with the classic triad of MTC, phaeochromocytoma, and hyperparathyroidism. Familial MTC is characterized by mutations that do not affect cysteines in exons 8, 13, 14, and 15 or by mutations in codons 609–620. The *RET* p.A883T mutation induced MTC in a family in a homozygous setting only. In about 2% of patients with MEN2, no mutation in the *RET* proto-oncogene can be detected, and therefore it is still unclear whether other genetic alterations can lead to MEN2 {3796}.

There are also correlations between genotype and the aggressiveness of MTC, which allowed the ATA to classify pathogenic sequence variants of *RET* into three different categories (highest, high, and moderate) based on the risk for aggressive MTC {4848}. Interestingly, in MEN2A, the closer to the cell membrane the mutant cysteine residue lies, the higher the transforming ability {2780,1427}. The highest-risk category (ATA-HST) includes patients with MEN2B and the *RET* p.M918T mutation; the high-risk category (ATA-H) includes patients with *RET* mutations at codon 634 (p.C634F, p.C634G, p.C634R, p.C634S, p.C634W, or p.C634Y) and/or the *RET* p.A883F mutation. The moderate-risk category (ATA-MOD) includes patients with all other listed *RET* mutations. The common *RET* mutations and their associated risk of aggressive MTC and development of phaeochromocytoma and hyperparathyroidism are described in Table 13.02.

The vast majority of patients with MEN2B carry the *RET* p.M918T mutation in the kinase domain, leading to a constitutive autophosphorylation. *RET* p.A883F is found in 2–3% of patients with MEN2B {1586}.

Usually, biallelic loss-of-function germline mutation of *RET* leads to a non-functioning RET receptor and is a cause of Hirschsprung disease. However, the association of Hirschsprung disease with MEN2 suggests that activation of this oncogene interferes with the normal development of the enteric plexuses.

Macroscopic appearance

MTC in this disorder is typically bilateral and multicentric; the cut surface is white to yellow and homogeneous {318}.

Phaeochromocytomas have a tan-white to dusky haemorrhagic appearance. The adrenals from patients with MEN2 can contain two or more separate phaeochromocytomas. Interposed adrenal medullary hyperplasia {2956} might or might not be apparent grossly. Patients with longstanding MEN2 can develop multiple tumours with a spectrum of degenerative changes.

Histopathology

Medullary thyroid carcinoma

MEN2-associated MTC appears histologically indistinguishable from sporadic MTC, but familial cases are more often multifocal, bilateral, and associated with C-cell hyperplasia {4909}. Complete sampling of prophylactically removed thyroids is important to identify medullary thyroid microcarcinomas. The junction of the upper third and lower two thirds of the lateral lobes has a high density of C cells and is a common location of microcarcinomas in this setting.

Histological patterns of MTC include solid, follicular (tubular/glandular), papillary, spindled, oxyphilic, paraganglioma-like, insular, angiosarcoma-like, and pleomorphic/anaplastic {1782, 3923,4245,620,2705,2936}. The tumour cells can be round, oval, plasmacytoid, or spindled and are often mixed. Occasional nuclear pleomorphism and scattered multinucleated cells can be seen. Rare melanotic, squamous, giant cell, clear cell, and small cell patterns exist {1250,4774,380,1134}. Amyloid is seen as many as 75–90% of MTCs, and calcifications may be identified with amyloid. Amyloid in MTC has been shown by mass spectrometry to be a deposition of a calcitonin precursor {1272}. Mucin production may also be seen {5104}. MTC cells have the traditional salt-and-pepper chromatin of neuroendocrine tumours (NETs) and may have a small eccentric nucleolus and amphophilic cytoplasm. Intranuclear pseudoinclusions, similar to those of papillary thyroid carcinoma, may be seen. Mitotic activity is generally low. MTC with increased mitotic activity, necrosis, small cell features, vascular invasion, and stromal desmoplasia may behave more aggressively. Mixed follicular–medullary thyroid carcinoma and mixed papillary–medullary thyroid carcinoma can also occur in MEN2 {3422,3046,3639}. MTC must be distinguished from follicular cell–derived thyroid carcinomas as well as from other NETs {2705}. MTC is immunoreactive for low-molecular-weight keratin, INSM1, chromogranin A, synaptophysin, calcitonin, CGRP, thyroid transcription factor 1 (TTF1), and monoclonal CEA, and it is negative for thyroglobulin and monoclonal PAX8 (clone MRQ-50) {1692}.

The progression of C-cell hyperplasia to neoplasia is a characteristic feature in the pathogenesis of MEN2-associated MTC. The term "hyperplasia" in this setting may not be appropriate, because the C cells in this setting are clonal proliferations {318}. Moreover, definitions of C-cell hyperplasia are controversial and numerous. These definitions have been based on various criteria: the number of C cells per area, of C-cell clusters, of complete follicles surrounded by C cells, and of C cells beyond their normal geographical distribution {2704,1723,3530,1722,1568}. C-cell hyperplasia was classically defined as ≥ 50 C cells per low-power field (an ambiguous measure) in areas of high C-cell concentration {2704}. C-cell clusters of at least 6–8 C cells per cluster in several foci with > 50 cells per low-power field have been used to define C-cell hyperplasia {2704,2956}. Some authors have suggested that the finding of MTC with concomitant C-cell hyperplasia does not distinguish sporadic from hereditary MTC {2219,2220}, because physiological or reactive/secondary C-cell hyperplasia can be seen in hypercalcaemia, hyperparathyroidism, increasing age, hypergastrinaemia, chronic lymphocytic thyroiditis, and adjacent non-medullary thyroid tumours {2704,1568,3372,1721,1723}. As noted by some authors, "The lower limit of C-cell hyperplasia and the upper limit of normal C-cell mass are not clear" {286}. It has been suggested that physiological C-cell hyperplasia is only seen on immunohistochemistry, whereas that associated with familial disease, particularly when nodular, may be more readily seen on H&E sections and may be associated with large cells and nuclear atypia {3530}.

Medullary thyroid microcarcinoma is ≤ 10 mm in size. The distinction of medullary thyroid microcarcinoma from C-cell hyperplasia can be difficult and several features have been suggested, including loss of organoid arrangement, extension beyond the basement membrane, desmoplastic stromal reaction, and surrounding infiltrating tumour cells {2220}; however, these features may be difficult to recognize {2956}. Even very small medullary microcarcinomas can behave aggressively. In a study of 233 individuals with medullary thyroid microcarcinomas (126 hereditary and 107 sporadic), lymph node metastasis increased with incremental tumour diameter {2778}: 8% of microcarcinomas measuring < 2 mm were associated with lymph node metastasis, as were 16% of tumours measuring 3–4 mm, 33% of tumours measuring 5–6 mm, and 43% of tumours measuring 7–10 mm {2778}. The important finding is that metastases occur even in tumours smaller than 2 mm. Hereditary medullary thyroid microcarcinomas were more often multifocal and more often had positive nodal status than sporadic medullary microcarcinomas {2778}. In a SEER Program database (1988–2007) study of 310 medullary thyroid microcarcinomas, 65 (37%) of 176 patients with any lymph nodes removed had metastases, including 23% with tumours measuring ≤ 5 mm {2247}.

Phaeochromocytoma

In MEN2 this may be indistinguishable from sporadic forms. However, in the setting of MEN2, phaeochromocytomas are often bilateral and associated with adrenal medullary hyperplasia. Progression of adrenal medullary hyperplasia to phaeochromocytoma is a characteristic of MEN2-associated phaeochromocytoma. In adrenal medullary hyperplasia, adrenal medullary tissue makes up more than one third of the thickness of the adrenal gland or the adrenal medulla extends beyond the normal location in the normal apex and body and is also found in the tail of the adrenal gland {2956,2977}. In MEN2, the term "microphaeochromocytoma" has replaced "nodular hyperplasia", because this is a clonal process. Phaeochromocytomas in MEN2 appear histologically similar to sporadic phaeochromocytomas, composed of nests (Zellballen) of polygonal tumour cells surrounded by capillaries, or they can have a trabecular or diffuse architecture. The nuclei are often vesicular with prominent nucleoli, and the cells have variably staining cytoplasm that can be granular, basophilic, or amphophilic. Phaeochromocytomas in MEN2 generally have a low risk of aggressive behaviour and produce both norepinephrine and epinephrine. Composite phaeochromocytomas can also be seen in MEN2 {5004,1203}.

Other tumours

Parathyroid proliferations associated with hyperparathyroidism can be seen in 15–30% of individuals with MEN2A but are not seen in MEN2B. They have been classified as adenomas and so-called hyperplasia when there is multiglandular disease that is more likely to be multiple neoplasms involving single or multiple glands.

Hirschsprung disease, affecting the gastrointestinal tract in 7% of MEN2A patients with mutations involving exon 10, is characterized by a complete absence of ganglion cells in the myenteric and submucosal plexus; this most often involves the rectosigmoid colon {1427,939}.

Mucosal neuromas in MEN2B can involve the oropharynx, lips, and eyelids. Additionally, corneal nerves may be thickened, and ganglioneuromatosis of the gastrointestinal tract may occur, characterized by neuroma or diffuse ganglioneuromatosis {4884,1639,2577,3098}.

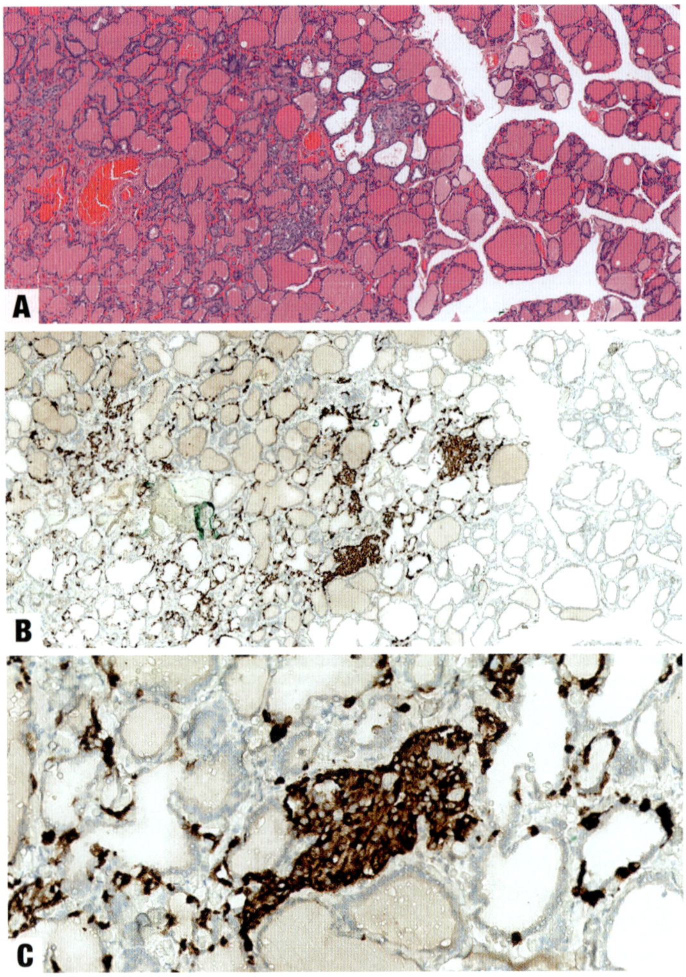

Fig. 13.10 C-cell hyperplasia in multiple endocrine neoplasia type 2. **A** Clusters of clear cells are seen at low magnification, disrupting the normal thyroid architecture. **B,C** Calcitonin staining identifies a markedly increased number of C cells arranged singly, in small groups, surrounding follicles, and forming solid nests.

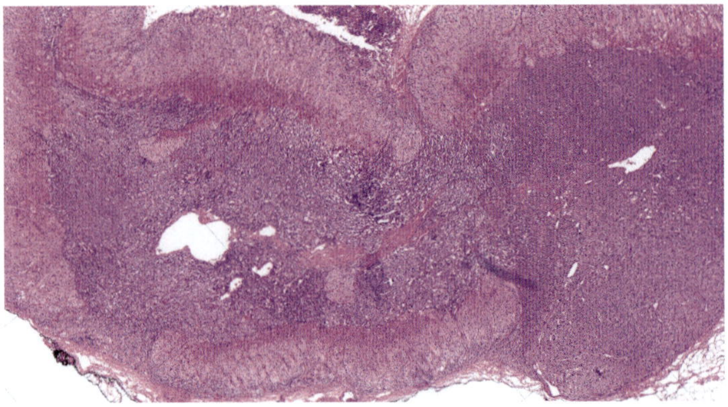

Fig. 13.09 The adrenal in multiple endocrine neoplasia type 2. This case contains multiple lesions and intervening medullary hyperplasia.

Cutaneous lichen amyloidosis, thought to be due to repeated scratching due to intense pruritus {1928,4686,3640}, is histologically characterized by globular deposits of amyloid in the papillary dermis with overlying epidermal hyperkeratosis and acanthosis.

Cytology

The cytopathological findings are presented in *Medullary thyroid carcinoma* (p. 174) and *Phaeochromocytoma* (p. 277).

Diagnostic molecular pathology

The diagnosis of MEN2 is confirmed by the identification of a germline mutation in *RET* that is known to be pathogenic. It is recommended that germline DNA testing be performed on any patient with MTC regardless of age, associated disorders, and family history.

Essential and desirable diagnostic criteria

Essential: a documented pathogenic variant of *RET* and/or manifestation of MTC associated with any of the other features of MEN2.

Desirable: C-cell hyperplasia; adrenal medullary hyperplasia; multifocal medullary carcinoma or phaeochromocytoma.

Staging

There is no uniformly accepted syndrome-specific staging system for MEN2. Malignant neoplasms associated with this syndrome generally follow the cancer staging suggested by Union for International Cancer Control (UICC) / American Joint Committee on Cancer (AJCC) criteria {132}.

Prognosis and prediction

The prognosis in MEN2 is determined by MTC, and much less or not at all by phaeochromocytoma, parathyroid disease, or other manifestations of MEN2B.

The prognosis for patients with MEN2-related MTC is superior to that for patients with sporadic MTC, with 10-year survival rates depending on disease stage: currently 100%, 93%, 71%, and 21% for stage I, II, III, and IV, respectively {3053}. This is likely to be the result of screening, early detection, and prophylactic surgery in this patient group. It has been firmly established that the various *RET* mutations confer a range of risk profiles to individuals and families carrying these mutations, with the p.M918T *RET* mutation (in MEN2B) carrying the highest risk, followed by

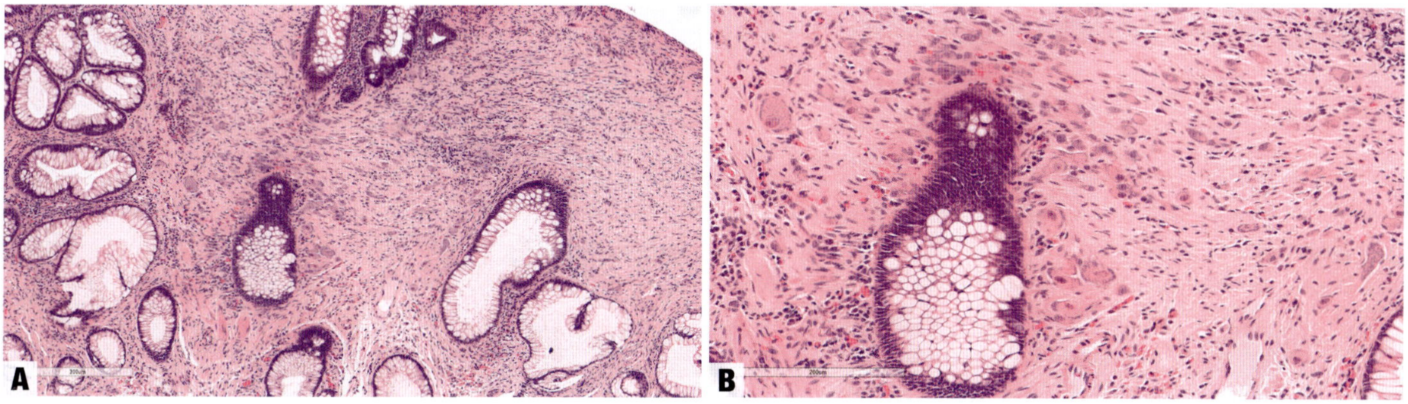

Fig. 13.11 Mucosal neuroma in multiple endocrine neoplasia type 2. **A,B** A tumour from a patient with multiple endocrine neoplasia type 2B. The gut mucosa is expanded by a proliferation with scattered trapped ganglion cells.

the p.A883P (in MEN2B) and p.C634 (in MEN2A) *RET* mutations (responsible for a high-risk profile), and then finally followed by the p.C609, p.C611, p.C618, and p.C620 mutations (which impart a moderate risk). Still other *RET* mutations result in an MTC-only phenotype, including p.G533, p.E768, p.L790, p.V804, and p.S891 {2779,1426,4847,3134}. An additional two *RET* sequence variants have been described as modifiers that result in a more aggressive clinical course {3152}. The risk profile has led to recommendations for prophylactic thyroidectomy in mutation carriers in MEN2 families, with surgery performed before the age of 1 year for the highest-risk group of MEN2B patients, and before the age of 5 years for those in the high-risk group with codon 634 mutations in MEN2A. For those in the moderate-risk group, surgery may be postponed until the age of 10 years {4743,4848}. Besides thyroid gland resection, central neck lymph node dissection is also performed, but lateral neck dissection is reserved for cases in which there would be suspicion of lymph node metastases, which in general is not the case in patients who undergo prophylactic surgery. C-cell hyperplasia is always found in thyroids of *RET* mutation carriers, and the occurrence of small MTC is not uncommon. Apart from surgical guidelines based on genetic risk status, biochemical screening for calcitonin levels plays an important role in the timing of surgery and postoperative follow-up. The latter is only necessary if an MTC has been found; for C-cell hyperplasia, no follow-up is indicated. In fact, postoperative biochemical cure is associated with very high 10-year survival rates, whereas short calcitonin doubling times are associated with a poor prognosis, except for the rare cases in which an MTC no longer produces calcitonin because of dedifferentiation.

Phaeochromocytoma development in patients with MEN2 is also determined by genotype, with the lifetime risk of phaeochromocytoma being almost 90% by the age of 80 years in patients with *RET* p.C634 mutations and 100% in patients with MEN2B with the p.M918 mutation {3152}. In contrast, the overall risk of phaeochromocytoma in patients with MEN2 is 40%, and some *RET* mutations, as mentioned above, are not associated at all with phaeochromocytoma in patients with MEN2 {4574}. Phaeochromocytoma is usually not the presenting tumour in patients with MEN2, although every patient needs to be screened for its presence in order to avoid life-threatening crises at thyroid surgery. In addition, biochemical screening for urinary metanephrines is imperative in the clinical follow-up of patients with MEN2 {4848}. Fewer than 5% of MEN2-related phaeochromocytomas give rise to metastasis {3054}.

Parathyroid disorders are also related to the specific genetic defect in *RET*, occurring most frequently with p.C634R mutations {3135,1249}. Screening for hyperparathyroidism is indicated from the age of 11 years for patients with ATA-HST and ATA-H *RET* mutations, and from the age of 16 years for those with ATA-MOD *RET* mutations {4848}. In MEN2B, no parathyroid disease has been described.

Multiple endocrine neoplasia type 4

Asa SL
Gimenez-Roqueplo A-P
Hernández-Ramírez LC
Osamura RY
Pellegata NS
Perren A
Valk GD

Definition

Multiple endocrine neoplasia type 4 (MEN4) is an autosomal dominant tumour syndrome caused by inactivating mutations in the *CDKN1B* gene.

MIM numbering

610755 Multiple endocrine neoplasia type 4; MEN4

ICD-11 coding

2F7A.0 Multiple polyglandular tumours

Table 13.03 Location of *CDKN1B* gene variants, the effect they have on the gene/protein function (if known), and corresponding clinical features (continued on next page)

CDKN1B variant	Codon	Amino acid	Family history	Predicted effect	Clinical manifestations	Reference
5′ UTR (RefSeq: NM_004064.5)						
c.-456_-453delCCTT	–	–	Negative	Reduced protein level	Acromegaly Well-differentiated non-functioning PanNET	{3312}
c.-80C>T	–	–	Negative	Transcription	Primary HPT	{481}
c.-29_-26delAGAG	–		Negative	Transcription	Gigantism	{3925}
c.-29_-26delAGAG	–	–	Negative	Transcription	Primary HPT	{481}
c.-29_-26delAGAG	–	–	Negative		Paediatric Cushing disease	{764}
c.-32_-29delGAGA		–	Negative	Reduced mRNA + protein level	Gastric NET Primary HPT	{2811}
c.-7G>C	–	–	Two asymptomatic variant-positive daughters	Transcription	Bilateral non-functioning adrenal masses Uterine fibroids Primary HPT	{41}
Exon 1						
c.25G>A	9	G9R	NA	Increased protein instability	Primary HPT	{929}
c.59_77dup19	25	K25fs	Negative	ND	Small cell neuroendocrine cervical carcinoma ACTH-dependent Cushing syndrome Primary HPT Multiple sclerosis	{1540}
c.121_122delTT	41	L41N*fs83	Positive	ND	Primary HPT Cushing disease	{1433}
c.163G>A	55	A55T	Negative	ND	ZES with gastrinoma and hepatic metastases Primary HPT	{371}
c.206C>T	69	P69L	Negative	No binding to CDK2, no growth suppression	PTC with neck lymph node metastases Bilateral multiple lung metastases from bronchial carcinoid Primary HPT Non-functioning pituitary microadenoma Subcutaneous epigastric lipoma Type 2 diabetes mellitus	{3064}
c.227G>A	76	W76X	Variant-positive sister with renal angiomyolipoma; her son (variant carrier) had testicular cancer	Mislocalization, no growth suppression	Acromegaly Primary HPT	{3494}

FIPA, familial isolated pituitary adenoma / pituitary neuroendocrine tumour; HPT, hyperparathyroidism; NA, not available; ND, not determined; NET, neuroendocrine tumour; PanNET, pancreatic neuroendocrine tumour; PTC, papillary thyroid carcinoma; SDS, sodium dodecyl sulfate; UTR, untranslated region; ZES, Zollinger–Ellison syndrome.

Related terminology

Not recommended: multiple endocrine neoplasia type 1–like syndrome.

Subtype(s)

None

Localization

Patients with germline inactivating mutations of *CDKN1B* develop a clinical phenotype that mimics multiple endocrine neoplasia type 1 (MEN1); they have tumours that arise in the pituitary, parathyroid, and pancreas. Parathyroid disease is the most prevalent, occurring in about 75% of patients. Pituitary tumours are identified in about one third of patients. Other neuroendocrine tumours (NETs) have also been reported, including those arising in the lung and stomach.

Clinical features

The diagnosis should be considered in a patient with primary hyperparathyroidism, diagnosed by an increase of serum levels

Table 13.03 Location of *CDKN1B* gene variants, the effect they have on the gene/protein function (if known), and corresponding clinical features (continued)

CDKN1B variant	Codon	Amino acid	Family history	Predicted effect	Clinical manifestations	Reference
c.283C>T	95	P95S	NA	No binding to GRB2	ZES with masses in duodenum and tail of pancreas Primary HPT	{41}
c.286A>C	96	K96Q	Asymptomatic variant-positive sister	No binding to GRB2	Hyperprolactinaemia due to a suspected prolactinoma Breast cancer at the age of 41 years	{4496}
c.320delA	107	Q107Rfs*12	Asymptomatic variant-positive mother, brother, children	Mislocalization, reduced RhoA binding	Paediatric Cushing disease	{764}
c.356T>C	119	I119T	The p.I119T change was found in 1 member of a 2-person FIPA family with somatotropinomas	Altered migration in SDS gels	Somatotropinoma	{4496}
c.356T>C	119	I119T	Negative	Reduced binding to RhoA and CDK2	Paediatric Cushing disease	{764}
c.374_375delCT	125	S125X	Asymptomatic variant-positive son		Gastrointestinal NET Primary HPT	{4521}
c.378G>C	126	E126D	Asymptomatic variant-positive mother and maternal grandfather		Early-onset primary HPT Recurrent renal calculi and hypercalcaemia	{1241}
c.378G>C	126	E126Q	Negative	Partial mislocalization, reduced binding to RhoA and CDK2	Paediatric Cushing disease	{764}
c.397C>A	133	P133T	NA	None identified	Primary HPT (1 parathyroid tumour)	{929}
c.397C>A	133	P133T	Negative	ND	Primary HPT Meningioma, papillary PTC Hürthle cell adenoma Cholesteatoma and uterine leiomyomas	{558}
c.397C>A	133	P133T	Negative	ND	Primary HPT	{481}
c.407A>G	136	D136G	Negative	Reduced binding to RhoA and CDK2	Paediatric Cushing disease	{764}
Exon 2						
c.595T>C	198	Stop>Q	Monozygotic twin sister variant-positive with primary HPT (1 parathyroid tumour) Aunt and cousin with primary HPT not tested	Reduced protein level	Primary HPT	{41}

FIPA, familial isolated pituitary adenoma / pituitary neuroendocrine tumour; HPT, hyperparathyroidism; NA, not available; ND, not determined; NET, neuroendocrine tumour; PanNET, pancreatic neuroendocrine tumour; PTC, papillary thyroid carcinoma; SDS, sodium dodecyl sulfate; UTR, untranslated region; ZES, Zollinger–Ellison syndrome.

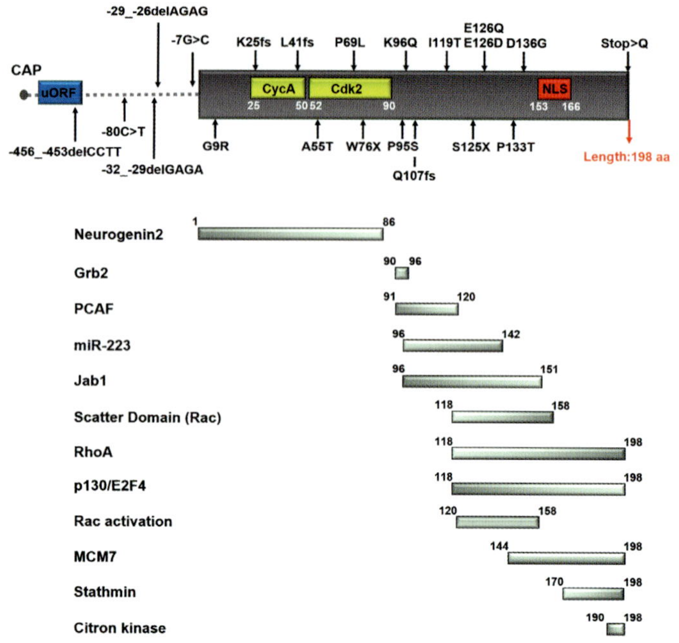

Fig. 13.12 Mutations of *CDKN1B* (*P27*) in multiple endocrine neoplasia type 4. Germline *CDKN1B* mutations so far identified in patients with multiple endocrine neoplasia type 4 span the coding sequence. They alter the protein's localization, its tumour-suppressor activity, or its binding with known partners. aa, amino acids; CycA, cyclin A; NLS, nuclear localization sequence; uORF, upstream open reading frame.

of calcium and of intact PTH, associated with NET(s) of the pituitary and/or gastroenteropancreatic system and a negative *MEN1* genetic test using a technique that is able to detect point mutations, small and large deletions, and mosaicism. Gastrointestinal NETs seem to be less prevalent in MEN4 than in MEN1 {109,1433}.

Epidemiology

With < 50 published cases worldwide, MEN4 is a very rare disease. It has been identified mainly in patients who were clinically suspected to have MEN1 but are negative for *MEN1* mutations; a significant female predominance is reported {3312,481, 3925,2811,41,929,3494,1540,371,3064,4496,4521,1241,558, 1433,764}.

Etiology

MEN4 is caused by heterozygous germline mutations in *CDKN1B* {3494,2576}. It is an autosomal dominant disorder with incomplete penetrance in some families.

Pathogenesis

CDKN1B (12p13.1) encodes the CDK inhibitor p27 (p27KIP1). The canonical role of p27 is the inhibition of CDK activity. Specifically, nuclear p27 binds to and inhibits cyclin E / CDK2 and cyclin A / CDK2 complexes that regulate the progression from the G1 phase to the S phase of the cell cycle. The main targets of CDK2 are members of the RB1 family. When these proteins are phosphorylated by CDK2, they release members of the E2F family, which in turn activate the transcription of genes responsible for G1-to-S progression {2576}. p27 mainly localizes to the nucleus in growth-arrested cells, but it is translocated to the cytoplasm when the cells progress through the cell cycle. When in the cytosol, p27 binds cyclin D / CDK4–6 complexes and acts as an essential assembly factor for such complexes. As opposed to cyclin E / CDK2, cyclin D / CDK4–6 complexes remain catalytically active when bound to p27. Sequestering p27 in the cytoplasm prevents the inhibition of nuclear cyclin/CDK complexes and ultimately promotes cell division {4183, 849}. In addition, p27 plays pro-oncogenic roles in the cytoplasm that are independent of cyclin/CDK inhibition. Indeed, cytosolic p27 plays a role in cell migration and invasion, apoptosis, and autophagy {383}.

Although p27 stops cell proliferation when overexpressed, and in mice it promotes tumour formation when deleted {1366, 3170,2328}, the rarity of somatic mutations in human cancers granted p27 the label of an atypical tumour suppressor. The identification of germline mutations in patients with MEN4 established p27 as a bona fide tumour suppressor {3587}.

The germline p27 mutations so far identified in patients with MEN4 span the coding sequence and the 5′ untranslated region of the gene without obvious mutation hotspots. Most of the reported changes in *CDKN1B* are missense mutations, followed by frameshift and nonsense alterations (see Table 13.03, p. 440). For some of these mutations, functional in vitro studies have been conducted, and the results have shown that they alter the protein's localization, its tumour-suppressor activity, or its binding with known partners. Altogether, the mutations so far identified behave as loss-of-function mutations, and this is in agreement with the tumour-suppressor role of p27.

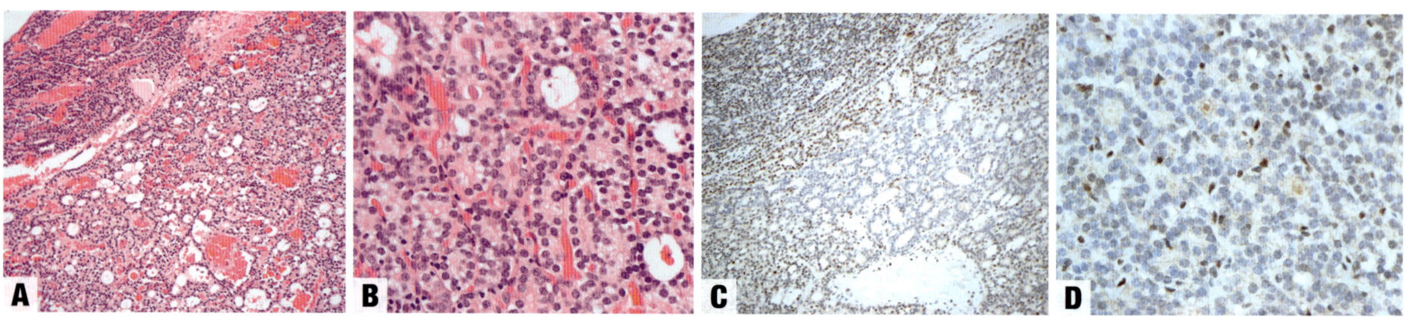

Fig. 13.13 Parathyroid adenoma in multiple endocrine neoplasia type 4. **A** The parathyroid contains a delineated nodule with surrounding non-neoplastic parenchyma. **B** The neoplastic parathyroid cells are crowded and the lesion is devoid of stromal fat. Pleomorphism is minimal. **C** Loss of nuclear p27. The non-tumorous parenchyma shows strong nuclear reactivity but the neoplasm lacks nuclear staining in the adenomatous cells. **D** Loss of nuclear p27. The neoplastic parathyroid cells lack nuclear p27 reactivity. The stromal cells provide an internal positive control.

Macroscopic appearance

The gross appearance of the tumours is not distinct from that of sporadic lesions.

Histopathology

Limited data are available on histopathological clues for a MEN4 diagnosis; no clear differences from sporadic cases are reported. The occurrence of multiple tumours of the spectrum is the only known hint {934}. Hyperparathyroidism is the most frequent symptom; uniglandular disease is frequent, and no relapse after parathyroidectomy has been reported so far {109}. Pituitary neuroendocrine tumours (PitNETs) include non-functioning lesions as well as tumours secreting growth hormone, prolactin, or ACTH. Pulmonary and ileal NETs have been reported in some patients, and adrenocortical tumours are rare.

Cytology

The cytopathological features of the various neoplasms related to MEN4 are indistinguishable from those of their sporadic counterparts, which are described elsewhere in this volume and in the other fifth-edition volumes of the WHO Classification of Tumours series.

Diagnostic molecular pathology

Because of the variable presentation of MEN4, this diagnosis can only be established by genetic testing. Such testing is recommended in patients with the MEN1 phenotype who are negative for *MEN1* mutations {1539}. Testing of patients with apparently sporadic isolated NETs is currently only carried out in research settings, because although deregulation of *CDKN1B* has been documented in multiple human neoplasms, somatic mutations are rare {4183,1422}.

Essential and desirable diagnostic criteria

Essential: documented germline pathogenic sequence variant of the *CDKN1B* gene; manifestation of pituitary, parathyroid, and/or pancreatic neuroendocrine neoplasia.

Desirable: manifestation of pituitary, parathyroid, and/or pancreatic neuroendocrine neoplasia in the absence of a pathogenic mutation in *MEN1*.

Staging

Staging follows the American Joint Committee on Cancer (AJCC) guidelines for the various neoplasms in this syndrome.

Prognosis and prediction

Given the small number of cases so far reported, no genotype–phenotype correlations have been established, and cases should be treated in accordance with the clinical guidelines for their individual tumours. Other than ruling out the presence of hyperparathyroidism, there are no data to guide the clinical screening and follow-up of *CDKN1B* mutation carriers.

Multiple endocrine neoplasia type 5 (*MAX*-related tumours)

Clifton-Bligh RJ
Duncan EL
Fuchs TL
Gimenez-Roqueplo A-P
Mete O
Osamura RY
Pellegata NS
Perren A
Taieb D
Valk GD

Definition

Multiple endocrine neoplasia type 5 (MEN5) is an inherited tumour syndrome caused by pathogenic germline sequence variants in the tumour suppressor gene *MAX*.

MIM numbering

None

ICD-11 coding

2F7A.0 Multiple polyglandular tumours

Related terminology

Acceptable: MAX-associated tumours.

Subtype(s)

None

Localization

Germline mutations in *MAX* manifest with multifocal endocrine neoplasms in the adrenal, pituitary, pancreas, and parathyroid glands {4047}. Tumours in non-endocrine organs have also

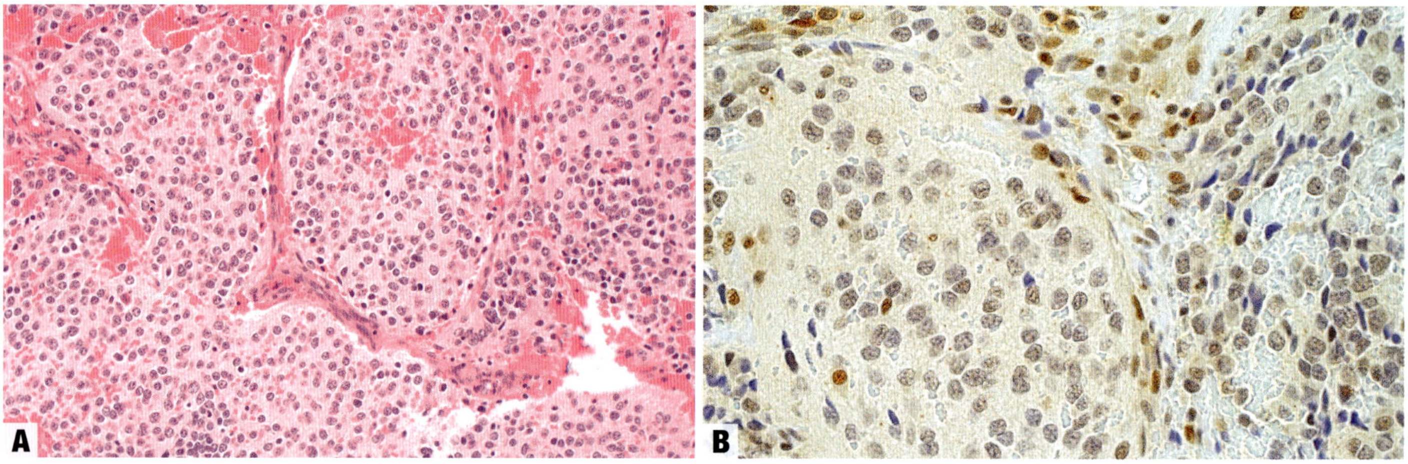

Fig. 13.14 Neuroblastoma. **A** A neuroblastoma from a patient with a known germline pathogenic *MAX* variant. This tumour is morphologically indistinguishable from a sporadic neoplasm. **B** MAX immunohistochemistry for the same tumour. The non-neoplastic inflammatory cells and endothelial cells demonstrate preserved positive staining for MAX, whereas there is loss of staining in the neoplastic cells of the neuroblastoma. Although some authors have found that MAX immunohistochemistry could have a role in triaging patients for genetic testing for *MAX* germline mutation, others have found that it lacks sensitivity and specificity, and it is not recommended in routine clinical practice.

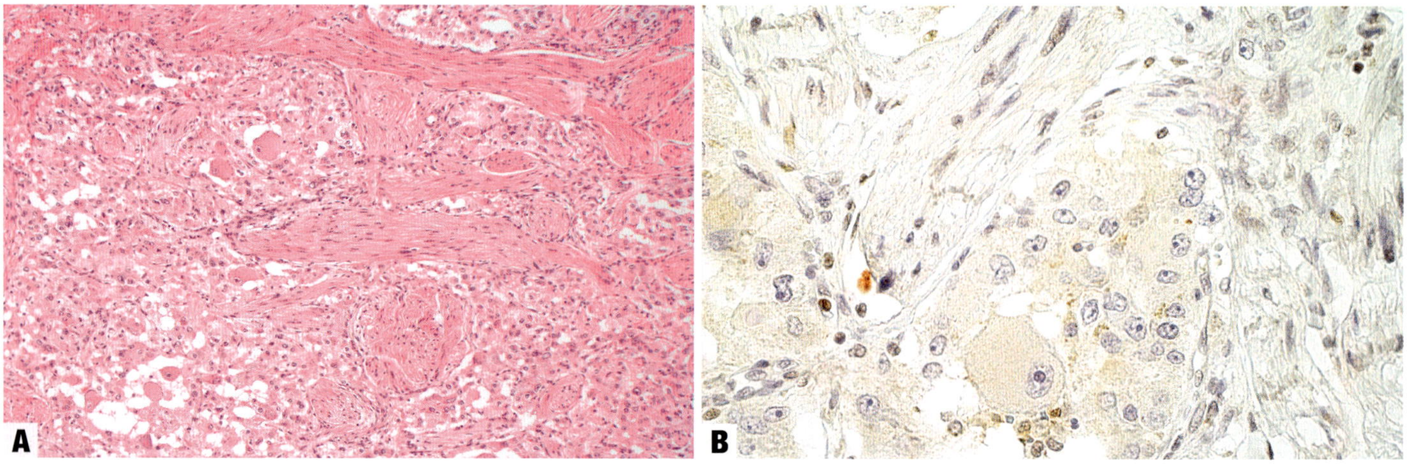

Fig. 13.15 Composite phaeochromocytoma-ganglioneuroma. **A** An example from a patient with a known germline pathogenic *MAX* variant. This tumour is morphologically indistinguishable from a sporadic neoplasm. **B** MAX immunohistochemistry in a section of the same tumour. The non-neoplastic inflammatory cells demonstrate preserved positive staining for MAX, whereas there is decreased expression in the neoplastic cells of the phaeochromocytoma component as well as in the Schwannian spindle cells and ganglion cells of the ganglioneuroma component. This tumour is morphologically indistinguishable from a sporadic neoplasm.

been reported, including renal cell carcinomas and oncocytomas, squamous cell carcinomas, and carcinomas of the breast, lung, and endometrium {573,693,2399,3798,621,4763}.

Clinical features

The clinical presentation of MEN5 syndrome encompasses the classic multiple endocrine neoplasia endocrinopathies such as paraganglioma and/or phaeochromocytoma (PPGL), pituitary neuroendocrine tumours (PitNETs) / pituitary adenomas, and multiglandular parathyroid adenomas, in addition to tumours of neural crest origin, such as ganglioneuroma and neuroblastoma {4047}.

Phaeochromocytomas in individuals with MEN5 are often bilateral at presentation, and metachronous paragangliomas are also common {573,351,1367,4112}. Affected individuals may present with symptoms of catecholamine excess, such as hypertension, heart palpitations, and diaphoresis. The tumours typically exhibit a mixed adrenergic and noradrenergic catecholamine secretory pattern {3644}.

MEN5-associated PitNETs / pituitary adenomas are usually functional, often presenting with acromegaly and/or hyperprolactinaemia {4047}, and are typically diagnosed later than PPGLs {973,3836,4047}. Secondary acromegaly due to GHRH secretion from other *MAX*-related tumours has also been reported {4047}.

Hypercalcaemia is also frequently reported in patients with MEN5, most often related to multiglandular parathyroid adenomas but occasionally arising from ectopic secretion of PTH or PTHrP by other *MAX*-associated tumours {3836}.

Recently, the phenotype of MEN5 has been extended to include other tumours of neural crest derivation, including ganglioneuroma and neuroblastoma {4047}, in addition to composite phaeochromocytoma-ganglioneuroma {3601}. A single case of a pancreatic neuroendocrine neoplasm (PanNEN) associated with a *MAX* pathogenic sequence variant has been reported {3537}.

Imaging

FDOPA PET is highly sensitive in the evaluation of *MAX*-related PPGL, both at initial diagnosis and during follow-up {4373}; 68Ga-DOTATATE PET and FDG PET are less sensitive in this setting. It is recommended that all individuals with germline *MAX* mutations undergo comprehensive baseline evaluation with an appropriate imaging modality to screen for PPGL, pituitary disease, and parathyroid disease.

Epidemiology

The prevalence and incidence of MEN5 has not yet been determined. Pathogenic germline *MAX* sequence variants are associated with < 1% of all phaeochromocytomas {573}. The median age at diagnosis of *MAX*-associated phaeochromocytoma is 34 years {4373}. The M:F ratio in reported kindreds is about 1:1 {4047}.

Etiology

MEN5 syndrome is caused by germline pathogenic variants in *MAX*, located on chromosome 14q23.3. There are no known environmental factors that increase the risk of tumour development.

Pathogenesis

The protein MAX is an essential component of the MYC/MAX/MXD1 network of transcription factors that regulate cell proliferation, differentiation, and apoptosis {689}. While heterodimerization of MAX with MYC results in transcriptional activation, heterodimerization with MXD1 (and other MXD family members) represses transcription through the same E-box DNA recognition sequences {689}. This cellular network maintains a complex equilibrium that controls the activation or repression of thousands of target genes {898}.

In individuals with MEN5, germline *MAX* sequence variants have been identified in all five of the gene's exons and include nonsense and missense variants as well as large deletions {898,573,351,693,4373,973,4626,3601}. Most pathogenic

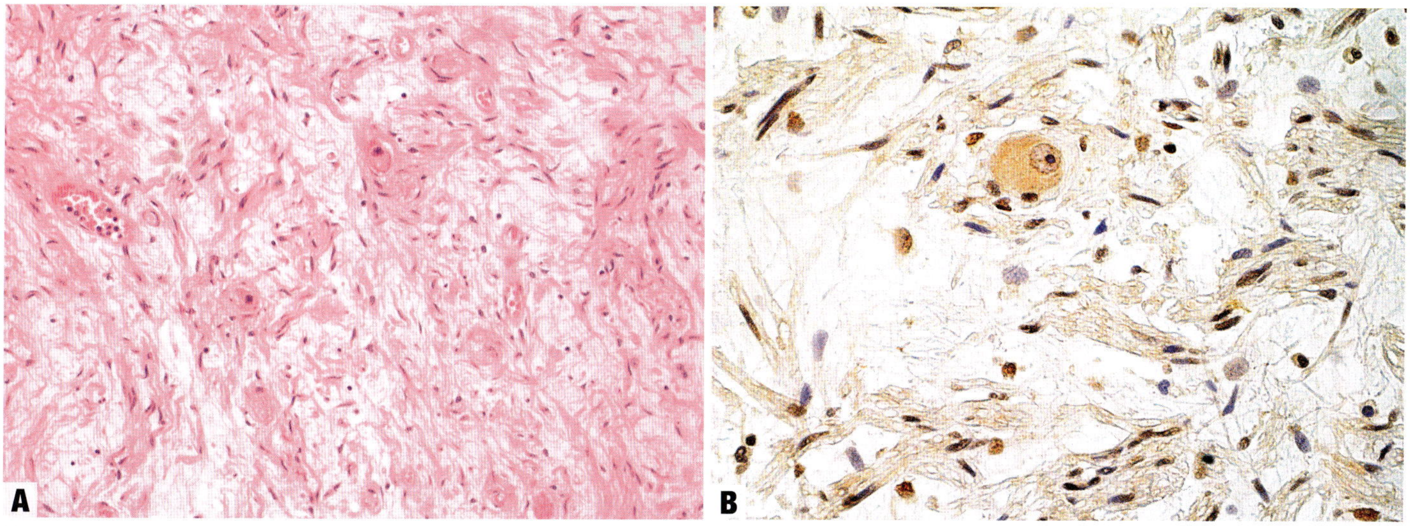

Fig. 13.16 Ganglioneuroma. **A** An example from a patient with a known germline pathogenic *MAX* variant. This tumour is morphologically indistinguishable from a sporadic neoplasm. **B** MAX immunohistochemistry in a section of the same tumour. The non-neoplastic inflammatory cells demonstrate preserved positive staining for MAX, whereas there is variable loss of staining in the ganglion cells and Schwannian stromal cells of the ganglioneuroma. The variable loss of expression in this case illustrates the difficulty in interpreting MAX immunohistochemistry in routine clinical practice.

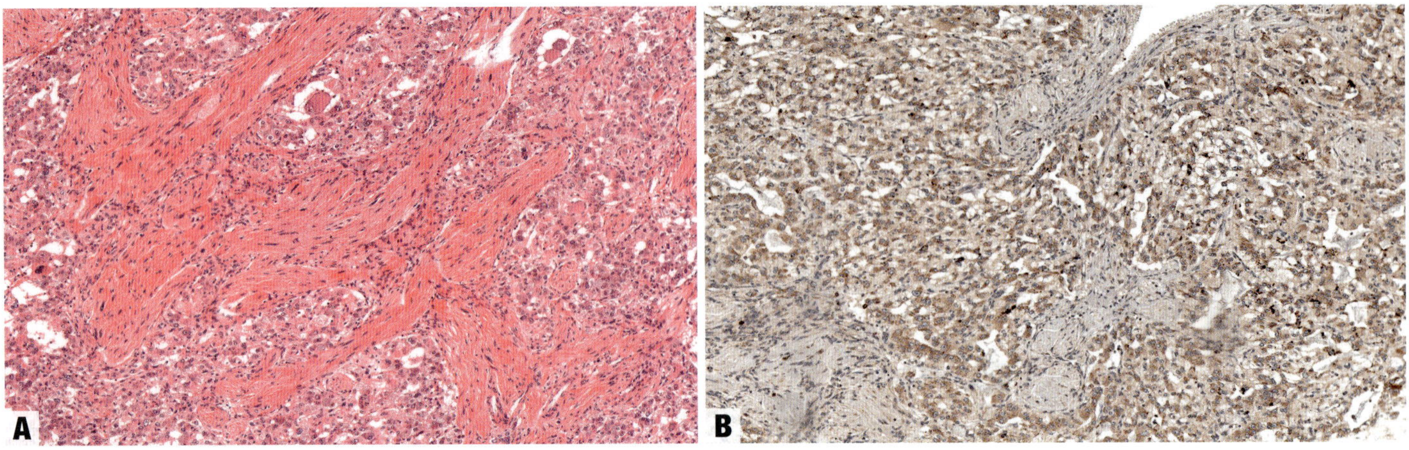

Fig. 13.17 Composite phaeochromocytoma-ganglioneuroma. **A** An example from a patient with acromegaly and a known pathogenic germline *MAX* variant. This tumour is morphologically indistinguishable from a sporadic neoplasm. **B** GHRH immunohistochemistry of the same tumour. The tumour cells are positive for GHRH, whereas the stromal cells are negative.

sequence variants affect highly conserved amino acids within the basic helix-loop-helix leucine zipper (bHLHZip) domain of MAX, which is the common structural element of the MYC/MAX/MXD1 axis {3157}. These mutations result in a protein incapable of homodimerization or heterodimerization and therefore incapable of repressing transcription and regulating MYC signalling through the aforementioned mechanisms {3733}. *MYC* itself is a well-known oncogene, with overexpression evident in many, if not most, human malignancies {689,2369,899}. Therefore, *MAX* acts as a tumour suppressor gene, whose constitutional loss of function highlights the importance of MYC regulation in hereditary malignancies and reveals that repression of the MYC/MAX/MXD1 axis may represent a common pathway of tumorigenesis for other PPGL susceptibility genes {3644}.

Macroscopic appearance

MAX-associated tumours are often bilateral and/or multicentric, but they are otherwise grossly indistinguishable from their sporadic counterparts.

Histopathology

Apart from their tendency towards multifocal/bilateral disease, individual *MAX*-associated tumours are histologically indistinguishable from their sporadic counterparts. Diffuse adrenal medullary hyperplasia can occur, although it is less common than in patients with MEN2 syndrome and succinate dehydrogenase–deficient PPGL {2400,1674,4373,3790}. In contrast, any distinct nodular medullary proliferations smaller than 10 mm represent microphaeochromocytomas {3790}. This designation is supported by several studies that have demonstrated similar molecular aberrations in these nodules to those seen in phaeochromocytomas, suggesting a common molecular origin for these entities {2400,1674}.

Recent studies have also described a number of neuroblastic tumours in patients with germline *MAX* variants, including ganglioneuroma, neuroblastoma, and composite PPGL tumours {3601,4047}. These tumours all share a common embryological origin from neural crest cells, from which the adrenal medulla and paraganglia are derived {4118}.

PIT1-lineage PitNETs / pituitary adenomas with somatotroph or lactotroph cell differentiation have been described in MEN5 {973,3537,4047,452}. These tumours are indistinguishable from their sporadic counterparts. Secondary acromegaly (due to somatotroph hyperplasia) has also been reported in the setting of GHRH-secreting phaeochromocytoma {4047}. Like in multiple endocrine neoplasia type 1, primary hyperparathyroidism with multiglandular parathyroid adenomas has also been described {4047}.

Although some studies have suggested that loss of MAX immunoreactivity may occur only in *MAX*-related tumours carrying truncating mutations {898,573}, others have reported poor sensitivity and specificity for MAX immunohistochemistry as a marker of *MAX* mutation {4587,808,4047}. At present, it appears that the overall utility of MAX immunohistochemistry in routine clinical practice is limited, and it is not recommended as a screening test for *MAX* mutation {4047}.

Cytology

The cytopathological features of the various neoplasms related to MEN5 are indistinguishable from those of their sporadic counterparts, which are described elsewhere in this volume and in the other fifth-edition volumes of the WHO Classification of Tumours series. It is important to remember that aspiration biopsy of functioning sympathetic PPGLs is not recommended, because of the risk of life-threatening catecholamine crisis.

Diagnostic molecular pathology

Germline pathogenic sequence variants occur in all five exons of the *MAX* gene but are most frequent in exons 3 and 4; these include nonsense and missense variants in addition to large deletions {898,351,693,4373,973,4626,3601}. Several studies have reported an apparent paternal transmission of the disease from loss of heterozygosity caused by uniparental disomy in some cases {898,573,3537}. This mode of transmission results in generation skipping and can complicate the identification of mutation carriers. Current recommendations for genetic testing of all individuals with PPGL and of all asymptomatic family members of individuals with germline *MAX* variants will facilitate further phenotypic characterization of MEN5 syndrome.

Essential and desirable diagnostic criteria

Essential: demonstration of a germline *MAX* pathogenic sequence variant.

Desirable: a personal or family history of MEN5 syndrome–related lesions.

Staging

PPGLs are staged according to the relevant American Joint Committee on Cancer (AJCC) staging schemes, whereas individual tumours other than PitNETs are staged according to the relevant Union for International Cancer Control (UICC) / AJCC staging schemes. PitNETs are currently staged using a standardized assessment of parasellar tumour invasiveness based on MRI Knosp criteria {2354}.

Prognosis and prediction

Prognostic data on specific *MAX*-related tumours are generally lacking, although a recent study reported a tendency towards more aggressive behaviour and greater metastatic potential in *MAX*-associated PPGL, which has not yet been confirmed in a larger population of *MAX* mutation carriers {898,573}.

Hyperparathyroidism–jaw tumour syndrome

Gill AJ
Asa SL
Erickson LA
Juhlin CC
Mete O
Morreau H

Definition

Hyperparathyroidism–jaw tumour syndrome (HPT-JT) is an autosomal dominant disorder caused by pathogenic germline sequence variants or deletions in *CDC73*. It is characterized predominantly by parathyroid adenoma and carcinoma, with a lower incidence of fibro-osseous jaw lesions.

MIM numbering

145001 Hyperparathyroidism–jaw tumour syndrome; HPT-JT

ICD-11 coding

5A51.0 Primary hyperparathyroidism

Related terminology

Acceptable: *CDC73*-related disorder.

Not recommended: familial cystic parathyroid adenomatosis; hyperparathyroidism 2 with jaw tumours.

Subtype(s)

None

Localization

In most kindreds, parathyroid tumours are the only feature {2011,3956,1580}. Jaw tumours are relatively uncommon, being found in as few as 2.5–20% of known *CDC73* mutation carriers {2928,2011,3956,4798,2863,1580,2019,2641}. Clinically significant renal and uterine tumours occur at an increased incidence, but are rare {2928,4720,511,2010,2641}.

Clinical features

Primary hyperparathyroidism is the usual presentation of HPT-JT. Contrasting with other forms of hereditary hyperparathyroidism where multigland involvement is very common, a single adenoma or carcinoma is found in 60–80% of cases at presentation {4589,4530}. Metachronous tumours

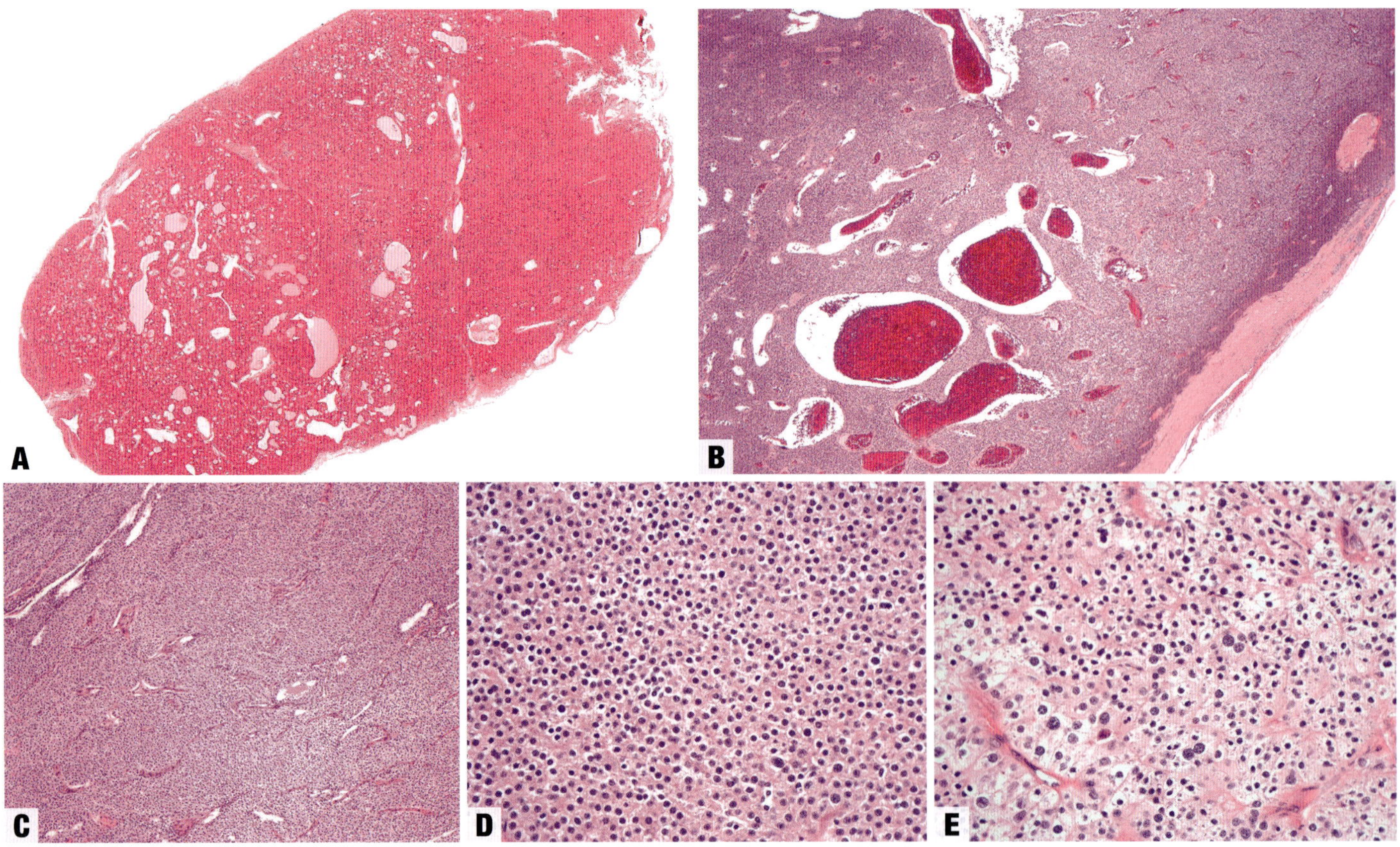

Fig. 13.18 Parafibromin-deficient parathyroid tumour. **A** Sheet-like growth pattern of cells with eosinophilic cytoplasm and microcystic change. **B** The morphological features of parafibromin-deficient parathyroid tumours are inconsistent but include a thickened and somewhat hyalinized fibrous capsule, a sheet-like growth pattern, eosinophilic cells, and prominent vasculature. A little microcystic change is noted. **C** In contrast to most usual parathyroid adenomas, which demonstrate a somewhat nested architecture, parafibromin-deficient parathyroid tumours commonly show a sheet-like architecture with prominent vasculature. **D** Cytological features include nuclear enlargement, perinuclear cytoplasmic clearing, and eosinophilic cells. **E** Cytological features include nuclear enlargement often with preserved N:C ratios, multinucleation, perinuclear cytoplasmic clearing, and eosinophilic cells, sometimes with a glassy quality.

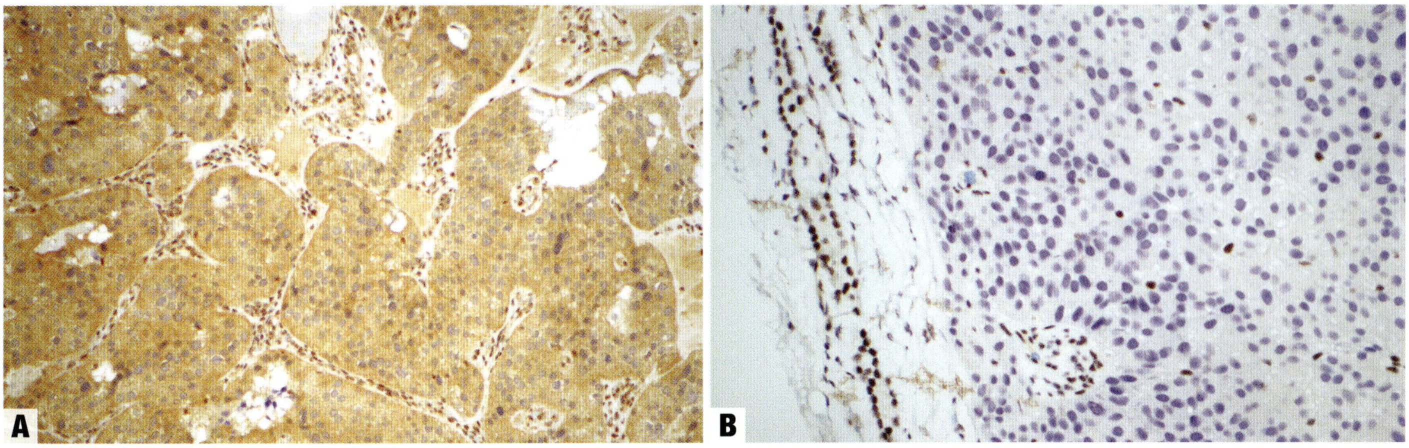

Fig. 13.19 Parafibromin-deficient parathyroid tumour. **A** Immunohistochemistry for parafibromin can be difficult to interpret. It is emphasized that significance is placed on nuclear expression only, and nonspecific cytoplasmic expression should be disregarded. In this case, all the neoplastic cells show loss of expression of parafibromin and there is preserved expression in non-neoplastic cells. Therefore, the tumour is considered parafibromin-deficient. **B** It is emphasized that for parafibromin immunohistochemistry to be considered negative there should be an internal positive control in non-neoplastic cells including non-neoplastic parathyroid tissue.

occur during long-term follow-up (decades) in the majority of patients in many series {3956,2073,2928,2011}. In addition to family history, clinical clues to the diagnosis of HPT-JT include a young age of onset (particularly if < 40 years), very large tumours, cystic change, markedly elevated serum PTH levels, and severe hypercalcaemia {2863,2011,530,1580,4826}. Parathyroid carcinoma is extremely rare outside the setting of germline or somatic *CDC73* mutation, whereas the lifetime risk of parathyroid carcinoma in HPT-JT may be as high as 15% {677,2928,2011,3956,530,1580}. Therefore, the possibility of HPT-JT should be considered in all patients with parathyroid carcinoma, even in the absence of a family history {1578,1574, 1580}. In fact, as many as 30% of patients with apparently sporadic parathyroid carcinomas have pathogenic germline sequence variants or deletions in *CDC73* indicating previously undiagnosed HPT-JT {723,4094,1580}. The jaw tumours arise more often in the mandible than the maxilla, and about 15% are multiple {4819,704,4803,2019}. They are commonly incidental findings on imaging, where they present as well-demarcated, usually radiolucent and unilocular lesions {4803, 3562}. They may present as an enlarging mass that interrupts dentition. Although clinically benign, they show a variable rate of growth and are usually slowly progressive. The incidence of germline *CDC73* mutations in patients with clinically sporadic ossifying fibromas has not been extensively studied. It is likely to be very low, given that even somatic-only *CDC73* mutations are found in only up to 5% {786}. Older reports suggested that a significant proportion of patients with HPT-JT develop renal pathology: predominantly simple cysts, but also adenomas, Wilms tumours, and mixed epithelial and stromal tumours {530,2928,1823,4720}. However, simple cysts are not uncommon in the general population, and in practice clinically significant renal pathology is very rare, being absent from many large series {2011,3956,4798,2379,1425,2863,1580}. Similarly, historically a significant proportion of female patients have been reported to have some form of uterine pathology {2928, 4720}. These are usually lesions that are also very common in the general community – particularly benign leiomyomas, but also endometrial hyperplasias, polyps, adenomyosis, or adenofibromas, which may represent incidental findings in patients under surveillance {2863,2928,4720}. However, a small number of uterine adenosarcomas (otherwise a rare pathology) have been reported {2928}, and adenosarcomas also arise in mouse models of *CDC73* mutation, suggesting a causal relationship and supporting an increased risk {4766}.

Epidemiology

HPT-JT is a rare cause of hyperparathyroidism, and it has been estimated that only 0.19% of unselected parathyroid tumours are associated with *CDC73* mutation {1580}. In contrast to sporadic hyperparathyroidism, there is an equal sex distribution for both parathyroid and jaw tumours {1580,2019}. The median age at presentation with either hyperparathyroidism or jaw tumours is in the third or fourth decade of life (reported age ranges: 7–66 years for parathyroid tumours and 10–66 years for jaw tumours) {2019,530,2928,1425,1580}. The estimated penetrance of primary hyperparathyroidism in non-index mutation carriers increases from 8% at 25 years, to 53% at 50 years, to 75% at 70 years, whereas the penetrance of any manifestation is 11% at 25 years, 65% at 50 years, and 83% at 70 years {4648}.

Etiology

HPT-JT is caused by heterozygous pathogenic germline sequence variants or deletions in *CDC73* (*HRPT2*), a 17-exon gene that maps to 1q25-q31 and encodes the 531-amino-acid protein parafibromin {4360,1574,677,1578}.

Pathogenesis

CDC73 is ubiquitously expressed in most tissues and functions as a bona fide tumour suppressor gene. A somatic second hit is usually, but not always, able to be demonstrated in neoplasms arising in the setting of HPT-JT {677,1574,5129}. Parafibromin is a critical component of the polymerase-associated factor 1 complex (PAF1C) that binds to RNA polymerase II and controls transcription {704,2116,4335}.

Macroscopic appearance

Parafibromin-deficient parathyroid tumours are usually larger than sporadic parathyroid tumours. In one study, the median weight was 1.84 g (range: 231 mg to 14 g) {1580}. Like sporadic

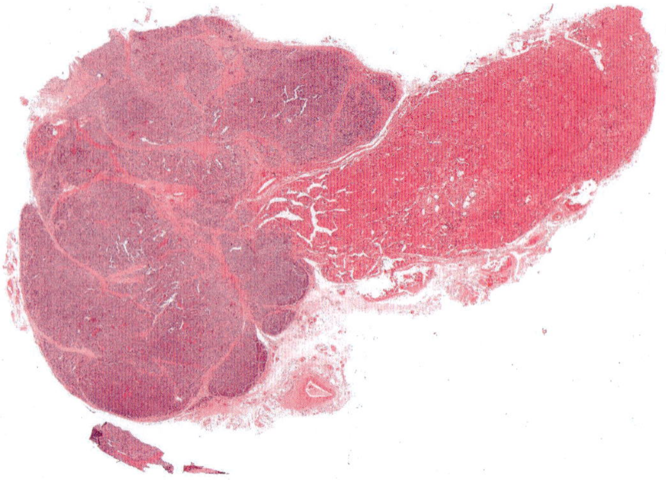

Fig. 13.20 Parathyroid carcinoma associated with hyperparathyroidism–jaw tumour syndrome. The diagnosis of carcinoma arising in the setting of hyperparathyroidism–jaw tumour syndrome relies on the same histological criteria as sporadic carcinomas: the demonstration of unequivocally invasive growth or vascular space invasion. In this instance, in addition to invasive growth, the neoplastic cells show typical cytological features of a parafibromin-deficient tumour.

parathyroid carcinomas, carcinomas arising in the setting of HPT-JT may appear to be stuck down or adherent to other structures {1580}.

Histopathology

Parathyroid tumours associated with biallelic *CDC73* mutation/inactivation (with or without a germline mutation) are termed parafibromin-deficient {1580}. There are morphological clues to a parafibromin-deficient parathyroid tumour, including a sheet-like (rather than acinar) growth pattern; eosinophilic cytoplasm; perinuclear cytoplasmic clearing; nuclear enlargement, occasionally with multinucleation; and a distinctive arborizing vasculature, often with staghorn vessels {4589,1580}. Cystic change was originally described as a common feature {677} but may be found in less than half of the parathyroid tumours {3956,1580}. Loss of immunohistochemical expression of parafibromin is usually seen in parafibromin-deficient parathyroid tumours {1574, 1580,1578,1960,2151}. It is emphasized that for a tumour to be considered parafibromin-deficient, there should be completely absent nuclear staining in all neoplastic cells, in the presence of preserved nuclear expression in non-neoplastic cells, which act as an internal positive control {1578,1580,2151}. Interpreted in this way, loss of nuclear expression of parafibromin is highly specific but not completely sensitive for biallelic *CDC73* inactivation. The significance of absent nucleolar expression of parafibromin with preserved expression elsewhere in the nucleus is uncertain, but some authors have suggested that this pattern is also associated with *CDC73* mutation {1918,2146,1271,1580, 2151}. Because some *CDC73* point mutations may be associated with preserved parafibromin expression, positive staining for parafibromin in parathyroid neoplasms does not exclude the diagnosis of HPT-JT {1960,1578,4904,2928}. In most cases, aberrant diffuse strong expression of PGP9.5 may serve as an adjunct to increase sensitivity, but on its own PGP9.5 overexpression lacks specificity for biallelic *CDC73* inactivation {1960, 1574,2438}. Although biallelic somatic-only mutations do occur, as many as two thirds of all parafibromin-deficient parathyroid tumours appear to be associated with pathogenic germline variants {1580}. Therefore, the identification of a parafibromin-deficient parathyroid tumour is considered an indication for genetic testing at any age and irrespective of family history {1580}.

The diagnosis of parathyroid carcinoma in HPT-JT is based on the standard criteria of unequivocal local invasion, vascular space invasion, and/or metastasis {4886}. Given the known high risk of malignancy, it has been argued that a lower threshold for invasive growth should be applied in parafibromin-deficient parathyroid tumours {1574,1580,2438}.

Although the terminology is not uniform, the jaw tumours are usually classified as ossifying fibromas {4803,3562,2019}. They are composed of a relatively avascular, cellular, fibroblast-rich stroma, sometimes with a prominent storiform pattern admixed with bony trabeculae and/or cementum-like spherules. The histological appearance is quite different from that of osteitis fibrosa cystica (brown tumours) associated with sporadic primary hyperparathyroidism, with which they may be confused clinically

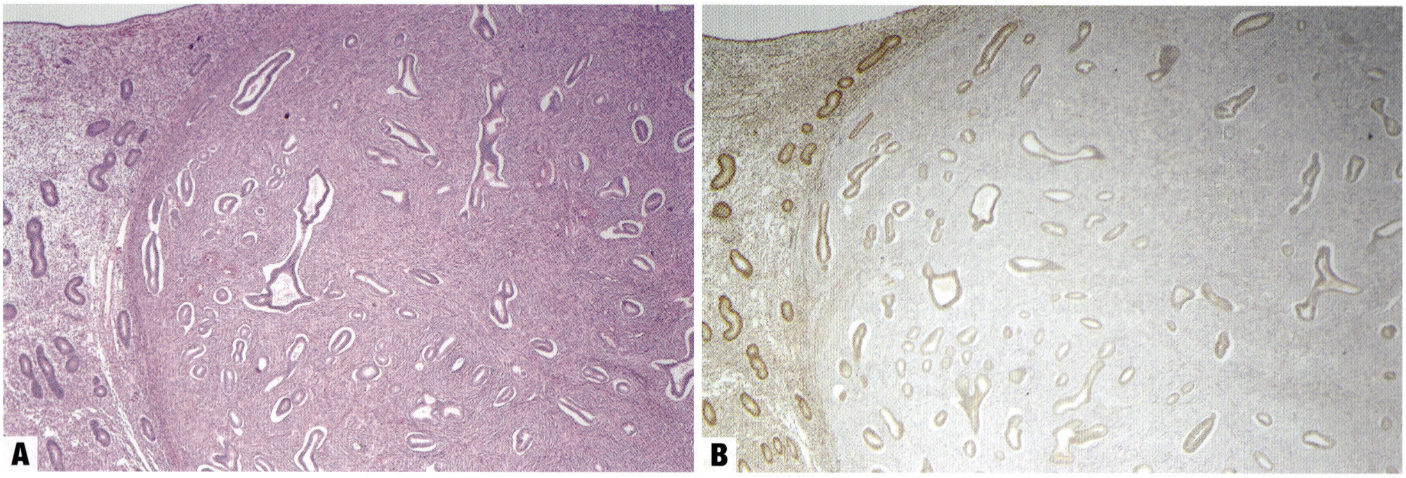

Fig. 13.21 Adenosarcoma of the uterus arising in hyperparathyroidism–jaw tumour syndrome. **A** There is a densely hypercellular stroma surrounding entrapped glands. **B** Parafibromin immunohistochemistry has not been well validated as a diagnostic marker of adenosarcoma in the setting of hyperparathyroidism–jaw tumour syndrome. However, in this case, the stromal component of the adenosarcoma demonstrates loss of nuclear expression that contrasts with the preserved expression in the glandular component and the adjacent non-neoplastic stroma.

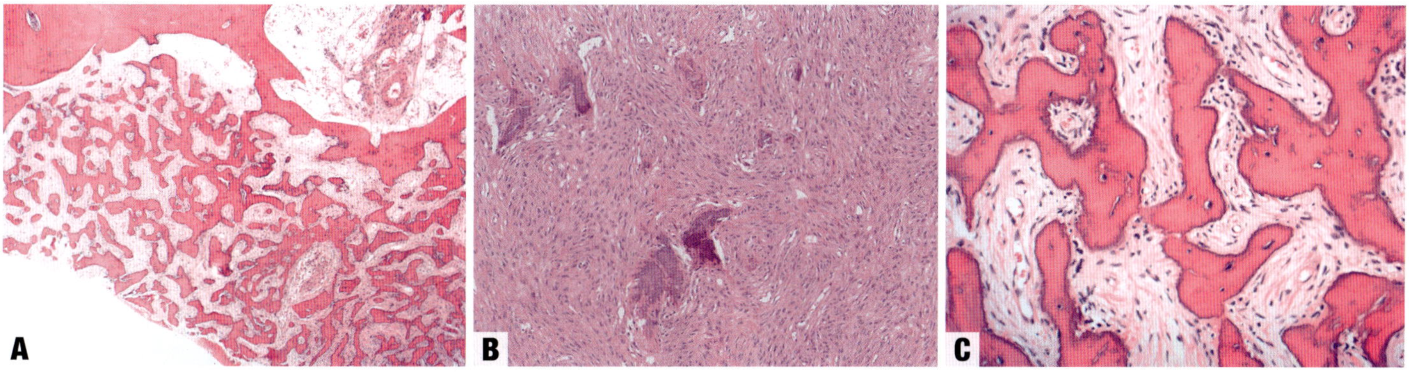
Fig. 13.22 Ossifying fibroma arising in hyperparathyroidism–jaw tumour syndrome. **A,B** There is a relatively avascular hypercellular stroma composed of bland spindled cells surrounding bony trabeculae. **C** A hypovascular stroma surrounds bony trabeculae.

{4803,3562}. Unlike in the parathyroid tumours, parafibromin immunohistochemistry does not appear to be effective in identifying HPT-JT–related ossifying fibromas {1574}. Being rare, the renal and uterine pathologies are less well described {530,2928, 1823,2011,3956,4798,2379,1425,2863}. Interestingly, an HPT-JT kindred with three family members with mixed epithelial and stromal tumour of the kidney was recently reported {4720} and, together with uterine adenosarcoma {2928,511}, these relatively rare tumours may be a clue to the diagnosis.

Cytology

Because the parathyroid tumours are often very large, they occasionally undergo FNAB if mistaken clinically for thyroid lesions. The cytopathological features of the parathyroid tumours are presented elsewhere in this volume.

Diagnostic molecular pathology

There are no true hotspots in *CDC73*, although mutations in exons 1, 2, and 7 are overrepresented {3218,2856,530,1580}. The majority of coding alterations are frameshift, nonsense, and splice-site mutations, which are predicted to encode a truncated protein {704,3476,4113,530}. As many as 35% of germline variants in *CDC73* are large-scale deletions and may not be detected unless specifically sought with multiplex ligation-dependent probe amplification or other dedicated studies {530,1580}. Unidentified deletions or mutations in the promoter, untranslated regions, or introns may account for the small proportion of otherwise typical HPT-JT cases for which no mutations are identified {3218,1743}. Recently it has been suggested that high-impact mutations in *CDC73* (defined as those that cause conformational disruption or loss of expression and always impact the C-terminal domain of parafibromin) are associated with a significantly higher risk of parathyroid carcinoma and jaw tumours, despite being associated with a similar risk of hyperparathyroidism to that associated with low-impact mutations {2641}.

Essential and desirable diagnostic criteria

Essential: demonstration of a germline pathogenic variant in *CDC73* or the presence of multiple histologically confirmed parafibromin-deficient neoplasms in an individual or kindred.

Staging

Staging of the individual tumours is based on the Union for International Cancer Control (UICC) / American Joint Committee on Cancer (AJCC) systems.

Prognosis and prediction

Lifelong surveillance is indicated for all patients with HPT-JT. This is primarily because of the risk of parathyroid adenoma and carcinoma {1580} but also because of the risk of jaw lesions and the much lower risk of gynaecological or renal pathology. The jaw lesions are benign, but they may be locally infiltrative and recur {4819,704}. The optimal surgical approach to patients with HPT-JT–related hyperparathyroidism is debated, and it is unclear whether subtotal parathyroidectomy {2928,3956} or selective parathyroidectomy should be offered when there is clear localization to one gland {2011,4530}. The majority of non-infiltrative parafibromin-deficient parathyroid tumours/adenomas are cured by surgery. Parafibromin-deficient parathyroid carcinomas may be at increased risk of recurrence and metastasis, as compared with non-*CDC73* related carcinomas {1578,1574,2438,1580}. Although metastasis of these tumours is a very rare event, it is worth noting that there are isolated case reports of unequivocally histologically benign parafibromin-deficient parathyroid tumours that have metastasized {3956,2658,1574,2438,1580}. However, the incidence of metastasis by an otherwise benign parafibromin-deficient parathyroid tumour is very low (estimated to be significantly less than 4% {1580}) and far exceeded by the risk of a new primary tumour in a different gland during long-term follow-up {2011,2928,1580,3956,4145}.

Von Hippel–Lindau syndrome

Asa SL
Erickson LA
Ezzat S
Favier J
Kasajima A

Definition

Von Hippel–Lindau syndrome (VHL) is an autosomal dominant tumour syndrome caused by inactivating mutations in the *VHL* gene. Patients with this disorder develop angiomas and haemangioblastomas; paragangliomas including phaeochromocytomas; renal cell carcinomas (RCCs); pancreatic serous cystadenomas and pancreatic neuroendocrine tumours (PanNETs); endolymphatic sac tumours (ELSTs); and cystadenomas of the epididymis, broad ligament, and mesosalpinx.

MIM numbering

193300 Von Hippel–Lindau syndrome; VHLS

ICD-11 coding

None

Related terminology

Acceptable: von Hippel–Lindau disease.

Subtype(s)

VHL types 1, 2A, 2B, and 2C have different manifestations and are associated with different genetic alterations in *VHL*.

Localization

The various lesions have distinct localizations.

Ears: About 10–15% of patients with VHL develop ELSTs {2829}; they are the initial manifestation of VHL in 32% of individuals with these lesions {352}. These benign cystadenomas arise in the vestibular aqueduct and may extend into the extraosseous portion of the endolymphatic sac, the petrous bone, and the inner ear {1605}. Large tumours may extend into the brain. They are bilateral in 30% of cases.

CNS: CNS haemangioblastomas occur in 80% of patients {4739} and are most commonly localized in the cerebellum (44–72%), followed by the spinal cord (most frequently in the posterior half of the spinal cord) and brainstem (usually in the posterior medulla oblongata). Supratentorial lesions are rare, accounting for about 2.9% of cases {4773}.

Retina: As many as 85% of individuals with VHL develop retinal haemangioblastomas (also known as retinal angioma or angiomatosis retinae) {810}, with an average age of 22.5 years at diagnosis {428}. Tumours are often multiple and are bilateral in about 50% of cases {3711}.

Kidney: Renal cysts and RCCs are usually multiple and bilateral in patients with VHL. As many as 40% of patients with VHL develop multicentric and bilateral clear cell RCC, and > 70% develop renal cysts {2784,2795}.

Adrenal gland and paraganglia: Approximately 30% of patients with VHL develop adrenal (phaeochromocytomas) and/or extra-adrenal paragangliomas, at a mean age of 30 years {4770}. Phaeochromocytomas are bilateral in about 40% of cases. Paragangliomas arise at various sites of the sympathetic or parasympathetic nervous systems, from the base of the skull to the urinary bladder. Head and neck paragangliomas arise in a number of locations along the carotid sheath and middle ear, including the carotid bifurcation (carotid body), vagal ganglia, jugular bulb, and tympanic plexus. Sympathetic paragangliomas may be located in the thorax, abdomen (organ of Zuckerkandl), and pelvis (bladder base).

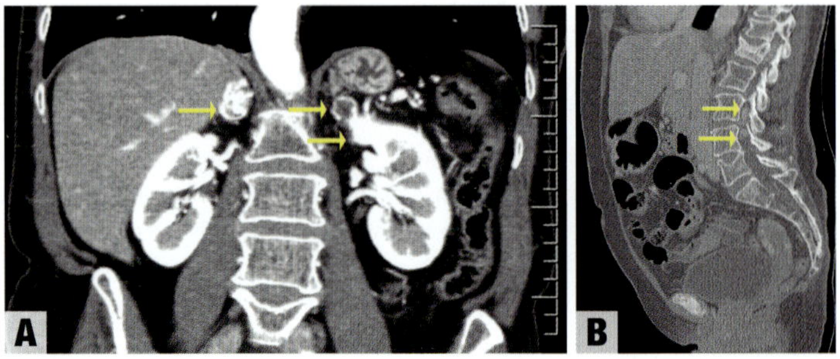

Fig. 13.23 Imaging of von Hippel–Lindau syndrome. Imaging of a patient with von Hippel–Lindau syndrome identifies multiple lesions. **A** The bilateral enhancing adrenal lesions (upper arrows) are suspicious for phaeochromocytoma, the left renal lesion (lower arrow) is most likely renal cell carcinoma, and there are multiple pancreatic cysts (not shown). **B** The central spinal canal enhancing mass lesions (arrows) are most likely haemangioblastomas.

Pancreas: Pancreatic manifestations of VHL include PanNETs, cysts, and serous cystadenomas. In patients with VHL, PanNETs are multiple in 50–56% of cases {2751,3522}. Pancreatic cystic lesions are frequent, occurring in as many as 91% of patients with VHL {1761,3522,3739}.

Duodenum, ampulla, and gallbladder / cystic duct: Neuroendocrine tumours (NETs) reported in patients with VHL include clear cell NETs of the ampulla and duodenum {1694,4166} and of the gallbladder and common bile duct {1349,2956}.

Reproductive organs: Epididymal papillary cystadenomas occur in as many as 60% of men with VHL. They arise from the efferent ductules of the epididymis and are often bilateral {3315}. Very rarely, papillary cystadenomas may manifest in the broad ligament and mesosalpinx in women {512,5119}.

Peripheral locations: Occasionally, haemangioblastomas identical to those seen in the CNS are found in peripheral nerves (e.g. the spinal nerve roots, cauda equina, and sciatic nerve) {3575,4336} or in extraneural tissues (e.g. adrenal glands, liver, lungs, and kidneys) {1043,1149,3285,3788}.

Clinical features

Clinical presentations of VHL can be broadly divided into three categories: neurological, obstructive, and hormone excess conditions. The neurological manifestations often begin with retinal disease; haemorrhages result in compromised visual acuity {185}. Extraocular problems include cerebellar ataxia and spinal cord compression from haemangioblastomas. Hearing loss can occur due to ELSTs. Obstructive features include those from outflow interruptions along the pancreaticobiliary or (more commonly) the genitourinary tract from expanding cysts or RCCs. Hormone excess symptoms are related directly to the cell lineage giving rise to the causative phaeochromocytomas or paragangliomas or PanNETs {1607,3903,800}. Of note, VHL-related NETs can also produce ectopic hormones, leading to further diagnostic challenges.

Epidemiology

VHL has an incidence of 1 in 36 000 births. Age at diagnosis varies from infancy to 60–70 years. There is no sex predilection.

Etiology

VHL is due to germline mutations in *VHL* that inactivate VHL protein. Type 1 VHL is associated with large deletion or truncation mutations of *VHL*; these generally yield a protein with very little or no biological activity. Type 2 VHL is usually due to missense mutations that result in a protein with limited activity.

Missense variants occur with the greatest frequency, with all variants localizing to the α- or β-domains of *VHL* {3903}. The most prevalent manifestations, including CNS, renal, and retinal neoplasms, are associated with frameshift variants and large deletions. Age-related penetrance is greater for CNS haemangioblastomas with truncating variants than for those with missense variants, whereas the reverse is true for phaeochromocytomas {3903}.

Somatic second hits of the wildtype allele inactivate the VHL protein in various tissues.

Pathogenesis

VHL protein is an E3 ligase that ubiquitinates for degradation HIF1α and HIF2α, subunits of a heterodimeric protein that regulates the transcription of the genes encoding VEGF, PDGFB, TGF-α, erythropoietin, and cyclin D1, as well as other genes that regulate cell metabolism and proliferation. VHL protein normally plays a role in the response to hypoxia, but loss of normal function in patients with VHL results in an unrestrained hypoxic response with upregulation of VEGF, PDGFB, TGF-α, erythropoietin, cyclin D1, and other substances that are pro-oncogenic.

Macroscopic appearance

ELSTs are red/brown, fibrous, highly vascularized nodules {2937,2255}.

Haemangioblastomas are usually well-circumscribed lesions but without true capsules. They are usually solid and cystic and highly vascular. The solid components are frequently in the wall of a cyst, which may be contiguous with the meninges. Cyst fluid may be either yellow (xanthochromic) or grey (proteinaceous). The cut surface of haemangioblastoma is usually beefy-red due to high vascularity and spongy with multiple cysts and cavernous spaces, but it may have bright yellow areas corresponding to lipid deposition {2000}. Retinal haemangioblastomas vary in size and shape {1736}.

RCC is usually encapsulated with well-defined borders. The cut surfaces are heterogeneous with variegated nodular growth and areas of necrosis and haemorrhage. A distinctive feature is the golden-yellow colour due to the abundant lipid content of tumour cells {2743}.

Paragangliomas (including intra-adrenal phaeochromocytomas) in patients with VHL are unusual macroscopically in that they have a thick vascular tumour capsule and they frequently have a variegated cut surface showing areas of haemorrhage and degenerative change {1489}, but they often also have areas of yellow parenchyma due to lipid accumulation; in the adrenal this can be mistaken for a cortical neoplasm {3676}.

Pancreaticoduodenal/ampullary and gallbladder NETs are usually solid, well-circumscribed nodules that may be red-brown, grey, or yellow in colour due to lipid storage. They may contain fibrotic foci, probably reflecting the profibrogenic role of HIF {910,1886}.

Pancreatic cysts are usually multiple and multicystic, and filled with serous fluid. They are usually small (< 5 mm) and may include papillary areas {3062,3522}.

In the reproductive organs, epididymal papillary cystadenomas are small tumours ranging from 10 to 40 mm. These are usually solid tumours with cystic spaces filled with colloid material, but they may be predominantly cystic {3315}. The reported size of cystadenoma of the broad ligament and mesosalpinx is 30–60 mm {3279}. Macroscopically, these tumours have a fibrous capsule and are partly cystic and lobulated, with haemorrhagic foci and stellate fibrous scars {3279}.

Histopathology

ELSTs have two growth patterns {2255}. The tumour may have a predominance of follicular-like architecture in which colloid-filled cysts are lined by a single layer of epithelium, mimicking thyroid follicular epithelium {2255}. The second pattern has more papillary architecture and a more glandular and solid pattern with only occasional cystic structures, and with a markedly

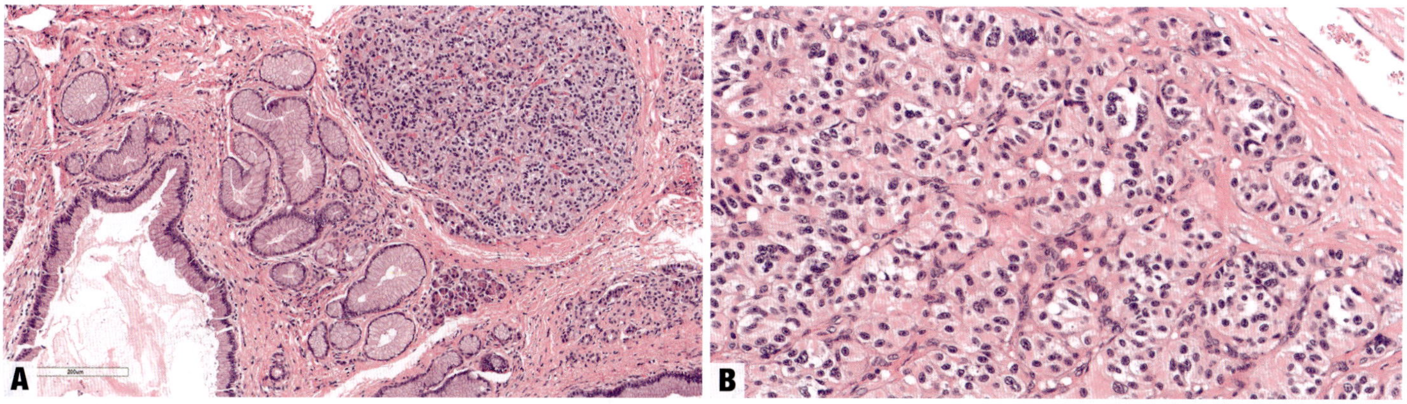

Fig. 13.24 The pancreas in von Hippel–Lindau syndrome. **A** The surrounding parenchyma contains prominent serous cysts lined by ductal epithelium, and there are often multiple smaller neuroendocrine tumours (NETs) associated with islet dysplasia and peliosis (not shown). **B** A pancreatic neuroendocrine tumour (PanNET) is composed of cells with striking clear cytoplasm.

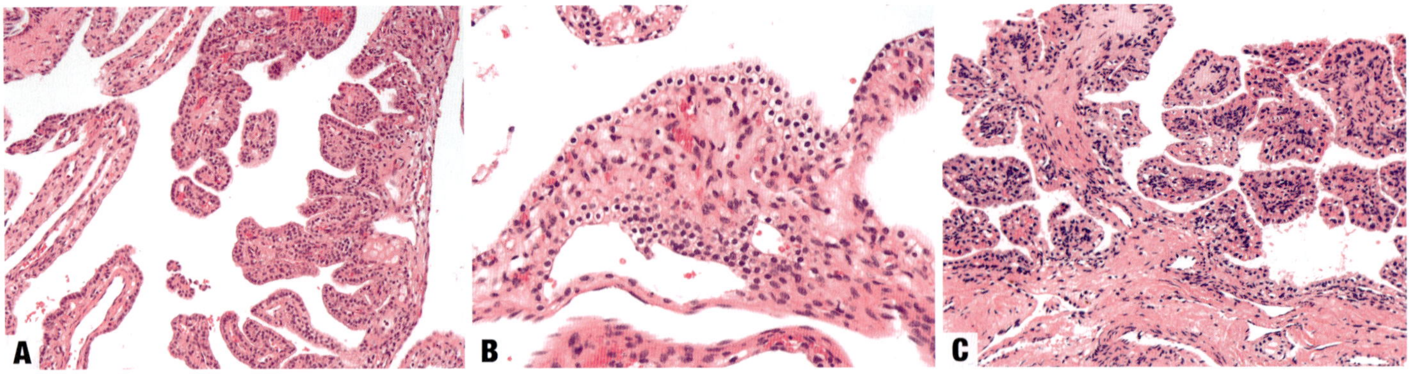

Fig. 13.25 Endolymphatic sac tumour in von Hippel–Lindau syndrome. **A** Broad interdigitating papillary projections composed of a single layer of cuboidal cells. **B** The neoplastic cells have a low cuboidal to tall cell appearance with round nuclei lining dilated cystic spaces. **C** Endolymphatic sac tumours exhibit a papillary architecture with a markedly vascular stroma.

vascular stroma {2255}. Small nests of plant cell–like cells with clear cytoplasm can be seen in the follicular pattern but are more prominent in the papillary pattern and can be mistaken for metastatic RCC {2255}. ELSTs are positive for keratin AE1/AE3, EMA, CK7, GLUT1, VEGF, CAIX, and PAX8 in the majority of cases and are negative for CD10 and RCCm {4486}.

Haemangioblastomas are circumscribed, often associated with a pseudocyst, and composed of variable proliferations of abundant mature vasculature thought to be reactive and the neoplastic so-called stromal cell component {4741,4739}. The so-called stromal cells may be haemangioblast progenitor cells, and these cells have deletion of *VHL* {1604,4741,4739}. There are two morphological patterns. Cellular (epithelioid) haemangioblastomas have prominent, larger, epithelioid so-called stromal cells with clear cytoplasm, that may be clustered in groups. The more common, and usually smaller, vascular-rich reticular (mesenchymal) haemangioblastomas have abundant vascularity and few scattered so-called stromal cells {1809,3740}. Cellular haemangioblastomas are more often positive for GFAP (80%) than are reticular haemangioblastomas (7%) {1809}. Ki-67 labelling indexes are higher in cellular haemangioblastomas than in reticular haemangioblastomas {1809}. Cellular and reticular haemangioblastomas also have different cytogenetic profiles, with loss of chromosomes 6, 22q, and 19 in the cellular pattern and loss of chromosomes 19, 22q, and 3 in the reticular pattern {3740}. Cellular haemangioblastomas recur more commonly than reticular haemangioblastomas (25% vs 8%) {1809}. Haemangioblastomas are benign but can cause neurological deficits similarly to other lesions in the brain. As many as 8% of CNS haemangioblastomas resected from individuals with VHL have been reported as being metastases, the most common primary site being the kidney (RCC) {2092}; haemangioblastomas are negative for PAX8, allowing the distinction from metastatic RCC {1205}. The histological features of retinal haemangioblastomas are identical to those of CNS haemangioblastomas.

Paragangliomas in patients with VHL may have a thick fibrous or vascular capsule and a myxoid, oedematous, or hyalinized stroma. The tumour cells lack nuclear atypia and mitoses; they often have clear vacuolated cytoplasm that can mimic adrenal cortex {3676,2361}, and they lack hyaline globules {2361}. VHL-related phaeochromocytomas are not associated with the medullary adrenal hyperplasia often seen in multiple endocrine neoplasia type 2–associated phaeochromocytomas {2361, 695}. Tumour cells are positive for the general neuroendocrine markers INSM1, chromogranin A, and synaptophysin {3676, 3823}, as well as for GATA3, tyrosine hydroxylase, and DBH, and they are generally negative for keratins (with rare exceptions {1092}). Intratumoural sustentacular cells express S100 and SOX10. CAIX is usually positive with a membranous staining pattern in the tumour cells of VHL-related phaeochromocytomas. Membranous CAIX expression in tumour cells occurs almost exclusively in VHL-related cases {3563,1344}.

Renal pathology in VHL is characterized by a spectrum of proliferative and cystic lesions. VHL-related RCCs are often multifocal, bilateral, and clear cell type {2258}. Other than being multifocal,

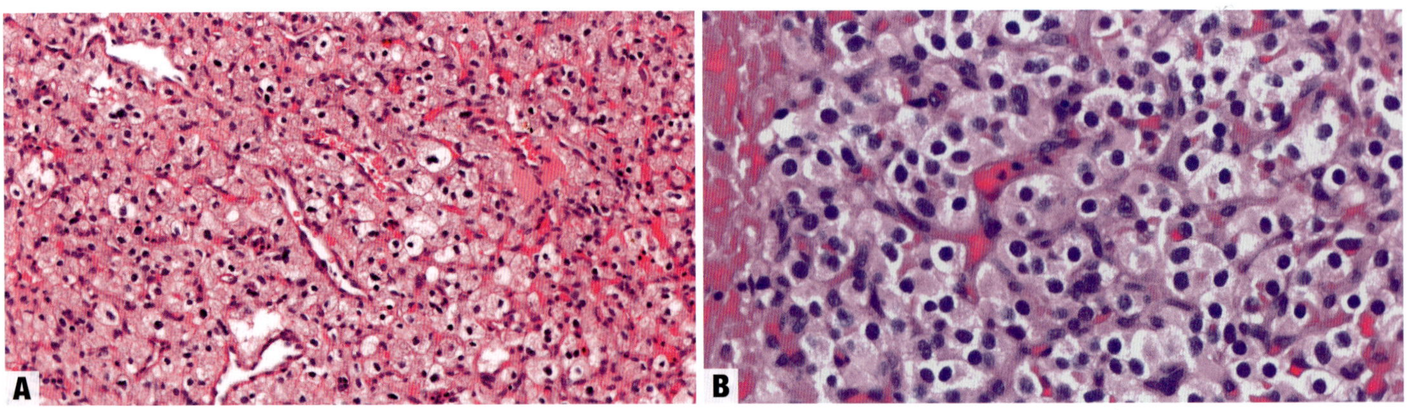

Fig. 13.26 Haemangioblastoma in von Hippel–Lindau syndrome. **A,B** The tumour is composed of a proliferation of neoplastic so-called stromal cells thought to be haemangioblast progenitor cells.

they are indistinguishable from sporadic tumours, although as many as 95% are cystic in this setting {2258}. Although clear cell RCC is the most common type of RCC in VHL, clear cell papillary-like RCC has also been reported {2258,22}. RCCs in VHL are often low stage at diagnosis {2258}. The RCCs are often surrounded by a thick fibrous capsule and often have a microcystic growth pattern. Like sporadic clear cell RCCs, those associated with VHL have an alveolar arrangement of nests of epithelial clear cells with a delicate vascular network {22}. The rare cases that have clear cell papillary-like RCC features have branching papillae, papillary tufts, and apical nuclei, but immunohistochemically do not show the characteristic CK7 and CAIX immunopositivity (basolateral) of clear cell papillary RCC {22}. Individuals with a known history of VHL may undergo surveillance imaging for RCC. Biopsies may be performed on masses identified through surveillance, many of which may be ablated after the diagnostic biopsy or subsequently removed {2258}. Early lesions show intratubular proliferations of clear cells. The kidneys may also show multiple small clear cell microtumours in the renal parenchyma, a feature seen in 44% of individuals with VHL-associated RCC {2258}. VHL-related RCC is often associated with numerous renal cysts {22}, including benign cysts lined by one or two layers of clear cells without atypia, atypical cysts with epithelial hyperplasia with or without cytological atypia, and cysts with a component of RCC {2258,22,4221}. A cyst-dependent progression for clear cell RCC has been suggested in VHL {3078}.

The pancreas in VHL exhibits a vast array of changes, including pancreatic cysts, pancreatic cystadenomas, NETs, and islet abnormalities {802,4091}. PanNETs are often multiple. Histologically, VHL-related PanNETs may appear identical to sporadic cases; however, they may have some distinctive features that have been attributed to a pseudohypoxic state due to the activation of HIF, such as nuclear atypia, clear cell change, oncocytic cytology, and hypervascularity {802}, and they may be cystic {4091}. They are also associated with precursor lesions that are seen in multiple endocrine neoplasia type 1 (islet dysplasia, microtumours, and peliosis {802}), emphasizing the importance of examining the non-tumorous parenchyma. Clear cell pancreatic neuroendocrine neoplasms (PanNENs) have been confused with metastatic RCC in the setting of VHL {1913}. PanNETs show similar immunohistochemical features to those of sporadic PanNETs, but they also may express inhibin {1694}.

Papillary cystadenoma of the epididymis is asymptomatic and may not be diagnosed, therefore the percentage of male patients with VHL who are reported to develop these lesions is variable {3315}; however, a detailed histological autopsy study of 5 male patients with VHL identified that half of the epididymes had papillary cystadenomas, and the other half without these lesions had multifocal epithelial cell proliferations (epithelial microtumours), with four architectural arrangements: complex epithelial change, papillary change, clear cell change, or cystic change {1606}. Like other lesions associated with VHL, papillary cystadenoma can be bilateral {936}. Histologically, this lesion features cystic spaces whose lining has intracystic papillary projections with fibrovascular cores and bland epithelial cells with glycogen-rich clear cytoplasm showing reverse polarity (i.e. the nuclei are oriented away from the basement membrane) {1715,3315,936}. The tumour cells are positive for CK7, usually positive for PAX8, and negative for RCCm {936}. The tumour cells are positive for CAIX {1715,936}.

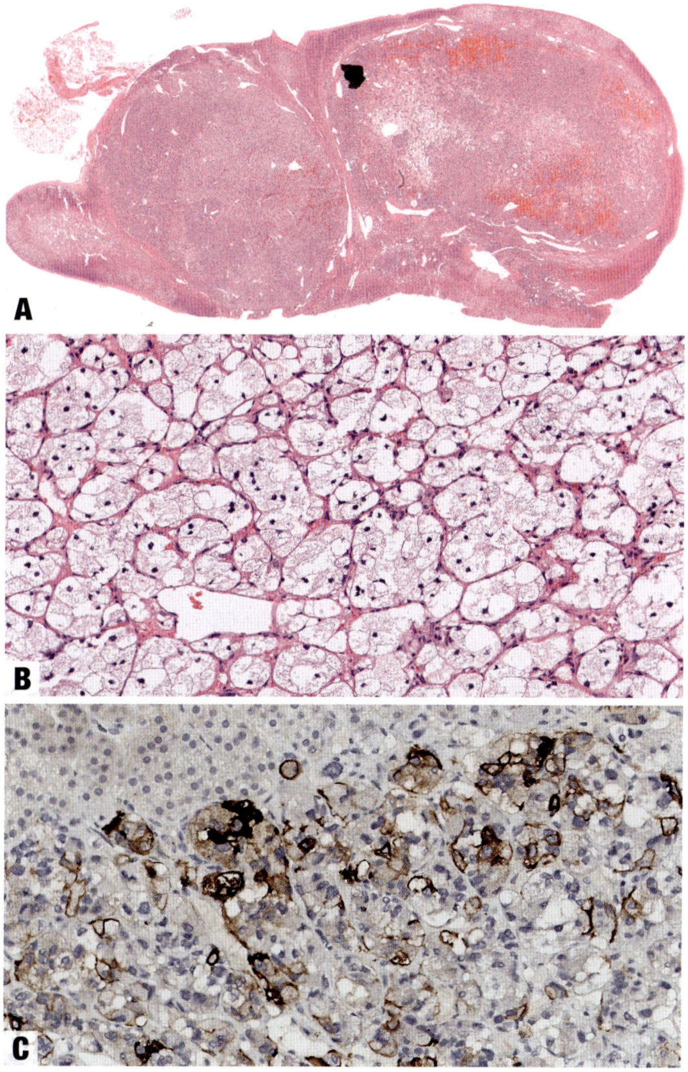

Fig. 13.27 Von Hippel–Lindau syndrome–related phaeochromocytoma. **A** The adrenal gland of a patient with von Hippel–Lindau syndrome contains multiple nodules of phaeochromocytoma. **B** The tumour cells have abundant clear, lipid-rich cytoplasm but are confirmed to be paraganglioma on the basis of their positivity for INSM1, chromogranin, GATA3, and tyrosine hydroxylase (not shown). **C** Tumours arising in patients with von Hippel–Lindau syndrome express CAIX (shown here), and they may have intact SDHB staining or loss of SDHB staining but also express inhibin (not shown).

Papillary cystadenoma of the mesosalpinx and broad ligament in female patients resembles papillary cystadenoma of the epididymis in male patients. Like papillary cystadenoma of the epididymis, papillary cystadenoma of the broad ligament in female patients appears to be a benign tumour in the setting of VHL {3279}, unlike sporadic cases that may be associated with more aggressive behaviour {3279}.

Cytology

The cytopathological features of the various neoplasms related to VHL are indistinguishable from those of their sporadic counterparts, which are described elsewhere in this volume and in the other fifth-edition volumes of the WHO Classification of Tumours series.

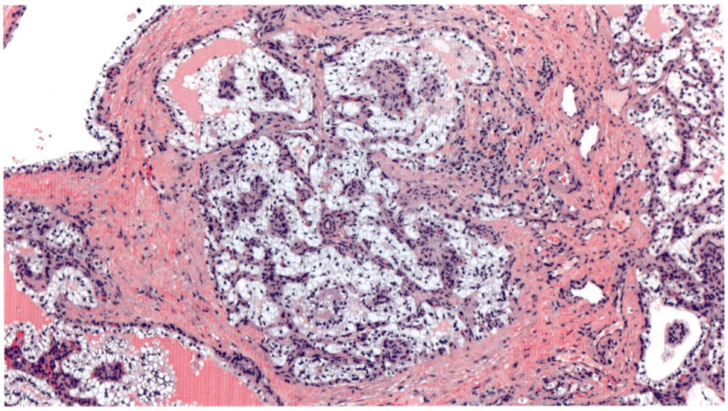

Fig. 13.28 Clear cell renal cell carcinoma in von Hippel–Lindau syndrome. The tumours have an alveolar arrangement of nests of epithelial clear cells with a delicate vascular network.

Diagnostic molecular pathology

The diagnosis of VHL is confirmed by the identification of a germline mutation in *VHL* that is known to be pathogenic.

Essential and desirable diagnostic criteria

Essential: documented pathogenic sequence variant of *VHL* and manifestation of any of the associated neoplasms.

Desirable: manifestation of haemangioblastomas of the retina and/or CNS and any other associated neoplasm in the absence of a pathogenic sequence variant in *VHL*.

Staging

There is no uniformly accepted syndrome-specific staging system for VHL. Malignant neoplasms associated with this syndrome generally follow cancer staging suggested by Union for International Cancer Control (UICC) / American Joint Committee on Cancer (AJCC) criteria. It is recognized, however, that neoplastic components of this syndrome may not be sufficiently separated from a prognostic standpoint. Such limitations have prompted some groups to offer modifications that may address this inherent weakness {4088}.

Prognosis and prediction

The prognosis for patients with VHL depends on the lesion(s) of each individual patient and kindred. Outcome is improved by screening that allows earlier detection of malignancies.

CNS haemangioblastoma as the initial presentation is associated with a higher risk of death from these lesions {4789}. Mutations in exon 2 of *VHL* confer a higher risk and younger age at diagnosis of CNS haemangioblastoma than mutations in other exons {3506}. Multicentric tumours, and particularly brainstem and spinal tumours, are difficult to treat and cause substantial morbidity. Surgical excision is the treatment of choice, and repeated surgical treatments are more frequently required in patients with VHL than in patients with sporadic haemangioblastomas {5091}; repeated surgery is associated with a younger age at presentation {2700}.

Retinal haemangioblastomas are rarely lethal but can cause blindness. Treatments include photocoagulation, cryotherapy, radiation, photodynamic therapy, and combinations of these modalities {739,1736}. Rarely, surgical excision is necessary.

RCC is the most frequent malignant neoplasm of patients with VHL and is therefore an important determinant of mortality. A larger tumour (> 30 mm) and/or bilateral tumours portend a worse prognosis {2474,3507}. VHL-associated RCCs seem to grow more slowly than sporadic clear cell RCCs {2645}. The mortality rates of VHL-associated RCC at 5 and 10 years are 4% and 7.5%, respectively {638}.

Phaeochromocytoma and paraganglioma are not usually a cause of mortality in patients with VHL unless there are cardiovascular complications of hypertension. Metastatic disease is not common in VHL-associated tumours, but multifocal disease can create problems. Bilateral adrenal lesions can result in adrenal insufficiency and the need for complex lifelong medical therapy, so cortical-sparing adrenalectomy should be considered {3215}. Some extra-adrenal paragangliomas may be surgically unresectable {1384}, creating a need for medical therapies.

The all-cause mortality risk of VHL-related PanNET is not higher than that of sporadic PanNET; however, the mortality rate is higher in VHL patients with PanNETs than in patients who have no pancreatic neoplasia {183}. Advanced tumour stage is associated with a higher mortality risk, emphasizing the importance of surveillance for these tumours in patients with VHL {183}. Mutations in exon 3, especially of codons 161/167, increase the risk of metastatic PanNETs {2428}. Surgical resection is advised for lesions larger than 25–28 mm {2428,49}, whereas a watch-and-wait approach is recommended for smaller tumours (< 20 mm) {49}.

Guidelines for clinical surveillance have been published {427A,3706A}.

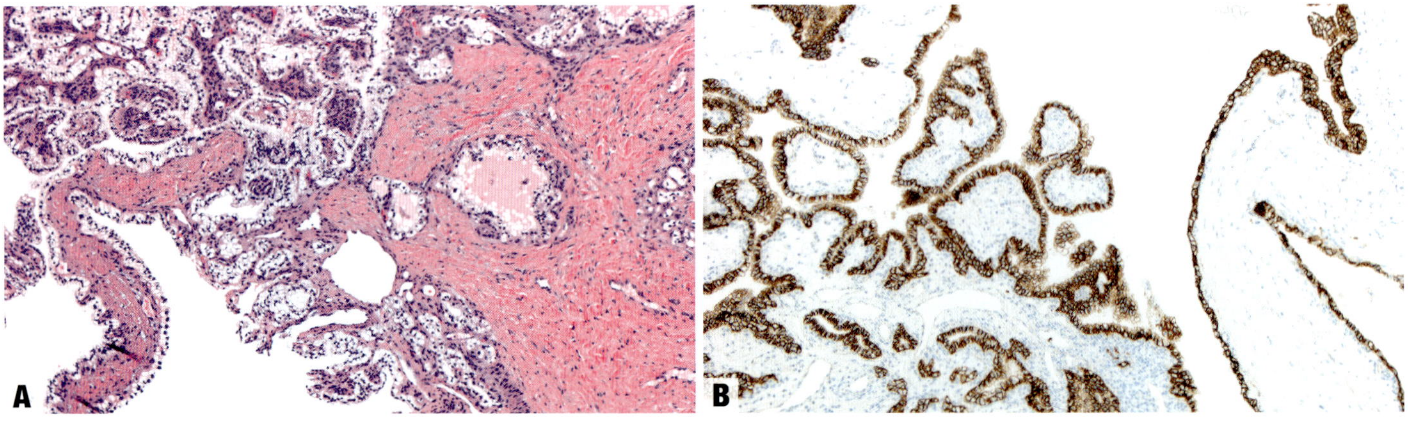

Fig. 13.29 Papillary cystadenoma of the epididymis. **A** This tumour is characterized by cystic spaces with intracystic papillary projections that have well-developed fibrovascular cores and are lined by bland epithelial cells with glycogen-rich clear cytoplasm showing reverse polarity. **B** The tumour cells stain for CAIX.

SDH-deficient tumour syndromes

Gill AJ
Agaimy A
Asa SL
de Krijger RR
Erickson LA
Gimenez-Roqueplo A-P
Juhlin CC
Mete O
Stratakis CA
Tischler AS

Definition

Succinate dehydrogenase (SDH)-deficient tumour syndromes are a group of syndromes characterized by SDH-deficient neoplasia, usually associated with pathogenic germline sequence variants in one of the SDH genes encoding the subunits of the protein SDH (*SDHA*, *SDHB*, *SDHC*, *SDHD*, *SDHAF2*) or with epimutation (promoter hypermethylation) of *SDHC*.

MIM numbering

600857 SDHA
185470 SDHB
602413 SDHC
602690 SDHD
613019 SDHAF2
604287 Carney triad

ICD-11 coding

None

Related terminology

Acceptable: paraganglioma syndrome types 1–5 (PGL1–5); familial paraganglioma phaeochromocytoma syndrome types 1–5; Carney triad (restricted to syndromic but non-hereditary disease).

Not recommended: Carney–Stratakis dyad/syndrome.

Subtype(s)

PGL1 (germline *SDHD* mutation); PGL2 (germline *SDHAF2* mutation); PGL3 (germline *SDHC* mutation); PGL4 (germline *SDHB* mutation); PGL5 (germline *SDHA* mutation); Carney triad (restricted to syndromic but non-hereditary disease in which no germline SDH mutation has been identified)

Localization

Paragangliomas and/or phaeochromocytomas are the most common manifestations, followed by SDH-deficient gastrointestinal stromal tumour (GIST) and SDH-deficient renal carcinomas. Pituitary neuroendocrine tumours (PitNETs)/adenomas, and pulmonary chondromas are recognized associations but are less common. There are strong but inconsistent genotype–phenotype correlations in that different genes are more commonly associated with certain tumour combinations and locations. However, there is overlap between all of the SDH-deficient tumour syndromes. SDH gene mutations are more commonly associated with extra-adrenal paragangliomas than adrenal phaeochromocytomas. The extra-adrenal tumours can be located in the head and neck, thorax, or abdomen and are associated with *SDHB*, *SDHD*, or *SDHC* mutation, as outlined in Table 13.04. *SDHB* mutations are most frequently identified in patients with intra-abdominal extra-adrenal paragangliomas and/or with metastatic paraganglioma, whereas mutations in *SDHD* are more common in patients with head and neck

Table 13.04 Clinicopathological features of succinate dehydrogenase (SDH)-deficient tumour syndromes

Syndrome	Gene	Locus	Inheritance	Sex	Adrenal PCC	Abdominal PGL	Thoracic PGL	Head and neck PGL	SDH-deficient GIST	SDH-deficient RCC	SDH-deficient PitNET	Pulmonary chondroma
PGL1	*SDHD*	11q23	AD;PT	M=F	+	++	+	+++	+	+/–	+	–
PGL2	*SDHAF2*	11q12.2	AD;PT	M=F	+/–	+/–	+/–	+	+/–	+/–	+	–
PGL3	*SDHC*	1q23.3	AD	M=F	+/–	+/–	+	++ (esp. carotid body)	+	++	+	–
PGL4	*SDHB*	1p36.1-p35	AD	M=F	+	++++	++	+	+	++	+	–
PGL5	*SDHA*	5p15	AD	M=F	+	++	+/–	+	+++ (30% of SDH-deficient GISTs)	+	++	–
Carney triad	*SDHC* promoter hyper-methylation	1q23.3	Not hereditary	F>>M	–	+++	+	++	++++ (50% of SDH-deficient GISTs)	–	–	++++

AD, autosomal dominant; AD;PT, autosomal dominant with paternal transmission (maternally imprinted, clinical disease is inherited only from paternal carrier); GIST, gastrointestinal stromal tumour; PCC, phaeochromocytoma; PGL, paraganglioma; PGL1–5, paraganglioma syndrome types 1–5; PitNET, pituitary neuroendocrine tumour / pituitary adenoma; RCC, renal cell carcinoma.

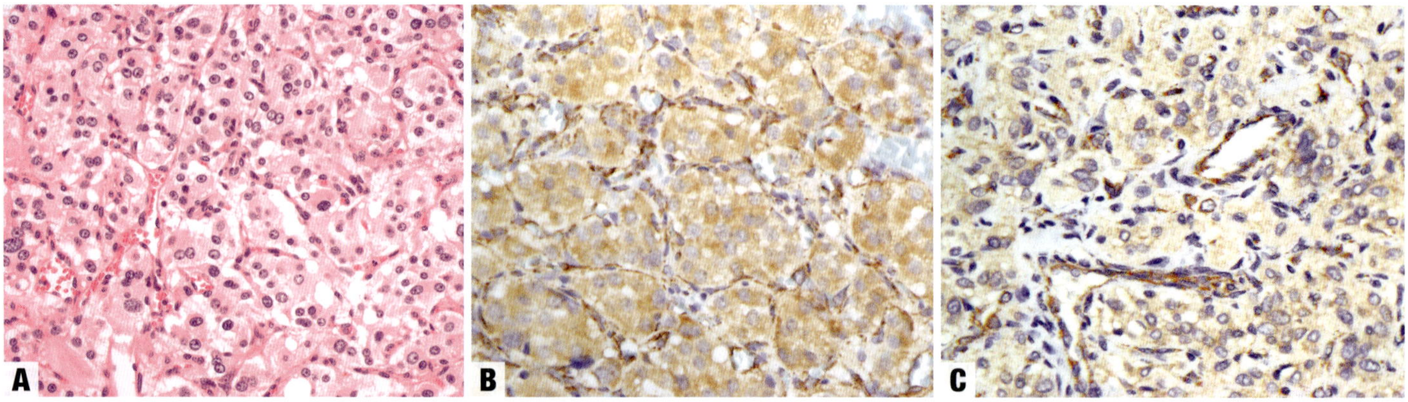

Fig. 13.30 Succinate dehydrogenase (SDH)-deficient paraganglioma. **A** Morphological clues to SDH-deficient paragangliomas are inconsistent but include well-developed, almost circular nests of epithelioid cells, sometimes with pale or vacuolated cytoplasm {4590}. **B,C** Immunohistochemistry for SDHB may be difficult to interpret. In these paragangliomas associated with germline mutation, there is a diffuse cytoplasmic blush in all the neoplastic cells. Because this staining contrasts with the intense granular expression in non-neoplastic internal controls, the tumours are still considered to be succinate dehydrogenase–deficient.

paragangliomas {1573}. SDH-deficient GISTs are most strongly associated with *SDHC* epimutation or *SDHA* mutation {1573}. With the exception of a single case report, all well-characterized SDH-deficient GISTs reported to date have arisen in the stomach {1576,2996,1242}. As their names indicate, renal cell carcinomas arise in the kidneys, PitNETs / pituitary adenomas in the sella turcica (with the exception of ectopic manifestations), and pulmonary chondromas in the lungs. SDH-deficient renal carcinomas usually harbour *SDHB* or *SDHC* mutation (less commonly, *SDHA*; and very rarely, if at all, *SDHD*) {4564}. Pulmonary chondromas are commonly associated with *SDHC* epimutation (Carney triad) but are very rare in other SDH-deficient syndromes.

Clinical features

Clinical features vary according to both genotype and tumour location {1572,1573,1582,1576,4590,4892}. In general, abdominal paragangliomas are more commonly associated with the production of norepinephrine (noradrenaline). Although they may be biochemically silent {4499,1154}, they are likely to give rise to the classic clinical symptoms. Head and neck paragangliomas usually present as mass lesions that are biochemically silent, although they frequently produce dopamine and, in a small minority of cases, norepinephrine (noradrenaline). Although tumours other than SDH-deficient phaeochromocytoma/paraganglioma, GIST, renal carcinoma, pulmonary chondroma, and PitNET / pituitary adenoma have been reported in SDH mutation carriers, it is likely that these are incidental findings in closely monitored populations {1573}. A family history of disease is commonly absent, and *SDHD* and *SDHAF2* usually behave as if they were maternally imprinted genes so that symptomatic disease is almost always only inherited from a paternal carrier {356,5057,354,574}.

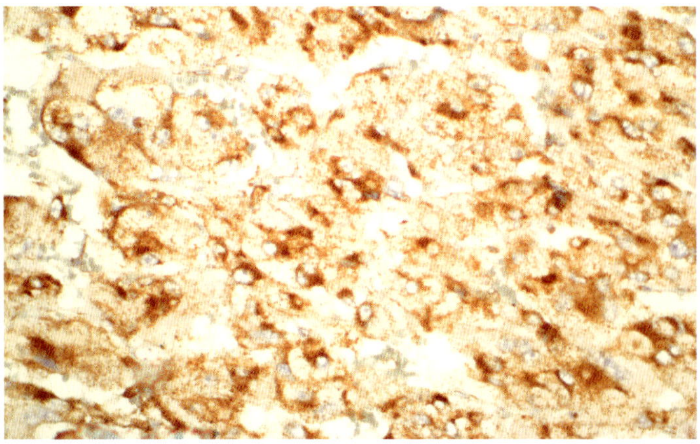

Fig. 13.31 Phaeochromocytoma. This phaeochromocytoma not associated with SDH mutation demonstrates diffuse strong SDHB expression. The cytoplasmic and distinctly granular (mitochondrial) pattern of expression is noted.

Epidemiology

At least 40% of paragangliomas and phaeochromocytomas in adults are hereditary {4587}, and close to half of all genetically determined cases are associated with one of the SDH deficiency syndromes – more if paraganglioma or phaeochromocytoma is diagnosed during childhood {1572,1573,2312,1040, 3705}. SDH-deficient GISTs account for 3% of all GISTs in an unselected adult population, but they account for the great majority of GISTs diagnosed in children {1576,2996}. SDH-deficient renal carcinoma accounts for less than 0.05–0.2% of all renal carcinomas {1579} but is overrepresented in young adults (median age: 35 years, range: 14–76 years) {1579,4891}. SDH-deficient PitNETs / pituitary adenomas are rare (< 0.3% of unselected tumours) {1582}. Pulmonary chondromas are typically found in young women and are very rare outside the setting of Carney triad {3778,765,662}.

Etiology

Contrasting with many other hereditary syndromes, biallelic somatic mutations of the SDH genes in tumours, although described, are very unusual in the absence of germline mutation, or (less commonly) postzygotic epimutation or mosaicism, of one of the SDH genes {1573}.

The term "Carney triad" is now restricted to syndromic but non-hereditary disease where no germline SDH mutation has been identified by clinically deployed testing methodologies. Carney triad is most commonly associated with postzygotic *SDHC* promoter hypermethylation (epimutation), but it may also be explained by other pathogenic genetic events not detected by some testing methodologies – for example, constitutional mosaicism not detected in DNA extracted from blood samples

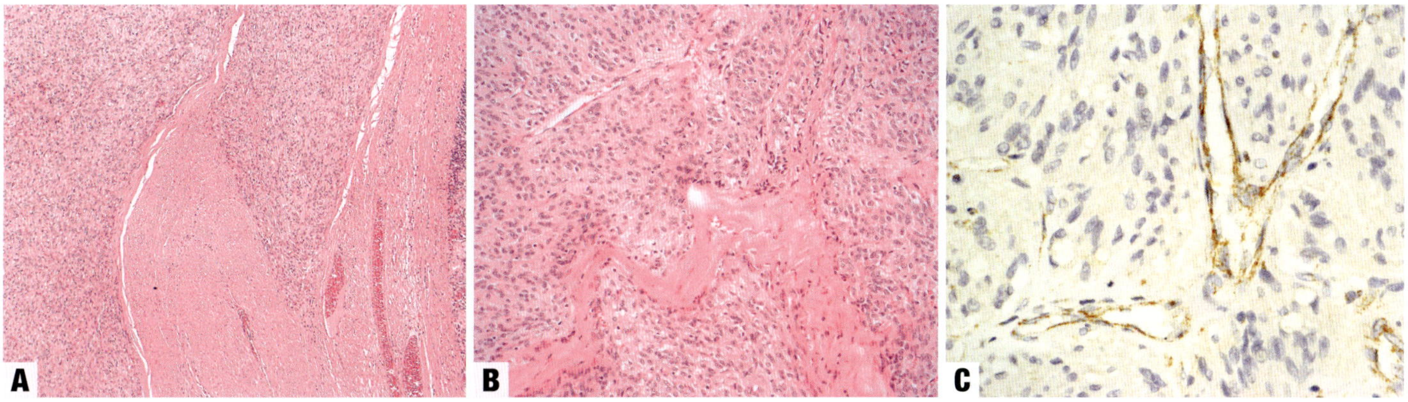

Fig. 13.32 Succinate dehydrogenase (SDH)-deficient gastrointestinal stromal tumour. **A** SDH-deficient gastrointestinal stromal tumour commonly demonstrates a multilobulated or plexiform growth pattern. **B** SDH-deficient gastrointestinal stromal tumour is usually epithelioid or epithelioid-predominant. Sometimes the epithelioid cells demonstrate a vaguely nested architecture. **C** Immunohistochemistry for SDHB in an SDH-deficient gastrointestinal stromal tumour. There is no expression of SDHB in any of the neoplastic cells. The granular cytoplasmic expression in the non-neoplastic cells, which acts as an internal positive control, is emphasized.

subjected to Sanger sequencing but potentially identifiable by massively parallel sequencing with many reads, or by deep intronic genetic variants not identified in some panels. It should be noted that Carney triad is unrelated to Carney complex, which is a different inherited neoplasia syndrome (discussed in *Carney complex*, p. 466) caused by germline variants in *PRKAR1A* {2744,494}.

Pathogenesis

Mitochondrial complex II, also known as the SDH complex, is a key mitochondrial enzyme that links the Krebs cycle and the electron transport chain {1572,1573}. It is encoded by four nuclear autosomal genes but assembled at the inner mitochondrial membrane. It is composed of four protein subunits: *SDHC* and *SDHD* (the anchoring components) and *SDHA* and *SDHB* (the catalytic components). Additionally, *SDHAF2* is required for the flavination of the SDHA protein. If any component of the SDH complex is lost or dysfunctional, the entire SDH complex becomes unstable, and the SDHB subunit is released into the cytoplasm, where it rapidly degrades, accounting for the loss of expression of SDHB protein {4654,1572,1573}. Dysfunction of this key enzyme causes the accumulation of succinate, which acts as an oncometabolite, behaving as a competitor of 2-oxoglutarate–dependent dioxygenases involved in a broad spectrum of tumorigenic pathways, including hypoxic regulation and epigenetic reprogramming {3585,3093}.

Table 13.05 Comparison of succinate dehydrogenase (SDH)-deficient and usual gastrointestinal stromal tumours (GISTs) {1576,2996,1577,1573}

Feature	Usual GIST	SDH-deficient GIST
Age group	Older adults	Children >> young adults >> older adults
Sex distribution	Equal	Female predominance
Associated syndromes	Rare Neurofibromatosis Germline *KIT* mutation Germline *PDGFRA* mutation	Almost always 30% germline *SDHA* mutation 50% *SDHC* epimutation (Carney triad) 20% *SDHB*, *SDHC*, *SDHD* mutation
Location	Throughout gastrointestinal tract	Stomach only[a]
Predominant cell type	Spindled	Epithelioid
Multifocality	Rare	Common
Multinodularity/lobulation	Rare	Usual
SDHB immunohistochemistry	Retained	Lost/deficient (definitional)
KIT or DOG1 immunohistochemistry	Usually positive for KIT and/or DOG1	Always positive for both KIT and DOG1
Somatic *KIT* or *PDGFRA* mutation	Usually	Never
Lymph node metastasis	Very rare	Common
Behaviour of metastasis	Aggressive	Commonly indolent
Response to imatinib	Usual	Usually primary resistance
Prognosis predicted by size and mitotic rate algorithm	Yes	No

[a]To date, a single SDH-deficient GIST arising in the duodenum has been reported {1242}.

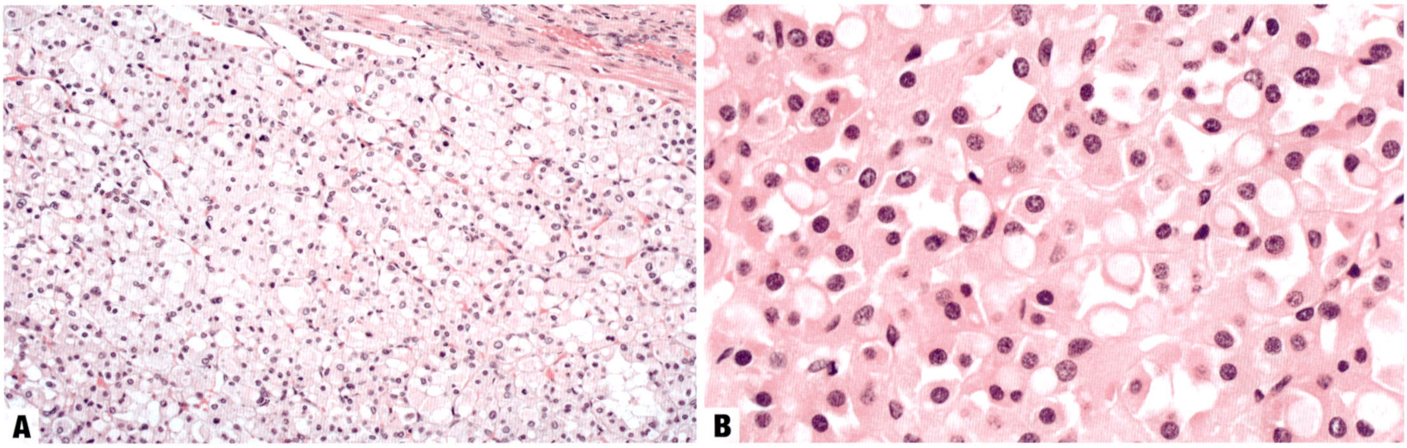

Fig. 13.33 Succinate dehydrogenase–deficient renal cell carcinoma. **A,B** Succinate dehydrogenase–deficient renal cell carcinoma composed of bland cells with eosinophilic (but not oncocytic) cytoplasm. Intracytoplasmic inclusions containing eosinophilic, flocculent, or pale material are a common and distinctive feature.

Macroscopic appearance

Although multifocality is an important clue, the phaeochromocytomas, paragangliomas, PitNETs / pituitary adenomas, and renal cell carcinomas associated with SDH mutation grossly resemble their sporadic counterparts. SDH-deficient GISTs are commonly multilobulated or plexiform and more frequently show lymph node metastases {1576,2996,1577}.

Histopathology

Loss of expression of SDHB (termed SDH deficiency) occurs whenever there is biallelic inactivation of any component of the SDH complex (i.e. *SDHA*, *SDHB*, *SDHC*, *SDHD*, or *SDHAF2*) {1572,1573,1582,1576,4590,4892}. Somatic-only mutations of both alleles of the SDH genes do occur but are extremely rare {4655}; therefore, SDH deficiency is clear evidence of an SDH-deficient tumour syndrome. Tumours with biallelic inactivation of *SDHA* show SDHA loss in addition to SDHB loss, whereas tumours associated with *SDHB*, *SDHC*, or *SDHD* mutation demonstrate preserved expression of SDHA {2398,1194}. SDHB and SDHA immunohistochemistry may be difficult to interpret in some cases, and a tumour should only be considered deficient if there is preserved expression in non-neoplastic cells, which act as internal controls. SDHB immunohistochemistry can be particularly valuable in assessing whether a particular tumour found in a patient with a germline SDH mutation is actually caused by tumoural loss of SDH {4954}, and whether a variant of unknown significance identified by genetic testing is pathogenic. Normal SDHA/SDHB immunostaining is granular and cytoplasmic (mitochondrial). In some SDH-deficient tumours, particularly *SDHD*-related tumours, interpretation may be particularly challenging, because a cytoplasmic blush is often retained. In this setting, weak diffuse expression in neoplastic cells which contrasts with the strong, distinctly granular expression in internal positive controls is a useful clue to the diagnosis of SDH deficiency {4654,1573}. Some phaeochromocytomas not associated with SDH mutation but arising in the setting of von Hippel–Lindau syndrome may show very weak expression of SDHB, which can be mistaken for SDH deficiency {1573}. Other markers of SDH deficiency may be useful when SDHB is difficult to interpret. For example, α-inhibin and CAIX are more commonly expressed in SDH-related and *VHL*-related (pseudohypoxic pathway–related cluster 1 disease) phaeochromocytomas and paragangliomas, respectively, than in other tumours, but these markers lack sensitivity and specificity {3563,1344,2975}.

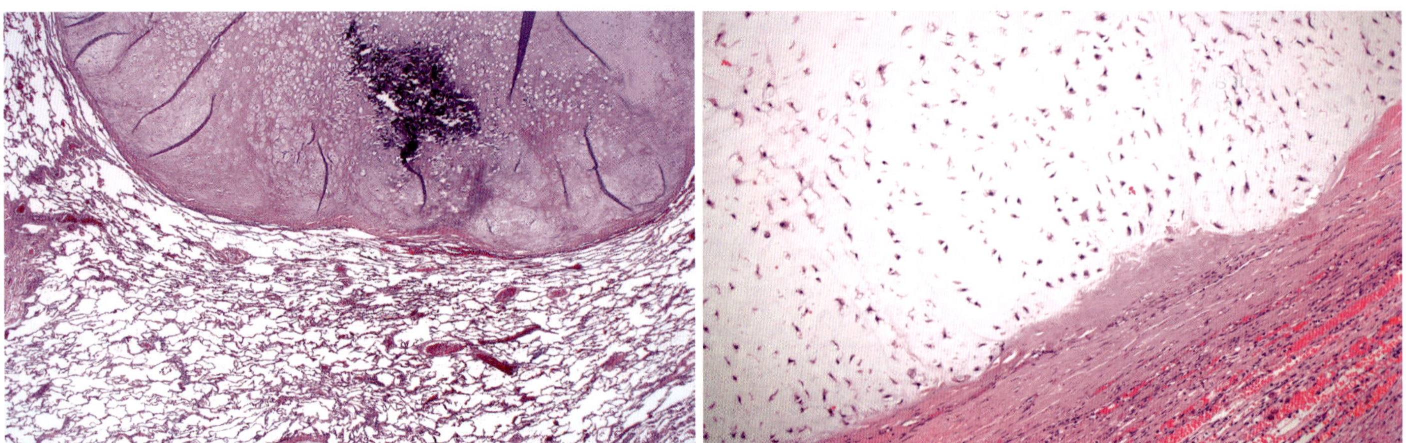

Fig. 13.34 Pulmonary chondroma arising in Carney triad. **A** In contrast to pulmonary hamartoma, the pulmonary chondromas associated with Carney triad do not show entrapped respiratory epithelium between the lobules of cartilage and do not contain other mesenchymal elements such as fat, smooth muscle, or myxoid spindle cells. **B** Instead, they show a smooth contour, lacking invaginations of entrapped respiratory epithelium between cartilage.

Some SDH-deficient paragangliomas are characterized by well-formed, almost circular, nests of epithelioid cells, sometimes with focally clear or vacuolated cytoplasm {4590}. However, this morphology is inconsistent and does not replace SDHB immunohistochemistry, which is recommended in all phaeochromocytomas and paragangliomas.

There are several morphological, clinical, and molecular clues to the identification of SDH-deficient GISTs. These include gastric location, multifocality, a plexiform or multinodular growth pattern, epithelioid cell–type predominance (sometimes with a vaguely nested architecture), and relatively frequent lymph node metastasis (summarized in Table 13.05, p. 459) {1576,1577,1573}. Although SDH-deficient GISTs are not associated with *KIT* or *PDGFRA* mutation, they virtually always show diffuse strong immunohistochemical expression of both KIT and DOG1 {1576,1577,1573}. This can be useful in the differential diagnosis with *PDGFRA*-mutant GISTs, which may resemble SDH-deficient GISTs because of their frequent gastric location and epithelioid cell predominance, but which commonly show patchy or absent KIT (c-KIT) expression. These morphological and immunohistochemical features can be subtle, and a low threshold for SDHB and SDHA immunohistochemistry is recommended for any gastric GIST {1576, 2996,1577}.

SDH-deficient renal carcinomas are now recognized as a distinct entity {1581,4891,1579,4564}. They usually show distinctive morphological features at least focally, being composed of sheets or compact nests of bland cells with eosinophilic cytoplasm. The eosinophilic cytoplasm lacks the fine homogeneous granularity of oncocytoma and may have a flocculent quality. Microcystic change is common {1581,1579,4891}. A characteristic but inconstant feature of SDH-deficient renal carcinoma is the presence of cytoplasmic inclusions containing eosinophilic or bubbly pale material {1581,4891,1579,4564}. Higher-grade transformation may occur in SDH-deficient renal carcinomas and is heralded by denser cytoplasm, increased nuclear atypia with prominent nucleoli, coagulative necrosis, and (occasionally) sarcomatoid changes. Other morphologies, including the presence of papillary architecture, are more frequently encountered in *SDHA*-related renal carcinomas {4564}. Non–SDH-related kidney tumours with very clear cytoplasm, such as clear cell renal cell carcinomas, may show markedly decreased expression of SDHB, a reflection of their cleared cytoplasm with few mitochondria, which should not be mistaken for SDH deficiency {4893,4565,4564}. In these cases, morphological correlation is key.

Experience with SDH-deficient PitNETs / pituitary adenomas is limited. According to some reports they may be larger at diagnosis and more frequently prolactin-producing {4956, 1582,3410,1195,1573}. However, suggestions of other morphological clues have not been confirmed {4956,1582,3410,1195, 1573}.

SDH-deficient pulmonary chondromas lack atypia and frequently show calcification. In contrast to pulmonary hamartomas, they usually demonstrate a smooth contour, do not show entrapped respiratory epithelium between the lobules of cartilage, and do not contain other mesenchymal elements such as fat, smooth muscle, or myxoid spindle cells. Although SDHB immunohistochemistry may assist in the diagnosis of syndromic chondromas, it is less reliable in this setting {765,1573}.

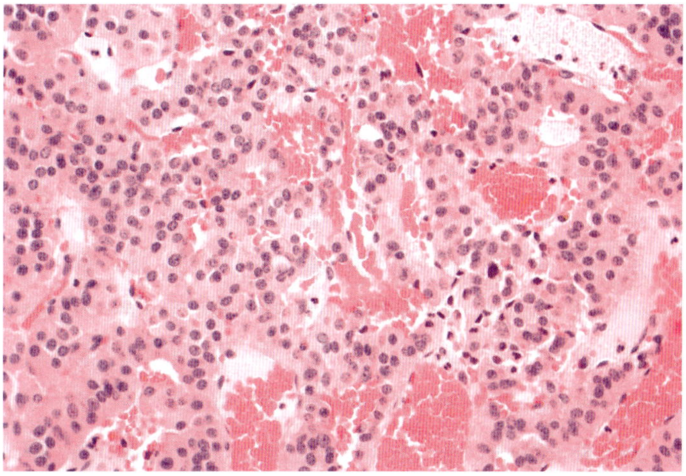

Fig. 13.35 Succinate dehydrogenase–deficient pituitary neuroendocrine tumour (PitNET)/adenoma. This succinate dehydrogenase–deficient PitNET is indistinguishable morphologically from a sporadic tumour.

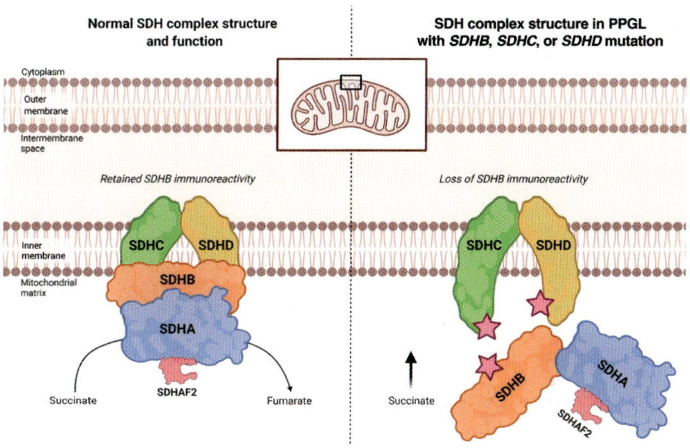

Fig. 13.36 Succinate dehydrogenase (SDH) complex. The SDH complex comprises two anchoring subunits, SDHC and SDHD; the catalytic components SDHA and SDHB; and SDHAF2, responsible for the flavination of the SDHA component of the complex. If any component of the SDH complex is lost, the complex becomes dysfunctional and SDHB immunohistochemistry becomes negative. PPGL, paraganglioma and/or phaeochromocytoma.

Cytology

The cytopathological features of paragangliomas, phaeochromocytomas, SDH-deficient GISTs, and renal cell carcinomas resemble those of related tumours described elsewhere in this volume and in the other fifth-edition volumes of the WHO Classification of Tumours series.

Diagnostic molecular pathology

Because biallelic somatic-only mutations are rare, the diagnosis of any SDH-deficient neoplasm is considered an indication for genetic counselling/testing {2603}. Close collaboration between geneticists and pathologists is important because various analyses based on tumoural tissues can strongly contribute to genetic diagnosis {379,2281,3226}. Immunohistochemistry for SDHB and SDHA can be very useful for assessing the pathogenicity of genetic variants of uncertain significance in the SDH genes {3412}. Germline pathogenic variants in *SDHA* appear to be relatively common (estimated to occur in up to 0.3% of the

Dutch population) {2398} but demonstrate a low lifetime penetrance (estimated as 1.7%) {386}. Therefore, the clinical significance of *SDHA* mutation, particularly if identified by large panel sequencing in the absence of SDH-deficient neoplasia, should be carefully considered and interpreted in the clinical context {2398,1194}. Given the low penetrance, recommendations for surveillance and cascade testing of family members in the setting of *SDHA* mutation vary {2821}.

The term "Carney triad" is appropriate when no germline SDH mutation is identified in an individual with syndromic, but not hereditary, disease. Given that somatic biallelic mutation in the SDH genes is rare, it is reasonable to assign a presumptive diagnosis of Carney triad to any patient with an SDH-deficient neoplasm and no proven germline SDH mutation, unless biallelic somatic-only mutation has been demonstrated. Current evidence suggests that Carney triad is usually associated with postzygotic mosaic epimutation (promoter hypermethylation) of *SDHC* {1755,2278,997}, which can only be identified by specific DNA methylation assays that are not widely available. However, it should be noted that mosaicism for constitutional SDH mutations also occurs and might not be detected by sequencing when the variant allelic ratio is low {654}. Some patients previously given the clinical diagnosis of Carney triad on the basis of syndromic SDH-deficient neoplasia in the absence of identifiable mutation may carry deep intronic pathogenic sequence variants that were previously unrecognized {1039}.

Essential and desirable diagnostic criteria

Essential: confirmed pathogenic or likely pathogenic sequence variant in one of the SDH genes or *SDHC* epimutation *or* the presence of more than one confirmed SDH-deficient neoplasm in an individual or family.

Desirable: identification of even a single SDH-deficient neoplasm is presumptive evidence of syndromic disease unless somatic-only biallelic mutation can be proved.

Staging

The individual tumours are staged according to the relevant Union for International Cancer Control (UICC) / American Joint Committee on Cancer (AJCC) staging schemes.

Prognosis and prediction

In view of the strongly syndromic nature of SDH-deficient neoplasia, surveillance and follow-up for other SDH-deficient neoplasms is indicated even in cases where no germline sequence variant has been identified {124}.

Neurofibromatosis type 1

Perren A
Mete O
Pacak K
Perry A

Definition

Neurofibromatosis type 1 (NF1) is an autosomal dominant hereditary tumour syndrome caused by germline variants of the *NF1* gene.

MIM numbering

162200 Neurofibromatosis, type 1; NF1

ICD-11 coding

LD2D.10 Neurofibromatosis type 1

Related terminology

Not recommended: von Recklinghausen disease; peripheral neurofibromatosis; von Recklinghausen's neurofibromatosis.

Subtype(s)

None

Localization

NF1 is characterized by multiple café-au-lait spots, axillary and inguinal freckling, multiple cutaneous neurofibromas, plexiform neurofibromas, Lisch nodules, optic nerve and other CNS gliomas, malignant peripheral nerve sheath tumours (MPNSTs), phaeochromocytoma (adrenal paraganglioma), duodenal and pancreatic neuroendocrine tumours (PanNETs), and choroidal freckling.

Clinical features

The presence of six or more café-au-lait spots supports a diagnosis of NF1 on clinical grounds {140}. The occurrence of multiple neurofibromas is one of the most typical clinical characteristics in both paediatric and adult patients with NF1. The presence of two or more neurofibromas or one plexiform neurofibroma further supports a diagnosis of NF1 {140}. Most are benign, but they can invade local structures, especially nerves, resulting in neurological manifestations. MPNST is rare, but neurofibromas often serve as precursor lesions, and the lifetime risk of transformation may be as high as 13% {4630,1296}. Most skin lesions appear during early childhood. Café-au-lait spots occur in > 95% of patients and skin freckling in about 50% of patients {2125}. Neurofibromas occur in about 40–60% of patients {1439,2918}.

Various skeletal dysplasias (sphenoid wing, orbital, and long bone dysplasias) are common. Ciliary bone cysts and giant cell granulomas may also occur, but much less frequently {140}.

Gastrointestinal stromal tumours (GISTs) occur in 5–25% of patients with NF1 and are often multifocal {2786}.

Growth hormone excess leading to clinical or subclinical gigantism or acromegaly is a rare but underrecognized phenomenon in patients with NF1 {1771}. NF1-related optic pathway tumours, especially those involving the hypothalamus and sellar region, are the common source of the growth hormone / IGF1 excess in children {601,1771,3944}, which may be transient. Tumour-related GHRH secretion and/or absence of somatostatinergic inhibition are potential mechanisms in NF1-related growth hormone excess {1771}. To date, no NF1-driven pituitary neuroendocrine tumours (PitNETs)/adenomas have been defined.

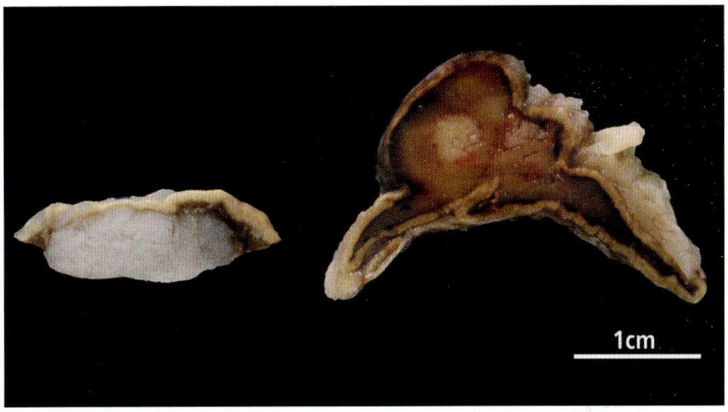

Fig. 13.37 Bilateral composite phaeochromocytoma of a patient with neurofibromatosis type 1. Bilateral phaeochromocytoma, whitish area corresponding to ganglioneuroma components.

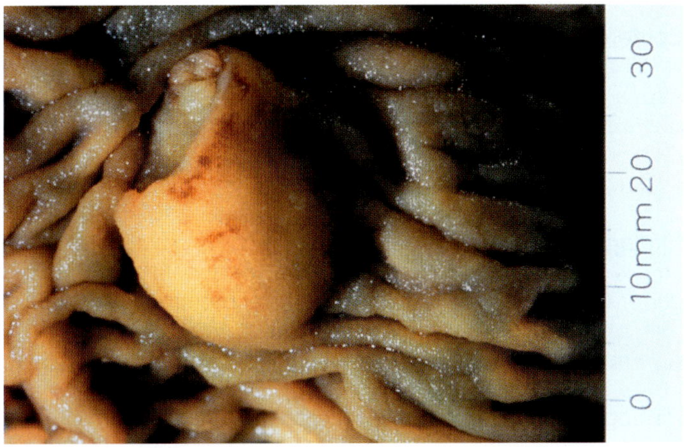

Fig. 13.38 Somatostatinoma of the ampulla of Vater in a patient with neurofibromatosis type 1. Ampullary somatostatinoma of a patient with neurofibromatosis type 1.

Ampullary-type duodenal somatostatinomas are the most common neuroendocrine tumours (NETs) associated with NF1. Other duodenal/ampullary NETs and composite gangliocytoma/neuroma and neuroendocrine tumour (CoGNET; formerly known as gangliocytic paraganglioma) are present in about 5% of patients {3721}. Very rarely, they can coexist {3721,4279}. These tumours most commonly present with signs and symptoms related to the anatomical presence of a tumour rather than with somatostatin-related or other hormone-related clinical syndromes. CoGNETs do not produce any catecholamines, because of their lack of tyrosine hydroxylase. Commonly, patients present with weight loss, abdominal pain, and gastrointestinal bleeding presenting as melaena and resulting in anaemia (especially those with CoGNET), or with clinical signs or symptoms related to pancreatic and gallbladder and pancreatic dysfunction due to the obstruction of the Vater papilla or (very rarely) elevated somatostatin levels. NF1-related duodenal NETs usually occur in adults, with a mean age between 40 and 50 years {3721}.

PanNETs have also been identified in patients with NF1 {176, 3263}. Phaeochromocytomas (adrenal paragangliomas) {350} are seen in 7% of patients with NF1, whereas extra-adrenal paragangliomas are very rare {1213,115,4769,350,3481,1999}. These tumours usually occur around the fourth or fifth decade of life {1214}. About 10% of patients presenting with NF1-related phaeochromocytomas and paragangliomas have multiple tumours. NF1-related phaeochromocytoma presents with a mature secretory phenotype characterized predominantly by the adrenergic biochemical phenotype (epinephrine [adrenaline] / metanephrine). Norepinephrine and normetanephrine may or may not be produced. NF1-related phaeochromocytomas present with classic symptoms and signs related to catecholamine excess, most commonly including hypertension, tachyarrhythmia, palpitations, sweating, nervousness, anxiety, and pallor {2602}.

Epidemiology

NF1 has an incidence of 1 case per 2500–3000 births {4889} and a prevalence of 1:4400 in Finland {3599}. The highest prevalence was described in 17-year-old Israeli military recruits, reaching 1:1000 (0.94:1000 for boys and 1.19:1000 for girls) {1512}.

Etiology

NF1 is caused by heterozygous germline variants of the tumour suppressor gene *NF1* encoding neurofibromin (NF1) {1365}. The second allele is typically inactivated in somatic cells that give rise to tumours.

Pathogenesis

Neurofibromin (NF1) is a RAS-GAP, and therefore NF1 is part of a group of human diseases that are collectively known as RASopathies {3687}. Its inactivation due to mutations leads to increased signalling by the RAS oncogenes {3687}. Neurofibromin (NF1) has multiple domains that interact and regulate multiple signalling pathways in addition to RAS signalling, such as the PKA pathway {4452}.

Although patients with larger deletions of the gene and surrounding genomic material have more severe phenotypes, there are few other genotype–phenotype correlations among patients with classic NF1 and pathogenic *NF1* sequence variants. This may be due to genetic modifiers on other chromosomal loci {3503}.

Macroscopic appearance

NF1-associated neoplasms are macroscopically similar to their sporadic counterparts. Bilateral phaeochromocytomas (adrenal paragangliomas) may occur {1030,2327}. NF1-related duodenal NETs are usually located in the ampulla and may be seen in association with synchronous non-neuroendocrine neoplasms {1668}. The data on gross correlates of NF1-related PanNETs are limited; however, cystic change may occur {4128}.

Histopathology

Endocrine manifestations in NF1

The histological growth pattern of ampullary-type duodenal NETs is typically tubular with psammoma bodies in the lumina in two thirds of the tumours. The psammoma bodies are composed of calcium apatite crystals {86}. Immunohistochemically, NF1-associated duodenal NETs express keratins, neuroendocrine markers (INSM1, synaptophysin, and chromogranin A), and somatostatin. The strong and diffuse labelling with somatostatin in patients with NF1 is in contrast to sporadic or multiple endocrine neoplasia type 1–associated duodenal NETs {568, 1501}. In patients with NF1, duodenal somatostatinomas may be combined with GISTs {3897} and adenoma/adenocarcinoma {1099,1668}. Duodenal CoGNETs can also occur in association with NF1 {3721,4279}.

NF1-associated phaeochromocytomas do not differ from their sporadic counterparts that harbour somatic *NF1* mutation, which occurs in about 20% of sporadic phaeochromocytomas {4846}. However, NF1 phaeochromocytomas may be more frequently of the composite type {2308} and may be associated with synchronous or asynchronous bilateral adrenal gland involvement {2327,1030}, which may also include subcentimetre tumours. By immunohistochemistry, NF1-related phaeochromocytomas and paragangliomas are positive for GATA3 and tyrosine hydroxylase, and negative for keratins and pseudohypoxia biomarkers, including α-inhibin and CAIX {2975}. They lack the high microvessel density typical of von Hippel–Lindau syndrome–associated phaeochromocytomas and paragangliomas.

At the morphological level, NF1-related PanNETs are largely indistinguishable from their sporadic counterparts. They express keratins and neuroendocrine differentiation markers (e.g. INSM1, chromogranin A, synaptophysin). Rare examples of functioning and non-functioning PanNETs have been documented in patients with NF1. (For literature reviews, see {3061,1704,4600}.)

Other manifestations in NF1

Café-au-lait spots are histologically characterized by basilar hyperpigmentation with or without superbasilar melanosis. A minor melanocytic hyperplasia may be observed.

All subtypes of neurofibroma (reviewed in {3779}) can be seen in patients with NF1. Localized cutaneous neurofibromas can affect the dermis or subcutis and show no site predilection. Like sporadic localized neurofibromas, the tumours are unencapsulated and round and are composed of a mixture of bland neoplastic Schwann cells and non-neoplastic perineural cells, entrapped axons, and fibroblasts, accompanied by a variable fibrous to myxoid matrix. Localized cutaneous neurofibromas do not bear a risk for malignancy. Diffuse cutaneous and subcutaneous neurofibroma is much less common and is characterized by a plaque-like tumour, usually in the head and neck region. Pseudomeissnerian corpuscles are frequent; about 10% arise in the setting of NF1. Malignant change is infrequent. Plexiform neurofibromas occur almost exclusively in patients with NF1. Involvement of multiple fascicles results in worm-like or rope-like tangles, referred to as a plexiform pattern. Many plexiform neurofibromas are present at birth or may continue to appear until adolescence. They occur in about 30% of patients with NF1. Plexiform neurofibromas and localized intraneural neurofibromas are precursor lesions of MPNST. MPNSTs are associated with a wide range of histological appearances. Pilocytic astrocytomas resemble their sporadic counterparts but may grow more diffusely.

GISTs in patients with NF1 belong to the group of wildtype GISTs without *KIT/PDGFRA* mutations {1122}.

Cytology

The cytopathological features of the various NF1-associated neoplasms are indistinguishable from those of their sporadic counterparts, which are described elsewhere in this volume and in the other fifth-edition volumes of the WHO Classification of Tumours series.

Diagnostic molecular pathology

NF1 defects are found in > 90% of individuals with a clinical diagnosis of NF1 {2948}. Genetic testing should include various methods to test for splicing defects, deletions, large chromosomal and smaller gene rearrangements, and other mutations. The disease is inherited as an autosomal dominant trait, and prenatal testing is routinely available for known carriers; however, about half of the patients have new (de novo) mutations, often due to paternal mosaicism. This complicates genetic counselling.

Essential and desirable diagnostic criteria

Essential: the diagnostic clinical criteria have been described in a US National Institutes of Health (NIH) consensus conference {3199} and are summarized in Box 13.01.

Box 13.01 Clinical diagnostic criteria for neurofibromatosis type 1

Two or more of the following criteria must be met for the diagnosis:

1. > 6 café-au-lait macules measuring > 5 mm in greatest diameter in prepubertal individuals and > 15 mm in greatest diameter after puberty
2. > 2 neurofibromas of any type or 1 plexiform neurofibroma
3. Axillary or inguinal freckling
4. Optic glioma
5. > 2 Lisch nodules (iris hamartomas)
6. A distinctive osseous lesion, such as sphenoid wing dysplasia or thinning of the cortex of long bones (with or without pseudarthrosis)
7. A first-degree relative (parent, sibling, or child) with neurofibromatosis type 1 diagnosed by the above criteria

References: {3199} {3217}.

Staging

None

Prognosis and prediction

By the age of 8 years, 97% of children with NF1 clinically fulfil the diagnostic criteria, and by the age of 20 years, 100% do {1044}. The phenotype, however, is highly variable {3684}. About 15% of patients with NF1 develop brain tumours {1177}. The lifetime risk for patients with NF1 of developing MPNST is reported as 8–13% {1295}; early detection and resection are essential. Patients with NF1 are at 5–7 times greater risk than the general population of developing leukaemia, brain tumours, and breast cancer. The prognosis of NF1-associated NETs and phaeochromocytomas and/or paragangliomas is comparable to that of their sporadic counterparts.

Carney complex

Kirschner LS
Mete O
Stratakis CA

Definition

Carney complex (CNC) is an autosomal dominant tumour predisposition syndrome whose cardinal features include spotty skin pigmentation, myxomatosis, secretory endocrine tumours, and pigmented schwannomas.

MIM numbering

160980 Carney complex, type 1; CNC1

ICD-11 coding

5A70.Y Other specified Cushing syndrome

Related terminology

Not recommended: NAME syndrome (naevi, atrial myxoma, myxoid neurofibromas, and ephelides); LAMB syndrome (lentigines, atrial myxoma, mucocutaneous myoma, and blue naevus).

Subtype(s)

None

Localization

The majority of patients with CNC have multisystem disease involving endocrine organs (e.g. pituitary, thyroid, adrenal) and non-endocrine organs (e.g. skin, mucosae, heart, gonads, peripheral nerve sheath, bone).

Clinical features

For most patients with CNC, the disease takes a variable but indolent course, with various manifestations (see below and Table 13.06) accumulating as the patient ages. Around one third of patients had no identifiable family history {3590}. Patients with CNC typically manifest pigmentation before puberty; this is usually the earliest physical manifestation, and it may become less prominent in patients as they age {4296}. Myxomatosis (including cardiac myxomas) and endocrine manifestations are often observed, beginning in the teenage years, although the endocrine manifestations may be subtle {3571}.

Skin pigmentation (lentiginosis and pigmented naevi): Lentigines are pigmented cutaneous macules with variable appearances. They are typically located on the central face but may involve the lips and other mucosal surfaces, such as the inside of the mouth, the sclera, and the genitalia {4296}. Pigmented or blue naevi are seen on the extremities and trunk, and less commonly on the head and neck {672}.

Myxomas: Cardiac myxomas in CNC are usually multifocal and are found in any cardiac chamber {2814,3571,1825}. By the age of 30 years, about 35% of female patients and 45% of male patients have one myxoma, and recurrence is more common in female patients {3571}. Myxomas may also occur in other sites, including the skin, external auditory canal, earlobe, eyelid, mucocutaneous boundaries, and breast {1371,4575,529}.

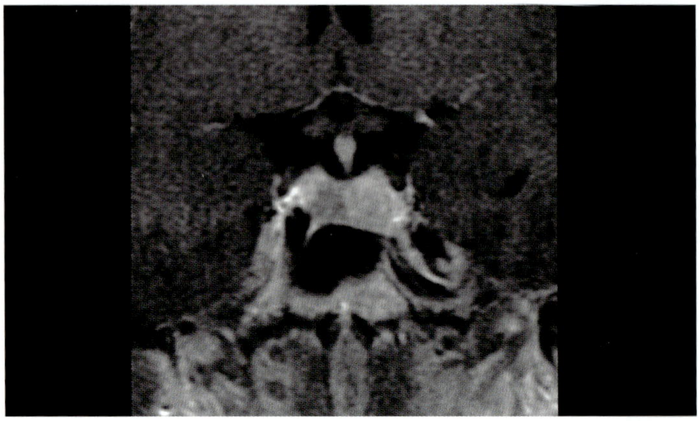

Fig. 13.39 Growth hormone–producing adenoma in a patient with Carney complex. MRI after gadolinium enhancement of the pituitary gland of a patient with Carney complex who had few obvious clinical signs of acromegaly. A developing microadenoma can be seen on the left side as a hypodense region with the gland. This is a common scenario among patients with the complex: biochemically, they meet all criteria of acromegaly, with elevated growth hormone levels and high IGF1. Yet in most patients, adenomas develop slowly within the background of hyperplasia. In this patient, who was followed for > 20 years, an obvious adenoma developed > 10 years after the first biochemical evidence of acromegaly.

Primary pigmented nodular adrenocortical disease (PPNAD): PPNAD causes ACTH-independent Cushing syndrome, and cortisol levels may paradoxically increase in response to dexamethasone {2742,2175,1285}. Patients may present with typical or cyclical symptoms of hypercortisolism {1167}. The adrenal glands are not notably enlarged on imaging studies. CT and MRI findings may underestimate the presence of bilateral adrenal gland involvement {1285,1916}. About 50% of affected patients may show an abnormal imaging finding {1285}, including bilateral multiple bead-like small nodules (2–5 mm) {3776}.

Pituitary neuroendocrine tumour (PitNET) / pituitary adenoma: CNC-related pituitary involvement may manifest with acromegaly (growth hormone excess) or with symptoms from mixed growth hormone and prolactin secretion {4429,452,932,214}. Patients may present with multiple pituitary adenomas / PitNETs or with pituitary hyperplasia {2728,4429,214}.

Thyroid nodules and cancer: Thyroid nodules are observed in 30–60% of patients with CNC {4298,407}. CNC joins the small group of dominantly inherited diseases, including Cowden syndrome, *DICER1* syndrome, and hereditary familial polyposis, in which non-medullary thyroid neoplasia occurs. However, in patients with CNC, follicular thyroid carcinoma is more common than papillary thyroid carcinoma {1146,3297,670}. Like in other populations with thyroid nodules, cancers are diagnosed in about 10% of these nodules {407,670}.

Gonadal tumours (large cell calcifying Sertoli cell tumour [LCCSCT] and ovarian cystadenoma or cystadenocarcinoma): LCCSCT occurs in a small percentage of male patients with CNC and presents as bilateral testicular masses {544,4822}.

The tumours may have palpable calcifications and cause infertility. Ovarian lesions in CNC range from ovarian cysts to serous cystadenomas and, rarely, to malignant tumours including endometroid and mucinous adenocarcinomas {4300}.

Nerve sheath tumours (psammomatous melanotic schwannoma): Psammomatous melanotic schwannomas are peripheral nerve sheath tumours that often affect the posterior spinal nerve roots, the alimentary tract (especially the oesophagus

Table 13.06 Clinical spectrum of Carney complex tumours

Manifestation	Prevalence	Notes
Skin findings		
Lentiginosis	70–80%	Lentiginosis may involve palpebral fissure, caruncle, or conjunctival semilunar fold
Blue naevi	40%	
Pigmented epithelioid melanocytoma	Rare	
Café-au-lait macules	Rare	
Spitz naevus	Rare	
Myxomatosis		
Cardiac	20–40%	
Skin	30–50%	
Breast	< 20%	Breast lesions may be myxomas (which may also involve the nipple) or myxoid fibroadenomas
Eyelid	~15%	
Uterine	Rare	
Adrenal		
PPNAD	25–60%	
Adrenocortical carcinoma	Rare	
Pituitary		
Acromegaly	10–12%	Acromegaly may be due to hyperplasia rather than discrete tumour
Prolactinoma	Rare	Subclinical hormonal abnormalities are seen in as many as 75% of patients when screened
Thyroid		
Benign disease (cysts, adenomas)	25–75%	
Thyroid cancer	2.5–10%	Thyroid cancer may be follicular or papillary histology, the former more frequent
Testes		
Large cell calcifying Sertoli cell tumours	~40% of male patients	
Other tumours (Leydig cell, adrenal rest tissue)	Rare	
Nerve sheath		
Pigmented melanotic schwannoma	10%	May be confused with melanoma on imaging, because of pigmentation
Ovaries		
Cysts	Rare	
Serous adenomas	Rare	
Cystic teratomas	Rare	
Bone		
Osteochondromyxoma	Rare	Typically seen in the young
Others	2.5%	
Pancreatic cancer	Rare	Pancreatic tumours may include acinar cell carcinoma, adenocarcinoma, or IPMN
Hepatic tumours, including fibrolamellar carcinoma	Rare	
Gastric/colon carcinoma	Rare	
Bronchogenic cyst	Rare	

IPMN, intraductal papillary mucinous neoplasm; PPNAD, primary pigmented nodular adrenocortical disease.
Note: Carney complex is a rare disease, so population-based studies of this condition and incidences of specific manifestations are lacking in the world literature. Major centres for the disease, including the US National Institutes of Health (NIH), Mayo Clinic (USA), and Hôpital Cochin (France), have collated data on > 750 cases of the disease, including subsets that have been reported previously {4299,407}. The table reflects an adaptation of these data {918}.

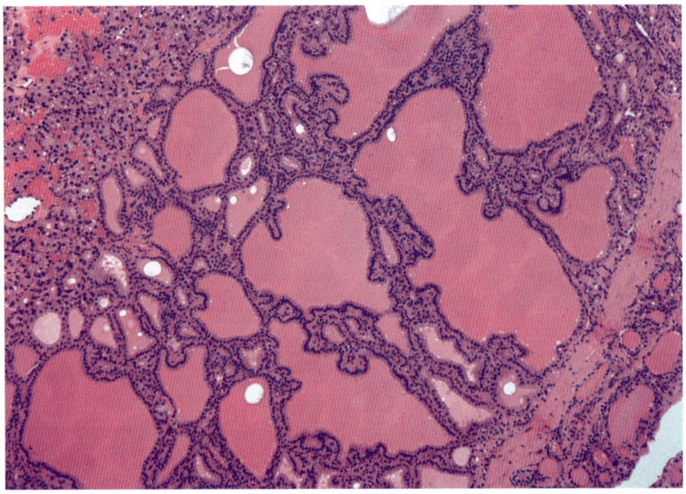

Fig. 13.40 Follicular thyroid adenoma with papillary architecture in a patient with Carney complex. This tumour has intrafollicular centripetal papillary projections. Consistent with the morphological findings, the patient had a suppressed TSH level.

and stomach), bone, and skin. The majority of the tumours are symptomatic, causing either neurological symptoms or mass effect {663,672}.

Osteochondromyxomas: These are bone tumours that tend to appear early in life in the craniofacial or long bones, and they may exhibit either a lytic or blastic appearance on imaging {665}.

Other manifestations: Tubular adenomas, ductal adenomas, myxomas, and myxoid fibroadenomas of the breast, as well as intraductal mucinous tumours of the pancreas and fibrolamellar hepatocellular carcinomas, may also be seen in adults with CNC {3535,1659}.

Epidemiology

CNC is a rare disease, with < 1000 patients described in the literature, and its true incidence and prevalence are unknown. An M:F ratio of 1:2 was documented in a large series of 353 patients {3590}. The median age of detection is about 20 years of age, although patients have been identified as early as 2 years of age and as late as the fifth decade of life {2167}.

Box 13.02 Clinical and histopathological thyroid findings in patients with Carney complex {670}

Clinical:
- Normal
- Diffuse enlargement (Graves disease)
- Bilateral multinodularity
- Unilateral or bilateral mass with or without hyperthyroidism
- Large mass, suspected carcinoma

Histopathological:
- Normal
- Benign
  - Unilateral
    - Adenoma, non-functioning and toxic, typical and atypical, follicular thyroid adenoma with papillary architecture
  - Bilateral
    - Thyroid follicular nodular disease, micronodular diffuse and papillary hyperplasia
    - Diffuse hyperplasia (Graves disease)
    - Thyroid follicular nodular disease
- Malignant
  - Unilateral or bilateral
    - Carcinoma (follicular and papillary)

Etiology

CNC is a genetic condition involving germline pathogenic mutation of *PRKAR1A* or, less commonly, of *PDE8B* or *PDE11A* {2167, 918}. Most patients present in their teenage years, although diagnosis can occur in the very young or in older individuals. Cascade testing from clinically identified index cases decreases the age at diagnosis for patients with this inherited disease.

Pathogenesis

In vitro and in vivo studies have determined that tumours in patients with CNC are caused by activation of the PKA signalling pathway {1678}. In many involved endocrine tissues, this signalling abnormality may result in the hormone hypersecretion that is seen clinically {4429,2141,214}. Because PKA functions in a tissue-specific fashion, tumours are limited to those tissues where this signalling pathway promotes growth {4429,2141,214, 2320}.

Macroscopic appearance

In PPNAD, the adrenal glands show no enlargement but the gross examination can highlight bilateral small pigmented cortical nodules (often < 5 mm) {1167,2963}. Pituitary adenomas / PitNETs of somatotroph cell lineage are soft with a white to grey cut surface. Pigmented melanotic schwannomas have a black, brown, or blue appearance and are usually encapsulated and solid or spongy. LCCSCTs may exhibit microcalcifications or macrocalcifications at the time of removal. Other tumours in CNC have a macroscopic appearance similar to that of their sporadic counterparts.

Histopathology

PPNAD is characterized by bilateral cortical micronodules (often < 5 mm) enriched in compact (lipid-poor) adrenocortical cells, typically located in the zona fasciculata layer or in the intersection of the zona reticularis and zona fasciculata layers. CNC-related PPNAD is indistinguishable from isolated PPNAD at the histological level. However, PPNAD is distinguished from isolated micronodular adrenocortical disease (a rare form of bilateral micronodular adrenocortical disease) by the presence of pigmented nodules and internodular cortical atrophy {2141, 2175,490}. Rarely, myelolipomas {2744}, adrenal cortical adenomas (> 10 mm) {5082,2744}, and adrenal cortical carcinomas {3094,161} have been described in the setting of CNC-related PPNAD. Cortical micronodules are positive for SF1, synaptophysin, α-inhibin, and melan-A {4101,669}.

PitNETs / pituitary adenomas are indistinguishable from their sporadic counterparts; however, most CNC-related PitNETs are often PIT1-lineage tumours with somatotroph or mammosomatotroph cell differentiation, often with densely granulated tumour cells {1725,4429,3996}. The rare occurrence of hyperprolactinaemia in CNC has an unknown etiology but may be related to a possible lactotroph cell pathology {3996,452}. In CNC, the detailed documentation of other PitNET subtypes using modern classification tools is lacking. Pituitary hyperplasia of somatotroph or mammosomatotroph cells, as well as multifocal PitNETs, can be identified in CNC {2728,4429,214}. Individual

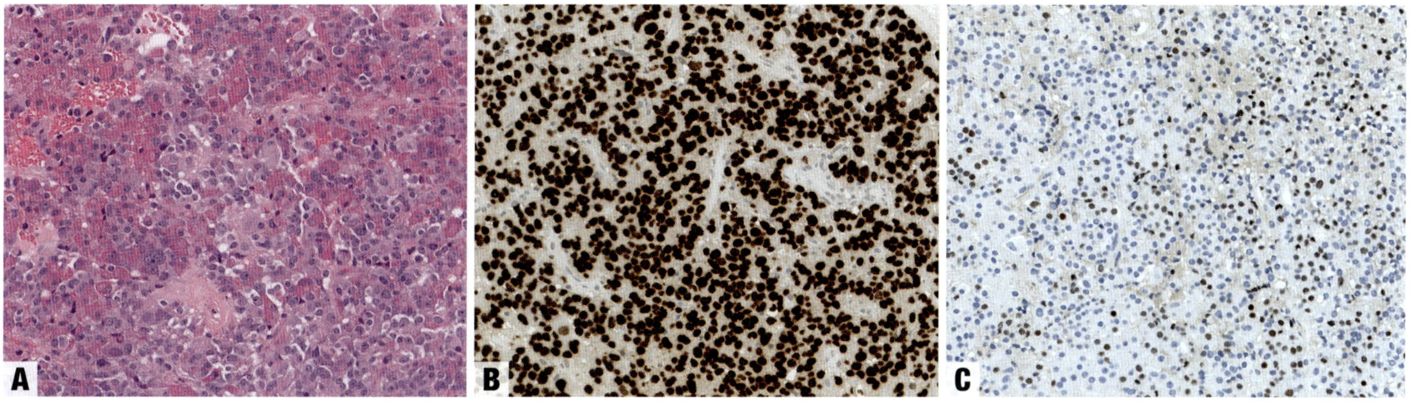

Fig. 13.41 Carney complex–related pituitary neuroendocrine tumour (PitNET)/adenoma consisting of a mixed somatotroph and lactotroph tumour. **A** The tumour consists of a mixture of acidophilic (densely granulated somatotroph tumour) and chromophobic (sparsely granulated lactotroph) cells. **B** There is diffuse PIT1 reactivity. **C** ERα is positive in the lactotroph tumour component, whereas the somatotroph tumour cells are negative for ERα.

tumours are subtyped according the criteria defined in the relevant sections within this volume.

Thyroid nodules typically appear as adenomatous nodules and follicular adenomas, including those with intrafollicular centripetal papillary growth (follicular thyroid adenoma with papillary architecture) that can manifest with hyperthyroidism {670, 3620,407}. Thyroid cancers may exhibit papillary or follicular histology {407,3297,1703} and are usually multicentric and bilateral, but they are not different to their sporadic counterparts (see Box 13.02).

LCCSCTs show various patterns, varying from solid to trabecular. An intratubular or in situ component may be present. The tumour cells are large, with abundant eosinophilic cytoplasm, and mitotic figures are uncommon. Distinctly laminated calcospherites are a common finding. Leydig cell tumours and adrenocortical rest tumours may also be seen {667}.

Lentiginosis exhibits localized hyperpigmentation of the basal layer epidermal keratinocytes and melanocyte hyperplasia. Other lesions may show coarse melanin granules in the epidermis. Hyperplasia of the epidermis with prominent rete pegs may also be present. Other pigmented naevi are poorly circumscribed, located in the dermis with two types of melanocytes: one heavily pigmented, globular, and fusiform; and the other lightly pigmented, polygonal, and spindle {666}. The melanocytes are usually located along the dermal collagen bundle.

Cardiac myxomas are hypocellular lesions with scattered polygonal and spindle tumour cells in a myxoid matrix. Extracardiac myxomas exhibit a similar appearance, with scattered polygonal cells, stellate cells, and spindle cells in a myxoid matrix. Capillaries are usually prominent. The cutaneous lesions, when in contact with the overlying epidermis, may induce epidermal proliferation into the dermis, which becomes incorporated into the myxoma.

Pigmented melanotic schwannoma presents microscopically as a well-circumscribed but incompletely encapsulated tumour composed of spindle and epithelioid cells with melanin pigment deposition, psammoma bodies, and adipose tissue. The spindle cells are arranged in interlacing fascicles and show whorling and occasionally nuclear palisading. They are usually positive for S100, SOX10, and vimentin, and negative for GFAP, actin, and keratin. Ultrastructural examination usually shows cells with elongated processes, continuous basal lamina, and melanosomes, as well as premelanosomes and intercellular long-spacing collagen.

Osteochondromyxomas exhibit a polymorphic histology, including areas of polygonal, stellate, or bipolar cells. Immature osteoid is present, with increased numbers of osteoclasts, indicating rapid bone remodelling. Areas of hyaline fibrosis may also be observed.

Box 13.03 Diagnostic criteria for Carney complex {4299,4296}

For a diagnosis of Carney complex, the patient must:

1. Exhibit two of the manifestations of the disease listed below

- Spotty skin pigmentation with a typical distribution: lips, conjunctiva and inner or outer canthi, vaginal and penile mucosa
- Myxomas, cutaneous and mucosal
- Cardiac myxoma
- Breast myxomatosis
- Primary pigmented nodular adrenocortical disease
- Acromegaly due to growth hormone–producing pituitary adenoma / pituitary neuroendocrine tumour (PitNET)
- Large cell calcifying Sertoli cell tumour or characteristic calcification on testicular ultrasonography
- Thyroid carcinoma or multiple hypoechoic nodules on thyroid ultrasonography
- Psammomatous melanotic schwannoma
- Blue naevus or epithelioid blue naevus, multiple
- Breast ductal adenomas, multiple
- Osteochondromyxoma of bone

2. OR exhibit one of the manifestations listed above and meet one of the supplemental criteria listed below

- Affected first-degree relative
- Inactivating mutation of *PRKAR1A*

Cytology

The cytopathological features of the various neoplasms related to Carney complex are indistinguishable from those of their sporadic counterparts, which are described elsewhere in this volume and in the other fifth-edition volumes of the WHO Classification of Tumours series.

Diagnostic molecular pathology

CNC can be diagnosed by the detection of pathogenic germline mutation of *PRKAR1A* or, less commonly, of *PDE8B* or *PDE11A*. Molecular diagnosis also includes gene copy testing for *PRKACA* or *PRKACB* {918}.

Essential and desirable diagnostic criteria

See Box 13.03 (p. 469).

Essential: at least two major criteria must be present to establish the diagnosis of CNC, and their occurrence must be confirmed biochemically, histologically, or by imaging, as indicated. In the presence of one supplemental criterion, a single clinical manifestation is sufficient to set the diagnosis.

Major diagnostic criteria:

- Typical skin pigmentation (lentiginosis, or multiple blue or epithelioid blue naevi)
- Myxomas (cutaneous, mucosal, breast, or cardiac)
- Specific endocrine tumours or endocrine hyperactivity (PPNAD, PitNET / pituitary adenoma leading to acromegaly or evidence of acromegaly, LCCSCT or characteristic calcification on ultrasound, thyroid cancer or multiple thyroid nodules in young patients)
- Any of the other rare tumours, including pigmented melanotic schwannoma, osteochondromyxoma, and breast adenomas

Supplemental criteria:

- An affected first-degree relative
- Pathogenic inactivating germline *PRKAR1A* mutation

Desirable (in patients with a clinicopathological diagnosis of CNC):

- Germline pathogenic *PRKAR1A* sequence variants
- Germline pathogenic *PDE8B* or *PDE11A* sequence variants in *PRKAR1A*-wildtype patients
- Gene copy testing for *PRKACA* or *PRKACB* in *PRKAR1A*-wildtype patients

Staging

Eighth-edition Union for International Cancer Control (UICC) / American Joint Committee on Cancer (AJCC) TNM staging is applicable to individual malignant tumours, like for their sporadic counterparts.

Prognosis and prediction

Most of the tumours associated with CNC are benign and slow-growing. The exceptions to this notion are the schwannomas, which can behave more aggressively, although not nearly as aggressively as melanomas, with which they can be confused radiologically owing to their striking melanotic pigmentation. The other tumour type that can cause catastrophic acute consequences is cardiac myxoma, although this is a feature of these tumours in general and is not due to malignancy per se. In families and/or patients with multiple cardiac myxomas, complications from open heart surgery may also lead to a decrease in overall lifespan.

McCune–Albright syndrome

Boyce AM
Asa SL
Ezzat S
Mete O
Stratakis CA

Definition

McCune–Albright syndrome (MAS) is a tumour disorder caused by somatic activating *GNAS* mutations resulting in mosaic disease with wide clinical variability and a broad spectrum of endocrine and non-endocrine manifestations.

MIM numbering

174800 McCune–Albright syndrome; MAS

ICD-11 coding

FB80.0 Fibrous dysplasia of bone

Related terminology

Not recommended: Albright syndrome; fibrous dysplasia (polyostotic and monostotic); Mazabraud syndrome.

Subtype(s)

The association of polyostotic fibrous dysplasia and intramuscular myxomas is categorized as Mazabraud syndrome.

Localization

MAS may involve any portion of the skin and/or skeleton. Endocrine manifestations involve the gonads, thyroid, pituitary, and adrenals.

Clinical features

The clinical spectrum of MAS is broad, ranging from asymptomatic findings to neonatal lethality. The phenotype reflects the distribution of *GNAS* mutations and the role of $G_s\alpha$ in mutation-bearing tissues. Penetrance is primarily determined by the number and location of mutant cells {1774}. Hyperpigmented macules are apparent at or shortly after birth {505}. Fibrous dysplasia lesions manifest during the first few years of life and expand during childhood {1801}. Most clinically significant bone lesions are detectable by the age of 10 years, and the final disease burden is close to established by the age of 15 years {1801}. Endocrinopathies are generally apparent in childhood, with the exception of FGF23-mediated hypophosphataemia, which may wax and wane {501,505}.

The presence of any feature of MAS should prompt evaluation for additional manifestations {2094}. In individuals with isolated monostotic fibrous dysplasia, the identification of a *GNAS* mutation is required to establish the diagnosis {2094}.

Precocious puberty is the most common endocrine manifestation in girls (accounting for ~80% of cases) {2872,392,505,503}. Precocious puberty is isosexual, due to peripheral estrogen and/or testosterone production {2872,392,3408}. One series revealed that the prevalence of gonadal involvement is equal between the sexes; however, precocious puberty is more frequent in girls than in boys (accounting for ~20%) {504}. In girls, precocity presents with episodic vaginal bleeding and breast budding, coinciding with the development of single or multiple

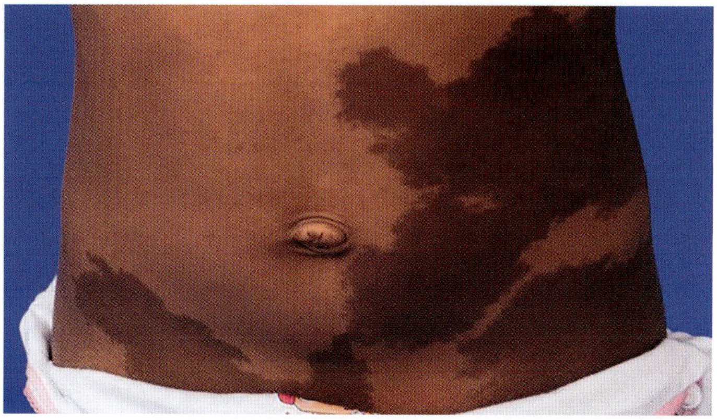

Fig. 13.42 McCune–Albright syndrome. Photograph showing characteristic skin hyperpigmentation, including irregular borders and location respecting the midline of the body.

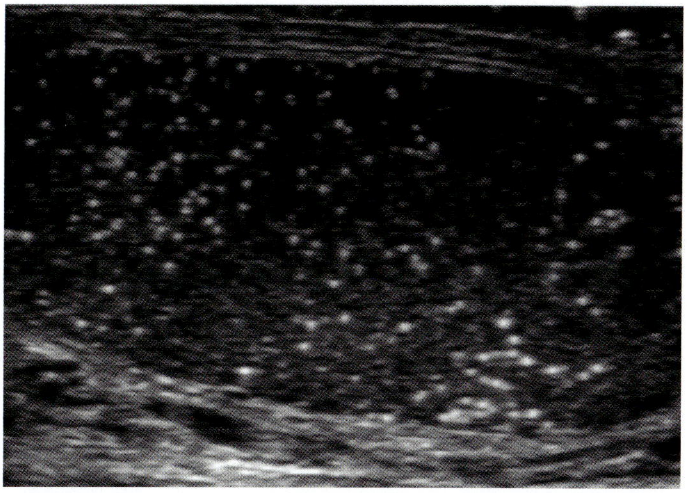

Fig. 13.43 McCune–Albright syndrome. Testicular ultrasonography in a patient with macro-orchidism demonstrates diffuse microlithiasis.

estrogen-producing ovarian cysts {913}. Affected boys develop enlarged testes with or without excess testosterone production {504}. Ultrasonography is useful for screening gonads in MAS. Ovarian cysts may be either present or absent, owing to the episodic nature of their development. Testicular microlithiasis, hyperechoic lesions, hypoechoic lesions, heterogeneity, and focal calcifications can be identified in most boys irrespective of precocity {504,2463}.

Hyperthyroidism is the second most common endocrine manifestation in MAS {505}. A comprehensive literature review identified subclinical or clinical hyperthyroidism in as many as 66% of patients with MAS-related goitre {714,896,4439}. Abnormal ultrasound findings have been reported in 54% of patients {714, 896}. Even in the absence of hyperthyroidism, affected patients have a higher triiodothyronine-to-thyroxine ratio, which is partially explained by cAMP-induced 5′-deiodinase activity {714}.

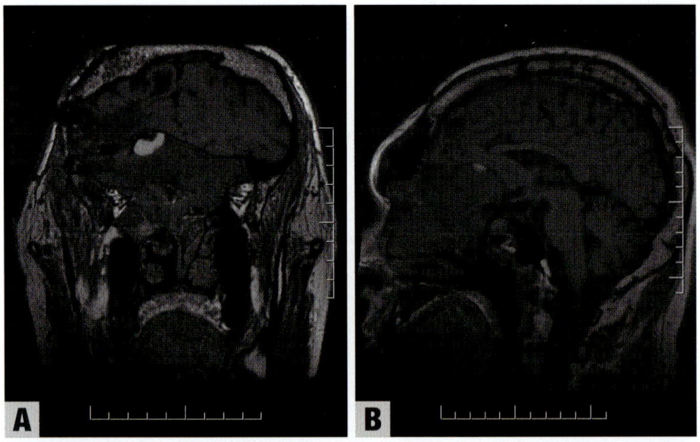

Fig. 13.44 Cranial MRI in McCune–Albright syndrome. Coronal (**A**) and sagittal (**B**) MRI shows extensive residual soft tissue tumour despite frontal craniotomy in a patient with McCune–Albright syndrome. Note the fibrous dysplasia throughout the cranium and skull base.

Growth hormone (GH) and prolactin excess gives rise to acromegaly/gigantism {3910}. Most patients with MAS-related acromegaly have a normal height, which may be attributable to fibrous dysplasia, precocity, and/or hyperthyroidism, and may lead to delayed diagnosis {3910}. Hyperprolactinaemia occurs in about 80% of patients with GH excess {3910}. Diffuse pituitary enlargement, microtumour, macrotumour, and multifocal microtumours have been reported {3910,4740}. Despite the presence of biochemical acromegaly, MRI fails to detect abnormalities in some cases {77,3910,4740}.

Adrenal Cushing syndrome typically manifests in the first year of life {549,3917} and affects 1.7–7.5% of patients {549, 2759}. Weight gain with decreasing growth velocity is characteristic of Cushing syndrome in childhood; however, neonates may develop failure to thrive and severe, life-threatening illness {1167,1621}. Spontaneous resolution has been described in some neonates {549}.

Renal phosphate wasting may lead to osteomalacia/rickets, with an increased risk of fractures and malformations {894,1048, 3398,397}. The phosphaturic factor FGF23 is released from fibrous dysplasia tissue {3746,3917}; as a result, hypophosphataemia is typically seen only in patients with significant skeletal disease {894}.

Hyperpigmented skin macules and fibrous dysplasia are characteristic non-endocrine manifestations of MAS {505}. Less common manifestations include oral pigmentation {3549}, gastrointestinal polyps {3770,4498}, hepatobiliary and pancreatic neoplasms {1519,3451,4933,2124}, and platelet dysfunction {272,4498}. An increased risk of breast cancer and other malignancies has been reported {1740,2801}.

Epidemiology

MAS with multisystem involvement is rare. There are no reliable data establishing disease prevalence; however, estimates range between 1 case per 1 million and 1 case per 100 000 population {506}. In contrast, fibrous dysplasia (particularly as monostotic disease) is not rare; it has been estimated to account for as many as 7% of all benign bone tumours {506}.

Etiology

MAS results from postzygotic somatic activating (gain-of-function) mutations in $G_s\alpha$, one of several transcripts encoded by *GNAS* at 20q13.2-q13.3 {4840}.

Pathogenesis

GNAS is a complex locus with an imprinted expression pattern. Multiple gene products, including maternal, paternal, and biallelic-expressed transcripts, are derived from four promoters and 5′ exons that splice onto a common set of downstream exons (exons 2–13) {4840}. Somatic *GNAS* mutations in MAS occur at one of two residues: R201 (accounting for > 95% of the mutations) {2759} and Q227 (accounting for < 5%) {2023}.

The major product of *GNAS* is $G_s\alpha$, which is generated by the most downstream promoter (exon 1). $G_s\alpha$ is the ubiquitously expressed heterotrimeric G protein α-subunit, which couples seven-transmembrane receptors to the cAMP-generating enzyme adenylyl cyclase and is required for the intracellular cAMP response to hormones and other extracellular signals. The *GNAS* variants at R201 and Q227 disrupt the intrinsic GTPase activity of $G_s\alpha$, causing constitutive activation and abnormal cAMP signalling {2522}.

There are no known genotype–phenotype correlations {5127}. Clinical presentation and disease severity are likely determined by the degree of mosaicism and by the location and extent of affected tissues.

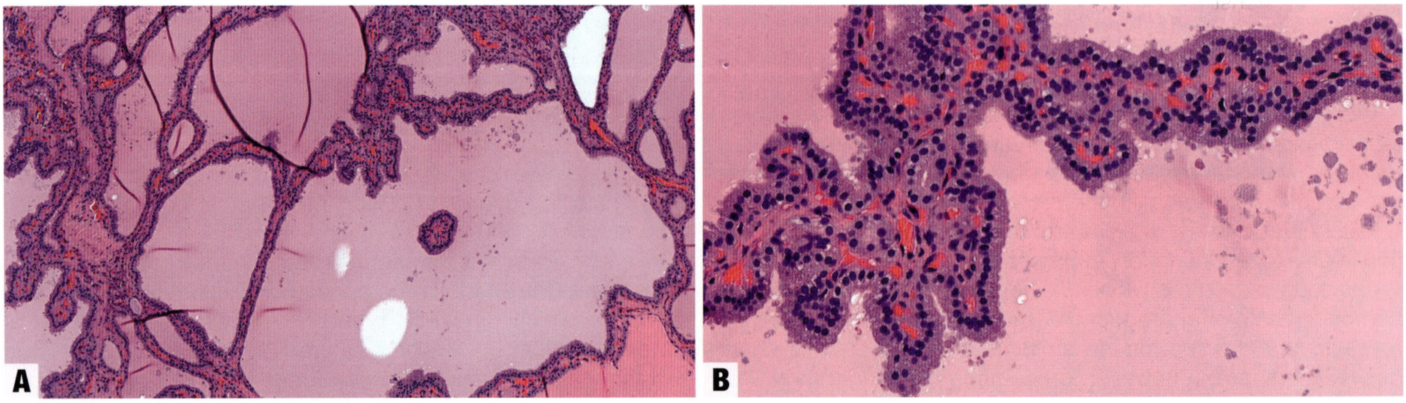

Fig. 13.45 Thyroid nodule in McCune–Albright syndrome. **A** The thyroid nodules exhibit a papillary architecture, with the formation of true papillae that have fibrovascular cores, but the papillae are organized in a centripetal fashion within the follicles and they are lined by uniform epithelial cells with bland, basally located nuclei. **B** Despite the formation of true papillae, the follicular epithelial cells forming the thyroid nodules have uniform, bland cytology with round basal nuclei that have dark chromatin.

Macroscopic appearance

See individual tumour types.

Histopathology

MAS-related gonadal disease: Ovarian follicular cysts lined by granulosa cells are frequently identified in girls with MAS-related precocity {986,2872}. A single case of borderline ovarian serous tumour {809} and another of virilizing sclerosing stromal tumour have been reported in MAS {492}. Testicular enlargement results from the maturation and growth of seminiferous tubules. Orchiectomy specimens reveal large foci of Leydig cell hyperplasia indistinguishable from Leydig cell tumours {504}. Sertoli cell proliferations (including Sertoli cell intraepithelial neoplasia), bilateral testicular germ cell tumours (including embryonal carcinoma), and testicular adrenal rests have also been reported {504}.

MAS-related thyroid disease: The thyroid in patients with MAS has multiple nodules that have been described as multinodular hyperplasia, papillary hyperplasia, or goitre; solitary nodules were interpreted as follicular adenoma with papillary architecture most frequently {714}. Like non-syndromic functioning thyroid nodules (which are typically associated with either *TSHR*-activating or *GNAS*-activating clonal mutations {3141,3394, 3580}, the solitary or multiple functioning nodules that occur in MAS appear warm or hot on scan {4104} and can cause subclinical or clinical hyperthyroidism. Regardless of size, such nodules are called follicular adenomas with papillary architecture and are histologically characterized by benign follicular proliferations with intrafollicular centripetal papillary projections. Rare cases of inflammatory thyroiditis and thyroid carcinomas have been described {895,1740}.

MAS-related pituitary disease: This is heterogeneous and typically involves a subset of PIT1-lineage adenohypophysial cells, including mammosomatotrophs and somatotrophs {1626, 4740,3878}. Some patients present with mammosomatotroph or somatotroph hyperplasia; others develop mammosomatotroph or somatotroph tumours {1626,2417,3910,4740}. Although findings of the non-tumorous anterior pituitary were largely unavailable in some reports, evidence suggests a hyperplasia-to-neoplasia progression sequence and multicentric microtumours in extended resection specimens {4740}. Given the heterogeneous nature of MAS-related pituitary disease, total hypophysectomy is required for surgical cure {3894,4740,5046}.

MAS-related adrenal disease: MAS-related Cushing syndrome typically demonstrates bilateral nodular hyperplasia, which also encompasses presentations with bilateral primary bimorphic adrenocortical disease {673,1167,3917,2141}. Although primary bimorphic adrenocortical disease is not specific to MAS, it is histologically characterized by diffuse nodular hyperplasia juxtaposed with areas of atrophic cortex, resulting in a bimorphic appearance {673}. Hyperplastic foci are distinguished by strong α-inhibin and synaptophysin expression, whereas the thin atrophic cortex reveals strong CD56 expression and lack of zona reticularis {673}. Rare examples of bilateral adenomas have also been described in MAS {673}.

Cytology

The cytopathological features of the various neoplasms associated with MAS-related disease are indistinguishable from those of their sporadic counterparts, which are described elsewhere in this volume and in the other fifth-edition volumes of the WHO Classification of Tumours series.

Box 13.04 Clinical features of McCune–Albright syndrome

Café-au-lait skin macules with characteristic features, including jagged borders and a distribution respecting the midline of the body

Polyostotic or monostotic fibrous dysplasia

Any of the following endocrinopathies:

- Gonadotropin-independent precocious puberty
- Testicular lesions with or without precocious puberty
- Thyroid lesions with or without non-autoimmune hyperthyroidism
- Growth hormone excess or mixed growth hormone and prolactin excess
- Renal phosphate wasting with or without hypophosphataemia
- Neonatal Cushing syndrome

Diagnostic molecular pathology

Documentation of a somatic activating mutation in *GNAS* confirms the diagnosis.

Essential and desirable diagnostic criteria

Essential: at least two of the three clinical features listed in Box 13.04 ***or*** monostotic fibrous dysplasia in a patient with demonstrated *GNAS* mutation.

Desirable: demonstration of *GNAS* mutation in addition to at least two of the three clinical criteria listed in Box 13.04.

Staging

Not relevant

Prognosis and prediction

The prognosis for individuals with MAS varies, depending on disease location and severity. Endocrinopathies persist throughout childhood and adulthood, with the exception of FGF23-mediated hypophosphataemia, which may worsen during periods of rapid linear growth and ameliorate in adulthood when fibrous dysplasia disease activity wanes {3144,1392}. Endocrinopathies can generally be controlled with pharmacotherapies or surgical removal of affected glands {505,2094}.

Optimizing the treatment of endocrinopathies may improve outcomes in fibrous dysplasia. Untreated GH excess is associated with expansion of craniofacial fibrous dysplasia, resulting in macrocephaly, vision loss, and hearing loss {4438,567,502}. Hyperthyroidism and hypophosphataemia increase fractures and malformations in patients with fibrous dysplasia {2595, 3398,397}.

GNAS mutations in MAS are weakly oncogenic, and affected tissues likely carry a small increased risk of malignant transformation {1740,2801}. Fibrous dysplasia rarely undergoes sarcomatous degeneration {3856,2644}, and additional cancers (summarized above) have been reported. Radiotherapy and uncontrolled GH excess may increase the risk of malignant transformation {505}.

This disorder is never inherited, presumably because germline mutations are probably lethal {1774}. Counselling should emphasize that although no pregnancy is at zero risk, the risk of recurrence appears to be no higher than in the general population.

DICER1 syndrome

de Kock L
Foulkes WD
Gill AJ
Mete O
Nosé V

Definition

DICER1 syndrome is an autosomal dominant tumour predisposition syndrome caused by heterozygous germline pathogenic variants in *DICER1*. It is characterized by an increased incidence of benign and malignant lesions involving multiple organ systems, including pleuropulmonary blastoma (PPB), cystic nephroma, embryonal rhabdomyosarcoma of the uterine cervix, and endocrine-related lesions such as multiple benign and malignant thyroid neoplasms, ovarian Sertoli–Leydig cell tumour (SLCT), and pituitary blastoma.

MIM numbering

601200 Pleuropulmonary blastoma familial tumour and dysplasia syndrome; PPBFTDS
606241 DICER1, ribonuclease III; DICER1

ICD-11 coding

None

Related terminology

Not recommended: pleuropulmonary blastoma familial tumour and dysplasia syndrome.

Subtype(s)

GLOW phenotype (global developmental delay, lung cysts, overgrowth, and Wilms tumour), associated with mosaic *DICER1* RNase IIIb hotspot mutations

Localization

Associated tumours arise in almost all major organ systems, including the thyroid, lungs and pleura, kidneys, urinary bladder, brain, liver, genitourinary tract (predominantly the ovaries, uterine corpus, and cervix in female patients, and the testes and paratestes in male patients), eye, and pituitary and pineal glands {1060,1631}. Individuals with clinically overt *DICER1* syndrome typically manifest one or two sites of disease in childhood or early adulthood; those with predisposing mosaic RNase IIIb hotspot mutations often develop numerous sites of disease, generally at an earlier age than those with germline variants {525}. Bilateral disease in paired organs is not unusual {2908}.

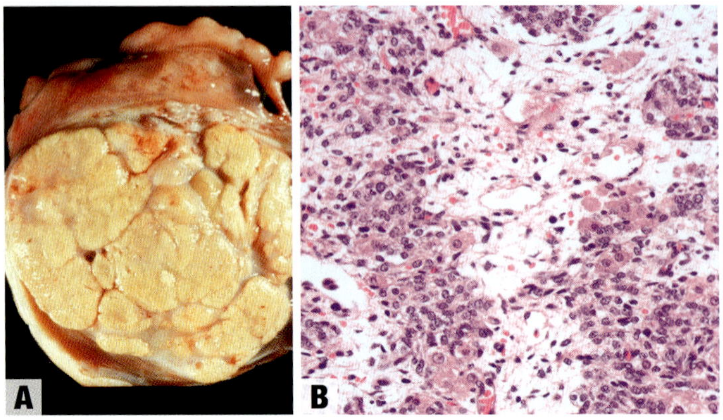

Fig. 13.46 Sertoli–Leydig cell tumour. **A** *DICER1*-related Sertoli–Leydig cell tumours are always moderately poorly differentiated, solid and cystic, and pale tan. **B** An example with intermediate differentiation. These tumours often grow in cellular lobules, as seen in this picture. The lobules are usually predominantly composed of dark-staining Sertoli cells with fewer Leydig cells. The latter are often conspicuous at the periphery of the lobules, as seen to some degree in this picture at the 3 o'clock position.

Clinical features

DICER1 syndrome features a number of characteristic tumours and dysplastic conditions {1060,1631}. Table 13.07

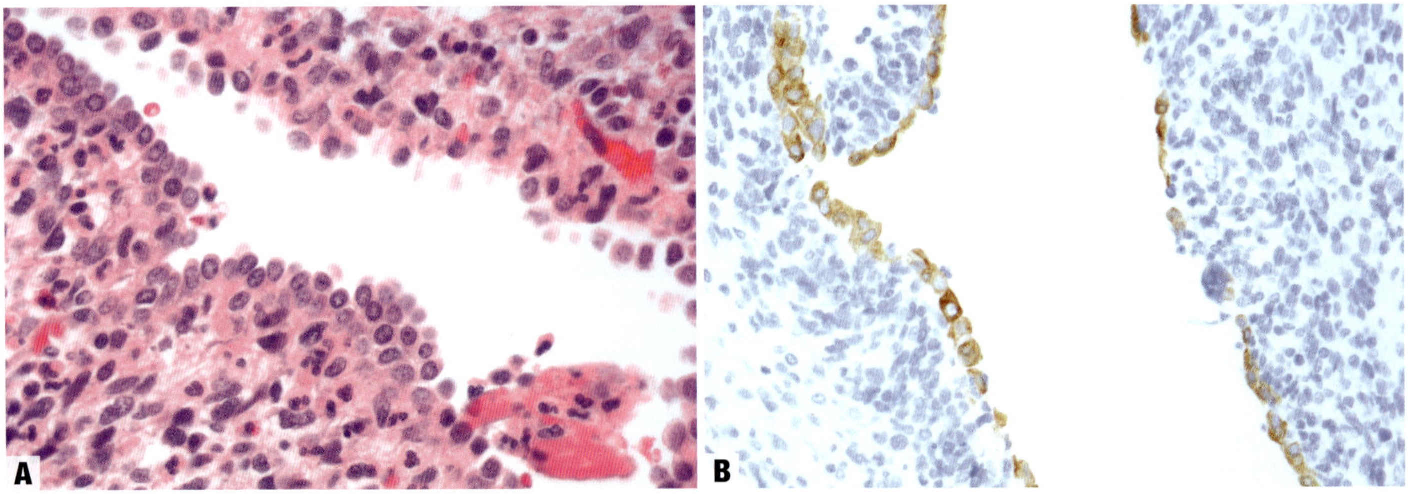

Fig. 13.47 *DICER1*-related pleuropulmonary blastoma. **A** Type I cysts are lined by epithelial cells, beneath which lie primitive mesenchymal tumour cells. **B** Type I cysts in pleuropulmonary blastoma are lined by keratin-positive epithelial cells.

summarizes the associated conditions, their age ranges, and their specificities for the syndrome; the syndrome phenotype is still emerging and may not be limited to the listed conditions. The most notable endocrine manifestations are multinodular goitre, differentiated thyroid carcinoma (DTC), and (more rarely) poorly differentiated thyroid carcinoma {794}, as well as ovarian sex cord stromal tumours, particularly SLCT. *DICER1*-related gynandroblastoma, juvenile granulosa cell tumours, and ovarian and testicular Sertoli cell tumours have also been reported {4811,269,1622}. These gonadal tumours may produce symptoms relating to abnormal hormone secretion. Pituitary blastoma is associated with Cushing disease in infants {2676}. Non-neoplastic syndrome manifestations include macrocephaly {2268} and ocular {1998}, structural renal {2270}, and dental abnormalities {833}. A subset of patients with mosaic RNase IIIb {2329} and germline RNase IIIa {3591} hotspot mutations also exhibit global developmental delay and/or overgrowth (GLOW phenotype [global developmental delay, lung cysts, overgrowth, and Wilms tumour]).

Table 13.07 *DICER1* syndrome phenotypes

Phenotypes	Age range in years (peak)	Specificity for *DICER1* syndrome
Most frequent phenotypes		
Pleuropulmonary blastoma[a]	0–8	High
Type I (cystic)	(0–2)	High
Type II (cystic and solid)	(1–5)	High
Type III (solid)	(1.5–6)	High
Type Ir (cystic)	Any age	High
Cystic nephroma	0–15 (0–4)	High
Ovarian Sertoli–Leydig cell tumour	2–40 (10–25)	High
Thyroid follicular nodular disease	2–40 (10–25)	Low, unless familial or age < 18 years
Moderately frequent phenotypes		
Embryonal rhabdomyosarcoma of the uterine cervix[a]	4–45 (10–20)	High
Nasal chondromesenchymal hamartoma	5–25 (8–20)	Moderate
Differentiated thyroid carcinoma	5–45 (10–30)	Low, unless age < 18 years
Rare phenotypes		
Pituitary blastoma	0–2	Very high
Anaplastic renal sarcoma[a]	2–20	High
Pineoblastoma	2–25 (2–10)	Moderate
Ciliary body medulloepithelioma	3–10	Moderate
Juvenile hamartomatous intestinal polyps	0–20 (0–4)	Low
Wilms tumour	3–8	Low
Embryonal rhabdomyosarcoma of the bladder[a]	0–12	Undetermined
Cerebral sarcoma[a]	Undetermined	Undetermined
Very rare phenotypes		
Infantile cerebellar embryonal tumour	0–1	High
Ovarian embryonal rhabdomyosarcoma[a]	Undetermined	High
Gynandroblastoma	Undetermined	High
Presacral malignant teratoid tumour	Undetermined	High
Pleuropulmonary blastoma–like peritoneal sarcoma[a]	Undetermined	Likely high
Well-differentiated fetal lung adenocarcinoma	Undetermined	Low
Paratesticular sarcoma[a]	Undetermined	Low
Poorly differentiated thyroid carcinoma	Undetermined	Undetermined
Testicular stromal cell tumour	Undetermined	Undetermined
Mesenchymal hamartoma of the liver	0–8 (0–3)	Undetermined

[a]*DICER1*-associated sarcomas, regardless of the site of origin, exhibit similar and characteristic histology and closely resemble pleuropulmonary blastoma. The use of a unified nomenclature to describe these lesions has been proposed {2910,2909}.

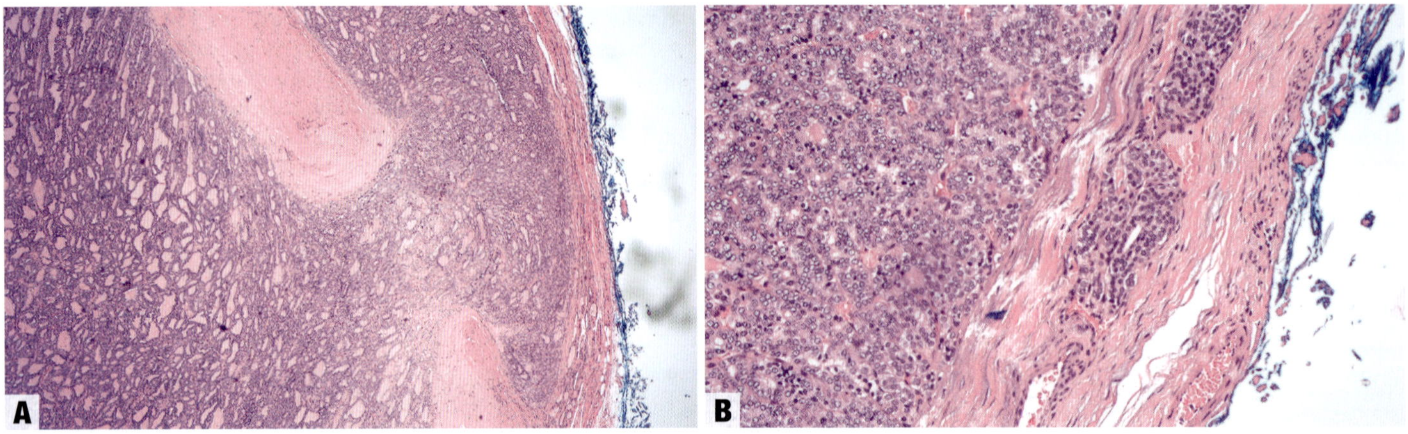

Fig. 13.48 Differentiated thyroid carcinoma arising in *DICER1* syndrome. **A** The diagnosis of thyroid carcinoma in *DICER1* syndrome should be restricted to lesions showing invasive growth. Here, a follicular carcinoma shows mushrooming growth into the adjacent thyroid. **B** The differentiated thyroid carcinomas arising in *DICER1* syndrome usually demonstrate a follicular or solid architecture. The nuclei may show subtle nuclear atypia.

Epidemiology

DICER1 syndrome is rare and exhibits incomplete penetrance that is dependent on both age and sex. In a recent study using the genome-first approach, it was determined that putative loss-of-function *DICER1* sequence variants are present in about 1 in 4000 individuals {3028}, which is more prevalent than the previous estimate of about 1 in 10 000 individuals {2286}. In this study, the penetrance of malignant tumours in *DICER1* heterozygotes was 16% by the age of 50 years {3028}. The most penetrant manifestation is multinodular goitre, occurring in about 75% of heterozygous women and 10–20% of heterozygous men by the age of 40 years {2269}. The risk of thyroid carcinoma is estimated to be increased 9-fold to 16-fold {3028, 2269}. Macrocephaly is documented in about 42% of patients with *DICER1* syndrome {2268}, and lung cysts (presumptively considered PPB type I/Ir) have been observed in about 45% of systematically screened at-risk patients {525}. The penetrance of other tumours is lower. *DICER1* syndrome disproportionately affects the female sex, a bias accounted for by the increased prevalence of thyroid disease and the presence of gynaecological manifestations in female patients {1060}.

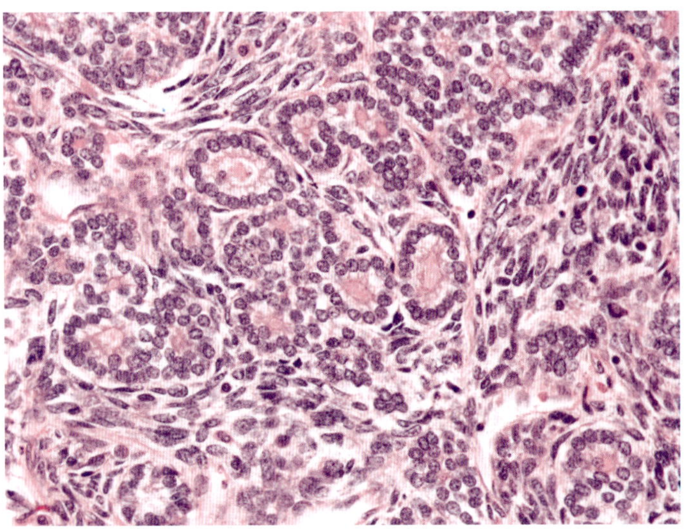

Fig. 13.49 Thyroblastoma. This is an underrecognized *DICER1*-associated tumour with primitive thyroid follicles surrounded by primitive spindle cell stroma, mimicking thyroid in development.

Etiology

DICER1 syndrome is caused by heterozygous germline pathogenic sequence variants in *DICER1*, located on chromosome 14q32 {1412}. Therapeutic or diagnostic radiation exposure in patients with *DICER1* syndrome may increase the risk of thyroid malignancy {1021}.

Pathogenesis

DICER1 functions canonically as an RNase III endoribonuclease central to microRNA biogenesis. DICER1 cleaves 20- to 22-nucleotide-long microRNAs from each strand of a hairpin-shaped precursor; the RNase IIIb domain cleaves the 5p microRNA from the 5′ arm, and the RNase IIIa domain cleaves the 3p microRNA from the 3′ arm. Mature microRNAs function to posttranscriptionally silence expression of target genes {1412}. *DICER1* syndrome tumours follow a two-hit model of pathogenesis whereby germline variants, which typically inactivate one allele, are coupled in tumours by highly characteristic second somatic hotspot missense mutations, which affect one of five metal-ion binding or adjacent residues in the RNase IIIb domain {1412}. RNase IIIb–mutated DICER1 exhibits impaired processing of 5p microRNAs, resulting in an altered 5p:3p microRNA ratio {152,3628,3151}, which, together with concomitant dysregulation of gene expression, is hypothesized to underlie tumorigenesis.

Macroscopic appearance

Other than showing a tendency towards multifocality, syndromic lesions are grossly indistinguishable from sporadic tumours.

Histopathology

DICER1-related endocrine manifestations

Pituitary blastoma is a characteristic *DICER1*-related neoplasm consisting of primitive blastemal cells, neuroendocrine cells, and Rathke pouch epithelium {3989}.

Most patients with *DICER1*-related thyroid disease feature thyroid follicular nodular disease that consists of multiple benign follicular nodules with variable architecture and subtle atypia, or follicular adenomas including those with intrafollicular centripetal papillary growth {4825,1706,794,614}. The diagnosis of malignancy is restricted to tumours with invasive growth and is enriched in low-risk follicular-patterned DTCs {4825,468,1855,614}. Poorly differentiated thyroid carcinomas arising in childhood or adolescence are less common but also strongly related to *DICER1* mutations {794}. In the appropriate morphological and clinical (e.g. absence of thyroid hormone administration or hyperthyroidism) context, the identification of variable involutional changes in the non-nodular thyroid parenchyma should raise suspicion of *DICER1*-related pathogenesis {4825,614}. Thyroblastoma, a rare *DICER1* gene–related thyroid manifestation, shows a primitive microfollicular structure surrounded by primitive spindle cells with or without heterologous elements {32,3809}.

Ovarian sex cord stromal tumours are almost always SLCT, but occasionally they are juvenile granulosa cell tumours or tumours of mixed forms (gynandroblastoma). *DICER1*-related SLCT are always moderately/poorly differentiated, and the presence of retiform and heterologous elements is highly predictive of *DICER1* mutation {1022,2228,2207}.

Other manifestations

PPB type I cysts are lined by epithelium, beneath which lie primitive mesenchymal tumour cells. The solid component of PPB type II/III is characterized by a high-grade sarcoma featuring at least two of the following: blastema, embryonal rhabdomyosarcoma, spindle cell sarcoma, and/or cartilage. Cystic nephroma is composed of variably sized cysts with a myxoid mesenchymal stroma, mimicking PPB type I. Embryonal rhabdomyosarcoma of the cervix or bladder shows primitive cells under an intact epithelium, likewise resembling PPB type I. Nasal chondromesenchymal hamartoma is composed of cysts lined by respiratory epithelium, immature cartilage, and mesenchyme.

Cytology

Because of the risk of thyroid neoplasia, thyroid nodules often require further investigation by FNAB {2269,1420}.

Diagnostic molecular pathology

Germline *DICER1* alterations are most often loss-of-function (frameshift, nonsense, or splice-site) mutations and are distributed across the entire coding region of the gene. A small minority are deletions of the entire *DICER1* locus, in-frame and out-of-frame intragenic deletions involving one or more exons, or (rarely) somatic mosaicism of loss-of-function variants or RNase IIIb hotspot mutations {1060}. In contrast to the wide distribution of germline variants, the second somatic mutations in *DICER1*-related lesions occur predominantly at hotspots within the RNase IIIb domain. Therefore, identification of an RNase IIIb hotspot mutation in a tumour should lead to broader testing of *DICER1* in the germline, because many panels designed to identify hotspot alterations may not identify the pathogenic germline variants. In a small percentage of tumours, the second mutation may be loss of the wildtype allele {1060,1059}.

In DTC, somatic *DICER1* alterations appear to be mutually exclusive with the most common somatic driver alterations, including *BRAF* p.V600E, RAS mutations, and *RET* rearrangements {4825,2590,1706,794}. Therefore, a useful clue to a *DICER1* etiology is the occurrence of a dark-matter thyroid malignancy (i.e. a thyroid tumour with no other known driver) occurring in a younger patient, particularly if the malignancy is poorly differentiated or a macrofollicular pattern of follicular thyroid carcinoma {468,1855,2590,794}.

Essential and desirable diagnostic criteria

Essential: demonstration of a germline *DICER1* pathogenic variant.

Desirable: a personal or family history of pathologically confirmed syndrome-related lesions, particularly those with a high specificity for *DICER1* syndrome, as detailed in Table 13.07 (p. 475).

Staging

Staging of individual tumours is based on the Union for International Cancer Control (UICC) / American Joint Committee on Cancer (AJCC) systems.

Prognosis and prediction

Presently, there are no data to suggest that the presence of a germline *DICER1* pathogenic variant influences the prognosis of syndrome-related tumours as compared with their sporadic counterparts. In general, outcome is favourable after diagnosis of multinodular goitre, DTC, ovarian sex cord stromal tumour, cystic nephroma, embryonal rhabdomyosarcoma of the uterine cervix, nasal chondromesenchymal hamartoma, and ciliary body medulloepithelioma. The prognosis is worse for poorly differentiated thyroid carcinoma {794}, and survival rates may be as low as 50% for PPB types II and III; pituitary blastoma; and anaplastic renal, peritoneal, and cerebral sarcomas {4745, 2949,2676,2173}.

Glucagon cell hyperplasia and neoplasia

Sipos B
Ezzat S
Gill AJ
Klöppel G
Mete O

Definition

Glucagon cell hyperplasia and neoplasia (GCHN) is an autosomal recessive syndrome usually attributable to pathogenic germline *GCGR* variants and characterized by widespread glucagon cell hyperplasia of the pancreas that progresses to multifocal neuroendocrine neoplasms (NENs) expressing glucagon almost exclusively.

MIM numbering

619290 Mahvash disease; MVAH

ICD-11 coding

2C10.1 Neuroendocrine neoplasms of pancreas

Related terminology

Not recommended: glucagon cell adenomatosis; Mahvash disease.

Subtype(s)

None

Localization

GCHN arises throughout the pancreas.

Clinical features

Patients present with nonspecific symptoms, such as abdominal pain, altered bowel habits, fatigue, diabetes, and/or acute pancreatitis. Serum glucagon levels are very high, but this is not accompanied by the anticipated actions of this hormone. Because of the receptor's deficient signalling, glucagonoma syndrome is not expected. However, 1 patient with wildtype *GCGR* presented with glucagonoma syndrome and necrolytic migratory erythema {3374,5096,2528}. A patient with PTH-independent hypercalcaemia has been reported {1571}. Abdominal imaging may reveal lesions of various sizes throughout the pancreas, which may also be SSTR-reactive on PET imaging {1862,4169,5098}. The only reported paediatric patient showed elevated levels of serum amino acids (e.g. glutamine, alanine, and arginine) at 2 months of age. During the first few years of life, the patient had anorexia and repeated emesis {2630}.

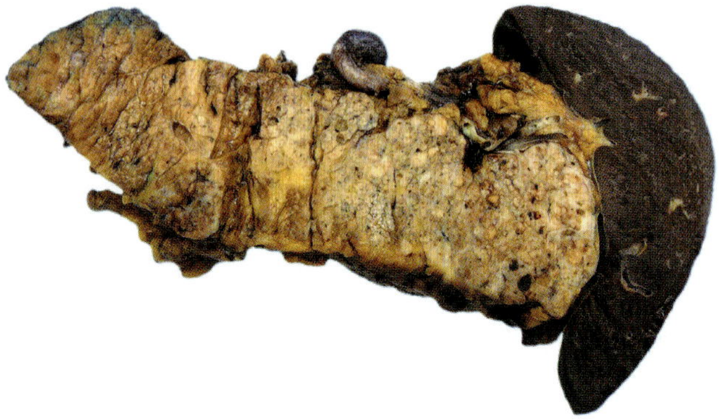

Fig. 13.50 Glucagon cell hyperplasia and neoplasia. The pancreas is diffusely enlarged. Its cut surface has a firm texture due to multiple coalescing glucagon-producing neoplasms.

Epidemiology

GCHN is an extremely rare disease; 14 cases have been reported to date. Both sexes seem to be equally affected. The age ranges from 7 to 68 years {5096}.

Etiology

More than 50% of the examined patients with GCHN showed germline sequence variants of *GCGR*, located on chromosome 17q25 {1862,4169,5098,3013}. Examinations in 1 index patient and his parents indicate that GCHN with *GCGR* mutation follows an autosomal recessive inheritance {4169}. The genetic disease

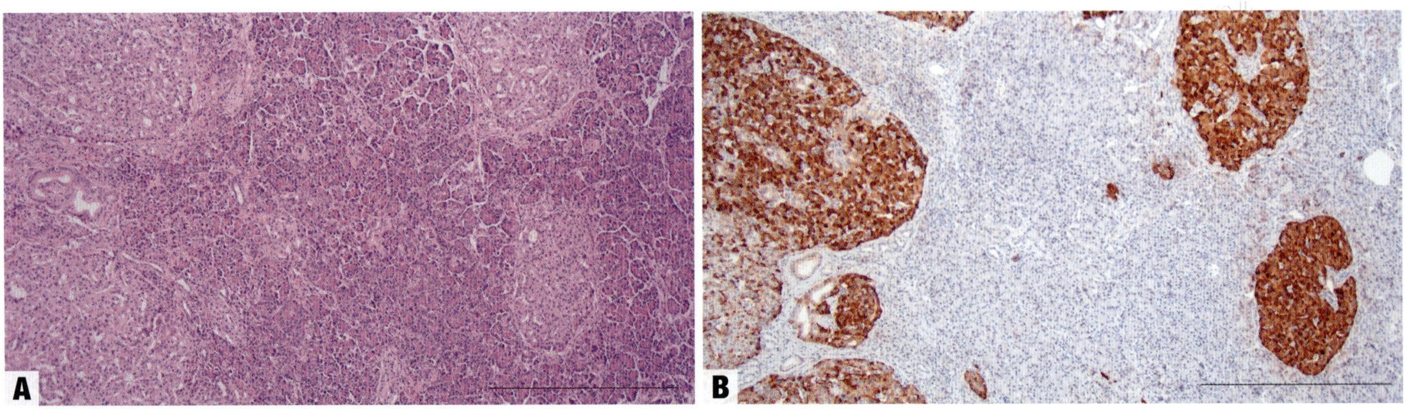

Fig. 13.51 Glucagon cell hyperplasia and neoplasia. **A** Multiple enlarged endocrine islets and microtumours are unevenly distributed throughout the entire pancreas. **B** By immunohistochemistry, hypertrophic islets and tumours exhibit glucagon expression almost exclusively.

mechanism in patients without *GCGR* mutation remains unclear {4169,112}. No alterations in *MEN1* or *VHL* have been identified.

Pathogenesis

GCHN harbours either homozygous *GCGR* sequence variants or at least two compound heterozygous sequence variants leading to premature stop codons or deficient protein expression. Deficient glucagon signalling in the liver causes a disturbance in a presumed feedback mechanism between the liver and the glucagon cells, which is probably mediated by amino acids {1571}. This leads to glucagon cell hyperplasia, elevated serum glucagon levels, and finally to neuroendocrine tumours (NETs).

Macroscopic appearance

Macroscopically, the pancreas can be normal-sized or enlarged. On the cut surface there are multiple white-yellow nodules ranging from a few millimetres to many centimetres in diameter {5098,1862,4169}.

Histopathology

Throughout the entire pancreatic tissue there are normal-sized and hypertrophic islets randomly distributed between microtumours, and in some cases also single macrotumours. Large tumours may undergo cystic transformation and focal calcification. The tumour cells are monomorphic and exhibit round or oval nuclei. The mitotic activity is very low. Micrometastases have been reported in regional lymph nodes but are rare {1862, 4169,1571}.

Immunohistochemically, the microtumours and macrotumours are almost exclusively composed of glucagon-positive cells, but they may occasionally also express PP {1571}. In the hypertrophic islets, glucagon-positive cells outnumber insulin cells and somatostatin cells. All endocrine cells express SSTR2A. Ki-67 labelling is very low (< 1%) {5098,1862,4169}. GCHN with *GCGR* mutation seems to have a more advanced phenotype regarding the number of hypertrophic islets and microtumours and the occurrence of macrotumours. Lymph node metastases were found in 1 patient with wildtype *GCGR* {4169}.

Cytology

Not clinically relevant

Diagnostic molecular pathology

Sequencing all exons of *GCGR*, including splice sites, is obligatory before *GCGR* mutation can be excluded. To date, sequence variants of *GCGR* have been reported in exons 2, 4, 8, 10, 11, and 12 {2630}.

Essential and desirable diagnostic criteria

Essential: markedly elevated serum glucagon levels; hypertrophic islets merging with multiple pancreatic neuroendocrine tumours (PanNETs), expressing glucagon predominantly or exclusively.

Desirable: identification of pathogenic germline *GCGR* variants; exclusion of multiple endocrine neoplasia type 1 and other syndromes associated with pancreatic neuroendocrine cell hyperplasia and microtumours.

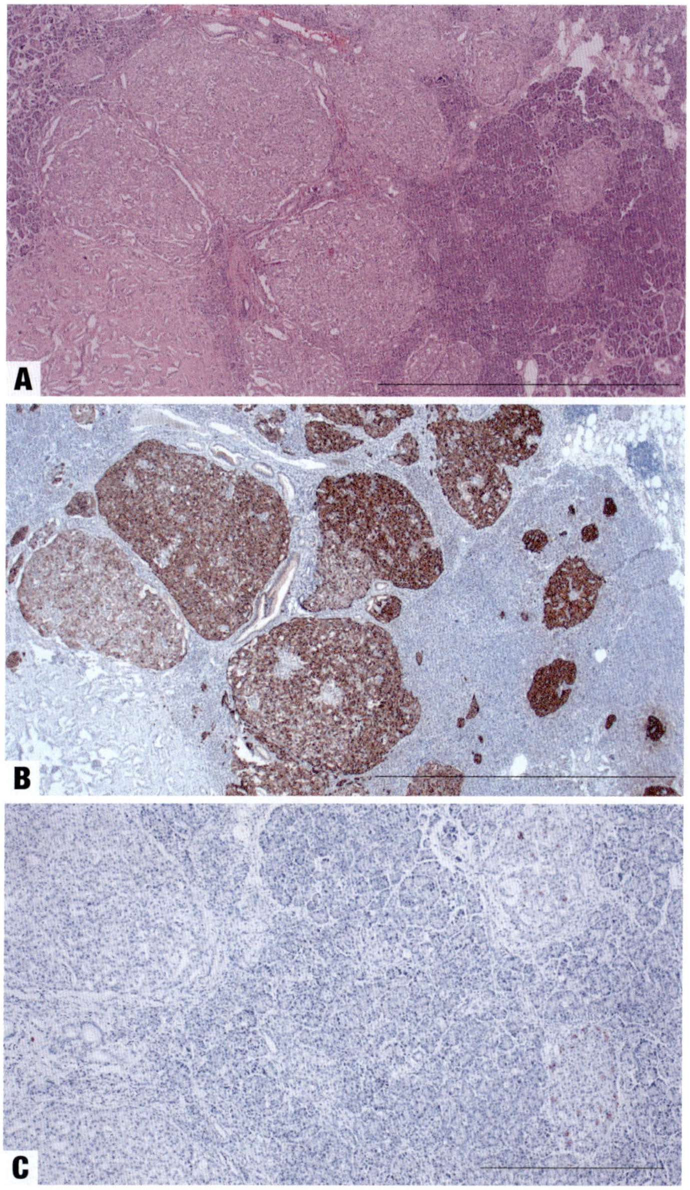

Fig. 13.52 Glucagon cell hyperplasia and neoplasia. **A** Numerous enlarged endocrine islets and microtumours are unevenly distributed throughout the entire pancreas. **B** Hypertrophic islets and tumours exhibit glucagon expression almost exclusively. **C** Minimal and focal insulin expression in the hypertrophic islets and tumours.

Staging

Staging follows the Union for International Cancer Control (UICC) / American Joint Committee on Cancer (AJCC) staging systems for PanNETs.

Prognosis and prediction

To date, all reported cases of GCHN have followed a benign clinical course except one. No recurrence of the disease has been noted in patients who underwent partial pancreatectomy {4169}. However, lifelong follow-up of these patients is indicated, because the tumours can metastasize. One patient died of severe migratory necrotizing erythema and sepsis {3374}.

MAFA-related familial insulinomatosis

Asa SL
Ezzat S
Gill AJ
Klöppel G
Mete O
Sipos B

Definition

MAFA-related familial insulinomatosis is an autosomal dominant syndrome caused by pathogenic *MAFA* sequence variants. It is characterized by multiple insulin-secreting pancreatic neuroendocrine tumours (PanNETs) that usually present as adult-onset hyperinsulinaemic hypoglycaemia.

MIM numbering

147630 Insulinomatosis and diabetes mellitus; INSDM

ICD-11 coding

2E92.9 Benign neoplasm of endocrine pancreas

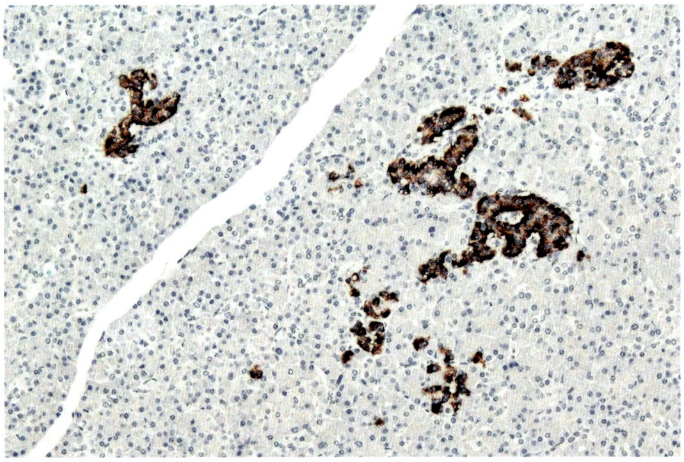

Fig. 13.53 *MAFA*-related familial insulinomatosis. The pancreas in *MAFA*-related insulinomatosis contains innumerable multicentric islet B-cell proliferations that stain for insulin.

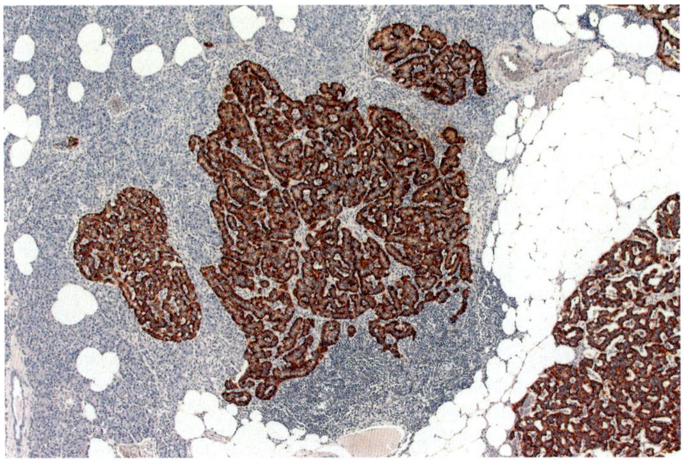

Fig. 13.54 *MAFA*-related familial insulinomatosis. There are multiple neuroendocrine trabecular microtumours (< 5 mm) and well-differentiated islet B-cell neuroendocrine tumours (> 5 mm) that are composed exclusively of insulin-positive cells.

Related terminology

Acceptable: familial insulinomatosis.

Subtype(s)

None

Localization

The disorder is restricted to the pancreas, where MAFA plays a critical role as a transcription factor regulating pancreatic B-cell function and proliferation.

Clinical features

Reflecting the role of MAFA as both an oncogene and an islet B-cell transcription factor, presentation is with either hyperinsulinaemic hypoglycaemia or diabetes, with the hypoglycaemic presentation being more common in female patients and the diabetic presentation being more common in male patients {2016}. Although the two manifestations are generally mutually exclusive, 1 patient with diabetes went on to develop hyperinsulinism and multifocal islet B-cell pancreatic proliferations {2016}. Onset is in adulthood, which distinguishes it from congenital hyperinsulinism. Clues to the diagnosis in patients presenting with diabetes include a normal body mass index, no other clinical features of insulin resistance, no history of diabetic ketoacidosis, and negative islet autoantibodies {2016}. Imaging identifies multicentric PanNETs that can measure > 10 mm {2016}.

Epidemiology

This disorder is too rare to determine the actual incidence and prevalence. Although the mutation is found equally in both sexes, hyperinsulinaemic hypoglycaemia has been reported to be more frequent in women, whereas men in the same kindreds develop diabetes more commonly. The onset of symptoms is usually in the fourth decade of life and there is no history of congenital hyperinsulinism {2016}.

Etiology

This disorder is attributed to a specific germline mutation, p.S64F, in the gene encoding the transcription factor MAFA. The presence of a *MAFA* mutation distinguishes this disorder from sporadic insulinomatosis {2016}.

Pathogenesis

MAFA is a bZIP-containing transcription factor that regulates glucose-stimulated insulin secretion {171,4266}; it also has oncogenic transformation potential in vitro. A specific mutation, p.S64F, impairs phosphorylation in the MAFA transactivation domain, resulting in increased protein stability that is insensitive to glucose concentrations, thereby interrupting the regulatory action of MAFA. In addition, MAFA p.S64F exhibits enhanced transactivation compared with wildtype MAFA {2016}.

Macroscopic appearance

The pancreas of patients with this disorder shows multifocal small tumours that vary in size and can reach > 10 mm.

Histopathology

The pancreas of patients with *MAFA*-related insulinomatosis contain innumerable multicentric islet B-cell proliferations, ranging from dysplastic B-cell cords to multifocal neuroendocrine trabecular microtumours (< 5 mm) and solitary well-differentiated tumours (> 5 mm) (Ki-67 index: < 2%). Although the islets contain insulin, glucagon, PP, and somatostatin-producing cells in normal distributions and numbers, the trabecular proliferations are exclusively positive for insulin, which helps distinguish the condition from multiple endocrine neoplasia type 1 and from glucagon cell adenomatosis and hyperplasia {153,2016}.

Cytology

PanNETs may come to FNAB, and their cytopathological features are described in the *WHO reporting system for pancreaticobiliary cytopathology*.

Diagnostic molecular pathology

A missense *MAFA* c.191C>T p.S64F sequence variant has been shown to segregate with the manifestations of both hyperinsulinism and diabetes. To date, other *MAFA* mutations have not been reported.

Essential and desirable diagnostic criteria

Essential: a pathogenic sequence variant of *MAFA*, with evidence of multifocal pancreatic trabecular islet B-cell proliferations staining for insulin.

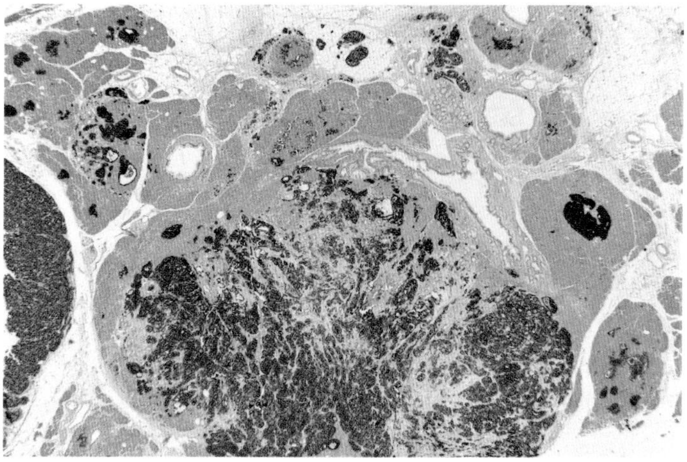

Fig. 13.55 *MAFA*-related familial insulinomatosis. Multicentric islet B-cell proliferations range from dysplastic B-cell cords to microtumours and well-differentiated tumours, all staining intensely and exclusively for insulin.

Staging

Not relevant

Prognosis and prediction

Medical therapy yields poor results with persistent hypoglycaemia {2016}. Most patients have undergone partial pancreatectomy, but this has not led to cure, and several patients have undergone multiple surgical procedures. The multifocal nature of the islet B-cell proliferations suggests that total pancreatectomy would be required for cure {4195}. Local or distant metastases have not been documented.

Syndromic familial follicular cell–derived thyroid tumours

Cameselle-Teijeiro JM
Erickson LA
LiVolsi V
Nosé V

Definition

Syndromic familial follicular cell–derived thyroid tumours are a heterogeneous group of familial follicular cell–derived carcinomas with a predominance of non-thyroid cancer.

MIM numbering

188550 Thyroid cancer, non-medullary, 1; NMTC1
188470 Thyroid cancer, non-medullary, 2; NMTC2
606240 Thyroid cancer, non-medullary, 3; NMTC3
616534 Thyroid cancer, non-medullary, 4; NMTC4
616535 Thyroid cancer, non-medullary, 5; NMTC5

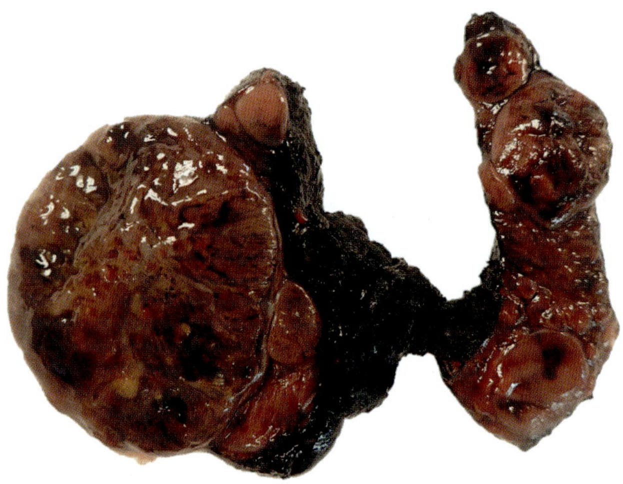

Fig. 13.56 *PTEN* hamartoma tumour syndrome. The thyroid gland in these patients typically shows multiple bilateral nodules.

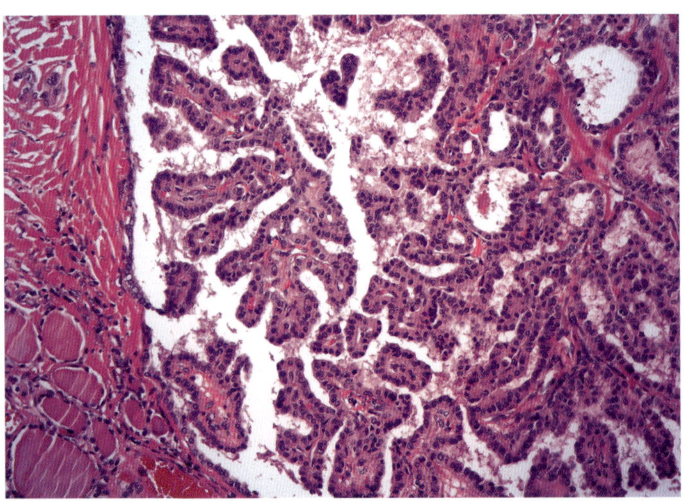

Fig. 13.57 *PTEN* hamartoma tumour syndrome. Conventional papillary thyroid carcinoma in a patient with known germline *PTEN* mutation.

ICD-11 coding

None

Related terminology

Acceptable: syndromic familial non-medullary thyroid carcinoma.

PTEN hamartoma tumour syndrome

Acceptable: Cowden syndrome; Cowden disease; Bannayan–Riley–Ruvalcaba syndrome; PTEN-related Proteus syndrome; PTEN-related Proteus-like syndrome.

Familial adenomatous polyposis

Not recommended: Gardner syndrome (almost all patients with familial adenomatous polyposis [FAP] have the same features).

DICER1 syndrome

Acceptable: pleuropulmonary blastoma familial tumour.

Carney complex

Acceptable: NAME syndrome (naevi, atrial myxoma, myxoid neurofibromas, and ephelides); LAMB syndrome (lentigines, atrial myxoma, mucocutaneous myoma, and blue naevus).

Werner syndrome

Acceptable: adult-onset progeria.

Subtype(s)

PTEN hamartoma tumour syndrome

Cowden syndrome; Cowden disease; Bannayan–Riley–Ruvalcaba syndrome; *PTEN*-related Proteus syndrome; *PTEN*-related Proteus-like syndrome.

Localization

Syndromic familial non-medullary thyroid carcinoma is often multifocal and usually affects both lobes at presentation {614}.

Clinical features

This is a heterogeneous group of familial cancer syndromes in which clinical manifestations of non-thyroid lesions predominate (see Table 13.08).

Epidemiology

The prevalence of *PTEN* hamartoma tumour syndrome (PHTS) is about 1 case per 200 000 population {5060}. The prevalence of FAP is 1 in 8 000–10 000 and it affects men and women equally {4673}; however, thyroid cancer in this setting is much more frequent in women (M:F ratio: 1:61) {615}. The prevalence of *DICER1* loss-of-function variants in population databases ranges from 1 in 2529 to 1 in 10 600 {2284}. Carney complex is a rare disease with an unknown prevalence {918,494} and a female predominance

{407}. Werner syndrome is thought to be underdiagnosed {1447}, and its prevalence is highly influenced by founder mutations and consanguinity {1644}. The frequency of pathogenic *WRN* variants was 2.12% among 9019 individuals in a recent study {1447}; in this group, the average age of patients with thyroid cancer was 39 years and the M:F ratio was 1:1–2.3 {2049,3365}.

Etiology

PHTS is caused by germline mutations in *PTEN* {5060}, in other genes (*PIK3CA*, *AKT1*, or SDH genes), or by germline *KLLN* methylation epimutation {3232,5061}; another 3–6% of individuals with PHTS have germline heterozygous *SEC23B* pathogenic variants, which are particularly associated with thyroid cancer {5062,5059}.

FAP is secondary to germline mutations in *APC* that result in a truncated or absent APC protein {1679}.

Over 70% of individuals with *DICER1* syndrome have a germline loss-of-function mutation with a second, tumour-specific missense mutation in the RNase IIIb domain; most mutations are inherited, but 10–20% appear to arise de novo {4031,1412, 3628}. Intronic mutations and large deletions have also been reported {4031,1874,2268}.

Most cases of Carney complex are due to germline heterozygous inactivating mutations of *PRKAR1A*, encoding the type I regulatory subunit of PKA {407,494}; *PRKAR1A* c.491-492del is associated with more frequent thyroid tumours {494}. Deleterious *PDE11A* variants have been described in patients with Carney complex associated with a *PRKAR1A* mutation {2651}.

Table 13.08 Syndromic familial non-medullary thyroid carcinoma

Syndrome	Gene (locus), inheritance	Gene MIM number	Thyroid lesions [incidence]	Other lesions
***PTEN* hamartoma tumour syndrome** {5060,5062,3224}	*PTEN* (10q23.31), AD	158350	PTC (classic and follicular variant) [60%]; FTC [14–45%]; HCC [~1%]; ATC [< 1%]; FTA (HCA, lipoadenoma, and microadenomas) [25%]; TFND [43–75%]; C-cell hyperplasia; lymphocytic thyroiditis [55%]	*Pathognomonic criteria:*[a] Adult Lhermitte–Duclos disease (cerebellar tumours), facial trichilemmomas, acral keratosis, papillomatous papules, autism spectrum disorder *Major criteria:*[a] Breast cancer, macrocephaly, endometrial carcinoma, multiple palmoplantar keratosis, multifocal cutaneous facial papules, macular pigmentation of the glans penis, multiple gastrointestinal hamartomas or ganglioneuromas *Minor criteria:*[a] Single gastrointestinal hamartoma or ganglioneuroma, fibrocystic breast disease, lipomas, fibromas, genitourinary tumours (particularly renal cell carcinoma), genitourinary malformations, uterine fibroids, intellectual disability (IQ ≤ 75)
Familial adenomatous polyposis {615,724,3242}	*APC* (5q22.2), AD	611731	Cribriform-morular thyroid carcinoma [16%]	Adenomatous polyps of the large bowel, colorectal adenocarcinoma, duodenal adenomas and carcinomas, GAPPS, desmoid tumours, hepatobiliary tree tumours, hepatoblastoma, adrenocortical adenomas and carcinomas, brain tumours, CHRPE
***DICER1* syndrome** {4284,2269,4030,4825}	*DICER1* (14q32.13), AD	606241	TC (PTC, FTC, PDTC)[b]; FTA; TFND	Macrocephaly, PPB, peritoneal PPB, pulmonary cysts and/or pneumothorax in a newborn or young child, ovarian tumours (Sertoli–Leydig cell tumour, gynandroblastoma, undifferentiated sarcomas, embryonal rhabdomyosarcoma), ciliary body medulloepithelioma, pituitary blastoma, CNS sarcoma, CNS embryonal tumours, pineoblastoma, nasal chondromesenchymal hamartoma, multicystic hepatic lesions, cystic nephroma, presacral teratoid neoplasm
Carney complex {407,494,4298,4295}	*PRKAR1A* (17q24.2), AD	188830	TC (FTC, PTC) [15%]; TFND (follicular adenomatosis); FTA	*Major criteria*: Spotty skin pigmentation (lips, conjunctiva and inner or outer canthi, vaginal and penile mucosa), myxoma (cutaneous, mucosal, cardiac, breast), growth hormone–producing pituitary adenoma, primary pigmented nodular adrenocortical disease, blue naevus and pigmented epithelioid melanocytoma (multiple), breast ductal adenoma (multiple), osteochondromyxoma, psammomatous melanotic schwannoma
Werner syndrome {2049,1644,3365}	*WRN* (8p12), AR	604611	TC (FTC, PTC, ATC) [18%]	Bilateral ocular cataracts, premature greying and/or thinning of scalp hair, short stature, chronic ulcers around the ankles, meningioma, melanoma, soft tissue sarcomas, osteosarcomas, leukaemia and preleukaemic disorders, atherosclerotic disease, diabetes mellitus, hypogonadism

AD, autosomal dominant; AR, autosomal recessive; ATC, anaplastic thyroid carcinoma; CHRPE, congenital hypertrophy of the retinal pigment epithelium; FTA, follicular thyroid adenoma; FTC, follicular thyroid carcinoma; GAPPS, gastric adenocarcinoma and proximal polyposis of the stomach; HCA, Hürthle cell adenoma; HCC, Hürthle cell carcinoma; PDTC, poorly differentiated thyroid carcinoma; PPB, pleuropulmonary blastoma; PTC, papillary thyroid carcinoma; TC, thyroid carcinoma; TFND, thyroid follicular nodular disease. [a]According to the International Cowden Consortium (ICC) operational diagnostic criteria, non-medullary thyroid cancer is a major criterion, and FTA and TFND are minor criteria {4405}. [b]Individuals with *DICER1* syndrome had a 16-fold increased risk of thyroid cancer {2269}.

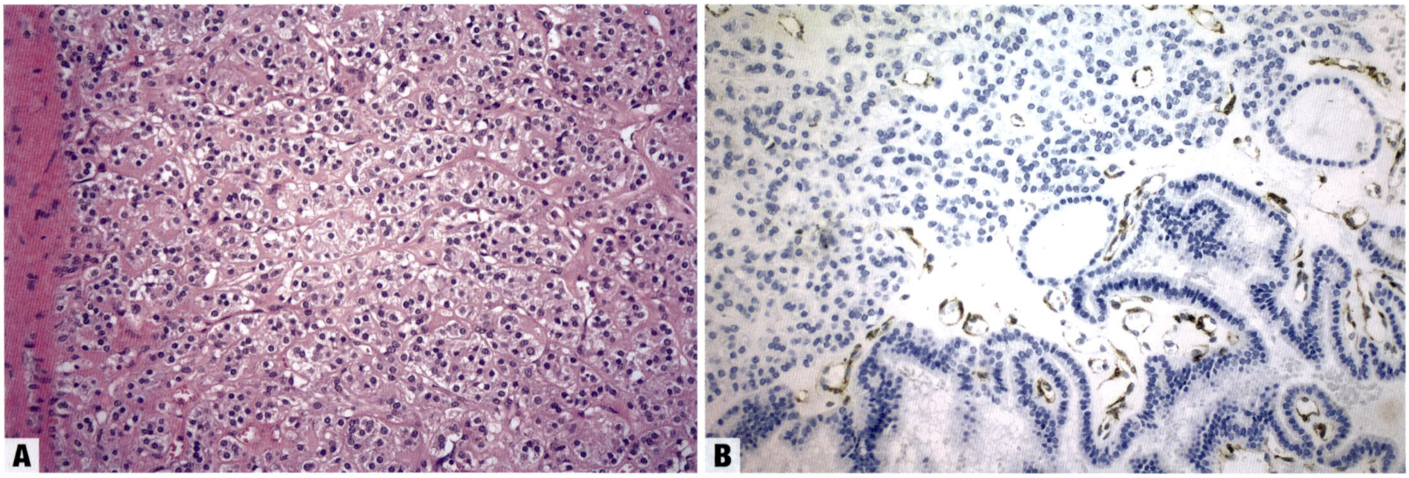

Fig. 13.58 *PTEN* hamartoma tumour syndrome. **A** Follicular thyroid adenoma with a solid histological pattern. **B** Follicular adenoma with a mixed microfollicular and papillary pattern. The staining for PTEN protein has been conserved only in the endothelial cells (internal control).

Germinal mutation of *PRKACB* has also been described in rare cases of Carney complex without *PRKAR1A* mutation {1409}. In other patients with clinical criteria of Carney complex without *PRKAR1A* mutation, another locus has been identified at 2p16 (*CNC2*) {2893}.

Werner syndrome is caused by pathogenic variants in the *WRN* gene, which encodes a multifunctional nuclear protein with exonuclease and helicase activities {5074,1447}.

Pathogenesis

PTEN regulates cell proliferation, cell migration, and apoptosis through inhibition of AKT via the PI3K/AKT pathway; inactivation of the second copy of the gene allows deregulation of the AKT pathway with upregulation of mTOR signalling {5059,4405}. Germline *PTEN* frameshift mutations seem overrepresented in thyroid cancer {3224}, but no correlation between specific mutations and thyroid pathological features has been evidenced {2545}. Germline mutations in non–PTEN pathway genes also associated with PHTS are SDH genes (*SDHB*, *SDHC*, *SDHD*), *KLLN* (epimutation), *SEC23B*, *USF3*, *TTN*, *PTK2*, and *RASAL1* {388,3224,5059,3225}. Some variants in SDH genes can act as modifiers of *PTEN*-associated thyroid cancer risk and tumour features {3232,5059}. Somatic *BRAF* p.V600E mutations and a large deletion in *MT-ND1* (encoded by mitochondrial DNA) were found in 1 papillary thyroid carcinoma (PTC) and 1 oncocytic cell carcinoma, respectively, in the thyroid of a patient with PHTS {3603}.

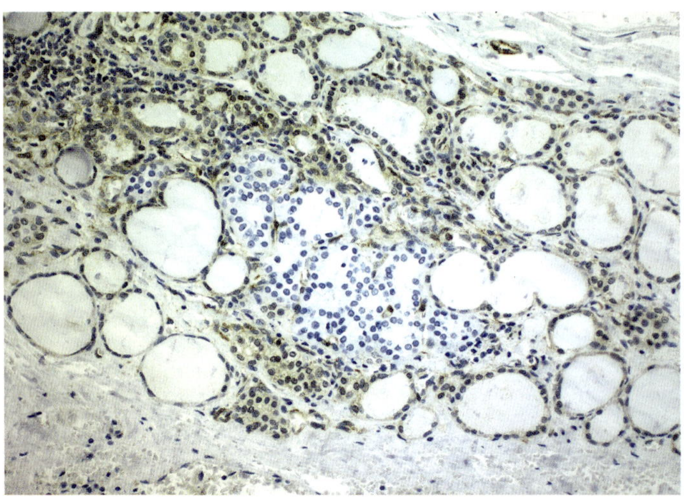

Fig. 13.59 *PTEN* hamartoma tumour syndrome. Characteristic loss of PTEN expression is found even in minute follicular clusters.

APC acts as a classic tumour suppressor gene, and the tumour phenotype appears when the non-mutant allele is spontaneously lost or mutated by a somatic event (second hit) {2516}. Most germline *APC* gene mutations in patients with thyroid cancer arise in exon 15 (codons 463–1387), the same genomic area associated with congenital hypertrophy of the retinal pigment epithelium {725}. Codon 1061 is a hotspot for thyroid cancer and hepatoblastoma {725}. Mutations predominate in the 5′ side of the *APC* gene, between codons 308 and 935 {4610}. Interestingly, in patients with FAP, thyroid cancer can even occur in the absence of biallelic inactivation of *APC* {724}. The truncated or absent APC protein produces an accumulation of cytoplasmic β-catenin that is then translocated to the nucleus, where it leads to the constitutive expression of WNT target genes. For this reason, strong cytoplasmic and nuclear staining for β-catenin is the hallmark of cribriform-morular thyroid carcinoma, which is the type of thyroid cancer affecting patients with FAP {2454,609, 615}. Thyroid cancer in FAP is often multifocal, with each tumour focus usually having a different somatic *APC* mutation (second hit) {3041}. Somatic *RET*::PTC rearrangements {4233,724,1560} and somatic mutations in the genes *AXIN1* {615}, *KMT2C*, or *KMT2D* {3242} (second hit) have also been reported. A role for estrogen and/or progesterone as tumour growth promoter(s) has also been suggested {615}.

DICER1 is an RNase III endoribonuclease involved in the maturation of several classes of small non-coding RNAs, such as microRNAs {4031,1412,3628}. In *DICER1* syndrome, alteration of DICER1 protein leads to aberrant posttranscriptional regulation of multiple cancer gene networks {494,407}.

Inactivating *PRKAR1A* mutations lead to dysregulation of the cAMP/PKA signalling pathway, resulting in the transcription of genes containing the cAMP response element (CRE) domain and tumour formation in Carney complex {494}.

WRN protein is thought to be involved in the optimization of various aspects of DNA metabolism, including DNA repair, recombination, and replication; telomere maintenance; and gene expression {5074,4415}. All of the variants thus far identified in patients with clinically ascertained Werner syndrome result in a null biochemical phenotype that abolishes the catalytic activities of the WRN protein {1903}, producing genetic instability, dysfunction, and senescence in many lineages and tissues {3366}. In Japanese individuals, follicular thyroid carcinoma (FTC) has been associated with the c.3139-1G>C mutation (exon 26 skip), whereas PTC was associated with the c.1105C>T p.R369* mutation, but the genotype–phenotype relationship seems different between Japanese and White patients {2049}.

Macroscopic appearance

In patients with PHTS, FAP, Werner syndrome, or *DICER1* syndrome, the thyroid gland is macroscopically multinodular with involvement of both lobes and isthmus {614}.

Histopathology

In PHTS, follicular cell–derived thyroid cancer usually appears in the context of multiple bilateral cellular adenomatous nodules and follicular adenomas that support an adenoma-to-carcinoma progression sequence {1781,607,4361,2545,4190,3299, 3002,1754,1703}. Lipoadenomas and/or numerous cellular adenomatous nodules (microadenomas) are also characteristic {1781,3297,607,317,4190}. Oncocytic or clear cells, as well as a hyalinizing trabecular adenoma-like pattern, are not uncommon {1781,4361,2545,3489}. Small foci of adipose tissue scattered throughout the gland and thyroiditis are also typical {4405,607, 4361,2545,1754}. Secondary (reactive) C-cell hyperplasia (but not medullary carcinoma) has been described {5114}. Loss of immunohistochemical expression of the PTEN protein in all nodules or in a subset of thyroid nodules is both sensitive and specific for PHTS {317,1703}; although tumour cells are negative for PTEN, positivity in normal follicular cells and endothelial cells can be used as a positive control {607,613,3298,1703}.

Thyroid cancer in FAP is typically cribriform-morular thyroid carcinoma, which is histologically characterized by a predominance of the cribriform component with a variable combination of follicular, papillary, trabecular, and solid growth patterns, with morular (squamoid) areas {1783,606,507}. Tumour cells are positive for thyroid transcription factor 1 (TTF1), weakly positive or negative for PAX8, and typically negative for thyroglobulin {507}, HBME1, calcitonin, and CK20 {615,507}. This is the only thyroid tumour with both nuclear and cytoplasmic reactivity for β-catenin {615, 507}. Tumour cells are also immunoreactive for pancytokeratins (AE1/AE3), EMA, vimentin, ERα, ERβ, and PR, sometimes showing focal staining for AR and PTEN {605,1560,2471,615,604}. The morular structures show strong nuclear positivity for β-catenin, as well as for CD5 and CK5 {507}, and selective positivity for CDX2, CA19-9, and CD10 {615,605,3900}. The differential diagnosis includes breast metastatic carcinoma, metastatic colon cancer, and the tall cell and columnar cell subtypes of PTC {615}.

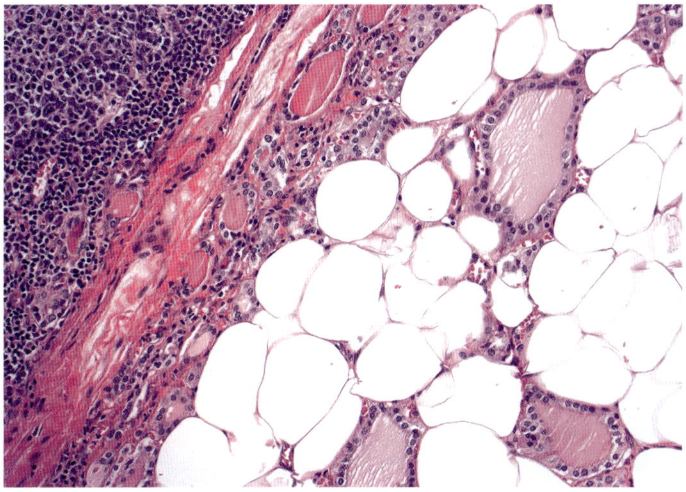

Fig. 13.60 *PTEN* hamartoma tumour syndrome. Lipoadenoma (adenolipoma) is not unusual in patients with *PTEN* hamartoma tumour syndrome. Note the chronic thyroiditis in the adjacent stroma.

Thyroid follicular nodular disease in patients with *DICER1* syndrome is characterized by nodules of follicular cells with frequent papillary growth pattern (follicular adenoma with papillary architecture), intermediate nuclei {1706}, and involutional changes {4825}. Most thyroid cancers are well differentiated, mainly the follicular variant of PTC and the minimally invasive FTC {1706}, but rare cases of the solid/trabecular subtype of PTC {3690} and high-grade follicular-derived carcinoma (poorly differentiated thyroid carcinoma of childhood) have also been

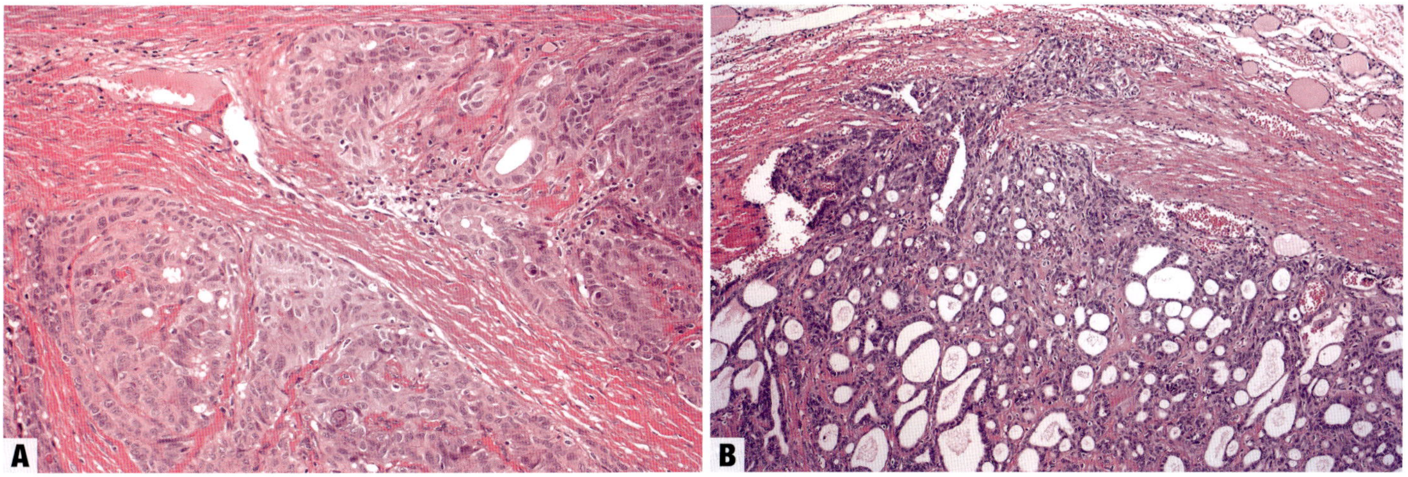

Fig. 13.61 Familial adenomatous polyposis. **A** Cribriform-morular thyroid carcinoma is usually circumscribed or encapsulated and lobulated due to fibrous septa. **B** In this cribriform-morular thyroid carcinoma, tumour cells penetrate through the full thickness of the capsule (capsular invasion).

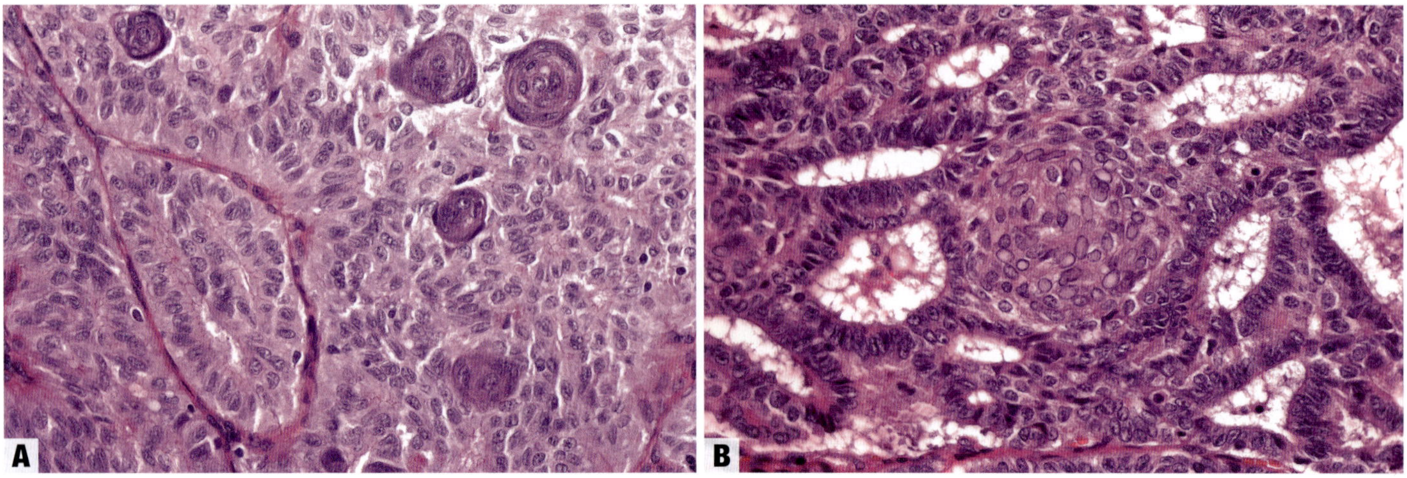

Fig. 13.62 Familial adenomatous polyposis. **A** Cribriform-morular thyroid carcinoma displays a variable combination of growth patterns. A solid/trabecular pattern with morules is shown here. **B** Cribriform-morular thyroid carcinoma displaying a cribriform pattern with morules. As can be appreciated in this image, morular structures frequently show a peculiar chromatin clearing.

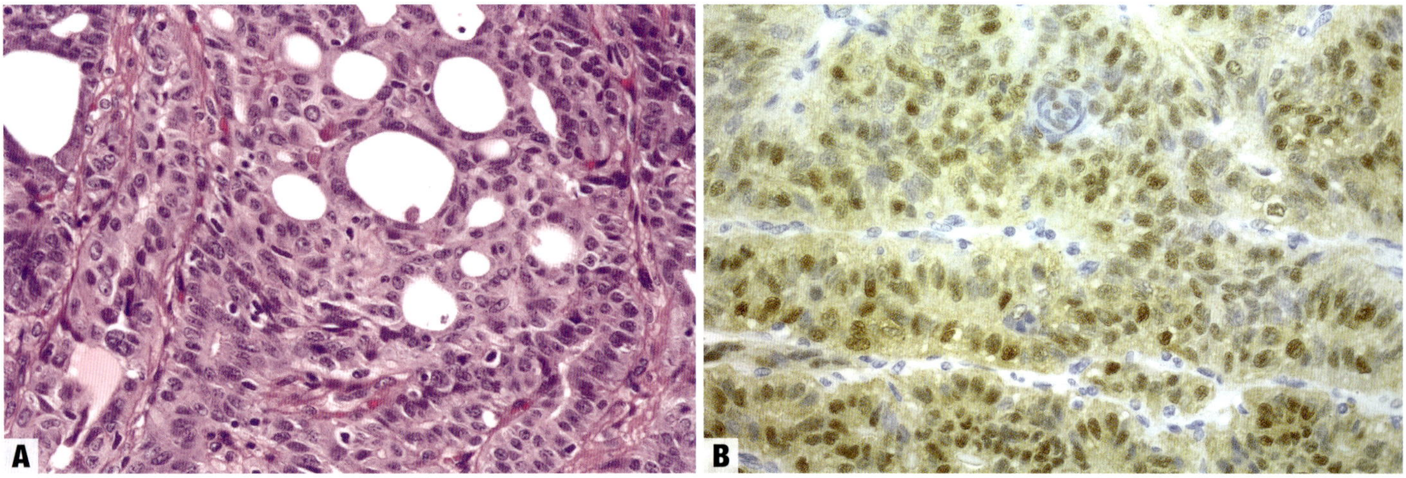

Fig. 13.63 Familial adenomatous polyposis. **A** Cribriform-morular thyroid carcinoma displaying a cribriform pattern. **B** The presence of both nuclear and cytoplasmic reactivity for β-catenin is a hallmark of cribriform-morular thyroid carcinoma.

reported {794}. The multinodularity, along with the description of some cases of PTC arising within one of these nodules {3861}, suggests a stepwise progression to malignancy {614,1706}.

In Carney complex the thyroid is typically multinodular, displaying encapsulated and unencapsulated follicular proliferations, sometimes with oncocytic change, distributed throughout the gland {4298,4295,1815}. This follicular adenomatosis {670} is analogous to the so-called microadenomas or adenomatous nodules described in PHTS. Papillary hyperfunctioning adenomas and oncocytic adenomas have also been reported {670, 931}. Both PTC and FTC have been described, generally in patients with a history of multiple adenomas {4295,4298,670, 3307,1749}. Lymphocytic thyroiditis and Graves disease have also been reported {5087}.

The most common thyroid cancer in Japanese patients with Werner syndrome is FTC, followed by PTC and anaplastic thyroid carcinoma {2049}; the presentation of anaplastic thyroid carcinoma at a younger age fits with the premature ageing of patients with Werner syndrome {614}.

Marfan syndrome {4898}, multiple endocrine neoplasia type 1 {3511}, and multiple endocrine neoplasia type 2A {2404,1558} can also present with follicular thyroid tumours. An unusual histological pattern of PTC exhibiting prominent long villous fronds has been reported in Marfan syndrome {4898}. Perhaps papillary microcarcinomas in patients with multiple endocrine neoplasia type 2A may not be related to the germline mutation of the *RET* gene but instead are the result of the careful study of the gland {614}. Some cases of familial paraganglioma phaeochromocytoma syndromes caused by SDH mutations have been associated with thyroid tumours {4908}.

Cytology

The cytological characteristics of thyroid tumours within a familial syndrome are not different from those of sporadic tumours. If suspected, β-catenin immunostaining of the cytology specimens can help to identify both the familial and sporadic forms of cribriform-morular thyroid carcinoma {1897,2156}.

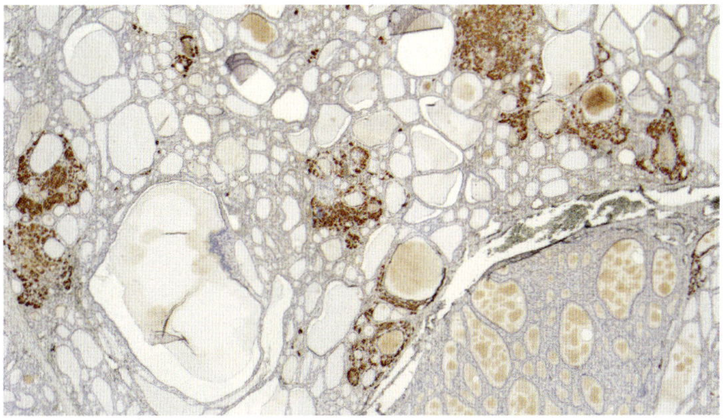

Fig. 13.64 *PTEN* hamartoma tumour syndrome. Reactive C-cell hyperplasia is highlighted by calcitonin staining adjacent to adenomatous nodules in *PTEN* hamartoma tumour syndrome.

Diagnostic molecular pathology

Germline pathogenic *PTEN* mutations cause PHTS, but rarely, other genes can be involved: *PIK3CA*, *AKT1*, SDH genes, *KLLN*, and *SEC23B* {5060}. In FAP patients with cribriform-morular thyroid carcinoma, about 85% of germline *APC* mutations occur in exon 15, usually outside the mutation cluster region {725,615}. When the suspicion of *DICER1* syndrome exists, the pathogenic mutation must be confirmed. The identification of a germline pathogenic *PRKAR1A* mutation helps to confirm the Carney complex diagnosis, but such a mutation may be absent in 20–30% of patients {407,4295}; rarely, germline mutations in *PRKACB* or *PDE11A* have been detected in some patients with Carney complex {1409,2651}. The definitive diagnosis of Werner syndrome can be achieved by molecular confirmation of biallelic loss-of-function mutations in *WRN* {3365}.

Essential and desirable diagnostic criteria

Essential: familial thyroid carcinoma of follicular origin usually with multiple benign bilateral follicular cell nodules (follicular microadenomas / adenomatous nodules / adenomatosis) in a patient with a non-thyroid cancer syndrome; cribriform-morular thyroid carcinoma with nuclear and cytoplasmic reactivity for β-catenin in a patient with FAP; loss of immunohistochemical expression of PTEN protein in more than one thyroid tumour fits with PHTS {317}.

Desirable: the identification of a pathogenic germline (constitutional) mutation in susceptibility genes.

Staging

See specific tumour types.

Prognosis and prediction

Pathologists play an important role in the recognition of these syndromes, facilitating cancer screening and genetic counselling {3297,5060,3299,607,603,1703}.

Total thyroidectomy is usually indicated, because of the frequent multicentricity of these lesions and the risk of recurrence and/or progression to carcinoma {5060,1781,3002}.

Non-syndromic familial follicular cell–derived thyroid tumours

Cameselle-Teijeiro JM
Erickson LA
LiVolsi V
Nosé V

Definition

Non-syndromic familial follicular cell–derived thyroid tumours are a heterogeneous group of hereditary thyroid cancers characterized by a predominance of follicular cell–derived or non-medullary thyroid carcinomas.

MIM numbering

None

ICD-11 coding

None

Related terminology

Acceptable: non-syndromic inherited follicular epithelial-derived thyroid carcinoma; familial papillary thyroid carcinoma; follicular cell–derived thyroid carcinoma; non-syndromic familial non-medullary thyroid carcinoma (NSFNMTC).

Subtype(s)

NSFNMTC is genetically heterogeneous {614}.

Localization

NSFNMTCs can occur anywhere in the gland and are often multifocal and bilateral, usually occurring in combination with thyroiditis and benign tumours {614,2061,2302,2901,2721,111, 4609,2765,2616,1146,4324,1675,565,3392,3295,4808,5144, 867}.

Clinical features

Patients with NSFNMTC usually present at a younger age (on average 5 years younger) than patients with sporadic thyroid cancer (~43 vs ~48 years) {4170,3101,2901,111,4309,4430}, although there is not always a significant difference between the two groups {2899,2061,3767,3146,4609,2917}. In families with NSFNMTCs, the second generation exhibits an earlier age at diagnosis (clinical anticipation), more extrathyroidal invasion, a higher recurrence rate, and shorter recurrence-free survival than the first generation {3443,635}; the possibility of bias, however, due to more frequent evaluations in the family group than in sporadic cases, cannot be excluded {3146}. No differences in the M:F ratio have been found between sporadic and familial follicular cell–derived thyroid cancers {2302,3146}.

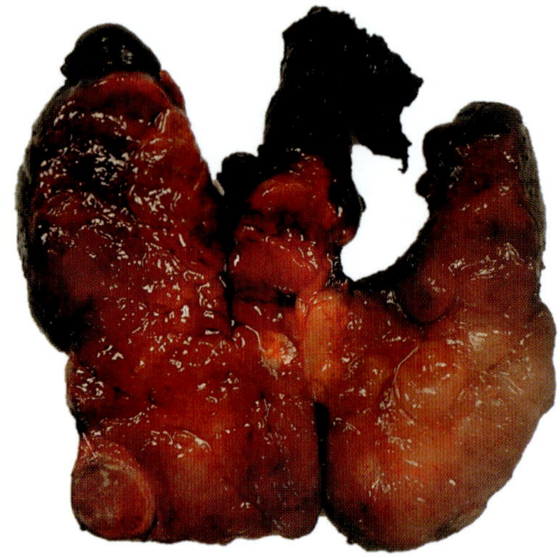

Fig. 13.65 Familial papillary thyroid carcinoma. Gross appearance of the gland of a patient with four foci of familial papillary carcinoma, one oncocytic adenoma, and lymphocytic thyroiditis.

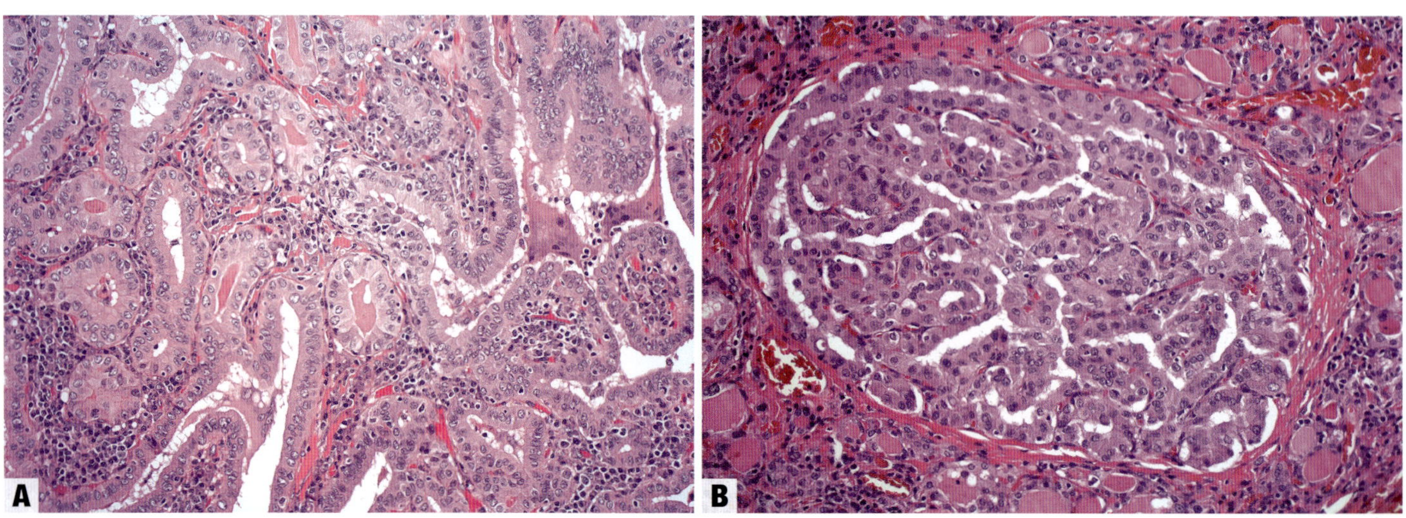

Fig. 13.66 Familial papillary thyroid carcinoma. **A** This papillary thyroid carcinoma includes oncocytic tall cells with a heavy lymphoid infiltrate (Warthin-like pattern). **B** Small papillary thyroid carcinoma. Both familial papillary thyroid carcinomas are not morphologically different from sporadic papillary thyroid carcinomas.

Epidemiology

The prevalence of NSFNMTC ranges between 4.5% and 10% of all thyroid tumours {3101,4170,2061,3767,3443}, in some series reaching as high as 13.5%, with 85% of patients having 2 affected relatives and 15% having ≥ 3 affected relatives {2302}.

Etiology

The genetic basis of NSFNMTC remains poorly understood. Most pedigrees are consistent with the inheritance of one autosomal dominant gene with reduced penetrance and variable expressivity, supporting a monogenic mode of inheritance (see Table 13.09); a polygenic mode of inheritance involving *CHEK2*, *EWSR1*, and *TIAM1* has also been recently proposed {4258}. Somatic mutations of *BRAF* (p.V600E), *NRAS*, *HRAS*, *KRAS*, *RET*/PTC1, *RET*/PTC3, *NTRK1*, and *TERT* have been identified in NSFNMTCs, so there appear to be no differences in the number or type of somatic mutations between sporadic and hereditary cases of papillary thyroid cancer {3101,306,867, 3514,5158,1514,705}.

Table 13.09 Non-syndromic familial non-medullary thyroid carcinoma

Gene (designation)	Chromosomal loci	MIM number	Thyroid lesions	Other lesions
ANXA3 {3955}	4q21.21	106490	PTC (classic and follicular variant)	
BROX {3455}	1q41	n/a	PTC (classic and follicular variant)	
CHEK2 {5158,1513,3568,4365}	22q12.1	604373	PTC	Breast cancer {4168}
DUOX2 {306}	15q21.1	606759	PTC, MNG	
FKBP10 {3955}	17q21.2	607063	PTC (classic and follicular variant)	
FOXE1 {473,2818,3514}	9q22.23	602617	PTC, FTC	
HABP2 {1499,5147}	10q25.3	603924	PTC, FTA	
MAP2K5 {5055}	15q23	602520	PTC	
NDUFA13 {2896}	19p13.11	609435	PTC (Hürthle cell variant), multiple benign Hürthle cell tumours	
NKX2-1 {3223,2647}	14q13.3	600635	PTC, MNG	
NOP53 {3360}	19q13.33	605691	PTC, HCC	
NTN4 {3955}	12q22	610401	PTC (classic and follicular variant)	
P2RX5 {3955}	17p13.2	602836	PTC (classic and follicular variant)	
PLCB1 {274,275,4882}	20p12.3	607120	PTC (follicular variant), MNG (papilloid adenomata)	
PLEKHG5 {3955}	1p36.31	611101	PTC (classic and follicular variant)	
POT1 {4896,3596,3738,4261}	7q31.33	606478	PTC (classic and follicular variant), HCC, HCA, MNG	Dysplastic naevi, melanoma {3596,3738}
SAPCD1 {3955}	6p21.33	603382	PTC (classic and follicular variant)	
SERPINA1 {3955}	14q32.13	107400	PTC	
SRGAP1 {1835}	12q14.2	606523	PTC	
SRRM2 {4518}	16p13.3	606032	PTC (classic and follicular variant)	
TIMM44 {471}	19p13.2	605058	PTC (classic and Hürthle cell variant), HCC, FTA with variable cell oxyphilia, multiple benign Hürthle cell tumours	
Unknown {4324}	6q22	n/a	PTC (classic and follicular variant), FTC[a], HCC[a], MTC[a]	
Unknown (fPTC/PRN) {4324,2812}	1q21	n/a	PTC, MNG	Papillary renal neoplasia {2812}
Unknown (*FTEN*) {706}	8p23.1-p22	n/a	PTC (classic and follicular variant)	
Unknown (*MNG1*)[b] {422}	14q32.13	138800	PTC, MNG	
Unknown (*NMTC3*) {2920,3607,2919}	2q21	606240	PTC (follicular variant)	
Unknown (*PTCSC1*) {1837}	8q24.22	617440	PTC, MNG, ATD	Melanoma {1837}
Unknown (*TCO*/*TCO1*) {414,626,1779,2422,2920,3607}	19p13.2	603386	PTC (classic and Hürthle cell variant), HCC, FTA with variable cell oxyphilia, multiple benign Hürthle cell tumours	

ATD, autoimmune thyroid disease (Hashimoto thyroiditis and Graves disease); FTA, follicular thyroid adenoma; FTC, follicular thyroid carcinoma; fPTC, familial papillary thyroid carcinoma; HCA, Hürthle cell adenoma; HCC, Hürthle cell carcinoma; MNG, multinodular goitre; MTC, medullary thyroid carcinoma; PRN, papillary renal neoplasia; PTC, papillary thyroid carcinoma.

[a]Concurrent FTC, HCC, and MTC were reported in some PTC cases. [b]Some of these cases are probably secondary to germline *DICER1* (MIM number: 606241) mutation.

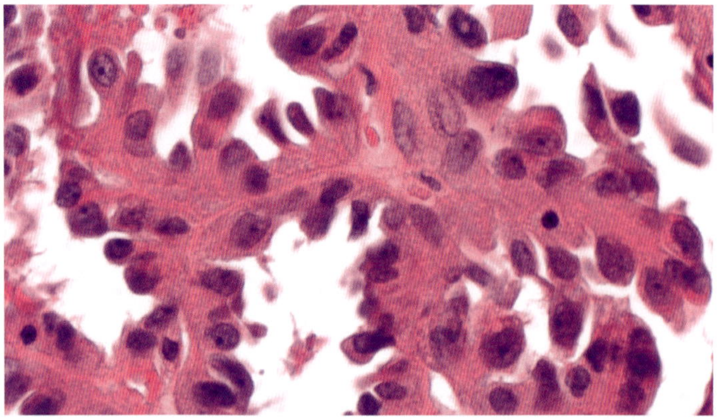

Fig. 13.67 Thyroid tumour associated with the *CHEK2* gene mutation. This papillary thyroid carcinoma consists of large follicular cells with oncocytic cytoplasm and large irregular nuclei.

Box 13.05 Essential[a] and supportive[b] clinical criteria for non-syndromic familial follicular cell–derived thyroid tumours

Essential:

Follicular cell–derived thyroid carcinoma in ≥ 3 first-degree relatives

OR

Papillary thyroid carcinoma in ≥ 2 first-degree relatives

AND

Absence of previous radiation exposure and inherited cancer syndromes

Supportive:

- Patient aged < 33 years
- Affected family member(s) aged < 45 years
- Papillary thyroid carcinoma multifocal and/or bilateral
- Papillary thyroid carcinoma in a male patient, particularly a young man
- Background thyroid with a combination of benign lesions

[a]References for essential criteria: {3146,636,4170,2902,2302,3276,3146,763,637,1703}.
[b]References for supportive criteria: {3146,1146,1857,637,1703}.

Pathogenesis

Whole-genome sequencing of NSFNMTC has shown the central role of MAPK/ERK and PI3K/AKT signalling pathways in this type of thyroid cancer {4260}, which would explain its similar morphological appearance to that of sporadic thyroid cancers. In addition, dysfunction of telomeres could in some cases be a mechanism predisposing individuals to familial papillary thyroid carcinoma {1836,634,4261}. The coexistence of NSFNMTC with multiple thyroid nodules, including the hyperplasia–neoplasia sequence, is consistent with a multistep model of tumour progression {111,565}.

Macroscopic appearance

Grossly, NSFNMTC may be indistinguishable from a multinodular goitre because of its frequent multicentricity, bilaterality, and/or association with benign nodules {614}.

Histopathology

NSFNMTC is mainly of the papillary type, including subcentimetre cases and the classic and follicular-type subtypes, but other subtypes of papillary carcinoma, oncocytic thyroid carcinoma, and other types of differentiated thyroid carcinoma have been reported as well (see Table 13.09, p. 489). No distinct morphological findings differentiate these carcinomas from their sporadic counterparts in most cases, but the multifocality and the combination with benign lesions (a background of hyperplastic nodules and/or follicular adenomas) and with Hashimoto thyroiditis {5144} suggest a hereditary origin {3297,614,1703}. In cases with germline *PLCB1* sequence variants there is a multinodular goitre of adolescent onset with an increased risk of progression to papillary thyroid carcinoma; this multinodular goitre is typically made up of sharply demarcated nodules lined by micropapillary projections (papilloid adenomata or so-called papillary hyperplasia) in a thyroid background of normal appearance {275,4882}. Overexpression of PLCB1, HABP2, EGFR, and NOP53, with lower immunostaining for CHK2, has been detected in thyroid tumour cells, associated with pathogenic germline variants of the genes *PLCB1*, *HABP2*, *BROX*, *NOP53*, and *CHEK2*, respectively {275,1499,3455,3360,5158}.

Cytology

No specific cytological features distinguish NSFNMTCs from their sporadic counterparts.

Diagnostic molecular pathology

The identification of pathological germline mutations in susceptibility genes is confirmatory, but some of these mutations have yet to be confirmed.

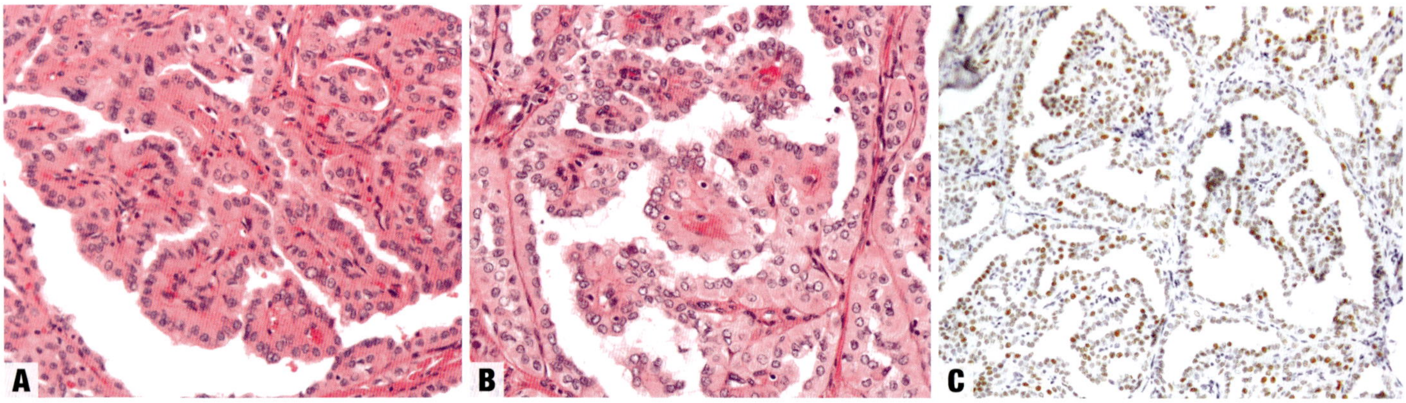

Fig. 13.68 Familial papillary thyroid carcinoma associated with renal papillary neoplasia. **A** This familial papillary thyroid carcinoma, associated with chromosomal region 1q21 (fPTC/PRN), shows a papillary arrangement with a glomeruloid appearance. **B** This hereditary papillary thyroid carcinoma is morphologically similar to renal papillary carcinoma. **C** The positivity for thyroid transcription factor 1 (TTF1) confirms the thyroid nature of the papillary tumour.

Essential and desirable diagnostic criteria

Essential: the clinical diagnosis of NSFNMTC has been defined by the presence of papillary thyroid carcinoma in ≥ 2 first-degree relatives, in the absence of previous ionizing radiation exposure and cancer syndromes {3146,636,637}, but this is controversial because of the high probability of including sporadic cases; other studies, however, indicate NSFNMTC when a follicular cell–derived thyroid carcinoma appears in ≥ 3 first-degree relatives {4170,2902,2302,3276,3146}, because the possibility of it being sporadic is therefore < 5% {763,3276}. The essential and supportive clinical criteria that can be used to identify patients with NSFNMTC are presented in Box 13.05.

Desirable: the identification of a pathogenic germline (constitutional) mutation in susceptibility genes.

Staging

See specific tumour types.

Prognosis and prediction

Although some studies have found no differences in clinical behaviour between sporadic and NSFNMTC {2899,763, 3767}, NSFNMTC is commonly associated with a higher rate of lymph node metastases {4170,2302,2901,635,2765,4808,5144}, extrathyroidal extension {2901,2917,4808,5144}, and recurrence {2901,2591} than sporadic cases, particularly in families with ≥ 3 affected members {3146,111,3296,2917,4553}. Despite the more aggressive presentation of NSFNMTC, appropriate treatment leads to an outcome similar to that observed for sporadic cases {867}. Screening of at-risk family members allows for early diagnosis of NSFNMTCs and less aggressive initial treatment {2348}. A less invasive surgical treatment could be considered in familial papillary carcinoma < 10 mm {4341}. Total thyroidectomy has been indicated, however, because of increased multifocality and the presence of benign nodules with an increased risk of recurrence and/or progression to carcinoma {2302,4430,4609,1779}.

Contributors

AGAIMY, Abbas
Erlangen University Hospital
Krankenhausstraße 8-10
91054 Erlangen

AKKARI, Yassmine
Nationwide Children's Hospital
575 Children's Crossroad
Columbus OH 43215

ARGANI, Pedram
Johns Hopkins Hospital
Weinberg 2242, 401 N Broadway
Baltimore MD 21231-2410

ARMON, Subasri
Hospital Kuala Lumpur
Pathology Department
Jalan Pahang 50586
Wilayah Persekutuan Kuala Lumpur

ASA, Sylvia L.*
Case Western Reserve University
11100 Euclid Ave
Cleveland OH 44106

ASSIÉ, Guillaume
Université Paris Cité; Inserm; Assistance
Publique Hôpitaux de Paris
27 Rue du Faubourg Saint-Jacques
75014 Paris

BALOCH, Zubair Wahid
Hospital of the University of Pennsylvania,
Perelman School of Medicine
6 Founders, Rm 6.043, 3400 Spruce St
Philadelphia PA 19104-4283

BARLETTA, Justine A.
Brigham and Women's Hospital
Harvard Medical School
75 Francis St
Boston MA 02115

BASTURK, Olca
Memorial Sloan Kettering Cancer Center
1275 York Ave
New York NY 10065

BEASLEY, Mary Beth
Icahn School of Medicine at Mount Sinai
1 Gustave L. Levy Place, Annenberg 15-265
New York NY 10025

BEISKE, Klaus Hermann
Oslo University Hospital, Radiumhospitalet
Ullernchausseen 64
0379 Oslo

BELL, Diana
City of Hope
Presbyterian Campus Suite A-616
200 Lothrop St
Pittsburgh PA 15213-2582

BONGIOVANNI, Massimo
Unilabs Switzerland
Rte de la Corniche 9A
1066 Epalinges

BOYCE, Alison M.*
National Institute of Dental and
Craniofacial Research
30 Convent Dr, Room 228, MSC 4320
Bethesda MD 20892

BRANDNER, Sebastian
UCL Queen Square Institute of Neurology and
National Hospital for Neurology and
Neurosurgery, University College London
Hospitals NHS Foundation Trust
Queen Square
London WC1N 3BG

BROSENS, Lodewijk A.A.
Department of Pathology
University Medical Center Utrecht
Heidelberglaan 100
3584 CX Utrecht

BUSAM, Klaus J.
Department of Pathology and
Laboratory Medicine
Memorial Sloan Kettering Cancer Center
1275 York Ave
New York NY 10065

BYCHKOV, Andrey
Kameda Medical Center
Department of Pathology
929 Higashi-cho
Kamogawa 296-8602

CALONJE, Jaime E.
St John's Institute of Dermatology
St Thomas' Hospital
Westminster Bridge Rd
London SE1 7EH

CAMESELLE-TEIJEIRO, José Manuel
University Clinical Hospital
University of Santiago de Compostela
Choupana s/n
15706 Santiago de Compostela

CASAR-BOROTA, Olivera
Uppsala University Hospital
Building C5
751 85 Uppsala

CHAN, John K.C.
Queen Elizabeth Hospital
30 Gascoigne Rd
Kowloon 000, Hong Kong SAR

CHENG, Liang
Department of Pathology
Brown University Warren Alpert Medical School
and the Legorreta Cancer Center
at Brown University
Brown University Health
593 Eddy St, APC 12, Room 105
Providence RI 02903

CLIFTON-BLIGH, Roderick J.
Royal North Shore Hospital
Pacific Hwy, St Leonards
Sydney NSW 2065

CREE, Ian A.
International Agency for Research on Cancer
25 Av. Tony Garnier, CS 90627
69366 Lyon, CEDEX 07

CULLINANE, Catherine
Department of Histopathology
St James's University Hospital
Beckett St, Level 5, Bexley Wing
Leeds LS9 7TF

de HERDER, Wouter W.*
Erasmus MC
Dr Molewaterplein 40
3015 GD Rotterdam

de KOCK, Leanne
Children's Hospital of Eastern Ontario
Research Institute
401 Smyth Rd
Ottawa ON K1H 5B2

de KRIJGER, Ronald R.
Princess Máxima Center for Pediatric
Oncology and Department of Pathology,
University Medical Center Utrecht
Heidelberglaan 25
3584 CS Utrecht

de la FOUCHARDIÈRE, Arnaud
Centre Léon Bérard
28 Rue Laennec
69008 Lyon

* Indicates disclosure of interests (see p. 499).

DEMICCO, Elizabeth G.
University of Toronto
Mount Sinai Hospital, 600 University Ave
Toronto ON M5G 1X5

DENTON, Erika R.E.
Norfolk and Norwich University Hospitals
NHS Foundation Trust
Colney Ln
Norwich NR4 7UY

DOYLE, Leona A.
St. Vincent's University Hospital
University College Dublin, School of Medicine
Elm Park
Dublin 4

DUNCAN, Emma L.
King's College London
St Thomas' Hospital Campus
3rd Floor, South Wing, Block D
Westminster Bridge Rd
London SE1 7EH

DURANTE, Cosimo
Sapienza University of Rome
Viale del Policlinico, 155
00161 Rome RM

ERICKSON, Lori A.
Mayo Clinic
200 1st St SW
Rochester MN 55905

EZZAT, Shereen
Princess Margaret Cancer Centre
585 University Ave
Toronto ON M5G 2N2

FACCHETTI, Fabio
University of Brescia
P.le Spedali Civili, 1
25123 Brescia BS

FADDA, Guido
University of Messina
Via Consolare Valeria, 1
98125 Messina ME

FALHAMMAR, Henrik
Karolinska University Hospital
QB85
171 76 Stockholm

FAVIER, Judith*
Centre de Recherche des Cordeliers
Inserm - Université Paris Cité
15 Rue de l'École de Médecine
75006 Paris

FIELD, Andrew S.
University of NSW Sydney and
University of Notre Dame Medical Schools
Department of Anatomical Pathology
St Vincent's Hospital Sydney
Victoria St
Darlinghurst, Sydney NSW 2010

FISCHER, Matthias
University Children's Hospital
Kerpener Str. 62
50937 Cologne

FOLPE, Andrew L.
Mayo Clinic
200 1st St SW
Rochester MN 55905

FONSECA, Anil Felix Angelo
Gandhi Medical College/TIMS
Hyderabad, Telangana

FONSECA, Daphne
Basavatarakam Indo American Cancer
Hospital and Research Institute
Banjara Hills
Hyderabad 500034

FOULKES, William D.
McGill University
Research Institute
McGill University Health Centre
1001 Bd Décarie
Montréal QC H4A 3J1

FRITCHIE, Karen J.
Cleveland Clinic
9500 Euclid Ave
Cleveland OH 44195

FUCHS, Talia L.
Douglass Hanly Moir Pathology
14 Giffnock Ave
Macquarie Park NSW 2113

GHOSSEIN, Ronald A.
Memorial Sloan Kettering Cancer Center
1275 York Ave
New York NY 10021

GILL, Anthony J.
Royal North Shore Hospital
Pacific Hwy
St Leonards NSW 2065

GIMENEZ-ROQUEPLO, Anne-Paule
Hôpital Européen Georges Pompidou AP-HP
20-40 Rue Leblanc
75015 Paris

GOLDMAN-LÉVY, Gabrielle
International Agency for Research on Cancer
25 Av. Tony Garnier, CS 90627
69366 Lyon, CEDEX 07

GROSSMAN, Ashley B.
University of Oxford
Churchill Hospital, Headington
Oxford OX3 7LE

GUJRAL, Sumeet
Tata Memorial Hospital, Mumbai
7, Charak, BPT Hospital Campus
Wadala East
Mumbai 400037

HERNÁNDEZ-RAMÍREZ, Laura C.
Red de Apoyo a la Investigación,
Coordinación de la Investigación Científica,
Universidad Nacional Autónoma de México,
and Instituto Nacional de Ciencias Médicas y
Nutrición Salvador Zubirán
Vasco de Quiroga 15
Radiation Oncology Building, 2nd Floor
14080 Mexico City

HICKS, M. John
Texas Children's Hospital
Baylor College of Medicine
6621 Fannin St, AB1195
Houston TX 77030

HIROSHIMA, Kenzo
Chiba University Graduate School of Medicine
1-8-1 Inohana, Chuo-ku
Chiba 260-8670

HODGE, Jennelle C.
Indiana University School of Medicine
975 W Walnut St, IB-354
Indianapolis IN 46202

HONG, Seung-Mo
Asan Medical Center
University of Ulsan College of Medicine
88 Olympic-ro 43 gil, Songpa-gu
Seoul 05505

HYRCZA, Martin D.*
University of Calgary
Arnie Charbonneau Cancer Institute
Rm 7566, McCaig Tower, 1403 29 St NW
Calgary AB T2N 2T9

INOMOTO, Chie
Tokai University Hachioji Hospital
1838 Ishikawa-machi, Hachioji
Tokyo 192-0032

INOSHITA, Naoko*
Tokyo Metropolitan Geriatric Hospital
35-2 Sakae-cho, Itabashi-ku
Tokyo 173-0015

INZANI, Frediano
Fondazione Policlinico Universitario Agostino
Gemelli IRCCS
Largo Agostino Gemelli, 8
00168 Rome RM

* Indicates disclosure of interests (see p. 499).

IRWIN, Meredith S.
Hospital for Sick Children
555 University Ave
Toronto ON M5G 1A8

JAIN, Deepali
All India Institute of Medical Sciences
Ansari Nagar
New Delhi 110029

JARZEMBOWSKI, Jason A.
Medical College of Wisconsin
8701 W Watertown Plank Rd
Milwaukee WI 53226

JOHNSON, Sarah J.
Newcastle upon Tyne Hospitals
NHS Foundation Trust
Royal Victoria Infirmary
Newcastle upon Tyne NE1 4LP

JUHLIN, C. Christofer
Karolinska University Hospital
Radiumhemmet, P1:02
171 76 Stockholm

JUNG, Chan Kwon
College of Medicine
Catholic University of Korea
Seoul St. Mary's Hospital
222 Banpo-daero, Seocho-gu
Seoul 06591

KAKKAR, Aanchal
Department of Pathology
All India Institute of Medical Sciences
New Delhi 110029

KAKUDO, Kennichi
Izumi City General Hospital
4-5-1 Wake-cho
Izumi, Osaka 594-0073

KARPATHIOU, Georgia
University Hospital of Saint-Etienne
42055 Saint-Etienne, CEDEX 02

KASAJIMA, Atsuko
TUM School of Medicine and Health
Technical University of Munich
Trogerstraße 18
81675 Munich

KATOH, Ryohei
Ito Hospital
4-3-6 Jingumae, Shibuya-ku
Tokyo 150-8308

KERR, Darcy A.
Dartmouth Hitchcock Medical Center
1 Medical Center Dr
Lebanon NH 03756

KHOURY, Joseph David
University of Nebraska Medical Center
985900 Nebraska Medical Center
Omaha NE 68198

KIMURA, Noriko
National Hospital Organization
Hakodate National Hospital
18-16 Kawahara
Hakodate, Hokkaido 041-8512

KIRSCHNER, Lawrence S.
Ohio State University College of Medicine
579 McCampbell Hall, 1581 Dodd Dr
Columbus OH 43210

KLEINSCHMIDT-DEMASTERS, Bette K.
University of Colorado
Anschutz Medical Campus
12605 E 16th Ave, Room 3017
Aurora CO 80045

KLIMSTRA, David S.*
Yale University School of Medicine
310 Cedar St
PO Box 208023
New Haven CT 06510

KLÖPPEL, Günter
Technical University of Munich
Trogerstraße 18
81675 Munich

KOHASHI, Kenichi
Graduate School of Medical Sciences
Kyushu University
3-1-1 Maidashi, Higashi-ku
Fukuoka 812-8582

KOMORI, Takashi
Tokyo Metropolitan Neurological Hospital
2-6-1 Musashidai, Fuchu
Tokyo 183-0042

KONDO, Tetsuo
University of Yamanashi
1110 Shimokato
Chuo, Yamanashi 409-3898

LA ROSA, Stefano
Unit of Pathology, Department of Medicine
and Technological Innovation
University of Insubria
Viale Luigi Borri, 57
21100 Varese VA

LAM, Alfred King-yin
Griffith University School of Medicine and
Dentistry
Gold Coast Campus
Gold Coast QLD 4222

LAX, Sigurd F.
General Hospital Graz II
Medical University of Graz
Göstinger Str. 22
8020 Graz

LAZAR, Alexander J.
University of Texas
MD Anderson Cancer Center
1515 Holcombe Blvd, Unit 85
Houston TX 77030

LIVOLSI, Virginia
University of Pennsylvania Medical Center
3400 Spruce St, Founders 6-040
Philadelphia PA 19104

LOKUHETTY, Dilani
International Agency for Research on Cancer
25 Av. Tony Garnier, CS 90627
69366 Lyon, CEDEX 07

LOOIJENGA, Leendert H.J.
Princess Máxima Center for Pediatric Oncology
and Department of Pathology, University
Medical Center Utrecht
Heidelberglaan 25
3584 CS Utrecht

LOPES, Maria Beatriz S.
University of Virginia School of Medicine
1215 Lee St
Charlottesville VA 22908-0214

McCLUGGAGE, W. Glenn
Belfast Health and Social Care Trust
Grosvenor Rd
Belfast BT12 6BA

McCUTCHEON, Ian E.
University of Texas
MD Anderson Cancer Center
1400 Holcombe Blvd
Houston TX 77030

MESSINA, Jane L.
Moffitt Cancer Center and Research Institute
12902 USF Magnolia Dr
Tampa FL 33612

METE, Ozgur
University Health Network and
University of Toronto
200 Elizabeth St, 11th Floor
Toronto General Hospital
Toronto ON M5G 2C4

MILIONE, Massimo
Fondazione IRCCS Istituto Nazionale dei
Tumori, Milan
Via Giacomo Venezian, 1
20133 Milan MI

* Indicates disclosure of interests (see p. 499).

MOCH, Holger
University of Zürich and
University Hospital Zürich
Schmelzbergstrasse 12
8091 Zürich

MORREAU, Hans
Department of Pathology
Leiden University Medical Center
Albinusdreef 2
3000 DR Leiden

MÜLLER, Hermann L.
University Children's Hospital
Klinikum Oldenburg AöR
Rahel-Straus-Straße 10
26133 Oldenburg

NAVARRO, Samuel
University of Valencia Medical School
Av. de Blasco Ibáñez
46010 Valencia

NISHIOKA, Hiroshi*
Toranomon Hospital
2-2-2 Toranomon, Minato-ku
Tokyo 105-8470

NOSÉ, Vania
Massachusetts General Hospital and
Harvard Medical School
55 Fruit St, Warren 214
Boston MA 02114-2696

OHIKE, Nobuyuki
St. Marianna University School of Medicine
2-16-1 Sugao, Miyamae-ku, Kawasaki
Kanagawa 216-8511

OKUBO, Yoichiro
Kanagawa Cancer Center
2-3-2 Nakao, Asahi-ku
Yokohama 241-8515

OSAMURA, Robert Y.
Nippon Koukan Hospital and
Keio University School of Medicine
1-2-1 Koukan-dori, Kawasaki-ku, Kawasaki-shi
Kanagawa 210-0852

OUDIJK, Lindsey
Erasmus MC University Medical Center
Dr Molewaterplein 40
3015 GD Rotterdam

OYAMA, Kenichi
Teikyo University School of Medicine
2-11-1 Kaga, Itabashi-ku
Tokyo 173-8605

PACAK, Karel
National Institutes of Health
Building 10, Room 1-3140, 10 Center Dr
Bethesda MD 20892

PAPOTTI, Mauro*
University of Turin
Via Santena, 7
10126 Turin TO

PARK, Sung-Hye
Seoul National University College of Medicine
Seoul National University Hospital
101 Daehak-ro, Jongno-gu
Seoul 03080

PAULUS, Werner
University Hospital Münster
Pottkamp 2
48149 Münster

PELLEGATA, Natalia Simona*
Dipartimento di Biologia e Biotecnologie
Universitá di Pavia
Via Ferrata, 9
27100 Pavia PV

PERREN, Aurel*
University of Bern
Murtenstrasse 31
3008 Bern

PERRY, Arie
University of California, San Francisco
505 Parnassus Ave, M551
San Francisco CA 94143-0102

PEUCHMAUR, Michel
Hôpital universitaire Robert-Debré AP-HP
Université Paris Cité
48 Bd Sérurier
75019 Paris

PIANA, Simonetta
Azienda USL-IRCCS Reggio Emilia
Viale Risorgimento, 80
42124 Reggio Emilia RE

PRASAD, Manju Lata
Yale School of Medicine
200 S Frontage Rd, PO Box 208070
New Haven CT 06520

REKHTMAN, Natasha
Memorial Sloan Kettering Cancer Center
1275 York Ave
New York NY 10065

RICHARDSON, Mary S.
Children's Hospital
Medical University of South Carolina
165 Ashley Ave, Room EH303D4
Charleston SC 29425

RIGHI, Alberto
IRCCS, Istituto Ortopedico Rizzoli
Via di Barbiano, 1/10
40136 Bologna BO

RINDI, Guido*
Università Cattolica del Sacro Cuore
Fondazione Policlinico Universitario Agostino
Gemelli IRCCS
Largo Agostino Gemelli, 8
00168 Rome RM

RONCAROLI, Federico R.
University of Manchester
Oxford Rd
Manchester M13 9PT

ROOPER, Lisa M.
Johns Hopkins University School of Medicine
401 N Broadway
Baltimore MD 21231

ROSSI, Esther D.
Fondazione Policlinico Universitario Agostino
Gemelli IRCCS
Largo Agostino Gemelli
00168 Rome RM

ROSSI, Sabrina
Bambino Gesù Children's Hospital
Piazza Sant'Onofrio, 4
00165 Rome RM

ROUS, Brian
NHS England
Victoria House, Capital Park
Fulbourn, Cambridge CB21 5XA

RUDZINSKI, Erin R.
Seattle Children's Hospital
4800 Sand Point Way NE
Seattle WA 98105

SADOW, Peter M.
Massachusetts General Hospital
Harvard Medical School
55 Fruit St, WRN219
Boston MA 02114

SAHM, Felix
Heidelberg University and
German Cancer Research Center (DKFZ)
Im Neuenheimer Feld 224
69120 Heidelberg

SANTAGATA, Sandro
Brigham and Women's Hospital
60 Fenwood Rd, Hale 8002P
Boston MA 02115

SARKAR, Chitra
All India Institute of Medical Sciences
Ansari Nagar
New Delhi 110029

SARTELET, Herve
CHRU de Nancy
Rue du Morvan
54511 Vandoeuvre-lès-Nancy

* Indicates disclosure of interests (see p. 499).

SASANO, Hironobu
Tohoku University School of Medicine
2-1 Seiryou-machi, Aoba-ku
Sendai 980-8575

SCHULTZ, Kris Ann P.
International PPB/DICER1 Registry
Cancer and Blood Disorders
Children's Minnesota
2530 Chicago Ave S
Minneapolis MN 55404

SCOAZEC, Jean-Yves
Gustave Roussy Cancer Campus
114 Rue Edouard Vaillant
94805 Villejuif

SCOLYER, Richard A.*
Royal Prince Alfred Hospital;
Melanoma Institute Australia; and
University of Sydney
Missenden Rd, Camperdown
Sydney NSW 2050

SEETHALA, Raja
UPMC Presbyterian Hospital
200 Lothrop St, Room A614
Pittsburgh PA 15213

SHIA, Jinru*
Memorial Sloan Kettering Cancer Center
1275 York Ave
New York NY 10065

SHIBUYA, Makoto
Tokyo Medical University
Hachioji Medical Center
1163 Tatemachi
Hachioji 193-0998

SHIMADA, Hiroyuki
Stanford University
300 Pasteur Dr
Stanford CA 94305

SIEVERS, Philipp
Heidelberg University and
German Cancer Research Center (DKFZ)
Im Neuenheimer Feld 224
69120 Heidelberg

SINGHI, Aatur D.
University of Pittsburgh Medical Center
200 Lothrop St, Scaife Hall A616.2
Pittsburgh PA 15213

SIPOS, Bence
University Hospital Tübingen
Otfried-Müller-Straße 14
72076 Tübingen

SOBRINHO-SIMOES, Manuel
Faculty of Medicine of Porto University /
IPATIMUP
Rua Dr. Roberto Frias s/n
4200-465 Porto

SRIGLEY, John R.
University of Toronto
Trillium Health Partners
2200 Eglinton Ave W
Mississauga ON L5M 2N1

STRATAKIS, Constantine A.
NICHD, National Institutes of Health
31 Center Dr, Room 2A46
Bethesda MD 20892

STRÖBEL, Philipp
University Medical Center Göttingen
Robert-Koch-Straße 40
37075 Göttingen

TAHARA, Shigeyuki
Nippon Medical School
1-1-5 Sendagi, Bunkyo-ku
Tokyo 113-8603

TAIEB, David
Aix-Marseille University
264 Rue Saint-Pierre
13005 Marseille

TALLINI, Giovanni
University of Bologna Medical Center
IRCCS Azienda Ospedaliero-Universitaria di
Bologna
Policlinico di Sant'Orsola
Via Giuseppe Massarenti, 9
40138 Bologna BO

TAN, Puay Hoon
Luma Medical Centre
Mount Elizabeth Medical Centre
3 Mount Elizabeth, #13-01
Singapore 228510

TANG, Laura H.
Memorial Sloan Kettering Cancer Center
1275 York Ave
New York NY 10065

TETZLAFF, Michael
University of California, San Francisco
1701 Divisadero St, Suite 271
San Francisco CA 94115

THOMPSON, Lester D.R.
Head and Neck Pathology Consultations
22543 Ventura Blvd, Ste 22, PMB1034
Woodland Hills CA 91364

TISCHLER, Arthur S.
Tufts Medical Center
800 Washington St, PO Box 802
Boston MA 02111

TONINI, Gian Paolo
Pediatric Research Institute
Corso Stati Uniti, 4
35127 Padua PD

TORNÓCZKY, Tamás
University of Pécs
Medical School and Clinical Centre
Szigeti út 12
Pécs 7625

TOURAINE, Philippe A.
Sorbonne Université, Faculté de Médecine
Hôpital Pitié Salpêtrière
83 Bd de l'Hôpital
75653 Paris, CEDEX 13

TRAVIS, William D.
Memorial Sloan Kettering Cancer Center
1275 York Ave
New York NY 10065

TSAI, Kenneth Y.*
H. Lee Moffitt Cancer Center
and Research Institute
12902 Magnolia Dr
Tampa FL 33612

TSUZUKI, Toyonori
Aichi Medical University Hospital
1-1 Yazakokarimata
Nagakute 480-1195

TUTTLE, R. Michael
Memorial Sloan Kettering Cancer Center
1275 York Ave
New York NY 10021

UCCELLA, Silvia
Humanitas University
IRCCS Humanitas Research Hospital
Via Rita Levi Montalcini, 4
20089 Pieve Emanuele MI

VALK, Gerlof D.*
University Medical Center Utrecht
Heidelberglaan 100
3584 CX Utrecht

VAN DER POL, Christian B.
Juravinski Hospital and Cancer Centre
Hamilton Health Sciences
711 Concession St
Hamilton ON L8V 1C3

VARLET, Pascale
GHU Paris, Site Hôpital Sainte-Anne
1 Rue Cabanis
75014 Paris

* Indicates disclosure of interests (see p. 499).

VOLANTE, Marco*
University of Turin, San Luigi Hospital
Regione Gonzole, 10
10043 Orbassano TO

WASHINGTON, Mary K.
Vanderbilt University Medical Center
C-3321 MCN
Nashville TN 37232

WENIG, Bruce M.
Moffitt Cancer Center
12902 Magnolia Dr
Tampa FL 33612

WESSELING, Pieter
Princess Máxima Center for Pediatric
Oncology, Utrecht, and
Amsterdam UMC / VUmc
De Boelelaan 1117
1081 HV Amsterdam

WHITE, Valerie A.
International Agency for Research on Cancer
25 Av. Tony Garnier, CS 90627
69366 Lyon, CEDEX 07

WIJESINGHE, Harshima
International Agency for Research on Cancer
25 Av. Tony Garnier, CS 90627
69366 Lyon, CEDEX 07

WILLIAMS, Michelle D.
University of Texas
MD Anderson Cancer Center
1515 Holcombe Blvd, Unit 085
Houston TX 77030

YAMADA, Shozo
Moriyama Neurological Center Hospital
7-12-7 Nishikasai, Edogawa-ku
Tokyo 134-0088

* Indicates disclosure of interests (see p. 499).

Declaration of interests

Dr Asa reports serving on the medical advisory boards of Leica Biosystems and Ibex Medical Analytics, receiving honoraria from Med Learning Group, and having received personal consultancy fees from Iron Mountain and PathAI.

Dr Boyce reports that her unit at National Institute of Dental and Craniofacial Research benefits from research funding from Amgen and Ultragenyx.

Dr de Herder reports that his unit at Erasmus MC benefits from research funding from Ipsen and Novartis/AAA.

Dr Favier reports holding patent EP2019/081848 on "Methods for predicting metastatic potential in patients suffering from *SDHB*-mutated paraganglioma".

Dr Hyrcza reports that his unit at the University of Calgary benefits from research funding from Bayer Canada.

Dr Inoshita reports that her research unit at Tokyo Metropolitan Geriatric Hospital benefited from research funding from Teijin Pharma, Eli Lilly Japan, and Astellas Pharma.

Dr Klimstra reports being a consultant for and equity holder in Paige AI and receiving royalties from UpToDate.

Dr Nishioka reports that his unit at Toranomon Hospital benefits from research funding from Teijin Pharma.

Dr Papotti reports receiving honoraria from Lilly, Roche, and Pfizer.

Dr Pellegata reports that her former unit at Helmholtz Zentrum München benefited from research funding from the German Research Foundation and the Wilhelm Sander Foundation.

Dr Perren reports receiving speaker fees from Novartis and Ipsen.

Dr Rindi reports having received personal consultancy fees from Novartis in his capacity as a speakers' bureau participant.

Dr Scolyer reports having received personal consultancy fees from a number of pharmaceutical companies.

Dr Shia reports being a consultant for Paige AI and conducting research supported by Paige AI.

Dr Tsai reports having received personal consultancy fees from EMD Serono and Merck.

Dr Valk reports that his unit at University Medical Center Utrecht benefits from research funding from Ipsen.

Dr Volante reports that his unit at the University of Turin benefited from research funding from Ipsen.

IARC/WHO Committee for the International Classification of Diseases for Oncology (ICD-O)

BRAY, Freddie
International Agency for Research on Cancer
25 Av. Tony Garnier, CS 90627
69366 Lyon, CEDEX 07

CREE, Ian A.
International Agency for Research on Cancer
25 Av. Tony Garnier, CS 90627
69366 Lyon, CEDEX 07

FERLAY, Jacques
International Agency for Research on Cancer
25 Av. Tony Garnier, CS 90627
69366 Lyon, CEDEX 07

GOLDMAN-LÉVY, Gabrielle
International Agency for Research on Cancer
25 Av. Tony Garnier, CS 90627
69366 Lyon, CEDEX 07

JAKOB, Robert
Classifications and Terminologies
World Health Organization (WHO)
Av. Appia 20
1211 Geneva

KRPELANOVA, Eva
Classifications and Terminologies
World Health Organization (WHO)
Av. Appia 20
1211 Geneva

LOKUHETTY, Dilani
International Agency for Research on Cancer
25 Av. Tony Garnier, CS 90627
69366 Lyon, CEDEX 07

ROUS, Brian
NHS England
Victoria House, Capital Park
Fulbourn, Cambridge CB21 5XA

WATANABE, Reiko
St. Marianna University School of Medicine
2-16-1 Sugao, Miyamae-ku, Kawasaki
Kanagawa 216-8511

ZNAOR, Ariana
International Agency for Research on Cancer
25 Av. Tony Garnier, CS 90627
69366 Lyon, CEDEX 07

Sources

Note: For any figure, table, or box not listed below, the original source is this volume; the suggested source citation is

WHO Classification of Tumours Editorial Board. Endocrine and neuroendocrine tumours. Lyon (France): International Agency for Research on Cancer; 2025. (WHO classification of tumours series, 5th ed.; vol. 10). https://publications.iarc.who.int/645.

Figures

1.01A	Mete O
1.01B	Asa SL
1.01C	Mete O
2.01	Adapted, by permission from Springer Nature, from: Asa SL, Mete O, Cusimano MD, et al. Pituitary neuroendocrine tumors: a model for neuroendocrine tumor classification. Mod Pathol. 2021 Sep;34(9):1634–50. doi: 10.1038/s41379-021-00820-y. PMID:34017065. Copyright 2021.
2.02A,B	Asa SL
2.03	Adapted, with permission, from: Di Ieva A, Rotondo F, Syro LV, et al. Aggressive pituitary adenomas--diagnosis and emerging treatments. Nat Rev Endocrinol. 2014;10(7):423–35. PMID:24821329.
2.04	Adapted, with permission, from: Asa SL, Mete O, Ezzat S. Genomics and epigenomics of pituitary tumors: What do pathologists need to know? Endocr Pathol. 2021 Mar;32(1):3–16. PMID:33433883.
2.05A–D	Yamada S
2.06A–D	Mete O
2.07A–C	Mete O
2.08A,B	Felipe Andreiuolo, Department of Neuropathology, Instituto Estadual do Cérebro Paulo Niemeyer, Rio de Janeiro
2.09A,B	Yamada S
2.10	Yamada S
2.11	Mete O
2.12	Mete O
2.13	Mete O
2.14	Mete O
2.15A–C	Mete O
2.16A,B	Nishioka H
2.17A–C	Perry A
2.18	Perry A
2.19A–C	Perry A
2.20	Perry A
2.21A,B	Perry A
2.22A,C,D	Lopes MBS
2.22B	Perry A
2.23	Perry A
2.24A–F	Perry A
2.25A–E	Perry A
2.26	Perry A
2.27A,B	Perry A
2.28A–E	Perry A
2.29A–D	Lopes MBS
2.30A–D	Lopes MBS
2.31	Casar-Borota O
2.32A–D	Yamada S
2.33A–D	Mete O
2.34A–C	Mete O
2.35A	Ulla Feldt-Rasmussen, Department of Nephrology and Endocrinology, Rigshospitalet, Copenhagen University Hospital, Copenhagen
2.35B–E	Casar-Borota O
2.36	Mete O
2.37A,B	Nishioka H
2.38A–D	Lopes MBS
2.39A–D	Lopes MBS
2.40A–E	Casar-Borota O
2.41A–D	Mete O
2.42A–D	Sofia Asioli and Raffaele Lodi, Department of Biomedical and Neuromotor Sciences (DIBINEM), University of Bologna, Bologna
2.42C,D	Ezzat S
2.43A–D	Tahara S; and Ryuji Ohashi, Nippon Medical School, Tokyo
2.44A–F	Perry A
2.45A,B	Nishioka H
2.46	Santagata S
2.47A–D	Santagata S
2.48A–C	Kleinschmidt-DeMasters BK
2.49A	Nishioka H
2.49B	WHO Classification of Tumours Editorial Board. Central nervous system tumours. Lyon (France): International Agency for Research on Cancer; 2021. (WHO classification of tumours series, 5th ed.; vol. 6). https://publications.iarc.who.int/601.
2.50A–F	Santagata S
2.51	Adapted, with permission, from: Nadaf J, de Kock L, Chong AS, et al. Molecular characterization of DICER1-mutated pituitary blastoma. Acta Neuropathol. 2021 Jun;141(6):929–44. PMID:33644822.
2.52A–F	Mete O
2.53	Mete O
2.54	Kleinschmidt-DeMasters BK
2.55A,B	Kleinschmidt-DeMasters BK
2.56A,B	David A. Ornan, Department of Radiology, University of Virginia, Charlottesville VA
2.57A–C	Shibuya M
2.58A–D	Kleinschmidt-DeMasters BK
2.59	Perry A
2.60A,B	Roncaroli FR
2.61	Asa SL
2.62	Roncaroli FR
2.63A–D	Knarik Arkun, Tufts University School of Medicine, Tufts Medical Center, Boston MA
2.64A,B	Ezzat S
2.65A–D	Asa SL
2.66A–C	Asa SL
2.67	Inomoto C
2.68	Inomoto C
2.69	Perry A
2.70A,B	Varlet P
2.70C	Roncaroli FR
3.01A–E	Reprinted, with permission from Elsevier, from: Cancer Genome Atlas Research Network. Integrated genomic characterization of papillary thyroid carcinoma. Cell. 2014 Oct 23;159(3):676–90. PMID:25417114.
3.02A–E	Reprinted, with permission from Elsevier, from: Cancer Genome Atlas Research Network. Integrated genomic characterization of papillary thyroid carcinoma. Cell. 2014 Oct 23;159(3):676–90. PMID:25417114.
3.03	Reprinted, with permission from Elsevier, from: Cancer Genome Atlas Research Network. Integrated genomic characterization of papillary thyroid carcinoma. Cell. 2014 Oct 23;159(3):676–90. PMID:25417114.
3.04	Reprinted, with permission, from: Haugen BR, Alexander EK, Bible KC, et al. 2015 American Thyroid Association management guidelines for adult patients with thyroid nodules and differentiated

	thyroid cancer: the American Thyroid Association Guidelines Task Force on Thyroid Nodules and Differentiated Thyroid Cancer. Thyroid. 2016 Jan;26(1):1–133. PMID:26462967.
3.05	Reprinted, with permission, from: Haugen BR, Alexander EK, Bible KC, et al. 2015 American Thyroid Association management guidelines for adult patients with thyroid nodules and differentiated thyroid cancer: the American Thyroid Association Guidelines Task Force on Thyroid Nodules and Differentiated Thyroid Cancer. Thyroid. 2016 Jan;26(1):1–133. PMID:26462967.
3.06A	Thompson LDR
3.06B	Richardson MS
3.07A–C	Thompson LDR
3.08A,B	Thompson LDR
3.09A,B	Thompson LDR
3.10A,B	Thompson LDR
3.10C–E	Baloch ZW
3.11A–C	Baloch ZW
3.12	Barletta JA
3.13A,C	Baloch ZW
3.13B,D	Barletta JA
3.14A–C	Baloch ZW
3.15A–D	Barletta JA
3.16A,B	Barletta JA
3.17A,B	Baloch ZW
3.18A	Asa SL
3.18B	Barletta JA
3.18C,D	Asa SL
3.19A,B	Baloch ZW
3.20	Baloch ZW
3.21A	Asa SL
3.21B–F	Barletta JA
3.22A,B	Baloch ZW
3.23	Ghossein RA
3.24A–C	Ghossein RA
3.25A–C	Ghossein RA
3.26A–C	Ghossein RA
3.27A,B	Tallini G
3.28	Tallini G
3.29A–D	Asa SL
3.30	Papotti M
3.31A–C	Volante M
3.32	Volante M
3.33A	Piana S
3.33B	Volante M
3.34	Adapted, with permission, from: Chan JKC. Tumors of the thyroid and parathyroid glands. In: Fletcher CDM, editor. Diagnostic histopathology of tumors. 3rd ed. London (UK): Churchill Livingstone; 2007. pp. 997–1078.
3.35A,B	Barletta JA
3.36	Juhlin CC
3.37	Barletta JA
3.38	Jung CK
3.39	Barletta JA
3.40A–C	Barletta JA
3.41	Ghossein RA
3.42	Barletta JA
3.43	Ghossein RA
3.44A	Baloch ZW
3.44B	Ghossein RA
3.45	Ghossein RA
3.46A	Baloch ZW
3.46B	Ghossein RA
3.47	Ghossein RA
3.48A	Asa SL
3.48B	Baloch ZW
3.49	Baloch ZW
3.50A,B	Asa SL
3.51	Ghossein RA
3.52A	Asa SL
3.52B	Baloch ZW
3.53A,B	Barletta JA
3.54A	Asa SL
3.54B,C	Barletta JA
3.55A,B	Mete O
3.55C,D	Ghossein RA
3.56A–C	Baloch ZW
3.57A,B	Baloch ZW
3.58	Baloch ZW
3.59A–C	Ghossein RA
3.60A,B	LiVolsi V
3.61	Baloch ZW
3.62A,B	Baloch ZW
3.63A	Piana S
3.63B	Barletta JA
3.64A–C	Ghossein RA
3.65A,B	Tallini G
3.66	Piana S
3.67A,B	Ghossein RA
3.68	Erickson LA
3.69A,B	Erickson LA
3.69C	Ghossein RA
3.70A,B	Ghossein RA
3.71	Erickson LA
3.72A,B	Baloch ZW
3.73	Adapted, with permission, from: Xu B, Fuchs T, Dogan S, et al. Dissecting anaplastic thyroid carcinoma: a comprehensive clinical, histologic, immunophenotypic, and molecular study of 360 cases. Thyroid. 2020 Oct;30(10):1505–17. PMID:32284020.
3.74A–D	Fuchs TL
3.75A–D	Fuchs TL
3.76A–F	Fuchs TL
3.77A	Fuchs TL
3.77B	Baloch ZW
3.78A–D	Volante M
3.79	Volante M
3.80A–D	Baloch ZW
3.81A–C	Baloch ZW
3.82A–D	Seethala R
3.83A,B	Seethala R
3.84	Seethala R
3.85A–C	Kerr DA
3.86A,B	Nosé V
3.87	Kerr DA
3.88	Cameselle-Teijeiro JM
3.89A,B	Erickson LA
3.90A,B	Erickson LA
3.91A,B	Nosé V
3.91C	Cameselle-Teijeiro JM
3.91D,E	Erickson LA
3.92	Chan JKC
3.93	Chan JKC
3.94A–D	Folpe AL
3.95A,B	Baloch ZW
3.96A,B,E	Cameselle-Teijeiro JM
3.96C,D	Papotti M
3.97A	Papotti M
3.97B,C	Cameselle-Teijeiro JM
3.98	Nosé V
3.99A,B	Nosé V
3.100A	Agaimy A
3.100B–D	Nosé V
3.101	Nosé V
4.01A,B	Johnson SJ
4.01C	Thompson LDR
4.02	Williams MD
4.03A,B	Gill AJ
4.04A,B	Juhlin CC
4.05	Perren A
4.06A,B	Asa SL
4.07A,B	Johnson SJ
4.08	Perren A
4.09A,B	Gill AJ
4.10A,B	Baloch ZW
4.11	Paul Komminoth, Zurich
4.12A–C	Juhlin CC
4.13	Gill AJ
4.14	Juhlin CC. Created in BioRender, 2021. https://BioRender.com/l87g919.
4.15A–C	Erickson LA
4.16A,B	Erickson LA
4.17	Juhlin CC
4.18A	Juhlin CC. Created in BioRender, 2021. https://BioRender.com/h68i408.
4.18B	Juhlin CC. Created in BioRender, 2021. https://BioRender.com/c03g277
4.19A,B	Mete O
4.20A	Reprinted, with permission, from: Duan K, Mete Ö. Parathyroid carcinoma: diagnosis and clinical implications. Turk Patoloji Derg. 2015;31 Suppl 1:80–97. doi: 10.5146/tjpath.2015.01316. PMID:26177319. The original article is available at http://www.turkjpath.org – http://www.turkjpath.org/text.php3?doi=10.5146/tjpath.2015.01316 © Federation of Turkish Pathology Societies
4.20B–D	Mete O
4.21A,D	Mete O
4.21B,C	Asa SL
5.01,inset	Papotti M
5.02	Papotti M
5.03	Falhammar H
5.04	Mete O
5.05A,B	Mete O
5.06A,B	Papotti M
5.07	Papotti M
5.08	Falhammar H
5.09	Mete O
5.10A	Mete O
5.10B	Papotti M
5.11	Juhlin CC. Created in BioRender, 2021. https://BioRender.com/k87i330.
5.12A–C	Erickson LA
5.13A,B	Erickson LA

5.14A–C	Erickson LA
5.15A,B	Mete O
5.16	Sasano H
5.17A–C	Mete O
5.18A,B	Sasano H
5.19	Mete O
5.20	Juhlin CC. Created in BioRender, 2024. https://BioRender.com/n04u186. Adapted, by permission from Springer, from: Juhlin CC, Bertherat J, Giordano TJ, et al. What did we learn from the molecular biology of adrenal cortical neoplasia? From histopathology to translational genomics. Endocr Pathol. 2021 Mar;32(1):102–33. PMID:33534120.
5.21	Juhlin CC. Created in BioRender, 2021. https://BioRender.com/a82s259. Adapted, by permission from Springer, from: Juhlin CC, Bertherat J, Giordano TJ, et al. What did we learn from the molecular biology of adrenal cortical neoplasia? From histopathology to translational genomics. Endocr Pathol. 2021 Mar;32(1):102–33. PMID:33534120.
5.22	Juhlin CC. Created in BioRender, 2020. https://BioRender.com/o15s485. Adapted, by permission from Springer, from: Juhlin CC, Bertherat J, Giordano TJ, et al. What did we learn from the molecular biology of adrenal cortical neoplasia? From histopathology to translational genomics. Endocr Pathol. 2021 Mar;32(1):102–33. PMID:33534120.
5.23A,B	Erickson LA
5.24A	Juhlin CC
5.24B	Erickson LA
5.25A	Erickson LA
5.25B	Mete O
5.26A–C	Erickson LA
5.27A,B	Juhlin CC
5.28	Juhlin CC. Created in BioRender, 2024. https://BioRender.com/n03u771. Adapted, by permission from Springer, from: Juhlin CC, Bertherat J, Giordano TJ, et al. What did we learn from the molecular biology of adrenal cortical neoplasia? From histopathology to translational genomics. Endocr Pathol. 2021 Mar;32(1):102–33. PMID:33534120.
5.29	Juhlin CC. Created in BioRender, 2024. https://BioRender.com/o08p295. Adapted, by permission from Springer, from: Juhlin CC, Bertherat J, Giordano TJ, et al. What did we learn from the molecular biology of adrenal cortical neoplasia? From histopathology to translational genomics. Endocr Pathol. 2021 Mar;32(1):102–33. PMID:33534120.
5.30	Juhlin CC. Created in BioRender, 2024. https://BioRender.com/w68f480. Adapted, by permission from Springer, from: Juhlin CC, Bertherat J, Giordano TJ, et al. What did we learn from the molecular biology of adrenal cortical neoplasia? From histopathology to translational genomics. Endocr Pathol. 2021 Mar;32(1):102–33. PMID:33534120.
5.31	Juhlin CC
5.32	Mete O
5.33	Mete O
5.34A,B	Mete O
5.35	Erickson LA
5.36A,B	Volante M
5.37A,B	Mete O
5.38A,B	Mete O
5.39	Mete O
5.40A–D	Gill AJ
5.41	Erickson LA
5.42A–D	Alison Potter, Tissue Pathology and Diagnostic Oncology, Royal Prince Alfred Hospital, Camperdown NSW; and Scolyer RA; and Stephen Mann, Histopath Diagnostic Specialists, Macquarie Park NSW
6.01	Reprinted, with permission from Elsevier, from: Fishbein L, Leshchiner I, Walter V, et al. Comprehensive molecular characterization of pheochromocytoma and paraganglioma. Cancer Cell. 2017 Feb 13;31(2):181–93. PMID:28162975.
6.02	Reprinted, with permission from Elsevier, from: Fishbein L, Leshchiner I, Walter V, et al. Comprehensive molecular characterization of pheochromocytoma and paraganglioma. Cancer Cell. 2017 Feb 13;31(2):181–93. PMID:28162975.
6.03	Shimada H
6.04A–D	Shimada H
6.05A,B	Shimada H
6.05C	Fischer M
6.06A,B	Fischer M
6.07	Beiske KH
6.08	Beiske KH
6.09A–D	Beiske KH
6.10	Shimada H
6.11	Shimada H
6.12	Shimada H
6.13	Shimada H
6.14A–E	Takao Sasaki, Department of Pediatric Surgery, Faculty of Medicine, University of Tsukuba, Ibaraki
6.15A,B	Arthur J.A.T. Braat, Department of Radiology and Nuclear Medicine, University Medical Center Utrecht, Utrecht
6.16A	Hicks MJ
6.16B	Mete O
6.17	de Krijger RR
6.18	de Krijger RR
6.19	Asa SL
6.20A,B	Mete O
6.21A–C	Kimura N
6.21D	Mete O
6.22A,B	Mete O
6.23A,E,F	Kimura N
6.23B–D	Mete O
6.24A,B	Mete O
6.25A,B	Kimura N
6.25C	Mete O
6.26A–C	Tischler AS
6.27A–D	Harry Kozakewich, General Pediatric Pathology, Department of Pathology, Boston Children's Hospital, Boston MA
6.28A–C	Tischler AS
6.29A–C	Arthur J.A.T. Braat, Department of Radiology and Nuclear Medicine, University Medical Center Utrecht, Utrecht
6.30	Tischler AS
6.31A–C	Tischler AS
6.32A,B	Tischler AS
6.33A–C	Tischler AS
6.34	Harry Kozakewich, General Pediatric Pathology, Department of Pathology, Boston Children's Hospital, Boston MA
6.35	Lam AK
6.36	Oudijk L
6.37	Lam AK
7.01A,B	Kasajima A
7.02A–D	Kasajima A
7.03A,C	Kasajima A
7.03B	La Rosa S
7.04	Kasajima A
7.05A,B	Kasajima A
7.06	Kasajima A
7.07A–H	Niklaus Schaefer and Sarah Boughdad, Department of Nuclear Medicine and Molecular Imaging, CHUV and University of Lausanne, Lausanne
7.08A,B	Reprinted, with permission, from: Hackeng WM, Schelhaas W, Morsink FHM, et al. Alternative lengthening of telomeres and differential expression of endocrine transcription factors distinguish metastatic and non-metastatic insulinomas. Endocr Pathol. 2020 Jun;31(2):108–18. PMID:32103422.
7.09A	Ohike N
7.09B–F	La Rosa S
7.10A,B	La Rosa S
7.11A–C	Brosens LAA

Figure	Source
7.12A–F	Reprinted, with permission, from: Hackeng WM, Schelhaas W, Morsink FHM, et al. Alternative lengthening of telomeres and differential expression of endocrine transcription factors distinguish metastatic and non-metastatic insulinomas. Endocr Pathol. 2020 Jun;31(2):108–18. PMID:32103422.
7.13	de Herder WW
7.14	de Herder WW
7.15	Brosens LAA
7.16A–C	Amedeo Sciarra, Department of Histopathology, Central Institute, Valais Hospital, Sion
7.17A,B	Singhi AD
7.18A–C	Singhi AD
7.18D	La Rosa S
7.19A,B	La Rosa S
7.20A–C	Basturk O
7.21A,B	de Herder WW
7.22A–E	La Rosa S
7.23	Anna Caterina Milanetto and Claudio Pasquali, Department of Surgery, Oncology and Gastroenterology, University of Padova, Padova
7.24A,C	Kasajima A
7.24B,D–F	La Rosa S
7.25A–C	Alessandro Vanoli, Department of Molecular Medicine, Unit of Anatomic Pathology, University of Pavia, Fondazione IRCCS Policlinico San Matteo, Pavia
7.26A,B	La Rosa S
7.27A,B	Basturk O
7.28A–C	Basturk O
7.29A–D	Alessandro Vanoli, Department of Molecular Medicine, Unit of Anatomic Pathology, University of Pavia, Fondazione IRCCS Policlinico San Matteo, Pavia
7.30A,B	Klimstra DS
7.31A–C	Adapted, with permission, from: Uccella S, La Rosa S. Looking into digestive mixed neuroendocrine – nonneuroendocrine neoplasms: subtypes, prognosis, and predictive factors. Histopathology. 2020 Nov;77(5):700–17. PMID:32538468.
8.01	Reprinted, with permission, from: Uccella S, La Rosa S, Metovic J, et al. Genomics of high-grade neuroendocrine neoplasms: well-differentiated neuroendocrine tumor with high-grade features (G3 NET) and neuroendocrine carcinomas (NEC) of various anatomic sites. Endocr Pathol. 2021;32(1):192–210. PMID:33433884.
8.02	Rindi G
8.03	Volante M
8.04A,B	Volante M
8.05A–C	Volante M
8.06A–C	Volante M
8.07	Uccella S
8.08A–F	Uccella S
8.09A–C	Osamura RY
8.10A–C	Tetzlaff M
8.11A–C	Milione M
8.12A–C	Uccella S
8.13	Gill AJ
8.14A–D	Fuchs TL
8.14E	Uccella S
8.15A–C	Fuchs TL
8.16	Fuchs TL
8.17	Francesco Carletti, Lysholm Department of Neuroradiology, National Hospital for Neurology and Neurosurgery, UCLH, London
8.18A–F	Brandner S
8.19	Perry A
9.01	Fritchie KJ
9.02A–D	Thompson LDR
9.03	Thompson LDR
9.04	Asa SL
9.05A–C	Catarina Eloy, IPATIMUP Pathology Laboratory, Porto
9.06	Erickson LA
9.07A–D	Doyle LA
9.08A,B	Doyle LA
9.09	Hyrcza MD
9.10	Hyrcza MD
9.11A–F	Erickson LA
9.12	Erickson LA
9.13	Erickson LA
9.14	Thompson LDR
9.15	Thompson LDR
9.16	Thompson LDR
9.17	Thompson LDR
9.18A–E	Thompson LDR
9.19A,B	Thompson LDR
9.20A,B	Thompson LDR
9.21	Thompson LDR
9.22A,B	Thompson LDR
9.23	Thompson LDR
9.24	Thompson LDR
9.25	Thompson LDR
9.26	Perry A
9.27	Perry A
9.28A,B	Perry A
9.29A–D	Thompson LDR
9.30A,B	Thompson LDR
10.01A,B	Lizhi Zhang, Division of Anatomic Pathology, May Clinic, Rochester MN
10.02A,B	Lizhi Zhang, Division of Anatomic Pathology, May Clinic, Rochester MN
10.03A,B	Tallini G
10.04A,B	Tallini G
10.05	Tallini G
10.06A,B	Tallini G
10.07A,B	Chan JKC
10.08A–D	Chan JKC
10.09	Touraine PA
10.10A–D	Shanop Shuangshoti, Department of Pathology, Faculty of Medicine, Chulalongkorn University, Bangkok
10.11A–D	Thompson LDR
10.11E	Bychkov A
10.12	Bychkov A
10.13	Facchetti F
10.14	Facchetti F
10.15	Facchetti F
10.16	Paulus W
10.17	Paulus W
10.18	Chan JKC
10.19	Chan JKC
10.20	Chan JKC
11.01	Thompson LDR
11.02	Thompson LDR
11.03	Thompson LDR
11.04	Thompson LDR
11.05	Rooper LM
11.06	Rooper LM
11.07	Rooper LM
12.01	Roncaroli FR
12.02	Roncaroli FR
12.03	Roncaroli FR
12.04A,B	Ghossein RA
12.05A,B	Ghossein RA
12.06	Ghossein RA
12.07A,B	Baloch ZW
12.08	Nosé V
12.09	Gill AJ
12.10A,B	Gill AJ
13.01A,B	Valk GD
13.02A,B	Ezzat S
13.03A,B	Toshihiko Masui, Division of Hepato-Biliary-Pancreatic Surgery and Transplantation, Department of Surgery, Graduate School of Medicine, Kyoto University, Kyoto
13.04A–C	Mete O
13.05A	Perren A
13.05B	Mete O
13.06	Mete O
13.07	Thompson LDR
13.08	Asa SL
13.09	de Krijger RR
13.10A–C	Erickson LA
13.11A,B	Asa SL
13.12	Pellegata NS
13.13A–D	Gill AJ
13.14A,B	Fuchs TL
13.15A,B	Fuchs TL
13.16A,B	Fuchs TL
13.17A,B	Mete O
13.18A–E	Gill AJ
13.19A,B	Gill AJ
13.20	Gill AJ
13.21A,B	Gill AJ
13.22A	Lloyd RV, Osamura RY, Klöppel G, Rosai J, editors. WHO classification of tumours of endocrine organs. Lyon (France): International Agency for Research on Cancer; 2017. (WHO classification of tumours series, 4th ed.; vol. 10). https://publications.iarc.who.int/554.
13.22B	Morreau H
13.22C	Gill AJ
13.23A,B	Ezzat S
13.24A	Asa SL
13.24B	Kasajima A
13.25A,B	Nosé V
13.25C	Erickson LA

13.26A,B Kasajima A
13.27A–C Asa SL
13.28 Erickson LA
13.29A,B Erickson LA
13.30A–C Gill AJ
13.31 Gill AJ
13.32A–C Gill AJ
13.33A,B Gill AJ
13.34A,B Jennifer M. Boland, Division of Anatomic Pathology, May Clinic, Rochester MN
13.35 Gill AJ
13.36 Juhlin CC. Created in BioRender, 2021. https://BioRender.com/q82v490.
13.37 Paul Komminoth, Zurich
13.38 Perren A
13.39 Stratakis CA
13.40 Mete O
13.41A–C Mete O
13.42 Boyce AM
13.43 Boyce AM
13.44A,B Ezzat S
13.45A,B Asa SL
13.46A,B Nosé V
13.47A,B Nosé V
13.48A,B Gill AJ
13.49 Nosé V
13.50 Gill AJ
13.51A,B Sipos B
13.52A–C Sipos B
13.53 Klöppel G
13.54 Klöppel G
13.55 Klöppel G
13.56 Cameselle-Teijeiro JM
13.57 Cameselle-Teijeiro JM
13.58A,B Cameselle-Teijeiro JM
13.59 Cameselle-Teijeiro JM
13.60 Cameselle-Teijeiro JM
13.61A,B Cameselle-Teijeiro JM
13.62A,B Cameselle-Teijeiro JM
13.63A Nosé V
13.63B Cameselle-Teijeiro JM
13.64 Nosé V
13.65 Cameselle-Teijeiro JM
13.66A,B Cameselle-Teijeiro JM
13.67 Nosé V
13.68A–C Nosé V

Tables

2.01 Asa SL
2.02 Adapted, with permission from Springer, from: Asa SL, Mete O, Ezzat S. Genomics and epigenomics of pituitary tumors: What do pathologists need to know? Endocr Pathol. 2021 Mar;32(1):3–16. PMID:33433883.
2.03 Adapted, with permission from Springer, from: Asa SL, Mete O, Ezzat S. Genomics and epigenomics of pituitary tumors: What do pathologists need to know? Endocr Pathol. 2021 Mar;32(1):3–16. PMID:33433883.

3.01 Tallini G
3.02 Tallini G
3.03 Volante M
3.04 Tallini G
3.05 Ghossein RA
3.06 Ghossein RA
3.07 Reprinted, with permission, from: Xu B, Fuchs TL, Ahmadi S, et al. International medullary thyroid carcinoma grading system: a validated grading system for medullary thyroid carcinoma. J Clin Oncol. 2022 Jan 1;40(1):96–104. PMID:34731032.
3.08 Cameselle-Teijeiro JM

4.01 Perren A

5.01 Erickson LA
5.02 Mete O
5.03 Mete O
5.04 Mete O
5.05 Mete O

6.01 Adapted from: Kleihues P, Cavenee WK, editors. Pathology and genetics of tumours of the nervous system. Lyon (France): International Agency for Research on Cancer; 2000. (WHO classification of tumours series, 3rd ed.; vol. 1). https://publications.iarc.who.int/1. and Lloyd RV, Osamura RY, Klöppel G, Rosai J, editors. WHO classification of tumours of endocrine organs. Lyon (France): International Agency for Research on Cancer; 2017. (WHO classification of tumours series, 4th ed.; vol. 10). https://publications.iarc.who.int/554.
6.02 Shimada H
6.03 Reprinted, with permission, from: Monclair T, Brodeur GM, Ambros PF, et al. The International Neuroblastoma Risk Group (INRG) staging system: an INRG Task Force report. J Clin Oncol. 2009 Jan 10;27(2):298–303. PMID:19047290.

7.01 Lloyd RV, Osamura RY, Klöppel G, Rosai J, editors. WHO classification of tumours of endocrine organs. Lyon (France): International Agency for Research on Cancer; 2017. (WHO classification of tumours series, 4th ed.; vol. 10). https://publications.iarc.who.int/554.
7.02 Lloyd RV, Osamura RY, Klöppel G, Rosai J, editors. WHO classification of tumours of endocrine organs. Lyon (France): International Agency for Research on Cancer; 2017. (WHO classification of tumours series, 4th ed.; vol. 10). https://publications.iarc.who.int/554.

8.01 Adapted, with permission from Springer Nature, from: Asa SL, Lloyd RV, Tischler AS. Neuroendocrine neoplasms: historical background and terminologies. In: Asa SL, La Rosa S, Mete O. The spectrum of neuroendocrine neoplasia: a practical approach to diagnosis, classification and therapy. Springer; 2020. pp. 1–14, Table 1.1.
8.02 Uccella S
8.03 Brandner S

9.01 Hyrcza MD

12.01 Thompson LDR

13.01 Nosé V; Lazar AJ
13.02 Gimenez-Roqueplo A-P
13.03 Pellegata NS
13.04 Gill AJ
13.05 Gill AJ
13.06 Kirschner LS
13.07 Foulkes WD
13.08 Cameselle-Teijeiro JM
13.09 Cameselle-Teijeiro JM

Boxes

5.01 Papotti M
5.02 Mete O
5.03 Mete O

8.01 La Rosa S

13.01 Perren A
13.02 Reprinted, with permission, from: Carney AJ, Lyssikatos C, Seethala RR, et al. The spectrum of thyroid gland pathology in Carney complex: the importance of follicular carcinoma. Am J Surg Pathol. 2018 May;42(5):587–94. PMID:29635258.
13.03 Adapted, with permission, from: Stratakis CA. Carney complex: a familial lentiginosis predisposing to a variety of tumors. Rev Endocr Metab Disord. 2016 Sep;17(3):36–71. PMID:27943004; and Stratakis CA, Kirschner LS, Carney JA. Clinical and molecular features of the Carney complex: diagnostic criteria and recommendations for patient evaluation. J Clin Endocrinol Metab. 2001 Sep;86(9):4041–6. PMID:11549623.
13.04 Bharat Rekhi, in: WHO Classification of Tumours Editorial Board. Genetic tumour syndromes [Internet; beta version ahead of print]. Lyon (France): International Agency for Research on Cancer; 2023. (WHO classification of tumours

	series, 5th ed.; vol. 14). https://tumourclassification.iarc.who.int/chapters/67.
13.05	Cameselle-Teijeiro JM

Images on the cover

Top left	Fig. 7.11A: Brosens LAA
Middle left	Fig. 7.09D: La Rosa S
Bottom left	Fig. 7.10A: La Rosa S
Top centre	Fig. 2.37B: Nishioka H
Middle centre	Fig. 2.38D: Lopes MBS
Bottom centre	Fig. 2.39C: Lopes MBS
Top right	Fig. 13.36: Juhlin CC. Created in BioRender, 2021. https://BioRender.com/q82v490.
Middle right	Fig. 13.33B: Gill AJ
Bottom right	Fig. 13.30C: Gill AJ

Images on the chapter title pages

Chapter 1	Fig. 1.01B: Asa SL
Chapter 2	Fig. 2.30B: Lopes MBS
Chapter 3	Fig. 3.11C: Baloch ZW
Chapter 4	Fig. 4.10B: Baloch ZW
Chapter 5	Fig. 5.12B: Erickson LA
Chapter 6	Fig. 6.18: de Krijger RR
Chapter 7	Fig. 7.18: Singhi AD
Chapter 8	Fig. 8.10: Tetzlaff M
Chapter 9	Fig. 9.11D: Erickson LA
Chapter 10	Fig. 10.08C: Chan JKC
Chapter 11	Fig. 11.06: Rooper LM
Chapter 12	Fig. 12.07B: Baloch ZW
Chapter 13	Fig. 13.18D: Gill AJ

References

1. Abbi KK, Hameed MK, Jiang Y, et al. Pulmonary collision tumor consisting of adenocarcinoma and typical carcinoid–a case report and review of literature. Am J Ther. 2014 Nov-Dec;21(6):e234–8. PMID:23689091
2. Abbosh PH, Zhang S, Maclennan GT, et al. Germ cell origin of testicular carcinoid tumors. Clin Cancer Res. 2008 Mar 1;14(5):1393–6. PMID:18316560
3. Abd-El Raouf SM, Ibrahim TR. Immunohistochemical expression of HBME-1 and galectin-3 in the differential diagnosis of follicular-derived thyroid nodules. Pathol Res Pract. 2014 Dec;210(12):971–8. PMID:25041837
4. Abe I, Lam AK. Anaplastic thyroid carcinoma: current issues in genomics and therapeutics. Curr Oncol Rep. 2021 Feb 13;23(3):31. PMID:33582932
5. Abe I, Lam AK. Anaplastic thyroid carcinoma: updates on WHO classification, clinicopathological features and staging. Histol Histopathol. 2021 Mar;36(3):239–48. PMID:33170501
6. Abedalthagafi M, Bi WL, Aizer AA, et al. Oncogenic PI3K mutations are as common as AKT1 and SMO mutations in meningioma. Neuro Oncol. 2016 May;18(5):649–55. PMID:26826201
7. Abiko Y, Ogawa I, Hattori Y, et al. Atypical carcinoid (neuroendocrine carcinoma) of the gingiva: counterpart of a laryngeal tumor. Pathol Int. 2004 Feb;54(2):97–100. PMID:14720139
8. Abla O, Jacobsen E, Picarsic J, et al. Consensus recommendations for the diagnosis and clinical management of Rosai-Dorfman-Destombes disease. Blood. 2018 Jun 28;131(26):2877–90. PMID:29720485
9. Abood A, Vestergaard P. Increasing incidence of primary hyperparathyroidism in Denmark. Dan Med J. 2013 Feb;60(2):A4567. PMID:23461985
10. Abou Saleh M, Mansoor E, Anindo M, et al. Prevalence of small intestine carcinoid tumors: a US Population-Based Study 2012-2017. Dig Dis Sci. 2019 May;64(5):1328–34. PMID:30519851
11. Abraham DT, Low TH, Messina M, et al. Medullary thyroid carcinoma: long-term outcomes of surgical treatment. Ann Surg Oncol. 2011 Jan;18(1):219–25. PMID:20878247
12. Abraham P, Ralston SH, Hewison M, et al. Presentation of a PTHrP-secreting pancreatic neuroendocrine tumour, with hypercalcaemic crisis, pre-eclampsia, and renal failure. Postgrad Med J. 2002 Dec;78(926):752–3. PMID:12509695
13. Abrosimov AY, LiVolsi VA. Spindle epithelial tumor with thymus-like differentiation (SETTLE) of the thyroid with neck lymph node metastasis: a case report. Endocr Pathol. 2005 Summer;16(2):139–43. PMID:16199899
14. Absher KJ, Truong LD, Khurana KK, et al. Parathyroid cytology: avoiding diagnostic pitfalls. Head Neck. 2002 Feb;24(2):157–64. PMID:11891946
15. Abu-Khudir R, Larrivée-Vanier S, Wasserman JD, et al. Disorders of thyroid morphogenesis. Best Pract Res Clin Endocrinol Metab. 2017 Mar;31(2):143–59. PMID:28648504
16. Abushamat LA, Kerr JM, Lopes MBS, et al. Very unusual sellar/suprasellar region masses: a review. J Neuropathol Exp Neurol. 2019 Aug 1;78(8):673–84. PMID:31233145
17. Acharya S, Sarafoglou K, LaQuaglia M, et al. Thyroid neoplasms after therapeutic radiation for malignancies during childhood or adolescence. Cancer. 2003 May 15;97(10):2397–403. PMID:12733137
18. Ackermann S, Cartolano M, Hero B, et al. A mechanistic classification of clinical phenotypes in neuroblastoma. Science. 2018 Dec 7;362(6419):1165–70. PMID:30523111
19. Adamson AR, Grahame-Smith DG, Bogomoletz V, et al. Malignant argentaffinoma with carcinoid syndrome and hypoglycaemia. Br Med J. 1971 Jul 10;3(5766):93–4. PMID:5314568
20. Adamson TE, Wiestler OD, Kleihues P, et al. Correlation of clinical and pathological features in surgically treated craniopharyngiomas. J Neurosurg. 1990 Jul;73(1):12–7. PMID:2352012
21. Adegun OK, Proctor I, Falzon M, et al. Spindle cell tumour with thymus-like differentiation (SETTLE) on fine needle aspiration cytology: a case report highlighting diagnostic pitfalls. Diagn Cytopathol. 2021 Aug;49(8):E325–8. PMID:33794064
22. Adeniran AJ, Shuch B, Humphrey PA. Hereditary renal cell carcinoma syndromes: clinical, pathologic, and genetic features. Am J Surg Pathol. 2015 Dec;39(12):e1–18. PMID:26559379
23. Adeniran AJ, Zhu Z, Gandhi M, et al. Correlation between genetic alterations and microscopic features, clinical manifestations, and prognostic characteristics of thyroid papillary carcinomas. Am J Surg Pathol. 2006 Feb;30(2):216–22. PMID:16434896
24. Adnan A, Basu S. Combined 177Lu-DOTATATE peptide receptor radionuclide therapy and platinum-based chemotherapy in recurrent, metastatic sinonasal neuroendocrine carcinoma: a promising therapeutic option. J Nucl Med Technol. 2020 Sep;48(3):292–4. PMID:32358042
25. Adriani KS, Stenvers DJ, Imanse JG. Pearls & oy-sters: Lumbar paraganglioma: can you see it in the eyes? Neurology. 2012 Jan 24;78(4):e27–8. PMID:22271522
26. Adsay NV, Andea A, Basturk O, et al. Secondary tumors of the pancreas: an analysis of a surgical and autopsy database and review of the literature. Virchows Arch. 2004 Jun;444(6):527–35. PMID:15057558
27. Afrogheh AH, Meserve E, Sadow PM, et al. Molecular characterization of an endometrial endometrioid adenocarcinoma metastatic to a thyroid Hürthle cell adenoma showing cancerization of follicles. Endocr Pathol. 2016 Sep;27(3):213–9. PMID:26687112
28. Agaimy A, Erlenbach-Wünsch K, Konukiewitz B, et al. ISL1 expression is not restricted to pancreatic well-differentiated neuroendocrine neoplasms, but is also commonly found in well and poorly differentiated neuroendocrine neoplasms of extrapancreatic origin. Mod Pathol. 2013 Jul;26(7):995–1003. PMID:23503646
29. Agaimy A, Hahn T, Schroeder J, et al. Follicular thyroid adenoma dominated by spindle cells: report of two unusual cases and literature review. Int J Clin Exp Pathol. 2012;5(2):143–51. PMID:22400075
30. Agaimy A, Lell M, Schaller T, et al. 'Neuroendocrine' middle ear adenomas: consistent expression of the transcription factor ISL1 further supports their neuroendocrine derivation. Histopathology. 2015 Jan;66(2):182–91. PMID:24766278
31. Agaimy A, Tögel L, Stoehr R, et al. NSD3-NUTM1-rearranged carcinoma of the median neck/thyroid bed developing after recent thyroidectomy for sclerosing mucoepidermoid carcinoma with eosinophilia: report of an extraordinary case. Virchows Arch. 2021 Dec;479(6):1095–9. PMID:33891143
32. Agaimy A, Witkowski L, Stoehr R, et al. Malignant teratoid tumor of the thyroid gland: an aggressive primitive multiphenotypic malignancy showing organotypical elements and frequent DICER1 alterations-is the term "thyroblastoma" more appropriate? Virchows Arch. 2020 Dec;477(6):787–98. PMID:32507920
33. Agaram NP, LaQuaglia MP, Alaggio R, et al. MYOD1-mutant spindle cell and sclerosing rhabdomyosarcoma: an aggressive subtype irrespective of age. A reappraisal for molecular classification and risk stratification. Mod Pathol. 2019 Jan;32(1):27–36. PMID:30181563
34. Agaram NP, Sung YS, Zhang L, et al. Dichotomy of genetic abnormalities in PEComas with therapeutic implications. Am J Surg Pathol. 2015 Jun;39(6):813–25. PMID:25651471
35. Agaram NP, Zhang L, Jungbluth AA, et al. A molecular reappraisal of glomus tumors and related pericytic neoplasms with emphasis on NOTCH-gene fusions. Am J Surg Pathol. 2020 Nov;44(11):1556–62. PMID:32604167
36. Agarwal C, Raychaudhuri S, Batra A, et al. Medullary carcinoma of thyroid mimicking Hurthle cell neoplasm on cytology: a diagnostic dilemma. Diagn Cytopathol. 2019 Sep;47(9):943–7. PMID:31190466
37. Agarwal S, Bychkov A, Jung CK, et al. The prevalence and surgical outcomes of Hürthle cell lesions in FNAs of the thyroid: a multi-institutional study in 6 Asian countries. Cancer Cytopathol. 2019 Mar;127(3):181–91. PMID:30668897
38. Agarwal S, Jindal I, Balazs A, et al. Catecholamine-secreting tumors in pediatric patients with cyanotic congenital heart disease. J Endocr Soc. 2019 Sep 5;3(11):2135–50. PMID:31687640
39. Agarwal SK. Multiple endocrine neoplasia type 1. Front Horm Res. 2013;41:1–15. PMID:23652667
40. Agarwal SK. The future: genetics advances in MEN1 therapeutic approaches and management strategies. Endocr Relat Cancer. 2017 Oct;24(10):T119–34. PMID:28899949
41. Agarwal SK, Mateo CM, Marx SJ. Rare germline mutations in cyclin-dependent kinase inhibitor genes in multiple endocrine neoplasia type 1 and related states. J Clin Endocrinol Metab. 2009 May;94(5):1826–34. PMID:19141585
42. Agate L, Lorusso L, Elisei R. New and old knowledge on differentiated thyroid cancer epidemiology and risk factors. J Endocrinol Invest. 2012;35(6 Suppl):3–9. PMID:23014067
43. Aggarwal G, Jackson L, Sharma S. Primary combined small cell carcinoma of larynx with lateralized histologic components and corresponding side-specific neck nodal metastasis: report of a unique case and review of literature. Int J Clin Exp Pathol. 2010 Dec 3;4(1):111–7. PMID:21228933
44. Aggarwal RR, Quigley DA, Huang J, et al. Whole-genome and transcriptional analysis of treatment-emergent small-cell neuroendocrine prostate cancer demonstrates intraclass heterogeneity. Mol Cancer Res. 2019 Jun;17(6):1235–40. PMID:30918106
45. Agnihotri S, Suppiah S, Tonge PD, et al. Therapeutic radiation for childhood cancer drives structural aberrations of NF2 in meningiomas. Nat Commun. 2017 Aug 4;8(1):186. PMID:28775249
46. Agrawal N, Jiao Y, Sausen M, et al. Exomic sequencing of medullary thyroid cancer reveals dominant and mutually exclusive oncogenic mutations in RET and RAS. J Clin Endocrinol Metab. 2013 Feb;98(2):E364–9. PMID:23264394
47. Aguirre P, Scully RE. Testosterone-secreting adrenal ganglioneuroma containing Leydig cells. Am J Surg Pathol. 1983 Oct;7(7):699–705. PMID:6685441
48. Agustsson TT, Baldvinsdottir T, Jonasson JG, et al. The epidemiology of pituitary adenomas in Iceland, 1955-2012: a nationwide population-based study. Eur J Endocrinol. 2015 Nov;173(5):655–64. PMID:26423473
49. Ahmad S, Naber MR, Giles RH, et al. Diagnostic and management strategies for pNETs in Von Hippel-Lindau: a systematic review. Endocr Relat Cancer. 2021 Mar;28(3):151–60. PMID:33512331
50. Ahmed AK, Dawood HY, Arnaout OM, et al. Presentation, treatment, and long-term outcome of intrasellar chordoma: a pooled analysis of institutional, SEER (Surveillance Epidemiology and End Results), and published data. World Neurosurg. 2018 Jan;109:e676–83. PMID:29061463
51. Ahmed FW, Majeed MS, Kirresh O. Multiple endocrine neoplasias type 4. 2023 Oct 18. In: StatPearls. Treasure Island (FL): StatPearls Publishing; 2024 Jan–. PMID:33760487
52. Ahn CH, Kim JH, Park MY, et al. Epidemiology and comorbidity of adrenal Cushing syndrome: a nationwide cohort study. J Clin Endocrinol Metab. 2021 Mar 8;106(3):e1362–72. PMID:33075802
53. Ahn D, Lee GJ, Sohn JH, et al. Fine-needle aspiration cytology versus core-needle biopsy for the diagnosis of extracranial head and neck schwannoma. Head Neck. 2018 Dec;40(12):2695–700. PMID:30457183
54. Ahn SH, Kim JH, Baek SH, et al. Characteristics of adrenal incidentalomas in a large, prospective computed tomography-based multicenter study: the COAR study in Korea. Yonsei Med J. 2018 Jun;59(4):501–10. PMID:29749133
55. Akaike K, Kurisaki-Arakawa A, Hara K, et al. Distinct clinicopathological features of NAB2-STAT6 fusion gene variants in solitary fibrous tumor with emphasis on the acquisition of highly malignant potential. Hum Pathol. 2015 Mar;46(3):347–56. PMID:25582503
56. Akaishi J, Kondo T, Sugino K, et al. Prognostic impact of the Turin criteria in poorly differentiated thyroid carcinoma. World J Surg. 2019

Sep;43(9):2235–44. PMID:31098668
57. Akbulut S. Incidentally detected hydatid cyst of the adrenal gland: a case report. World J Clin Cases. 2016 Sep 16;4(9):269–72. PMID:27672642
58. Aker FV, Bas Y, Ozkara S, et al. Spindle cell metaplasia in follicular adenoma of the thyroid gland: case report and review of the literature. Endocr J. 2004 Oct;51(5):457–61. PMID:15516778
59. Akerström G, Malmaeus J, Bergström R. Surgical anatomy of human parathyroid glands. Surgery. 1984 Jan;95(1):14–21. PMID:6691181
60. Akerström G, Malmaeus J, Grimelius L, et al. Histological changes in parathyroid glands in subclinical and clinical renal disease. An autopsy investigation. Scand J Urol Nephrol. 1984;18(1):75–84. PMID:6719054
61. Åkerström T, Maharjan R, Sven Willenberg H, et al. Activating mutations in CTNNB1 in aldosterone producing adenomas. Sci Rep. 2016 Jan 27;6:19546. PMID:26815163
62. Akhavanfard S, Yehia L, Padmanabhan R, et al. Germline EGFR variants are over-represented in adolescents and young adults (AYA) with adrenocortical carcinoma. Hum Mol Genet. 2021 Jan 21;29(22):3679–90. PMID:33326033
63. Akın O, Ataş E, Atasoy İA, et al. Two subsequent metachroneus solid tumors: oncocytic variant adrenocortical carcinoma and rhabdomyosarcoma of childhood: case report and literature review. J Clin Res Pediatr Endocrinol. 2021 Jun 2;13(2):225–31. PMID:32539319
64. Akirov A, Asa SL, Amer L, et al. The clinicopathological spectrum of acromegaly. J Clin Med. 2019 Nov 13;8(11):1962. PMID:31766255
65. Akirov A, Asa SL, Larouche V, et al. The clinicopathological spectrum of parathyroid carcinoma. Front Endocrinol (Lausanne). 2019 Oct 23;10:731. PMID:31708875
66. Akirov A, Larouche V, Shimon I, et al. Significance of Crooke's hyaline change in nontumorous corticotrophs of patients with Cushing disease. Front Endocrinol (Lausanne). 2021 Mar 18;12:620005. PMID:33815279
67. Akishima-Fukasawa Y, Yoshihara A, Ishikawa Y, et al. Malignant adrenal rest tumor of the retroperitoneum producing adrenocortical steroids. Endocr Pathol. 2011 Jun;22(2):112–7. PMID:21374072
68. Akramipour R, Zargooshi J, Rahimi Z. Infant with concomitant presence of hernia/hydrocele and primary paratesticular neuroblastoma: a diagnostic and therapeutic challenge. J Pediatr Hematol Oncol. 2009 May;31(5):349. PMID:19415016
69. Al Badi MK, Al-Alwan I, Al-Dubayee M, et al. Testosterone- and cortisol-secreting oncocytic adrenocortical adenoma in the pediatric age-group. Pediatr Dev Pathol. 2018 Nov-Dec;21(6):568–73. PMID:29426273
70. Al Khaldi M, Mesbah A, Dubé P, et al. Neuroendocrine carcinoma arising in a tailgut cyst. Int J Surg Case Rep. 2018;49:91–5. PMID:29966957
71. Al Qahtani MS, Bojal SA, Alqarzaie AA, et al. Insulinoma in tuberous sclerosis: an entity not to be missed. Saudi Med J. 2021 Mar;42(3):332–7. PMID:33632913
72. Alaggio R, Zhang L, Sung YS, et al. A molecular study of pediatric spindle and sclerosing rhabdomyosarcoma: identification of novel and recurrent VGLL2-related fusions in infantile cases. Am J Surg Pathol. 2016 Feb;40(2):224–35. PMID:26501226
73. Alagoz E, Okuyucu K, Ince S, et al. Prognostic risk factors for rare oncocytic variantin 101 cases of papillary thyroid carcinoma. Hell J Nucl Med. 2019 May-Aug;22(2):116–22. PMID:31273353
74. Alahmadi H, Lee D, Wilson JR, et al. Clinical features of silent corticotroph adenomas. Acta Neurochir (Wien). 2012 Aug;154(8):1493–8. PMID:22619024
75. Al Alawi AM, Nordenström A, Falhammar H. Clinical perspectives in congenital adrenal hyperplasia due to 3β-hydroxysteroid dehydrogenase type 2 deficiency. Endocrine. 2019 Mar;63(3):407–21. PMID:30719691
76. Alanazi SM, Limaiem F. Ectopic thyroid. 2023 Jan 1. In: StatPearls. Treasure Island (FL): StatPearls Publishing; 2024 Jan–. PMID:30969714
77. Alband N, Korbonits M. Familial pituitary tumors. Handb Clin Neurol. 2014;124:339–60. PMID:25248598
78. Albano D, Agnello F, Midiri F, et al. Imaging features of adrenal masses. Insights Imaging. 2019 Jan 25;10(1):1. PMID:30684056
79. Al-Bazzaz S, Karamchandani J, Mocarski E, et al. Ectopic prolactin-producing pituitary adenoma in a benign ovarian cystic teratoma. Endocr Pathol. 2014 Sep;25(3):321–3. PMID:24584638
80. Albores-Saavedra J, Batich K, Hossain S, et al. Carcinoid tumors and small-cell carcinomas of the gallbladder and extrahepatic bile ducts: a comparative study based on 221 cases from the Surveillance, Epidemiology, and End Results Program. Ann Diagn Pathol. 2009 Dec;13(6):378–83. PMID:19917473
81. Albores-Saavedra J, Gorraez de la Mora T, de la Torre-Rendon F, et al. Mixed medullary-papillary carcinoma of the thyroid: a previously unrecognized variant of thyroid carcinoma. Hum Pathol. 1990 Nov;21(11):1151–5. PMID:2227923
82. Albores-Saavedra J, Gu X, Luna MA. Clear cells and thyroid transcription factor I reactivity in sclerosing mucoepidermoid carcinoma of the thyroid gland. Ann Diagn Pathol. 2003 Dec;7(6):348–53. PMID:15018117
83. Albores-Saavedra J, Monforte H, Nadji M, et al. C-cell hyperplasia in thyroid tissue adjacent to follicular cell tumors. Hum Pathol. 1988 Jul;19(7):795–9. PMID:2900208
84. Albores-Saavedra J, Sharma S. Poorly differentiated follicular thyroid carcinoma with rhabdoid phenotype: a clinicopathologic, immunohistochemical and electron microscopic study of two cases. Mod Pathol. 2001 Feb;14(2):98–104. PMID:11235911
85. Albores-Saavedra J, Wu J. The many faces and mimics of papillary thyroid carcinoma. Endocr Pathol. 2006 Spring;17(1):1–18. PMID:16760576
86. Albrecht S, Gardiner GW, Kovacs K, et al. Duodenal somatostatinoma with psammoma bodies. Arch Pathol Lab Med. 1989 May;113(5):517–20. PMID:2565711
87. Albuquerque FC, Weiss MH, Kovacs K, et al. A functioning composite 'corticotroph' pituitary adenoma with interspersed adrenocortical cells. Pituitary. 1999 May;1(3-4):279–84. PMID:11081209
88. Al-Dahmani K, Mohammad S, Imran F, et al. Sellar masses: an epidemiological study. Can J Neurol Sci. 2016 Mar;43(2):291–7. PMID:26522017
89. Alese OB, Jiang R, Shaib W, et al. High-grade gastrointestinal neuroendocrine carcinoma management and outcomes: a National Cancer Database study. Oncologist. 2019 Jul;24(7):911–20. PMID:30482824
90. Alexander EK, Kennedy GC, Baloch ZW, et al. Preoperative diagnosis of benign thyroid nodules with indeterminate cytology. N Engl J Med. 2012 Aug 23;367(8):705–15. PMID:22731672
91. Alexander N, Sullivan K, Shaikh F, et al. Characteristics and management of ganglioneuroma and ganglioneuroblastoma-intermixed in children and adolescents. Pediatr Blood Cancer. 2018 May;65(5):e26964. PMID:29369484
92. Alexander VR, Manjaly JG, Pepper CM, et al. Head and neck teratomas in children–a series of 23 cases at Great Ormond Street Hospital. Int J Pediatr Otorhinolaryngol. 2015 Dec;79(12):2008–14. PMID:26611341
93. Alexandraki KI, Grossman AB. The ectopic ACTH syndrome. Rev Endocr Metab Disord. 2010 Jun;11(2):117–26. PMID:20544290
94. Alexandraki KI, Kaltsas GA, Karavitaki N, et al. The medical therapy of craniopharyngiomas: the way ahead. J Clin Endocrinol Metab. 2019 Dec 1;104(12):5751–64. PMID:31369091
95. Alexandrescu S, Brown RE, Tandon N, et al. Neuron precursor features of spindle cell oncocytoma of adenohypophysis. Ann Clin Lab Sci. 2012 Spring;42(2):123–9. PMID:22585606
96. Alharbi N, Asa SL, Szybowska M, et al. Intrathyroidal parathyroid carcinoma: an atypical thyroid lesion. Front Endocrinol (Lausanne). 2018 Nov 1;9:641. PMID:30455668
97. Aliyev E, Ladra-González MJ, Sánchez-Ares M, et al. Thyroid papillary microtumor: validation of the (updated) Porto proposal assessing sex hormone receptor expression and mutational BRAF gene status. Am J Surg Pathol. 2020 Sep;44(9):1161–72. PMID:32804453
98. Allard RH. The thyroglossal cyst. Head Neck Surg. 1982 Nov-Dec;5(2):134–46. PMID:7169333
99. Allen CE, Merad M, McClain KL. Langerhans-cell histiocytosis. N Engl J Med. 2018 Aug 30;379(9):856–68. PMID:30157397
100. Allison KH, Mann GN, Norwood TH, et al. An unusual case of multiple giant myelolipomas: clinical and pathogenetic implications. Endocr Pathol. 2003 Spring;14(1):93–100. PMID:12746567
101. Allolio B, Fassnacht M. Clinical review: Adrenocortical carcinoma: clinical update. J Clin Endocrinol Metab. 2006 Jun;91(6):2027–37. PMID:16551738
102. Allolio B, Hahner S, Weismann D, et al. Management of adrenocortical carcinoma. Clin Endocrinol (Oxf). 2004 Mar;60(3):273–87. PMID:15008991
103. AlMalki MH, Alotaibi M, Ahmad MM, et al. Schwannoma misdiagnosed as adrenal adenoma: a case report and review of the literature. Case Rep Endocrinol. 2020 Jan 30;2020:8020761. PMID:32082650
104. Al-Mefty O, Holoubi A, Rifai A, et al. Microsurgical removal of suprasellar meningiomas. Neurosurgery. 1985 Mar;16(3):364–72. PMID:3982616
105. Almeida JP, Stephens CC, Eschbacher JM, et al. Clinical, pathologic, and imaging characteristics of pituitary null cell adenomas as defined according to the 2017 World Health Organization criteria: a case series from two pituitary centers. Pituitary. 2019 Oct;22(5):514–9. PMID:31401793
106. Almeida MQ, Kaupert LC, Brito LP, et al. Increased expression of ACTH (MC2R) and androgen (AR) receptors in giant bilateral myelolipomas from patients with congenital adrenal hyperplasia. BMC Endocr Disord. 2014 May 12;14:42. PMID:24884994
107. Alos L, Hakim S, Larque AB, et al. p16 overexpression in high-grade neuroendocrine carcinomas of the head and neck: potential diagnostic pitfall with HPV-related carcinomas. Virchows Arch. 2016 Sep;469(3):277–84. PMID:27392929
108. Al-Qurayshi Z, Sullivan CB, Pagedar N, et al. Prevalence and risk of metastatic thyroid cancers and management outcomes: a national perspective. Laryngoscope. 2021 Jan;131(1):237–44. PMID:32574405
109. Alrezk R, Hannah-Shmouni F, Stratakis CA. MEN4 and CDKN1B mutations: the latest of the MEN syndromes. Endocr Relat Cancer. 2017 Oct;24(10):T195–208. PMID:28824003
110. Al-Salameh A, Cadiot G, Calender A, et al. Clinical aspects of multiple endocrine neoplasia type 1. Nat Rev Endocrinol. 2021 Apr;17(4):207–24. PMID:33564173
111. Alsanea O, Wada N, Ain K, et al. Is familial non-medullary thyroid carcinoma more aggressive than sporadic thyroid cancer? A multicenter series. Surgery. 2000 Dec;128(6):1043–50. PMID:11114641
112. Al-Sarireh B, Haidermota M, Verbeke C, et al. Glucagon cell adenomatosis without glucagon receptor mutation. Pancreas. 2013 Mar;42(2):360–2. PMID:23407487
113. Alshaikh OM, Asa SL, Mete O, et al. An institutional experience of tumor progression to pituitary carcinoma in a 15-year cohort of 1055 consecutive pituitary neuroendocrine tumors. Endocr Pathol. 2019 Jun;30(2):118–27. PMID:30706322
114. Alshaikh OM, Yoon JY, Chan BA, et al. Pancreatic neuroendocrine tumor producing insulin and vasopressin. Endocr Pathol. 2018 Mar;29(1):15–20. PMID:28718084
115. Al-Sharefi A, Javaid U, Perros P, et al. Clinical presentation and outcomes of phaeochromocytomas/paragangliomas in neurofibromatosis type 1. Eur Endocrinol. 2019 Aug;15(2):95–100. PMID:31616500
116. AlSufyani MH, Alzahrani AM, Allah AA, et al. Prevalence of painful diabetic peripheral neuropathy and its impact on quality of life among diabetic patients in Western region, Saudi Arabia. J Family Med Prim Care. 2020 Sep 30;9(9):4897–903. PMID:33209819
117. Alvarado-Cabrero I, Young RH, Vamvakas EC, et al. Carcinoma of the fallopian tube: a clinicopathological study of 105 cases with observations on staging and prognostic factors. Gynecol Oncol. 1999 Mar;72(3):367–79. PMID:10053109
118. Alwaheeb S, Rambaldini G, Boerner S, et al. Worrisome histologic alterations following fine-needle aspiration of the parathyroid. J Clin Pathol. 2006 Oct;59(10):1094–6. PMID:17021134
119. Alwan H, La Rosa S, Andreas Kopp P, et al. Incidence trends of lung and gastroenteropancreatic neuroendocrine neoplasms in Switzerland. Cancer Med. 2020 Dec;9(24):9454–61. PMID:33078908
120. Alzouebi M, Goepel JR, Horsman JM, et al. Primary thyroid lymphoma: the 40 year experience of a UK lymphoma treatment centre. Int J Oncol. 2012 Jun;40(6):2075–80. PMID:22367111
121. Alzumaili B, Xu B, Spanheimer PM, et al. Grading of medullary thyroid carcinoma on the basis of tumor necrosis and high mitotic rate is an independent predictor of poor outcome. Mod Pathol. 2020 Sep;33(9):1690–701. PMID:32313184
122. Amacher AM, Goyal B, Lewis JS Jr, et al. Prevalence of a hobnail pattern in papillary, poorly differentiated, and anaplastic thyroid carcinoma: a possible manifestation of high-grade transformation. Am J Surg Pathol. 2015 Feb;39(2):260–5. PMID:25321328
123. Amano K, Kubo O, Komori T, et al. Clinicopathological features of sellar region xanthogranuloma: correlation with Rathke's cleft cyst. Brain Tumor Pathol. 2013 Oct;30(4):233–41. PMID:23322180
124. Amar L, Pacak K, Steichen O, et al. International consensus on initial screening and follow-up of asymptomatic SDHx mutation carriers. Nat Rev Endocrinol. 2021 Jul;17(7):435–44. PMID:34021277
125. Ambros IM, Zellner A, Roald B, et al. Role of ploidy, chromosome 1p, and Schwann cells in the maturation of neuroblastoma. N Engl J Med. 1996 Jun 6;334(23):1505–11. PMID:8618605

126. Ambrosi F, Righi A, Ricci C, et al. Hobnail variant of papillary thyroid carcinoma: a literature review. Endocr Pathol. 2017 Dec;28(4):293–301. PMID:29019044
127. Ambrosini V, Kunikowska J, Baudin E, et al. Consensus on molecular imaging and theranostics in neuroendocrine neoplasms. Eur J Cancer. 2021 Mar;146:56–73. PMID:33588146
128. Amérigo J, Roig J, Pulido F, et al. Primary malignant melanoma of the adrenal gland. Surgery. 2000 Jan;127(1):107–11. PMID:10660767
129. Ames E, Campbell MJ, Afify A, et al. Sclerosing mucoepidermoid carcinoma with eosinophilia: cytologic characterization of a rare distinct entity in the thyroid. Diagn Cytopathol. 2018 Jul;46(7):632–5. PMID:29479842
130. Amiel J, Laudier B, Attié-Bitach T, et al. Polyalanine expansion and frameshift mutations of the paired-like homeobox gene PHOX2B in congenital central hypoventilation syndrome. Nat Genet. 2003 Apr;33(4):459–61. PMID:12640453
132. Amin MB, Edge S, Greene F, et al., editors. AJCC cancer staging manual. 8th ed. New York (NY): Springer; 2017.
133. Amin SM, Albrechtsen NW, Forster J, et al. Gangliocytic paraganglioma of duodenum metastatic to lymph nodes and liver and extending into the retropancreatic space. Pathologica. 2013 Jun;105(3):90–3. PMID:24047035
134. Amine MM, Mohamed B, Mourad H, et al. Neuroendocrine testicular tumors: a systematic review and meta-analysis. Curr Urol. 2017 Apr;10(1):15–25. PMID:28559773
135. Amirbaigloo A, Esfahanian F, Mouodi M, et al. IgG4-related hypophysitis. Endocrine. 2021 Aug;73(2):270–91. PMID:33837927
136. Amouri W, Charfeddine S, Charfi S, et al. Clinicopathological features and outcomes after radioactive iodine treatment of oncocytic well-differentiated thyroid carcinomas. Nucl Med Commun. 2019 Sep;40(9):888–93. PMID:31343615
137. Anagnostouli M, Piperingos G, Yapijakis C, et al. Thyroid gland neurofibroma in a NF1 patient. Acta Neurol Scand. 2002 Jul;106(1):58–61. PMID:12067331
138. Anand VK, Osborne CM, Harkey HL 3rd. Infiltrative clival pituitary adenoma of ectopic origin. Otolaryngol Head Neck Surg. 1993 Feb;108(2):178–83. PMID:8441545
139. Andea AA, Coit DG, Amin B, et al. Merkel cell carcinoma: histologic features and prognosis. Cancer. 2008 Nov 1;113(9):2549–58. PMID:18798233
140. Anderson JL, Gutmann DH. Neurofibromatosis type 1. Handb Clin Neurol. 2015;132:75–86. PMID:26564071
141. Andoniadou CL, Gaston-Massuet C, Reddy R, et al. Identification of novel pathways involved in the pathogenesis of human adamantinomatous craniopharyngioma. Acta Neuropathol. 2012 Aug;124(2):259–71. PMID:22349813
142. Andoniadou CL, Matsushima D, Mousavy Gharavy SN, et al. Sox2(+) stem/progenitor cells in the adult mouse pituitary support organ homeostasis and have tumor-inducing potential. Cell Stem Cell. 2013 Oct 3;13(4):433–45. PMID:24094324
143. Andrion A, Bellis D, Delsedime L, et al. Leiomyoma and neurilemoma: report of two unusual non-epithelial tumours of the thyroid gland. Virchows Arch A Pathol Anat Histopathol. 1988;413(4):367–72. PMID:3140480
144. Andruska N, Fischer-Valuck BW, Mahapatra L, et al. Association between surgical margins larger than 1 cm and overall survival in patients with Merkel cell carcinoma. JAMA Dermatol. 2021 May 1;157(5):540–8. PMID:33760021
145. Anene C, Thompson JS, Saigh J, et al. Somatostatinoma: atypical presentation of a rare pancreatic tumor. Am J Gastroenterol. 1995 May;90(5):819–21. PMID:7733095
146. Angeletti S, Corleto VD, Schillaci O, et al. Use of the somatostatin analogue octreotide to localise and manage somatostatin-producing tumours. Gut. 1998 Jun;42(6):792–4. PMID:9691916
147. Angelini P, London WB, Cohn SL, et al. Characteristics and outcome of patients with ganglioneuroblastoma, nodular subtype: a report from the INRG project. Eur J Cancer. 2012 May;48(8):1185–91. PMID:22137163
148. Angelousi A, Alexandraki K, Tsoli M, et al. Hypophysitis (including IgG4 and immunotherapy). Neuroendocrinology. 2020;110(9-10):822–35. PMID:32126548
149. Angelousi A, Alexandraki KI, Kyriakopoulos G, et al. Neoplastic metastases to the endocrine glands. Endocr Relat Cancer. 2020 Jan;27(1):R1–20. PMID:31645015
150. Angelousi A, Koffas A, Grozinsky-Glasberg S, et al. Diagnostic and management challenges in vasoactive intestinal peptide secreting tumors: a series of 15 patients. Pancreas. 2019 Aug;48(7):934–42. PMID:31268974
151. Angelousi A, Peppa M, Chrisoulidou A, et al. Malignant pheochromocytomas/paragangliomas and ectopic hormonal secretion: a case series and review of the literature. Cancers (Basel). 2019 May 24;11(5):724. PMID:31137729
152. Anglesio MS, Wang Y, Yang W, et al. Cancer-associated somatic DICER1 hotspot mutations cause defective miRNA processing and reverse-strand expression bias to predominantly mature 3p strands through loss of 5p strand cleavage. J Pathol. 2013 Feb;229(3):400–9. PMID:23132766
153. Anlauf M, Bauersfeld J, Raffel A, et al. Insulinomatosis: a multicentric insulinoma disease that frequently causes early recurrent hyperinsulinemic hypoglycemia. Am J Surg Pathol. 2009 Mar;33(3):339–46. PMID:19011561
154. Anlauf M, Enosawa T, Henopp T, et al. Primary lymph node gastrinoma or occult duodenal microgastrinoma with lymph node metastases in a MEN1 patient: the need for a systematic search for the primary tumor. Am J Surg Pathol. 2008 Jul;32(7):1101–5. PMID:18520436
155. Anlauf M, Garbrecht N, Henopp T, et al. Sporadic versus hereditary gastrinomas of the duodenum and pancreas: distinct clinico-pathological and epidemiological features. World J Gastroenterol. 2006 Sep 14;12(34):5440–6. PMID:17006979
156. Anlauf M, Perren A, Meyer CL, et al. Precursor lesions in patients with multiple endocrine neoplasia type 1-associated duodenal gastrinomas. Gastroenterology. 2005 May;128(5):1187–98. PMID:15887103
157. Anlauf M, Schlenger R, Perren A, et al. Microadenomatosis of the endocrine pancreas in patients with and without the multiple endocrine neoplasia type 1 syndrome. Am J Surg Pathol. 2006 May;30(5):560–74. PMID:16699310
158. Annamalai AK, Dean AF, Kandasamy N, et al. Temozolomide responsiveness in aggressive corticotroph tumours: a case report and review of the literature. Pituitary. 2012 Sep;15(3):276–87. PMID:22076588
159. Annapurni A, Rathi M. Acidophil stem cell pituitary adenoma: a case report and literature review. Hormones (Athens). 2019 Dec;18(4):507–12. PMID:31721135
160. Ansell SM, Grant CS, Habermann TM. Primary thyroid lymphoma. Semin Oncol. 1999 Jun;26(3):316–23. PMID:10375088
161. Anselmo J, Medeiros S, Carneiro V, et al. A large family with Carney complex caused by the S147G PRKAR1A mutation shows a unique spectrum of disease including adrenocortical cancer. J Clin Endocrinol Metab. 2012 Feb;97(2):351–9. PMID:22112814
162. Apel RL, Alpert LC, Rizzo A, et al. A metastasizing composite carcinoma of the thyroid with distinct medullary and papillary components. Arch Pathol Lab Med. 1994 Nov;118(11):1143–7. PMID:7979902
163. Apel RL, Asa SL, LiVolsi VA. Papillary Hürthle cell carcinoma with lymphocytic stroma. "Warthin-like tumor" of the thyroid. Am J Surg Pathol. 1995 Jul;19(7):810–4. PMID:7793479
164. Apel RL, Ezzat S, Bapat BV, et al. Clonality of thyroid nodules in sporadic goiter. Diagn Mol Pathol. 1995 Jun;4(2):113–21. PMID:7551291
165. Apel RL, Wilson RJ, Asa SL. A composite somatotroph-corticotroph pituitary adenoma. Endocr Pathol. 1994 Dec;5(4):240–6. PMID:32370421
166. Apps JR, Carreno G, Gonzalez-Meljem JM, et al. Tumour compartment transcriptomics demonstrates the activation of inflammatory and odontogenic programmes in human adamantinomatous craniopharyngioma and identifies the MAPK/ERK pathway as a novel therapeutic target. Acta Neuropathol. 2018 May;135(5):757–77. PMID:29541918
167. Apps JR, Martinez-Barbera JP. Genetically engineered mouse models of craniopharyngioma: an opportunity for therapy development and understanding of tumor biology. Brain Pathol. 2017 May;27(3):364–9. PMID:28414891
168. Apps JR, Stache C, Gonzalez-Meljem JM, et al. CTNNB1 mutations are clonal in adamantinomatous craniopharyngioma. Neuropathol Appl Neurobiol. 2020 Aug;46(5):510–4. PMID:32125720
169. Arai K, Muro H, Suzuki M, et al. Adrenal rest tumor of the liver: a case report with immunohistochemical investigation of steroidogenesis. Pathol Int. 2000 Mar;50(3):244–8. PMID:10792789
170. Araki Y, Sakai N, Andoh T, et al. Central neurocytoma presenting with gigantism: case report. Surg Neurol. 1992 Aug;38(2):141–5. PMID:1509347
171. Aramata S, Han SI, Kataoka K. Roles and regulation of transcription factor MafA in islet beta-cells. Endocr J. 2007 Dec;54(5):659–66. PMID:17785922
172. Araujo-Castro M, Pascual-Corrales E, Molina-Cerrillo J, et al. Immunotherapy in adrenocortical carcinoma: predictors of response, efficacy, safety, and mechanisms of resistance. Biomedicines. 2021 Mar 16;9(3):304. PMID:33809752
173. Ares Valdés Y, Ares Valdés N. [Adrenal gland cyst. Report of one case and review of the literature]. Arch Esp Urol. 2004 Sep;57(7):751–3. Spanish. PMID:15536959
174. Argani P, Aulmann S, Illei PB, et al. A distinctive subset of PEComas harbors TFE3 gene fusions. Am J Surg Pathol. 2010 Oct;34(10):1395–406. PMID:20871214
175. Argani P, Zhong M, Reuter VE, et al. TFE3-fusion variant analysis defines specific clinicopathologic associations among Xp11 translocation cancers. Am J Surg Pathol. 2016 Jun;40(6):723–37. PMID:26975036
176. Arif AA, Kim PTW, Melck A, et al. Pancreatic gastrinoma, gastrointestinal stromal tumor (GIST), pheochromocytoma, and Hürthle cell neoplasm in a patient with neurofibromatosis type 1: a case report and literature review. Am J Case Rep. 2021 Jan 16;22:e927761. PMID:33452231
177. Armin A, Castelli M. Congenital adrenal tissue in the lung with adrenal cytomegaly. Case report and review of the literature. Am J Clin Pathol. 1984 Aug;82(2):225–8. PMID:6465087
178. Armstrong MJ, Yang H, Yip L, et al. PAX8/PPARγ rearrangement in thyroid nodules predicts follicular-pattern carcinomas, in particular the encapsulated follicular variant of papillary carcinoma. Thyroid. 2014 Sep;24(9):1369–74. PMID:24798894
179. Armstrong R, Greenhalgh KL, Rattenberry E, et al. Succinate dehydrogenase subunit B (SDHB) gene deletion associated with a composite paraganglioma/neuroblastoma. J Med Genet. 2009 Mar;46(3):215–6. PMID:19251979
180. Arnaud L, Hervier B, Néel A, et al. CNS involvement and treatment with interferon-α are independent prognostic factors in Erdheim-Chester disease: a multicenter survival analysis of 53 patients. Blood. 2011 Mar 10;117(10):2778–82. PMID:21239701
181. Arndt A, Steinestel K, Rump A, et al. Anaplastic lymphoma kinase (ALK) gene rearrangements in radiation-related human papillary thyroid carcinoma after the Chernobyl accident. J Pathol Clin Res. 2018 Jul;4(3):175–83. PMID:29633575
182. Arnold A, Brown MF, Ureña P, et al. Monoclonality of parathyroid tumors in chronic renal failure and in primary parathyroid hyperplasia. J Clin Invest. 1995 May;95(5):2047–53. PMID:7738171
183. Arnon L, Halperin R, Tirosh A. Impact of pancreatic neuroendocrine tumor on mortality in patients with von Hippel-Lindau Disease. Endocr Pract. 2021 Oct;27(10):1040–5. PMID:33737209
184. Arola J, Salmenkivi K, Liu J, et al. p53 and Ki67 in adrenocortical tumors. Endocr Res. 2000 Nov;26(4):861–5. PMID:11196463
185. Aronow ME, Wiley HE, Gaudric A, et al. Von Hippel-Lindau disease: update on pathogenesis and systemic aspects. Retina. 2019 Dec;39(12):2243–53. PMID:31095066
186. Arpin D, Charpentier MC, Bernardi M, et al. PD-L1-expression patterns in large-cell neuroendocrine carcinoma of the lung: potential implications for use of immunotherapy in these patients: the GFPC 03-2017 "EPNEC" study. Ther Adv Med Oncol. 2020 Jul 7;12:1758835920937972. PMID:32684990
187. Arps H, Dietel M, Schulz A, et al. Pancreatic endocrine carcinoma with ectopic PTH-production and paraneoplastic hypercalcaemia. Virchows Arch A Pathol Anat Histopathol. 1986;408(5):497–503. PMID:3082066
188. Arribas B, Cristobal E, Alcazar JA, et al. p53/MDM2 pathway aberrations in parathyroid tumors: p21(WAF-1) and MDM2 are frequently overexpressed in parathyroid adenomas. Endocr Pathol. 2000 Autumn;11(3):251–7. PMID:12114697
189. Arya AK, Bhadada SK, Singh P, et al. Promoter hypermethylation inactivates CDKN2A, CDKN2B and RASSF1A genes in sporadic parathyroid adenomas. Sci Rep. 2017 Jun 9;7(1):3123. PMID:28600574
190. Asa SL. Challenges in the diagnosis of pituitary neuroendocrine tumors. Endocr Pathol. 2021 Jun;32(2):222–7. PMID:33866514
191. Asa SL, Arkun K, Tischler AS, et al. Middle ear "adenoma": a neuroendocrine tumor with predominant L cell differentiation. Endocr Pathol. 2021 Dec;32(4):433–41. PMID:34041698
192. Asa SL, Bamberger AM, Cao B, et al. The transcription activator steroidogenic factor-1 is preferentially expressed in the human pituitary gonadotroph. J Clin Endocrinol Metab. 1996 Jun;81(6):2165–70. PMID:8964846
193. Asa SL, Casar-Borota O, Chanson P, et al. From pituitary adenoma to pituitary neuroendocrine tumor (PitNET): an International Pituitary Pathology Club proposal. Endocr Relat Cancer. 2017 Apr;24(4):C5–8. PMID:28264912
194. Asa SL, Dardick I, Van Nostrand AW,

et al. Primary thyroid thymoma: a distinct clinicopathologic entity. Hum Pathol. 1988 Dec;19(12):1463–7. PMID:3056830
195. Asa SL, Digiovanni R, Jiang J, et al. A growth hormone receptor mutation impairs growth hormone autofeedback signaling in pituitary tumors. Cancer Res. 2007 Aug 1;67(15):7505–11. PMID:17671221
196. Asa SL, Ezzat S. Aggressive pituitary tumors or localized pituitary carcinomas: defining pituitary tumors. Expert Rev Endocrinol Metab. 2016 Mar;11(2):149–62. PMID:30058871
197. Asa SL, Ezzat S. An update on pituitary neuroendocrine tumors leading to acromegaly and gigantism. J Clin Med. 2021 May 22;10(11):2254. PMID:34067494
198. Asa SL, Ezzat S. Genomic approaches to problems in pituitary neoplasia. Endocr Pathol. 2014 Sep;25(3):209–13. PMID:24272682
199. Asa SL, Ezzat S. Hypothalamic hormone-producing tumors. Handb Clin Neurol. 2021;181:67–74. PMID:34238480
200. Asa SL, Ezzat S. The pathogenesis of pituitary tumors. Annu Rev Pathol. 2009;4:97–126. PMID:19400692
201. Asa SL, Ezzat S. The pathogenesis of pituitary tumours. Nat Rev Cancer. 2002 Nov;2(11):836–49. PMID:12415254
202. Asa SL, Ezzat S, Kelly DF, et al. Hypothalamic vasopressin-producing tumors: often inappropriate diuresis but occasionally Cushing disease. Am J Surg Pathol. 2019 Feb;43(2):251–60. PMID:30379651
203. Asa SL, Ezzat S, Mete O. The diagnosis and clinical significance of paragangliomas in unusual locations. J Clin Med. 2018 Sep 13;7(9):280. PMID:30217041
204. Asa SL, Kovacs K, Horvath E, et al. Sellar glomangioma. Ultrastruct Pathol. 1984;7(1):49–54. PMID:6097000
205. Asa SL, Kovacs K, Killinger DW, et al. Pancreatic islet cell carcinoma producing gastrin, ACTH, alpha-endorphin, somatostatin and calcitonin. Am J Gastroenterol. 1980 Jul;74(1):30–5. PMID:6107042
206. Asa SL, Kovacs K, Tindall GT, et al. Cushing's disease associated with an intrasellar gangliocytoma producing corticotrophin-releasing factor. Ann Intern Med. 1984 Dec;101(6):789–93. PMID:6333843
207. Asa SL, La Rosa S, Basturk O, et al. Molecular pathology of well-differentiated gastro-entero-pancreatic neuroendocrine tumors. Endocr Pathol. 2021 Mar;32(1):169–91. PMID:33459926
208. Asa SL, Mete O. Cytokeratin profiles in pituitary neuroendocrine tumors. Hum Pathol. 2021 Jan;107:87–95. PMID:33098891
209. Asa SL, Mete O. Endocrine pathology: past, present and future. Pathology. 2018 Jan;50(1):111–8. PMID:29132721
210. Asa SL, Mete O. Hypothalamic endocrine tumors: an update. J Clin Med. 2019 Oct 20;8(10):1741. PMID:31635149
211. Asa SL, Mete O. Immunohistochemical biomarkers in pituitary pathology. Endocr Pathol. 2018 Jun;29(2):130–6. PMID:29453601
212. Asa SL, Mete O. Oncocytic change in thyroid pathology. Front Endocrinol (Lausanne). 2021 May 3;12:678119. PMID:34012422
213. Asa SL, Mete O, Cusimano MD, et al. Pituitary neuroendocrine tumors: a model for neuroendocrine tumor classification. Mod Pathol. 2021 Sep;34(9):1634–50. PMID:34017065
214. Asa SL, Mete O, Ezzat S. Genomics and epigenomics of pituitary tumors: What do pathologists need to know? Endocr Pathol. 2021 Mar;32(1):3–16. PMID:33433883
215. Asa SL, Mete O, Schüller U, et al. Cauda equina neuroendocrine tumors: distinct epithelial neuroendocrine neoplasms of spinal origin. Am J Surg Pathol. 2023 Apr 1;47(4):469–75. PMID:36543154
216. Asa SL, Perry A. Tumors of the pituitary gland. Rockville (MD): American Registry of Pathology; 2020. (AFIP atlas of tumor and non-tumor pathology, series 5; fascicle 1).
217. Asa SL, Puy LA, Lew AM, et al. Cell type-specific expression of the pituitary transcription activator pit-1 in the human pituitary and pituitary adenomas. J Clin Endocrinol Metab. 1993 Nov;77(5):1275–80. PMID:8077321
218. Asa SL, Scheithauer BW, Bilbao JM, et al. A case for hypothalamic acromegaly: a clinicopathological study of six patients with hypothalamic gangliocytomas producing growth hormone-releasing factor. J Clin Endocrinol Metab. 1984 May;58(5):796–803. PMID:6423659
219. Asa SL, Singer W, Kovacs K, et al. Pancreatic endocrine tumour producing growth hormone-releasing hormone associated with multiple endocrine neoplasia type I syndrome. Acta Endocrinol (Copenh). 1987 Jul;115(3):331–7. PMID:2887080
220. Asanuma K, Sugenoya A, Ohashi T, et al. Pure clear cell papillary thyroid carcinoma with chronic thyroiditis: report of a case. Surg Today. 1998;28(4):464–6. PMID:9590722
221. Asare EA, Silva-Figueroa A, Hess KR, et al. Risk of distant metastasis in parathyroid carcinoma and its effect on survival: a retrospective review from a high-volume center. Ann Surg Oncol. 2019 Oct;26(11):3593–9. PMID:31111352
222. Asare EA, Sturgeon C, Winchester DJ, et al. Parathyroid carcinoma: an update on treatment outcomes and prognostic factors from the National Cancer Data Base (NCDB). Ann Surg Oncol. 2015 Nov;22(12):3990–5. PMID:26077914
223. Aschebrook-Kilfoy B, Grogan RH, Ward MH, et al. Follicular thyroid cancer incidence patterns in the United States, 1980-2009. Thyroid. 2013 Aug;23(8):1015–21. PMID:23360496
224. Aschebrook-Kilfoy B, Ward MH, Sabra MM, et al. Thyroid cancer incidence patterns in the United States by histologic type, 1992-2006. Thyroid. 2011 Feb;21(2):125–34. PMID:21186939
225. Asgharian B, Chen YJ, Patronas NJ, et al. Meningiomas may be a component tumor of multiple endocrine neoplasia type 1. Clin Cancer Res. 2004 Feb 1;10(3):869–80. PMID:14871962
226. Asgharian B, Turner ML, Gibril F, et al. Cutaneous tumors in patients with multiple endocrine neoplasm type 1 (MEN1) and gastrinomas: prospective study of frequency and development of criteria with high sensitivity and specificity for MEN1. J Clin Endocrinol Metab. 2004 Nov;89(11):5328–36. PMID:15531478
227. Asioli S, Erickson LA, Righi A, et al. Papillary thyroid carcinoma with hobnail features: histopathologic criteria to predict aggressive behavior. Hum Pathol. 2013 Mar;44(3):320–8. PMID:23036367
228. Asioli S, Erickson LA, Righi A, et al. Poorly differentiated carcinoma of the thyroid: validation of the Turin proposal and analysis of IMP3 expression. Mod Pathol. 2010 Sep;23(9):1269–78. PMID:20562850
229. Asioli S, Erickson LA, Sebo TJ, et al. Papillary thyroid carcinoma with prominent hobnail features: a new aggressive variant of moderately differentiated papillary carcinoma. A clinicopathologic, immunohistochemical, and molecular study of eight cases. Am J Surg Pathol. 2010 Jan;34(1):44–52. PMID:19956062
230. Asioli S, Foschini MP, Masetti R, et al. Working formulation of neuroendocrine tumors of the skin and breast. Endocr Pathol. 2014 Jun;25(2):141–50. PMID:24729037
231. Asioli S, Maletta F, Pagni F, et al. Cytomorphologic and molecular features of hobnail variant of papillary thyroid carcinoma: case series and literature review. Diagn Cytopathol. 2014 Jan;42(1):78–84. PMID:23913779
232. Asioli S, Righi A, de Biase D, et al. Expression of p63 is the sole independent marker of aggressiveness in localised (stage I-II) Merkel cell carcinomas. Mod Pathol. 2011 Nov;24(11):1451–61. PMID:21765392
233. Asioli S, Righi A, Iommi M, et al. Validation of a clinicopathological score for the prediction of post-surgical evolution of pituitary adenoma: retrospective analysis on 566 patients from a tertiary care centre. Eur J Endocrinol. 2019 Feb 1;180(2):127–34. PMID:30481158
234. Asioli S, Righi A, Volante M, et al. p63 expression as a new prognostic marker in Merkel cell carcinoma. Cancer. 2007 Aug 1;110(3):640–7. PMID:17599745
235. Asioli S, Zoli M, Guaraldi F, et al. Peculiar pathological, radiological and clinical features of skull-base de-differentiated chordomas. Results from a referral centre case-series and literature review. Histopathology. 2020 Apr;76(5):731–9. PMID:31652338
236. Assié G, Jouinot A, Fassnacht M, et al. Value of molecular classification for prognostic assessment of adrenocortical carcinoma. JAMA Oncol. 2019 Oct 1;5(10):1440–7. PMID:31294750
237. Assié G, Letouzé E, Fassnacht M, et al. Integrated genomic characterization of adrenocortical carcinoma. Nat Genet. 2014 Jun;46(6):607–12. PMID:24747642
238. Assié G, Libé R, Espiard S, et al. ARMC5 mutations in macronodular adrenal hyperplasia with Cushing's syndrome. N Engl J Med. 2013 Nov 28;369(22):2105–14. PMID:24283224
239. Asteria C, Anagni M, Persani L, et al. Loss of heterozygosity of the MEN1 gene in a large series of TSH-secreting pituitary adenomas. J Endocrinol Invest. 2001 Nov;24(10):796–801. PMID:11765049
240. Astrom K, Cohen JE, Willett-Brozick JE, et al. Altitude is a phenotypic modifier in hereditary paraganglioma type 1: evidence for an oxygen-sensing defect. Hum Genet. 2003 Aug;113(3):228–37. PMID:12811540
241. Atienza-Amores M, Guerini-Rocco E, Soslow RA, et al. Small cell carcinoma of the gynecologic tract: a multifaceted spectrum of lesions. Gynecol Oncol. 2014 Aug;134(2):410–8. PMID:24875120
242. Attiyeh EF, London WB, Mossé YP, et al. Chromosome 1p and 11q deletions and outcome in neuroblastoma. N Engl J Med. 2005 Nov 24;353(21):2243–53. PMID:16306521
243. Aubert S, Wacrenier A, Leroy X, et al. Weiss system revisited: a clinicopathologic and immunohistochemical study of 49 adrenocortical tumors. Am J Surg Pathol. 2002 Dec;26(12):1612–9. PMID:12459628
244. Avgerinos DV, Nazarian M, Scherr DS, et al. Primary adrenal melanoma with inferior vena caval thrombus. Ann Thorac Surg. 2012 Dec;94(6):2108–10. PMID:23176924
245. Awad SS, Miskulin J, Thompson N. Parathyroid adenomas versus four-gland hyperplasia as the cause of primary hyperparathyroidism in patients with prolonged lithium therapy. World J Surg. 2003 Apr;27(4):486–8. PMID:12658498
246. Axiotis CA, Merino MJ, Ain K, et al. Papillary endothelial hyperplasia in the thyroid following fine-needle aspiration. Arch Pathol Lab Med. 1991 Mar;115(3):240–2. PMID:2001162
247. Aydin H, Magi-Galluzzi C, Lane BR, et al. Renal angiomyolipoma: clinicopathologic study of 194 cases with emphasis on the epithelioid histology and tuberous sclerosis association. Am J Surg Pathol. 2009 Feb;33(2):289–97. PMID:18852677
248. Aysal A, Agalar C, Egeli T, et al. Reconsideration of clinicopathologic prognostic factors in pancreatic neuroendocrine tumors for better determination of adverse prognosis. Endocr Pathol. 2021 Dec;32(4):461–72. PMID:34283399
249. Azizan EA, Lam BY, Newhouse SJ, et al. Microarray, qPCR, and KCNJ5 sequencing of aldosterone-producing adenomas reveal differences in genotype and phenotype between zona glomerulosa- and zona fasciculata-like tumors. J Clin Endocrinol Metab. 2012 May;97(5):E819–29. PMID:22442279
250. Azizan EA, Poulsen H, Tuluc P, et al. Somatic mutations in ATP1A1 and CACNA1D underlie a common subtype of adrenal hypertension. Nat Genet. 2013 Sep;45(9):1055–60. PMID:23913004
251. Baas EJ, Bontrop RE, Otting N, et al. Molecular analysis of HLA-DP specificities HLA-DPw1, -DPw2 and -DPw4: DP beta chain heterogeneity correlates with PLT subtyping. Tissue Antigens. 1988 Jan;31(1):5–13. PMID:2829386
252. Baba S, Miyoshi A, Obara S, et al. A case of Williams syndrome with suspected coexisting ectopic aldosterone-producing tumor in the liver. Endocrinol Diabetes Metab Case Rep. 2020 Sep 23;2020:20-0057. PMID:33434178
253. Baba Y, Beppu T, Imai K, et al. A case of adrenal rest tumor of the liver: radiological imaging and immunohistochemical study of steroidogenic enzymes. Hepatol Res. 2008;38(11):1154–8. PMID:18564144
254. Babakoohi S, Fu P, Yang M, et al. Combined SCLC clinical and pathologic characteristics. Clin Lung Cancer. 2013 Mar;14(2):113–9. PMID:23010092
255. Babic B, Patel D, Aufforth R, et al. Pediatric patients with pheochromocytoma and paraganglioma should have routine preoperative genetic testing for common susceptibility genes in addition to imaging to detect extra-adrenal and metastatic tumors. Surgery. 2017 Jan;161(1):220–7. PMID:27865588
256. Babin E, Rouleau V, Vedrine PO, et al. Small cell neuroendocrine carcinoma of the nasal cavity and paranasal sinuses. J Laryngol Otol. 2006 Apr;120(4):289–97. PMID:16526967
257. Badalian-Very G. A common progenitor cell in LCH and ECD. Blood. 2014 Aug 14;124(7):991–2. PMID:25124781
258. Badalian-Very G, Vergilio JA, Degar BA, et al. Recurrent BRAF mutations in Langerhans cell histiocytosis. Blood. 2010 Sep 16;116(11):1919–23. PMID:20519626
259. Badarna M, Percik R, Aharon-Hananel G, et al. Anatomic site as prognostic marker of pancreatic neuroendocrine tumors: a cohort study. Eur J Endocrinol. 2019 Sep;181(3):325–30. PMID:31299638
260. Baek SK, Lee MC, Hah JH, et al. Role of surgery in the management of anaplastic thyroid carcinoma: Korean nationwide multicenter study of 329 patients with anaplastic thyroid carcinoma, 2000 to 2012. Head Neck. 2017 Jan;39(1):133–9. PMID:27534388
261. Bahar A, Torabizadeh Z, Movahedi Rad M, et al. Papillary carcinoma in correlation to thyroidal duct cyst: a case series. Caspian J Intern Med. 2020 Winter;11(1):110–5. PMID:32042395
262. Bahn RS, Castro MR. Approach to the patient with nontoxic multinodular goiter. J Clin Endocrinol Metab. 2011 May;96(5):1202–12. PMID:21543434
263. Bahrami A, Lee S, Schaefer IM, et al. TERT promoter mutations and prognosis in solitary fibrous tumor. Mod Pathol. 2016 Dec;29(12):1511–22. PMID:27562490
264. Bai J, Shi J, Li C, et al. Whole genome sequencing of skull-base chordoma reveals

genomic alterations associated with recurrence and chordoma-specific survival. Nat Commun. 2021 Feb 3;12(1):757. PMID:33536423
265. Bai J, Zhao F, Pan S. Clinicopathological characteristics and survival of small cell carcinoma of the salivary gland: a population-based study. Cancer Manag Res. 2019 Dec 24;11:10749–57. PMID:31920384
266. Bai S, Baloch ZW, Samulski TD, et al. Poorly differentiated oncocytic (Hürthle cell) follicular carcinoma: an institutional experience. Endocr Pathol. 2015 May;26(2):164–9. PMID:25898815
267. Bai S, LiVolsi VA, Fraker DL, et al. Water-clear parathyroid adenoma: report of two cases and literature review. Endocr Pathol. 2012 Sep;23(3):196–200. PMID:22638654
268. Bai Y, Kakudo K, Jung CK. Updates in the pathologic classification of thyroid neoplasms: a review of the World Health Organization Classification. Endocrinol Metab (Seoul). 2020 Dec;35(4):696–715. PMID:33261309
269. Baillard P, Genestie C, Croce S, et al. Rare DICER1 and absent FOXL2 mutations characterize ovarian juvenile granulosa cell tumors. Am J Surg Pathol. 2021 Feb 1;45(2):223–9. PMID:32910017
270. Baine MK, Hsieh MS, Lai WV, et al. SCLC subtypes defined by ASCL1, NEUROD1, POU2F3, and YAP1: a comprehensive immunohistochemical and histopathologic characterization. J Thorac Oncol. 2020 Dec;15(12):1823–35. PMID:33011388
271. Baisakh MR, Mohapatra N, Adhikary SD, et al. Malignant peripheral nerve sheath tumor of adrenal gland with heterologus osseous differentiation in a case of Von Recklinghausen's disease. Indian J Pathol Microbiol. 2014 Jan-Mar;57(1):130–2. PMID:24739852
272. Bajpai A, Greenway A, Zacharin M. Platelet dysfunction and increased bleeding tendency in McCune-Albright syndrome. J Pediatr. 2008 Aug;153(2):287–9. PMID:18639732
273. Baker PM, Oliva E, Young RH, et al. Ovarian mucinous carcinoids including some with a carcinomatous component: a report of 17 cases. Am J Surg Pathol. 2001 May;25(5):557–68. PMID:11342766
274. Bakhsh A, Kirov G, Gregory JW, et al. A new form of familial multi-nodular goitre with progression to differentiated thyroid cancer. Endocr Relat Cancer. 2006 Jun;13(2):475–83. PMID:16728575
275. Bakhsh AD, Ladas I, Hamshere ML, et al. An InDel in phospholipase-C-B-1 is linked with euthyroid multinodular goiter. Thyroid. 2018 Jul;28(7):891–901. PMID:29897006
276. Bakhtiar Y, Arita K, Hirano H, et al. Prolactin-producing pituitary adenoma with abundant spherical amyloid deposition masquerading as extensive calcification. Neurol Med Chir (Tokyo). 2010;50(11):1023–6. PMID:21123991
277. Bakhtiar Y, Hirano H, Arita K, et al. Relationship between cytokeratin staining patterns and clinico-pathological features in somatotropinomae. Eur J Endocrinol. 2010 Oct;163(4):531–9. PMID:20688896
278. Bakuła-Zalewska E, Cameron R, Gałczyński JP, et al. Hyaline matrix in hyalinizing trabecular tumor: findings in fine-needle aspiration smears. Diagn Cytopathol. 2015 Sep;43(9):710–3. PMID:25352467
279. Balachandar S, La Quaglia M, Tuttle RM, et al. Pediatric differentiated thyroid carcinoma of follicular cell origin: prognostic significance of histologic subtypes. Thyroid. 2016 Feb;26(2):219–26. PMID:26854950
280. Balakumar T, Perry LA, Savage MO. Adrenocortical adenoma–an unusual presentation with hypersecretion of oestradiol, androgens and cortisol. J Pediatr Endocrinol Metab. 1997 Mar-Apr;10(2):227–9. PMID:9364358
281. Balasubramanyam S, O'Donnell BP, Musher BL, et al. Evaluating treatment patterns for small cell carcinoma of the colon using the National Cancer Database (NCDB). J Gastrointest Cancer. 2019 Jun;50(2):244–53. PMID:29354876
282. Baldari S, Ferraù F, Alafaci C, et al. First demonstration of the effectiveness of peptide receptor radionuclide therapy (PRRT) with 111In-DTPA-octreotide in a giant PRL-secreting pituitary adenoma resistant to conventional treatment. Pituitary. 2012 Dec;15 Suppl 1:S57–60. PMID:22222543
283. Balineni P, Arcot R, Devygounder K, et al. Malignant peripheral nerve sheath tumor of the pancreas-a case report. Int J Surg Case Rep. 2019;55:239–42. PMID:30785006
284. Baloch Z, Mete O, Asa SL. Immunohistochemical biomarkers in thyroid pathology. Endocr Pathol. 2018 Jun;29(2):91–112. PMID:29744727
285. Baloch ZW, Gupta PK, Yu GH, et al. Follicular variant of papillary carcinoma. Cytologic and histologic correlation. Am J Clin Pathol. 1999 Feb;111(2):216–22. PMID:9930143
286. Baloch ZW. LiVolsi VA. C-cells and their associated lesions and conditions: a pathologists perspective. Turk Patoloji Derg. 2015;31 Suppl 1:60–79. PMID:26177318
287. Baloch ZW, LiVolsi VA. Clonality in thyroid nodules: the hyperplasia-neoplasia sequence. Endocr Pathol. 1998 Winter;9(1):287–92. PMID:12114776
288. Baloch ZW, LiVolsi VA. Cytologic and architectural mimics of papillary thyroid carcinoma. Diagnostic challenges in fine-needle aspiration and surgical pathology specimens. Am J Clin Pathol. 2006 Jun;125 Suppl:S135–44. PMID:16830963
289. Baloch ZW, LiVolsi VA. Encapsulated follicular variant of papillary thyroid carcinoma with bone metastases. Mod Pathol. 2000 Aug;13(8):861–5. PMID:10955452
290. Baloch ZW, LiVolsi VA. Intravascular Kaposi's-like spindle cell proliferation of the capsular vessels of follicular-derived thyroid carcinomas. Mod Pathol. 1998 Oct;11(10):995–8. PMID:9796729
291. Baloch ZW, LiVolsi VA. Microcarcinoma of the thyroid. Adv Anat Pathol. 2006 Mar;13(2):69–75. PMID:16670460
292. Baloch ZW, LiVolsi VA. Our approach to follicular-patterned lesions of the thyroid. J Clin Pathol. 2007 Mar;60(3):244–50. PMID:16798933
293. Baloch ZW, LiVolsi VA. Post fine-needle aspiration histologic alterations of thyroid revisited. Am J Clin Pathol. 1999 Sep;112(3):311–6. PMID:10478135
294. Baloch ZW, LiVolsi VA. Special types of thyroid carcinoma. Histopathology. 2018 Jan;72(1):40–52. PMID:29239042
295. Baloch ZW, LiVolsi VA. Tumor-to-tumor metastasis to follicular variant of papillary carcinoma of thyroid. Arch Pathol Lab Med. 1999 Aug;123(8):703–6. PMID:10420227
296. Baloch ZW, LiVolsi VA. Unusual tumors of the thyroid gland. Endocrinol Metab Clin North Am. 2008 Jun;37(2):297–310, vii. PMID:18502328
297. Baloch ZW, LiVolsi VA. Warthin-like papillary carcinoma of the thyroid. Arch Pathol Lab Med. 2000 Aug;124(8):1192–5. PMID:10923082
298. Baloch ZW, Solomon AC, LiVolsi VA. Primary mucoepidermoid carcinoma and sclerosing mucoepidermoid carcinoma with eosinophilia of the thyroid gland: a report of nine cases. Mod Pathol. 2000 Jul;13(7):802–7. PMID:10912941
299. Balogun JA, Monsalves E, Juraschka K, et al. Null cell adenomas of the pituitary gland: an institutional review of their clinical imaging and behavioral characteristics. Endocr Pathol. 2015 Mar;26(1):63–70. PMID:25403448
300. Balsamo A, Baronio F, Ortolano R, et al. Congenital adrenal hyperplasias presenting in the newborn and young infant. Front Pediatr. 2020 Dec 22;8:593315. PMID:33415088
301. Ban A, Satapara J, Rathod K, et al. Teratoma involving adrenal gland - a case report and review of literature. Indian J Radiol Imaging. 2019 Oct-Dec;29(4):472–6. PMID:31949356
302. Bancos I, Tamhane S, Shah M, et al. Diagnosis of endocrine disease: The diagnostic performance of adrenal biopsy: a systematic review and meta-analysis. Eur J Endocrinol. 2016 Aug;175(2):R65–80. PMID:27257146
303. Bando H, Iguchi G, Fukuoka H, et al. The prevalence of IgG4-related hypophysitis in 170 consecutive patients with hypopituitarism and/or central diabetes insipidus and review of the literature. Eur J Endocrinol. 2013 Dec 21;170(2):161–72. PMID:24165017
304. Bando H, Sano T, Ohshima T, et al. Differences in pathological findings and growth hormone responses in patients with growth hormone-producing pituitary adenoma. Endocrinol Jpn. 1992 Aug;39(4):355–63. PMID:1446651
305. Bang JY, Hebert-Magee S, Varadarajulu S. Diagnosis of bilateral adrenal metastases secondary to malignant melanoma by EUS-guided FNA. Am J Gastroenterol. 2011 Oct;106(10):1862–3. PMID:21979216
306. Bann DV, Jin Q, Sheldon KE, et al. Genetic variants implicate dual oxidase-2 in familial and sporadic nonmedullary thyroid cancer. Cancer Res. 2019 Nov 1;79(21):5490–9. PMID:31501191
307. Bannykh S, Strugar J, Baehring J. Paraganglioma of the lumbar spinal canal. J Neurooncol. 2005 Nov;75(2):119. PMID:16283440
308. Bao PP, Li K, Wu CX, et al. [Recent incidences and trends of childhood malignant solid tumors in Shanghai, 2002-2010]. Zhonghua Er Ke Za Zhi. 2013 Apr;51(4):288–94. Chinese. PMID:23927803
309. Barabadze E, Munjishvili V, Burkadze G. BRAF antibody expression in different types of thyroid nodular lesions. Georgian Med News. 2017 Oct; (271):107–13. PMID:29099711
310. Barazeghi E, Gill AJ, Sidhu S, et al. 5-Hydroxymethylcytosine discriminates between parathyroid adenoma and carcinoma. Clin Epigenetics. 2016 Mar 12;8:31. PMID:26973719
311. Barazeghi E, Gill AJ, Sidhu S, et al. A role for TET2 in parathyroid carcinoma. Endocr Relat Cancer. 2017 Jul;24(7):329–38. PMID:28642344
312. Barbeaux A, Duck L, Weynand B, et al. Primary combined squamous and small cell carcinoma of the larynx: report of two cases and discussion of treatment modalities. Eur Arch Otorhinolaryngol. 2006 Aug;263(8):786–90. PMID:16718502
313. Barbieri A, Prasad ML, Gilani SM. Thyroid tissue outside the thyroid gland: differential diagnosis and associated diagnostic challenges. Ann Diagn Pathol. 2020 Oct;48:151584. PMID:32871503
314. Barghorn A, Komminoth P, Bachmann D, et al. Deletion at 3p25.3-p23 is frequently encountered in endocrine pancreatic tumours and is associated with metastatic progression. J Pathol. 2001 Aug;194(4):451–8. PMID:11523053
315. Barghorn A, Speel EJ, Farspour B, et al. Putative tumor suppressor loci at 6q22 and 6q23-q24 are involved in the malignant progression of sporadic endocrine pancreatic tumors. Am J Pathol. 2001 Jun;158(6):1903–11. PMID:11395364
316. Barham HP, Said S, Ramakrishnan VR. Colliding tumor of the paranasal sinus. Allergy Rhinol (Providence). 2013 Spring;4(1):e13–6. PMID:23772319
317. Barletta JA, Bellizzi AM, Hornick JL. Immunohistochemical staining of thyroidectomy specimens for PTEN can aid in the identification of patients with Cowden syndrome. Am J Surg Pathol. 2011 Oct;35(10):1505–11. PMID:21921783
318. Barletta JA, Nosé V, Sadow PM. Genomics and epigenomics of medullary thyroid carcinoma: from sporadic disease to familial manifestations. Endocr Pathol. 2021 Mar;32(1):35–43. PMID:33492588
319. Barmpari ME, Savvidis C, Dede AD, et al. Adrenal malignant melanoma masquerading as a pheochromocytoma in a patient with a history of a multifocal papillary and medullary thyroid carcinoma. Hormones (Athens). 2016 Apr;15(2):283–90. PMID:27376430
320. Barr FG, Galili N, Holick J, et al. Rearrangement of the PAX3 paired box gene in the paediatric solid tumour alveolar rhabdomyosarcoma. Nat Genet. 1993 Feb;3(2):113–7. PMID:8098985
321. Barr FG, Qualman SJ, Macris MH, et al. Genetic heterogeneity in the alveolar rhabdomyosarcoma subset without typical gene fusions. Cancer Res. 2002 Aug 15;62(16):4704–10. PMID:12183429
322. Barrea L, Fonderico F, DI Somma C, et al. Papillary thyroid carcinoma arising in ectopic thyroid tissue within sternocleidomastoid muscle: a review of current literature. Minerva Endocrinol. 2020 Dec;45(4):318–25. PMID:32744438
323. Barreau O, Assié G, Wilmot-Roussel H, et al. Identification of a CpG island methylator phenotype in adrenocortical carcinomas. J Clin Endocrinol Metab. 2013 Jan;98(1):E174–84. PMID:23093492
324. Barresi V, Simbolo M, Gessi M, et al. Clinical-pathological, immunohistochemical, and genetic characterization of a series of posterior pituitary tumors. J Neuropathol Exp Neurol. 2021 Jan 1;80(1):45–51. PMID:33212494
325. Barry S, Korbonits M. Update on the genetics of pituitary tumors. Endocrinol Metab Clin North Am. 2020 Sep;49(3):433–52. PMID:32741481
326. Bartosch C, Afonso M, Pires-Luís AS, et al. Distant metastases in uterine leiomyosarcomas: the wide variety of body sites and time intervals to metastatic relapse. Int J Gynecol Pathol. 2017 Jan;36(1):31–41. PMID:27015437
327. Bartsch D, Hahn SA, Danichevski KD, et al. Mutations of the DPC4/Smad4 gene in neuroendocrine pancreatic tumors. Oncogene. 1999 Apr 8;18(14):2367–71. PMID:10327057
328. Bartsch DK, Albers MB, Lopez CL, et al. Bronchopulmonary neuroendocrine neoplasms and their precursor lesions in multiple endocrine neoplasia type 1. Neuroendocrinology. 2016;103(3-4):240–7. PMID:26113081
329. Bartsch DK, Slater EP, Albers M, et al. Higher risk of aggressive pancreatic neuroendocrine tumors in MEN1 patients with MEN1 mutations affecting the CHES1 interacting MENIN domain. J Clin Endocrinol Metab. 2014 Nov;99(11):E2387–91. PMID:25210877
330. Bartsch DK, Waldmann J, Fendrich V, et al. Impact of lymphadenectomy on survival after surgery for sporadic gastrinoma. Br J Surg. 2012 Sep;99(9):1234–40. PMID:22864882
331. Baser H, Topaloglu O, Tam AA, et al. Comparing clinicopathologic and radiographic findings between TT-UMP, classical, and non-encapsulated follicular variants of papillary thyroid carcinomas. Endocr Pathol. 2016 Sep;27(3):233–42. PMID:27256097
332. Basili T, Dopeso H, Kim SH, et al. Oncogenic properties and signaling basis of the

PAX8-GLIS3 fusion gene. Int J Cancer. 2020 Oct 15;147(8):2253–64. PMID:32383186
333. Bassett JH, Forbes SA, Pannett AA, et al. Characterization of mutations in patients with multiple endocrine neoplasia type 1. Am J Hum Genet. 1998 Feb;62(2):232–44. PMID:9463336
334. Bassiouni H, Asgari S, Stolke D. Tuberculum sellae meningiomas: functional outcome in a consecutive series treated microsurgically. Surg Neurol. 2006 Jul;66(1):37–44. PMID:16793435
335. Baste Subia MN, Digoy P, Hum M, et al. Cytologic findings of spindle epithelial tumor with thymus-like elements. Laryngoscope. 2018 Feb;128(2):E78–82. PMID:29193099
336. Bastide C, Arroua F, Carcenac A, et al. Primary malignant melanoma of the adrenal gland. Int J Urol. 2006 May;13(5):608–10. PMID:16771734
337. Bastos AU, de Jesus AC, Cerutti JM. ETV6-NTRK3 and STRN-ALK kinase fusions are recurrent events in papillary thyroid cancer of adult population. Eur J Endocrinol. 2018 Jan;178(1):83–91. PMID:29046324
338. Basturk O, Adsay V, Hruban RH, et al. Pancreatic acinar cell carcinomas with prominent neuroendocrine differentiation: clinicopathologic analysis of a distinct and diagnostically challenging neoplasm. Mod Pathol. 2014 Feb 7;27(Suppl 2):447A. Abstract no. 1837. doi:10.1038/modpathol.2014.24.
339. Basturk O, Tang L, Hruban RH, et al. Poorly differentiated neuroendocrine carcinomas of the pancreas: a clinicopathologic analysis of 44 cases. Am J Surg Pathol. 2014 Apr;38(4):437–47. PMID:24503751
340. Basturk O, Yang Z, Tang LH, et al. The high-grade (WHO G3) pancreatic neuroendocrine tumor category is morphologically and biologically heterogenous and includes both well differentiated and poorly differentiated neoplasms. Am J Surg Pathol. 2015 May;39(5):683–90. PMID:25723112
341. Bates AS, Farrell WE, Bicknell EJ, et al. Allelic deletion in pituitary adenomas reflects aggressive biological activity and has potential value as a prognostic marker. J Clin Endocrinol Metab. 1997 Mar;82(3):818–24. PMID:9062489
342. Bates T, McQueen A, Iqbal MS, et al. Small cell neuroendocrine carcinoma of the oropharynx harbouring oncogenic HPV-infection. Head Neck Pathol. 2014 Mar;8(1):127–31. PMID:23838856
343. Batista RL, Trarbach EB, Marques MD, et al. Nonfunctioning pituitary adenoma recurrence and its relationship with sex, size, and hormonal immunohistochemical profile. World Neurosurg. 2018 Dec;120:e241–6. PMID:30138730
344. Batsakis JG, el-Naggar AK, Luna MA. Teratomas of the head and neck with emphasis on malignancy. Ann Otol Rhinol Laryngol. 1995 Jun;104(6):496–500. PMID:7771726
345. Batten PJ, Kamara SG. The descriptive epidemiology of unnatural deaths in Oregon's state institutions: a 25-year (1963-1987) study. II. Analysis of the incidence rate and its many variations. Am J Forensic Med Pathol. 1992 Jun;13(2):154–8. PMID:1510067
346. Baudin E, Bidart JM, Rougier P, et al. Screening for multiple endocrine neoplasia type 1 and hormonal production in apparently sporadic neuroendocrine tumors. J Clin Endocrinol Metab. 1999 Jan;84(1):69–75. PMID:9920064
347. Bauer AJ. Thyroid nodules and differentiated thyroid cancer. Endocr Dev. 2014;26:183–201. PMID:25231453
348. Bauer JL, Toluie S, Thompson LDR. Metastases to the parathyroid glands: a comprehensive literature review of 127 reported cases. Head Neck Pathol. 2018 Dec;12(4):534–41. PMID:28875280
349. Baumgarten J, Happel C, Sabet A, et al. MIBI scintigraphy in a patient with hyalinizing trabecular tumor of the thyroid. Nuklearmedizin. 2020 Dec;59(6):438–9. PMID:32691403
350. Bausch B, Koschker AC, Fassnacht M, et al. Comprehensive mutation scanning of NF1 in apparently sporadic cases of pheochromocytoma. J Clin Endocrinol Metab. 2006 Sep;91(9):3478–81. PMID:16787982
351. Bausch B, Schiavi F, Ni Y, et al. Clinical characterization of the pheochromocytoma and paraganglioma susceptibility genes SDHA, TMEM127, MAX, and SDHAF2 for gene-informed prevention. JAMA Oncol. 2017 Sep 1;3(9):1204–12. PMID:28384794
352. Bausch B, Wellner U, Peyre M, et al. Characterization of endolymphatic sac tumors and von Hippel-Lindau disease in the International Endolymphatic Sac Tumor Registry. Head Neck. 2016 Apr;38 Suppl 1:E673–9. PMID:25867206
353. Bayer Y, Neumann S, Meyer B, et al. Genome-wide linkage analysis reveals evidence for four new susceptibility loci for familial euthyroid goiter. J Clin Endocrinol Metab. 2004 Aug;89(8):4044–52. PMID:15292347
354. Bayley JP, Oldenburg RA, Nuk J, et al. Paraganglioma and pheochromocytoma upon maternal transmission of SDHD mutations. BMC Med Genet. 2014 Oct 10;15:111. PMID:25300370
355. Bayraktar F, Kebapcilar L, Kocdor MA, et al. Cushing's syndrome due to ectopic CRH secretion by adrenal pheochromocytoma accompanied by renal infarction. Exp Clin Endocrinol Diabetes. 2006 Sep;114(8):444–7. PMID:17039427
356. Baysal BE, McKay SE, Kim YJ, et al. Genomic imprinting at a boundary element flanking the SDHD locus. Hum Mol Genet. 2011 Nov 15;20(22):4452–61. PMID:21862453
357. Beaty NB, Ahn E. Images in clinical medicine. Adamantinomatous craniopharyngioma containing teeth. N Engl J Med. 2014 Feb 27;370(9):860. PMID:24571758
358. Beauchesne P, Trouillas J, Barral F, et al. Gonadotropic pituitary carcinoma: case report. Neurosurgery. 1995 Oct;37(4):810–5. PMID:8559312
359. Beccaria K, Tauziède-Espariat A, Monnien F, et al. Pediatric chordomas: results of a multicentric study of 40 children and proposal for a histopathological prognostic grading system and new therapeutic strategies. J Neuropathol Exp Neurol. 2018 Mar 1;77(3):207–15. PMID:29361006
360. Becker JC, Stang A, DeCaprio JA, et al. Merkel cell carcinoma. Nat Rev Dis Primers. 2017 Oct 26;3:17077. PMID:29072302
361. Beckers A, Aaltonen LA, Daly AF, et al. Familial isolated pituitary adenomas (FIPA) and the pituitary adenoma predisposition due to mutations in the aryl hydrocarbon receptor interacting protein (AIP) gene. Endocr Rev. 2013 Apr;34(2):239–77. PMID:23371967
362. Beckers A, Abs R, Willems PJ, et al. Aldosterone-secreting adrenal adenoma as part of multiple endocrine neoplasia type 1 (MEN1): loss of heterozygosity for polymorphic chromosome 11 deoxyribonucleic acid markers, including the MEN1 locus. J Clin Endocrinol Metab. 1992 Aug;75(2):564–70. PMID:1639957
363. Beckers A, Lodish MB, Trivellin G, et al. X-linked acrogigantism syndrome: clinical profile and therapeutic responses. Endocr Relat Cancer. 2015 Jun;22(3):353–67. PMID:25712922
364. Beck-Peccoz P, Giavoli C, Lania A. A 2019 update on TSH-secreting pituitary adenomas. J Endocrinol Invest. 2019 Dec;42(12):1401–6. PMID:31175617
365. Beck-Peccoz P, Lania A, Beckers A, et al. 2013 European thyroid association guidelines for the diagnosis and treatment of thyrotropin-secreting pituitary tumors. Eur Thyroid J. 2013 Jun;2(2):76–82. PMID:24783044
366. Beck-Peccoz P, Persani L. Medical management of thyrotropin-secreting pituitary adenomas. Pituitary. 2002;5(2):83–8. PMID:12675505
367. Beck-Peccoz P, Persani L, Mannavola D, et al. Pituitary tumours: TSH-secreting adenomas. Best Pract Res Clin Endocrinol Metab. 2009 Oct;23(5):597–606. PMID:19945025
368. Beggs RE, Kelly ME, Eltayeb O, et al. Large cell neuroendocrine carcinoma of the ampulla of Vater. JOP. 2012 Sep 10;13(5):470–5. PMID:22964952
369. Begum S, Emami N, Cheung A, et al. Cell-type-specific regulation of distinct sets of gene targets by Pax3 and Pax3/FKHR. Oncogene. 2005 Mar 10;24(11):1860–72. PMID:15688035
370. Bejarano PA, Nikiforov YE, Swenson ES, et al. Thyroid transcription factor-1, thyroglobulin, cytokeratin 7, and cytokeratin 20 in thyroid neoplasms. Appl Immunohistochem Mol Morphol. 2000 Sep;8(3):189–94. PMID:10981870
371. Belar O, De La Hoz C, Pérez-Nanclares G, et al. Novel mutations in MEN1, CDKN1B and AIP genes in patients with multiple endocrine neoplasia type 1 syndrome in Spain. Clin Endocrinol (Oxf). 2012 May;76(5):719–24. PMID:22026581
372. Belei OA, Heredea ER, Boeriu E, et al. Verner-Morrison syndrome. Literature review. Rom J Morphol Embryol. 2017;58(2):371–6. PMID:28730220
373. Bell D, El-Naggar AK, Gidley PW. Middle ear adenomatous neuroendocrine tumors: a 25-year experience at MD Anderson Cancer Center. Virchows Arch. 2017 Nov;471(5):667–72. PMID:28547535
374. Bellantone R, Ferrante A, Raffaelli M, et al. Adrenal cystic lesions: report of 12 surgically treated cases and review of the literature. J Endocrinol Invest. 1998 Feb;21(2):109–14. PMID:9585385
375. Bellevicine C, Migliatico I, Sgariglia R, et al. Evaluation of BRAF, RAS, RET/PTC, and PAX8/PPARg alterations in different Bethesda diagnostic categories: a multicentric prospective study on the validity of the 7-gene panel test in 1172 thyroid FNAs deriving from different hospitals in South Italy. Cancer Cytopathol. 2020 Feb;128(2):107–18. PMID:31821746
376. Bellizzi AM. Immunohistochemistry in the diagnosis and classification of neuroendocrine neoplasms: What can brown do for you? Hum Pathol. 2020 Feb;96:8–33. PMID:31857137
377. Bellizzi AM. SATB2 in neuroendocrine neoplasms: strong expression is restricted to well-differentiated tumours of lower gastrointestinal tract origin and is most frequent in Merkel cell carcinoma among poorly differentiated carcinomas. Histopathology. 2020 Jan;76(2):251–64. PMID:31233624
378. Bellizzi AM, Montgomery EA, Hornick JL. American Registry of Pathology Expert Opinions: evaluation of poorly differentiated malignant neoplasms on limited samples - gastrointestinal mucosal biopsies. Ann Diagn Pathol. 2020 Feb;44:151419. PMID:31786484
379. Ben Aim L, Pigny P, Castro-Vega LJ, et al. Targeted next-generation sequencing detects rare genetic events in pheochromocytoma and paraganglioma. J Med Genet. 2019 Aug;56(8):513–20. PMID:30877234
380. Ben Romdhane K, Khattech R, Ben Othman M, et al. Melanin production in medullary thyroid carcinoma. Histopathology. 1995 Dec;27(6):569–71. PMID:8838338
381. Ben Salah R, Mekni A, Doghri R, et al. A mixed medullary-follicular thyroid carcinoma discovered by fine needle aspiration. Tunis Med. 2012 Jun;90(6):488–90. PMID:22693094
382. Benali K, Aarab J, Benmessaoud H, et al. Intrathyroidal parathyroid carcinoma: a case report and literature review. Radiat Oncol J. 2021 Jun;39(2):145–51. PMID:33857367
383. Bencivenga D, Caldarelli I, Stampone E, et al. p27Kip1 and human cancers: a reappraisal of a still enigmatic protein. Cancer Lett. 2017 Sep 10;403:354–65. PMID:28687353
384. Bengtsson D, Joost P, Aravidis C, et al. Corticotroph pituitary carcinoma in a patient with Lynch syndrome (LS) and pituitary tumors in a nationwide LS cohort. J Clin Endocrinol Metab. 2017 Nov 1;102(11):3928–32. PMID:28938458
385. Bengtsson D, Schrøder HD, Andersen M, et al. Long-term outcome and MGMT as a predictive marker in 24 patients with atypical pituitary adenomas and pituitary carcinomas given treatment with temozolomide. J Clin Endocrinol Metab. 2015 Apr;100(4):1689–98. PMID:25646794
386. Benn DE, Zhu Y, Andrews KA, et al. Bayesian approach to determining penetrance of pathogenic SDH variants. J Med Genet. 2018 Nov;55(11):729–34. PMID:30201732
387. Bennett JA, Braga AC, Pinto A, et al. Uterine PEComas: a morphologic, immunohistochemical, and molecular analysis of 32 tumors. Am J Surg Pathol. 2018 Oct;42(10):1370–83. PMID:30001237
388. Bennett KL, Mester J, Eng C. Germline epigenetic regulation of KILLIN in Cowden and Cowden-like syndrome. JAMA. 2010 Dec 22;304(24):2724–31. PMID:21177507
389. Bennicelli JL, Edwards RH, Barr FG. Mechanism for transcriptional gain of function resulting from chromosomal translocation in alveolar rhabdomyosarcoma. Proc Natl Acad Sci U S A. 1996 May 28;93(11):5455–9. PMID:8643596
390. Benzerdjeb N, Traverse-Glehen A, Philouze P, et al. Poorly differentiated neuroendocrine carcinoma of the head and neck: human papillomavirus tumour status/p16 status and impact on overall survival. Histopathology. 2020 Mar;76(4):581–91. PMID:31463946
391. Berbegall AP, Villamón E, Piqueras M, et al. Comparative genetic study of intratumoral heterogenous MYCN amplified neuroblastoma versus aggressive genetic profile neuroblastic tumors. Oncogene. 2016 Mar 17;35(11):1423–32. PMID:26119945
392. Bercaw-Pratt JL, Moorjani TP, Santos XM, et al. Diagnosis and management of precocious puberty in atypical presentations of McCune-Albright syndrome: a case series review. J Pediatr Adolesc Gynecol. 2012 Feb;25(1):e9–13. PMID:22051789
393. Berends AMA, Buitenwerf E, de Krijger RR, et al. Incidence of pheochromocytoma and sympathetic paraganglioma in the Netherlands: a nationwide study and systematic review. Eur J Intern Med. 2018 May;51:68–73. PMID:29361475
394. Berezin M, Shimon I, Hadani M. Prolactinoma in 53 men: clinical characteristics and modes of treatment (male prolactinoma). J Endocrinol Invest. 1995 Jun;18(6):436–41. PMID:7594238
395. Bergamini M, Tonelli P. [Nimesulide in oral surgery. Clinical experience in postoperative treatment]. Minerva Stomatol. 1988 Oct;37(10):793–6. Italian. PMID:3216840
396. Bergero N, De Pompa R, Sacerdote C, et al. Galectin-3 expression in parathyroid carcinoma: immunohistochemical study of 26 cases. Hum Pathol. 2005 Aug;36(8):908–14. PMID:16112008
397. Berglund JA, Tella SH, Tuthill KF, et al. Scoliosis in fibrous dysplasia/McCune-Albright syndrome: factors associated with curve

progression and effects of bisphosphonates. J Bone Miner Res. 2018 Sep;33(9):1641–8. PMID:29669167
398. Berho M, Suster S. The oncocytic variant of papillary carcinoma of the thyroid: a clinicopathologic study of 15 cases. Hum Pathol. 1997 Jan;28(1):47–53. PMID:9013831
399. Berna MJ, Annibale B, Marignani M, et al. A prospective study of gastric carcinoids and enterochromaffin-like cell changes in multiple endocrine neoplasia type 1 and Zollinger-Ellison syndrome: identification of risk factors. J Clin Endocrinol Metab. 2008 May;93(5):1582–91. PMID:18270260
400. Bernardo-Castiñeira C, Valdés N, Sierra MI, et al. SDHC promoter methylation, a novel pathogenic mechanism in parasympathetic paragangliomas. J Clin Endocrinol Metab. 2018 Jan 1;103(1):295–305. PMID:29126304
401. Bernini GP, Moretti A, Mannelli M, et al. Unique association of non-functioning pheochromocytoma, ganglioneuroma, adrenal cortical adenoma, hepatic and vertebral hemangiomas in a patient with a new intronic variant in the VHL gene. J Endocrinol Invest. 2005 Dec;28(11):1032–7. PMID:16483185
402. Bernstein ML, Buchino JJ. The histologic similarity between craniopharyngioma and odontogenic lesions: a reappraisal. Oral Surg Oral Med Oral Pathol. 1983 Nov;56(5):502–11. PMID:6196702
403. Berry T, Luther W, Bhatnagar N, et al. The ALK(F1174L) mutation potentiates the oncogenic activity of MYCN in neuroblastoma. Cancer Cell. 2012 Jul 10;22(1):117–30. PMID:22789543
404. Bertagna F, Biasiotto G, Rodella C, et al. Massive bilateral adrenal gland metastases from melanoma diagnosed by F18-FDG-PET/CT. Jpn J Radiol. 2009 Nov;27(9):392–3. PMID:19943154
405. Bertherat J. Adrenocortical cancer in Carney complex: a paradigm of endocrine tumor progression or an association of genetic predisposing factors? J Clin Endocrinol Metab. 2012 Feb;97(2):387–90. PMID:22312093
406. Bertherat J, Groussin L, Sandrini F, et al. Molecular and functional analysis of PRKAR1A and its locus (17q22-24) in sporadic adrenocortical tumors: 17q losses, somatic mutations, and protein kinase A expression and activity. Cancer Res. 2003 Sep 1;63(17):5308–19. PMID:14500362
407. Bertherat J, Horvath A, Groussin L, et al. Mutations in regulatory subunit type 1A of cyclic adenosine 5'-monophosphate-dependent protein kinase (PRKAR1A): phenotype analysis in 353 patients and 80 different genotypes. J Clin Endocrinol Metab. 2009 Jun;94(6):2085–91. PMID:19293268
408. Bertoin F, Letouzé E, Grignani P, et al. Genome-wide paternal uniparental disomy as a cause of Beckwith-Wiedemann syndrome associated with recurrent virilizing adrenocortical tumors. Horm Metab Res. 2015 Jun;47(7):497–503. PMID:25365508
409. Beshay M, Gutierrez F, Windmöller BA, et al. Huge typical pulmonary carcinoid presented with gigantism syndrome. Gen Thorac Cardiovasc Surg. 2021 Feb;69(2):371–4. PMID:32725474
410. Betônico CC, Rodrigues R, Mendonça SC, et al. [Primary hypothyroidism mimicking pituitary macroadenoma]. Arq Bras Endocrinol Metabol. 2004 Jun;48(3):423–6. Portugese. PMID:15640908
411. Beuschlein F, Boulkroun S, Osswald A, et al. Somatic mutations in ATP1A1 and ATP2B3 lead to aldosterone-producing adenomas and secondary hypertension. Nat Genet. 2013 Apr;45(4):440–4, 444e1–2. PMID:23416519
412. Beuschlein F, Fassnacht M, Assié G, et al. Constitutive activation of PKA catalytic subunit in adrenal Cushing's syndrome. N Engl J Med. 2014 Mar 13;370(11):1019–28. PMID:24571724
413. Beuschlein F, Weigel J, Saeger W, et al. Major prognostic role of Ki67 in localized adrenocortical carcinoma after complete resection. J Clin Endocrinol Metab. 2015 Mar;100(3):841–9. PMID:25559399
414. Bevan S, Pal T, Greenberg CR, et al. A comprehensive analysis of MNG1, TCO1, fPTC, PTEN, TSHR, and TRKA in familial nonmedullary thyroid cancer: confirmation of linkage to TCO1. J Clin Endocrinol Metab. 2001 Aug;86(8):3701–4. PMID:11502798
415. Bhatnagar P, Bhatnagar A, Kishan S, et al. Unusual widespread metastatic presentation of mixed medullary-follicular thyroid carcinoma. Clin Nucl Med. 2004 May;29(5):303–5. PMID:15069329
416. Bhayana S, Booth GL, Asa SL, et al. The implication of somatotroph adenoma phenotype to somatostatin analog responsiveness in acromegaly. J Clin Endocrinol Metab. 2005 Nov;90(11):6290–5. PMID:16118335
417. Bholah R, Bunchman TE. Review of pediatric pheochromocytoma and paraganglioma. Front Pediatr. 2017 Jul 13;5:155. PMID:28752085
418. Bi WL, Horowitz P, Greenwald NF, et al. Landscape of genomic alterations in pituitary adenomas. Clin Cancer Res. 2017 Apr 1;23(7):1841–51. PMID:27707790
419. Biankin SA, Cachia AR. Leiomyoma of the thyroid gland. Pathology. 1999 Feb;31(1):64–6. PMID:10212928
420. Bielle F, Fréneaux P, Jeanne-Pasquier C, et al. PHOX2B immunolabeling: a novel tool for the diagnosis of undifferentiated neuroblastomas among childhood small round blue-cell tumors. Am J Surg Pathol. 2012 Aug;36(8):1141–9. PMID:22790854
421. Bigard MA, Boissel P, Regent D, et al. Intrapancreatic lipoma. First case in the literature. Gastroenterol Clin Biol. 1989 May;13(5):505–7. PMID:2753287
422. Bignell GR, Canzian F, Shayeghi M, et al. Familial nontoxic multinodular thyroid goiter locus maps to chromosome 14q but does not account for familial nonmedullary thyroid cancer. Am J Hum Genet. 1997 Nov;61(5):1123–30. PMID:9345104
423. Bilbao Garay I, Daly AF, Egaña Zunzunegi N, et al. Pituitary disease in AIP mutation-positive familial isolated pituitary adenoma (FIPA): a kindred-based overview. J Clin Med. 2020 Jun 26;9(6):2003. PMID:32604740
424. Bílek R, Vlček P, Šafařík L, et al. Chromogranin A in the laboratory diagnosis of pheochromocytoma and paraganglioma. Cancers (Basel). 2019 Apr 25;11(4):586. PMID:31027285
425. Bilezikian JP, Brandi ML, Eastell R, et al. Guidelines for the management of asymptomatic primary hyperparathyroidism: summary statement from the Fourth International Workshop. J Clin Endocrinol Metab. 2014 Oct;99(10):3561–9. PMID:25162665
426. Bilodeau S, Vallette-Kasic S, Gauthier Y, et al. Role of Brg1 and HDAC2 in GR trans-repression of the pituitary POMC gene and misexpression in Cushing disease. Genes Dev. 2006 Oct 15;20(20):2871–86. PMID:17043312
427. Bin X, Qing Y, Linhui W, et al. Adrenal incidentalomas: experience from a retrospective study in a Chinese population. Urol Oncol. 2011 May-Jun;29(3):270–4. PMID:19481963
427A. Binderup ML, Bisgaard ML, Harbud V, et al. Von Hippel-Lindau disease (vHL). National clinical guideline for diagnosis and surveillance in Denmark. 3rd edition. Dan Med J. 2013 Dec;60(12):B4763. PMID:24355456
428. Binderup MLM, Stendell AS, Galanakis M, et al. Retinal hemangioblastoma: prevalence, incidence and frequency of underlying von Hippel-Lindau disease. Br J Ophthalmol. 2018 Jul;102(7):942–7. PMID:28972023
429. Birnbaum DJ, Gaujoux S, Cherif R, et al. Sporadic nonfunctioning pancreatic neuroendocrine tumors: prognostic significance of incidental diagnosis. Surgery. 2014 Jan;155(1):13–21. PMID:24238123
430. Bisceglia M, Carosi I, Scillitani A, et al. Cystic lymphangioma-like adenomatoid tumor of the adrenal gland: case presentation and review of the literature. Adv Anat Pathol. 2009 Nov;16(6):424–32. PMID:19851133
431. Bisceglia M, Ludovico O, Di Mattia A, et al. Adrenocortical oncocytic tumors: report of 10 cases and review of the literature. Int J Surg Pathol. 2004 Jul;12(3):231–43. PMID:15306935
432. Bishop E, Eble JN, Cheng L, et al. Adrenal myelolipomas show nonrandom X-chromosome inactivation in hematopoietic elements and fat: support for a clonal origin of myelolipomas. Am J Surg Pathol. 2006 Jul;30(7):838–43. PMID:16819325
433. Bishop JA, Westra WH. Human papillomavirus-related small cell carcinoma of the oropharynx. Am J Surg Pathol. 2011 Nov;35(11):1679–84. PMID:21997688
434. Bishop JA, Wu G, Tufano RP, et al. Histological patterns of locoregional recurrence in Hürthle cell carcinoma of the thyroid gland. Thyroid. 2012 Jul;22(7):690–4. PMID:22524498
435. Bisi H, Fernandes VS, de Camargo RY, et al. The prevalence of unsuspected thyroid pathology in 300 sequential autopsies, with special reference to the incidental carcinoma. Cancer. 1989 Nov 1;64(9):1888–93. PMID:2676140
436. Bisi H, Ruggeri GB, Longatto Filho A, et al. Neoplastic and non-neoplastic thyroid lesions in autopsy material: historical review of six decades in São Paulo, Brazil. Tumori. 1998 Jul-Aug;84(4):499–503. PMID:9825004
437. Bismar TA, Basturk O, Gerald WL, et al. Desmoplastic small cell tumor in the pancreas. Am J Surg Pathol. 2004 Jun;28(6):808–12. PMID:15166674
438. Bittencourt AG, Tsuji RK, Cabral F, et al. Middle ear adenoma with neuroendocrine differentiation: relate of two cases and literature review. Int Arch Otorhinolaryngol. 2013 Jul;17(3):340–3. PMID:25992031
439. Bizzarro T, Martini M, Capodimonti S, et al. Young investigator challenge: the morphologic analysis of noninvasive follicular thyroid neoplasm with papillary-like nuclear features on liquid-based cytology: some insights into their identification. Cancer Cytopathol. 2016 Oct;124(10):699–710. PMID:27717284
440. Black BK. Carcinoma of the parathyroid. Ann Surg. 1954 Mar;139(3):355–63. PMID:13149082
441. Blakeley JO, Plotkin SR. Therapeutic advances for the tumors associated with neurofibromatosis type 1, type 2, and schwannomatosis. Neuro Oncol. 2016 May;18(5):624–38. PMID:26851632
442. Blansfield JA, Choyke L, Morita SY, et al. Clinical, genetic and radiographic analysis of 108 patients with von Hippel-Lindau disease (VHL) manifested by pancreatic neuroendocrine neoplasms (PNETs). Surgery. 2007 Dec;142(6):814–8. PMID:18063061
443. Bleeker JS, Quevedo JF, Folpe AL. "Malignant" perivascular epithelioid cell neoplasm: risk stratification and treatment strategies. Sarcoma. 2012;2012:541626. PMID:22619565
444. Block GA, Klassen PS, Lazarus JM, et al. Mineral metabolism, mortality, and morbidity in maintenance hemodialysis. J Am Soc Nephrol. 2004 Aug;15(8):2208–18. PMID:15284307
445. Blum M, Shenkman L, Hollander CS. The autonomous nodule of the thyroid: correlation of patient age, nodule size and functional status. Am J Med Sci. 1975 Jan-Feb;269(1):43–50. PMID:1130435
446. Bobos M, Hytiroglou P, Kostopoulos I, et al. Immunohistochemical distinction between Merkel cell carcinoma and small cell carcinoma of the lung. Am J Dermatopathol. 2006 Apr;28(2):99–104. PMID:16625069
447. Boccara G, Mann C, Guillon G. Secretion of vasopressin from a human pheochromocytoma. Ann Intern Med. 1998 Jun 15;128(12 Pt 1):1049. PMID:9625677
448. Bockhorn M, Sheu SY, Frilling A, et al. Paraganglioma-like medullary thyroid carcinoma: a rare entity. Thyroid. 2005 Dec;15(12):1363–7. PMID:16405409
449. Bockmayr M, Körner M, Schweizer L, et al. Cauda equina paragangliomas express HOXB13. Neuropathol Appl Neurobiol. 2021 Oct;47(6):889–90. PMID:33768604
450. Boekhoff S, Bison B, Eveslage M, et al. Craniopharyngiomas presenting as incidentalomas: results of KRANIOPHARYNGEOM 2007. Pituitary. 2019 Oct;22(5):532–41. PMID:31440945
451. Bogolyubova AV, Abrosimov AY, Selivanova LS, et al. [Histopatological and molecular genetic characteristics of clinically aggressive variants of papillary thyroid carcinoma]. Arkh Patol. 2019;81(1):46–51. Russian. PMID:30830105
452. Bogusławska A, Korbonits M. Genetics of acromegaly and gigantism. J Clin Med. 2021 Mar 29;10(7):1377. PMID:33805450
453. Bogusz A, Boekhoff S, Warmuth-Metz M, et al. Posterior hypothalamus-sparing surgery improves outcome after childhood craniopharyngioma. Endocr Connect. 2019 May 1;8(5):481–92. PMID:30925462
454. Bohnenberger H, Dinter H, König A, et al. Neuroendocrine tumors of the thymus and mediastinum. J Thorac Dis. 2017 Nov;9(Suppl 15):S1448–57. PMID:29201448
455. Bohnenberger H, Ströbel P. Recent advances and conceptual changes in the classification of neuroendocrine tumors of the thymus. Virchows Arch. 2021 Jan;478(1):129–35. PMID:33555458
456. Boichard A, Croux L, Al Ghuzlan A, et al. Somatic RAS mutations occur in a large proportion of sporadic RET-negative medullary thyroid carcinomas and extend to a previously unidentified exon. J Clin Endocrinol Metab. 2012 Oct;97(10):E2031–5. PMID:22865907
457. Boman F, Gultekin H, Dickman PS. Latent Epstein-Barr virus infection demonstrated in low-grade leiomyosarcomas of adults with acquired immunodeficiency syndrome, but not in adjacent Kaposi's lesion or smooth muscle tumors in immunocompetent patients. Arch Pathol Lab Med. 1997 Aug;121(8):834–8. PMID:9278611
458. Bonato M, Frigerio B, Capelia C, et al. Composite enteric-type adenocarcinoma-carcinoid of the nasal mucosa. Endocr Pathol. 1993 Mar;4(1):40–7. PMID:32138448
459. Bondeson L, Bondeson AG. Cytologic features in fine-needle aspirates from a sclerosing mucoepidermoid thyroid carcinoma with eosinophilia. Diagn Cytopathol. 1996 Nov;15(4):301–5. PMID:8982585
460. Bondeson L, Bondeson AG, Thompson NW. Papillary carcinoma of the thyroid with mucoepidermoid features. Am J Clin Pathol. 1991 Feb;95(2):175–9. PMID:1992608
461. Bondeson L, Sandelin K, Grimelius L. Histopathological variables and DNA cytometry in parathyroid carcinoma. Am J Surg Pathol. 1993 Aug;17(8):820–9. PMID:8338192

462. Bonetti F, Martignoni G, Colato C, et al. Abdominopelvic sarcoma of perivascular epithelioid cells. Report of four cases in young women, one with tuberous sclerosis. Mod Pathol. 2001 Jun;14(6):563–8. PMID:11406657

463. Bongers PJ, Kluijfhout WP, Verzijl R, et al. Papillary thyroid cancers with focal tall cell change are as aggressive as tall cell variants and should not be considered as low-risk disease. Ann Surg Oncol. 2019 Aug;26(8):2533–9. PMID:31115855

464. Bongiovanni M, Bloom L, Krane JF, et al. Cytomorphologic features of poorly differentiated thyroid carcinoma: a multi-institutional analysis of 40 cases. Cancer. 2009 Jun 25;117(3):185–94. PMID:19365842

465. Bongiovanni M, Giovanella L, Romanelli F, et al. Cytological diagnoses associated with noninvasive follicular thyroid neoplasms with papillary-like nuclear features according to the Bethesda System for Reporting Thyroid Cytopathology: a systematic review and meta-analysis. Thyroid. 2019 Feb;29(2):222–8. PMID:30426887

466. Bongiovanni M, Mazzucchelli L, Giovanella L, et al. Well-differentiated follicular patterned tumors of the thyroid with high-grade features can metastasize in the absence of capsular or vascular invasion: report of a case. Int J Surg Pathol. 2014 Dec;22(8):749–56. PMID:24788527

467. Bongiovanni M, Mermod M, Canberk S, et al. Columnar cell variant of papillary thyroid carcinoma: cytomorphological characteristics of 11 cases with histological correlation and literature review. Cancer Cytopathol. 2017 Jun;125(6):389–97. PMID:28374549

468. Bongiovanni M, Sykiotis GP, La Rosa S, et al. Macrofollicular variant of follicular thyroid carcinoma: a rare underappreciated pitfall in the diagnosis of thyroid carcinoma. Thyroid. 2020 Jan;30(1):72–80. PMID:31701808

469. Bonnavion R, Teinturier R, Gherardi S, et al. Foxa2, a novel protein partner of the tumour suppressor menin, is deregulated in mouse and human MEN1 glucagonomas. J Pathol. 2017 May;242(1):90–101. PMID:28188614

470. Bonomi M, Ahmed T, Warner D, et al. Human papillomavirus-related small cell carcinoma of the oropharynx: a case report and literature review. Cancers Head Neck. 2017 Feb 6;2:3. PMID:31093350

471. Bonora E, Evangelisti C, Bonichon F, et al. Novel germline variants identified in the inner mitochondrial membrane transporter TIMM44 and their role in predisposition to oncocytic thyroid carcinomas. Br J Cancer. 2006 Dec 4;95(11):1529–36. PMID:17088905

472. Bonora E, Porcelli AM, Gasparre G, et al. Defective oxidative phosphorylation in thyroid oncocytic carcinoma is associated with pathogenic mitochondrial DNA mutations affecting complexes I and III. Cancer Res. 2006 Jun 15;66(12):6087–96. PMID:16778181

473. Bonora E, Rizzato C, Diquigiovanni C, et al. The FOXE1 locus is a major genetic determinant for familial nonmedullary thyroid carcinoma. Int J Cancer. 2014 May 1;134(9):2098–107. PMID:24127282

474. Boos LA, Dettmer M, Schmitt A, et al. Diagnostic and prognostic implications of the PAX8-PPARγ translocation in thyroid carcinomas-a TMA-based study of 226 cases. Histopathology. 2013 Aug;63(2):234–41. PMID:23738683

475. Booth GL, Smyth HS, Kovacs K, et al. Clinicopathological variations in Cushing's syndrome. Endocr Pathol. 1999 Jun;10(2):165–71. PMID:27519220

476. Borchert DH, Massmann A, Kim YJ, et al. Recurrent high-flow arterio-venous malformation of the thyroid gland. Thyroid. 2015 Sep;25(9):1060–3. PMID:26061261

477. Bordi C, Corleto VD, Azzoni C, et al. The antral mucosa as a new site for endocrine tumors in multiple endocrine neoplasia type 1 and Zollinger-Ellison syndromes. J Clin Endocrinol Metab. 2001 May;86(5):2236–42. PMID:11344233

478. Borges MT, Lillehei KO, Kleinschmidt-DeMasters BK. Spindle cell oncocytoma with late recurrence and unique neuroimaging characteristics due to recurrent subclinical intratumoral bleeding. J Neurooncol. 2011 Jan;101(1):145–54. PMID:20495848

479. Borrelli N, Panebianco F, Condello V, et al. Characterization of activating mutations of the MEK1 gene in papillary thyroid carcinomas. Thyroid. 2019 Sep;29(9):1279–85. PMID:31407636

480. Borrill R, Cheesman E, Stivaros S, et al. Papillary craniopharyngioma in a 4-year-old girl with BRAF V600E mutation: a case report and review of the literature. Childs Nerv Syst. 2019 Jan;35(1):169–73. PMID:30069716

481. Borsari S, Pardi E, Pellegata NS, et al. Loss of p27 expression is associated with MEN1 gene mutations in sporadic parathyroid adenomas. Endocrine. 2017 Feb;55(2):386–97. PMID:27038812

482. Borson-Chazot F, Garby L, Raverot G, et al. Acromegaly induced by ectopic secretion of GHRH: a review 30 years after GHRH discovery. Ann Endocrinol (Paris). 2012 Dec;73(6):497–502. PMID:23122576

484. Bosman FT, Carneiro F, Hruban RH, et al., editors. WHO classification of tumours of the digestive system. Lyon (France): International Agency for Research on Cancer; 2010. (WHO classification of tumours series, 4th ed.; vol. 3). https://publications.iarc.who.int/13.

485. Bothra S, Chekavar A, Mayilvaganan S. Prognostic significance of the proportion of tall cell components in papillary thyroid carcinoma. World J Surg. 2017 Oct;41(10):2644. PMID:28265727

486. Botling J, Lamarca A, Bajic D, et al. High-grade progression confers poor survival in pancreatic neuroendocrine tumors. Neuroendocrinology. 2020;110(11-12):891–8. PMID:31658459

487. Böttcher Y, Eszlinger M, Tönjes A, et al. The genetics of euthyroid familial goiter. Trends Endocrinol Metab. 2005 Sep;16(7):314–9. PMID:16054835

488. Bouchaala H, Mejdoub I, Mseddi MA, et al. Giant primary hydatid cyst of the adrenal gland: a rare case report. Urol Case Rep. 2021 Jan 26;36:101580. PMID:33643845

489. Bourdeau I, Matyakhina L, Stergiopoulos SG, et al. 17q22-24 chromosomal losses and alterations of protein kinase a subunit expression and activity in adrenocorticotropin-independent macronodular adrenal hyperplasia. J Clin Endocrinol Metab. 2006 Sep;91(9):3626–32. PMID:16772351

490. Bourdeau I, Parisien-La Salle S, Lacroix A. Adrenocortical hyperplasia: a multifaceted disease. Best Pract Res Clin Endocrinol Metab. 2020 May;34(3):101386. PMID:32115357

491. Bourgois B, Boman F, Nelken B, et al. [Intractable diarrhoea revealing a neuroblastoma hypersecreting the vasoactive intestinal peptide]. Arch Pediatr. 2004 Apr;11(4):340–3. French. PMID:15051093

492. Boussaïd K, Meduri G, Maiza JC, et al. Virilizing sclerosing-stromal tumor of the ovary in a young woman with McCune Albright syndrome: clinical, pathological, and immunohistochemical studies. J Clin Endocrinol Metab. 2013 Feb;98(2):E314–20. PMID:23365131

493. Boutross-Tadross O, Saleh R, Asa SL. Follicular variant papillary thyroid carcinoma arising in struma ovarii. Endocr Pathol. 2007 Fall;18(3):182–6. PMID:18058267

494. Bouys L, Bertherat J. Management of endocrine disease: Carney complex: clinical and genetic update 20 years after the identification of the CNC1 (PRKAR1A) gene. Eur J Endocrinol. 2021 Mar;184(3):R99–109. PMID:33444222

495. Bouzidi L, Triki M, Charfi S, et al. Incidental finding of bilateral ovarian adrenal rest tumor in a patient with congenital adrenal hyperplasia: a case report and brief review. Pediatr Dev Pathol. 2021 Mar-Apr;24(2):137–41. PMID:33433255

496. Bovio S, Cataldi A, Reimondo G, et al. Prevalence of adrenal incidentaloma in a contemporary computerized tomography series. J Endocrinol Invest. 2006 Apr;29(4):298–302. PMID:16699294

497. Bowers DC, Moskowitz CS, Chou JF, et al. Morbidity and mortality associated with meningioma after cranial radiotherapy: a report from the childhood cancer survivor study. J Clin Oncol. 2017 May 10;35(14):1570–6. PMID:28339329

498. Bowers DC, Nathan PC, Constine L, et al. Subsequent neoplasms of the CNS among survivors of childhood cancer: a systematic review. Lancet Oncol. 2013 Jul;14(8):e321–8. PMID:23816298

499. Bown N, Cotterill S, Lastowska M, et al. Gain of chromosome arm 17q and adverse outcome in patients with neuroblastoma. N Engl J Med. 1999 Jun 24;340(25):1954–61. PMID:10379019

500. Boyar Cetinkaya R, Aagnes B, Thiis-Evensen E, et al. Trends in incidence of neuroendocrine neoplasms in Norway: a report of 16,075 cases from 1993 through 2010. Neuroendocrinology. 2017;104(1)1–10. PMID:26562558

501. Boyce AM, Bhattacharyya N, Collins MT. Fibrous dysplasia and fibroblast growth factor-23 regulation. Curr Osteoporos Rep. 2013 Jun;11(2):65–71. PMID:23532406

502. Boyce AM, Brewer C, DeKlotz TR, et al. Association of hearing loss and otologic outcomes with fibrous dysplasia. JAMA Otolaryngol Head Neck Surg. 2018 Feb 1;144(2):102–7. PMID:29192304

503. Boyce AM, Casey RK, Ovejero Crespo D, et al. Gynecologic and reproductive outcomes in fibrous dysplasia/McCune-Albright syndrome. Orphanet J Rare Dis. 2019 Apr 29;14(1):90. PMID:31036049

504. Boyce AM, Chong WH, Shawker TH, et al. Characterization and management of testicular pathology in McCune-Albright syndrome. J Clin Endocrinol Metab. 2012 Sep;97(9):E1782–90. PMID:22745241

505. Boyce AM, Collins MT. Fibrous dysplasia/McCune-Albright syndrome: a rare, mosaic disease of Gαs activation. Endocr Rev. 2020 Apr 1;41(2):345–70. PMID:31673695

506. Boyce AM, Florenzano P, de Castro LF, et al. Collins MT fibrous dysplasia / McCune-Albright syndrome. In: Adam MP, Everman DB, Mirzaa GM, et al., editors. GeneReviews. Seattle (WA): University of Washington, Seattle; 2015 Feb 26 [updated 2024 Feb 8]. PMID:25719192

507. Boyraz B, Sadow PM, Asa SL, et al. Cribriform-morular thyroid carcinoma is a distinct thyroid malignancy of uncertain cytogenesis. Endocr Pathol. 2021 Sep;32(3):327–35. PMID:34019236

508. Bozdogan N, Dilek GB, Benzer E, et al. Transducing-like enhancer of split 1: a potential immunohistochemical marker for glomus tumor. Am J Dermatopathol. 2017 Jul;39(7):524–7. PMID:28632567

509. Brabander T, van der Zwan WA, Teunissen JJM, et al. Long-term efficacy, survival, and safety of [177Lu-DOTA0,Tyr3]octreotate in patients with gastroenteropancreatic and bronchial neuroendocrine tumors. Clin Cancer Res. 2017 Aug 15;23(16):4617–24. PMID:28428192

510. Bradley KJ, Bowl MR, Williams SE, et al. Parafibromin is a nuclear protein with a functional monopartite nuclear localization signal. Oncogene. 2007 Feb 22;26(8):1213–21. PMID:16964291

511. Bradley KJ, Hobbs MR, Buley ID, et al. Uterine tumours are a phenotypic manifestation of the hyperparathyroidism-jaw tumour syndrome. J Intern Med. 2005 Jan;257(1):18–26. PMID:15606373

512. Brady A, Nayar A, Cross P, et al. A detailed immunohistochemical analysis of 2 cases of papillary cystadenoma of the broad ligament: an extremely rare neoplasm characteristic of patients with von Hippel-Lindau disease. Int J Gynecol Pathol. 2012 Mar;31(2):133–40. PMID:22317868

513. Brady S, Lechan RM, Schwaitzberg SD, et al. Composite pheochromocytoma/ganglioneuroma of the adrenal gland associated with multiple endocrine neoplasia 2A: case report with immunohistochemical analysis. Am J Surg Pathol. 1997 Jan;21(1):102–8. PMID:8990146

514. Braham E, Ben Rejeb H, Marghli A, et al. A rare and particular form of goiter to recognize. Ann Transl Med. 2013 Jul;1(2):21. PMID:25332965

515. Brandi ML, Agarwal SK, Perrier ND, et al. Multiple endocrine neoplasia type 1: latest insights. Endocr Rev. 2021 Mar 15;42(2):133–70. PMID:33249439

516. Brandi ML, Gagel RF, Angeli A, et al. Guidelines for diagnosis and therapy of MEN type 1 and type 2. J Clin Endocrinol Metab. 2001 Dec;86(12):5658–71. PMID:11739416

517. Brandler TC, Liu CZ, Cho M, et al. Does noninvasive follicular thyroid neoplasm with papillary-like nuclear features (NIFTP) have a unique molecular profile? Am J Clin Pathol. 2018 Oct 1;150(5):451–60. PMID:30052723

518. Brandwein-Gensler MS, Wang BY, Urken ML. Spindle cell transformation of papillary carcinoma: an aggressive entity distinct from anaplastic thyroid carcinoma. Arch Pathol Lab Med. 2004 Jan;128(1):87–9. PMID:14692805

519. Brastianos PK, Shankar GM, Gill CM, et al. Dramatic response of BRAF V600E mutant papillary craniopharyngioma to targeted therapy. J Natl Cancer Inst. 2015 Oct 23;108(2):djv310. PMID:26498373

520. Brastianos PK, Taylor-Weiner A, Manley PE, et al. Exome sequencing identifies BRAF mutations in papillary craniopharyngiomas. Nat Genet. 2014 Feb;46(2):161–5. PMID:24413733

521. Brat DJ, Scheithauer BW, Eberhart CG, et al. Extraventricular neurocytomas: pathologic features and clinical outcome. Am J Surg Pathol. 2001 Oct;25(10):1252–60. PMID:11688459

522. Brat DJ, Scheithauer BW, Staugaitis SM, et al. Pituicytoma: a distinctive low-grade glioma of the neurohypophysis. Am J Surg Pathol. 2000 Mar;24(3):362–8. PMID:10716149

523. Brems H, Park C, Maertens O, et al. Glomus tumors in neurofibromatosis type 1: genetic, functional, and clinical evidence of a novel association. Cancer Res. 2009 Sep 15;69(18):7393–401. PMID:19738042

524. Brennan SM, Gregory DL, Stillie A, et al. Should extrapulmonary small cell cancer be managed like small cell lung cancer? Cancer. 2010 Feb 15;116(4):888–95. PMID:20052730

525. Brenneman M, Field A, Yang J, et al. Temporal order of RNase IIIb and loss-of-function mutations during development determines phenotype in pleuropulmonary blastoma / DICER1 syndrome: a unique variant of the two-hit tumor suppression model. F1000Res. 2015 Jul 10;4:214. PMID:26925222

526. Brenner B, Tang LH, Klimstra DS, et al. Small-cell carcinomas of the gastrointestinal tract: a review. J Clin Oncol. 2004 Jul 1;22(13):2730–9. PMID:15226341
527. Bresler SC, Weiser DA, Huwe PJ, et al. ALK mutations confer differential oncogenic activation and sensitivity to ALK inhibition therapy in neuroblastoma. Cancer Cell. 2014 Nov 10;26(5):682–94. PMID:25517749
528. Brewer K, Costa-Guda J, Arnold A. Molecular genetic insights into sporadic primary hyperparathyroidism. Endocr Relat Cancer. 2019 Feb 1;26(2):R53–72. PMID:30475215
529. Briassoulis G, Quezado M, Lee CC, et al. Myxoma of the ear lobe in a 23-month-old girl with Carney complex. J Cutan Pathol. 2012 Jan;39(1):68–71. PMID:21880053
530. Bricaire L, Odou MF, Cardot-Bauters C, et al. Frequent large germline HRPT2 deletions in a French National cohort of patients with primary hyperparathyroidism. J Clin Endocrinol Metab. 2013 Feb;98(2):E403–8. PMID:23293331
531. Bricaire L, Villa C, Brière M, et al. Pituitary lesion of unknown origin: think epithelioid angiosarcoma. J Endocr Soc. 2017 Jan 12;1(1):72–4. PMID:29264447
532. Brierley JD, Gospodarowicz MK, Wittekind C, editors. TNM classification of malignant tumours. 8th ed. Oxford (UK): Wiley-Blackwell; 2017.
533. Brignardello E, Manti R, Papotti M, et al. Ectopic secretion of LH by an endocrine pancreatic tumor. J Endocrinol Invest. 2004 Apr;27(4):361–5. PMID:15233557
534. Brimo F, Robinson B, Guo C, et al. Renal epithelioid angiomyolipoma with atypia: a series of 40 cases with emphasis on clinicopathologic prognostic indicators of malignancy. Am J Surg Pathol. 2010 May;34(5):715–22. PMID:20410812
535. Brinkmeier ML, Bando H, Camarano AC, et al. Rathke's cleft-like cysts arise from Isl1 deletion in murine pituitary progenitors. J Clin Invest. 2020 Aug 3;130(8):4501–15. PMID:32453714
536. Brochier S, Galland F, Kujas M, et al. Factors predicting relapse of nonfunctioning pituitary macroadenomas after neurosurgery: a study of 142 patients. Eur J Endocrinol. 2010 Aug;163(2):193–200. PMID:20460423
537. Brodeur GM, Pritchard J, Berthold F, et al. Revisions of the international criteria for neuroblastoma diagnosis, staging, and response to treatment. J Clin Oncol. 1993 Aug;11(8):1466–77. PMID:8336186
538. Brodeur GM, Seeger RC, Barrett A, et al. International criteria for diagnosis, staging, and response to treatment in patients with neuroblastoma. J Clin Oncol. 1988 Dec;6(12):1874–81. PMID:3199170
539. Brodeur GM, Seeger RC, Schwab M, et al. Amplification of N-myc in untreated human neuroblastomas correlates with advanced disease stage. Science. 1984 Jun 8;224(4653):1121–4. PMID:6719137
540. Brondani VB, Lacombe AMF, Mariani BMP, et al. Low protein expression of both ATRX and ZNRF3 as novel negative prognostic markers of adult adrenocortical carcinoma. Int J Mol Sci. 2021 Jan 27;22(3):1238. PMID:33513905
541. Bronner MP, LiVolsi VA. Spindle cell squamous carcinoma of the thyroid: an unusual anaplastic tumor associated with tall cell papillary cancer. Mod Pathol. 1991 Sep;4(5):637–43. PMID:1722043
542. Broughan TA, Leslie JD, Soto JM, et al. Pancreatic islet cell tumors. Surgery. 1986 Jun;99(6):671–8. PMID:2424108
543. Brouillard P, Ghassibé M, Penington A, et al. Four common glomulin mutations cause two thirds of glomuvenous malformations ("familial glomangiomas"): evidence for a founder effect. J Med Genet. 2005 Feb;42(2):e13. PMID:15689436
544. Brown B, Ram A, Clayton P, et al. Conservative management of bilateral Sertoli cell tumors of the testicle in association with the Carney complex: a case report. J Pediatr Surg. 2007 Sep;42(9):E13–5. PMID:17848226
545. Brown FM, Gaffey TA, Wold LE, et al. Myxoid neoplasms of the adrenal cortex: a rare histologic variant. Am J Surg Pathol. 2000 Mar;24(3):396–401. PMID:10716153
546. Brown HM, Komorowski RA, Wilson SD, et al. Predicting metastasis of pheochromocytomas using DNA flow cytometry and immunohistochemical markers of cell proliferation: a positive correlation between MIB-1 staining and malignant tumor behavior. Cancer. 1999 Oct 15;86(8):1583–9. PMID:10526289
547. Brown K, Kristopaitis T, Yong S, et al. Cystic glucagonoma: a rare variant of an uncommon neuroendocrine pancreas tumor. J Gastrointest Surg. 1998 Nov-Dec;2(6):533–6. PMID:10457311
548. Brown NA, Furtado LV, Betz BL, et al. High prevalence of somatic MAP2K1 mutations in BRAF V600E-negative Langerhans cell histiocytosis. Blood. 2014 Sep 4;124(10):1655–8. PMID:24982505
549. Brown RJ, Kelly MH, Collins MT. Cushing syndrome in the McCune-Albright syndrome. J Clin Endocrinol Metab. 2010 Apr;95(4):1508–15. PMID:20157193
550. Brown RJ, Szymula NJ, Loré JM Jr. Neuroblastoma of the head and neck. Arch Otolaryngol. 1978 Jul;104(7):395–8. PMID:666647
551. Brown RL, Muzzafar T, Wollman R, et al. A pituitary carcinoma secreting TSH and prolactin: a non-secreting adenoma gone awry. Eur J Endocrinol. 2006 May;154(5):639–43. PMID:16645009
552. Brown S, O'Neill C, Suliburk J, et al. Parathyroid carcinoma: increasing incidence and changing presentation. ANZ J Surg. 2011 Jul-Aug;81(7-8):528–32. PMID:22295377
553. Bruford EA, Antonescu CR, Carroll AJ, et al. HUGO Gene Nomenclature Committee (HGNC) recommendations for the designation of gene fusions. Leukemia. 2021 Nov;35(11):3040–3. PMID:34615987
554. Buckingham M, Relaix F. PAX3 and PAX7 as upstream regulators of myogenesis. Semin Cell Dev Biol. 2015 Aug;44:115–25. PMID:26424495
555. Budan RM, Georgescu CE. Multiple pituitary adenomas: a systematic review. Front Endocrinol (Lausanne). 2016 Feb 1;7:1. PMID:26869991
556. Buffa R, Rindi G, Sessa F, et al. Synaptophysin immunoreactivity and small clear vesicles in neuroendocrine cells and related tumours. Mol Cell Probes. 1987 Dec;1(4):367–81. PMID:3134611
557. Buffolo F, Monticone S, Williams TA, et al. Subtype diagnosis of primary aldosteronism: is adrenal vein sampling always necessary? Int J Mol Sci. 2017 Apr 17;18(4):848. PMID:28420172
558. Bugalho MJ, Domingues R. Uncommon association of cerebral meningioma, parathyroid adenoma and papillary thyroid carcinoma in a patient harbouring a rare germline variant in the CDKN1B gene. BMJ Case Rep. 2016 Jan 13;2016:bcr2015213934. PMID:26762354
559. Bujko M, Kober P, Boresowicz J, et al. USP8 mutations in corticotroph adenomas determine a distinct gene expression profile irrespective of functional tumour status. Eur J Endocrinol. 2019 Dec;181(6):615–27. PMID:31581124
560. Bullock M, O'Neill C, Chou A, et al. Utilization of a MAB for BRAF(V600E) detection in papillary thyroid carcinoma. Endocr Relat Cancer. 2012 Nov 9;19(6):779–84. PMID:22997209
561. Bumpers HL, Hassett JM Jr, Penetrante RB, et al. Endocrine organ metastases in subjects with lobular carcinoma of the breast. Arch Surg. 1993 Dec;128(12):1344–7. PMID:8250706
562. Bunin GR, Surawicz TS, Witman PA, et al. The descriptive epidemiology of craniopharyngioma. J Neurosurg. 1998 Oct;89(4):547–51. PMID:9761047
563. Buonocore F, McGlacken-Byrne SM, Del Valle I, et al. Current insights into adrenal insufficiency in the newborn and young infant. Front Pediatr. 2020 Dec 14;8:619041. PMID:33381483
564. Burel-Vandenbos F, Cardot-Leccia N, Effi B, et al. [An unusual tumor of the adrenal gland]. Ann Pathol. 2005 Oct;25(5):386–8. French. PMID:16498291
565. Burgess JR, Duffield A, Wilkinson SJ, et al. Two families with an autosomal dominant inheritance pattern for papillary carcinoma of the thyroid. J Clin Endocrinol Metab. 1997 Feb;82(2):345–8. PMID:9024215
566. Burgess JR, Harle RA, Tucker P, et al. Adrenal lesions in a large kindred with multiple endocrine neoplasia type 1. Arch Surg. 1996 Jul;131(7):699–702. PMID:8678766
567. Burke AB, Collins MT, Boyce AM. Fibrous dysplasia of bone: craniofacial and dental implications. Oral Dis. 2017 Sep;23(6):697–708. PMID:27493082
568. Burke AP, Federspiel BH, Sobin LH, et al. Carcinoids of the duodenum. A histologic and immunohistochemical study of 65 tumors. Am J Surg Pathol. 1989 Oct;13(10):828–37. PMID:2476943
569. Burke AP, Helwig EB. Gangliocytic paraganglioma. Am J Clin Pathol. 1989 Jul;92(1):1–9. PMID:2750701
570. Burkeen G, Chauhan A, Agrawal R, et al. Gynecologic large cell neuroendocrine carcinoma: a review. Rare Tumors. 2020 Oct 29;12:2036361320968401. PMID:33194158
571. Burlacu MC, Tichomirowa M, Daly A, et al. [Familial pituitary adenomas]. Presse Med. 2009 Jan;38(1):112–6. French. PMID:18990538
572. Burman P, Falhammar H, Waldenström E, et al. 11C-metomidate PET/CT detected multiple ectopic adrenal rest tumors in a woman with congenital adrenal hyperplasia. J Clin Endocrinol Metab. 2021 Jan 23;106(2):e675–9. PMID:33245336
573. Burnichon N, Cascón A, Schiavi F, et al. MAX mutations cause hereditary and sporadic pheochromocytoma and paraganglioma. Clin Cancer Res. 2012 May 15;18(10):2828–37. PMID:22452945
574. Burnichon N, Mazzella JM, Drui D, et al. Risk assessment of maternally inherited SDHD paraganglioma and phaeochromocytoma. J Med Genet. 2017 Feb;54(2):125–33. PMID:27856506
575. Busaidy NL, Jimenez C, Habra MA, et al. Parathyroid carcinoma: a 22-year experience. Head Neck. 2004 Aug;26(8):716–26. PMID:15287039
576. Busam KJ, Jungbluth AA, Rekthman N, et al. Merkel cell polyomavirus expression in Merkel cell carcinomas and its absence in combined tumors and pulmonary neuroendocrine carcinomas. Am J Surg Pathol. 2009 Sep;33(9):1378–85. PMID:19609205
577. Bush K, Bateman DE. Papilloedema secondary to a spinal paraganglioma. Pract Neurol. 2014 Jun;14(3):179–81. PMID:23918468
578. Buslei R, Hölsken A, Hofmann B, et al. Nuclear beta-catenin accumulation associates with epithelial morphogenesis in craniopharyngiomas. Acta Neuropathol. 2007 May;113(5):585–90. PMID:17221204
579. Buslei R, Nolde M, Hofmann B, et al. Common mutations of beta-catenin in adamantinomatous craniopharyngiomas but not in other tumours originating from the sellar region. Acta Neuropathol. 2005 Jun;109(6):589–97. PMID:15891929
580. Bussières V, Roy S, Deladoey J, et al. Prophylactic thyroidectomies in MEN2 syndrome: management and outcomes. J Pediatr Surg. 2018 Feb;53(2):283–5. PMID:29336779
581. Butler JR, Fohtung TM, Sandrasegaran K, et al. The natural history of pancreatic lipoma: Does it need observation. Pancreatology. 2016 Jan-Feb;16(1):95–8. PMID:26682506
582. Buurman H, Saeger W. Subclinical adenomas in postmortem pituitaries: classification and correlations to clinical data. Eur J Endocrinol. 2006 May;154(5):753–8. PMID:16645024
583. Buys TP, Aviel-Ronen S, Waddell TK, et al. Defining genomic alteration boundaries for a combined small cell and non-small cell lung carcinoma. J Thorac Oncol. 2009 Feb;4(2):227–39. PMID:19179901
584. Buza N, Cohen PJ, Pei Hui, et al. Inverse p16 and p63 expression in small cell carcinoma and high-grade urothelial cell carcinoma of the urinary bladder. Int J Surg Pathol. 2010 Apr;18(2):94–102. PMID:20164052
585. Bychkov A, Jung CK, Liu Z, et al. Noninvasive follicular thyroid neoplasm with papillary-like nuclear features in Asian practice: perspectives for surgical pathology and cytopathology. Endocr Pathol. 2018 Sep;29(3):276–88. PMID:29476382
586. Cabibi D, Mondello A, Florena AM, et al. A case of follicular tumor of uncertain malignant potential (FT-UMP) with glomeruloid features showing capsular mucinous degeneration. Case Rep Pathol. 2021 Mar 11;2021:1686025. PMID:33833889
587. Cadiñanos J, Llorente JL, de la Rosa J, et al. Novel germline SDHD deletion associated with an unusual sympathetic head and neck paraganglioma. Head Neck. 2011 Aug;33(8):1233–40. PMID:20310044
588. Cai M, He H, Zhang B, et al. An ectopic recurrent craniopharyngioma of the temporal lobe: case report and review of the literature. World Neurosurg. 2019 Jun;126:216–22. PMID:30877004
589. Cai WY, Alexander JM, Hedley-Whyte ET, et al. ras mutations in human prolactinomas and pituitary carcinomas. J Clin Endocrinol Metab. 1994 Jan;78(1):89–93. PMID:8288721
590. Cai Z, Lin M, Blanco AI, et al. Epstein-Barr virus-positive large cell neuroendocrine carcinoma of the nasopharynx: report of one case and review of the literature. Head Neck Pathol. 2019 Sep;13(3):313–7. PMID:30191506
591. Caimari F, Korbonits M. Novel genetic causes of pituitary adenomas. Clin Cancer Res. 2016 Oct 15;22(20):5030–42. PMID:27742789
592. Caimari F, Kumar AV, Kurzawinski T, et al. A novel DICER1 mutation in familial multinodular goitre. Clin Endocrinol (Oxf). 2018 Jul;89(1):110–2. PMID:29633305
593. Cakir M, Altunbas H, Balci MK, et al. Medullary thyroid carcinoma, follicular variant. Endocr Pathol. 2002 Spring;13(1):75–9. PMID:12114753
594. Calabrò D, Argalia G, Ambrosini V. Role of PET/CT and therapy management of pancreatic neuroendocrine tumors. Diagnostics (Basel). 2020 Dec 7;10(12):1059. PMID:33297381
595. Calebiro D, Grassi ES, Eszlinger M, et al. Recurrent EZH1 mutations are a second hit in autonomous thyroid adenomas. J Clin Invest. 2016 Sep 1;126(9):3383–8. PMID:27500488
596. Caleo A, Vitale M, Valvano L, et al. Fine needle cytology pre-surgical differentiation of parathyroid neoplasms: Is it reliable? Cytopathology. 2017 Aug;28(4):273–9.

PMID:28217943
597. Caliò A, Warfel KA, Eble JN. Papillary adenomas and other small epithelial tumors in the kidney: an autopsy study. Am J Surg Pathol. 2019 Feb;43(2):277–87. PMID:30418186
598. Calzolari F, Sartori PV, Talarico C, et al. Surgical treatment of intrathyroid metastases: preliminary results of a multicentric study. Anticancer Res. 2008 Sep-Oct;28 5B:2885–8. PMID:19031929
599. Camargo RY, Gross JL, Silveiro SP, et al. Pathological findings in dyshormonogenetic goiter with defective iodide transport. Endocr Pathol. 1998 Autumn;9(3):225–33. PMID:12114713
600. Cambiaso P, Amodio D, Procaccini E, et al. Pituicytoma and Cushing's disease in a 7-year-old girl: a mere coincidence? Pediatrics. 2015 Dec;136(6):e1632–6. PMID:26553184
601. Cambiaso P, Galassi S, Palmiero M, et al. Growth hormone excess in children with neurofibromatosis type-1 and optic glioma. Am J Med Genet A. 2017 Sep;173(9):2353–8. PMID:28631895
602. Cameselle-García S, Abdulkader-Sande S, Sánchez-Ares M, et al. PD-L1 expression and immune cells in anaplastic carcinoma and poorly differentiated carcinoma of the human thyroid gland: a retrospective study. Oncol Lett. 2021 Jul;22(1):553. PMID:34093774
603. Cameselle-Teijeiro J. The pathologist's role in familial nonmedullary thyroid tumors. Int J Surg Pathol. 2010 Jun;18(3 Suppl):194S–200S. PMID:20484290
604. Cameselle-Teijeiro J, Alberte-Lista L, Chiarelli S, et al. CD10 is a characteristic marker of tumours forming morules with biotin-rich, optically clear nuclei that occur in different organs. Histopathology. 2008 Feb;52(3):389–92. PMID:18081818
605. Cameselle-Teijeiro J, Alberte-Lista L, Peteiro-González D, et al. CDX2 expression in some variants of papillary thyroid carcinoma. Am J Clin Pathol. 2012 Dec;138(6):907–9. PMID:23161723
606. Cameselle-Teijeiro J, Chan JK. Cribriform-morular variant of papillary carcinoma: a distinctive variant representing the sporadic counterpart of familial adenomatous polyposis-associated thyroid carcinoma? Mod Pathol. 1999 Apr;12(4):400–11. PMID:10229505
607. Cameselle-Teijeiro J, Fachal C, Cabezas-Agrícola JM, et al. Thyroid pathology findings in Cowden syndrome: a clue for the diagnosis of the PTEN hamartoma tumor syndrome. Am J Clin Pathol. 2015 Aug;144(2):322–8. PMID:26185318
608. Cameselle-Teijeiro J, Febles-Pérez C, Sobrinho-Simões M. Cytologic features of fine needle aspirates of papillary and mucoepidermoid carcinoma of the thyroid with anaplastic transformation. A case report. Acta Cytol. 1997 Jul-Aug;41(4 Suppl):1356–60. PMID:9990275
609. Cameselle-Teijeiro J, Menasce LP, Yap BK, et al. Cribriform-morular variant of papillary thyroid carcinoma: molecular characterization of a case with neuroendocrine differentiation and aggressive behavior. Am J Clin Pathol. 2009 Jan;131(1):134–42. PMID:19095577
610. Cameselle-Teijeiro J, Pardal F, Eloy C, et al. Follicular thyroid carcinoma with an unusual glomeruloid pattern of growth. Hum Pathol. 2008 Oct;39(10):1540–7. PMID:18602667
611. Cameselle-Teijeiro J, Preto A, Soares P, et al. A stem cell role for thyroid solid cell nests. Hum Pathol. 2005 May;36(5):590–1. PMID:15948129
612. Cameselle-Teijeiro J, Ruiz-Ponte C, Loidi L, et al. Somatic but not germline mutation of the APC gene in a case of cribriform-morular variant of papillary thyroid carcinoma. Am J Clin Pathol. 2001 Apr;115(4):486–93. PMID:11293895
613. Cameselle-Teijeiro JM, Eloy C, Sobrinho-Simões M. Pitfalls in challenging thyroid tumors: emphasis on differential diagnosis and ancillary biomarkers. Endocr Pathol. 2020 Sep;31(3):197–217. PMID:32632840
614. Cameselle-Teijeiro JM, Mete O, Asa SL, et al. Inherited follicular epithelial-derived thyroid carcinomas: from molecular biology to histological correlates. Endocr Pathol. 2021 Mar;32(1):77–101. PMID:33495912
615. Cameselle-Teijeiro JM, Peteiro-González D, Caneiro-Gómez J, et al. Cribriform-morular variant of thyroid carcinoma: a neoplasm with distinctive phenotype associated with the activation of the WNT/β-catenin pathway. Mod Pathol. 2018 Aug;31(8):1168–79. PMID:29785019
616. Cameselle-Teijeiro JM, Rodríguez-Pérez I, Celestino R, et al. Hobnail variant of papillary thyroid carcinoma: clinicopathologic and molecular evidence of progression to undifferentiated carcinoma in 2 cases. Am J Surg Pathol. 2017 Jun;41(6):854–60. PMID:28009606
617. Cameselle-Teijeiro JM, Sobrinho-Simões M. Cribriform-morular variant of thyroid carcinoma. Pathologica. 2019 Mar;111(1):1–3. PMID:31217615
618. Canberk S, Griffin AC, Goyal A, et al. Oncocytic follicular nodules of the thyroid with or without chronic lymphocytic thyroiditis: an institutional experience. Cytojournal. 2013 Jan 31;10:2. PMID:23599721
619. Canberk S, LiVolsi VA, Baloch Z. Oncocytic lesions of the neuroendocrine system. Adv Anat Pathol. 2014 Mar;21(2):69–82. PMID:24508690
620. Canberk S, Onenerk M, Gunes P, et al. Oncocytic variant of medullary thyroid carcinoma. Endocr Pathol. 2015 Dec;26(4):320–3. PMID:26293669
621. Cancer Genome Atlas Research Network. Comprehensive molecular profiling of lung adenocarcinoma. Nature. 2014 Jul 31;511(7511):543–50. PMID:25079552
622. Cancer Genome Atlas Research Network. Integrated genomic characterization of papillary thyroid carcinoma. Cell. 2014 Oct 23;159(3):676–90. PMID:25417114
623. Candrina R, Sleiman I, Zorzi F. ACTH-secreting pituitary adenoma within an ovarian teratoma. Eur J Intern Med. 2005 Sep;16(5):359–60. PMID:16137552
624. Candrlić B, Pusić M, Kukuljan M, et al. Patient with lingual thyroid and squamous cell carcinoma of the tongue base–case report. Coll Antropol. 2012 Nov;36 Suppl 2:227–9. PMID:23397793
625. Canu GL, Bulla JS, Lai ML, et al. Primary thyroid leiomyosarcoma: a case report and review of the literature. G Chir. 2018 Jan-Feb;39(1):51–6. PMID:29549682
626. Canzian F, Amati P, Harach HR, et al. A gene predisposing to familial thyroid tumors with cell oxyphilia maps to chromosome 19p13.2. Am J Hum Genet. 1998 Dec;63(6):1743–8. PMID:9837827
627. Cao C, Dou C, Chen F, et al. An unusual mediastinal parathyroid carcinoma coproducing PTH and PTHrP: a case report. Oncol Lett. 2016 Jun;11(6):4113–6. PMID:27313750
628. Cao L, Yu Y, Bilke S, et al. Genome-wide identification of PAX3-FKHR binding sites in rhabdomyosarcoma reveals candidate target genes important for development and cancer. Cancer Res. 2010 Aug 15;70(16):6497–508. PMID:20663909
629. Cao Y, Gao Z, Li L, et al. Whole exome sequencing of insulinoma reveals recurrent T372R mutations in YY1. Nat Commun. 2013;4:2810. PMID:24326773
630. Capdevila J, Arqués O, Hernández Mora JR, et al. Epigenetic EGFR gene repression confers sensitivity to therapeutic BRAFV600E blockade in colon neuroendocrine carcinomas. Clin Cancer Res. 2020 Feb 15;26(4):902–9. PMID:31672771
631. Capdevila J, Wirth LJ, Ernst T, et al. PD-1 blockade in anaplastic thyroid carcinoma. J Clin Oncol. 2020 Aug 10;38(23):2620–7. PMID:32364844
632. Capella C, Riva C, Leutner M, et al. Pituitary lesions in multiple endocrine neoplasia syndrome (MENS) type 1. Pathol Res Pract. 1995 May;191(4):345–7. PMID:7479350
633. Capelli M, Bertino G, Morbini P, et al. Neuroendocrine carcinomas of the upper airways: a small case series with histopathological considerations. Tumori. 2007 Sep-Oct;93(5):499–503. PMID:18038886
634. Capezzone M, Cantara S, Marchisotta S, et al. Telomere length in neoplastic and nonneoplastic tissues of patients with familial and sporadic papillary thyroid cancer. J Clin Endocrinol Metab. 2011 Nov;96(11):E1852–6. PMID:21865371
635. Capezzone M, Marchisotta S, Cantara S, et al. Familial non-medullary thyroid carcinoma displays the features of clinical anticipation suggestive of a distinct biological entity. Endocr Relat Cancer. 2008 Dec;15(4):1075–81. PMID:18832444
636. Capezzone M, Robenshtok E, Cantara S, et al. Familial non-medullary thyroid cancer: a critical review. J Endocrinol Invest. 2021 May;44(5):943–50. PMID:33025555
637. Capezzone M, Sagnella A, Pilli T, et al. Role of age at diagnosis in defining potential familial nonmedullary thyroid cancer in kindreds with two affected members. J Clin Endocrinol Metab. 2021 Jan 23;106(2):e855–65. PMID:33175120
638. Capitanio U, Rosiello G, Erdem S, et al. Clinical, surgical, pathological and follow-up features of kidney cancer patients with Von Hippel-Lindau syndrome: novel insights from a large consortium. World J Urol. 2021 Aug;39(8):2969–75. PMID:33416974
639. Caplin ME, Pavel M, Ćwikła JB, et al. Lanreotide in metastatic enteropancreatic neuroendocrine tumors. N Engl J Med. 2014 Jul 17;371(3):224–33. PMID:25014687
640. Cappabianca P, Cirillo S, Alfieri A, et al. Pituitary macroadenoma and diaphragma sellae meningioma: differential diagnosis on MRI. Neuroradiology. 1999 Jan;41(1):22–6. PMID:9987763
641. Capper D, Jones DTW, Sill M, et al. DNA methylation-based classification of central nervous system tumours. Nature. 2018 Mar 22;555(7697):469–74. PMID:29539639
642. Cappola AR, Mandel SJ. Molecular testing in thyroid cancer: BRAF mutation status and mortality. JAMA. 2013 Apr 10;309(14):1529–30. PMID:23571594
643. Căpraru OM, Gaillard C, Vasiljevic A, et al. Diagnosis, pathology, and management of TSH-secreting pituitary tumors. A single-center retrospective study of 20 patients from 1981 to 2014. Ann Endocrinol (Paris). 2019 Sep;80(4):216–24. PMID:31400861
644. Capriotti G, Duatti A. Adding 64Cu radiopharmaceuticals to the toolkit of molecular imaging. Q J Nucl Med Mol Imaging. 2020 Dec;64(4):327–8. PMID:33073559
645. Caputo M, Prencipe N, Bisceglia A, et al. Primary pituitary lymphoma as rare cause of a pituitary mass and hypopituitarism in adulthood. Endocr Pract. 2020 Nov;26(11):1337–50. PMID:33471665
646. Carcangiu ML. Hürthle cell carcinoma: clinic-pathological and biological aspects. Tumori. 2003 Sep-Oct;89(5):529–32. PMID:14870778
647. Carcangiu ML, Sibley RK, Rosai J. Clear cell change in primary thyroid tumors. A study of 38 cases. Am J Surg Pathol. 1985 Oct;9(10):705–22. PMID:4061729
648. Carcangiu ML, Zampi G, Pupi A, et al. Papillary carcinoma of the thyroid. A clinicopathologic study of 241 cases treated at the University of Florence, Italy. Cancer. 1985 Feb 15;55(4):805–28. PMID:3967175
649. Carcangiu ML, Zampi G, Rosai J. Papillary thyroid carcinoma: a study of its many morphologic expressions and clinical correlates. Pathol Annu. 1985;20(Pt 1):1–44. PMID:3887295
650. Carcangiu ML, Zampi G, Rosai J. Poorly differentiated ("insular") thyroid carcinoma. A reinterpretation of Langhans' "wuchernde Struma". Am J Surg Pathol. 1984 Sep;8(9):655–68. PMID:6476195
651. Carda C, Ferrer J, Vilanova M, et al. Anaplastic carcinoma of the thyroid with rhabdomyosarcomatous differentiation: a report of two cases. Virchows Arch. 2005 Jan;446(1):46–51. PMID:15517365
652. Cardinalli IA, de Oliveira-Filho AG, Mastellaro MJ, et al. A unique case of synchronous functional adrenocortical adenoma and myelolipoma within the ectopic adrenal cortex in a child with Beckwith-Wiedemann syndrome. Pathol Res Pract. 2012 Mar 15;208(3):189–94. PMID:22309953
653. Cardoso L, Stevenson M, Thakker RV. Molecular genetics of syndromic and non-syndromic forms of parathyroid carcinoma. Hum Mutat. 2017 Dec;38(12):1621–48. PMID:28881068
654. Cardot-Bauters C, Carnaille B, Aubert S, et al. A full phenotype of paraganglioma linked to a germline SDHB mosaic mutation. J Clin Endocrinol Metab. 2019 Aug 1;104(8):3362–6. PMID:31046099
655. Carén H, Kryh H, Nethander M, et al. High-risk neuroblastoma tumors with 11q-deletion display a poor prognostic, chromosome instability phenotype with later onset. Proc Natl Acad Sci U S A. 2010 Mar 2;107(9):4323–8. PMID:20145112
656. Carić T, Bilić M, Bilić LK, et al. Neuroendocrine tumors of larynx–two case reports and literature review. Coll Antropol. 2012 Nov;36 Suppl 2:173–8. PMID:23397781
657. Carlberg M, Hedendahl L, Ahonen M, et al. Increasing incidence of thyroid cancer in the Nordic countries with main focus on Swedish data. BMC Cancer. 2016 Jul 7;16:426. PMID:27388603
658. Carlé A, Pedersen IB, Knudsen N, et al. Epidemiology of subtypes of hyperthyroidism in Denmark: a population-based study. Eur J Endocrinol. 2011 May;164(5):801–9. PMID:21357288
659. Carleton-Bland N, Kilday JP, Pathmanaban ON, et al. Ventricular metastatic dissemination of a paediatric craniopharyngioma: case report and literature review. Br J Neurosurg. 2017 Aug;31(4):474–7. PMID:27310220
660. Carling T, Du Y, Fang W, et al. Intragenic allelic loss and promoter hypermethylation of the RIZ1 tumor suppressor gene in parathyroid tumors and pheochromocytomas. Surgery. 2003 Dec;134(6):932–9. PMID:14668725
661. Carmina E, Dewailly D, Escobar-Morreale HF, et al. Non-classic congenital adrenal hyperplasia due to 21-hydroxylase deficiency revisited: an update with a special focus on adolescent and adult women. Hum Reprod Update. 2017 Sep 1;23(5):580–99. PMID:28582566
662. Carney JA. Carney triad: a syndrome featuring paraganglionic, adrenocortical, and possibly other endocrine tumors. J Clin Endocrinol Metab. 2009 Oct;94(10):3656–62. PMID:19723753
663. Carney JA. Psammomatous melanotic schwannoma. A distinctive, heritable tumor with

special associations, including cardiac myxoma and the Cushing syndrome. Am J Surg Pathol. 1990 Mar;14(3):206–22. PMID:2305928
664. Carney JA. Unusual tumefactive spindle-cell lesions in the adrenal glands. Hum Pathol. 1987 Oct;18(10):980–5. PMID:3653882
665. Carney JA, Boccon-Gibod L, Jarka DE, et al. Osteochondromyxoma of bone: a congenital tumor associated with lentigines and other unusual disorders. Am J Surg Pathol. 2001 Feb;25(2):164–76. PMID:11176065
666. Carney JA, Ferreiro JA. The epithelioid blue nevus. A multicentric familial tumor with important associations, including cardiac myxoma and psammomatous melanotic schwannoma. Am J Surg Pathol. 1996 Mar;20(3):259–72. PMID:8772778
667. Carney JA, Gordon H, Carpenter PC, et al. The complex of myxomas, spotty pigmentation, and endocrine overactivity. Medicine (Baltimore). 1985 Jul;64(4):270–83. PMID:4010501
668. Carney JA, Hirokawa M, Lloyd RV, et al. Hyalinizing trabecular tumors of the thyroid gland are almost all benign. Am J Surg Pathol. 2008 Dec;32(12):1877–89. PMID:18813121
669. Carney JA, Libé R, Bertherat J, et al. Primary pigmented nodular adrenocortical disease: the original 4 cases revisited after 30 years for follow-up, new investigations, and molecular genetic findings. Am J Surg Pathol. 2014 Sep;38(9):1266–73. PMID:24805858
670. Carney JA, Lyssikatos C, Seethala RR, et al. The spectrum of thyroid gland pathology in Carney complex: the importance of follicular carcinoma. Am J Surg Pathol. 2018 May;42(5):587–94. PMID:29635258
671. Carney JA, Ryan J, Goellner JR. Hyalinizing trabecular adenoma of the thyroid gland. Am J Surg Pathol. 1987 Aug;11(8):583–91. PMID:2441614
672. Carney JA, Stratakis CA. Epithelioid blue nevus and psammomatous melanotic schwannoma: the unusual pigmented skin tumors of the Carney complex. Semin Diagn Pathol. 1998 Aug;15(3):216–24. PMID:9711672
673. Carney JA, Young WF, Stratakis CA. Primary bimorphic adrenocortical disease: cause of hypercortisolism in McCune-Albright syndrome. Am J Surg Pathol. 2011 Sep;35(9):1311–26. PMID:21836496
674. Caron P, Maiza JC, Renaud C, et al. High third generation/second generation PTH ratio in a patient with parathyroid carcinoma: clinical utility of third generation/second generation PTH ratio in patients with primary hyperparathyroidism. Clin Endocrinol (Oxf). 2009 Apr;70(4):533–8. PMID:18782355
675. Carpenter EL, Mossé YP. Targeting ALK in neuroblastoma–preclinical and clinical advancements. Nat Rev Clin Oncol. 2012 May 15;9(7):391–9. PMID:22585002
676. Carpenter GR, Emery JL. Inclusions in the human thyroid. J Anat. 1976 Sep;122(Pt 1):77–89. PMID:185189
677. Carpten JD, Robbins CM, Villablanca A, et al. HRPT2, encoding parafibromin, is mutated in hyperparathyroidism-jaw tumor syndrome. Nat Genet. 2002 Dec;32(4):676–80. PMID:12434154
678. Carr AA, Yen TWF, Ortiz DI, et al. Patients with oncocytic variant papillary thyroid carcinoma have a similar prognosis to matched classical papillary thyroid carcinoma controls. Thyroid. 2018 Nov;28(11):1462–7. PMID:30215297
679. Carrasco CA, Rojas-Z D, Chiorino R, et al. Primary pituitary lymphoma in immunocompetent patient: diagnostic problems and prolonged follow-up. Pituitary. 2012 Mar;15(1):93–6. PMID:20146099
680. Carroll PV, Joshi MN. Acromegaly. In: Feingold KR, Anawalt B, Blackman MR, et al., editors. Endotext. South Dartmouth (MA): MDText.com, Inc.; 2000 [updated 2022 Sep 7]. PMID:25905322
681. Carroll RS, Zhang J, Dashner K, et al. Androgen receptor expression in meningiomas. J Neurosurg. 1995 Mar;82(3):453–60. PMID:7861224
682. Carroll RS, Zhang J, Dashner K, et al. Progesterone and glucocorticoid receptor activation in meningiomas. Neurosurgery. 1995 Jul;37(1):92–7. PMID:8587697
683. Carstens PH, Kuhns JG, Ghazi C. Primary malignant melanomas of the lung and adrenal. Hum Pathol. 1984 Oct;15(10):910–4. PMID:6479972
684. Carter JM, Wenger DE, Rose PS, et al. Atypical notochordal cell tumors: a series of notochordal-derived tumors that defy current classification schemes. Am J Surg Pathol. 2017 Jan;41(1):39–48. PMID:27819871
685. Carter SL, Cibulskis K, Helman E, et al. Absolute quantification of somatic DNA alterations in human cancer. Nat Biotechnol. 2012 May;30(5):413–21. PMID:22544022
686. Caruso ML, Pilato FP, D'Adda T, et al. Composite carcinoid-adenocarcinoma of the stomach associated with multiple gastric carcinoids and nonantral gastric atrophy. Cancer. 1989 Oct 1;64(7):1534–9. PMID:2776113
687. Casar-Borota O, Boldt HB, Engström BE, et al. Corticotroph aggressive pituitary tumors and carcinomas frequently harbor ATRX mutations. J Clin Endocrinol Metab. 2021 Mar 25;106(4):1183–94. PMID:33106857
688. Casar-Borota O, Botling J, Granberg D, et al. Serotonin, ATRX, and DAXX expression in pituitary adenomas: markers in the differential diagnosis of neuroendocrine tumors of the sellar region. Am J Surg Pathol. 2017 Sep;41(9):1238–46. PMID:28719461
689. Cascón A, Robledo M. MAX and MYC: a heritable breakup. Cancer Res. 2012 Jul 1;72(13):3119–24. PMID:22706201
690. Casey MB, Sebo TJ, Carney JA. Hyalinizing trabecular adenoma of the thyroid gland identification through MIB-1 staining of fine-needle aspiration biopsy smears. Am J Clin Pathol. 2004 Oct;122(4):506–10. PMID:15487446
691. Casey MB, Sebo TJ, Carney JA. Hyalinizing trabecular adenoma of the thyroid gland: cytologic features in 29 cases. Am J Surg Pathol. 2004 Jul;28(7):859–67. PMID:15223954
692. Casey R, Neumann HPH, Maher ER. Genetic stratification of inherited and sporadic phaeochromocytoma and paraganglioma: implications for precision medicine. Hum Mol Genet. 2020 Oct 20;29 R2:R128–37. PMID:33059362
693. Casey RT, Warren AY, Martin JE, et al. Clinical and molecular features of renal and pheochromocytoma/paraganglioma tumor association syndrome (RAPTAS): case series and literature review. J Clin Endocrinol Metab. 2017 Nov 1;102(11):4013–22. PMID:28973655
694. Cassarino DS, Auerbach A, Rushing EJ. Widely invasive solitary fibrous tumor of the sphenoid sinus, cavernous sinus, and pituitary fossa. Ann Diagn Pathol. 2003 Jun;7(3):169–73. PMID:12808569
695. Cassol C, Mete O. Endocrine manifestations of von Hippel-Lindau disease. Arch Pathol Lab Med. 2015 Feb;139(2):263–8. PMID:25611110
696. Castelblanco E, Gallel P, Ros S, et al. Thyroid paraganglioma. Report of 3 cases and description of an immunohistochemical profile useful in the differential diagnosis with medullary thyroid carcinoma, based on complementary DNA array results. Hum Pathol. 2012 Jul;43(7):1103–12. PMID:22209341
697. Castellana M, Grani G, Radzina M, et al. Performance of EU-TIRADS in malignancy risk stratification of thyroid nodules: a meta-analysis. Eur J Endocrinol. 2020 Sep;183(3):255–64. PMID:32544875
698. Castellana M, Piccardo A, Virili C, et al. Can ultrasound systems for risk stratification of thyroid nodules identify follicular carcinoma? Cancer Cytopathol. 2020 Apr;128(4):250–9. PMID:31899594
699. Castellana M, Trimboli P, Piccardo A, et al. Performance of 18F-FDG PET/CT in selecting thyroid nodules with indeterminate fine-needle aspiration cytology for surgery. a systematic review and a meta-analysis. J Clin Med. 2019 Aug 28;8(9):1333. PMID:31466411
700. Castinetti F, Dufour H, Gaillard S, et al. Non-functioning pituitary adenoma: when and how to operate? What pathologic criteria for typing? Ann Endocrinol (Paris). 2015 Jul;76(3):220–7. PMID:26070464
701. Castle-Kirszbaum M, Goldschlager T, Ho B, et al. Twelve cases of pituitary metastasis: a case series and review of the literature. Pituitary. 2018 Oct;21(5):463–73. PMID:29974330
702. Castoldi L, De Rai P, Marini A, et al. Neurofibromatosis-1 and ampullary gangliocytic paraganglioma causing biliary and pancreatic obstruction. Int J Pancreatol. 2001;29(2):93–7. PMID:11876254
703. Castro P, Rebocho AP, Soares RJ, et al. PAX8-PPARgamma rearrangement is frequently detected in the follicular variant of papillary thyroid carcinoma. J Clin Endocrinol Metab. 2006 Jan;91(1):213–20. PMID:16219715
704. Cavaco BM, Barros L, Pannett AA, et al. The hyperparathyroidism-jaw tumour syndrome in a Portuguese kindred. QJM. 2001 Apr;94(4):213–22. PMID:11294964
705. Cavaco BM, Batista PF, Martins C, et al. Familial non-medullary thyroid carcinoma (FNMTC): analysis of fPTC/PRN, NMTC1, MNG1 and TCO susceptibility loci and identification of somatic BRAF and RAS mutations. Endocr Relat Cancer. 2008 Mar;15(1):207–15. PMID:18310288
706. Cavaco BM, Batista PF, Sobrinho LG, et al. Mapping a new familial thyroid epithelial neoplasia susceptibility locus to chromosome 8p23.1-p22 by high-density single-nucleotide polymorphism genome-wide linkage analysis. J Clin Endocrinol Metab. 2008 Nov;93(11):4426–30. PMID:18765515
707. Cavaco BM, Santos R, Félix A, et al. Identification of de novo germline mutations in the HRPT2 gene in two apparently sporadic cases with challenging parathyroid tumor diagnoses. Endocr Pathol. 2011 Mar;22(1):44–52. PMID:21360064
708. Cavalcanti MS, Schultheis AM, Ho C, et al. Mixed mesonephric adenocarcinoma and high-grade neuroendocrine carcinoma of the uterine cervix: case description of a previously unreported entity with insights into its molecular pathogenesis. Int J Gynecol Pathol. 2017 Jan;36(1):76–89. PMID:27532149
709. Cavalier E, Betea D, Schleck ML, et al. The third/second generation PTH assay ratio as a marker for parathyroid carcinoma: evaluation using an automated platform. J Clin Endocrinol Metab. 2014 Mar;99(3):E453–7. PMID:24423313
710. Cavalier E, Daly AF, Betea D, et al. The ratio of parathyroid hormone as measured by third- and second-generation assays as a marker for parathyroid carcinoma. J Clin Endocrinol Metab. 2010 Aug;95(8):3745–9. PMID:20519352
711. Cavallaro G, Crocetti D, Paliotta A, et al. Cystic adrenal lesions: clinical and surgical management. The experience of a referral centre. Int J Surg. 2015 Jan;13:23–6. PMID:25447606
712. Cazes A, Lopez-Delisle L, Tsarovina K, et al. Activated Alk triggers prolonged neurogenesis and Ret upregulation providing a therapeutic target in ALK-mutated neuroblastoma. Oncotarget. 2014 May 15;5(9):2688–702. PMID:24811913
713. Cejas P, Drier Y, Dreijerink KMA, et al. Enhancer signatures stratify and predict outcomes of non-functional pancreatic neuroendocrine tumors. Nat Med. 2019 Aug;25(8):1260–5. PMID:31263286
714. Celi FS, Coppotelli G, Chidakel A, et al. The role of type 1 and type 2 5'-deiodinase in the pathophysiology of the 3,5,3'-triiodothyronine toxicosis of McCune-Albright syndrome. J Clin Endocrinol Metab. 2008 Jun;93(6):2383–9. PMID:18349068
715. Celio MR, Pasi A, Bürgisser E, et al. 'Proopiocortin fragments' in normal human adult pituitary. Distribution and ultrastructural characterization of immunoreactive cells. Acta Endocrinol (Copenh). 1980 Sep;95(1):27–40. PMID:6257006
716. Centeno PP, Herberger A, Mun HC, et al. Phosphate acts directly on the calcium-sensing receptor to stimulate parathyroid hormone secretion. Nat Commun. 2019 Oct 16;10(1):4693. PMID:31619668
717. Cerami E, Gao J, Dogrusoz U, et al. The cBio cancer genomics portal: an open platform for exploring multidimensional cancer genomics data. Cancer Discov. 2012 May;2(5):401–4. PMID:22588877
718. Cerecer-Gil NY, Figuera LE, Llamas FJ, et al. Mutation of SDHB is a cause of hypoxia-related high-altitude paraganglioma. Clin Cancer Res. 2010 Aug 15;16(16):4148–54. PMID:20592014
719. Cerhan JR, Habermann TM. Epidemiology of marginal zone lymphoma. Ann Lymphoma. 2021 Mar;5(Mar):5. PMID:33829216
720. Cetani F, Ambrogini E, Viacava P, et al. Should parafibromin staining replace HRTP2 gene analysis as an additional tool for histologic diagnosis of parathyroid carcinoma? Eur J Endocrinol. 2007 May;156(5):547–54. PMID:17468190
721. Cetani F, Frustaci G, Torregrossa L, et al. A nonfunctioning parathyroid carcinoma misdiagnosed as a follicular thyroid nodule. World J Surg Oncol. 2015 Sep 8;13:270. PMID:26350418
722. Cetani F, Marcocci C, Torregrossa L, et al. Atypical parathyroid adenomas: challenging lesions in the differential diagnosis of endocrine tumors. Endocr Relat Cancer. 2019 Jul;26(7):R441–64. PMID:31085770
723. Cetani F, Pardi E, Borsari S, et al. Genetic analyses of the HRPT2 gene in primary hyperparathyroidism: germline and somatic mutations in familial and sporadic parathyroid tumors. J Clin Endocrinol Metab. 2004 Nov;89(11):5583–91. PMID:15531515
724. Cetta F, Curia MC, Montalto G, et al. Thyroid carcinoma usually occurs in patients with familial adenomatous polyposis in the absence of biallelic inactivation of the adenomatous polyposis coli gene. J Clin Endocrinol Metab. 2001 Jan;86(1):427–32. PMID:11232035
725. Cetta F, Montalto G, Gori M, et al. Germline mutations of the APC gene in patients with familial adenomatous polyposis-associated thyroid carcinoma: results from a European cooperative study. J Clin Endocrinol Metab. 2000 Jan;85(1):286–92. PMID:10634400
726. Cetta F, Ugolini G, Barellini L, et al. FAP associated cribriform morular variant of PTC: striking female prevalence and indolent course. Endocr J. 2011;58(9):817–8. PMID:21878742
727. Cevizci R, Karakullukçu B, van den Brekel MW, et al. Laser excision of a typical carcinoid tumor of the larynx: a case report. Kulak Burun Bogaz Ihtis Derg. 2010 Nov-Dec;20(6):305–8.

PMID:20961285
728. Ceyran AB, Senol S, Bayraktar B, et al. Langerhans cell histiocytosis of the thyroid with multiple cervical lymph node involvement accompanying metastatic thyroid papillary carcinoma. Case Rep Pathol. 2014;2014:184237. PMID:25349760
729. Cha H, Pyo JY, Hong SW. The usefulness of immunocytochemistry of CD56 in determining malignancy from indeterminate thyroid fine-needle aspiration cytology. J Pathol Transl Med. 2018 Nov;52(6):404–10. PMID:30317844
730. Chabre O, Libé R, Assie G, et al. Serum miR-483-5p and miR-195 are predictive of recurrence risk in adrenocortical cancer patients. Endocr Relat Cancer. 2013 Jul 5;20(4):579–94. PMID:23756429
731. Chai L, Ying HF, Wu TT, et al. Clinical features and hypoxic marker expression of primary sinonasal and laryngeal small-cell neuroendocrine carcinoma: a small case series. World J Surg Oncol. 2014 Jul 1;12:199. PMID:24980293
732. Chainey J, Chan VK, Au K, et al. Multiple recurrences of spindle cell oncocytoma: a case report and literature review. Clin Neuropathol. 2020 Jan/Feb;39(1):32–9. PMID:31496509
733. Chakraborty PP, Bhattacharjee R, Mukhopadhyay P, et al. Bilateral adrenal myelolipoma in Cushing's disease: a relook into the role of corticotropin in adrenal tumourigenesis. BMJ Case Rep. 2016 Jun 15;2016:bcr2016214965. PMID:27307426
734. Chakraborty R, Abdel-Wahab O, Durham BH. MAP-kinase-driven hematopoietic neoplasms: a decade of progress in the molecular age. Cold Spring Harb Perspect Med. 2021 May 3;11(5):a034892. PMID:32601132
735. Chakraborty R, Hampton OA, Shen X, et al. Mutually exclusive recurrent somatic mutations in MAP2K1 and BRAF support a central role for ERK activation in LCH pathogenesis. Blood. 2014 Nov 6;124(19):3007–15. PMID:25202140
736. Chamberlain BK, McClain CM, Gonzalez RS, et al. Alveolar soft part sarcoma and granular cell tumor: an immunohistochemical comparison study. Hum Pathol. 2014 May;45(5):1039–44. PMID:24746209
737. Chambers M, Nosé V, Sadow PM, et al. Salivary-like tumors of the thyroid: a comprehensive review of three rare carcinomas. Head Neck Pathol. 2021 Mar;15(1):212–24. PMID:32562215
738. Chambers M, Tafe LJ, Gutmann EJ, et al. Cytologic features of a case of mixed medullary and follicular cell-derived thyroid carcinoma with review of the literature. Diagn Cytopathol. 2021 Mar;49(3):E125–9. PMID:32936534
739. Chan CC, Collins AB, Chew EY. Molecular pathology of eyes with von Hippel-Lindau (VHL) Disease: a review. Retina. 2007 Jan;27(1):1–7. PMID:17218907
740. Chan CS, Laddha SV, Lewis PW, et al. ATRX, DAXX or MEN1 mutant pancreatic neuroendocrine tumors are a distinct alpha-cell signature subgroup. Nat Commun. 2018 Oct 12;9(1):4158. PMID:30315258
741. Chan H, Zhang L, Choti MA, et al. Recurrence patterns after surgical resection of gastroenteropancreatic neuroendocrine tumors: analysis from the National Comprehensive Cancer Network Oncology Outcomes Database. Pancreas. 2021 Apr 1;50(4):506–12. PMID:33939661
742. Chan JK. Papillary carcinoma of thyroid: classical and variants. Histol Histopathol. 1990 Apr;5(2):241–57. PMID:2134378
743. Chan JK, Albores-Saavedra J, Battifora H, et al. Sclerosing mucoepidermoid thyroid carcinoma with eosinophilia. A distinctive low-grade malignancy arising from the metaplastic follicles of Hashimoto's thyroiditis. Am J Surg Pathol. 1991 May;15(5):438–48. PMID:2035738
744. Chan JK, Rosai J. Tumors of the neck showing thymic or related branchial pouch differentiation: a unifying concept. Hum Pathol. 1991 Apr;22(4):349–67. PMID:2050369
745. Chan JK, Suster S, Wenig BM, et al. Cytokeratin 20 immunoreactivity distinguishes Merkel cell (primary cutaneous neuroendocrine) carcinomas and salivary gland small cell carcinomas from small cell carcinomas of various sites. Am J Surg Pathol. 1997 Feb;21(2):226–34. PMID:9042291
746. Chan JK, Tse CC. Mucin production in metastatic papillary carcinoma of the thyroid. Hum Pathol. 1988 Feb;19(2):195–200. PMID:3277907
747. Chan LP, Chiang FY, Lee KW, et al. Carcinoma showing thymus-like differentiation (CASTLE) of thyroid: a case report and literature review. Kaohsiung J Med Sci. 2008 Nov;24(11):591–7. PMID:19239992
748. Chandra RK, Maddalozzo J, Kovarik P. Histological characterization of the thyroglossal tract: implications for surgical management. Laryngoscope. 2001 Jun;111(6):1002–5. PMID:11404612
749. Chandramohan A, Sathyakumar K, John RA, et al. Atypical ultrasound features of parathyroid tumours may bear a relationship to their clinical and biochemical presentation. Insights Imaging. 2014 Feb;5(1):103–11. PMID:24293304
750. Chandrasekharappa SC, Guru SC, Manickam P, et al. Positional cloning of the gene for multiple endocrine neoplasia-type 1. Science. 1997 Apr 18;276(5311):404–7. PMID:9103196
751. Chang CF, Li WY, Shu CH, et al. Sino-nasal neuro-endocrine carcinoma. Acta Otolaryngol. 2010 Mar;130(3):392–7. PMID:19685359
752. Chang EF, Zada G, Kim S, et al. Long-term recurrence and mortality after surgery and adjuvant radiotherapy for nonfunctional pituitary adenomas. J Neurosurg. 2008 Apr;108(4):736–45. PMID:18377253
753. Chang KC, Chen PI, Huang ZH, et al. Adrenal myelolipoma with translocation (3;21)(q25;p11). Cancer Genet Cytogenet. 2002 Apr 1;134(1):77–80. PMID:11996801
754. Chang KTE, Tay AZE, Kuick CH, et al. ALK-positive histiocytosis: an expanded clinicopathologic spectrum and frequent presence of KIF5B-ALK fusion. Mod Pathol. 2019 May;32(5):598–608. PMID:30573850
755. Chang MT, Penson A, Desai NB, et al. Small-cell carcinomas of the bladder and lung are characterized by a convergent but distinct pathogenesis. Clin Cancer Res. 2018 Apr 15;24(8):1965–73. PMID:29180607
756. Chang ST, Chuang SS. Ectopic cervical thymoma: a mimic of T-lymphoblastic lymphoma. Pathol Res Pract. 2003;199(9):633–5. PMID:14621201
757. Chang YS, Chang CC, Huang HY, et al. Detection of molecular alterations in Taiwanese patients with medullary thyroid cancer using whole-exome sequencing. Endocr Pathol. 2018 Dec;29(4):324–31. PMID:30120715
758. Chang-Chretien K, Chew JT, Judge DP. Reversible dilated cardiomyopathy associated with glucagonoma. Heart. 2004 Jul;90(7):e44. PMID:15201270
759. Chapman MC, Soares BP, Li Y, et al. Congenital oral masses: an anatomic approach to diagnosis. Radiographics. 2019 Jul-Aug;39(4):1143–60. PMID:31283464
760. Chapurin N, Totten DJ, Louis PC, et al. Sinonasal small cell carcinoma-case series of a rare malignancy. Ear Nose Throat J. 2022 Jul;101(6):392–5. PMID:33090899
761. Chapuy B, Stewart C, Dunford AJ, et al. Molecular subtypes of diffuse large B cell lymphoma are associated with distinct pathogenic mechanisms and outcomes. Nat Med. 2018 May;24(5):679–90. PMID:29713087
762. Charfi S, Ayadi L, Ellouze S, et al. [Composite pheochromocytoma associated with multiple endocrine neoplasia type 2B]. Ann Pathol. 2008 Jun;28(3):225–8. French. PMID:18706367
763. Charkes ND. On the prevalence of familial nonmedullary thyroid cancer in multiply affected kindreds. Thyroid. 2006 Feb;16(2):181–6. PMID:16613533
764. Chasseloup F, Pankratz N, Lane J, et al. Germline CDKN1B loss-of-function variants cause pediatric Cushing's disease with or without an MEN4 phenotype. J Clin Endocrinol Metab. 2020 Jun 1;105(6):1983–2005. PMID:32232325
765. Chatzopoulos K, Fritchie KJ, Aubry MC, et al. Loss of succinate dehydrogenase B immunohistochemical expression distinguishes pulmonary chondromas from hamartomas. Histopathology. 2019 Dec;75(6):825–32. PMID:31236950
766. Chau C, Rimmer Frcr Y, Choudhury PhD A, et al. Treatment outcomes for small cell carcinoma of the bladder: results from a UK patient retrospective cohort study. Int J Radiat Oncol Biol Phys. 2021 Jul 15;110(4):1143–50. PMID:33561506
767. Chebib I, Hornicek FJ, Nielsen GP, et al. Cytomorphologic features that distinguish schwannoma from other low-grade spindle cell lesions. Cancer Cytopathol. 2015 Mar;123(3):171–9. PMID:25641870
768. Chen B, Shi Y, Xu Y, et al. The predictive value of coexisting BRAFV600E and TERT promoter mutations on poor outcomes and high tumour aggressiveness in papillary thyroid carcinoma: a systematic review and meta-analysis. Clin Endocrinol (Oxf). 2021 May;94(5):731–42. PMID:32816325
769. Chen BB, Yeh CC, Chang TC, et al. Computed tomography diagnosis of primary thyroid teratoma. J Formos Med Assoc. 2005 Jul;104(7):514–7. PMID:16091830
770. Chen CH, Boag AH, Beiko DT, et al. Composite paraganglioma-ganglioneuroma of the urinary bladder: a rare neoplasm causing hemodynamic crisis at tumour resection. Can Urol Assoc J. 2009 Oct;3(5):E45–8. PMID:19829717
771. Chen DA, Mandell-Brown M, Moore SF, et al. "Composite" tumor–mixed squamous cell and small-cell anaplastic carcinoma of the larynx. Otolaryngol Head Neck Surg. 1986 Jul;95(1):99–103. PMID:3033580
772. Chen ED, Cheng P, Cai YF, et al. Ultrasonographic features of Langerhans cell histiocytosis of the thyroid. Int J Clin Exp Pathol. 2014 Feb 15;7(3):1229–35. PMID:24696742
773. Chen G, Liu Z, Su C, et al. Primary peripheral nerve sheath tumors of the thyroid gland: a case report and literature review. Mol Clin Oncol. 2016 Feb;4(2):209–10. PMID:26893864
774. Chen H, Li Y, Gao X, et al. Clinical value of 99mTc-HYNIC-TOC SPECT/CT for the diagnosis primary small cell neuroendocrine carcinomas of the nasal cavity and paranasal sinuses. Clin Imaging. 2018 Nov-Dec 52:365–9. PMID:30248495
775. Chen H, Sippel RS, O'Dorisio MS, et al. The North American Neuroendocrine Tumor Society consensus guideline for the diagnosis and management of neuroendocrine tumors: pheochromocytoma, paraganglioma, and medullary thyroid cancer. Pancreas. 2010 Aug;39(6):775–83. PMID:20664475
776. Chen HD, Huang LE, Zhong ZH, et al. Ovarian adrenal rest tumors undetected by imaging studies and identified at surgery in three females with congenital adrenal hyperplasia unresponsive to increased hormone therapy dosage. Endocr Pathol. 2017 Jun;28(2):146–51. PMID:28032206
777. Chen J, Jian X, Deng S, et al. Identification of recurrent USP48 and BRAF mutations in Cushing's disease. Nat Commun. 2018 Aug 9;9(1):3171. PMID:30093687
778. Chen J, Tward JD, Shrieve DC, et al. Surgery and radiotherapy improves survival in patients with anaplastic thyroid carcinoma: analysis of the Surveillance, Epidemiology, and End Results 1983-2002. Am J Clin Oncol. 2008 Oct;31(5):460–4. PMID:18838882
779. Chen JH, Faquin WC, Lloyd RV, et al. Clinicopathological and molecular characterization of nine cases of columnar cell variant of papillary thyroid carcinoma. Mod Pathol. 2011 May;24(5):739–49. PMID:21358618
780. Chen KT, Papavasiliou P, Edwards K, et al. A better prognosis for Merkel cell carcinoma of unknown primary origin. Am J Surg. 2013 Nov;206(5):752–7. PMID:23835211
781. Chen P, Jin L, Yang Y, et al. Bilateral primary adrenal diffuse large B cell lymphoma without adrenal insufficiency: a case report and review of the literature. Mol Clin Oncol. 2017 Jul;7(1):145–7. PMID:28685093
782. Chen PP, Ramalingam P, Alvarado-Cabrero I, et al. High-grade neuroendocrine carcinomas of the vulva: a clinicopathologic study of 16 cases. Am J Surg Pathol. 2021 Mar 1;45(3):304–16. PMID:32826525
783. Chen S, Zheng Y, Chen L, et al. A broad ligament solitary fibrous tumor with Doege-Potter syndrome. Medicine (Baltimore). 2018 Sep;97(39):e12564. PMID:30278559
784. Chen TY, Lorch JH, Wong KS, et al. Histological features of BRAF V600E-mutant anaplastic thyroid carcinoma. Histopathology. 2020 Aug;77(2):314–20. PMID:32428249
785. Chen W, Wang J, Wang E, et al. Detection of clonal lymphoid receptor gene rearrangements in langerhans cell histiocytosis. Am J Surg Pathol. 2010 Jul;34(7):1049–57. PMID:20551822
786. Chen Y, Hu DY, Wang TT, et al. CDC73 gene mutations in sporadic ossifying fibroma of the jaws. Diagn Pathol. 2016 Sep 22;11(1):91. PMID:27658992
787. Chen Y, Takita J, Choi YL, et al. Oncogenic mutations of ALK kinase in neuroblastoma. Nature. 2008 Oct 16;455(7215):971–4. PMID:18923524
788. Chen Y, Wang F, Han A. Fat-forming solitary fibrous tumor of the kidney: a case report and literature review. Int J Clin Exp Pathol. 2015 Jul 1;8(7):8632–5. PMID:26339447
789. Cheng JY, Gill AJ, Kumar SK. Granulosa cell tumour of the adrenal. Pathology. 2015 Aug;47(5):487–9. PMID:26126046
790. Cheng S, Al-Agha R, Araujo PB, et al. Metabolic glucose status and pituitary pathology portend therapeutic outcomes in acromegaly. PLoS One. 2013 Sep 9;8(9):e73543. PMID:24039977
791. Cheng V, Brainard J, Nasr C. Co-occurrence of papillary thyroid carcinoma and primary lymphoma of the thyroid in a patient with long-standing Hashimoto's thyroiditis. Thyroid. 2012 Jun;22(6):647–50. PMID:22568399
792. Chentli F, Belhimer F, Kessaci F, et al. Congenital craniopharyngioma: a case report and literature review. J Pediatr Endocrinol Metab. 2012;25(11-12):1181–3. PMID:23329768
793. Cheon T, Song YJ, Kim JI, et al. Aggressive thyroid carcinoma showing thymus-like differentiation (CASTLE) with lung metastasis and carotid artery invasion. Ear Nose Throat J. 2019 Oct-Nov;98(9):557–9. PMID:31284751
794. Chernock RD, Rivera B, Borrelli N, et al. Poorly differentiated thyroid carcinoma of childhood and adolescence: a distinct

entity characterized by DICER1 mutations. Mod Pathol. 2020 Jul;33(7):1264–74. PMID:31937902

795. Cheson BD, Fisher RI, Barrington SF, et al. Recommendations for initial evaluation, staging, and response assessment of Hodgkin and non-Hodgkin lymphoma: the Lugano classification. J Clin Oncol. 2014 Sep 20;32(27):3059–68. PMID:25113753

796. Chetty R. Cytokeratin expression in cauda equina paragangliomas. Am J Surg Pathol. 1999 Apr;23(4):491. PMID:10199484

797. Chetty R. Follicular patterned lesions of the thyroid gland: a practical algorithmic approach. J Clin Pathol. 2011 Sep;64(9):737–41. PMID:21593347

798. Chetty R, Capo-Chichi JM, Serra S. Colorectal large-cell neuroendocrine carcinoma with lymphoid stroma: further evidence confirming a unique subtype associated with MLH1/PMS2 loss, BRAF mutation, Epstein-Barr virus negativity, and the possibility of a better prognosis. Histopathology. 2019 Aug;75(2):247–53. PMID:30990915

799. Chetty R, Duhig JD. Bilateral pheochromocytoma-ganglioneuroma of the adrenal in type 1 neurofibromatosis. Am J Surg Pathol. 1993 Aug;17(8):837–41. PMID:8338194

800. Chetty R, Ezzat S, Asa SL. Microadenomatosis of the pancreas in von Hippel-Lindau disease. Am J Surg Pathol. 2006 Dec;30(12):1630. PMID:17122523

801. Chetty R, Goetsch S, Nayler S, et al. Spindle epithelial tumour with thymus-like element (SETTLE): the predominantly monophasic variant. Histopathology. 1998 Jul;33(1):71–4. PMID:9726052

802. Chetty R, Kennedy M, Ezzat S, et al. Pancreatic endocrine pathology in von Hippel-Lindau disease: an expanding spectrum of lesions. Endocr Pathol. 2004 Summer;15(2):141–8. PMID:15299200

803. Cheuk W, Jacobson AA, Chan JK. Spindle epithelial tumor with thymus-like differentiation (SETTLE): a distinctive malignant thyroid neoplasm with significant metastatic potential. Mod Pathol. 2000 Oct;13(10):1150–5. PMID:11048811

804. Cheuk W, Kwan MY, Suster S, et al. Immunostaining for thyroid transcription factor 1 and cytokeratin 20 aids the distinction of small cell carcinoma from Merkel cell carcinoma, but not pulmonary from extrapulmonary small cell carcinomas. Arch Pathol Lab Med. 2001 Feb;125(2):228–31. PMID:11175640

805. Cheung CC, Boerner SL, MacMillan CM, et al. Hyalinizing trabecular tumor of the thyroid: a variant of papillary carcinoma proved by molecular genetics. Am J Surg Pathol. 2000 Dec;24(12):1622–6. PMID:11117782

806. Cheung NK, Dyer MA. Neuroblastoma: developmental biology, cancer genomics and immunotherapy. Nat Rev Cancer. 2013 Jun;13(6):397–411. PMID:23702928

807. Cheung NK, Zhang J, Lu C, et al. Association of age at diagnosis and genetic mutations in patients with neuroblastoma. JAMA. 2012 Mar 14;307(10):1062–71. PMID:22416102

808. Cheung VKY, Gill AJ, Chou A. Old, new, and emerging immunohistochemical markers in pheochromocytoma and paraganglioma. Endocr Pathol. 2018 Jun;29(2):169–75. PMID:29779206

809. Chevalier N, Paris F, Fontana S, et al. Postpubertal persistent hyperestrogenemia in McCune-Albright syndrome: unilateral oophorectomy improved fertility but detected an unexpected borderline epithelial ovarian tumor. J Pediatr Adolesc Gynecol. 2015 Dec;28(6):e169–72. PMID:26321108

810. Chew EY. Ocular manifestations of von Hippel-Lindau disease: clinical and genetic investigations. Trans Am Ophthalmol Soc. 2005;103:495–511. PMID:17057815

811. Chew KT, Abu MA, Arifuddin Y, et al. Ectopic adrenal tissue associated with borderline mucinous cystadenoma of ovary: a case report with review of the literature. Horm Mol Biol Clin Investig. 2017 Sep 20;32(3):/j/hmbci.2017.32.issue-3/hmbci-2017-0021/hmbci-2017-0021.xml. PMID:28930625

812. Chey WY, Frankel WL, Roy S, et al. Primary pancreatic secretinoma: further evidence supporting secretin as a diarrheogenic hormone. Ann Surg. 2017 Aug;266(2):346–52. PMID:27501174

813. Chhabra S, Agarwal R, Garg S, et al. Rosai-Dorfman disease: a case report with extranodal thyroid involvement. Diagn Cytopathol. 2012 May;40(5):447–9. PMID:21630484

814. Chhuon Y, Weon YC, Park G, et al. Pituitary blastoma in a 19-year-old woman: a case report and review of literature. World Neurosurg. 2020 Jul;139:310–3. PMID:32339726

815. Chiacchiarini M, Trocchianesi S, Besharat ZM, et al. Role of tissue and circulating microRNAs and DNA as biomarkers in medullary thyroid cancer. Pharmacol Ther. 2021 Mar;219:107708. PMID:33091426

816. Chiale F, Abrigo E, Lonati L, et al. Severe arterial hypertension and hyperandrogenism in a boy: a rare case of catecholamine- and β-HCG-secreting pheochromocytoma. J Pediatr Endocrinol Metab. 2019 Oct 25;32(10):1193–7. PMID:31490776

817. Chiang CS, Shyr BU, Chen SC, et al. Periampullary gangliocytic paraganglioma. J Gastrointest Surg. 2019 Nov;23(11):2247–54. PMID:30565068

818. Chien HP, Chang YS, Hsu PS, et al. Adrenal cystic lesions: a clinicopathological analysis of 25 cases with proposed histogenesis and review of the literature. Endocr Pathol. 2008 Winter;19(4):274–81. PMID:18972224

819. Chinezu L, Vasiljevic A, Jouanneau E, et al. Expression of somatostatin receptors, SSTR2A and SSTR5, in 108 endocrine pituitary tumors using immunohistochemical detection with new specific monoclonal antibodies. Hum Pathol. 2014 Jan;45(1):71–7. PMID:24182563

820. Chiosea S, Nikiforova M, Zuo H, et al. A novel complex BRAF mutation detected in a solid variant of papillary thyroid carcinoma. Endocr Pathol. 2009 Summer;20(2):122–6. PMID:19370421

821. Chmielecki J, Crago AM, Rosenberg M, et al. Whole-exome sequencing identifies a recurrent NAB2-STAT6 fusion in solitary fibrous tumors. Nat Genet. 2013 Feb;45(2):131–2. PMID:23313954

822. Chmielecki J, Hutchinson KE, Frampton GM, et al. Comprehensive genomic profiling of pancreatic acinar cell carcinomas identifies recurrent RAF fusions and frequent inactivation of DNA repair genes. Cancer Discov. 2014 Dec;4(12):1398–405. PMID:25266736

823. Ch'ng ES, Hoshida Y, Iizuka N, et al. Composite malignant pheochromocytoma with malignant peripheral nerve sheath tumour: a case with 28 years of tumour-bearing history. Histopathology. 2007 Sep;51(3):420–2. PMID:17727489

824. Cho HR, Sugihara J, Shimizu H, et al. Pathogenesis of multinodular goiter in elderly XB130-deficient mice: alteration of thyroperoxidase affinity with iodide and hydrogen peroxide. Thyroid. 2022 Apr;32(4):385–96. PMID:34915750

825. Cho J, Kinsey D, Kimchi ET, et al. Retroperitoneal extra-adrenal myelolipoma misdiagnosed as liposarcoma: a case report. Radiol Case Rep. 2020 Dec 5;16(2):364–8. PMID:33532014

826. Cho J, Shin JH, Hahn SY, et al. Columnar cell variant of papillary thyroid carcinoma: ultrasonographic and clinical differentiation between the indolent and aggressive types. Korean J Radiol. 2018 Sep-Oct;19(5):1000–5. PMID:30174490

827. Cho JH, Park YH, Kim WS, et al. High incidence of mucosa-associated lymphoid tissue in primary thyroid lymphoma: a clinicopathologic study of 18 cases in the Korean population. Leuk Lymphoma. 2006 Oct;47(10):2128–31. PMID:17071486

828. Cho SJ, Suh CH, Baek JH, et al. Active surveillance for small papillary thyroid cancer: a systematic review and meta-analysis. Thyroid. 2019 Oct;29(10):1399–408. PMID:31368412

829. Cho U, Mete O, Kim MH, et al. Molecular correlates and rate of lymph node metastasis of non-invasive follicular thyroid neoplasm with papillary-like nuclear features and invasive follicular variant papillary thyroid carcinoma: the impact of rigid criteria to distinguish non-invasive follicular thyroid neoplasm with papillary-like nuclear features. Mod Pathol. 2017 Jun;30(6):810–25. PMID:28281551

830. Choi H, Kim S, Moon JH, et al. Multiple endocrine neoplasia type 1 with multiple leiomyomas linked to a novel mutation in the MEN1 gene. Yonsei Med J. 2008 Aug 30;49(4):655–61. PMID:18729310

831. Choi M, Scholl UI, Yue P, et al. K+ channel mutations in adrenal aldosterone-producing adenomas and hereditary hypertension. Science. 2011 Feb 11;331(6018):768–72. PMID:21311022

832. Choi NY, Kim BS, Oh ST, et al. Comparative outcomes in patients with small- and large-cell neuroendocrine carcinoma (NEC) and mixed neuroendocrine-non-neuroendocrine neoplasm (MiNEN) of the stomach. Am Surg. 2021 Apr;87(4):631–7. PMID:33142079

833. Choi S, Lee JS, Bassim CW, et al. Dental abnormalities in individuals with pathogenic germline variation in DICER1. Am J Med Genet A. 2019 Sep;179(9):1820–5. PMID:31313479

834. Choi WJ, Baek JH, Ha EJ, et al. The ultrasonography features of hyalinizing trabecular tumor of the thyroid gland and the role of fine needle aspiration cytology and core needle biopsy in its diagnosis. Acta Radiol. 2015 Sep;56(9):1113–8. PMID:25232186

835. Choi YM, Kim TY, Song DE, et al. Papillary thyroid carcinoma arising from a thyroglossal duct cyst: a single institution experience. Endocr J. 2013;60(5):665–70. PMID:23318645

836. Chong AS, Han H, Albrecht S, et al. DICER1 syndrome in a young adult with pituitary blastoma. Acta Neuropathol. 2021 Dec;142(6):1071–6. PMID:34677675

837. Chong AS, Nikiforov YE, Condello V, et al. Prevalence and spectrum of DICER1 mutations in adult-onset thyroid nodules with indeterminate cytology. J Clin Endocrinol Metab. 2021 Mar 25;106(4):968–77. PMID:33460435

838. Chong Y, Shin JH, Oh YL, et al. Cribriform-morular variant of papillary thyroid carcinoma: ultrasonographic and clinical characteristics. Thyroid. 2013 Jan;23(1):45–9. PMID:22892017

839. Chou A, Fraser S, Toon CW, et al. A detailed clinicopathologic study of ALK-translocated papillary thyroid carcinoma. Am J Surg Pathol. 2015 May;39(5):652–9. PMID:25501013

840. Chou A, Itchins M, de Reuver PR, et al. ATRX loss is an independent predictor of poor survival in pancreatic neuroendocrine tumors. Hum Pathol. 2018 Dec;82:249–57. PMID:30081149

841. Chou A, Qiu MR, Crayton H, et al. A detailed histologic and molecular assessment of the diffuse sclerosing variant of papillary thyroid carcinoma. Mod Pathol. 2023 Dec;36(12):100329. PMID:37716505

842. Chou J, Walters A, Hage R, et al. Thyroglossal duct cysts: anatomy, embryology and treatment. Surg Radiol Anat. 2013 Dec;35(10):875–81. PMID:23689821

843. Chow LT, Metreweli C, King WW, et al. Histological changes of parathyroid adenoma after percutaneous injection of ethanol. Histopathology. 1997 Jan;30(1):87–9. PMID:9023564

844. Chow SM, Chan JK, Tse LL, et al. Carcinoma showing thymus-like element (CASTLE) of thyroid: combined modality treatment in 3 patients with locally advanced disease. Eur J Surg Oncol. 2007 Feb;33(1):83–5. PMID:17085008

845. Chrisoulidou A, Iliadou P, Doumala E, et al. Thyroglossal duct cyst carcinomas: is there a need for thyroidectomy? Hormones (Athens). 2013 Oct-Dec;12(4):522–8. PMID:24457400

846. Christ E, Antwi K, Fani M, et al. Innovative imaging of insulinoma: the end of sampling? A review. Endocr Relat Cancer. 2020 Apr;27(4):R79–92. PMID:31951592

847. Christison-Lagay ER, Baertschiger RM, Dinauer C, et al. Pediatric differentiated thyroid carcinoma: an update from the APSA Cancer Committee. J Pediatr Surg. 2020 Nov;55(11):2273–83. PMID:32553450

848. Christmas TJ, Chapple CR, Noble JG, et al. Hyperparathyroidism after neck irradiation. Br J Surg. 1988 Sep;75(9):873–4. PMID:3179662

849. Chu IM, Hengst L, Slingerland JM. The Cdk inhibitor p27 in human cancer: prognostic potential and relevance to anticancer therapy. Nat Rev Cancer. 2008 Apr;8(4):253–67. PMID:18354415

850. Chun YS, Pawlik TM, Vauthey JN. 8th edition of the AJCC Cancer Staging Manual: pancreas and hepatobiliary cancers. Ann Surg Oncol. 2018 Apr;25(4):845–7. PMID:28752469

851. Chung AY, Tran TB, Brumund KT, et al. Metastases to the thyroid: a review of the literature from the last decade. Thyroid. 2012 Mar;22(3):258–68. PMID:22313412

852. Chung DH, Kang GH, Kim WH, et al. Clonal analysis of a solitary follicular nodule of the thyroid with the polymerase chain reaction method. Mod Pathol. 1999 Mar;12(3):265–71. PMID:10102611

853. Chung DH, Kim NR, Kim T, et al. Malignant glomus tumor of the thyroid gland where is heretofore an unreported organ: a case report and literature review. Endocr Pathol. 2015 Mar;26(1):37–44. PMID:25544269

854. Chung SM, Kim KJ, Moon JS, et al. Fever of unknown origin caused by intrathyroidal thymic carcinoma. Korean J Intern Med. 2019 May;34(3):683–4. PMID:30099866

855. Chung-Park M, Yang JT, McHenry CR, et al. Adenomatoid tumor of the adrenal gland with micronodular adrenal cortical hyperplasia. Hum Pathol. 2003 Aug;34(8):818–21. PMID:14506647

856. Ciampi R, Romei C, Cosci B, et al. Chromosome 10 and RET gene copy number alterations in hereditary and sporadic medullary thyroid carcinoma. Mol Cell Endocrinol. 2012 Jan 2;348(1):176–82. PMID:21867742

857. Ciampi R, Romei C, Ramone T, et al. Genetic landscape of somatic mutations in a large cohort of sporadic medullary thyroid carcinomas studied by next-generation targeted sequencing. iScience. 2019 Oct 25;20:324–36. PMID:31605946

858. Cibas ES, Ali SZ. The 2017 Bethesda System for Reporting Thyroid Cytopathology. Thyroid. 2017 Nov;27(11):1341–6. PMID:29091573

859. Cichoń S, Anielski R, Konturek A, et al. Metastases to the thyroid gland: seventeen cases operated on in a single clinical center. Langenbecks Arch Surg. 2006 Nov;391(6):581–7. PMID:16983577

860. Cignarelli M, Ambrosi A, Marino A, et al. Three cases of papillary carcinoma and three of adenoma in thyroglossal duct cysts: clinical-diagnostic comparison with benign thyroglossal duct cysts. J Endocrinol Invest. 2002 Dec;25(11):947–54. PMID:12553553
861. Cimbek EA, Polat R, Sönmez B, et al. Clinical, sonographical, and pathological findings of pediatric thyroid nodules. Eur J Pediatr. 2021 Sep;180(9):2823–9. PMID:33772338
862. Cingolani N, Shaco-Levy R, Farruggio A, et al. Alpha-fetoprotein production by pancreatic tumors exhibiting acinar cell differentiation: study of five cases, one arising in a mediastinal teratoma. Hum Pathol. 2000 Aug;31(8):938–44. PMID:10987254
863. Cinque L, Pugliese F, Clemente C, et al. Rare somatic MEN1 gene pathogenic variant in a patient affected by atypical parathyroid adenoma. Int J Endocrinol. 2020 Apr 27;2020:2080797. PMID:32411220
864. Cipriani C, Biamonte F, Costa AG, et al. Prevalence of kidney stones and vertebral fractures in primary hyperparathyroidism using imaging technology. J Clin Endocrinol Metab. 2015 Apr;100(4):1309–15. PMID:25646791
865. Cipriani NA. Prognostic parameters in differentiated thyroid carcinomas. Surg Pathol Clin. 2019 Dec;12(4):883–900. PMID:31672296
866. Cipriani NA, Agarwal S, Dias-Santagata D, et al. Clear cell change in thyroid carcinoma: a clinicopathologic and molecular study with identification of variable genetic anomalies. Thyroid. 2017 Jun;27(6):819–24. PMID:28293986
867. Cirello V, Colombo C, Karapanou O, et al. Clinical and genetic features of a large monocentric series of familial non-medullary thyroid cancers. Front Endocrinol (Lausanne). 2021 Jan 7;11:589340. PMID:33488516
868. Cisco RM, Norton JA. Surgery for gastrinoma. Adv Surg. 2007;41:165–76. PMID:17972563
869. Claahsen-van der Grinten HL, Speiser PW, Ahmed SF, et al. Congenital adrenal hyperplasia-current insights in pathophysiology, diagnostics, and management. Endocr Rev. 2022 Jan 12;43(1):91–159. PMID:33961029
870. Claahsen-van der Grinten HL, Stikkelbroeck N, Falhammar H, et al. Management of endocrine disease: gonadal dysfunction in congenital adrenal hyperplasia. Eur J Endocrinol. 2021 Mar;184(3):R85–97. PMID:33320831
871. Clark ES, Carney JA. Pancreatic islet cell tumor associated with Cushing's syndrome. Am J Surg Pathol. 1984 Dec;8(12):917–24. PMID:6097131
872. Clark VE, Erson-Omay EZ, Serin A, et al. Genomic analysis of non-NF2 meningiomas reveals mutations in TRAF7, KLF4, AKT1, and SMO. Science. 2013 Mar 1;339(6123):1077–80. PMID:23348505
873. Clarke CN, Katsonis P, Hsu TK, et al. Comprehensive genomic characterization of parathyroid cancer identifies novel candidate driver mutations and core pathways. J Endocr Soc. 2018 Sep 3;3(3):544–59. PMID:30788456
874. Classe M, Yao H, Mouawad R, et al. Integrated multi-omic analysis of esthesioneuroblastomas identifies two subgroups linked to cell ontogeny. Cell Rep. 2018 Oct 16;25(3):811–821.e5. PMID:30332658
875. Claus EB, Calvocoressi L, Bondy ML, et al. Exogenous hormone use, reproductive factors, and risk of intracranial meningioma in females. J Neurosurg. 2013 Mar;118(3):649–56. PMID:23101448
876. Clay MR, Martinez AP, Weiss SW, et al. MDM2 amplification in problematic lipomatous tumors: analysis of FISH testing criteria. Am J Surg Pathol. 2015 Oct;39(10):1433–9. PMID:26146760
877. Clemente M, Caracseghi F, Gussinyer M, et al. Macroorchidism and panhypopituitarism: two different forms of presentation of FSH-secreting pituitary adenomas in adolescence. Horm Res Paediatr. 2011;75(3):225–30. PMID:21196695
878. ClinicalTrials.gov [Internet]. Bethesda (MD): U.S. National Library of Medicine; 2022. Identifier NCT03084770, Asymptomatic small pancreatic endocrine neoplasms (ASPEN); first posted 2017 Mar 21 [updated 2022 Mar 7]. Available from: https://clinicaltrials.gov/ct2/show/NCT03084770.
879. Coca-Pelaz A, Shah JP, Hernandez-Prera JC, et al. Papillary thyroid cancer-aggressive variants and impact on management: a narrative review. Adv Ther. 2020 Jul;37(7):3112–28. PMID:32488657
880. Cohen JB, Troxell M, Kong CS, et al. Ectopic intrathyroidal thymoma: a case report and review. Thyroid. 2003 Mar;13(3):305–8. PMID:12729482
881. Cohen M, Persky R, Stegemann R, et al. Germline USP8 mutation associated with pediatric Cushing disease and other clinical features: a new syndrome. J Clin Endocrinol Metab. 2019 Oct 1;104(10):4676–82. PMID:31162547
882. Cohen-Cohen S, Brown DA, Himes BT, et al. Pituitary adenomas in the setting of multiple endocrine neoplasia type 1: a single-institution experience. J Neurosurg. 2020 Apr 3;134(3):1132–8. PMID:32244213
883. Cohen-Kerem R, Schachter P, Sheinfeld M, et al. Multinodular goiter: the surgical procedure of choice. Otolaryngol Head Neck Surg. 2000 Jun;122(6):848–50. PMID:10828797
884. Cohn SL, Pearson AD, London WB, et al. The International Neuroblastoma Risk Group (INRG) classification system: an INRG Task Force report. J Clin Oncol. 2009 Jan 10;27(2):289–97. PMID:19047291
885. Coindre JM, de Mascarel A, Trojani M, et al. Immunohistochemical study of rhabdomyosarcoma. Unexpected staining with S100 protein and cytokeratin. J Pathol. 1988 Jun;155(2):127–32. PMID:2455782
886. Coiré CI, Horvath E, Kovacs K, et al. A composite silent corticotroph pituitary adenoma with interspersed adrenocortical cells: case report. Neurosurgery. 1998 Mar;42(3):650–4. PMID:9527001
887. Coiré CI, Horvath E, Smyth HS, et al. Rapidly recurring folliculostellate cell tumor of the adenohypophysis with the morphology of a spindle cell oncocytoma: case report with electron microscopic studies. Clin Neuropathol. 2009 Jul-Aug;28(4):303–8. PMID:19642510
888. Coleman KD, Wright JA, Ghosh M, et al. Estradiol modulation of hepatocyte growth factor by stromal fibroblasts in the female reproductive tract. Fertil Steril. 2009 Sep;92(3):1107–9. PMID:19423096
889. Coli A, Asa SL, Fadda G, et al. Minichromosome maintenance protein 7 as prognostic marker of tumor aggressiveness in pituitary adenoma patients. Eur J Endocrinol. 2016 Mar;174(3):307–14. PMID:26620390
890. Collazo-Gutiérrez N, de Jesús O, Villamil-Jarauta M, et al. Double pituitary adenomas with synchronous somatotroph and corticotroph clinical presentation of acromegaly and Cushing's disease. World Neurosurg. 2019 Dec;132:161–4. PMID:31505284
891. Collina G, Eusebi V, Capella C, et al. Merkel cell differentiation in trichoblastoma. Virchows Arch. 1998 Oct;433(4):291–6. PMID:9808429
892. Collini P, Negri T, Barisella M, et al. High-grade sarcomatous overgrowth in solitary fibrous tumors: a clinicopathologic study of 10 cases. Am J Surg Pathol. 2012 Aug;36(8):1202–15. PMID:22613995
893. Collins JA, Ping B, Bishop JA, et al. Carcinoma showing thymus-like differentiation (CASTLE): cytopathological features and differential diagnosis. Acta Cytol. 2016;60(5):421–8. PMID:27643719
894. Collins MT, Chebli C, Jones J, et al. Renal phosphate wasting in fibrous dysplasia of bone is part of a generalized renal tubular dysfunction similar to that seen in tumor-induced osteomalacia. J Bone Miner Res. 2001 May;16(5):806–13. PMID:11341325
895. Collins MT, Sarlis NJ, Merino MJ, et al. Thyroid carcinoma in the McCune-Albright syndrome: contributory role of activating Gs alpha mutations. J Clin Endocrinol Metab. 2003 Sep;88(9):4413–7. PMID:12970318
896. Collins MT, Singer FR, Eugster E. McCune-Albright syndrome and the extraskeletal manifestations of fibrous dysplasia. Orphanet J Rare Dis. 2012 May 24;7 Suppl 1 (Suppl 1):S4. PMID:22640971
897. Colonna M, Guizard AV, Schvartz C, et al. A time trend analysis of papillary and follicular cancers as a function of tumour size: a study of data from six cancer registries in France (1983-2000). Eur J Cancer. 2007 Mar;43(5):891–900. PMID:17289376
898. Comino-Méndez I, Gracia-Aznárez FJ, Schiavi F, et al. Exome sequencing identifies MAX mutations as a cause of hereditary pheochromocytoma. Nat Genet. 2011 Jun 19;43(7):663–7. PMID:21685915
899. Comino-Méndez I, Leandro-García LJ, Montoya G, et al. Functional and in silico assessment of MAX variants of unknown significance. J Mol Med (Berl). 2015 Nov;93(11):1247–55. PMID:26070438
900. Comstock JM, Willmore-Payne C, Holden JA, et al. Composite pheochromocytoma: a clinicopathologic and molecular comparison with ordinary pheochromocytoma and neuroblastoma. Am J Clin Pathol. 2009 Jul;132(1):69–73. PMID:19864235
901. Concolino P, Costella A, Capoluongo E. Multiple endocrine neoplasia type 1 (MEN1): an update of 208 new germline variants reported in the last nine years. Cancer Genet. 2016 Jan-Feb;209(1-2):36–41. PMID:26767918
902. Conemans EB, Brosens LAA, Raicu-Ionita GM, et al. Prognostic value of WHO grade in pancreatic neuro-endocrine tumors in multiple endocrine neoplasia type 1: results from the DutchMEN1 Study Group. Pancreatology. 2017 Sep-Oct;17(5):766–72. PMID:28811081
903. Coons SW, Estrada SI, Gamez R, et al. Cytokeratin CK 7 and CK 20 expression in pituitary adenomas. Endocr Pathol. 2005 Fall;16(3):201–10. PMID:16299403
904. Cooper CL, Wills EJ, Awad N, et al. Incidental meningioma in the adrenal gland: report of a case. Pathology. 2007 Oct;39(5):520–2. PMID:17886105
905. Cooper DS, Wenig BM. Hyperthyroidism caused by an ectopic TSH-secreting pituitary tumor. Thyroid. 1996 Aug;6(4):337–43. PMID:8875757
906. Cooper O. Silent corticotroph adenomas. Pituitary. 2015 Apr;18(2):225–31. PMID:25534889
907. Coopmans EC, Schneiders JJ, El-Sayed N, et al. T2-signal intensity, SSTR expression, and somatostatin analogs efficacy predict response to pasireotide in acromegaly. Eur J Endocrinol. 2020 Jun;182(6):595–605. PMID:32375119
908. Corbetta S, Peracchi M, Cappiello V, et al. Circulating ghrelin levels in patients with pancreatic and gastrointestinal neuroendocrine tumors: identification of one pancreatic ghrelinoma. J Clin Endocrinol Metab. 2003 Jul;88(7):3117–20. PMID:12843152
909. Corbetta S, Pizzocaro A, Peracchi M, et al. Multiple endocrine neoplasia type 1 in patients with recognized pituitary tumours of different types. Clin Endocrinol (Oxf). 1997 Nov;47(5):507–12. PMID:9425388
910. Corcos O, Couvelard A, Giraud S, et al. Endocrine pancreatic tumors in von Hippel-Lindau disease: clinical, histological, and genetic features. Pancreas. 2008 Jul;37(1):85–93. PMID:18580449
911. Corean J, Furtado LV, Kadri S, et al. Cribriform-morular variant of papillary thyroid carcinoma with poorly differentiated features: a case report with immunohistochemical and molecular genetic analysis. Int J Surg Pathol. 2019 May;27(3):294–304. PMID:30176755
912. Corenblum B, Sirek AM, Horvath E, et al. Human mixed somatotrophic and lactotrophic pituitary adenomas. J Clin Endocrinol Metab. 1976 May;42(5):857–63. PMID:773951
913. Corica D, Aversa T, Pepe G, et al. Peculiarities of precocious puberty in boys and girls with McCune-Albright syndrome. Front Endocrinol (Lausanne). 2018 Jun 22;9:337. PMID:29988390
914. Corica D, Bottari A, Aversa T, et al. An unusual epididymal localization of testicular adrenal rest tumor in an adolescent with congenital adrenal hyperplasia. Endocrine. 2019 Dec;66(3):695–8. PMID:31227992
915. Cormier EM, Wolf MF, Jordan VC. Decrease in estradiol-stimulated progesterone receptor production in MCF-7 cells by epidermal growth factor and possible clinical implication for paracrine-regulated breast cancer growth. Cancer Res. 1989 Feb 1;49(3):576–80. PMID:2783381
916. Cornejo KM, Afari HA, Sadow PM. Adrenocortical carcinoma arising in an adrenal rest: a case report and review of the literature. Endocr Pathol. 2017 Jun;28(2):165–70. PMID:28258518
917. Correa H. Li-Fraumeni syndrome. J Pediatr Genet. 2016 Jun;5(2):84–8. PMID:27617148
918. Correa R, Salpea P, Stratakis CA. Carney complex: an update. Eur J Endocrinol. 2015 Oct;173(4):M85–97. PMID:26130139
919. Corrin B, Gilby ED, Jones NF, et al. Oat cell carcinoma of the pancreas with ectopic ACTH secretion. Cancer. 1973 Jun;31(6):1523–7. PMID:4350960
920. Cortés JMR, Zerón HM. Genetics of thyroid disorders. Folia Med (Plovdiv). 2019 Jun 1;61(2):172–9. PMID:31301652
921. Cortet-Rudelli C, Bonneville JF, Borson-Chazot F, et al. Post-surgical management of non-functioning pituitary adenoma. Ann Endocrinol (Paris). 2015 Jul;76(3):228–38. PMID:26116412
922. Cortez GM, Monteiro A, Agnoletto G, et al. Aggressive pituitary tumor with Crooke's cells and invasion of the posterior fossa. World Neurosurg. 2020 Jun;138:530–534.e1. PMID:32145418
923. Corver WE, Demmers J, Oosting J, et al. ROS-induced near-homozygous genomes in thyroid cancer. Endocr Relat Cancer. 2018 Jan;25(1):83–97. PMID:29066502
924. Corver WE, Ruano D, Weijers K, et al. Genome haploidisation with chromosome 7 retention in oncocytic follicular thyroid carcinoma. PLoS One. 2012;7(6):e38287. PMID:22675538
925. Cosby WN, Babin RW. Simultaneous oat cell and squamous cell carcinoma of the larynx. Mil Med. 1988 Apr;153(4):196–8. PMID:2838769
926. Cossu G, Daniel RT, Messerer M. Gangliocytomas of the sellar region: a challenging diagnosis. Clin Neurol Neurosurg. 2016 Oct;149:122–35. PMID:27521460
927. Costa LJ, Xavier AC. Features and outcomes of diffuse large B-cell lymphoma of

the thyroid in a large contemporary cohort. Leuk Lymphoma. 2014 Feb;55(2):283–7. PMID:23647064
928. Costa V, Esposito R, Pallante P, et al. The "next-generation" knowledge of papillary thyroid carcinoma. Cell Cycle. 2018-21;201514(13). PMID:26030480
929. Costa-Guda J, Marinoni I, Molatore S, et al. Somatic mutation and germline sequence abnormalities in CDKN1B, encoding p27Kip1, in sporadic parathyroid adenomas. J Clin Endocrinol Metab. 2011 Apr;96(4):E701–6. PMID:21289244
930. Cote DJ, Smith TR, Sandler CN, et al. Functional gonadotroph adenomas: case series and report of literature. Neurosurgery. 2016 Dec;79(6):823–31. PMID:26692108
931. Courcoutsakis N, Patronas N, Filie AC, et al. Ectopic thymus presenting as a thyroid nodule in a patient with the Carney complex. Thyroid. 2009 Mar;19(3):293–6. PMID:19265501
932. Courcoutsakis NA, Tatsi C, Patronas NJ, et al. The complex of myxomas, spotty skin pigmentation and endocrine overactivity (Carney complex): imaging findings with clinical and pathological correlation. Insights Imaging. 2013 Feb;4(1):119–33. PMID:23315333
933. Courtillot C, Laugier Robiolle S, Cohen Aubart F, et al. Endocrine manifestations in a monocentric cohort of 64 patients with Erdheim-Chester disease. J Clin Endocrinol Metab. 2016 Jan;101(1):305–13. PMID:26565949
934. Couvelard A, Scoazec JY. [Inherited tumor syndromes of gastroenteropancreatic and thoracic neuroendocrine neoplasms]. Ann Pathol. 2020 Apr;40(2):120–33. French. PMID:32035641
935. Covington MF, Chin SS, Osborn AG. Pituicytoma, spindle cell oncocytoma, and granular cell tumor: clarification and meta-analysis of the world literature since 1893. AJNR Am J Neuroradiol. 2011 Dec;32(11):2067–72. PMID:21960498
936. Cox R, Vang R, Epstein JI. Papillary cystadenoma of the epididymis and broad ligament: morphologic and immunohistochemical overlap with clear cell papillary renal cell carcinoma. Am J Surg Pathol. 2014 May;38(5):713–8. PMID:24441657
937. Coy S, Du Z, Sheu SH, et al. Distinct patterns of primary and motile cilia in Rathke's cleft cysts and craniopharyngioma subtypes. Mod Pathol. 2016 Dec;29(12):1446–59. PMID:27562488
938. Coy S, Rashid R, Lin JR, et al. Multiplexed immunofluorescence reveals potential PD-1/PD-L1 pathway vulnerabilities in craniopharyngioma. Neuro Oncol. 2018 Jul 5;20(8):1101–12. PMID:29509940
939. Coyle D, Friedmacher F, Puri P. The association between Hirschsprung's disease and multiple endocrine neoplasia type 2a: a systematic review. Pediatr Surg Int. 2014 Aug;30(8):751–6. PMID:24972642
940. Cracolici V, Kadri S, Ritterhouse LL, et al. Clinicopathologic and molecular features of metastatic follicular thyroid carcinoma in patients presenting with a thyroid nodule versus a distant metastasis. Am J Surg Pathol. 2019 Apr;43(4):514–22. PMID:30557173
941. Cracolici V, Parilla M, Henriksen KJ, et al. An evaluation of CD61 immunohistochemistry in identification of vascular invasion in follicular thyroid neoplasms. Head Neck Pathol. 2020 Jun;14(2):399–405. PMID:31218593
942. Cracolici V, Ritterhouse LL, Segal JP, et al. Follicular thyroid neoplasms: comparison of clinicopathologic and molecular features of atypical adenomas and follicular thyroid carcinomas. Am J Surg Pathol. 2020 Jul;44(7):881–92. PMID:32282345
943. Cree IA, Tan PH, Travis WD, et al. Counting mitoses: SI(ze) matters! Mod Pathol. 2021 Sep;34(9):1651–7. PMID:34079071
944. Cromer MK, Starker LF, Choi M, et al. Identification of somatic mutations in parathyroid tumors using whole-exome sequencing. J Clin Endocrinol Metab. 2012 Sep;97(9):E1774–81. PMID:22740705
945. Crona J, Lamarca A, Ghosal S, et al. Genotype-phenotype correlations in pheochromocytoma and paraganglioma: a systematic review and individual patient meta-analysis. Endocr Relat Cancer. 2019 May;26(5):539–50. PMID:30893643
946. Crona J, Norlén O, Antonodimitrakis P, et al. Multiple and secondary hormone secretion in patients with metastatic pancreatic neuroendocrine tumours. J Clin Endocrinol Metab. 2016 Feb;101(2):445–52. PMID:26672633
947. Crosetti E, Arrigoni G, Cerutti M, et al. Atypical carcinoid of the larynx. Ear Nose Throat J. 2020 Jul;99(6):369–70. PMID:31012344
948. Crotty TB, Scheithauer BW, Young WF Jr, et al. Papillary craniopharyngioma: a clinicopathological study of 48 cases. J Neurosurg. 1995 Aug;83(2):206–14. PMID:7616262
949. Crowley RK, Al-Derazi Y, Lynch K, et al. Acromegaly associated with gangliocytoma. Ir J Med Sci. 2012 Sep;181(3):353–5. PMID:19789938
950. Cryer PE, Axelrod L, Grossman AB, et al. Evaluation and management of adult hypoglycemic disorders: an Endocrine Society clinical practice guideline. J Clin Endocrinol Metab. 2009 Mar;94(3):709–28. PMID:19088155
951. Cryns VL, Rubio MP, Thor AD, et al. p53 abnormalities in human parathyroid carcinoma. J Clin Endocrinol Metab. 1994 Jun;78(6):1320–4. PMID:8200932
952. Cryns VL, Thor A, Xu HJ, et al. Loss of the retinoblastoma tumor-suppressor gene in parathyroid carcinoma. N Engl J Med. 1994 Mar 17;330(11):757–61. PMID:7906387
953. Csiszkó A, László I, Palatka K, et al. Primary angiosarcoma of the pancreas mimicking severe acute pancreatitis–case report. Pancreatology. 2015 Jan-Feb;15(1):84–7. PMID:25541144
954. Cuevas-Ocampo AK, Bollen AW, Goode B, et al. Genetic confirmation that ependymoma can arise as part of multiple endocrine neoplasia type 1 (MEN1) syndrome. Acta Neuropathol. 2017 Apr;133(4):661–3. PMID:28238068
955. Cui Y, Li C, Jiang Z, et al. Single-cell transcriptome and genome analyses of pituitary neuroendocrine tumors. Neuro Oncol. 2021 Nov 2;23(11):1859–71. PMID:33908609
956. Cui Y, Yao J, Wang S, et al. The clinical and pathological characteristics of malignant struma ovarii: an analysis of 144 published patients. Front Oncol. 2021 Mar 5;11:645156. PMID:33763376
957. Cunningham J, Locatelli F, Rodriguez M. Secondary hyperparathyroidism: pathogenesis, disease progression, and therapeutic options. Clin J Am Soc Nephrol. 2011 Apr;6(4):913–21. PMID:21454719
958. Cuny T, Pertuit M, Sahnoun-Fathallah M, et al. Genetic analysis in young patients with sporadic pituitary macroadenomas: besides AIP don't forget MEN1 genetic analysis. Eur J Endocrinol. 2013 Mar 15;168(4):533–41. PMID:23321498
959. Cupisti K, Lehwald N, Anlauf M, et al. Encapsulation status of papillary thyroid microcarcinomas is associated with the risk of lymph node metastases and tumor multifocality. Horm Metab Res. 2014 Feb;46(2):138–44. PMID:24356791
960. Cyprich J, Donoho DA, Brunswick A, et al. Surgical management of clinically silent thyrotropin pituitary adenomas: a single center series of 20 patients. J Clin Neurosci. 2020 Jan;71:70–5. PMID:31668712
961. Czarnywojtek A, Zgorzalewicz-Stachowiak M, Czarnocka B, et al. Effect of lithium carbonate on the function of the thyroid gland: mechanism of action and clinical implications. J Physiol Pharmacol. 2020 Apr;71(2). PMID:32633237
962. da Costa VR, Bim LV, Pacheco E Silva LDP, et al. Advances in detecting low prevalence somatic TERT promoter mutations in papillary thyroid carcinoma. Front Endocrinol (Lausanne). 2021 Mar 12;12:643151. PMID:33776938
963. Dagrada GP, Spagnuolo RD, Mauro V, et al. Solitary fibrous tumors: loss of chimeric protein expression and genomic instability mark dedifferentiation. Mod Pathol. 2015 Aug;28(8):1074–83. PMID:26022454
964. Dahan H, Bèges C, Weiss L, et al. Leiomyoma of the adrenal gland in a patient with AIDS. Abdom Imaging. 1994 May-Jun;19(3):259–61. PMID:8019358
965. Dahia PL, Aguiar RC, Honegger J, et al. Mutation and expression analysis of the p27/kip1 gene in corticotrophin-secreting tumours. Oncogene. 1998 Jan 8;16(1):69–76. PMID:9467944
966. Dahia PL, Ross KN, Wright ME, et al. A HIF1alpha regulatory loop links hypoxia and mitochondrial signals in pheochromocytomas. PLoS Genet. 2005 Jul;1(1):72–80. PMID:16103922
967. Dahl LD, Myssiorek D, Heller KS. Hurthle cell neoplasms of the thyroid. Laryngoscope. 2002 Dec;112(12):2178–80. PMID:12461336
968. Dahl NA, Luebbert T, Loi M, et al. Chordoma occurs in young children with tuberous sclerosis. J Neuropathol Exp Neurol. 2017 Jun 1;76(6):418–23. PMID:28498973
969. d'Alessandro AF, Montenegro FL, Brandão LG, et al. Supernumerary parathyroid glands in hyperparathyroidism associated with multiple endocrine neoplasia type 1. Rev Assoc Med Bras (1992). 2012 May-Jun;58(3):323–7. PMID:22735224
970. Dalia S, Shao H, Sagatys E, et al. Dendritic cell and histiocytic neoplasms: biology, diagnosis, and treatment. Cancer Control. 2014 Oct;21(4):290–300. PMID:25310210
971. Daly AF, Beckers A. The epidemiology of pituitary adenomas. Endocrinol Metab Clin North Am. 2020 Sep;49(3):347–55. PMID:32741475
972. Daly AF, Beckers A. Update on the treatment of pituitary adenomas: familial and genetic considerations. Acta Clin Belg. 2008 Nov-Dec;63(6):418–24. PMID:19170361
973. Daly AF, Castermans E, Oudijk L, et al. Pheochromocytomas and pituitary adenomas in three patients with MAX exon deletions. Endocr Relat Cancer. 2018 May;25(5):L37–42. PMID:29535143
974. Daly AF, Rixhon M, Adam C, et al. High prevalence of pituitary adenomas: a cross-sectional study in the province of Liege, Belgium. J Clin Endocrinol Metab. 2006 Dec;91(12):4769–75. PMID:16968795
975. Daly AF, Tichomirowa MA, Beckers A. Update on familial pituitary tumors: from multiple endocrine neoplasia type 1 to familial isolated pituitary adenoma. Horm Res. 2009 Jan;71 Suppl 1:105–11. PMID:19153518
976. Daly AF, Tichomirowa MA, Petrossians P, et al. Clinical characteristics and therapeutic responses in patients with germ-line AIP mutations and pituitary adenomas: an international collaborative study. J Clin Endocrinol Metab. 2010 Nov;95(11):E373–83. PMID:20685857
977. Damiani L, Riccioni L, Nuzzi D, et al. Two cases of double pituitary adenomas in a surgical series over 16 years in a single centre. Endocr Metab Immune Disord Drug Targets. 2021;21(8):1518–23. PMID:33538680
978. Danau T, Verfaillie G, Gordts F, et al. Thyroglossal duct cysts in children: a 30-year survey with emphasis on clinical presentation, surgical treatment, and outcome. Acta Chir Belg. 2019 Dec;119(6):357–62. PMID:30388395
979. Dandpat SK, Rai SKR, Shah A, et al. Silent stellate ganglion paraganglioma masquerading as schwannoma: a surgical nightmare. J Craniovertebr Junction Spine. 2020 Jul-Sep;11(3):240–2. PMID:33100776
980. D'Andrea N, Romano V, Mattioli F, et al. Pulmonary artery leiomyosarcoma with thyroid metastases. Monaldi Arch Chest Dis. 2003 Oct-Dec;59(4):304–7. PMID:15148841
981. Dandurand C, Sepehry AA, Asadi Lari MH, et al. Adult craniopharyngioma: case series, systematic review, and meta-analysis. Neurosurgery. 2018 Oct 1;83(4):631–41. PMID:29267973
982. Daneshbod Y, Daneshbod K, Rasekhi AR, et al. Cytologic differentiation of struma ovarii from other ovarian neoplasms. Acta Cytol. 2008 Jan-Feb;52(1):72–6. PMID:18323278
983. D'Angelo D, Palmieri D, Mussnich P, et al. Altered microRNA expression profile in human pituitary GH adenomas: down-regulation of miRNA targeting HMGA1, HMGA2, and E2F1. J Clin Endocrinol Metab. 2012 Jul;97(7):E1128–38. PMID:22564666
984. Danish MH, Wasif M, Ud Din N, et al. Malignant peripheral nerve sheath tumour of thyroid: a diagnostic dilemma. BMJ Case Rep. 2020 Apr 22;13(4):e234374. PMID:32327463
985. Dannenberg H, van Nederveen FH, Abbou M, et al. Clinical characteristics of pheochromocytoma patients with germline mutations in SDHD. J Clin Oncol. 2005 Mar 20;23(9):1894–901. PMID:15774781
986. Danon M, Robboy SJ, Kim S, et al. Cushing syndrome, sexual precocity, and polyostotic fibrous dysplasia (Albright syndrome) in infancy. J Pediatr. 1975 Dec;87(6 Pt 1):917–21. PMID:171361
987. Dao AH, Page DL, Reynolds VH, et al. Primary malignant melanoma of the adrenal gland. A report of two cases and review of the literature. Am Surg. 1990 Apr;56(4):199–203. PMID:2194410
988. Darbà J, Marsà A. Exploring the current status of neuroendocrine tumours: a population-based analysis of epidemiology, management and use of resources. BMC Cancer. 2019 Dec 16;19(1):1226. PMID:31842791
989. Darré T, Tchaou M, Tchangaï B, et al. Primary angiosarcoma pancreas: a case report of an exceptional localization. J Gastrointest Cancer. 2019 Dec;50(4):935–8. PMID:29858730
990. Das DK, Mallik MK, Sharma P, et al. Papillary thyroid carcinoma and its variants in fine needle aspiration smears. A cytomorphologic study with special reference to tall cell variant. Acta Cytol. 2004 May-Jun;48(3):325–36. PMID:15192947
991. Das DK, Pathan SK, Francis IM, et al. Cytoplasmic colloid inclusions in thyroid lesions: a cytomorphological study based on fine needle aspiration. Cytopathology. 2005 Oct;16(5):233–9. PMID:16181309
992. Das P, Soni P, Jones J, et al. Descriptive epidemiology of chordomas in the United States. J Neurooncol. 2020 May;148(1):173–8. PMID:32342333
993. Das S, Ang LC, Ramsay D. Intrasellar cavernous hemangioma presenting as pituitary adenoma: a report of two cases and review of the literature. Clin Neuropathol. 2018 Mar/Apr;37(2):64–7. PMID:29189199
994. Dasari A, Mehta K, Byers LA, et al. Comparative study of lung and extrapulmonary poorly differentiated neuroendocrine carcinomas: a SEER database analysis of 162,983

cases. Cancer. 2018 Feb 15;124(4):807–15. PMID:29211313
995. Dasari A, Shen C, Halperin D, et al. Trends in the incidence, prevalence, and survival outcomes in patients with neuroendocrine tumors in the United States. JAMA Oncol. 2017 Oct 1;3(10):1335–42. PMID:28448665
996. Dasgupta A, Teerthanath S, Jayakumar M, et al. Primary cavernous haemangioma of the thyroid - a case report. J Clin Diagn Res. 2014 Feb;8(2):151–2. PMID:24701513
997. Daumova M, Svajdler M, Fabian P, et al. SDHC methylation pattern in patients with Carney triad. Appl Immunohistochem Mol Morphol. 2021 Sep 1;29(8):599–605. PMID:33624983
998. D'Avanzo A, Treseler P, Ituarte PH, et al. Follicular thyroid carcinoma: histology and prognosis. Cancer. 2004 Mar 15;100(6):1123–9. PMID:15022277
999. Dave B, Shet T, Ramadwar M, et al. Cytological evaluation of head and neck tumors in children–a pattern analysis. Diagn Cytopathol. 2006 Jun;34(6):434–46. PMID:16680771
1000. Davenport C, Agha A. The role of menin in parathyroid tumorigenesis. Adv Exp Med Biol. 2009;668:79–86. PMID:20175455
1001. Davenport E, Lennard T. Acute hypercortisolism: what can the surgeon offer? Clin Endocrinol (Oxf). 2014 Oct;81(4):498–502. PMID:24802156
1002. Davies L, Hoang JK. Thyroid cancer in the USA: current trends and outstanding questions. Lancet Diabetes Endocrinol. 2021 Jan;9(1):11–2. PMID:33220765
1003. Davies MP, John Evans TW, Tahir F, et al. Parathyroid cancer: a systematic review of diagnostic biomarkers. Surgeon. 2021 Dec;19(6):e536–48. PMID:33642204
1004. Davies-Husband CR, Montgomery P, Premachandra D, et al. Primary, combined, atypical carcinoid and squamous cell carcinoma of the larynx: a new variety of composite tumour. J Laryngol Otol. 2010 Feb;124(2):226–9. PMID:19930775
1005. Davila JI, Starr JS, Attia S, et al. Comprehensive genomic profiling of a rare thyroid follicular dendritic cell sarcoma. Rare Tumors. 2017 Sep 15;9(2):6834. PMID:28975018
1006. Davis DA, Medline NM. Spironolactone (aldactone) bodies: concentric lamellar formations in the adrenal cortices of patients treated with spironolactone. Am J Clin Pathol. 1970 Jul;54(1):22–32. PMID:5504616
1007. Davis RJ, D'Cruz CM, Lovell MA, et al. Fusion of PAX7 to FKHR by the variant t(1;13)(p36;q14) translocation in alveolar rhabdomyosarcoma. Cancer Res. 1994 Jun 1;54(11):2869–72. PMID:8187070
1008. Dawood NB, Yan KL, Shieh A, et al. Normocalcaemic primary hyperparathyroidism: an update on diagnostic and management challenges. Clin Endocrinol (Oxf). 2020 Nov;93(5):519–27. PMID:32803770
1009. Dayan CM, Daniels GH. Chronic autoimmune thyroiditis. N Engl J Med. 1996 Jul 11;335(2):99–107. PMID:8649497
1010. de Almeida Verdolin A, Lamback EB, Ventura N, et al. Collision sellar lesions: coexistence of pituitary adenoma and Rathke cleft cyst-a single-center experience. Endocrine. 2020 Apr;68(1):174–81. PMID:31802354
1011. De Bernardi B, Gambini C, Haupt R, et al. Retrospective study of childhood ganglioneuroma. J Clin Oncol. 2008 Apr 1;26(10):1710–6. PMID:18375900
1012. de Biase D, Ragazzi M, Asioli S, et al. Extracutaneous Merkel cell carcinomas harbor polyomavirus DNA. Hum Pathol. 2012 Jul;43(7):980–5. PMID:22204708
1013. de Biase D, Torricelli F, Ragazzi M, et al. Not the same thing: metastatic PTCs have a different background than ATCs. Endocr Connect. 2018 Dec;7(12):1370–9. PMID:30400028
1014. de Chadarévian JP, MaePascasio J, Halligan GE, et al. Malignant peripheral nerve sheath tumor arising from an adrenal ganglioneuroma in a 6-year-old boy. Pediatr Dev Pathol. 2004 May-Jun;7(3):277–84. PMID:15022069
1015. De Crea C, Raffaelli M, Sessa L, et al. Actual incidence and clinical behaviour of follicular thyroid carcinoma: an institutional experience. ScientificWorldJournal. 2014 Mar 4;2014:952095. PMID:24741369
1016. De Felice F, Moscatelli E, Orelli S, et al. Primary thyroid angiosarcoma: a systematic review. Oral Oncol. 2018 Jul;82:48–52. PMID:29909901
1017. de Fraipont F, El Atifi M, Cherradi N, et al. Gene expression profiling of human adrenocortical tumors using complementary deoxyribonucleic Acid microarrays identifies several candidate genes as markers of malignancy. J Clin Endocrinol Metab. 2005 Mar;90(3):1819–29. PMID:15613424
1018. de Herder WW, Kwekkeboom DJ, Valkema R, et al. Neuroendocrine tumors and somatostatin: imaging techniques. J Endocrinol Invest. 2005;28(11 Suppl International):132–6. PMID:16625862
1019. de Herder WW, Niederle B, Scoazec JY, et al. Well-differentiated pancreatic tumor/carcinoma: insulinoma. Neuroendocrinology. 2006;84(3):183–8. PMID:17312378
1020. de Kock L, Sabbaghian N, Plourde F, et al. Pituitary blastoma: a pathognomonic feature of germ-line DICER1 mutations. Acta Neuropathol. 2014 Jul;128(1):111–22. PMID:24839956
1021. de Kock L, Sabbaghian N, Soglio DB, et al. Exploring the association between DICER1 mutations and differentiated thyroid carcinoma. J Clin Endocrinol Metab. 2014 Jun;99(6):E1072–7. PMID:24617712
1022. de Kock L, Terzic T, McCluggage WG, et al. DICER1 mutations are consistently present in moderately and poorly differentiated Sertoli-Leydig cell tumors. Am J Surg Pathol. 2017 Sep;41(9):1178–87. PMID:28654427
1023. de Laat JM, Dekkers OM, Pieterman CR, et al. Long-term natural course of pituitary tumors in patients with MEN1: results from the DutchMEN1 Study Group (DMSG). J Clin Endocrinol Metab. 2015 Sep;100(9):3288–96. PMID:26126205
1024. de Laat JM, Pieterman CR, van den Broek MF, et al. Natural course and survival of neuroendocrine tumors of thymus and lung in MEN1 patients. J Clin Endocrinol Metab. 2014 Sep;99(9):3325–33. PMID:24915123
1025. de Laat JM, van der Luijt RB, Pieterman CR, et al. MEN1 redefined, a clinical comparison of mutation-positive and mutation-negative patients. BMC Med. 2016 Nov 15;14(1):182. PMID:27842554
1026. De Las Casas LE, Williams HJ, Strausbauch PH, et al. Hurthle cell adenoma of the mediastinum: intraoperative cytology and differential diagnosis with correlative gross, histology, and ancillary studies. Diagn Cytopathol. 2000 Jan;22(1):16–20. PMID:10613966
1027. De Los Santos-Aguilar RG, Chávez-Villa M, Contreras AG, et al. Successful multimodal treatment of an IGF2-producing solitary fibrous tumor with acromegaloid changes and hypoglycemia. J Endocr Soc. 2019 Jan 8;3(3):537–43. PMID:30788455
1028. de Matos LL, Del Giglio AB, Matsubayashi CO, et al. Expression of CK-19, galectin-3 and HBME-1 in the differentiation of thyroid lesions: systematic review and diagnostic meta-analysis. Diagn Pathol. 2012 Aug 13;7:97. PMID:22888980
1029. de Mestier L, Hentic O, Cros J, et al. Metachronous hormonal syndromes in patients with pancreatic neuroendocrine tumors: a case-series study. Ann Intern Med. 2015 May 19;162(10):682–9. PMID:25984844
1030. de Miguel V, Paissan A, García Marchiñena P, et al. Bilateral pheochromocytoma after kidney transplantation in neurofibromatosis type 1. Endocrinol Diabetes Metab Case Rep. 2019 May 23;2019:18-0162. PMID:31125973
1031. de Montpréville VT, Mussot S, Gharbi N, et al. Paraganglioma with ganglioneuromatous component located in the posterior mediastinum. Ann Diagn Pathol. 2005 Apr;9(2):110–4. PMID:15806520
1032. de Morais Fernandes FCG, de Souza DLB, Curado MP, et al. Incidence and mortality from thyroid cancer in Latin America. Trop Med Int Health. 2021 Jul;26(7):800–9. PMID:33837603
1033. de Pontual L, Kettaneh D, Gordon CT, et al. Germline gain-of-function mutations of ALK disrupt central nervous system development. Hum Mutat. 2011 Mar;32(3):272–6. PMID:21972109
1034. De Raedt T, Beert E, Pasmant E, et al. PRC2 loss amplifies Ras-driven transcription and confers sensitivity to BRD4-based therapies. Nature. 2014 Oct 9;514(7521):247–51. PMID:25119042
1035. de Reyniès A, Assié G, Rickman DS, et al. Gene expression profiling reveals a new classification of adrenocortical tumors and identifies molecular predictors of malignancy and survival. J Clin Oncol. 2009 Mar 1;27(7):1108–15. PMID:19139432
1036. de Ridder M, Nieveen van Dijkum E, Engelsman A, et al. Anaplastic thyroid carcinoma: a nationwide cohort study on incidence, treatment and survival in the Netherlands over 3 decades. Eur J Endocrinol. 2020 Aug;183(2):203–9. PMID:32460234
1037. de Silva AC, Rodriguez FJ, Aldecoa I, et al. Compound gonadotrophic pituitary adenoma and rhabdomyosarcoma. Histopathology. 2016 Jun;68(7):1111–4. PMID:26462864
1038. De Sousa SMC, McCabe MJ, Wu K, et al. Germline variants in familial pituitary tumour syndrome genes are common in young patients and families with additional endocrine tumours. Eur J Endocrinol. 2017 May;176(5):635–44. PMID:28220018
1039. De Sousa SMC, Toubia J, Hardy TSE, et al. Aberrant splicing of SDHC in families with unexplained succinate dehydrogenase-deficient paragangliomas. J Endocr Soc. 2020 Jun 16;4(12):bvaa071. PMID:33195952
1040. de Tersant M, Généré L, Freyçon C, et al. Pheochromocytoma and paraganglioma in children and adolescents: experience of the French Society of Pediatric Oncology (SFCE). J Endocr Soc. 2020 Apr 3;4(5):bvaa039. PMID:32432211
1041. de Waal YR, Thomas CM, Oei AL, et al. Secondary ovarian malignancies: frequency, origin, and characteristics. Int J Gynecol Cancer. 2009 Oct;19(7):1160–5. PMID:19823050
1042. Dean PG, van Heerden JA, Farley DR, et al. Are patients with multiple endocrine neoplasia type I prone to premature death? World J Surg. 2000 Nov;24(11):1437–41. PMID:11038219
1043. Deb P, Pal S, Dutta V, et al. Adrenal haemangioblastoma presenting as phaeochromocytoma: a rare manifestation of extraneural hemangioblastoma. Endocr Pathol. 2012 Sep;23(3):187–90. PMID:22544391
1044. DeBella K, Szudek J, Friedman JM. Use of the national institutes of health criteria for diagnosis of neurofibromatosis 1 in children. Pediatrics. 2000 Mar;105(3 Pt 1):608–14. PMID:10699117
1045. Debol SM, Stanley MW, Mallery S, et al. Glomus tumor of the stomach: cytologic diagnosis by endoscopic ultrasound-guided fine-needle aspiration. Diagn Cytopathol. 2003 Jun;28(6):316–21. PMID:12768637
1046. DeCaprio JA. Merkel cell polyomavirus and Merkel cell carcinoma. Philos Trans R Soc Lond B Biol Sci. 2017 Oct 19;372(1732):372. PMID:28893943
1047. Decarolis B, Simon T, Krug B, et al. Treatment and outcome of ganglioneuroma and ganglioneuroblastoma intermixed. BMC Cancer. 2016 Jul 27;16:542. PMID:27465021
1048. de Castro LF, Ovejero D, Boyce AM. Diagnosis of endocrine disease: Mosaic disorders of FGF23 excess: fibrous dysplasia/McCune-Albright syndrome and cutaneous skeletal hypophosphatemia syndrome. Eur J Endocrinol. 2020 May;182(5):R83–99. PMID:32069220
1049. Decaussin-Petrucci M. [Hereditary predispositions to follicular thyroid tumors]. Ann Pathol. 2020 Apr;40(2):142–7. French. PMID:32192806
1050. Decmann Á, Perge P, Tóth M, et al. Adrenal myelolipoma: a comprehensive review. Endocrine. 2018 Jan;59(1):7–15. PMID:29164520
1051. Deeken-Draisey A, Yang GY, Gao J, et al. Anaplastic thyroid carcinoma: an epidemiologic, histologic, immunohistochemical, and molecular single-institution study. Hum Pathol. 2018 Dec;82:140–8. PMID:30075157
1052. Deep NL, Ekbom DC, Hinni ML, et al. High-grade neuroendocrine carcinoma of the larynx: the Mayo Clinic experience. Ann Otol Rhinol Laryngol. 2016 Jun;125(6):464–9. PMID:26611246
1053. De Felice M, Di Lauro R. Thyroid development and its disorders: genetics and molecular mechanisms. Endocr Rev. 2004 Oct;25(5):722–46. PMID:15466939
1054. de Herder WW, Hofland J. CCKoma. In: Feingold KR, Anawalt B, Blackman MR, et al., editors. Endotext. South Dartmouth (MA): MDText.com, Inc.; 2000 [updated 2021 Jan 23]. PMID:25905295
1055. De Herder WW, Lamberts SW. Octapeptide somatostatin-analogue therapy of Cushing's syndrome. Postgrad Med J. 1999 Feb;75(880):65–6. PMID:10448463
1056. Dehner LP, Chen KT. Primary tumors of the external and middle ear. III. A clinicopathologic study of embryonal rhabdomyosarcoma. Arch Otolaryngol. 1978 Jul;104(7):399–403. PMID:666648
1057. Dehner LP, Hill DA. Adrenal cortical neoplasms in children: why so many carcinomas and yet so many survivors? Pediatr Dev Pathol. 2009 Jul-Aug;12(4):284–91. PMID:19326954
1058. Dei Tos AP, Seregard S, Calonje E, et al. Giant cell angiofibroma. A distinctive orbital tumor in adults. Am J Surg Pathol. 1995 Nov;19(11):1286–93. PMID:7573691
1059. de Kock L, Rivera B, Foulkes WD. Pineoblastoma is uniquely tolerant of mutually exclusive loss of DICER1, DROSHA or DGCR8. Acta Neuropathol. 2020 Jun;139(6):1115–8. PMID:32124011
1060. de Kock L, Wu MK, Foulkes WD. Ten years of DICER1 mutations: provenance, distribution, and associated phenotypes. Hum Mutat. 2019 Nov;40(11):1939–53. PMID:31342592
1061. de Krijger RE, Bertherat J. 5th International ACC Symposium: Classification of adrenocortical cancers from pathology to integrated genomics: real advances or lost in translation? Horm Cancer. 2016 Feb;7(1):3–8. PMID:26676358
1062. de Krijger RR, Papathomas TG. Adrenocortical neoplasia: evolving concepts in tumorigenesis with an emphasis on adrenal cortical carcinoma variants. Virchows Arch. 2012

Jan;460(1):9–18. PMID:22086150
1063. del Pozo C, García-Pascual L, Balsells M, et al. Parathyroid carcinoma in multiple endocrine neoplasia type 1. Case report and review of the literature. Hormones (Athens). 2011 Oct-Dec;10(4):326–31. PMID:22281890
1064. Delcore R Jr, Cheung LY, Friesen SR. Outcome of lymph node involvement in patients with the Zollinger-Ellison syndrome. Ann Surg. 1988 Sep;208(3):291–8. PMID:3421754
1065. DeLellis RA. Parathyroid tumors and related disorders. Mod Pathol. 2011 Apr;24 Suppl 2:S78–93. PMID:21455204
1066. DeLellis RA, May L, Tashjian AH Jr, et al. C-cell granule heterogeneity in man. An ultrastructural immunocytochemical study. Lab Invest. 1978 Mar;38(3):263–9. PMID:633851
1067. DeLellis RA, Nunnemacher G, Wolfe HJ. C-cell hyperplasia. An ultrastructural analysis. Lab Invest. 1977 Mar;36(3):237–48. PMID:839736
1068. DeLellis RA, Wolfe HJ, Gagel RF, et al. Adrenal medullary hyperplasia. A morphometric analysis in patients with familial medullary thyroid carcinoma. Am J Pathol. 1976 Apr;83(1):177–96. PMID:1275056
1069. De Leo S, Trevisan M, Fugazzola L. Recent advances in the management of anaplastic thyroid cancer. Thyroid Res. 2020 Nov 24;13(1):17. PMID:33292371
1070. Delgado J, Jaramillo D, Ho-Fung V, et al. MRI features of plexiform neurofibromas involving the liver and pancreas in children with neurofibromatosis type 1. Clin Radiol. 2014 Jun;69(6):e280–4. PMID:24594377
1071. Delgado S, Smith SM, Mehra S, et al. Composite paraganglioma: pioneering in the head and neck. Int J Surg Pathol. 2019 May;27(3):282–9. PMID:30222023
1072. Delgrange E, Trouillas J, Maiter D, et al. Sex-related difference in the growth of prolactinomas: a clinical and proliferation marker study. J Clin Endocrinol Metab. 1997 Jul;82(7):2102–7. PMID:9215279
1073. Delgrange E, Vasiljevic A, Wierinckx A, et al. Expression of estrogen receptor alpha is associated with prolactin pituitary tumor prognosis and supports the sex-related difference in tumor growth. Eur J Endocrinol. 2015 Jun;172(6):791–801. PMID:25792376
1074. Deligeorgi-Politi H. Nuclear crease as a cytodiagnostic feature of papillary thyroid carcinoma in fine-needle aspiration biopsies. Diagn Cytopathol. 1987 Dec;3(4):307–10. PMID:3428064
1075. Dell'Aquila M, Gravina C, Cocomazzi A, et al. A large series of hyalinizing trabecular tumors: cytomorphology and ancillary techniques on fine needle aspiration. Cancer Cytopathol. 2019 Jun;127(6):390–8. PMID:31135104
1076. Dellatolas G, Annesi I, Jallon P, et al. An epidemiological reconsideration of the Geschwind-Galaburda theory of cerebral lateralization. Arch Neurol. 1990 Jul;47(7):778–82. PMID:2357158
1077. Delle Fave G, O'Toole D, Sundin A, et al. ENETS consensus guidelines update for gastroduodenal neuroendocrine neoplasms. Neuroendocrinology. 2016;103(2):119–24. PMID:26784901
1078. Delprat C, Aricò M. Blood spotlight on Langerhans cell histiocytosis. Blood. 2014 Aug 7;124(6):867–72. PMID:24894775
1079. Demicco EG, Griffin AM, Gladdy RA, et al. Comparison of published risk models for prediction of outcome in patients with extrameningeal solitary fibrous tumour. Histopathology. 2019 Nov;75(5):723–37. PMID:31206727
1080. Demicco EG, Harms PW, Patel RM, et al. Extensive survey of STAT6 expression in a large series of mesenchymal tumors. Am J Clin Pathol. 2015 May;143(5):672–82. PMID:25873501
1081. Demicco EG, Park MS, Araujo DM, et al. Solitary fibrous tumor: a clinicopathological study of 110 cases and proposed risk assessment model. Mod Pathol. 2012 Sep;25(9):1298–306. PMID:22575866
1082. Demicco EG, Wagner MJ, Maki RG, et al. Risk assessment in solitary fibrous tumors: validation and refinement of a risk stratification model. Mod Pathol. 2017 Oct;30(10):1433–42. PMID:28731041
1083. Demicco EG, Wani K, Ingram D, et al. TERT promoter mutations in solitary fibrous tumour. Histopathology. 2018 Nov;73(5):843–51. PMID:29985536
1084. Demir OM, Paschou SA, Ellis HC, et al. Reversal of dilated cardiomyopathy after glucagonoma excision. Hormones (Athens). 2015 Jan-Mar;14(1):172–3. PMID:25553769
1085. Demirçivi Ozer F, Aydin M, Bezircioğlu H, et al. Paraganglioma of the cauda equina: a highly vascular tumour. J Clin Neurosci. 2010 Nov;17(11):1445–7. PMID:20637630
1086. Dénes J, Kasuki L, Trivellin G, et al. Regulation of aryl hydrocarbon receptor interacting protein (AIP) protein expression by MiR-34a in sporadic somatotropinomas. PLoS One. 2015 Feb 6;10(2):e0117107. PMID:25658813
1087. Dénes J, Korbonits M. The clinical aspects of pituitary tumour genetics. Endocrine. 2021 Mar;71(3):663–74. PMID:33543431
1088. Dénes J, Swords F, Rattenberry E, et al. Heterogeneous genetic background of the association of pheochromocytoma/paraganglioma and pituitary adenoma: results from a large patient cohort. J Clin Endocrinol Metab. 2015 Mar;100(3):E531–41. PMID:25494863
1089. Denzinger S, Burger M, Hartmann A, et al. Spontaneous rupture of a benign giant adrenal adenoma. APMIS. 2007 Apr;115(4):381–4. PMID:17504308
1090. Derks JL, Dingemans AC, van Suylen RJ, et al. Is the sum of positive neuroendocrine immunohistochemical stains useful for diagnosis of large cell neuroendocrine carcinoma (LCNEC) on biopsy specimens? Histopathology. 2019 Mar;74(4):555–66. PMID:30485478
1091. Derks JL, Leblay N, Thunnissen E, et al. Molecular subtypes of pulmonary large-cell neuroendocrine carcinoma predict chemotherapy treatment outcome. Clin Cancer Res. 2018 Jan 1;24(1):33–42. PMID:29066508
1092. Dermawan JK, Mukhopadhyay S, Shah AA. Frequency and extent of cytokeratin expression in paraganglioma: an immunohistochemical study of 60 cases from 5 anatomic sites and review of the literature. Hum Pathol. 2019 Nov;93:16–22. PMID:31442521
1093. Derringer GA, Thompson LD, Frommelt RA, et al. Malignant lymphoma of the thyroid gland: a clinicopathologic study of 108 cases. Am J Surg Pathol. 2000 May;24(5):623–39. PMID:10800981
1094. Derwahl M, Studer H. Hyperplasia versus adenoma in endocrine tissues: are they different? Trends Endocrinol Metab. 2002 Jan-Feb;13(1):23–8. PMID:11750859
1095. Derwahl M, Studer H. Multinodular goitre: 'much more to it than simply iodine deficiency'. Baillieres Best Pract Res Clin Endocrinol Metab. 2000 Dec;14(4):577–600. PMID:11289736
1096. Derwahl M, Studer H. Nodular goiter and goiter nodules: where iodine deficiency falls short of explaining the facts. Exp Clin Endocrinol Diabetes. 2001;109(5):250–60. PMID:11507648
1097. Desai MA, Mehrad M, Ely KA, et al. Secretory carcinoma of the thyroid gland: report of a highly aggressive case clinically mimicking undifferentiated carcinoma and review of the literature. Head Neck Pathol. 2019 Dec;13(4):562–72. PMID:30564997
1098. Desai SS, Sarkar S, Borges AM. A study of histopathological features of medullary carcinoma of the thyroid: cases from a single institute in India. Indian J Cancer. 2005 Jan-Mar;42(1):25–9. PMID:15805688
1099. Deschamps L, Dokmak S, Guedj N, et al. Mixed endocrine somatostatinoma of the ampulla of vater associated with a neurofibromatosis type 1: a case report and review of the literature. JOP. 2010 Jan 8;11(1):64–8. PMID:20065557
1100. Deshmukh SD, Khandeparkar SG, Gulati HK, et al. Microfollicular adenoma of ectopic thyroid gland masquerading as salivary gland tumor - a diagnostic and therapeutic challenge: a case report. J Med Case Rep. 2014 Aug 7;8:270. PMID:25103611
1101. Deshpande AH, Bobhate SK. Cytological features of dyshormonogenetic goiter: case report and review of the literature. Diagn Cytopathol. 2005 Oct;33(4):252–4. PMID:16138369
1102. Deshpande V, Fernandez-del Castillo C, Muzikansky A, et al. Cytokeratin 19 is a powerful predictor of survival in pancreatic endocrine tumors. Am J Surg Pathol. 2004 Sep;28(9):1145–53. PMID:15316313
1103. Deshpande V, Zen Y, Chan JK, et al. Consensus statement on the pathology of IgG4-related disease. Mod Pathol. 2012 Sep;25(9):1181–92. PMID:22596100
1104. Dettloff J, Seethala RR, Stevens TM, et al. Mammary analog secretory carcinoma (MASC) involving the thyroid gland: a report of the first 3 cases. Head Neck Pathol. 2017 Jun;11(2):124–30. PMID:27400918
1105. Dettmer M, Schmitt A, Steinert H, et al. Poorly differentiated oncocytic thyroid carcinoma–diagnostic implications and outcome. Histopathology. 2012 Jun;60(7):1045–51. PMID:22348590
1106. Devaney K, Snyder R, Norris HJ, et al. Proliferative and histologically malignant struma ovarii: a clinicopathologic study of 54 cases. Int J Gynecol Pathol. 1993 Oct;12(4):333–43. PMID:8253550
1107. Deveci MS, Deveci G, LiVolsi VA, et al. Concordance between thyroid nodule sizes measured by ultrasound and gross pathology examination: effect on patient management. Diagn Cytopathol. 2007 Sep;35(9):579–83. PMID:17703450
1108. Dhanasekar K, Visakan V, Tahir F, et al. Composite phaeochromocytomas-a systematic review of published literature. Langenbecks Arch Surg. 2022 Mar;407(2):517–27. PMID:33651160
1109. Dhingra R, Tse JY, Saif MW. Cutaneous metastasis of gastroenteropancreatic neuroendocrine tumors (GEP-Nets). JOP. 2018 Sep;19(5):http://pancreas.imedpub.com/cutaneous-metastasis-of-gastroenteropancreatic-neuroendocrine-tumors-gepnets.pdf. PMID:30405324
1110. Di Dalmazi G, Altieri B, Scholz C, et al. RNA sequencing and somatic mutation status of adrenocortical tumors: novel pathogenetic insights. J Clin Endocrinol Metab. 2020 Dec 1;105(12):dgaa616. PMID:32875319
1111. Di Dalmazi G, Kisker C, Calebiro D, et al. Novel somatic mutations in the catalytic subunit of the protein kinase A as a cause of adrenal Cushing's syndrome: a European multicentric study. J Clin Endocrinol Metab. 2014 Oct;99(10):E2093–100. PMID:25057884
1112. Di Ieva A, Davidson JM, Syro LV, et al. Crooke's cell tumors of the pituitary. Neurosurgery. 2015 May;76(5):616–22. PMID:25635886
1113. Di Martino M, García Sanz I, Mora-Guzmán I, et al. Surgery in late melanoma adrenal metastasis. BMJ Case Rep. 2017 May 22;2017:bcr2016218681. PMID:28536111
1114. Diamond EL, Durham BH, Haroche J, et al. Diverse and targetable kinase alterations drive histiocytic neoplasms. Cancer Discov. 2016 Feb;6(2):154–65. PMID:26566875
1115. Dias T, Santos A, Mesquita C, et al. Acute airway obstruction due to benign multinodular goitre. BMJ Case Rep. 2019 Apr 16;12(4):e228095. PMID:30996065
1116. Dibelius G, Mehra S, Clain JB, et al. Noninvasive anaplastic thyroid carcinoma: report of a case and literature review. Thyroid. 2014 Aug;24(8):1319–24. PMID:24865498
1117. Dick JC, Ritchie GM, Thompson H. Histological differentiation between phaeochromocytoma and melanoma of the suprarenal gland. J Clin Pathol. 1955 May;8(2):89–98. PMID:14367536
1118. Dikbas O, Duman AA, Guvendi GF. Medullary thyroid carcinoma and papillary thyroid carcinoma in the same patient as a collision tumour. Case Rep Endocrinol. 2019 Mar 12;2019:4038628. PMID:30993022
1119. Dinesh U, Pervatikar SK, Rao R. FNAC diagnosis of pancreatic somatostatinoma. J Cytol. 2009 Oct;26(4):153–5. PMID:21938182
1120. Dinter H, Bohnenberger H, Beck J, et al. Molecular classification of neuroendocrine tumors of the thymus. J Thorac Oncol. 2019 Aug;14(8):1472–83. PMID:31042566
1121. Diskin SJ, Hou C, Glessner JT, et al. Copy number variation at 1q21.1 associated with neuroblastoma. Nature. 2009 Jun 18;459(7249):987–91. PMID:19536264
1122. Djerouni M, Dumont SN. [Wild-type gastrointestinal stromal tumors]. Bull Cancer. 2020 Apr;107(4):499–505. French. PMID:32063345
1123. Doerfler WR, Nikitski AV, Morariu EM, et al. Molecular alterations in Hürthle cell nodules and preoperative cancer risk. Endocr Relat Cancer. 2021 Apr 27;28(5):301–9. PMID:33792557
1124. Dogan S, Vasudevaraja V, Xu B, et al. DNA methylation-based classification of sinonasal undifferentiated carcinoma. Mod Pathol. 2019 Oct;32(10):1447–59. PMID:31186531
1125. Dogan S, Wang L, Ptashkin RN, et al. Mammary analog secretory carcinoma of the thyroid gland: a primary thyroid adenocarcinoma harboring ETV6-NTRK3 fusion. Mod Pathol. 2016 Sep;29(9):985–95. PMID:27282352
1126. Doğanşen SÇ, Bilgiç B, Yalin GY, et al. Clinical significance of granulation pattern in corticotroph pituitary adenomas. Turk Patoloji Derg. 2019;35(1):9–14. PMID:30035294
1127. Dogansen SC, Yalin GY, Tanrikulu S, et al. Clinicopathological significance of baseline T2-weighted signal intensity in functional pituitary adenomas. Pituitary. 2018 Aug;21(4):347–54. PMID:29460202
1128. Doghri R, Znaidi N, Blel A, et al. Thyroid oncocytic neoplasms. Tunis Med. 2018 Mar;96(3):219–23. PMID:30325491
1129. Dogru S, Wilkinson EP, Robinson RA, et al. Middle ear adenoma with neuroendocrine differentiation (MEA-ND) in the pediatric population. Int J Pediatr Otorhinolaryngol. 2009 Jun;73(6):895–8. PMID:19303146
1130. Doherty GM, Lairmore TC, DeBenedetti MK. Multiple endocrine neoplasia type 1 parathyroid adenoma development over time. World J Surg. 2004 Nov;28(11):1139–42. PMID:15490065
1131. Doi M, Imai T, Shichiri M, et al. Octreotide-sensitive ectopic ACTH production by islet cell carcinoma with multiple liver metastases. Endocr J. 2003 Apr;50(2):135–43. PMID:12803233
1132. Domènech M, Grau E, Solanes A, et al. Characteristics of adrenocortical carcinoma associated with Lynch syndrome. J Clin Endocrinol Metab. 2021 Jan 23;106(2):318–25. PMID:33185660

1133. Domingue ME, Marbaix E, Do Rego JL, et al. Infrasellar pituitary gangliocytoma causing Cushing's syndrome. Pituitary. 2015 Oct;18(5):738–44. PMID:25183169
1134. Dominguez-Malagon H, Delgado-Chavez R, Torres-Najera M, et al. Oxyphil and squamous variants of medullary thyroid carcinoma. Cancer. 1989 Mar 15;63(6):1183–8. PMID:2917321
1135. Dominguez-Malagon H, Guerrero-Medrano J, Suster S. Ectopic poorly differentiated (insular) carcinoma of the thyroid. Report of a case presenting as an anterior mediastinal mass. Am J Clin Pathol. 1995 Oct;104(4):408–12. PMID:7572790
1136. Dominguez-Malagon H, Macias-Martinez V, Molina-Cardenas H, et al. Amphicrine medullary carcinoma of the thyroid with luminal differentiation: report of an immunohistochemical and ultrastructural study. Ultrastruct Pathol. 1997 Nov-Dec;21(6):569–74. PMID:9355239
1137. Donangelo I, Araújo PB, Antenuzi D, et al. Tumor deletion mapping of chromosomal region 13q14 in 43 growth hormone secreting pituitary adenomas. Endocrine. 2005 Nov;28(2):131–6. PMID:16388084
1138. Dong W, Zhang P, Li J, et al. Outcome of thyroid carcinoma showing thymus-like differentiation in patients undergoing radical resection. World J Surg. 2018 Jun;42(6):1754–61. PMID:29134304
1139. Donow C, Pipeleers-Marichal M, Schröder S, et al. Surgical pathology of gastrinoma. Site, size, multicentricity, association with multiple endocrine neoplasia type 1, and malignancy. Cancer. 1991 Sep 15;68(6):1329–34. PMID:1678681
1140. Doppman JL, Nieman LK, Travis WD, et al. CT and MR imaging of massive macronodular adrenocortical disease: a rare cause of autonomous primary adrenal hypercortisolism. J Comput Assist Tomogr. 1991 Sep-Oct;15(5):773–9. PMID:1653280
1141. D'Orazio JA. Inherited cancer syndromes in children and young adults. J Pediatr Hematol Oncol. 2010 Apr;32(3):195–228. PMID:20186103
1142. Dorfman DM, Shahsafaei A, Miyauchi A. Immunohistochemical staining for bcl-2 and mcl-1 in intrathyroidal epithelial thymoma (ITET)/carcinoma showing thymus-like differentiation (CASTLE) and cervical thymic carcinoma. Mod Pathol. 1998 Oct;11(10):989–94. PMID:9796728
1143. Dorfman DM, Shahsafaei A, Miyauchi A. Intrathyroidal epithelial thymoma (ITET)/carcinoma showing thymus-like differentiation (CASTLE) exhibits CD5 immunoreactivity: new evidence for thymic differentiation. Histopathology. 1998 Feb;32(2):104–9. PMID:9543665
1144. Doria MI Jr, Attal H, Wang HH, et al. Fine needle aspiration cytology of the oxyphil variant of papillary carcinoma of the thyroid. A report of three cases. Acta Cytol. 1996 Sep-Oct;40(5):1007–11. PMID:8842184
1145. Doshi SV, Cruz RM, Hilsinger RL Jr. Thyroglossal duct carcinoma: a large case series. Ann Otol Rhinol Laryngol. 2001 Aug;110(8):734–8. PMID:11510730
1146. Dotto J, Nosé V. Familial thyroid carcinoma: a diagnostic algorithm. Adv Anat Pathol. 2008 Nov;15(6):332–49. PMID:18948764
1147. Dotto RS, Marx G, Bastos M, et al. A rare case of virilizing adult ectopic adrenal tumor. Urol Case Rep. 2019 Aug 6;27:100907. PMID:31467854
1148. Doulias T, Papaziogas B, Rosser JH, et al. Thyroid neurofibroma in a female patient with neurofibromatosis type I: report of a case. BMJ Case Rep. 2013 Jun 5;2013:bcr2012008216. PMID:23744851
1149. Doyle LA, Fletcher CD. Peripheral hemangioblastoma: clinicopathologic characterization in a series of 22 cases. Am J Surg Pathol. 2014 Jan;38(1):119–27. PMID:24145646
1150. Doyle LA, Hornick JL, Fletcher CD. PEComa of the gastrointestinal tract: clinicopathologic study of 35 cases with evaluation of prognostic parameters. Am J Surg Pathol. 2013 Dec;37(12):1769–82. PMID:24061520
1151. Doyle LA, Vivero M, Fletcher CD, et al. Nuclear expression of STAT6 distinguishes solitary fibrous tumor from histologic mimics. Mod Pathol. 2014 Mar;27(3):390–5. PMID:24030747
1152. Dreijerink KM, Derks JL, Cataldo I, et al. Genetics and epigenetics of pancreatic neuroendocrine tumors and pulmonary carcinoids. Front Horm Res. 2015;44:115–38. PMID:26303708
1153. Dreijerink KM, Goudet P, Burgess JR, et al. Breast-cancer predisposition in multiple endocrine neoplasia type 1. N Engl J Med. 2014 Aug 7;371(6):583–4. PMID:25099597
1154. Dreijerink KMA, Rijken JA, Compaijen CJ, et al. Biochemically silent sympathetic paraganglioma, pheochromocytoma, or metastatic disease in SDHD mutation carriers. J Clin Endocrinol Metab. 2019 Nov 1;104(11):5421–6. PMID:31194241
1155. Drouet C, Morel O, Boulahdour H. Bilateral huge incidentalomas of isolated adrenal metastases from unknown primary melanoma revealed by 18F-FDG PET/CT. Clin Nucl Med. 2017 Jan;42(1):e51–3. PMID:27775937
1156. Drucker DJ, Asa SL, Henderson J, et al. The parathyroid hormone-like peptide gene is expressed in the normal and neoplastic human endocrine pancreas. Mol Endocrinol. 1989 Oct;3(10):1589–95. PMID:2691879
1157. Drummond J, Roncaroli F, Grossman AB, et al. Clinical and pathological aspects of silent pituitary adenomas. J Clin Endocrinol Metab. 2019 Jul 1;104(7):2473–89. PMID:30020466
1158. Drut R, Quijano G, Altamirano ME, et al. Vascular malformation and choroid plexus adrenal heterotopia: new findings in Beckwith-Wiedemann syndrome? Fetal Pediatr Pathol. 2006 Jul-Aug;25(4):191–7. PMID:17162526
1159. Du J, Ji H, Jin J, et al. Pituitary adenoma secondary to primary hypothyroidism: two case reports. Medicine (Baltimore). 2020 Feb;99(8):e19222. PMID:32080117
1160. Du L, Wang Y, Sun X, et al. Thyroid cancer: trends in incidence, mortality and clinical-pathological patterns in Zhejiang Province, Southeast China. BMC Cancer. 2018 Mar 15;18(1):291. PMID:29544469
1161. Du Z, Santagata S. Uncovering the links between systemic hormones and oncogenic signaling in the pathogenesis of meningioma. Ann Oncol. 2018 Mar 1;29(3):537–40. PMID:29346520
1162. Duan F, Smith LM, Gustafson DM, et al. Genomic and clinical analysis of fusion gene amplification in rhabdomyosarcoma: a report from the Children's Oncology Group. Genes Chromosomes Cancer. 2012 Jul;51(7):662–74. PMID:22447499
1163. Duan H, Li Y, Hu P, et al. Mutational profiling of poorly differentiated and anaplastic thyroid carcinoma by the use of targeted next-generation sequencing. Histopathology. 2019 Dec;75(6):890–9. PMID:31230400
1164. Duan H, Liu X, Ren X, et al. Mutation profiles of follicular thyroid tumors by targeted sequencing. Diagn Pathol. 2019 May 10;14(1):39. PMID:31077238
1165. Duan K, Asa SL, Winer D, et al. Xanthomatous hypophysitis is associated with ruptured Rathke's cleft cyst. Endocr Pathol. 2017 Mar;28(1):83–90. PMID:28120170
1166. Duan K, Giordano TJ, Mete O. Adrenal cortical proliferations. In: Mete O, Asa SL, editors. Endocrine pathology. Cambridge (UK): Cambridge University Press; 2016. pp. 602–27.
1167. Duan K, Gomez Hernandez K, Mete O. Clinicopathological correlates of adrenal Cushing's syndrome. J Clin Pathol. 2015 Mar;68(3):175–86. PMID:25425660
1168. Duan K, Gomez Hernandez K, Mete O. Clinicopathological correlates of hyperparathyroidism. J Clin Pathol. 2015 Oct;68(10):771–87. PMID:26163537
1169. Duan K, Hernandez KG, Mete O. Clinicopathological correlates of adrenal Cushing's syndrome. Postgrad Med J. 2015 Jun;91(1076):331–42. PMID:26045561
1170. Duan K, Mete O. Algorithmic approach to neuroendocrine tumors in targeted biopsies: practical applications of immunohistochemical markers. Cancer Cytopathol. 2016 Dec;124(12):871–84. PMID:27529763
1171. Duan K, Mete O. Clinicopathologic correlates of primary aldosteronism. Arch Pathol Lab Med. 2015 Jul;139(7):948–54. PMID:26125435
1172. Duan K, Mete Ö. Parathyroid carcinoma: diagnosis and clinical implications. Turk Patoloji Derg. 2015;31 Suppl 1:80–97. PMID:26177319
1173. Dubois S, Guyétant S, Menei P, et al. Relevance of Ki-67 and prognostic factors for recurrence/progression of gonadotropic adenomas after first surgery. Eur J Endocrinol. 2007 Aug;157(2):141–7. PMID:17656591
1174. Dubois SG, London WB, Zhang Y, et al. Lung metastases in neuroblastoma at initial diagnosis: a report from the International Neuroblastoma Risk Group (INRG) project. Pediatr Blood Cancer. 2008 Nov;51(5):589–92. PMID:18649370
1175. Duet M, Sauvaget E, Pételle B, et al. Clinical impact of somatostatin receptor scintigraphy in the management of paragangliomas of the head and neck. J Nucl Med. 2003 Nov;44(11):1767–74. PMID:14602858
1176. Duff J, Meyer FB, Ilstrup DM, et al. Long-term outcomes for surgically resected craniopharyngiomas. Neurosurgery. 2000 Feb;46(2):291–302. PMID:10690718
1177. Duffner PK, Cohen ME, Seidel FG, et al. The significance of MRI abnormalities in children with neurofibromatosis. Neurology. 1989 Mar;39(3):373–8. PMID:2494565
1178. Dugan JM, Atkinson BF, Avitabile A, et al. Psammoma bodies in fine needle aspirate of the thyroid in lymphocytic thyroiditis. Acta Cytol. 1987 May-Jun;31(3):330–4. PMID:3473869
1179. Dulfer RR, Franssen GJH, Hesselink DA, et al. Systematic review of surgical and medical treatment for tertiary hyperparathyroidism. Br J Surg. 2017 Jun;104(7):804–13. PMID:28518414
1180. Duncan VE, Nabors LB, Warren PP, et al. Primary sellar rhabdomyosarcoma arising in association with a pituitary adenoma. Int J Surg Pathol. 2016 Dec;24(8):753–6. PMID:27422470
1181. Dundr P, Dudorkinová D, Povýsil C, et al. Pigmented composite paraganglioma-ganglioneuroma of the urinary bladder. Pathol Res Pract. 2003;199(11):765–9. PMID:14708645
1182. Duò D, Gasverde S, Benech F, et al. MIB-1 immunoreactivity in craniopharyngiomas: a clinico-pathological analysis. Clin Neuropathol. 2003 Sep-Oct;22(5):229–34. PMID:14531547
1183. Duregon E, Cappellesso R, Maffeis V, et al. Validation of the prognostic role of the "Helsinki Score" in 225 cases of adrenocortical carcinoma. Hum Pathol. 2017 Apr;62:1–7. PMID:27916625
1184. Duregon E, Fassina A, Volante M, et al. The reticulin algorithm for adrenocortical tumor diagnosis: a multicentric validation study on 245 unpublished cases. Am J Surg Pathol. 2013 Sep;37(9):1433–40. PMID:23774167
1185. Duregon E, Molinaro L, Volante M, et al. Comparative diagnostic and prognostic performances of the hematoxylin-eosin and phospho-histone H3 mitotic count and Ki-67 index in adrenocortical carcinoma. Mod Pathol. 2014 Sep;27(9):1246–54. PMID:24434900
1186. Duregon E, Volante M, Bollito E, et al. Pitfalls in the diagnosis of adrenocortical tumors: a lesson from 300 consultation cases. Hum Pathol. 2015 Dec;46(12):1799–807. PMID:26472162
1187. Duregon E, Volante M, Giorcelli J, et al. Diagnostic and prognostic role of steroidogenic factor 1 in adrenocortical carcinoma: a validation study focusing on clinical and pathologic correlates. Hum Pathol. 2013 May;44(5):822–8. PMID:23158211
1188. Duregon E, Volante M, Guzzetti S, et al. Images in endocrine pathology: unique composite adrenal adenomatoid tumor, ganglioneuroma, myelolipoma, and cortical nodular hyperplasia. Endocr Pathol. 2017 Sep;28(3):276–9. PMID:28382483
1189. Durham BH, Lopez Rodrigo E, Picarsic J, et al. Activating mutations in CSF1R and additional receptor tyrosine kinases in histiocytic neoplasms. Nat Med. 2019 Dec;25(12):1839–42. PMID:31768065
1190. Durham BH, Roos-Weil D, Baillou C, et al. Functional evidence for derivation of systemic histiocytic neoplasms from hematopoietic stem/progenitor cells. Blood. 2017 Jul 13;130(2):176–80. PMID:28566492
1191. Dusková J, Janotová D, Svobodová E, et al. Fine needle aspiration biopsy of mixed medullary-follicular thyroid carcinoma. A report of two cases. Acta Cytol. 2003 Jan-Feb;47(1):71–7. PMID:12585034
1192. Dustin SM, Atkins KA, Shami VM, et al. The cytologic diagnosis of gangliocytic paraganglioma: a case report. Diagn Cytopathol. 2013 Jul;41(7):650–3. PMID:22102547
1193. Dutta M, Chatterjee I, Roy S, et al. Primary embryonal rhabdomyosarcoma of the anterior neck and thyroid: report of a new case with review of the literature. Laryngoscope. 2013 Aug;123(8):2072–6. PMID:23625578
1194. Dwight T, Benn DE, Clarkson A, et al. Loss of SDHA expression identifies SDHA mutations in succinate dehydrogenase-deficient gastrointestinal stromal tumors. Am J Surg Pathol. 2013 Feb;37(2):226–33. PMID:23060355
1195. Dwight T, Mann K, Benn DE, et al. Familial SDHA mutation associated with pituitary adenoma and pheochromocytoma/paraganglioma. J Clin Endocrinol Metab. 2013 Jun;98(6):E1103–8. PMID:23633203
1196. Dworakowska D, Grossman AB. The molecular pathogenesis of corticotroph tumours. Eur J Clin Invest. 2012 Jun;42(6):665–76. PMID:22098190
1197. Dyer EH, Civit T, Abecassis JP, et al. Functioning ectopic supradiaphragmatic pituitary adenomas. Neurosurgery. 1994 Mar;34(3):529–32. PMID:7832831
1198. Ebbehoj A, Stochholm K, Jacobsen SF, et al. Incidence and clinical presentation of pheochromocytoma and sympathetic paraganglioma: a population-based study. J Clin Endocrinol Metab. 2021 Apr 23;106(5):e2251–61. PMID:33479747
1199. Ebbo M, Daniel L, Pavic M, et al. IgG4-related systemic disease: features and treatment response in a French cohort: results of a multicenter registry. Medicine (Baltimore). 2012 Jan;91(1):49–56. PMID:22198501
1200. Ebinu JO, Shahideh M, Ibrahim GM, et al. Sellar glomangioma. Endocr Pathol. 2011 Dec;22(4):218–21. PMID:21912963
1201. Economides KD, Zeltser L, Capecchi MR. Hoxb13 mutations cause overgrowth of

caudal spinal cord and tail vertebrae. Dev Biol. 2003 Apr 15;256(2):317–30. PMID:12679105
1202. Efanov AA, Brenner AV, Bogdanova TI, et al. Investigation of the relationship between radiation dose and gene mutations and fusions in post-Chernobyl thyroid cancer. J Natl Cancer Inst. 2018 Apr 1;110(4):371–8. PMID:29165687
1203. Efared B, Atsame-Ebang G, Tahirou S, et al. Bilateral pheochromocytoma with ganglioneuroma component associated with multiple neuroendocrine neoplasia type 2A: a case report. J Med Case Rep. 2017 Aug 1;11(1):208. PMID:28760150
1204. Egashira A, Morita M, Kumagai R, et al. Neuroendocrine carcinoma of the esophagus: clinicopathological and immunohistochemical features of 14 cases. PLoS One. 2017 Mar 13;12(3):e0173501. PMID:28288180
1205. Eichberg DG, Buttrick S, White K, et al. PAX8 expression variability in cerebellar hemangioblastoma: case series and review of the literature. Appl Immunohistochem Mol Morphol. 2019 Jul;27(6):477–81. PMID:29629948
1206. Eichhorn F, Harms A, Warth A, et al. PD-L1 expression in large cell neuroendocrine carcinoma of the lung. Lung Cancer. 2018 Apr;118:76–82. PMID:29572007
1207. Eichhorn JH, Young RH, Scully RE. Primary ovarian small cell carcinoma of pulmonary type. A clinicopathologic, immunohistologic, and flow cytometric analysis of 11 cases. Am J Surg Pathol. 1992 Oct;16(10):926–38. PMID:1384368
1208. Eieland AK, Normann KR, Sundaram AYM, et al. Distinct pattern of endoplasmic reticulum protein processing and extracellular matrix proteins in functioning and silent corticotroph pituitary adenomas. Cancers (Basel). 2020 Oct 14;12(10):2980. PMID:33066652
1209. Eisenhofer G, Goldstein DS, Kopin IJ, et al. Pheochromocytoma: rediscovery as a catecholamine-metabolizing tumor. Endocr Pathol. 2003 Fall;14(3):193–212. PMID:14586065
1210. Eisenhofer G, Klink B, Richter S, et al. Metabologenomics of phaeochromocytoma and paraganglioma: an integrated approach for personalised biochemical and genetic testing. Clin Biochem Rev. 2017 Apr;38(2):69–100. PMID:29332973
1211. Eisenhofer G, Kopin IJ, Goldstein DS. Catecholamine metabolism: a contemporary view with implications for physiology and medicine. Pharmacol Rev. 2004 Sep;56(3):331–49. PMID:15317907
1212. Eisenhofer G, Lenders JW, Timmers H, et al. Measurements of plasma methoxytyramine, normetanephrine, and metanephrine as discriminators of different hereditary forms of pheochromocytoma. Clin Chem. 2011 Mar;57(3):411–20. PMID:21262951
1213. Eisenhofer G, Pacak K, Huynh TT, et al. Catecholamine metabolomic and secretory phenotypes in phaeochromocytoma. Endocr Relat Cancer. 2010 Dec 21;18(1):97–111. PMID:21051559
1214. Eisenhofer G, Timmers HJ, Lenders JW, et al. Age at diagnosis of pheochromocytoma differs according to catecholamine phenotype and tumor location. J Clin Endocrinol Metab. 2011 Feb;96(2):375–84. PMID:21147885
1215. Ejaz S, Shawa H, Henderson SA, et al. Melanoma of unknown primary origin presenting as a rapidly enlarging adrenal mass. BMJ Case Rep. 2013 Jun 19;2013:bcr2013009727. PMID:23784764
1216. Ejlsmark-Svensson H, Bislev LS, Rolighed L, et al. Predictors of renal function and calcifications in primary hyperparathyroidism: a nested case-control study. J Clin Endocrinol Metab. 2018 Sep 1;103(9):3574–83. PMID:29955845
1217. El Khatib N, Aoun C, Zbibo R, et al. Follicular carcinoma arising in a large ectopic lingual thyroid: a case report and review of literature. J Surg Case Rep. 2018 Oct 22;2018(10):rjy196. PMID:30364552
1218. El Lakis M, Nockel P, Gaitanidis A, et al. Probability of positive genetic testing results in patients with family history of primary hyperparathyroidism. J Am Coll Surg. 2018 May;226(5):933–8. PMID:29408534
1219. Eldor R, Glaser B, Fraenkel M, et al. Glucagonoma and the glucagonoma syndrome - cumulative experience with an elusive endocrine tumour. Clin Endocrinol (Oxf). 2011 May;74(5):593–8. PMID:21470282
1220. Elhassan YS, Idkowiak J, Smith K, et al. Causes, patterns, and severity of androgen excess in 1205 consecutively recruited women. J Clin Endocrinol Metab. 2018 Mar 1;103(3):1214–23. PMID:29342266
1221. El Hussein S, Vincentelli C. Pituicytoma: review of commonalities and distinguishing features among TTF-1 positive tumors of the central nervous system. Ann Diagn Pathol. 2017 Aug;29:57–61. PMID:28807344
1222. Elisei R, Cosci B, Romei C, et al. Prognostic significance of somatic RET oncogene mutations in sporadic medullary thyroid cancer: a 10-year follow-up study. J Clin Endocrinol Metab. 2008 Mar;93(3):682–7. PMID:18073307
1223. Elisei R, Tacito A, Ramone T, et al. Twenty-five years experience on RET genetic screening on hereditary MTC: an update on the prevalence of germline RET mutations. Genes (Basel). 2019 Sep 10;10(9):698. PMID:31510104
1224. Elliott DD, Pitman MB, Bloom L, et al. Fine-needle aspiration biopsy of Hurthle cell lesions of the thyroid gland: a cytomorphologic study of 139 cases with statistical analysis. Cancer. 2006 Apr 25;108(2):102–9. PMID:16453320
1225. Ellis CL, Banerjee P, Carney E, et al. Adrenal lymphangioma: clinicopathologic and immunohistochemical characteristics of a rare lesion. Hum Pathol. 2011 Jul;42(7):1013–8. PMID:21315417
1226. Ellis PD, van Nostrand AW. The applied anatomy of thyroglossal tract remnants. Laryngoscope. 1977 May;87(5 Pt 1):765–70. PMID:850454
1227. Ellis RJ, Patel D, Prodanov T, et al. The presence of SDHB mutations should modify surgical indications for carotid body paragangliomas. Ann Surg. 2014 Jul;260(1):158–62. PMID:24169168
1228. Ellison DW, Aldape KD, Capper D, et al. cIMPACT-NOW update 7: advancing the molecular classification of ependymal tumors. Brain Pathol. 2020 Sep;30(5):863–6. PMID:32502305
1229. Ellison E, Lapuerta P, Martin SE. Psammoma bodies in fine-needle aspirates of the thyroid: predictive value for papillary carcinoma. Cancer. 1998 Jun 25;84(3):169–75. PMID:9678732
1230. El-Maouche D, Arlt W, Merke DP. Congenital adrenal hyperplasia. Lancet. 2017 Nov 11;390(10108):2194–210. PMID:28576284
1231. Elms AF, Carlan SJ, Rich AE, et al. Ovarian tumor-derived ectopic hyperprolactinemia. Pituitary. 2012 Dec;15(4):552–5. PMID:22105889
1232. Elowe-Gruau E, Beltrand J, Brauner R, et al. Childhood craniopharyngioma: hypothalamus-sparing surgery decreases the risk of obesity. J Clin Endocrinol Metab. 2013 Jun;98(6):2376–82. PMID:23633208
1233. Eloy C, Oliveira M, Vieira J, et al. Carcinoma of the thyroid with ewing family tumor elements and favorable prognosis: report of a second case. Int J Surg Pathol. 2014 May;22(3):260–5. PMID:23637256
1234. Eloy JA, Mortensen M, Gupta S, et al. Metastasis of uterine leiomyosarcoma to the thyroid gland: case report and review of the literature. Thyroid. 2007 Dec;17(12):1295–7. PMID:17988195
1235. Else T, Kim AC, Sabolch A, et al. Adrenocortical carcinoma. Endocr Rev. 2014 Apr;35(2):282–326. PMID:24423978
1236. Else T, Lerario AM, Everett J, et al. Adrenocortical carcinoma and succinate dehydrogenase gene mutations: an observational case series. Eur J Endocrinol. 2017 Nov;177(5):439–44. PMID:28819017
1237. Else T, Rodriguez-Galindo C. 5th International ACC Symposium: hereditary predisposition to childhood ACC and the associated molecular phenotype: 5th International ACC Symposium Session: Not just for kids! Horm Cancer. 2016 Feb;7(1):36–9. PMID:26660147
1238. Elsheikh TM, Asa SL, Chan JK, et al. Interobserver and intraobserver variation among experts in the diagnosis of thyroid follicular lesions with borderline nuclear features of papillary carcinoma. Am J Clin Pathol. 2008 Nov;130(5):736–44. PMID:18854266
1239. Elster AD. Modern imaging of the pituitary. Radiology. 1993 Apr;187(1):1–14. PMID:8451394
1240. Elston MS, Meyer-Rochow GY, Conaglen HM, et al. Increased SSTR2A and SSTR3 expression in succinate dehydrogenase-deficient pheochromocytomas and paragangliomas. Hum Pathol. 2015 Mar;46(3):390–6. PMID:25554089
1241. Elston MS, Meyer-Rochow GY, Dray M, et al. Early onset primary hyperparathyroidism associated with a novel germline mutation in CDKN1B. Case Rep Endocrinol. 2015;2015:510985. PMID:26257968
1242. Elston MS, Sehgal S, Dray M, et al. A duodenal SDH-deficient gastrointestinal stromal tumor in a patient with a germline SDHB mutation. J Clin Endocrinol Metab. 2017 May 1;102(5):1447–50. PMID:28324028
1243. Emile JF, Abla O, Fraitag S, et al. Revised classification of histiocytoses and neoplasms of the macrophage-dendritic cell lineages. Blood. 2016 Jun 2;127(22):2672–81. PMID:26966089
1244. Emile JF, Diamond EL, Hélias-Rodzewicz Z, et al. Recurrent RAS and PIK3CA mutations in Erdheim-Chester disease. Blood. 2014 Nov 6;124(19):3016–9. PMID:25150293
1245. Emmerich D, Zemojtel T, Hecht J, et al. Somatic neurofibromatosis type 1 (NF1) inactivation events in cutaneous neurofibromas of a single NF1 patient. Eur J Hum Genet. 2015 Jun;23(6):870–3. PMID:25293717
1246. Emy P, Michenet P, Saint-Marc O. [Microscopic thyroid papillary cancers presenting as cervical lymph node metastases]. Ann Chir. 1998;52(5):461–4. French. PMID:9752488
1247. Ende K, Henkel B, Brodhun M, et al. A 45-year-old female with hypokalemic rhabdomyolysis due to VIP-producing composite pheochromocytoma. Z Gastroenterol. 2012 Jun;50(6):589–94. PMID:22660994
1248. Eng C, Clayton D, Schuffenecker I, et al. The relationship between specific RET proto-oncogene mutations and disease phenotype in multiple endocrine neoplasia type 2. International RET mutation consortium analysis. JAMA. 1996 Nov 20;276(19):1575–9. PMID:8918855
1249. Eng C, Mulligan LM, Smith DP, et al. Low frequency of germline mutations in the RET proto-oncogene in patients with apparently sporadic medullary thyroid carcinoma. Clin Endocrinol (Oxf). 1995 Jul;43(1):123–7. PMID:7641404
1250. Eng HL, Chen WJ. Melanin-producing medullary carcinoma of the thyroid gland. Arch Pathol Lab Med. 1989 Apr;113(4):377–80. PMID:2705868
1251. Engels EA, Frisch M, Goedert JJ, et al. Merkel cell carcinoma and HIV infection. Lancet. 2002 Feb 9;359(9305):497–8. PMID:11853800
1252. Engels M, Span PN, van Herwaarden AE, et al. Testicular adrenal rest tumors: current insights on prevalence, characteristics, origin, and treatment. Endocr Rev. 2019 Aug 1;40(4):973–87. PMID:30882882
1253. Enjoji M, Sanada K, Seki R, et al. Adrenal rest tumor of the liver preoperatively diagnosed as hepatocellular carcinoma. Case Rep Surg. 2017;2017:8231943. PMID:28706747
1254. Enriquez ML, Baloch ZW, Montone KT, et al. CDX2 expression in columnar cell variant of papillary thyroid carcinoma. Am J Clin Pathol. 2012 May;137(5):722–6. PMID:22523209
1255. Enríquez-Vega ME, Muñoz-Paredes JG, Cossío-Zazueta A, et al. [SDHD gene mutation in Mexican population whit carotid body tumor]. Cir Cir. 2018;86(1):38–42. Spanish. PMID:29681642
1256. Epstein JI, Amin MB, Beltran H, et al. Proposed morphologic classification of prostate cancer with neuroendocrine differentiation. Am J Surg Pathol. 2014 Jun;38(6):756–67. PMID:24705311
1257. Erber R, Warth A, Muley T, et al. BAP1 loss is a useful adjunct to distinguish malignant mesothelioma including the adenomatoid-like variant from benign adenomatoid tumors. Appl Immunohistochem Mol Morphol. 2020 Jan;28(1):67–73. PMID:30640754
1258. Erbil Y, Salmaslioğlu A, Barbaros U, et al. Clinical and radiological features of adrenal cysts. Urol Int. 2008;80(1):31–6. PMID:18204230
1259. Ercolino T, Becherini L, Valeri A, et al. Uncommon clinical presentations of pheochromocytoma and paraganglioma in two different patients affected by two distinct novel VHL germline mutations. Clin Endocrinol (Oxf). 2008 May;68(5):762–8. PMID:18031321
1260. Erdenebaatar C, Yamaguchi M, Saito F, et al. An ovarian carcinoid tumor with peptide YY-positive insular component: a case report and review of the literature. Int J Gynecol Pathol. 2016 Jul;35(4):362–8. PMID:26630222
1261. Erdogan-Durmus S, Ozcan D, Yarikkaya E, et al. CD56, HBME-1 and cytokeratin 19 expressions in papillary thyroid carcinoma and nodular thyroid lesions. J Res Med Sci. 2016 Jun 14;21:49. PMID:27904595
1262. Ergul E, Gozetlik EO. Does percutaneous thyroid laser ablation induce mixed papillary and medullary thyroid carcinoma? Acta Chir Belg. 2010 Mar-Apr;110(2):228–31. PMID:20514841
1263. Erickson D, Kudva YC, Ebersold MJ, et al. Benign paragangliomas: clinical presentation and treatment outcomes in 236 patients. J Clin Endocrinol Metab. 2001 Nov;86(11):5210–6. PMID:11701678
1264. Erickson D, Scheithauer B, Atkinson J, et al. Silent subtype 3 pituitary adenoma: a clinicopathologic analysis of the Mayo Clinic experience. Clin Endocrinol (Oxf). 2009 Jul;71(1):92–9. PMID:19170710
1265. Erickson LA. Angiosarcoma of the adrenal gland. Mayo Clin Proc. 2021 May;96(5):1376–8. PMID:33958072
1266. Erickson LA, Jalal SM, Goellner JR, et al. Analysis of Hurthle cell neoplasms of the thyroid by interphase fluorescence in situ hybridization. Am J Surg Pathol. 2001 Jul;25(7):911–7. PMID:11420462
1267. Erickson LA, Jin L, Papotti M, et al. Oxyphil parathyroid carcinomas: a clinicopathologic and immunohistochemical study of 10 cases. Am J Surg Pathol. 2002 Mar;26(3):344–9. PMID:11859206

1268. Erickson LA, Jin L, Wollan P, et al. Parathyroid hyperplasia, adenomas, and carcinomas: differential expression of p27Kip1 protein. Am J Surg Pathol. 1999 Mar;23(3):288–95. PMID:10078919

1269. Erickson LA, Jin L, Wollan PC, et al. Expression of p27kip1 and Ki-67 in benign and malignant thyroid tumors. Mod Pathol. 1998 Feb;11(2):169–74. PMID:9504687

1270. Erickson LA, Lloyd RV, Hartman R, et al. Cystic adrenal neoplasms. Cancer. 2004 Oct 1;101(7):1537–44. PMID:15378490

1271. Erickson LA, Mete O. Immunohistochemistry in diagnostic parathyroid pathology. Endocr Pathol. 2018 Jun;29(2):113–29. PMID:29626276

1272. Erickson LA, Vrana JA, Theis J, et al. Analysis of amyloid in medullary thyroid carcinoma by mass spectrometry-based proteomic analysis. Endocr Pathol. 2015 Dec;26(4):291–5. PMID:26304852

1273. Eriksson B, Orlefors H, Oberg K, et al. Developments in PET for the detection of endocrine tumours. Best Pract Res Clin Endocrinol Metab. 2005 Jun;19(2):311–24. PMID:15763703

1274. Erkiliç S, Erkiliç A, Bayazit YA. Primary leiomyoma of the thyroid gland. J Laryngol Otol. 2003 Oct;117(10):832–4. PMID:14653931

1275. Erovic BM, Goldstein DP, Kim D, et al. Parathyroid cancer: outcome analysis of 16 patients treated at the Princess Margaret Hospital. Head Neck. 2013 Jan;35(1):35–9. PMID:22290780

1276. Erovic BM, Harris L, Jamali M, et al. Biomarkers of parathyroid carcinoma. Endocr Pathol. 2012 Dec;23(4):221–31. PMID:23001705

1277. Erovic BM, Kim D, Cassol C, et al. Prognostic and predictive markers in medullary thyroid carcinoma. Endocr Pathol. 2012 Dec;23(4):232–42. PMID:23150029

1278. Erşen A, Durak MG, Canda T, et al. Warthin-like papillary carcinoma of the thyroid: a case series and review of the literature. Turk Patoloji Derg. 2013;29(2):150–5. PMID:23661355

1279. Erstine EM, Tetzlaff MT, Jia X, et al. Prognostic significance of "nonsolid" microscopic metastasis in Merkel cell carcinoma sentinel lymph nodes. Am J Surg Pathol. 2019 Jul;43(7):907–19. PMID:31094923

1280. Esapa CT, Johnson SJ, Kendall-Taylor P, et al. Prevalence of Ras mutations in thyroid neoplasia. Clin Endocrinol (Oxf). 1999 Apr;50(4):529–35. PMID:10468914

1281. Eschbacher JM, Coons SW. Cytokeratin CK20 is a sensitive marker for Crooke's cells and the early cytoskeletal changes associated with hypercortisolism within pituitary corticotrophs. Endocr Pathol. 2006 Winter;17(4):365–76. PMID:17525485

1282. Espiard S, Bertherat J. Carney complex. Front Horm Res. 2013;41:50–62. PMID:23652670

1283. Espiard S, Drougat L, Libé R, et al. ARMC5 mutations in a large cohort of primary macronodular adrenal hyperplasia: clinical and functional consequences. J Clin Endocrinol Metab. 2015 Jun;100(6):E926–35. PMID:25853793

1284. Espiard S, Knape MJ, Bathon K, et al. Activating PRKACB somatic mutation in cortisol-producing adenomas. JCI Insight. 2018 Apr 19;3(8):e98296. PMID:29669941

1285. Espiard S, Vantyghem MC, Assié G, et al. Frequency and incidence of Carney complex manifestations: a prospective multicenter study with a three-year follow-up. J Clin Endocrinol Metab. 2020 Mar 1;105(3):dgaa002. PMID:31912137

1286. Espiritu GAM, Malana JT, Dumasis AJGV, et al. High preponderance of BRAF V600E mutation in papillary thyroid carcinoma among Filipinos: a clinicopathologic study. J Glob Oncol. 2019 Jan;5:1–6. PMID:30694737

1287. Esposito I, Segler A, Steiger K, et al. Pathology, genetics and precursors of human and experimental pancreatic neoplasms: an update. Pancreatology. 2015 Nov-Dec;15(6):598–610. PMID:26365060

1288. Esteves C, Neves C, Augusto L, et al. Pituitary incidentalomas: analysis of a neuroradiological cohort. Pituitary. 2015 Dec;18(6):777–81. PMID:25800168

1289. Estrella JS, Broaddus RR, Mathews A, et al. Progesterone receptor and PTEN expression predict survival in patients with low- and intermediate-grade pancreatic neuroendocrine tumors. Arch Pathol Lab Med. 2014 Aug;138(8):1027–36. PMID:25076292

1290. Eusebi V, Betts CM, Giangaspero F. Primary oat-cell carcinoma of the larynx. Virchows Arch A Pathol Anat Histol. 1978 Dec 4;380(4):349–54. PMID:214939

1291. Eusebi V, Carcangiu ML, Dina R, et al. Keratin-positive epithelioid angiosarcoma of thyroid. A report of four cases. Am J Surg Pathol. 1990 Aug;14(8):737–47. PMID:1696070

1292. Evang JA, Berg JP, Casar-Borota O, et al. Reduced levels of E-cadherin correlate with progression of corticotroph pituitary tumours. Clin Endocrinol (Oxf). 2011 Dec;75(6):811–8. PMID:21595730

1293. Evangelisti C, de Biase D, Kurelac I, et al. A mutation screening of oncogenes, tumor suppressor gene TP53 and nuclear encoded mitochondrial complex I genes in oncocytic thyroid tumors. BMC Cancer. 2015 Mar 21;15:157. PMID:25880213

1294. Evans AJ, Humphrey PA, Belani J, et al. Large cell neuroendocrine carcinoma of prostate: a clinicopathologic summary of 7 cases of a rare manifestation of advanced prostate cancer. Am J Surg Pathol. 2006 Jun;30(6):684–93. PMID:16723845

1295. Evans DG, Baser ME, McGaughran J, et al. Malignant peripheral nerve sheath tumours in neurofibromatosis 1. J Med Genet. 2002 May;39(5):311–4. PMID:12011145

1296. Evans DG, Huson SM, Birch JM. Malignant peripheral nerve sheath tumours in inherited disease. Clin Sarcoma Res. 2012 Oct 4;2(1):17. PMID:23036231

1297. Evans HL. Columnar-cell carcinoma of the thyroid. A report of two cases of an aggressive variant of thyroid carcinoma. Am J Clin Pathol. 1986 Jan;85(1):77–80. PMID:3940424

1298. Eveslage M, Calaminus G, Warmuth-Metz M, et al. The postopera tive quality of life in children and adolescents with craniopharyngioma. Dtsch Arztebl Int. 2019 May 3;116(18):321–8. PMID:31219033

1299. Evranos B, Polat SB, Baser H, et al. Bethesda classification is a valuable guide for fine needle aspiration reports and highly predictive especially for diagnosing aggressive variants of papillary thyroid carcinoma. Cytopathology. 2017 Aug;28(4):259–67. PMID:27666595

1300. Eytan S, Kim KY, Bleich D, et al. Isolated double pituitary adenomas: a silent corticotroph adenoma and a microprolactinoma. J Clin Neurosci. 2015 Oct;22(10):1676–8. PMID:26067545

1301. Ezzat S, Asa SL. Mechanisms of disease: the pathogenesis of pituitary tumors. Nat Clin Pract Endocrinol Metab. 2006 Apr;2(4):220–30. PMID:16932287

1302. Ezzat S, Asa SL, Couldwell WT, et al. The prevalence of pituitary adenomas: a systematic review. Cancer. 2004 Aug 1;101(3):613–9. PMID:15274075

1303. Ezzat S, Asa SL, Stefaneanu L, et al. Somatotroph hyperplasia without pituitary adenoma associated with a long standing growth hormone-releasing hormone-producing bronchial carcinoid. J Clin Endocrinol Metab. 1994 Mar;78(3):555–60. PMID:8126126

1304. Ezzat S, Caspar-Bell GM, Chik CL, et al. Predictive markers for postsurgical medical management of acromegaly: a systematic review and consensus treatment guideline. Endocr Pract. 2019 Apr;25(4):379–93. PMID:30657362

1305. Ezzat S, Ezrin C, Yamashita S, et al. Recurrent acromegaly resulting from ectopic growth hormone gene expression by a metastatic pancreatic tumor. Cancer. 1993 Jan 1;71(1):66–70. PMID:8416728

1306. Ezzat S, Forster MJ, Berchtold P, et al. Acromegaly. Clinical and biochemical features in 500 patients. Medicine (Baltimore). 1994 Sep;73(5):233–40. PMID:7934807

1307. Ezzat S, Horvath E, Kovacs K, et al. Basic fibroblast growth factor expression by two prolactin and thyrotropin-producing pituitary adenomas. Endocr Pathol. 1995 Summer;6(2):125–34. PMID:12114648

1308. Ezzat S, Kontogeorgos G, Redelmeier DA, et al. In vivo responsiveness of morphological variants of growth hormone-producing pituitary adenomas to octreotide. Eur J Endocrinol. 1995 Dec;133(6):686–90. PMID:8548053

1309. Ezzat S, Mader R, Fischer S, et al. An essential role for the hematopoietic transcription factor Ikaros in hypothalamic-pituitary-mediated somatic growth. Proc Natl Acad Sci U S A. 2006 Feb 14;103(7):2214–9. PMID:16467156

1310. Ezzat S, Yu S, Asa SL. Ikaros isoforms in human pituitary tumors: distinct localization, histone acetylation, and activation of the 5' fibroblast growth factor receptor-4 promoter. Am J Pathol. 2003 Sep;163(3):1177–84. PMID:12937159

1311. Ezzat S, Zheng L, Winer D, et al. Targeting N-cadherin through fibroblast growth factor receptor-4: distinct pathogenetic and therapeutic implications. Mol Endocrinol. 2006 Nov;20(11):2965–75. PMID:16857743

1312. Facchetti F, Lorenzi L. Follicular dendritic cells and related sarcoma. Semin Diagn Pathol. 2016 Sep;33(5):262–76. PMID:27318412

1313. Facchetti F, Pileri SA, Lorenzi L, et al. Histiocytic and dendritic cell neoplasms: what have we learnt by studying 67 cases. Virchows Arch. 2017 Oct;471(4):467–89. PMID:28695297

1314. Fadul CE, Kominsky AL, Meyer LP, et al. Long-term response of pituitary carcinoma to temozolomide. Report of two cases. J Neurosurg. 2006 Oct;105(4):621–6. PMID:17044568

1315. Fahlbusch R, Schott W. Pterional surgery of meningiomas of the tuberculum sellae and planum sphenoidale: surgical results with special consideration of ophthalmological and endocrinological outcomes. J Neurosurg. 2002 Feb;96(2):235–43. PMID:11838796

1316. Fahrenkamp AG, Wibbeke C, Winde G, et al. Immunohistochemical distribution of chromogranins A and B and secretogranin II in neuroendocrine tumours of the gastrointestinal tract. Virchows Arch. 1995;426(4):361–7. PMID:7599788

1317. Fahrenkrug J. Transmitter role of vasoactive intestinal peptide. Pharmacol Toxicol. 1993 Jun;72(6):354–63. PMID:8103215

1318. Faillot S, Foulonneau T, Néou M, et al. Genomic classification of benign adrenocortical lesions. Endocr Relat Cancer. 2021 Jan;28(1):79–95. PMID:33151900

1319. Falco EC, Daniele L, Metovic J, et al. Adrenal rests in the uro-genital tract of an adult population. Endocr Pathol. 2021 Sep;32(3):375–84. PMID:34095993

1320. Falconi M, Bartsch DK, Eriksson B, et al. ENETS consensus guidelines for the management of patients with digestive neuroendocrine neoplasms of the digestive system: well-differentiated pancreatic non-functioning tumors. Neuroendocrinology. 2012;95(2):120–34. PMID:22261872

1321. Falconi M, Eriksson B, Kaltsas G, et al. ENETS consensus guidelines update for the management of patients with functional pancreatic neuroendocrine tumors and non-functional pancreatic neuroendocrine tumors. Neuroendocrinology. 2016;103(2):153–71. PMID:26742109

1322. Falhammar H, Nyström HF, Ekström U, et al. Fertility, sexuality and testicular adrenal rest tumors in adult males with congenital adrenal hyperplasia. Eur J Endocrinol. 2012 Mar;166(3):441–9. PMID:22157069

1323. Falto Aizpurua LA, Wang M, Ruiz HA, et al. A case of combined Merkel cell carcinoma and squamous cell carcinoma: molecular insights and diagnostic pitfalls. JAAD Case Rep. 2018 Nov 3;4(10):996–9. PMID:30417062

1324. Falvo L, Catania A, D'Andrea V, et al. Prognostic importance of histologic vascular invasion in papillary thyroid carcinoma. Ann Surg. 2005 Apr;241(4):640–6. PMID:15798466

1325. Famini P, Maya MM, Melmed S. Pituitary magnetic resonance imaging for sellar and parasellar masses: ten-year experience in 2598 patients. J Clin Endocrinol Metab. 2011 Jun;96(6):1633–41. PMID:21470998

1326. Fan S, Jiang Y, Yao Y, et al. Pituitary ACTH-secreting adenoma in Addison's disease: a case report. Clin Neurol Neurosurg. 2013 Dec;115(12):2543–6. PMID:24216004

1327. Fanburg-Smith JC, Meis-Kindblom JM, Fante R, et al. Malignant granular cell tumor of soft tissue: diagnostic criteria and clinicopathologic correlation. Am J Surg Pathol. 1998 Jul;22(7):779–94. PMID:9669341

1328. Fang J, Dagenais SL, Erickson RP, et al. Mutations in FOXC2 (MFH-1), a forkhead family transcription factor, are responsible for the hereditary lymphedema-distichiasis syndrome. Am J Hum Genet. 2000 Dec;67(6):1382–8. PMID:11078474

1329. Faquin WC. The thyroid gland: recurring problems in histologic and cytologic evaluation. Arch Pathol Lab Med. 2008 Apr;132(4):622–32. PMID:18384214

1330. Farber LJ, Kort EJ, Wang P, et al. The tumor suppressor parafibromin is required for posttranscriptional processing of histone mRNA. Mol Carcinog. 2010 Mar;49(3):215–23. PMID:19908240

1331. Farhat NA, Faquin WC, Sadow PM. Primary mucoepidermoid carcinoma of the thyroid gland: a report of three cases and review of the literature. Endocr Pathol. 2013 Dec;24(4):229–33. PMID:24096806

1332. Faria A, Lopes F, Figueira A, et al. Pancreas angiosarcoma-case report of a rare cause of abdominal pain. Int J Surg Case Rep. 2020;76:116–20. PMID:33032040

1333. Fariduddin MM, Mathias PM, Syed W. Hurthle cell thyroid carcinoma. 2023 Feb 13. In: StatPearls. Treasure Island (FL): StatPearls Publishing; 2024 Jan–. PMID:33760495

1334. Farley CR, Perez MC, Soelling SJ, et al. Merkel cell carcinoma outcomes: Does AJCC8 underestimate survival? Ann Surg Oncol. 2020 Jun;27(6):1978–85. PMID:32103415

1335. Farooqui ZA, Chauhan A. Neuroendocrine tumors in pediatrics. Glob Pediatr Health. 2019 Jul 22;6:2333794X19862712. PMID:31384627

1336. Farrell JM, Pang JC, Kim GE, et al. Pancreatic neuroendocrine tumors: accurate grading with Ki-67 index on fine-needle aspiration specimens using the WHO 2010/ENETS criteria. Cancer Cytopathol. 2014 Oct;122(10):770–8. PMID:25044931

1337. Fasano M, Della Corte CM, Papaccio

F, et al. Pulmonary large-cell neuroendocrine carcinoma: from epidemiology to therapy. J Thorac Oncol. 2015 Aug;10(8):1133–41. PMID:26039012
1338. Fassnacht M, Allolio B. Clinical management of adrenocortical carcinoma. Best Pract Res Clin Endocrinol Metab. 2009 Apr;23(2):273–89. PMID:19500769
1339. Fassnacht M, Dekkers OM, Else T, et al. European Society of Endocrinology clinical practice guidelines on the management of adrenocortical carcinoma in adults, in collaboration with the European Network for the Study of Adrenal Tumors. Eur J Endocrinol. 2018 Oct 1;179(4):G1–46. PMID:30299884
1340. Fassnacht M, Libé R, Kroiss M, et al. Adrenocortical carcinoma: a clinician's update. Nat Rev Endocrinol. 2011 Jun;7(6):323–35. PMID:21386792
1341. Fatemi N, Dusick JR, de Paiva Neto MA, et al. The endonasal microscopic approach for pituitary adenomas and other parasellar tumors: a 10-year experience. Neurosurgery. 2008 Oct;63(4 Suppl 2):244–56. PMID:18981830
1342. Faucz FR, Tirosh A, Tatsi C, et al. Somatic USP8 gene mutations are a common cause of pediatric Cushing disease. J Clin Endocrinol Metab. 2017 Aug 1;102(8):2836–43. PMID:28505279
1343. Favier J, Amar L, Gimenez-Roqueplo AP. Paraganglioma and phaeochromocytoma: from genetics to personalized medicine. Nat Rev Endocrinol. 2015 Feb;11(2):101–11. PMID:25385035
1344. Favier J, Meatchi T, Robidel E, et al. Carbonic anhydrase 9 immunohistochemistry as a tool to predict or validate germline and somatic VHL mutations in pheochromocytoma and paraganglioma-a retrospective and prospective study. Mod Pathol. 2020 Jan;33(1):57–64. PMID:31383958
1345. Febrero B, Oviedo I, Ríos A, et al. Primary rhabdomyosarcoma of the thyroid in an adult with auricular thrombosis. Eur Ann Otorhinolaryngol Head Neck Dis. 2017 Feb;134(1):49–51. PMID:27595524
1346. Febrero B, Rodríguez JM, Ríos A, et al. Prophylactic thyroidectomy in multiple endocrine neoplasia 2 (MEN2) patients with the C634Y mutation: a long-term follow-up in a large single-center cohort. Eur J Surg Oncol. 2019 Apr;45(4):625–30. PMID:30366876
1347. Feldmeyer L, Hudgens CW, Ray-Lyons G, et al. Density, distribution, and composition of immune infiltrates correlate with survival in Merkel cell carcinoma. Clin Cancer Res. 2016 Nov 15;22(22):5553–63. PMID:27166398
1348. Fellegara G, Rosai J. Signet ring cells in a poorly differentiated Hurthle cell carcinoma of the thyroid combined with two papillary microcarcinomas. Int J Surg Pathol. 2007 Oct;15(4):388–90. PMID:17913947
1349. Fellows IW, Leach IH, Smith PG, et al. Carcinoid tumour of the common bile duct–a novel complication of von Hippel-Lindau syndrome. Gut. 1990 Jun;31(6):728–9. PMID:2379881
1350. Fendrich V, Langer P, Waldmann J, et al. Management of sporadic and multiple endocrine neoplasia type 1 gastrinomas. Br J Surg. 2007 Nov;94(11):1331–41. PMID:17939142
1351. Fendrich V, Ramerth R, Waldmann J, et al. Sonic hedgehog and pancreatic-duodenal homeobox 1 expression distinguish between duodenal and pancreatic gastrinomas. Endocr Relat Cancer. 2009 Jun;16(2):613–22. PMID:19240184
1352. Feng H, Shuda M, Chang Y, et al. Clonal integration of a polyomavirus in human Merkel cell carcinoma. Science. 2008 Feb 22;319(5866):1096–100. PMID:18202256
1353. Feola T, Centello R, Sesti F, et al. Neuroendocrine carcinomas with atypical proliferation index and clinical behavior: a systematic review. Cancers (Basel). 2021 Mar 12;13(6):1247. PMID:33809007
1354. Ferlay J, Ervik M, Lam F, et al. Global Cancer Observatory: Cancer Today [Internet]. Lyon (France): International Agency for Research on Cancer; 2020. Available from: https://gco.iarc.who.int/today.
1355. Ferlito A, Recher G, Caruso G. Primary combined small cell carcinoma of the larynx. Am J Otolaryngol. 1985 Jul-Aug;6(4):302–8. PMID:2994505
1356. Ferlito A, Rinaldo A, Bishop JA, et al. Paraneoplastic syndromes in patients with laryngeal neuroendocrine carcinomas: clinical manifestations and prognostic significance. Eur Arch Otorhinolaryngol. 2016 Mar;273(3):533–6. PMID:25351497
1357. Fernandes-Rosa FL, Daniil G, Orozco IJ, et al. A gain-of-function mutation in the CLCN2 chloride channel gene causes primary aldosteronism. Nat Genet. 2018 Mar;50(3):355–61. PMID:29403012
1358. Fernandez A, Conrad M, Gill RM, et al. Solitary fibrous tumor in the abdomen and pelvis: a case series with radiological findings and treatment recommendations. Clin Imaging. 2018 Mar-Apr;48:48–54. PMID:29028514
1359. Fernandez A, Karavitaki N, Wass JA. Prevalence of pituitary adenomas: a community-based, cross-sectional study in Banbury (Oxfordshire, UK). Clin Endocrinol (Oxf). 2010 Mar;72(3):377–82. PMID:19650784
1360. Fernandez FG, Battafarano RJ. Large-cell neuroendocrine carcinoma of the lung. Cancer Control. 2006 Oct;13(4):270–5. PMID:17075564
1361. Fernandez JF, Ordoñez NG, Schultz PN, et al. Thyroglossal duct carcinoma. Surgery. 1991 Dec;110(6):928–34. PMID:1745980
1362. Fernandez-Ranvier GG, Jensen K, Khanafshar E, et al. Nonfunctioning parathyroid carcinoma: case report and review of literature. Endocr Pract. 2007 Nov-Dec;13(7):750–7. PMID:18194932
1363. Fernandez-Ranvier GG, Khanafshar E, Jensen K, et al. Parathyroid carcinoma, atypical parathyroid adenoma, or parathyromatosis? Cancer. 2007 Jul 15;110(2):255–64. PMID:17559137
1364. Fernandez-Ranvier GG, Khanafshar E, Tacha D, et al. Defining a molecular phenotype for benign and malignant parathyroid tumors. Cancer. 2009 Jan 15;115(2):334–44. PMID:19107770
1365. Ferner RE, Huson SM, Thomas N, et al. Guidelines for the diagnosis and management of individuals with neurofibromatosis 1. J Med Genet. 2007 Feb;44(2):81–8. PMID:17105749
1366. Fero ML, Rivkin M, Tasch M, et al. A syndrome of multiorgan hyperplasia with features of gigantism, tumorigenesis, and female sterility in p27(Kip1)-deficient mice. Cell. 1996 May 31;85(5):733–44. PMID:8646781
1367. Ferrara AM, Lombardi G, Pambuku A, et al. Temozolomide treatment of a malignant pheochromocytoma and an unresectable MAX-related paraganglioma. Anticancer Drugs. 2018 Jan;29(1):102–5. PMID:29099418
1368. Ferrari SM, Fallahi P, Ruffilli I, et al. Molecular testing in the diagnosis of differentiated thyroid carcinomas. Gland Surg. 2018 Aug;7(Suppl 1):S19–29. PMID:30175060
1369. Ferraro V, Sgaramella LI, Di Meo G, et al. Current concepts in parathyroid carcinoma: a single centre experience. BMC Endocr Disord. 2019 May 29;19(Suppl 1):46. PMID:31142320
1370. Ferraz-Filho JR, Torres US, Teixeira AC, et al. Ectopic growth hormone-secreting pituitary adenoma involving the clivus treated with octreotide: role of magnetic resonance imaging in the diagnosis and clinical follow-up. Arq Neuropsiquiatr. 2012 Sep;70(9):744–5. PMID:22990736
1371. Ferreiro JA, Carney JA. Myxomas of the external ear and their significance. Am J Surg Pathol. 1994 Mar;18(3):274–80. PMID:8116795
1372. Ferreiro JA, Hay ID, Lloyd RV. Columnar cell carcinoma of the thyroid: report of three additional cases. Hum Pathol. 1996 Nov;27(11):1156–60. PMID:8912824
1373. Ferrell RE. Research perspectives in inherited lymphatic disease. Ann N Y Acad Sci. 2002 Dec;979:39–51. PMID:12543715
1374. Ferrell RE, Levinson KL, Esman JH, et al. Hereditary lymphedema: evidence for linkage and genetic heterogeneity. Hum Mol Genet. 1998 Dec;7(13):2073–8. PMID:9817924
1375. Ferrigno R, Hasenmajer V, Caiulo S, et al. Paediatric Cushing's disease: epidemiology, pathogenesis, clinical management and outcome. Rev Endocr Metab Disord. 2021 Dec;22(4):817–35. PMID:33515368
1376. Ferrone CR, Tang LH, Tomlinson J, et al. Determining prognosis in patients with pancreatic endocrine neoplasms: Can the WHO classification system be simplified? J Clin Oncol. 2007 Dec 10;25(35):5609–15. PMID:18065733
1377. Fesinmeyer MD, Austin MA, Li CI, et al. Differences in survival by histologic type of pancreatic cancer. Cancer Epidemiol Biomarkers Prev. 2005 Jul;14(7):1766–73. PMID:16030115
1378. Feuillan PP, Shawker T, Rose SR, et al. Thyroid abnormalities in the McCune-Albright syndrome: ultrasonography and hormonal studies. J Clin Endocrinol Metab. 1990 Dec;71(6):1596–601. PMID:2229316
1379. Fidler WJ. Ovarian thecal metaplasia in adrenal glands. Am J Clin Pathol. 1977 Apr;67(4):318–23. PMID:851092
1380. Filetti S, Durante C, Hartl D, et al. Thyroid cancer: ESMO clinical practice guidelines for diagnosis, treatment and follow-up. Ann Oncol. 2019 Dec 1;30(12):1856–83. PMID:31549998
1381. Filie AC, Lage JM, Azumi N. Immunoreactivity of S100 protein, alpha-1-antitrypsin, and CD68 in adult and congenital granular cell tumors. Mod Pathol. 1996 Sep;9(9):888–92. PMID:8878020
1382. Filosso PL, Guerrera F, Evangelista A, et al. Adjuvant chemotherapy for large-cell neuroendocrine lung carcinoma: results from the European Society for Thoracic Surgeons Lung Neuroendocrine Tumours Retrospective Database. Eur J Cardiothorac Surg. 2017 Aug 1;52(2):339–45. PMID:28459956
1383. Finzi G, Cerati M, Marando A, et al. Mixed pituitary adenoma/craniopharyngioma: clinical, morphological, immunohistochemical and ultrastructural study of a case, review of the literature, and pathogenetic and nosological considerations. Pituitary. 2014 Feb;17(1):53–9. PMID:23344977
1384. Fishbein L, Del Rivero J, Else T, et al. The North American Neuroendocrine Tumor Society consensus guidelines for surveillance and management of metastatic and/or unresectable pheochromocytoma and paraganglioma. Pancreas. 2021 Apr 1;50(4):469–93. PMID:33939658
1385. Fishbein L, Leshchiner I, Walter V, et al. Comprehensive molecular characterization of pheochromocytoma and paraganglioma. Cancer Cell. 2017 Feb 13;31(2):181–93. PMID:28162975
1386. Fite JJ, Maleki Z. Paraganglioma: cytomorphologic features, radiologic and clinical findings in 12 cases. Diagn Cytopathol. 2018 Jun;46(6):473–81. PMID:29575826
1387. Fitko R, Roth SI, Hines JR, et al. Parathyromatosis in hyperparathyroidism. Hum Pathol. 1990 Feb;21(2):234–7. PMID:2307452
1388. Fitzgerald TL, Dennis S, Kachare SD, et al. Dramatic increase in the incidence and mortality from Merkel cell carcinoma in the United States. Am Surg. 2015 Aug;81(8):802–6. PMID:26215243
1389. Fleming KE, Ly TY, Pasternak S, et al. Support for p63 expression as an adverse prognostic marker in Merkel cell carcinoma: report on a Canadian cohort. Hum Pathol. 2014 May;45(5):952–60. PMID:24746200
1390. Fleury A, Fléjou JF, Sauvanet A, et al. Calcitonin-secreting tumors of the pancreas: about six cases. Pancreas. 1998 May;16(4):545–50. PMID:9598818
1391. Floreani A, Okazaki K, Uchida K, et al. IgG4-related disease: changing epidemiology and new thoughts on a multisystem disease. J Transl Autoimmun. 2020 Dec 19;4:100074. PMID:33490938
1392. Florenzano P, Pan KS, Brown SM, et al. Age-related changes and effects of bisphosphonates on bone turnover and disease progression in fibrous dysplasia of bone. J Bone Miner Res. 2019 Apr;34(4):653–60. PMID:30645769
1393. Flores-Carrillo VM, Santaella-Torres F, Sánchez-Martínez LC, et al. [Rosai-Dorfman disease presented with involvement of the adrenal gland. A clinical case reported]. Rev Med Inst Mex Seguro Soc. 2014 Mar-Apr;52(2):224–7. Spanish. PMID:24758864
1394. Florez JC, Burton DW, Arnell PM, et al. Hypercalcemia and local production of parathyroid hormone-related protein by a perisellar rhabdomyosarcoma after remote pituitary irradiation. Endocr Pract. 2005 May-Jun;11(3):184–9. PMID:16239205
1395. Folpe AL, Devaney K, Weiss SW. Lipomatous hemangiopericytoma: a rare variant of hemangiopericytoma that may be confused with liposarcoma. Am J Surg Pathol. 1999 Oct;23(10):1201–7. PMID:10524520
1396. Folpe AL, Fanburg-Smith JC, Miettinen M, et al. Atypical and malignant glomus tumors: analysis of 52 cases, with a proposal for the reclassification of glomus tumors. Am J Surg Pathol. 2001 Jan;25(1):1–12. PMID:11145243
1397. Folpe AL, Goodman ZD, Ishak KG, et al. Clear cell myomelanocytic tumor of the falciform ligament/ligamentum teres: a novel member of the perivascular epithelioid clear cell family of tumors with a predilection for children and young adults. Am J Surg Pathol. 2000 Sep;24(9):1239–46. PMID:10976698
1398. Folpe AL, Kwiatkowski DJ. Perivascular epithelioid cell neoplasms: pathology and pathogenesis. Hum Pathol. 2010 Jan;41(1):1–15. PMID:19604538
1399. Folpe AL, Lloyd RV, Bacchi CE, et al. Spindle epithelial tumor with thymus-like differentiation: a morphologic, immunohistochemical, and molecular genetic study of 11 cases. Am J Surg Pathol. 2009 Aug;33(8):1179–86. PMID:19417583
1400. Folpe AL, Mentzel T, Lehr HA, et al. Perivascular epithelioid cell neoplasms of soft tissue and gynecologic origin: a clinicopathologic study of 26 cases and review of the literature. Am J Surg Pathol. 2005 Dec;29(12):1558–75. PMID:16327428
1401. Fong MHY, Feng M, McConkey DJ, et al. Update on bladder cancer molecular subtypes. Transl Androl Urol. 2020 Dec;9(6):2881–9. PMID:33457262
1402. Fonseca AL, Kugelberg J, Starker LF, et al. Comprehensive DNA methylation analysis of benign and malignant adrenocortical tumors. Genes Chromosomes Cancer. 2012 Oct;51(10):949–60. PMID:22733721
1403. Fonseca D, Bhuyan S, Murthy SS, et al. Noninvasive follicular thyroid neoplasm with papillary-like nuclear features: a distinct clinicopathologic entity. Indian J Pathol Microbiol.

2018 Jul-Sep;61(3):380–2. PMID:30004059
1404. Fonseca D, Murthy SS, Tagore KR, et al. Diagnosis of adrenocortical tumors by reticulin algorithm. Indian J Endocrinol Metab. 2017 Sep-Oct;21(5):734–7. PMID:28989884
1405. Fontana E, Gaillard R. [Epidemiology of pituitary adenoma: results of the first Swiss study]. Rev Med Suisse. 2009 Oct 28;5(223):2172–4. French. PMID:19968031
1406. Foote M, Veness M, Zarate D, et al. Merkel cell carcinoma: the prognostic implications of an occult primary in stage IIIB (nodal) disease. J Am Acad Dermatol. 2012 Sep;67(3):395–9. PMID:22030017
1407. Forest VI, Murali R, Clark JR. Thyroglossal duct cyst carcinoma: case series. J Otolaryngol Head Neck Surg. 2011 Apr;40(2):151–6. PMID:21453651
1408. Foresti M, Parmiggiani A. Adrenal adenoma-hemangioma collision tumor: description of two cases. J Radiol Case Rep. 2019 Jun 30;13(6):1–12. PMID:31558958
1409. Forlino A, Vetro A, Garavelli L, et al. PRKACB and Carney complex. N Engl J Med. 2014 Mar 13;370(11):1065–7. PMID:24571725
1410. Foster DG. Adrenal cysts. Review of literature and report of case. Arch Surg. 1966 Jan;92(1):131–43. PMID:5901251
1411. Fougner SL, Casar-Borota O, Heck A, et al. Adenoma granulation pattern correlates with clinical variables and effect of somatostatin analogue treatment in a large series of patients with acromegaly. Clin Endocrinol (Oxf). 2012 Jan;76(1):96–102. PMID:21722151
1412. Foulkes WD, Priest JR, Duchaine TF. DICER1: mutations, microRNAs and mechanisms. Nat Rev Cancer. 2014 Oct;14(10):662–72. PMID:25176334
1413. Fountas A, Giotaki Z, Ligkros N, et al. Cushing's syndrome due to CRH and ACTH co-secreting pancreatic tumor–presentation of a new case focusing on diagnostic pitfalls. Endocr Pathol. 2015 Sep;26(3):239–42. PMID:26202047
1414. Fountas A, Lavrentaki A, Subramanian A, et al. Recurrence in silent corticotroph adenomas after primary treatment: a systematic review and meta-analysis. J Clin Endocrinol Metab. 2018 Dec 21. PMID:30590584
1415. Fraenkel M, Kim M, Faggiano A, et al. Incidence of gastroenteropancreatic neuroendocrine tumours: a systematic review of the literature. Endocr Relat Cancer. 2014 May 6;21(3):R153–63. PMID:24322304
1416. Fraga J, Caetano Oliveira R, Alexandrino H, et al. Neuroendocrine carcinoma and intracystic papillary neoplasm: a rare association in the gallbladder. GE Port J Gastroenterol. 2019 Aug;26(5):356–61. PMID:31559326
1417. Fraker DL, Travis WD, Merendino JJ Jr, et al. Locally recurrent parathyroid neoplasms as a cause for recurrent and persistent primary hyperparathyroidism. Ann Surg. 1991 Jan;213(1):58–65. PMID:1985539
1418. Franchi A, Rocchetta D, Palomba A, et al. Primary combined neuroendocrine and squamous cell carcinoma of the maxillary sinus: report of a case with immunohistochemical and molecular characterization. Head Neck Pathol. 2015 Mar;9(1):107–13. PMID:24327102
1419. Franchi A, Sardi I, Cetica V, et al. Pediatric sinonasal neuroendocrine carcinoma after treatment of retinoblastoma. Hum Pathol. 2009 May;40(5):750–5. PMID:19157501
1420. Francis GL, Waguespack SG, Bauer AJ, et al. Management guidelines for children with thyroid nodules and differentiated thyroid cancer. Thyroid. 2015 Jul;25(7):716–59. PMID:25900731
1421. Francis IM, Das DK, Sheikh ZA, et al. Role of nuclear grooves in the diagnosis of papillary thyroid carcinoma. A quantitative assessment on fine needle aspiration smears. Acta Cytol. 1995 May-Jun;39(3):409–15. PMID:7539202
1422. Francis JM, Kiezun A, Ramos AH, et al. Somatic mutation of CDKN1B in small intestine neuroendocrine tumors. Nat Genet. 2013 Dec;45(12):1483–6. PMID:24185511
1423. Franko J, Feng W, Yip L, et al. Non-functional neuroendocrine carcinoma of the pancreas: incidence, tumor biology, and outcomes in 2,158 patients. J Gastrointest Surg. 2010 Mar;14(3):541–8. PMID:19997980
1424. Frank-Raue K, Döhring J, Scheumann G, et al. New mutations in the RET protooncogene-L881V - associated with medullary thyroid carcinoma and -R770Q - in a patient with mixed medullar/follicular thyroid tumour. Exp Clin Endocrinol Diabetes. 2010 Aug;118(8):550–3. PMID:20013610
1425. Frank-Raue K, Haag C, Schulze E, et al. CDC73-related hereditary hyperparathyroidism: five new mutations and the clinical spectrum. Eur J Endocrinol. 2011 Sep;165(3):477–83. PMID:21652691
1426. Frank-Raue K, Machens A, Scheuba C, et al. Difference in development of medullary thyroid carcinoma among carriers of RET mutations in codons 790 and 791. Clin Endocrinol (Oxf). 2008 Aug;69(2):259–63. PMID:18248648
1427. Frank-Raue K, Rybicki LA, Erlic Z, et al. Risk profiles and penetrance estimations in multiple endocrine neoplasia type 2A caused by germline RET mutations located in exon 10. Hum Mutat. 2011 Jan;32(1):51–8. PMID:20979234
1428. Franquemont DW, Mills SE, Lack EE. Immunohistochemical detection of neuroblastomatous foci in composite adrenal pheochromocytoma-neuroblastoma. Am J Clin Pathol. 1994 Aug;102(2):163–70. PMID:8042583
1429. Franssila KO, Harach HR, Wasenius VM. Mucoepidermoid carcinoma of the thyroid. Histopathology. 1984 Sep;8(5):847–60. PMID:6083973
1430. Franz IW. [Blood pressure under stress in hypertensive patients and sports]. Fortschr Med. 1988 Feb 29;106(6):107–10. German. PMID:3371825
1431. Fraser WD. Hyperparathyroidism. Lancet. 2009 Jul 11;374(9684):145–58. PMID:19595349
1432. Freda PU, Post KD. Differential diagnosis of sellar masses. Endocrinol Metab Clin North Am. 1999 Mar;28(1):81–117, vi. PMID:10207686
1433. Frederiksen A, Rossing M, Hermann P, et al. Clinical features of multiple endocrine neoplasia type 4: novel pathogenic variant and review of published cases. J Clin Endocrinol Metab. 2019 Sep 1;104(9):3637–46. PMID:30990521
1434. French B, Hattier G, Mardekian SK. Utility of tumor capsule thickness as a predictor of invasion in encapsulated follicular variant of papillary thyroid carcinoma and a diagnostic tool for noninvasive follicular thyroid neoplasm with papillary-like nuclear features. Int J Surg Pathol. 2020 Feb;28(1):13–9. PMID:31256687
1435. French CA, Alexander EK, Cibas ES, et al. Genetic and biological subgroups of low-stage follicular thyroid cancer. Am J Pathol. 2003 Apr;162(4):1053–60. PMID:12651598
1436. Frey S, Caillard C, Toulgoat F, et al. Non-adrenal tumors of the adrenal area; what are the pitfalls? J Visc Surg. 2020 Jun;157(3):217–30. PMID:32201083
1437. Fridman M, Lam AK, Krasko O. Characteristics of young adults of Belarus with post-Chernobyl papillary thyroid carcinoma: a long-term follow-up of patients with early exposure to radiation at the 30th anniversary of the accident. Clin Endocrinol (Oxf). 2016 Dec;85(6):971–8. PMID:27314225
1438. Friedman E, Sakaguchi K, Bale AE, et al. Clonality of parathyroid tumors in familial multiple endocrine neoplasia type 1. N Engl J Med. 1989 Jul 27;321(4):213–8. PMID:2568586
1439. Friedman JM, Birch PH. Type 1 neurofibromatosis: a descriptive analysis of the disorder in 1,728 patients. Am J Med Genet. 1997 May 16;70(2):138–43. PMID:9128932
1440. Friend KE, Chiou YK, Lopes MB, et al. Estrogen receptor expression in human pituitary: correlation with immunohistochemistry in normal tissue, and immunohistochemistry and morphology in macroadenomas. J Clin Endocrinol Metab. 1994 Jun;78(6):1497–504. PMID:7515390
1441. Friis RB, Safwat A, Baad-Hansen T, et al. Solitary fibrous tumour: a single institution retrospective study and further validation of a prognostic risk assessment system. Clin Oncol (R Coll Radiol). 2018 Dec;30(12):798–804. PMID:30206022
1442. Fritz A, Percy C, Jack A, et al., editors. International classification of diseases for oncology (ICD-O). 3rd ed. 1st rev. Geneva (Switzerland): World Health Organization; 2013.
1443. Fritzsche FR, Bode PK, Koch S, et al. Radiological and pathological findings of a metastatic composite paraganglioma with neuroblastoma in a man: a case report. J Med Case Rep. 2010 Nov 19;4:374. PMID:21092109
1444. Frizziero M, Chakrabarty B, Nagy B, et al. Mixed neuroendocrine non-neuroendocrine neoplasms: a systematic review of a controversial and underestimated diagnosis. J Clin Med. 2020 Jan 19;9(1):273. PMID:31963850
1445. Frizziero M, Wang X, Chakrabarty B, et al. Retrospective study on mixed neuroendocrine non-neuroendocrine neoplasms from five European centres. World J Gastroenterol. 2019 Oct 21;25(39):5991–6005. PMID:31660035
1446. Frost AR, Tenner S, Tenner M, et al. ACTH-producing pituitary carcinoma presenting as the cauda equina syndrome. Arch Pathol Lab Med. 1995 Jan;119(1):93–6. PMID:7802565
1447. Fu W, Ligabue A, Rogers KJ, et al. Human RECQ helicase pathogenic variants, population variation and "missing" diseases. Hum Mutat. 2017 Feb;38(2):193–203. PMID:27859906
1448. Fuchs TL, Bell SE, Chou A, et al. Revisiting the significance of prominent c cells in the thyroid. Endocr Pathol. 2019 Jun;30(2):113–7. PMID:30694510
1449. Fuchs TL, Luxford C, Clarkson A, et al. A clinicopathologic and molecular analysis of fumarate hydratase-deficient pheochromocytoma and paraganglioma. Am J Surg Pathol. 2023 Jan 1;47(1):25–36. PMID:35993574
1450. Fuchs TL, Nassour AJ, Glover A, et al. A proposed grading scheme for medullary thyroid carcinoma based on proliferative activity (Ki-67 and mitotic count) and coagulative necrosis. Am J Surg Pathol. 2020 Oct;44(10):1419–28. PMID:32452872
1451. Fujio S, Juratli TA, Arita K, et al. A clinical rule for preoperative prediction of BRAF mutation status in craniopharyngiomas. Neurosurgery. 2019 Aug 1;85(2):204–10. PMID:30481321
1452. Fujiwara S, Sposto R, Shiraki M, et al. Levels of parathyroid hormone and calcitonin in serum among atomic bomb survivors. Radiat Res. 1994 Jan;137(1):96–103. PMID:8265793
1453. Fujiyoshi Y, Kuhara H, Eimoto T. Composite glandular-endocrine cell carcinoma of the stomach. Report of two cases with goblet cell carcinoid component. Pathol Res Pract. 2005;200(11-12):823–9. PMID:15792127
1454. Fukahori M, Yoshida A, Hayashi H, et al. The associations between RAS mutations and clinical characteristics in follicular thyroid tumors: new insights from a single center and a large patient cohort. Thyroid. 2012 Jul;22(7):683–9. PMID:22650231
1455. Fukuhara N, Iwata T, Inoshita N, et al. Immunohistochemistry or molecular analysis: Which method is better for subtyping craniopharyngioma? Endocr Pathol. 2021 Jun;32(2):262–8. PMID:32965631
1456. Fukui T, Tsuta K, Furuta K, et al. Epidermal growth factor receptor mutation status and clinicopathological features of combined small cell carcinoma with adenocarcinoma of the lung. Cancer Sci. 2007 Nov;98(11):1714–9. PMID:17784875
1457. Fukunaga M, Ishibashi T, Koyama T, et al. Malignant struma ovarii with a predominant component of anaplastic carcinoma. Int J Gynecol Pathol. 2016 Jul;35(4):357–61. PMID:26630220
1458. Fuminari K, Hideki A, Manabu O, et al. Extended endoscopic endonasal surgery using three-dimensional endoscopy in the intra-operative MRI suite for supra-diaphragmatic ectopic pituitary adenoma. Turk Neurosurg. 2015;25(3):503–7. PMID:26037197
1459. Funayama T, Sakane M, Yoshizawa T, et al. Tanycytic ependymoma of the filum terminale associated with multiple endocrine neoplasia type 1: first reported case. Spine J. 2013 Aug;13(8):e49–54. PMID:23562332
1460. Fundakowski CE, Chapman JR, Thomas G. Middle ear carcinoid with distant osseous metastasis. Laryngoscope. 2013 Mar;123(3):779–82. PMID:22777694
1461. Funder JW, Carey RM, Mantero F, et al. The management of primary aldosteronism: case detection, diagnosis, and treatment: an Endocrine Society Clinical Practice Guideline. J Clin Endocrinol Metab. 2016 May;101(5):1889–916. PMID:26934393
1462. Fung AD, Cohen C, Kavuri S, et al. Phosphohistone H3 and Ki-67 labeling indices in cytologic specimens from well-differentiated neuroendocrine tumors of the gastrointestinal tract and pancreas: a comparative analysis using automated image cytometry. Acta Cytol. 2013;57(5):501–8. PMID:24021213
1463. Furlan A, Dyachuk V, Kastriti ME, et al. Multipotent peripheral glial cells generate neuroendocrine cells of the adrenal medulla. Science. 2017 Jul 7;357(6346):eaal3753. PMID:28684471
1464. Furlan D, Cerutti R, Genasetti A, et al. Microallelotyping defines the monoclonal or the polyclonal origin of mixed and collision endocrine-exocrine tumors of the gut. Lab Invest. 2003 Jul;83(7):963–71. PMID:12861036
1465. Furlan D, Sahnane N, Bernasconi B, et al. APC alterations are frequently involved in the pathogenesis of acinar cell carcinoma of the pancreas, mainly through gene loss and promoter hypermethylation. Virchows Arch. 2014 May;464(5):553–64. PMID:24590585
1466. Furlan JC, Bedard YC, Rosen IB. Clinicopathologic significance of histologic vascular invasion in papillary and follicular thyroid carcinomas. J Am Coll Surg. 2004 Mar;198(3):341–8. PMID:14992733
1467. Furlanetto TW, Pinheiro CF, Oppitz PP, et al. Solitary fibrous tumor of the sella mimicking pituitary adenoma: an uncommon tumor in a rare location-a case report. Endocr Pathol. 2009 Spring;20(1):56–61. PMID:19224406
1468. Furtado LV, Leventaki V, Layfield LJ, et al. Yolk sac tumor of the thyroid gland: a case report. Pediatr Dev Pathol. 2011 Nov-Dec;14(6):475–9. PMID:21793665
1469. Furze AD, Lehman DA, Roy S. Rhabdomyosarcoma presenting as an anterior neck mass and possible thyroid malignancy in a seven-month-old. Int J Pediatr Otorhinolaryngol.

2005 Feb;69(2):267–70. PMID:15656963
1470. Gaal J, Stratakis CA, Carney JA, et al. SDHB immunohistochemistry: a useful tool in the diagnosis of Carney-Stratakis and Carney triad gastrointestinal stromal tumors. Mod Pathol. 2011 Jan;24(1):147–51. PMID:20890271
1471. Gabel BC, Cleary DR, Martin JR, et al. Unusual and rare locations for craniopharyngiomas: clinical significance and review of the literature. World Neurosurg. 2017 Feb;98:381–7. PMID:27908738
1472. Gadelha MR, Wildemberg LE, Bronstein MD, et al. Somatostatin receptor ligands in the treatment of acromegaly. Pituitary. 2017 Feb;20(1):100–8. PMID:28176162
1473. Gadner H, Grois N, Arico M, et al. A randomized trial of treatment for multisystem Langerhans' cell histiocytosis. J Pediatr. 2001 May;138(5):728–34. PMID:11343051
1474. Gadner H, Minkov M, Grois N, et al. Therapy prolongation improves outcome in multisystem Langerhans cell histiocytosis. Blood. 2013 Jun 20;121(25):5006–14. PMID:23589673
1475. Gaffey MJ, Mills SE, Fechner RE, et al. Vascular adrenal cysts. A clinicopathologic and immunohistochemical study of endothelial and hemorrhagic (pseudocystic) variants. Am J Surg Pathol. 1989 Sep;13(9):740–7. PMID:2504065
1476. Gaffey TA, Scheithauer BW, Lloyd RV, et al. Corticotroph carcinoma of the pituitary: a clinicopathological study. Report of four cases. J Neurosurg. 2002 Feb;96(2):352–60. PMID:11838811
1477. Gaffney EF, Doorly T, Dinn JJ. Aggressive oncocytic neuroendocrine tumour ('oncocytic paraganglioma') of the cauda equina. Histopathology. 1986 Mar;10(3):311–9. PMID:2422107
1478. Gaffney RL, Carney JA, Sebo TJ, et al. Galectin-3 expression in hyalinizing trabecular tumors of the thyroid gland. Am J Surg Pathol. 2003 Apr;27(4):494–8. PMID:12657934
1479. Gahr N, Darge K, Hahn G, et al. Diffusion-weighted MRI for differentiation of neuroblastoma and ganglioneuroblastoma/ganglioneuroma. Eur J Radiol. 2011 Sep;79(3):443–6. PMID:20462716
1480. Galati LT, Barnes EL, Myers EN. Dendritic cell sarcoma of the thyroid. Head Neck. 1999 May;21(3):273–5. PMID:10208672
1481. Galili N, Davis RJ, Fredericks WJ, et al. Fusion of a fork head domain gene to PAX3 in the solid tumour alveolar rhabdomyosarcoma. Nat Genet. 1993 Nov;5(3):230–5. PMID:8275086
1482. Galland F, Lacroix L, Saulnier P, et al. Differential gene expression profiles of invasive and non-invasive non-functioning pituitary adenomas based on microarray analysis. Endocr Relat Cancer. 2010 Apr 21;17(2):361–71. PMID:20228124
1483. Gallo M, Campione S, Di Vito V, et al. Primary neuroendocrine neoplasms of the breast: still open issues. Front Endocrinol (Lausanne). 2021 Jan 26;11:610230. PMID:33584543
1484. Galluzzi F, Pignataro L, Gaini RM, et al. Risk of recurrence in children operated for thyroglossal duct cysts: a systematic review. J Pediatr Surg. 2013 Jan;48(1):222–7. PMID:23331819
1485. Gambardella C, Offi C, Patrone R, et al. Calcitonin negative medullary thyroid carcinoma: a challenging diagnosis or a medical dilemma? BMC Endocr Disord. 2019 May 29;19(Suppl 1):45. PMID:31142313
1486. Gambella A, Falco EC, Metovic J, et al. Amyloid-rich pancreatic neuroendocrine tumors: a potential diagnostic pitfall in endoscopic ultrasound-guided fine needle aspiration cytology (EUS-FNAC). Endocr Pathol. 2021 Jun;32(2):318–25. PMID:32399832
1487. Gan HW, Bulwer C, Jeelani O, et al. Treatment-resistant pediatric giant prolactinoma and multiple endocrine neoplasia type 1. Int J Pediatr Endocrinol. 2015;2015(1):15. PMID:26180530
1488. Gandolfi G, Ragazzi M, de Biase D, et al. Genome-wide profiling identifies the THYT1 signature as a distinctive feature of widely metastatic papillary thyroid carcinomas. Oncotarget. 2017 Dec 1;9(2):1813–25. PMID:29416733
1489. Ganeshan D, Menias CO, Pickhardt PJ, et al. Tumors in von Hippel-Lindau syndrome: from head to toe-comprehensive state-of-the-art review. Radiographics. 2018 May-Jun;38(3):849–66. PMID:29601266
1490. Ganly I, Makarov V, Deraje S, et al. Integrated genomic analysis of Hürthle cell cancer reveals oncogenic drivers, recurrent mitochondrial mutations, and unique chromosomal landscapes. Cancer Cell. 2018 Aug 13;34(2):256–270.e5. PMID:30107176
1491. Ganly I, McFadden DG. Short review: genomic alterations in Hürthle cell carcinoma. Thyroid. 2019 Apr;29(4):471–9. PMID:30848171
1492. Ganly I, Ricarte Filho J, Eng S, et al. Genomic dissection of Hurthle cell carcinoma reveals a unique class of thyroid malignancy. J Clin Endocrinol Metab. 2013 May;98(5):E962–72. PMID:23543667
1493. Ganly I, Wang L, Tuttle RM, et al. Invasion rather than nuclear features correlates with outcome in encapsulated follicular tumors: further evidence for the reclassification of the encapsulated papillary thyroid carcinoma follicular variant. Hum Pathol. 2015 May;46(5):657–64. PMID:25721865
1494. Gao J, Aksoy BA, Dogrusoz U, et al. Integrative analysis of complex cancer genomics and clinical profiles using the cBioPortal. Sci Signal. 2013 Apr 2;6(269):pl1. PMID:23550210
1495. Gao R, Jia X, Ji T, et al. Management and prognostic factors for thyroid carcinoma showing thymus-like elements (CASTLE): a case series study. Front Oncol. 2018 Oct 26;8:477. PMID:30416983
1496. Gao S, Shi X, Wang Y, et al. Malignant transformation of craniopharyngioma: case report and review of the literature. J Neurooncol. 2011 Jul;103(3):719–25. PMID:20872276
1497. Gao X, Zhang X, Zhang Y, et al. Is papillary thyroid microcarcinoma an indolent tumor?: A retrospective study on 280 cases treated with radioiodine. Medicine (Baltimore). 2016 Oct;95(40):e5067. PMID:27749574
1498. Gao XL, Zhang KW, Tang MB, et al. Pooled analysis for surgical treatment for isolated adrenal metastasis and non-small cell lung cancer. Interact Cardiovasc Thorac Surg. 2017 Jan;24(1):1–7. PMID:27664424
1499. Gara SK, Jia L, Merino MJ, et al. Germline HABP2 mutation causing familial nonmedullary thyroid cancer. N Engl J Med. 2015 Jul 30;373(5):448–55. PMID:26222560
1500. Garbicz F, Mehlich D, Rak B, et al. Increased expression of the microRNA 106b~25 cluster and its host gene MCM7 in corticotroph pituitary adenomas is associated with tumor invasion and Crooke's cell morphology. Pituitary. 2017 Aug;20(4):450–63. PMID:28432562
1501. Garbrecht N, Anlauf M, Schmitt A, et al. Somatostatin-producing neuroendocrine tumors of the duodenum and pancreas: incidence, types, biological behavior, association with inherited syndromes, and functional activity. Endocr Relat Cancer. 2008 Mar;15(1):229–41. PMID:18310290
1502. Garby L, Caron P, Claustrat F, et al. Clinical characteristics and outcome of acromegaly induced by ectopic secretion of growth hormone-releasing hormone (GHRH): a French nationwide series of 21 cases. J Clin Endocrinol Metab. 2012 Jun;97(6):2093–104. PMID:22442262
1503. Garces S, Medeiros LJ, Patel KP, et al. Mutually exclusive recurrent KRAS and MAP2K1 mutations in Rosai-Dorfman disease. Mod Pathol. 2017 Oct;30(10):1367–77. PMID:28664935
1504. Garcés Visier C, Espinoza Vega M, Guillén Redondo P, et al. Prophylactic thyroidectomy in multiple endocrine neoplasia type 2A in children: a single centre experience. J Pediatr Endocrinol Metab. 2019 Aug 27;32(8):889–93. PMID:31343983
1505. Garces-Descovich A, Callery MP, Anderson KR, et al. Synchronous granular cell tumors of the pancreas and cecum. Clin Imaging. 2018 Nov-Dec;52:95–9. PMID:30036783
1506. Garcia E, Osterbauer B, Parham D, et al. The incidence of microscopic thyroglossal duct tissue superior to the hyoid bone. Laryngoscope. 2019 May;129(5):1215–7. PMID:30194760
1507. Garcia-Lavandeira M, Saez C, Diaz-Rodriguez E, et al. Craniopharyngiomas express embryonic stem cell markers (SOX2, OCT4, KLF4, and SOX9) as pituitary stem cells but do not coexpress RET/GFRA3 receptors. J Clin Endocrinol Metab. 2012 Jan;97(1):E80–7. PMID:22031517
1508. Gardner DF, Frable WJ. Primary lymphangioma of the thyroid gland. Arch Pathol Lab Med. 1989 Sep;113(9):1084–5. PMID:2774858
1509. Garg K, Lee P, Ro JY, et al. Adenomatoid tumor of the adrenal gland: a clinicopathologic study of 3 cases. Ann Diagn Pathol. 2005 Feb;9(1):11–5. PMID:15692945
1510. Garg K, Soslow RA, Rivera M, et al. Histologically bland "extremely well differentiated" thyroid carcinomas arising in struma ovarii can recur and metastasize. Int J Gynecol Pathol. 2009 May;28(3):222–30. PMID:19620939
1511. Garren B, Stephan M, Hogue JS. NRAS associated RASopathy and embryonal rhabdomyosarcoma. Am J Med Genet A. 2020 Jan;182(1):195–200. PMID:31697451
1512. Garty BZ, Laor A, Danon YL. Neurofibromatosis type 1 in Israel: survey of young adults. J Med Genet. 1994 Nov;31(11):853–7. PMID:7853369
1513. Gąsior-Perczak D, Kowalik A, Gruszczyński K, et al. Incidence of the CHEK2 germline mutation and its impact on clinicopathological features, treatment responses, and disease course in patients with papillary thyroid carcinoma. Cancers (Basel). 2021 Jan 26;13(3):470. PMID:33530461
1514. Gąsior-Perczak D, Kowalik A, Walczyk A, et al. Coexisting germline CHEK2 and somatic BRAFV600E mutations in papillary thyroid cancer and their association with clinicopathological features and disease course. Cancers (Basel). 2019 Nov 7;11(11):1744. PMID:31703344
1515. Gasparre G, Porcelli AM, Bonora E, et al. Disruptive mitochondrial DNA mutations in complex I subunits are markers of oncocytic phenotype in thyroid tumors. Proc Natl Acad Sci U S A. 2007 May 22;104(21):9001–6. PMID:17517629
1516. Gaston-Massuet C, Andoniadou CL, Signore M, et al. Increased Wingless (Wnt) signaling in pituitary progenitor/stem cells gives rise to pituitary tumors in mice and humans. Proc Natl Acad Sci U S A. 2011 Jul 12;108(28):11482–7. PMID:21636786
1517. Gatta-Cherifi B, Chabre O, Murat A, et al. Adrenal involvement in MEN1. Analysis of 715 cases from the Groupe d'etude des Tumeurs Endocrines database. Eur J Endocrinol. 2012 Feb;166(2):269–79. PMID:22084155
1518. Gaujoux S, Pinson S, Gimenez-Roqueplo AP, et al. Inactivation of the APC gene is constant in adrenocortical tumors from patients with familial adenomatous polyposis but not frequent in sporadic adrenocortical cancers. Clin Cancer Res. 2010 Nov 1;16(21):5133–41. PMID:20978149
1519. Gaujoux S, Salenave S, Ronot M, et al. Hepatobiliary and pancreatic neoplasms in patients with McCune-Albright syndrome. J Clin Endocrinol Metab. 2014 Jan;99(1):E97–101. PMID:24170100
1520. Gaur P, Leary C, Yao JC. Thymic neuroendocrine tumors: a SEER database analysis of 160 patients. Ann Surg. 2010 Jun;251(6):1117–21. PMID:20485130
1521. Gauthé M, Testart Dardel N, Nascimento C, et al. Uterine leiomyosarcoma metastatic to thyroid shown by 18F-FDG PET/CT imaging. Rev Esp Med Nucl Imagen Mol. 2017 Mar-Apr;36(2):113–5. PMID:27777040
1522. Ge W, Yao YZ, Chen G, et al. Clinical analysis of 82 cases of carcinoma showing thymus-like differentiation of the thyroid. Oncol Lett. 2016 Feb;11(2):1321–6. PMID:26893738
1523. Ge Y, Luna MA, Cowan DF, et al. Thyrolipoma and thyrolipomatosis: 5 case reports and historical review of the literature. Ann Diagn Pathol. 2009 Dec;13(6):384–9. PMID:19917474
1524. Gebresellassie HW, Mohammed Y, Kotiso B, et al. A giant solitary fibrous tumor of the adrenal gland in a 13-year old: a case report and review of the literature. J Med Case Rep. 2019 Aug 8;13(1):246. PMID:31391097
1525. Gelabert-González M. Paragangliomas of the lumbar region. Report of two cases and review of the literature. J Neurosurg Spine. 2005 Mar;2(3):354–65. PMID:15796363
1526. Geller KA, Cohen D, Koempel JA. Thyroglossal duct cyst and sinuses: a 20-year Los Angeles experience and lessons learned. Int J Pediatr Otorhinolaryngol. 2014 Feb;78(2):264–7. PMID:24332664
1527. Gempt J, Baldawa SS, Weirich G, et al. Recurrent multiple spinal paragangliomas as a manifestation of a metastatic composite paraganglioma-ganglioneuroblastoma. Acta Neurochir (Wien). 2013 Jul;155(7):1241–2. PMID:23532344
1528. Genç CG, Falconi M, Partelli S, et al. Recurrence of pancreatic neuroendocrine tumors and survival predicted by Ki67. Ann Surg Oncol. 2018 Aug;25(8):2467–74. PMID:29789972
1529. Geng H, Ye Y, Jin Y, et al. Malignant solitary fibrous tumor of the pancreas with systemic metastasis: a case report and review of the literature. World J Clin Cases. 2020 Jan 26;8(2):343–52. PMID:32047784
1530. Genpeng L, Jianyong L, Jiaying Y, et al. Independent predictors and lymph node metastasis characteristics of multifocal papillary thyroid cancer. Medicine (Baltimore). 2018 Feb;97(5):e9619. PMID:29384841
1531. Geoerger B, Hero B, Harms D, et al. Metabolic activity and clinical features of primary ganglioneuromas. Cancer. 2001 May 15;91(10):1905–13. PMID:11346873
1532. Georgantzoglou N, Kokkali S, Tsourouflis G, et al. Tumor microenvironment in adrenocortical carcinoma: barrier to immunotherapy success? Cancers (Basel). 2021 Apr 9;13(8):1798. PMID:33918733
1533. George DH, Scheithauer BW, Kovacs K, et al. Crooke's cell adenoma of the pituitary: an aggressive variant of corticotroph adenoma. Am J Surg Pathol. 2003 Oct;27(10):1330–6. PMID:14508394
1534. George DJ, Watermeyer GA, Levin D, et al. Composite adrenal phaeochromocytoma-ganglioneuroma causing watery diarrhoea, hypokalaemia and achlorhydria syndrome. Eur

J Gastroenterol Hepatol. 2010 May;22(5):632–4. PMID:20216072
1535. George J, Walter V, Peifer M, et al. Integrative genomic profiling of large-cell neuroendocrine carcinomas reveals distinct subtypes of high-grade neuroendocrine lung tumors. Nat Commun. 2018 Mar 13;9(1):1048. PMID:29535388
1536. George MM, Eugster EA, Chernausek SD. Pituitary gigantism. In: Feingold KR, Anawalt B, Blackman MR, et al., editors. Endotext. South Dartmouth (MA): MDText.com, Inc.; 2000 [updated 2022 Jun 22]. PMID:25905378
1537. George RE, London WB, Cohn SL, et al. Hyperdiploidy plus nonamplified MYCN confers a favorable prognosis in children 12 to 18 months old with disseminated neuroblastoma: a Pediatric Oncology Group study. J Clin Oncol. 2005 Sep 20;23(27):6466–73. PMID:16116152
1538. Georgiesh T, Boye K, Bjerkehagen B. A novel risk score to predict early and late recurrence in solitary fibrous tumour. Histopathology. 2020 Jul;77(1):123–32. PMID:31991494
1539. Georgitsi M. MEN-4 and other multiple endocrine neoplasias due to cyclin-dependent kinase inhibitors (p27(Kip1) and p18(INK4C)) mutations. Best Pract Res Clin Endocrinol Metab. 2010 Jun;24(3):425–37. PMID:20833334
1540. Georgitsi M, Raitila A, Karhu A, et al. Germline CDKN1B/p27Kip1 mutation in multiple endocrine neoplasia. J Clin Endocrinol Metab. 2007 Aug;92(8):3321–5. PMID:17519308
1541. Gerhard R, Kanashiro EH, Kliemann CM, et al. Fine-needle aspiration biopsy of ectopic cervical spindle-cell thymoma: a case report. Diagn Cytopathol. 2005 Jun;32(6):358–62. PMID:15880711
1542. Gerson JN, Witteles RM, Chang DT, et al. Carcinoid syndrome complicating a pancreatic neuroendocrine tumor: a case report. Pancreas. 2017 Nov/Dec;46(10):1381–5. PMID:29040196
1543. Ghaferi AA, Chojnacki KA, Long WD, et al. Pancreatic VIPomas: subject review and one institutional experience. J Gastrointest Surg. 2008 Feb;12(2):382–93. PMID:17510774
1544. Ghazi AA, Amirbaigloo A, Dezfooli AA, et al. Ectopic acromegaly due to growth hormone releasing hormone. Endocrine. 2013 Apr;43(2):293–302. PMID:22983831
1545. Ghazi AA, Boustani I, Amouzegar A, et al. Postpartum hypercalcemia secondary to a neuroendocrine tumor of pancreas; a case report and review of literature. Iran J Med Sci. 2011 Sep;36(3):217–21. PMID:23358529
1546. Ghazi AA, Dezfooli AA, Mohamadi F, et al. Cushing syndrome secondary to a thymic carcinoid tumor due to multiple endocrine neoplasia type 1. Endocr Pract. 2011 Jul-Aug;17(4):e92–6. PMID:21550948
1547. Ghazi AA, Rotondo F, Kovacs K, et al. Treatment of invasive silent somatotroph pituitary adenoma with temozolomide. Report of a case and review of the literature. Endocr Pathol. 2015 May;26(2):135–9. PMID:25716461
1548. Gholami S, Cassidy MR, Kirane A, et al. Size and location are the most important risk factors for malignant behavior in resected solitary fibrous tumors. Ann Surg Oncol. 2017 Dec;24(13):3865–71. PMID:29039030
1549. Ghossein CA, Khimraj A, Dogan S, et al. Metastasis to the thyroid gland: a single-institution 16-year experience. Histopathology. 2021 Mar;78(4):508–19. PMID:32897542
1550. Ghossein R. Encapsulated malignant follicular cell-derived thyroid tumors. Endocr Pathol. 2010 Dec;21(4):212–8. PMID:21088998
1551. Ghossein R, Barletta JA, Bullock M, et al. Data set for reporting carcinoma of the thyroid: recommendations from the International Collaboration on Cancer Reporting. Hum Pathol. 2021 Apr;110:62–72. PMID:32920035
1552. Ghossein R, Ganly I, Biagini A, et al. Prognostic factors in papillary microcarcinoma with emphasis on histologic subtyping: a clinicopathologic study of 148 cases. Thyroid. 2014 Feb;24(2):245–53. PMID:23745671
1553. Ghossein R, Livolsi VA. Papillary thyroid carcinoma tall cell variant. Thyroid. 2008 Nov;18(11):1179–81. PMID:18925842
1554. Ghossein RA, Hiltzik DH, Carlson DL, et al. Prognostic factors of recurrence in encapsulated Hurthle cell carcinoma of the thyroid gland: a clinicopathologic study of 50 cases. Cancer. 2006 Apr 15;106(8):1669–76. PMID:16534796
1555. Ghossein RA, Leboeuf R, Patel KN, et al. Tall cell variant of papillary thyroid carcinoma without extrathyroid extension: biologic behavior and clinical implications. Thyroid. 2007 Jul;17(7):655–61. PMID:17696836
1556. Ghossein RA, Rosai J, Heffess C. Dyshormonogenetic goiter: a clinicopathologic study of 56 cases. Endocr Pathol. 1997 Winter;8(4):283–92. PMID:12114789
1557. Giacomazzi J, Graudenz MS, Osorio CA, et al. Prevalence of the TP53 p.R337H mutation in breast cancer patients in Brazil. PLoS One. 2014 Jun 17;9(6):e99893. PMID:24936644
1558. Giacomelli L, Guerriero G, Falvo L, et al. Simultaneous occurrence of medullary carcinoma and papillary microcarcinoma of thyroid in a patient with MEN 2A syndrome. report of a case. Tumori. 2007 Jan-Feb;93(1):109–11. PMID:17455883
1559. Gianella P, Dulguerov N, Arnoux G, et al. Thyroid Rosai-Dorfman disease with infiltration of IgG4-bearing plasma cells associated with multiple small pulmonary cysts. BMC Pulm Med. 2019 May 3;19(1):83. PMID:31053123
1560. Giannelli SM, McPhaul L, Nakamoto J, et al. Familial adenomatous polyposis-associated, cribriform morular variant of papillary thyroid carcinoma harboring a K-RAS mutation: case presentation and review of molecular mechanisms. Thyroid. 2014 Jul;24(7):1184–9. PMID:24702198
1561. Giannetta E, Guarnotta V, Rota F, et al. A rare rarity: neuroendocrine tumor of the esophagus. Crit Rev Oncol Hematol. 2019 May;137:92–107. PMID:31014519
1562. Giannikaki E, Mantadakis E, Mamalaki E, et al. Metastatic uterine leiomyosarcoma coexisting with papillary carcinoma of the thyroid gland. Int J Gynecol Cancer. 2006 Jan-Feb;16(1):442–5. PMID:16445675
1563. Gianoli GJ, Butcher RB, Martin EJ 3rd. Composite tumor of the larynx. Ear Nose Throat J. 1992 Feb;71(2):81–2, 85–7. PMID:1315242
1564. Giantini Larsen AM, Cote DJ, Zaidi HA, et al. Spindle cell oncocytoma of the pituitary gland. J Neurosurg. 2018 Oct 19;131(2):517–25. PMID:30485213
1565. Giardina E, Capon F, D'Apice MR, et al. Mutational analysis of peroxiredoxin IV: exclusion of a positional candidate for multinodular goitre. BMC Med Genet. 2002 Jul 23;3:5. PMID:12135533
1566. Gibril F, Jensen RT. Zollinger-Ellison syndrome revisited: diagnosis, biologic markers, associated inherited disorders, and acid hypersecretion. Curr Gastroenterol Rep. 2004 Dec;6(6):454–63. PMID:15527675
1567. Gibril F, Schumann M, Pace A, et al. Multiple endocrine neoplasia type 1 and Zollinger-Ellison syndrome: a prospective study of 107 cases and comparison with 1009 cases from the literature. Medicine (Baltimore). 2004 Jan;83(1):43–83. PMID:14747767
1568. Gibson WG, Peng TC, Croker BP. Age-associated C-cell hyperplasia in the human thyroid. Am J Pathol. 1982 Mar;106(3):388–93. PMID:6175219
1569. Gicquel C, Bertagna X, Schneid H, et al. Rearrangements at the 11p15 locus and overexpression of insulin-like growth factor-II gene in sporadic adrenocortical tumors. J Clin Endocrinol Metab. 1994 Jun;78(6):1444–53. PMID:7911125
1570. Gil-Carcedo LM, Coca MC. [First structure of the olfactory pathway. The olfactory cilium]. An Otorrinolaringol Ibero Am. 1988;15(1):85–96. Spanish. PMID:3281503
1571. Gild ML, Tsang V, Samra J, et al. Hypercalcemia in glucagon cell hyperplasia and neoplasia (Mahvash syndrome): a new association. J Clin Endocrinol Metab. 2018 Sep 1;103(9):3119–23. PMID:30032256
1572. Gill AJ. Succinate dehydrogenase (SDH) and mitochondrial driven neoplasia. Pathology. 2012 Jun;44(4):285–92. PMID:22544211
1573. Gill AJ. Succinate dehydrogenase (SDH)-deficient neoplasia. Histopathology. 2018 Jan;72(1):106–16. PMID:29239034
1574. Gill AJ. Understanding the genetic basis of parathyroid carcinoma. Endocr Pathol. 2014 Mar;25(1):30–4. PMID:24402736
1575. Gill AJ, Benn DE, Chou A, et al. Immunohistochemistry for SDHB triages genetic testing of SDHB, SDHC, and SDHD in paraganglioma-pheochromocytoma syndromes. Hum Pathol. 2010 Jun;41(6):805–14. PMID:20236688
1576. Gill AJ, Chou A, Vilain R, et al. Immunohistochemistry for SDHB divides gastrointestinal stromal tumors (GISTs) into 2 distinct types. Am J Surg Pathol. 2010 May;34(5):636–44. PMID:20305538
1577. Gill AJ, Chou A, Vilain RE, et al. "Pediatric-type" gastrointestinal stromal tumors are SDHB negative ("type 2") GISTs. Am J Surg Pathol. 2011 Aug;35(8):1245–7. PMID:21753704
1578. Gill AJ, Clarkson A, Gimm O, et al. Loss of nuclear expression of parafibromin distinguishes parathyroid carcinomas and hyperparathyroidism-jaw tumor (HPT-JT) syndrome-related adenomas from sporadic parathyroid adenomas and hyperplasias. Am J Surg Pathol. 2006 Sep;30(9):1140–9. PMID:16931959
1579. Gill AJ, Hes O, Papathomas T, et al. Succinate dehydrogenase (SDH)-deficient renal carcinoma: a morphologically distinct entity: a clinicopathologic series of 36 tumors from 27 patients. Am J Surg Pathol. 2014 Dec;38(12):1588–602. PMID:25025441
1580. Gill AJ, Lim G, Cheung VKY, et al. Parafibromin-deficient (HPT-JT Type, CDC73 Mutated) parathyroid tumors demonstrate distinctive morphologic features. Am J Surg Pathol. 2019 Jan;43(1):35–46. PMID:29324469
1581. Gill AJ, Pachter NS, Chou A, et al. Renal tumors associated with germline SDHB mutation show distinctive morphology. Am J Surg Pathol. 2011 Oct;35(10):1578–85. PMID:21934479
1582. Gill AJ, Toon CW, Clarkson A, et al. Succinate dehydrogenase deficiency is rare in pituitary adenomas. Am J Surg Pathol. 2014 Apr;38(4):560–6. PMID:24625421
1583. Gill CM, Orfanelli T, Yoxtheimer L, et al. Histology-specific FGFR2 alterations and FGFR2-TACC2 fusion in mixed adenoid cystic and neuroendocrine small cell carcinoma of the uterine cervix. Gynecol Oncol Rep. 2020 Nov 2;34:100668. PMID:33241100
1584. Gillenwater A, Lewin J, Roberts D, et al. Moderately differentiated neuroendocrine carcinoma (atypical carcinoid) of the larynx: a clinically aggressive tumor. Laryngoscope. 2005 Jul;115(7):1191–5. PMID:15995505
1585. Gilliland FD, Hunt WC, Morris DM, et al. Prognostic factors for thyroid carcinoma. A population-based study of 15,698 cases from the Surveillance, Epidemiology and End Results (SEER) program 1973-1991. Cancer. 1997 Feb 1;79(3):564–73. PMID:9028369
1586. Gimm O, Marsh DJ, Andrew SD, et al. Germline dinucleotide mutation in codon 883 of the RET proto-oncogene in multiple endocrine neoplasia type 2B without codon 918 mutation. J Clin Endocrinol Metab. 1997 Nov;82(11):3902–4. PMID:9360560
1587. Giner J, Esteban I, Carceller F, et al. Spinal adrenal cortical adenoma associated with Beckwith-Wiedemann syndrome: case report and review of the literature. Childs Nerv Syst. 2017 Jun;33(6):1009–13. PMID:28365908
1588. Ginter PS, Scognamiglio T. Papillary thyroid carcinoma with nodular fasciitis-like stroma: a usual entity with distinctive morphology. Int J Surg Pathol. 2015 Jun;23(4):305–7. PMID:25663334
1589. Giordano G, Corcione L, Giordano D, et al. Primary moderately differentiated neuroendocrine carcinoma (atypical carcinoid) of the larynx: a case report with immunohistochemical and molecular study. Auris Nasus Larynx. 2009 Apr;36(2):228–31. PMID:18617341
1590. Giordano TJ. The argument for mitotic rate-based grading for the prognostication of adrenocortical carcinoma. Am J Surg Pathol. 2011 Apr;35(4):471–3. PMID:21383612
1591. Giordano TJ, Berney D, de Krijger RR, et al. Data set for reporting of carcinoma of the adrenal cortex: explanations and recommendations of the guidelines from the International Collaboration on Cancer Reporting. Hum Pathol. 2021 Apr;110:50–61. PMID:33058949
1592. Giordano TJ, Kuick R, Else T, et al. Molecular classification and prognostication of adrenocortical tumors by transcriptome profiling. Clin Cancer Res. 2009 Jan 15;15(2):668–76. PMID:19147773
1593. Giordano TJ, Kuick R, Thomas DG, et al. Molecular classification of papillary thyroid carcinoma: distinct BRAF, RAS, and RET/PTC mutation-specific gene expression profiles discovered by DNA microarray analysis. Oncogene. 2005 Oct 6;24(44):6646–56. PMID:16007166
1594. Giordano TJ, Thomas DG, Kuick R, et al. Distinct transcriptional profiles of adrenocortical tumors uncovered by DNA microarray analysis. Am J Pathol. 2003 Feb;162(2):521–31. PMID:12547710
1595. Giovanella L, Bacigalupo L, Treglia G, et al. Will 18F-fluorocholine PET/CT replace other methods of preoperative parathyroid imaging? Endocrine. 2021 Feb;71(2):285–97. PMID:32892309
1596. Giovanella L, Ceriani L, Crippa S, et al. Imaging in endocrinology: Langherans cell histiocytosis of the thyroid gland detected by 18FDG-PET/CT. J Clin Endocrinol Metab. 2007 Aug;92(8):2866–7. PMID:17682085
1597. Giovanella L, Crippa S, Cariani L. Serum calcitonin-negative medullary thyroid carcinoma: role of CgA and CEA as complementary markers. Int J Biol Markers. 2008 Apr-Jun;23(2):129–31. PMID:18629788
1598. Giraldi L, Vecchioni A, Carioli G, et al. Risk factors for pancreas and lung neuroendocrine neoplasms: a case-control study. Endocrine. 2021 Jan;71(1):233–41. PMID:32869113
1599. Girardi DM, Silva ACB, Rêgo JFM, et al. Unraveling molecular pathways of poorly differentiated neuroendocrine carcinomas of the gastroenteropancreatic system: a systematic review. Cancer Treat Rev. 2017 May;56:28–35. PMID:28456055
1600. Giri D, Roncaroli F, Sinha A, et al. Silent Crooke's cell corticotroph adenoma of the pituitary gland presenting as delayed puberty. Endocrinol Diabetes Metab Case Rep. 2017 Mar 31;2017:16-0153. PMID:28458905
1601. Giusiano-Courcambeck S,

Denizot A, Secq V, et al. Pure spindle cell follicular carcinoma of the thyroid. Thyroid. 2008 Sep;18(9):1023–5. PMID:18788926
1602. Giusti F, Cianferotti L, Boaretto F, et al. Multiple endocrine neoplasia syndrome type 1: institution, management, and data analysis of a nationwide multicenter patient database. Endocrine. 2017 Nov;58(2):349–59. PMID:28132167
1603. Giustina A, Gola M, Doga M, et al. Clinical review 136: Primary lymphoma of the pituitary: an emerging clinical entity. J Clin Endocrinol Metab. 2001 Oct;86(10):4567–75. PMID:11600505
1604. Gläsker S, Li J, Xia JB, et al. Hemangioblastomas share protein expression with embryonal hemangioblast progenitor cell. Cancer Res. 2006 Apr 15;66(8):4167–72. PMID:16618738
1605. Gläsker S, Lonser RR, Tran MG, et al. Effects of VHL deficiency on endolymphatic duct and sac. Cancer Res. 2005 Dec 1;65(23):10847–53. PMID:16322231
1606. Gläsker S, Tran MG, Shively SB, et al. Epididymal cystadenomas and epithelial tumourlets: effects of VHL deficiency on the human epididymis. J Pathol. 2006 Sep;210(1):32–41. PMID:16841375
1607. Gläsker S, Vergauwen E, Koch CA, et al. Von Hippel-Lindau disease: current challenges and future prospects. Onco Targets Ther. 2020 Jun 16;13:5669–90. PMID:32606780
1608. Glatz K, Wegmann W. Papillary adenomatoid tumour of the adrenal gland. Histopathology. 2000 Oct;37(4):376–7. PMID:11184184
1609. Glenn ST, Jones CA, Sexton S, et al. Conditional deletion of p53 and Rb in the renin-expressing compartment of the pancreas leads to a highly penetrant metastatic pancreatic neuroendocrine carcinoma. Oncogene. 2014 Dec 11;33(50):5706–15. PMID:24292676
1610. Gnemmi V, Renaud F, Do Cao C, et al. Poorly differentiated thyroid carcinomas: application of the Turin proposal provides prognostic results similar to those from the assessment of high-grade features. Histopathology. 2014 Jan;64(2):263–73. PMID:24164362
1611. Gnepp DR, Ferlito A, Hyams V. Primary anaplastic small cell (oat cell) carcinoma of the larynx. Review of the literature and report of 18 cases. Cancer. 1983 May 1;51(9):1731–45. PMID:6299507
1612. Gnepp DR, Ogorzalek JM, Heffess CS. Fat-containing lesions of the thyroid gland. Am J Surg Pathol. 1989 Jul;13(7):605–12. PMID:2660611
1613. Goasguen N, Chirica M, Roger N, et al. Primary hyperparathyroidism from parathyroid microadenoma: specific features and implications for a surgical strategy in the era of minimally invasive parathyroidectomy. J Am Coll Surg. 2010 Apr;210(4):456–62. PMID:20347738
1614. Goel D, Enny L, Rana C, et al. Cystic adrenal lesions: a report of five cases. Cancer Rep (Hoboken). 2021 Feb;4(1):e1314. PMID:33295135
1615. Goffredo P, Roman SA, Sosa JA. Hurthle cell carcinoma: a population-level analysis of 3311 patients. Cancer. 2013 Feb 1;119(3):504–11. PMID:22893587
1616. Goffredo P, Sawka AM, Pura J, et al. Malignant struma ovarii: a population-level analysis of a large series of 68 patients. Thyroid. 2015 Feb;25(2):211–5. PMID:25375817
1617. Gogna S, Goldberg M, Samson D, et al. Medullary thyroid cancer in patients older than 45-epidemiologic trends and predictors of survival. Cancers (Basel). 2020 Oct 26;12(11):3124. PMID:33114488
1618. Goh G, Scholl UI, Healy JM, et al. Recurrent activating mutation in PRKACA in cortisol-producing adrenal tumors. Nat Genet. 2014 Jun;46(6):613–7. PMID:24747643
1619. Goh G, Walradt T, Markarov V, et al. Mutational landscape of MCPyV-positive and MCPyV-negative Merkel cell carcinomas with implications for immunotherapy. Oncotarget. 2016 Jan 19;7(3):3403–15. PMID:26655088
1620. Gokden M, Mrak RE. Pituitary adenoma with craniopharyngioma component. Hum Pathol. 2009 Aug;40(8):1189–93. PMID:19427020
1621. Goldinger JM, Hong RB, Lee SH, et al. Lack of interaction between atrial natriuretic factor and renal organic anion transport system. Proc Soc Exp Biol Med. 1986 Jul;182(3):358–63. PMID:2940600
1622. Golmard L, Vasta LM, Duflos V, et al. Testicular Sertoli cell tumour and potentially testicular Leydig cell tumour are features of DICER1 syndrome. J Med Genet. 2022 Apr;59(4):346–50. PMID:33782093
1623. Golouh R, Us-Krasovec M, Auersperg M, et al. Amphicrine–composite calcitonin and mucin-producing–carcinoma of the thyroid. Ultrastruct Pathol. 1985;8(2-3):197–206. PMID:4060258
1624. Golovko A, Kuryk O, Tkachenko R, et al. Thyroid metastasis of vaginal leiomyosarcoma: a case report and review of the literature. Exp Oncol. 2020 Sep;42(3):242–4. PMID:32996738
1625. Gómez-Ferrer M, Villanueva-Badenas E, Sánchez-Sánchez R, et al. HIF-1α and pro-inflammatory signaling improves the immunomodulatory activity of MSC-derived extracellular vesicles. Int J Mol Sci. 2021 Mar 26;22(7):3416. PMID:33810359
1626. Gomez-Hernandez K, Ezzat S, Asa SL, et al. Clinical implications of accurate subtyping of pituitary adenomas: perspectives from the treating physician. Turk Patoloji Derg. 2015;31 Suppl 1:4–17. PMID:26177314
1627. Gomez-Sanchez CE, Kuppusamy M, Reincke M, et al. Disordered CYP11B2 expression in primary aldosteronism. Horm Metab Res. 2017 Dec;49(12):957–62. PMID:29202495
1628. Gong J, Wang X, Chen X, et al. Adrenal and extra-adrenal nonfunctioning composite pheochromocytoma/paraganglioma with immunohistochemical ectopic hormone expression: comparison of two cases. Urol Int. 2010;85(3):368–72. PMID:20829582
1629. Gong X, Yu Y, Zhan W. Ultrasonographic findings of 1385 adrenal masses: a retrospective study of 1319 benign and 66 malignant masses. J Ultrasound Med. 2019 Sep;38(9):2249–57. PMID:29194699
1630. Gonzales-Laguado E, Guerra-Miller H, García-Ruiz L, et al. Intrathyroidal thymic carcinoma misdiagnosed as a medullary thyroid carcinoma. Cir Cir. 2020;88(Suppl 1):35–8. PMID:32963401
1631. González IA, Stewart DR, Schultz KAP, et al. DICER1 tumor predisposition syndrome: an evolving story initiated with the pleuropulmonary blastoma. Mod Pathol. 2022 Jan;35(1):4–22. PMID:34599283
1632. Gonzalez-Crussi F, Winkler RF, Mirkin DL. Sacrococcygeal teratomas in infants and children: relationship of histology and prognosis in 40 cases. Arch Pathol Lab Med. 1978 Aug;102(8):420–5. PMID:580884
1633. Gonzalez-Meljem JM, Haston S, Carreno G, et al. Stem cell senescence drives age-attenuated induction of pituitary tumours in mouse models of paediatric craniopharyngioma. Nat Commun. 2017 Nov 28;8(1):1819. PMID:29180744
1634. González-Sáez L, Pita-Fernández S, Lorenzo-Patiño MJ, et al. Primary melanoma of the adrenal gland: a case report and review of the literature. J Med Case Rep. 2011 Jul 2;5:273. PMID:21722390
1635. Goode B, Joseph NM, Stevers M, et al. Adenomatoid tumors of the male and female genital tract are defined by TRAF7 mutations that drive aberrant NF-kB pathway activation. Mod Pathol. 2018 Apr;31(4):660–73. PMID:29148537
1636. Gopal PP, Montone KT, Baloch Z, et al. The variable presentations of anaplastic spindle cell squamous carcinoma associated with tall cell variant of papillary thyroid carcinoma. Thyroid. 2011 May;21(5):493–9. PMID:21309723
1637. Gopal RK, Kübler K, Calvo SE, et al. Widespread chromosomal losses and mitochondrial DNA alterations as genetic drivers in Hürthle cell carcinoma. Cancer Cell. 2018 Aug 13;34(2):242–255.e5. PMID:30107175
1638. Gorelyshev A, Mazerkina N, Medvedeva O, et al. Second-hit APC mutation in a familial adamantinomatous craniopharyngioma. Neuro Oncol. 2020 Jun 9;22(6):889–91. PMID:32170310
1639. Gorlin RJ, Sedano HO, Vickers RA, et al. Multiple mucosal neuromas, pheochromocytoma and medullary carcinoma of the thyroid–a syndrome. Cancer. 1968 Aug;22(2):293–9. PMID:5660196
1640. Gosain R, Alexander JS, Gill A, et al. Radioactive iodine-refractory differentiated thyroid cancer in the elderly. Curr Oncol Rep. 2018 Sep 11;20(10):82. PMID:30206719
1641. Goschzik T, Gessi M, Dreschmann V, et al. Genomic alterations of adamantinomatous and papillary craniopharyngioma. J Neuropathol Exp Neurol. 2017 Feb 1;76(2):126–34. PMID:28069929
1642. Goto J, Otsuka F, Kodera R, et al. A rare tumor in the adrenal region: neuron-specific enolase (NSE)-producing leiomyosarcoma in an elderly hypertensive patient. Endocr J. 2008 Mar;55(1):175–81. PMID:18250540
1643. Goto K, Anan T, Nakatsuka T, et al. Low-grade neuroendocrine carcinoma of the skin (primary cutaneous carcinoid tumor) as a distinctive entity of cutaneous neuroendocrine tumors: a clinicopathologic study of 3 cases with literature review. Am J Dermatopathol. 2017 Apr;39(4):250–8. PMID:28169866
1644. Goto M, Miller RW, Ishikawa Y, et al. Excess of rare cancers in Werner syndrome (adult progeria). Cancer Epidemiol Biomarkers Prev. 1996 Apr;5(4):239–46. PMID:8722214
1645. Goudet P, Bonithon C, Costa A, et al. [A Multiple endocrine neoplasia type-1 observatory in a French-speaking area. A tool from the Endocrine Tumor study Group (GTE)]. Ann Endocrinol (Paris). 2007 Jun;68(2-3):154–9. French. PMID:17379178
1646. Goudet P, Bonithon-Kopp C, Murat A, et al. Gender-related differences in MEN1 lesion occurrence and diagnosis: a cohort study of 734 cases from the Groupe d'etude des Tumeurs Endocrines. Eur J Endocrinol. 2011 Jul;165(1):97–105. PMID:21551167
1647. Goudet P, Dalac A, Le Bras M, et al. MEN1 disease occurring before 21 years old: a 160-patient cohort study from the Groupe d'étude des Tumeurs Endocrines. J Clin Endocrinol Metab. 2015 Apr;100(4):1568–77. PMID:25594862
1648. Goudet P, Murat A, Binquet C, et al. Risk factors and causes of death in MEN1 disease. A GTE (Groupe d'Etude des Tumeurs Endocrines) cohort study among 758 patients. World J Surg. 2010 Feb;34(2):249–55. PMID:19949948
1649. Goujon A, Schoentgen N, Betari R, et al. Prognostic factors after adrenalectomy for adrenal metastasis. Int Urol Nephrol. 2020 Oct;52(10):1869–76. PMID:32419066
1650. Gould TJ, Johnson LN, Colapinto EV, et al. Intrasellar vascular malformation mimicking a pituitary macroadenoma. J Neuroophthalmol. 1996 Sep;16(3):199–203. PMID:8865015
1651. Gowrishankar S, Pai SA, Carney JA. Hyalinizing trabecular carcinoma of the thyroid gland. Histopathology. 2008 Mar;52(4):529–31. PMID:18315612
1652. Goyal G, Heaney ML, Collin M, et al. Erdheim-Chester disease: consensus recommendations for evaluation, diagnosis, and treatment in the molecular era. Blood. 2020 May 28;135(22):1929–45. PMID:32187362
1653. Goyal M, Batra S, Singh P, et al. Swyer syndrome with heterotopic adrenal cortical tissue in streak gonads: a rare case and review of literature. J Hum Reprod Sci. 2019 Oct-Dec;12(4):345–7. PMID:32038087
1654. Goyal R, Nada R, Rao KL, et al. Mixed medullary and follicular cell carcinoma of the thyroid with lymph node metastasis in a 7-year-old child. Pathol Int. 2006 Feb;56(2):84–8. PMID:16445820
1655. Gozu HI, Bircan R, Krohn K, et al. Similar prevalence of somatic TSH receptor and Gsalpha mutations in toxic thyroid nodules in geographical regions with different iodine supply in Turkey. Eur J Endocrinol. 2006 Oct;155(4):535–45. PMID:16990652
1656. Graceffa G, Cipolla C, Florena AM, et al. Primary schwannoma of the thyroid gland involving the isthmus: report of a case. Surg Today. 2013 Jan;43(1):106–9. PMID:22623175
1657. Graf H. [Thyroid nodular disease]. Arq Bras Endocrinol Metabol. 2004 Feb;48(1):93–104. Portuguese. PMID:15611822
1658. Graff-Baker A, Roman SA, Thomas DC, et al. Prognosis of primary thyroid lymphoma: demographic, clinical, and pathologic predictors of survival in 1,408 cases. Surgery. 2009 Dec;146(6):1105–15. PMID:19958938
1659. Graham RP, Lackner C, Terracciano L, et al. Fibrolamellar carcinoma in the Carney complex: PRKAR1A loss instead of the classic DNAJB1-PRKACA fusion. Hepatology. 2018 Oct;68(4):1441–7. PMID:29222914
1660. Graham RP, Shrestha B, Caron BL, et al. Islet-1 is a sensitive but not entirely specific marker for pancreatic neuroendocrine neoplasms and their metastases. Am J Surg Pathol. 2013 Mar;37(3):399–405. PMID:23348208
1661. Graillon T, Castinetti F, Chabert-Orsini V, et al. Functioning gonadotroph adenoma with severe ovarian hyperstimulation syndrome: A new emergency in pituitary adenoma surgery? Surgical considerations and literature review. Ann Endocrinol (Paris). 2019 Apr;80(2):122–7. PMID:30825998
1662. Grand B, Cazes A, Mordant P, et al. High grade neuroendocrine lung tumors: pathological characteristics, surgical management and prognostic implications. Lung Cancer. 2013 Sep;81(3):404–9. PMID:23769675
1663. Granero LE, Al-Lawati T, Bobin JY. Primary melanoma of the adrenal gland, a continuous dilemma: report of a case. Surg Today. 2004;34(6):554–6. PMID:15170557
1664. Grani G, Lamartina L, Durante C, et al. Follicular thyroid cancer and Hürthle cell carcinoma: challenges in diagnosis, treatment, and clinical management. Lancet Diabetes Endocrinol. 2018 Jun;6(6):500–14. PMID:29102432
1665. Granter SR, Badizadegan K, Fletcher CD. Myofibromatosis in adults, glomangiopericytoma, and myopericytoma: a spectrum of tumors showing perivascular myoid differentiation. Am J Surg Pathol. 1998 May;22(5):513–25. PMID:9591720
1666. Greco C, Brigante G, Taliani E, et al. Concomitant medullary thyroid carcinoma with paraganglioma-like pattern and papillary thyroid carcinoma. Endocrinol Diabetes Metab Case Rep. 2019 Nov 28;2019:19-0094. PMID:31778356
1667. Greenberg SE, Jacobs MF, Wachtel H, et al. Tumor detection rates in screening of

individuals with SDHx-related hereditary paraganglioma-pheochromocytoma syndrome. Genet Med. 2020 Dec;22(12):2101–7. PMID:32741965
1668. Gregório C, Rosset C, Alves LDS, et al. Synchronous periampullary tumors in a patient with pancreas divisum and neurofibromatosis type 1. Front Genet. 2020 Apr 28;11:395. PMID:32425982
1669. Griffin AC, Kelz R, LiVolsi VA. Aldosterone-secreting adrenal cortical carcinoma. A case report and review of the literature. Endocr Pathol. 2014 Sep;25(3):344–9. PMID:24682757
1670. Griffin GK, Sholl LM, Lindeman NI, et al. Targeted genomic sequencing of follicular dendritic cell sarcoma reveals recurrent alterations in NF-κB regulatory genes. Mod Pathol. 2016 Jan;29(1):67–74. PMID:26564005
1671. Grimm F, Maurus R, Beschorner R, et al. Ki-67 labeling index and expression of p53 are non-predictive for invasiveness and tumor size in functional and nonfunctional pituitary adenomas. Acta Neurochir (Wien). 2019 Jun;161(6):1149–56. PMID:31037500
1672. Griniatsos JE, Dimitriou N, Zilos A, et al. Bilateral adrenocortical carcinoma in a patient with multiple endocrine neoplasia type 1 (MEN1) and a novel mutation in the MEN1 gene. World J Surg Oncol. 2011 Jan 25;9:6. PMID:21266030
1673. Groeschl RT, Christians KK, Turaga KK, et al. Management of primary hepatopancreatobiliary small cell carcinoma. J Surg Oncol. 2013 Jun;107(7):692–5. PMID:23280574
1674. Grogan RH, Pacak K, Pasche L, et al. Bilateral adrenal medullary hyperplasia associated with an SDHB mutation. J Clin Oncol. 2011 Mar 10;29(8):e200–2. PMID:21172883
1675. Grossman RF, Tu SH, Duh QY, et al. Familial nonmedullary thyroid cancer. An emerging entity that warrants aggressive treatment. Arch Surg. 1995 Aug;130(8):892–7. PMID:7632152
1676. Grothey A. Risk assessment in stage II colon cancer: to treat or not to treat? Oncology (Williston Park). 2010 Jan;24(1 Suppl 1):1–2. PMID:20225604
1677. Groussin L, Jullian E, Perlemoine K, et al. Mutations of the PRKAR1A gene in Cushing's syndrome due to sporadic primary pigmented nodular adrenocortical disease. J Clin Endocrinol Metab. 2002 Sep;87(9):4324–9. PMID:12213893
1678. Groussin L, Kirschner LS, Vincent-Dejean C, et al. Molecular analysis of the cyclic AMP-dependent protein kinase A (PKA) regulatory subunit 1A (PRKAR1A) gene in patients with Carney complex and primary pigmented nodular adrenocortical disease (PPNAD) reveals novel mutations and clues for pathophysiology: augmented PKA signaling is associated with adrenal tumorigenesis in PPNAD. Am J Hum Genet. 2002 Dec;71(6):1433–42. PMID:12424709
1679. Groves C, Lamlum H, Crabtree M, et al. Mutation cluster region, association between germline and somatic mutations and genotype-phenotype correlation in upper gastrointestinal familial adenomatous polyposis. Am J Pathol. 2002 Jun;160(6):2055–61. PMID:12057910
1680. Grubbs EG, Ng PK, Bui J, et al. RET fusion as a novel driver of medullary thyroid carcinoma. J Clin Endocrinol Metab. 2015 Mar;100(3):788–93. PMID:25546157
1681. Grubbs EG, Williams MD, Scheet P, et al. Role of CDKN2C copy number in sporadic medullary thyroid carcinoma. Thyroid. 2016 Nov;26(11):1553–62. PMID:27610696
1682. Gruppetta M, Mercieca C, Vassallo J. Prevalence and incidence of pituitary adenomas: a population based study in Malta. Pituitary. 2013 Dec;16(4):545–53. PMID:23239049
1683. Gryder BE, Yohe ME, Chou HC, et al. PAX3-FOXO1 establishes myogenic super enhancers and confers BET bromodomain vulnerability. Cancer Discov. 2017 Aug;7(8):884–99. PMID:28446439
1684. Guadagno E, Cervasio M, Di Somma A, et al. Essential role of ultrastructural examination for spindle cell oncocytoma: case report of a rare neoplasm and review of the literature. Ultrastruct Pathol. 2016;40(2):121–4. PMID:27031178
1685. Guan H, Matonis D, Toraldo G, et al. Clinical significance of thyroid-stimulating hormone receptor gene mutations and/or sodium-iodine symporter gene overexpression in indeterminate thyroid fine needle biopsies. Front Endocrinol (Lausanne). 2018 Sep 25;9:566. PMID:30319546
1686. Guan H, Vandenbussche CJ, Erozan YS, et al. Can the tall cell variant of papillary thyroid carcinoma be distinguished from the conventional type in fine needle aspirates? A cytomorphologic study with assessment of diagnostic accuracy. Acta Cytol. 2013;57(5):534–42. PMID:24021475
1687. Guaraldi F, Zoli M, Righi A, et al. A practical algorithm to predict postsurgical recurrence and progression of pituitary neuroendocrine tumours (PitNET)s. Clin Endocrinol (Oxf). 2020 Jul;93(1):36–43. PMID:32306401
1688. Guarda LA, Ordonez NG, del Junco GW, et al. Gangliocytic paraganglioma of the duodenum: an immunocytochemical study. Am J Gastroenterol. 1983 Dec;78(12):794–8. PMID:6139954
1689. Guastamacchia E, Triggiani V, Tafaro E, et al. Evolution of a prolactin-secreting pituitary microadenoma into a fatal carcinoma: a case report. Minerva Endocrinol. 2007 Sep;32(3):231–6. PMID:17912159
1690. Gubbiotti MA, Livolsi V, Montone K, et al. Papillary thyroid microcarcinomas: does subtyping predict aggressive clinical behavior? Hum Pathol. 2021 Aug;114:28–35. PMID:33971214
1691. Gucer H, Bagci P, Bedir R, et al. The value of HBME-1 and Claudin-1 expression profile in the distinction of BRAF-like and RAS-like phenotypes in papillary thyroid carcinoma. Endocr Pathol. 2016 Sep;27(3):224–32. PMID:27153840
1692. Gucer H, Caliskan S, Kefeli M, et al. Do you know the details of your PAX8 antibody? Monoclonal PAX8 (MRQ-50) is not expressed in a series of 45 medullary thyroid carcinomas. Endocr Pathol. 2020 Mar;31(1):33–8. PMID:31912298
1693. Gucer H, Mete O. Endobronchial gangliocytic paraganglioma: not all keratin-positive endobronchial neuroendocrine neoplasms are pulmonary carcinoids. Endocr Pathol. 2014 Sep;25(3):356–8. PMID:23912549
1694. Gucer H, Szentgyorgyi E, Ezzat S, et al. Inhibin-expressing clear cell neuroendocrine tumor of the ampulla: an unusual presentation of von Hippel-Lindau disease. Virchows Arch. 2013 Oct;463(4):593–7. PMID:23913169
1695. Gudsoorkar PS, Asa SL, Silverman M. Syndrome of inappropriate antidiuresis in a young adult-searching for the causative needle in the proverbial haystack. Kidney Int Rep. 2019 Nov 6;5(2):231–4. PMID:32043038
1696. Guerges M, Slama E, Maskoni B, et al. Gangliocytic paraganglioma treated with ampullectomy, a case report. Ann Med Surg (Lond). 2016 Aug 16;11:16–20. PMID:27656281
1697. Guerrero MA, Suh I, Vriens MR, et al. Age and tumor size predicts lymph node involvement in Hürthle cell carcinoma. J Cancer. 2010 Jun 2;1:23–6. PMID:20842220
1698. Guerrero-Pérez F, Marengo AP, Vidal N, et al. Primary tumors of the posterior pituitary: a systematic review. Rev Endocr Metab Disord. 2019 Jun;20(2):219–38. PMID:30864049
1699. Guerrero-Pérez F, Vidal N, López-Vázquez M, et al. Sarcomas of the sellar region: a systematic review. Pituitary. 2021 Feb;24(1):117–29. PMID:32785833
1700. Guerrero-Pérez F, Vidal N, Marengo AP, et al. Posterior pituitary tumours: the spectrum of a unique entity. A clinical and histological study of a large case series. Endocrine. 2019 Jan;63(1):36–43. PMID:30276594
1701. Guillou L, Gebhard S, Coindre JM. Lipomatous hemangiopericytoma: a fat-containing variant of solitary fibrous tumor? Clinicopathologic, immunohistochemical, and ultrastructural analysis of a series in favor of a unifying concept. Hum Pathol. 2000 Sep;31(9):1108–15. PMID:11014579
1702. Guillou L, Gebhard S, Coindre JM. Orbital and extraorbital giant cell angiofibroma: a giant cell-rich variant of solitary fibrous tumor? Clinicopathologic and immunohistochemical analysis of a series in favor of a unifying concept. Am J Surg Pathol. 2000 Jul;24(7):971–9. PMID:10895819
1703. Guilmette J, Nosé V. Hereditary and familial thyroid tumours. Histopathology. 2018 Jan;72(1):70–81. PMID:29239041
1704. Guilmette JM, Nosé V. Neoplasms of the neuroendocrine pancreas: an update in the classification, definition, and molecular genetic advances. Adv Anat Pathol. 2019 Jan;26(1):13–30. PMID:29912000
1705. Gul S, Bahadir B, Dusak A, et al. Spherical amyloid deposition in a prolactin-producing pituitary adenoma. Neuropathology. 2009 Feb;29(1):81–4. PMID:18498287
1706. Gullo I, Batista R, Rodrigues-Pereira P, et al. Multinodular goiter progression toward malignancy in a case of DICER1 syndrome: histologic and molecular alterations. Am J Clin Pathol. 2018 Mar 29;149(5):379–86. PMID:29538609
1707. Gumbs AA, Moore PS, Falconi M, et al. Review of the clinical, histological, and molecular aspects of pancreatic endocrine neoplasms. J Surg Oncol. 2002 Sep;81(1):45–53. PMID:12210027
1708. Guo F, Song L, Meng Y. Malignant peripheral nerve sheath tumour following radiotherapy for pituitary adenoma. J Clin Neurosci. 2014 Jan;21(1):184–5. PMID:23830587
1709. Guo F, Wang G, Wang F, et al. Identification of novel genes involved in the pathogenesis of an ACTH-secreting pituitary carcinoma: a case report and literature review. Front Oncol. 2018 Nov 6;8:510. PMID:30460199
1710. Guo X, Chen H, Fu H, et al. Hereditary leiomyomatosis and renal cell carcinoma syndrome combined with adrenocortical carcinoma on 18F-FDG PET/CT. Clin Nucl Med. 2017 Sep;42(9):692–4. PMID:28737576
1711. Gupta G, Saran RK, Godhi S, et al. Composite pheochromocytoma masquerading as solid-pseudopapillary neoplasm of pancreas. World J Clin Cases. 2015 May 16;3(5):474–8. PMID:25984524
1712. Gupta P, Aggarwal R, Sarangi R. Solitary neurofibroma of the adrenal gland not associated with type-1 neurofibromatosis. Urol Ann. 2015 Jan-Mar;7(1):124–6. PMID:25657564
1713. Gupta R, Sharma A, Arora R, et al. Composite phaeochromocytoma with malignant peripheral nerve sheath tumour and rhabdomyosarcomatous differentiation in a patient without von Recklinghausen disease. J Clin Pathol. 2009 Jul;62(7):659–61. PMID:19561238
1714. Gupta S, Ajise O, Dultz L, et al. Follicular variant of papillary thyroid cancer: encapsulated, nonencapsulated, and diffuse: distinct biologic and clinical entities. Arch Otolaryngol Head Neck Surg. 2012 Mar;138(3):227–33. PMID:22431868
1715. Gupta S, Erickson LA. Paratesticular papillary cystadenoma of the epididymis in the setting of von Hippel-Lindau. Mayo Clin Proc. 2021 Mar;96(3):828–9. PMID:33673939
1716. Gupta S, Thompson RH, Boorjian SA, et al. High grade neuroendocrine carcinoma of the urinary bladder treated by radical cystectomy: a series of small cell, mixed neuroendocrine and large cell neuroendocrine carcinoma. Pathology. 2015 Oct;47(6):533–42. PMID:26308137
1717. Gupta S, Zhang J, Erickson LA. Composite pheochromocytoma/paraganglioma-ganglioneuroma: a clinicopathologic study of eight cases with analysis of succinate dehydrogenase. Endocr Pathol. 2017 Sep;28(3):269–75. PMID:28752484
1718. Gurazada K, Ihuoma A, Galloway M, et al. Nasally located ectopic ACTH-secreting pituitary adenoma (EAPA) causing Nelson's syndrome: diagnostic challenges. Pituitary. 2014 Oct;17(5):423–9. PMID:24065616
1719. Gurkan E, Gurbuz Y, Tarkun I, et al. Mixed medullary-papillary carcinoma of the thyroid: report of two cases and review of the literature. Indian J Pathol Microbiol. 2014 Oct-Dec;57(4):598–602. PMID:25308015
1720. Gururaj S, Nisal K, Davies Q, et al. Ectopic prolactin secretion secondary to an ovarian tumour. Endocrinol Diabetes Metab Case Rep. 2013;2013:130016. PMID:24616762
1721. Guyétant S, Bléchet C, Saint-André JP. C-cell hyperplasia. Ann Endocrinol (Paris). 2006 Jun;67(3):190–7. PMID:16840909
1722. Guyétant S, Rousselet MC, Durigon M, et al. Sex-related C cell hyperplasia in the normal human thyroid: a quantitative autopsy study. J Clin Endocrinol Metab. 1997 Jan;82(1):42–7. PMID:8989230
1723. Guyetant S, Wion-Barbot N, Rousselet MC, et al. C-cell hyperplasia associated with chronic lymphocytic thyroiditis: a retrospective quantitative study of 112 cases. Hum Pathol. 1994 May;25(5):514–21. PMID:8200646
1724. Guzel A, Tatli M, Senturk S, et al. Pituitary carcinoma presenting with multiple metastases: case report. J Child Neurol. 2008 Dec;23(12):1467–71. PMID:19073854
1725. Gyo K. Benign paroxysmal positional vertigo as a complication of postoperative bedrest. Laryngoscope. 1988 Mar;98(3):332–3. PMID:3343883
1726. Ha HJ, Kim EJ, Kim JS, et al. Major clues and pitfalls in the differential diagnosis of parathyroid and thyroid lesions using fine needle aspiration cytology. Medicina (Kaunas). 2020 Oct 24;56(11):558. PMID:33114338
1727. Ha LN, Iravani A, Nhung NT, et al. Relationship between clinicopathologic factors and FDG avidity in radioiodine-negative recurrent or metastatic differentiated thyroid carcinoma. Cancer Imaging. 2021 Jan 7;21(1):8. PMID:33413689
1728. Haas RL, Walraven I, Lecointe-Artzner E, et al. Extrameningeal solitary fibrous tumors-surgery alone or surgery plus perioperative radiotherapy: a retrospective study from the global solitary fibrous tumor initiative in collaboration with the Sarcoma Patients EuroNet. Cancer. 2020 Jul 1;126(13):3002–12. PMID:32315454
1729. Haase GM, O'Leary MC, Stram DO, et al. Pelvic neuroblastoma–implications for a new favorable subgroup: a Children's Cancer Group experience. Ann Surg Oncol. 1995 Nov;2(6):516–23. PMID:8591082
1730. Habra MA, Sukkari MA, Hasan A, et al. Epidemiological risk factors for adrenocortical carcinoma: a hospital-based case-control

study. Int J Cancer. 2020 Apr 1;146(7):1836–40. PMID:31241762
1731. Habu M, Tokimura H, Hirano H, et al. Pituitary metastases: current practice in Japan. J Neurosurg. 2015 Oct;123(4):998–1007. PMID:26186025
1732. Hackeng WM, Brosens LAA, Kim JY, et al. Non-functional pancreatic neuroendocrine tumours: ATRX/DAXX and alternative lengthening of telomeres (ALT) are prognostically independent from ARX/PDX1 expression and tumour size. Gut. 2022 May;71(5):961–73. PMID:33849943
1733. Hackeng WM, Dreijerink KMA, Offerhaus GJA, et al. A parathyroid-gut axis: hypercalcemia and the pathogenesis of gastrinoma in multiple endocrine neoplasia 1. Mol Cancer Res. 2021 Jun;19(6):946–9. PMID:33771883
1734. Hackeng WM, Schelhaas W, Morsink FHM, et al. Alternative lengthening of telomeres and differential expression of endocrine transcription factors distinguish metastatic and non-metastatic insulinomas. Endocr Pathol. 2020 Jun;31(2):108–18. PMID:32103422
1735. Haddad AF, Young JS, Oh T, et al. Clinical characteristics and outcomes of null-cell versus silent gonadotroph adenomas in a series of 1166 pituitary adenomas from a single institution. Neurosurg Focus. 2020 Jun;48(6):E13. PMID:32480370
1736. Haddad NM, Cavallerano JD, Silva PS. Von Hippel-Lindau disease: a genetic and clinical review. Semin Ophthalmol. 2013 Sep-Nov;28(5-6):377–86. PMID:24138046
1737. Haddy N, Andriamboavonjy T, Paoletti C, et al. Thyroid adenomas and carcinomas following radiotherapy for a hemangioma during infancy. Radiother Oncol. 2009 Nov;93(2):377–82. PMID:19515442
1738. Hafez MT, Hegazy MA, Abd Elwahab K, et al. Metastatic rhabdomyosarcoma of the thyroid gland, a case report. Head Neck Oncol. 2012 May 29;4:27. PMID:22642938
1739. Hagel C, Buslei R, Buchfelder M, et al. Immunoprofiling of glial tumours of the neurohypophysis suggests a common pituicytic origin of neoplastic cells. Pituitary. 2017 Apr;20(2):211–7. PMID:27744503
1740. Hagelstein-Rotman M, Meier ME, Majoor BCJ, et al. Increased prevalence of malignancies in fibrous dysplasia/McCune-Albright syndrome (FD/MAS): data from a national referral center and the Dutch National Pathology Registry (PALGA). Calcif Tissue Int. 2021 Mar;108(3):346–53. PMID:33226445
1741. Hagen C, Schroeder HD, Hansen S, et al. Temozolomide treatment of a pituitary carcinoma and two pituitary macroadenomas resistant to conventional therapy. Eur J Endocrinol. 2009 Oct;161(4):631–7. PMID:19654234
1742. Haglund F, Juhlin CC, Brown T, et al. TERT promoter mutations are rare in parathyroid tumors. Endocr Relat Cancer. 2015 Jun;22(3):L9–11. PMID:25876648
1743. Hahn MA, Howell VM, Gill AJ, et al. CDC73/HRPT2 CpG island hypermethylation and mutation of 5'-untranslated sequence are uncommon mechanisms of silencing parafibromin in parathyroid tumors. Endocr Relat Cancer. 2010 Feb 18;17(1):273–82. PMID:20026646
1744. Hahn MA, Marsh DJ. Identification of a functional bipartite nuclear localization signal in the tumor suppressor parafibromin. Oncogene. 2005 Sep 15;24(41):6241–8. PMID:16116486
1745. Hahn MA, Marsh DJ. Nucleolar localization of parafibromin is mediated by three nucleolar localization signals. FEBS Lett. 2007 Oct 30;581(26):5070–4. PMID:17923126
1746. Hahn SY, Shin JH, Lim HK, et al. Follicular variant of papillary thyroid carcinoma: comparison of ultrasound-guided core needle biopsy and ultrasound-guided fine needle aspiration in a multicentre study. Clin Endocrinol (Oxf). 2017 Jan;86(1):113–9. PMID:27338864
1747. Hahn SY, Shin JH, Oh YL, et al. Role of ultrasound in predicting tumor invasiveness in follicular variant of papillary thyroid carcinoma. Thyroid. 2017 Sep;27(9):1177–84. PMID:28699414
1748. Hakeem AH, Pradhan S, Bhele S, et al. Primary calcitonin-secreting neuroendocrine carcinoma of the supraglottic larynx. Ear Nose Throat J. 2015 Jan;94(1):E34–5. PMID:25606844
1749. Halászlaki C, Takács I, Butz H, et al. Novel genetic mutation in the background of Carney complex. Pathol Oncol Res. 2012 Apr;18(2):149–52. PMID:22297707
1750. Halfdanarson TR, Bamlet WR, McWilliams RR, et al. Risk factors for pancreatic neuroendocrine tumors: a clinic-based case-control study. Pancreas. 2014 Nov;43(8):1219–22. PMID:25291526
1751. Halfdanarson TR, Rabe KG, Rubin J, et al. Pancreatic neuroendocrine tumors (PNETs): incidence, prognosis and recent trend toward improved survival. Ann Oncol. 2008 Oct;19(10):1727–33. PMID:18515795
1752. Halfdanarson TR, Rubin J, Farnell MB, et al. Pancreatic endocrine neoplasms: epidemiology and prognosis of pancreatic endocrine tumors. Endocr Relat Cancer. 2008 Jun;15(2):409–27. PMID:18508996
1753. Hall BJ, Pincus LB, Yu SS, et al. Immunohistochemical prognostication of Merkel cell carcinoma: p63 expression but not polyomavirus status correlates with outcome. J Cutan Pathol. 2012 Oct;39(10):911–7. PMID:22882157
1754. Hall JE, Abdollahian DJ, Sinard RJ. Thyroid disease associated with Cowden syndrome: a meta-analysis. Head Neck. 2013 Aug;35(8):1189–94. PMID:22431287
1755. Haller F, Moskalev EA, Faucz FR, et al. Aberrant DNA hypermethylation of SDHC: a novel mechanism of tumor development in Carney triad. Endocr Relat Cancer. 2014 Aug;21(4):567–77. PMID:24859990
1756. Hama Y, Sugenoya A, Kobayashi S, et al. Squamous cell carcinoma arising from thyroglossal duct remnants: report of a case and results of immunohistochemical studies. Surg Today. 1997;27(11):1077–81. PMID:9413065
1757. Hamazaki M, Saito A. Beckwith-Wiedemann's syndrome–a report of an autopsied case–. Acta Pathol Jpn. 1979 Jan;29(1):99–107. PMID:433592
1758. Hamidi O, Raman R, Lazik N, et al. Clinical course of adrenal myelolipoma: a long-term longitudinal follow-up study. Clin Endocrinol (Oxf). 2020 Jul;93(1):11–8. PMID:32275787
1759. Hamilton NA, Liu TC, Cavatiao A, et al. Ki-67 predicts disease recurrence and poor prognosis in pancreatic neuroendocrine neoplasms. Surgery. 2012 Jul;152(1):107–13. PMID:22503317
1760. Hammarstedt L, Muth A, Wängberg B, et al. Adrenal lesion frequency: a prospective, cross-sectional CT study in a defined region, including systematic re-evaluation. Acta Radiol. 2010 Dec;51(10):1149–56. PMID:20969508
1761. Hammel PR, Vilgrain V, Terris B, et al. Pancreatic involvement in von Hippel-Lindau disease. The Groupe Francophone d'Etude de la Maladie de von Hippel-Lindau. Gastroenterology. 2000 Oct;119(4):1087–95. PMID:11040195
1762. Han F, Zhang L, Zhang S, et al. Occult oncocytic papillary thyroid carcinoma with lymphoid stroma (Warthin-like tumor): report of a case with concomitant mutations of BRAF V600E and V600K. Int J Clin Exp Pathol. 2015 May 1;8(5):5896–901. PMID:26191315
1763. Hanafy AK, Mujtaba B, Roman-Colon AM, et al. Imaging features of adrenal gland masses in the pediatric population. Abdom Radiol (NY). 2020 Apr;45(4):964–81. PMID:31538225
1764. Handra-Luca A, Belleannee G, Straub B. Psammomatoid calcification-rich oncocytic thyroid adenoma with clear-cell change. Clin Pathol. 2019 Mar 18;12:2632010X19829251. PMID:30911738
1765. Hang JF, Siddiqui MT, Ali SZ. Fine needle aspiration of langerhans cell histiocytosis: a cytopathologic study of 37 cases. Acta Cytol. 2017;61(2):96–102. PMID:28407623
1766. Hänggi D, Adams H, Hans VH, et al. Recurrent glomus tumor of the sellar region with malignant progression. Acta Neuropathol. 2005 Jul;110(1):93–6. PMID:15952045
1767. Hanna AN, Michael CW, Jing X. Mixed medullary-follicular carcinoma of the thyroid: diagnostic dilemmas in fine-needle aspiration cytology. Diagn Cytopathol. 2011 Nov;39(11):862–5. PMID:21994201
1768. Hanna FW, Ardill JE, Johnston CF, et al. Regulatory peptides and other neuroendocrine markers in medullary carcinoma of the thyroid. J Endocrinol. 1997 Feb;152(2):275–81. PMID:9071985
1769. Hannah-Shmouni F, Faucz FR, Stratakis CA. Alterations of phosphodiesterases in adrenocortical tumors. Front Endocrinol (Lausanne). 2016 Aug 30;7:111. PMID:27625633
1770. Hannah-Shmouni F, Morissette R, Sinaii N, et al. Revisiting the prevalence of nonclassic congenital adrenal hyperplasia in US Ashkenazi Jews and Caucasians. Genet Med. 2017 Nov;19(11):1276–9. PMID:28541281
1771. Hannah-Shmouni F, Stratakis CA. Growth hormone excess in neurofibromatosis 1. Genet Med. 2019 May;21(5):1254–5. PMID:30283094
1772. Hannah-Shmouni F, Trivellin G, Stratakis CA. Genetics of gigantism and acromegaly. Growth Horm IGF Res. 2016 Oct-Dec;30-31:37–41. PMID:27657986
1773. Hapke MR, Dehner LP. The optically clear nucleus. A reliable sign of papillary carcinoma of the thyroid? Am J Surg Pathol. 1979 Feb;3(1):31–8. PMID:534382
1774. Happle R. The McCune-Albright syndrome: a lethal gene surviving by mosaicism. Clin Genet. 1986 Apr;29(4):321–4. PMID:3720010
1775. Haque S, Modlin IM, West AB. Multiple glomus tumors of the stomach with intravascular spread. Am J Surg Pathol. 1992 Mar;16(3):291–9. PMID:1317998
1776. Hara T, Akutsu H, Takano S, et al. Clinical and biological significance of adamantinomatous craniopharyngioma with CTNNB1 mutation. J Neurosurg. 2019 Jul 1;131(1):217–26. PMID:30074466
1777. Harach HR, Escalante DA, Onativia A, et al. Thyroid carcinoma and thyroiditis in an endemic goitre region before and after iodine prophylaxis. Acta Endocrinol (Copenh). 1985 Jan;108(1):55–60. PMID:3969810
1778. Harach HR, Franssila KO. Thyroglobulin immunostaining in follicular thyroid carcinoma: relationship to the degree of differentiation and cell type. Histopathology. 1988 Jul;13(1):43–54. PMID:3061922
1779. Harach HR, Lesueur F, Amati P, et al. Histology of familial thyroid tumours linked to a gene mapping to chromosome 19p13.2. J Pathol. 1999 Nov;189(3):387–93. PMID:10547601
1780. Harach HR, Sánchez SS, Williams ED. Pathology of the autonomously functioning (hot) thyroid nodule. Ann Diagn Pathol. 2002 Feb;6(1):10–9. PMID:11842375
1781. Harach HR, Soubeyran I, Brown A, et al. Thyroid pathologic findings in patients with Cowden disease. Ann Diagn Pathol. 1999 Dec;3(6):331–40. PMID:10594284
1782. Harach HR, Williams ED. Glandular (tubular and follicular) variants of medullary carcinoma of the thyroid. Histopathology. 1983 Jan;7(1):83–97. PMID:6840715
1783. Harach HR, Williams GT, Williams ED. Familial adenomatous polyposis associated thyroid carcinoma: a distinct type of follicular cell neoplasm. Histopathology. 1994 Dec;25(6):549–61. PMID:7698732
1784. Harada K, Yasuda M, Hasegawa K, et al. A novel case of myxoid variant of adrenocortical carcinoma in a patient with multiple endocrine neoplasia type 1. Endocr J. 2019 Aug 29;66(8):739–44. PMID:31118348
1785. Harari A, Waring A, Fernandez-Ranvier G, et al. Parathyroid carcinoma: a 43-year outcome and survival analysis. J Clin Endocrinol Metab. 2011 Dec;96(12):3679–86. PMID:21937626
1786. Hardy J. Transsphenoidal surgery of hypersecreting pituitary tumours. In: Kohler PO, Ross GT, editors. Diagnosis and treatment of pituitary tumors. International Congress Series No. 303. Amsterdam (Netherlands): Exerpta Medica; 1973. pp. 179–98.
1787. Haresh KP, Prabhakar R, Anand Rajan KD, et al. A rare case of paraganglioma of the sella with bone metastases. Pituitary. 2009;12(3):276–9. PMID:18320326
1788. Hargreaves HK, Wright TC Jr. A large functioning parathyroid lipoadenoma found in the posterior mediastinum. Am J Clin Pathol. 1981 Jul;76(1):89–93. PMID:7258157
1789. Harmon CM, Brown N. Langerhans cell histiocytosis: a clinicopathologic review and molecular pathogenetic update. Arch Pathol Lab Med. 2015 Oct;139(10):1211–4. PMID:26414464
1790. Harms KL, Healy MA, Nghiem P, et al. Analysis of prognostic factors from 9387 Merkel cell carcinoma cases forms the basis for the new 8th edition AJCC Staging System. Ann Surg Oncol. 2016 Oct;23(11):3564–71. PMID:27198511
1791. Harms KL, Zhao L, Johnson B, et al. Virus-positive Merkel cell carcinoma is an independent prognostic group with distinct predictive biomarkers. Clin Cancer Res. 2021 May 1;27(9):2494–504. PMID:33547200
1792. Harms PW. Update on Merkel cell carcinoma. Clin Lab Med. 2017 Sep;37(3):485–501. PMID:28802497
1793. Harms PW, Vats P, Verhaegen ME, et al. The distinctive mutational spectra of polyomavirus-negative Merkel cell carcinoma. Cancer Res. 2015 Sep 15;75(18):3720–7. PMID:26238782
1794. Harms PW, Verhaegen ME, Hu K, et al. Genomic evidence suggests that cutaneous neuroendocrine carcinomas can arise from squamous dysplastic precursors. Mod Pathol. 2022 Apr;35(4):506–14. PMID:34593967
1795. Haroche J, Charlotte F, Arnaud L, et al. High prevalence of BRAF V600E mutations in Erdheim-Chester disease but not in other non-Langerhans cell histiocytoses. Blood. 2012 Sep 27;120(13):2700–3. PMID:22879539
1796. Harrer P, Bröcker M, Zint A, et al. The clonality of nodules in recurrent goiters at second surgery. Langenbecks Arch Surg. 1998 Dec;383(6):453–5. PMID:9921946
1797. Harrington F, Greenslade M, Talaulikar D, et al. Genomic characterisation of diffuse large B-cell lymphoma. Pathology. 2021 Apr;53(3):367–76. PMID:33642095
1798. Harrington KJ, Michalaki VJ, Vini L, et al. Management of non-Hodgkin's lymphoma of the thyroid: the Royal Marsden Hospital experience. Br J Radiol. 2005 May;78(929):405–10. PMID:15845932
1799. Harrison B, Moore AM, Calfee R, et al. The association between glomus tumors and

neurofibromatosis. J Hand Surg Am. 2013 Aug;38(8):1571–4. PMID:23849732
1800. Harrison B, Sammer D. Glomus tumors and neurofibromatosis: a newly recognized association. Plast Reconstr Surg Glob Open. 2014 Oct 7;2(9):e214. PMID:25426397
1801. Hart ES, Kelly MH, Brillante B, et al. Onset, progression, and plateau of skeletal lesions in fibrous dysplasia and the relationship to functional outcome. J Bone Miner Res. 2007 Sep;22(9):1468–74. PMID:17501668
1802. Hartl DM, Al Ghuzlan A, Chami L, et al. High rate of multifocality and occult lymph node metastases in papillary thyroid carcinoma arising in thyroglossal duct cysts. Ann Surg Oncol. 2009 Sep;16(9):2595–601. PMID:19565286
1803. Hartlieb SA, Sieverling L, Nadler-Holly M, et al. Alternative lengthening of telomeres in childhood neuroblastoma from genome to proteome. Nat Commun. 2021 Feb 24;12(1):1269. PMID:33627664
1804. Hasan M, Siddiqui F, Al-Ajmi M. FNA diagnosis of adrenal myelolipoma: a rare entity. Diagn Cytopathol. 2008 Dec;36(12):925–6. PMID:18855887
1805. Hasan R, Marshall MC Jr, Medhi M, et al. Meningioma metastatic to thyroid gland. Endocr Pract. 2001 Sep-Oct;7(5):370–4. PMID:11585373
1806. Hasegawa H, Van Gompel JJ, Oushy SH, et al. A comprehensive study of spindle cell oncocytoma of the pituitary gland: series of 6 cases and meta-analysis of 85 cases. World Neurosurg. 2021 May;149:e197–216. PMID:33610869
1807. Hashimoto S, Hayasaka K, Suzuki K, et al. Thymic small cell carcinoma associated with lambert-eaton myasthenic syndrome. Ann Thorac Surg. 2020 May;109(5):e347–8. PMID:31586614
1808. Hasney CP, Amedee RG. Mixed medullary-papillary carcinoma of the thyroid: a case report. Laryngoscope. 2010;120 Suppl 4:S153. PMID:21225751
1809. Hasselblatt M, Jeibmann A, Gerss J, et al. Cellular and reticular variants of haemangioblastoma revisited: a clinicopathologic study of 88 cases. Neuropathol Appl Neurobiol. 2005 Dec;31(6):618–22. PMID:16281910
1810. Hasselblatt M, Thomas C, Hovestadt V, et al. Poorly differentiated chordoma with SMARCB1/INI1 loss: a distinct molecular entity with dismal prognosis. Acta Neuropathol. 2016 Jul;132(1):149–51. PMID:27067307
1811. Hassoun AA, Hay ID, Goellner JR, et al. Insular thyroid carcinoma in adolescents: a potentially lethal endocrine malignancy. Cancer. 1997 Mar 1;79(5):1044–8. PMID:9041169
1812. Haston S, Pozzi S, Carreno G, et al. MAPK pathway control of stem cell proliferation and differentiation in the embryonic pituitary provides insights into the pathogenesis of papillary craniopharyngioma. Development. 2017 Jun 15;144(12):2141–52. PMID:28506993
1813. Hata JL, Correa H, Krishnan C, et al. Diagnostic utility of PHOX2B in primary and treated neuroblastoma and in neuroblastoma metastatic to the bone marrow. Arch Pathol Lab Med. 2015 Apr;139(4):543–6. PMID:25822764
1814. Hatano K, Horii S, Nakai Y, et al. The outcomes of adrenalectomy for solitary adrenal metastasis: a 17-year single-center experience. Asia Pac J Clin Oncol. 2020 Apr;16(2):e86–90. PMID:30270570
1815. Hattori S, Yamane Y, Shimomura R, et al. Carney complex: a case with thyroid follicular adenoma without a PRKAR1A mutation. Surg Case Rep. 2018 Apr 17;4(1):34. PMID:29666959
1816. Hauffa BP, Menzel D, Stolecke H. Age-related changes in adrenal size during the first year of life in normal newborns, infants and patients with congenital adrenal hyperplasia due to 21-hydroxylase deficiency: comparison of ultrasound and hormonal parameters. Eur J Pediatr. 1988 Oct;148(1):43–9. PMID:2973986
1817. Haugen BR, Alexander EK, Bible KC, et al. 2015 American Thyroid Association management guidelines for adult patients with thyroid nodules and differentiated thyroid cancer: the American Thyroid Association Guidelines Task Force on Thyroid Nodules and Differentiated Thyroid Cancer. Thyroid. 2016 Jan;26(1):1–133. PMID:26462967
1818. Haugen BR, Sawka AM, Alexander EK, et al. American Thyroid Association guidelines on the management of thyroid nodules and Differentiated Thyroid Cancer Task Force review and recommendation on the proposed renaming of encapsulated follicular variant papillary thyroid carcinoma without invasion to noninvasive follicular thyroid neoplasm with papillary-like nuclear features. Thyroid. 2017 Apr;27(4):481–3. PMID:28114862
1819. Haugen BR, Sherman SI. Evolving approaches to patients with advanced differentiated thyroid cancer. Endocr Rev. 2013 Jun;34(3):439–55. PMID:23575762
1820. Hautzel H, Alnajdawi Y, Fendler WP, et al. N-staging in large cell neuroendocrine carcinoma of the lung: diagnostic value of [18F] FDG PET/CT compared to the histopathology reference standard. EJNMMI Res. 2021 Jul 22;11(1):68. PMID:34292419
1821. Haven CJ, van Puijenbroek M, Karperien M, et al. Differential expression of the calcium sensing receptor and combined loss of chromosomes 1q and 11q in parathyroid carcinoma. J Pathol. 2004 Jan;202(1):86–94. PMID:14694525
1822. Haven CJ, van Puijenbroek M, Tan MH, et al. Identification of MEN1 and HRPT2 somatic mutations in paraffin-embedded (sporadic) parathyroid carcinomas. Clin Endocrinol (Oxf). 2007 Sep;67(3):370–6. PMID:17555500
1823. Haven CJ, Wong FK, van Dam EW, et al. A genotypic and histopathological study of a large Dutch kindred with hyperparathyroidism-jaw tumor syndrome. J Clin Endocrinol Metab. 2000 Apr;85(4):1449–54. PMID:10770180
1824. Håvik AL, Bruland O, Myrseth E, et al. Genetic landscape of sporadic vestibular schwannoma. J Neurosurg. 2018 Mar;128(3):911–22. PMID:28409725
1825. Havrankova E, Stenova E, Olejarova I, et al. Carney complex with biatrial cardiac myxoma. Ann Thorac Cardiovasc Surg. 2014;20 Suppl:890–2. PMID:24088910
1826. Hawkins DS, Gupta AA, Rudzinski ER. What is new in the biology and treatment of pediatric rhabdomyosarcoma? Curr Opin Pediatr. 2014 Feb;26(1):50–6. PMID:24326270
1827. Hay ID, Hutchinson ME, Gonzalez-Losada T, et al. Papillary thyroid microcarcinoma: a study of 900 cases observed in a 60-year period. Surgery. 2008 Dec;144(6):980–7. PMID:19041007
1828. Hay ID, Johnson TR, Kaggal S, et al. Papillary thyroid carcinoma (PTC) in children and adults: comparison of initial presentation and long-term postoperative outcome in 4432 patients consecutively treated at the Mayo Clinic during eight decades (1936-2015). World J Surg. 2018 Feb;42(2):329–42. PMID:29030676
1829. Hayashi D, Kusutani N, Sowa-Osako J, et al. Combined Merkel cell carcinoma and sebaceous carcinoma in the eyelid with cervical lymph node metastasis of both components. J Dermatol. 2021 Apr;48(4):e175–7. PMID:33533503
1830. Hayashi K, Inoshita N, Kawaguchi K, et al. The USP8 mutational status may predict drug susceptibility in corticotroph adenomas of Cushing's disease. Eur J Endocrinol. 2016 Feb;174(2):213–26. PMID:26578638
1831. Hayashi T, Gucer H, Mete O. A mimic of sarcomatoid adrenal cortical carcinoma: epithelioid angiosarcoma occurring in adrenal cortical adenoma. Endocr Pathol. 2014 Dec;25(4):404–9. PMID:25246132
1832. Haydar Ali Tajuddin A, Kamaruddin N, Sukor N, et al. Estrogen receptors in nonfunctioning pituitary neuroendocrine tumors: review on expression and gonadotroph functions. J Endocr Soc. 2020 Oct 19;4(12):bvaa157. PMID:33241169
1833. Haymerle G, Janik S, Fochtmann A, et al. Expression of Merkelcell polyomavirus (MCPyV) large T-antigen in Merkel cell carcinoma lymph node metastases predicts poor outcome. PLoS One. 2017 Aug 1;12(8):e0180426. PMID:28763479
1834. He C, Yang Y, Yang Y, et al. Teratoma of the adrenal gland: clinical experience and literature review. Gland Surg. 2020 Aug;9(4):1056–64. PMID:32953615
1835. He H, Bronisz A, Liyanarachchi S, et al. SRGAP1 is a candidate gene for papillary thyroid carcinoma susceptibility. J Clin Endocrinol Metab. 2013 May;98(5):E973–80. PMID:23539728
1836. He H, Li W, Comiskey DF, et al. A truncating germline mutation of TINF2 in individuals with thyroid cancer or melanoma results in longer telomeres. Thyroid. 2020 Feb;30(2):204–13. PMID:31928178
1837. He H, Nagy R, Liyanarachchi S, et al. A susceptibility locus for papillary thyroid carcinoma on chromosome 8q24. Cancer Res. 2009 Jan 15;69(2):625–31. PMID:19147577
1838. He MX, Cuoco MS, Crowdis J, et al. Transcriptional mediators of treatment resistance in lethal prostate cancer. Nat Med. 2021 Mar;27(3):426–33. PMID:33664492
1839. He W, Chen F, Dalm B, et al. Metastatic involvement of the pituitary gland: a systematic review with pooled individual patient data analysis. Pituitary. 2015 Feb;18(1):159–68. PMID:24445565
1840. He WG, Yan Y, Tang W, et al. Clinical and biological features of neuroblastic tumors: a comparison of neuroblastoma and ganglioneuroblastoma. Oncotarget. 2017 Jun 6;8(23):37730–9. PMID:28465480
1841. He X, Wang L, Yan J, et al. Menin localization in cell membrane compartment. Cancer Biol Ther. 2016;17(1):114–22. PMID:26560942
1842. He YQ, Lu HZ, Li DZ, et al. Recurrent granular cell tumor of the thyroid: a case report and literature review. BMC Surg. 2020 Jul 14;20(1):154. PMID:32669088
1843. Heaphy CM, Bi WL, Coy S, et al. Telomere length alterations and ATRX/DAXX loss in pituitary adenomas. Mod Pathol. 2020 Aug;33(8):1475–81. PMID:32203094
1844. Heaphy CM, de Wilde RF, Jiao Y, et al. Altered telomeres in tumors with ATRX and DAXX mutations. Science. 2011 Jul 22;333(6041):425. PMID:21719641
1845. Heath H 3rd, Edis AJ. Pheochromocytoma associated with hypercalcemia and ectopic secretion of calcitonin. Ann Intern Med. 1979 Aug;91(2):208–10. PMID:464464
1846. Heath M, Jaimes N, Lemos B, et al. Clinical characteristics of Merkel cell carcinoma at diagnosis in 195 patients: the AEIOU features. J Am Acad Dermatol. 2008 Mar;58(3):375–81. PMID:18280333
1847. Heck A, Ringstad G, Fougner SL, et al. Intensity of pituitary adenoma on T2-weighted magnetic resonance imaging predicts the response to octreotide treatment in newly diagnosed acromegaly. Clin Endocrinol (Oxf). 2012 Jul;77(1):72–8. PMID:22066905
1848. Heck JE, Lee PC, Wu CK, et al. Gestational risk factors and childhood cancers: a cohort study in Taiwan. Int J Cancer. 2020 Sep 1;147(5):1343–53. PMID:32020595
1849. Hedgire SS, McDermott S, Borczuk D, et al. The spectrum of IgG4-related disease in the abdomen and pelvis. AJR Am J Roentgenol. 2013 Jul;201(1):14–22. PMID:23789654
1850. Heetfeld M, Chougnet CN, Olsen IH, et al. Characteristics and treatment of patients with G3 gastroenteropancreatic neuroendocrine neoplasms. Endocr Relat Cancer. 2015 Aug;22(4):657–64. PMID:26113608
1851. Heffess CS, Wenig BM, Thompson LD. Metastatic renal cell carcinoma to the thyroid gland: a clinicopathologic study of 36 cases. Cancer. 2002 Nov 1;95(9):1869–78. PMID:12404280
1852. Hegedüs L, Bonnema SJ, Bennedbaek FN. Management of simple nodular goiter: current status and future perspectives. Endocr Rev. 2003 Feb;24(1):102–32. PMID:12588812
1853. Heide S, Masliah-Planchon J, Isidor B, et al. Oncologic phenotype of peripheral neuroblastic tumors associated with PHOX2B non-polyalanine repeat expansion mutations. Pediatr Blood Cancer. 2016 Jan;63(1):71–7. PMID:26375764
1854. Heilmann AM, Subbiah V, Wang K, et al. Comprehensive genomic profiling of clinically advanced medullary thyroid carcinoma. Oncology. 2016;90(6):339–46. PMID:27207748
1855. Hellgren LS, Hysek M, Jatta K, et al. Macrofollicular variant of follicular thyroid carcinoma (MV-FTC) with a somatic DICER1 gene mutation: case report and review of the literature. Head Neck Pathol. 2021 Jun;15(2):668–75. PMID:32712880
1856. Helton M, Abu-Rmaileh M, Thomas K, et al. Pituitary metastatic composite tumors: a case report with next-generation sequencing and review of the literature. Case Rep Oncol Med. 2020 Jul 21;2020:5073236. PMID:32774962
1857. Hemminki K, Eng C, Chen B. Familial risks for nonmedullary thyroid cancer. J Clin Endocrinol Metab. 2005 Oct;90(10):5747–53. PMID:16030170
1858. Hemminki K, Liu X, Ji J, et al. Kaposi sarcoma and Merkel cell carcinoma after autoimmune disease. Int J Cancer. 2012 Aug 1;131(3):E326–8. PMID:22120659
1859. Hempenstall LE, Siriwardana AR, Desai DJ. Investigation of a renal mass: diagnosing renal paraganglioma. Urol Case Rep. 2018 Aug 9;21:8–9. PMID:30116720
1860. Hendrick JW. Leiomyoma of thyroid gland; report of case. Surgery. 1957 Sep;42(3):597–9. PMID:13467621
1861. Heng LJ, Jia D, Gong L, et al. Endoscopic endonasal resection of a mixed lesion of gangliocytoma and nonfunctioning pituitary adenoma. World Neurosurg. 2017 Oct;106:1050.e1–6. PMID:28532920
1862. Henopp T, Anlauf M, Schmitt A, et al. Glucagon cell adenomatosis: a newly recognized disease of the endocrine pancreas. J Clin Endocrinol Metab. 2009 Jan;94(1):213–7. PMID:18957496
1863. Henry I, Jeanpierre M, Couillin P, et al. Molecular definition of the 11p15.5 region involved in Beckwith-Wiedemann syndrome and probably in predisposition to adrenocortical carcinoma. Hum Genet. 1989 Feb;81(3):273–7. PMID:2921038
1864. Héritier S, Saffroy R, Radosevic-Robin N, et al. Common cancer-associated PIK3CA activating mutations rarely occur in Langerhans cell histiocytosis. Blood. 2015 Apr 9;125(15):2448–9. PMID:25858893
1865. Hermann G, Konukiewitz B, Schmitt A, et al. Hormonally defined pancreatic and

duodenal neuroendocrine tumors differ in their transcription factor signatures: expression of ISL1, PDX1, NGN3, and CDX2. Virchows Arch. 2011 Aug;459(2):147–54. PMID:21739268
1866. Hermans BCM, Derks JL, Thunnissen E, et al. Prevalence and prognostic value of PD-L1 expression in molecular subtypes of metastatic large cell neuroendocrine carcinoma (LCNEC). Lung Cancer. 2019 Apr;130:179–86. PMID:30885341
1867. Hernández García J, Negro Alvarez JM, García Sellés FJ, et al. [Adverse reactions to food preservatives]. Allergol Immunopathol (Madr). 1986 Jan-Feb;14(1):55–63. Spanish. PMID:2421566
1868. Hernandez KG, Ezzat S, Morel CF, et al. Familial pheochromocytoma and renal cell carcinoma syndrome: TMEM127 as a novel candidate gene for the association. Virchows Arch. 2015 Jun;466(6):727–32. PMID:25800244
1869. Hernandez-Prera JC, Machado RA, Asa SL, et al. Pathologic reporting of tall-cell variant of papillary thyroid cancer: Have we reached a consensus? Thyroid. 2017 Dec;27(12):1498–504. PMID:29020884
1870. Hernandez-Prera JC, Valderrabano P, Creed JH, et al. Molecular determinants of thyroid nodules with indeterminate cytology and RAS mutations. Thyroid. 2021 Jan;31(1):36–49. PMID:32689909
1871. Hernández-Ramírez LC, Gabrovska P, Dénes J, et al. Landscape of familial isolated and young-onset pituitary adenomas: prospective diagnosis in AIP mutation carriers. J Clin Endocrinol Metab. 2015 Sep;100(9):E1242–54. PMID:26186299
1872. Hernández-Ramírez LC, Gam R, Valdés N, et al. Loss-of-function mutations in the CABLES1 gene are a novel cause of Cushing's disease. Endocr Relat Cancer. 2017 Aug;24(8):379–92. PMID:28533356
1873. Herndon J, Nadeau AM, Davidge-Pitts CJ, et al. Primary adrenal insufficiency due to bilateral infiltrative disease. Endocrine. 2018 Dec;62(3):721–8. PMID:30178435
1874. Herriges JC, Brown S, Longhurst M, et al. Identification of two 14q32 deletions involving DICER1 associated with the development of DICER1-related tumors. Eur J Med Genet. 2019 Jan;62(1):9–14. PMID:29698806
1875. Hervier B, Haroche J, Arnaud L, et al. Association of both Langerhans cell histiocytosis and Erdheim-Chester disease linked to the BRAFV600E mutation. Blood. 2014 Aug 14;124(7):1119–26. PMID:24894769
1876. Heseltine D, White MC, Kendall-Taylor P, et al. Testicular enlargement and elevated serum inhibin concentrations occur in patients with pituitary macroadenomas secreting follicle stimulating hormone. Clin Endocrinol (Oxf). 1989 Oct;31(4):411–23. PMID:2627747
1877. Heshmati HM, Fatourechi V, van Heerden JA, et al. Thyroglossal duct carcinoma: report of 12 cases. Mayo Clin Proc. 1997 Apr;72(4):315–9. PMID:9121176
1878. Hess KR, Varadhachary GR, Taylor SH, et al. Metastatic patterns in adenocarcinoma. Cancer. 2006 Apr 1;106(7):1624–33. PMID:16518827
1879. Heukamp LC, Thor T, Schramm A, et al. Targeted expression of mutated ALK induces neuroblastoma in transgenic mice. Sci Transl Med. 2012 Jul 4;4(141):141ra91. PMID:22764207
1880. Hibbitts E, Chi YY, Hawkins DS, et al. Refinement of risk stratification for childhood rhabdomyosarcoma using FOXO1 fusion status in addition to established clinical outcome predictors: a report from the Children's Oncology Group. Cancer Med. 2019 Oct;8(14):6437–48. PMID:31456361
1881. Hickman RA, Bruce JN, Otten M, et al. Gonadotroph tumours with a low SF-1 labelling index are more likely to recur and are associated with enrichment of the PI3K-AKT pathway. Neuropathol Appl Neurobiol. 2021 Apr;47(3):415–27. PMID:33128255
1882. Hickman RA, Gionco JT, Faust PL, et al. Pituitary corticotroph tumour with adrenocortical cells: a distinct clinicopathologic entity with unique morphology and methylation profile. Neuropathol Appl Neurobiol. 2022 Feb;48(2):e12754. PMID:34296770
1883. Hicks DG, LiVolsi VA, Neidich JA, et al. Clonal analysis of solitary follicular nodules in the thyroid. Am J Pathol. 1990 Sep;137(3):553–62. PMID:1975986
1884. Hier J, Avior G, Pusztaszeri M, et al. Molecular testing for cytologically suspicious and malignant (Bethesda V and VI) thyroid nodules to optimize the extent of surgical intervention: a retrospective chart review. J Otolaryngol Head Neck Surg. 2021 Apr 28;50(1):29. PMID:33910629
1885. Higaki-Mori H, Kuwamoto S, Iwasaki T, et al. Association of Merkel cell polyomavirus infection with clinicopathological differences in Merkel cell carcinoma. Hum Pathol. 2012 Dec;43(12):2282–91. PMID:22795182
1886. Higgins DF, Kimura K, Bernhardt WM, et al. Hypoxia promotes fibrogenesis in vivo via HIF-1 stimulation of epithelial-to-mesenchymal transition. J Clin Invest. 2007 Dec;117(12):3810–20. PMID:18037992
1887. Hijioka S, Hosoda W, Matsuo K, et al. Rb loss and KRAS mutation are predictors of the response to platinum-based chemotherapy in pancreatic neuroendocrine neoplasm with grade 3: a Japanese multicenter pancreatic NEN-G3 study. Clin Cancer Res. 2017 Aug 15;23(16):4625–32. PMID:28455360
1888. Hillman RT, Cardnell R, Fujimoto J, et al. Comparative genomics of high grade neuroendocrine carcinoma of the cervix. PLoS One. 2020 Jun 16;15(6):e0234505. PMID:32544169
1889. Hiltzik D, Carlson DL, Tuttle RM, et al. Poorly differentiated thyroid carcinomas defined on the basis of mitosis and necrosis: a clinicopathologic study of 58 patients. Cancer. 2006 Mar 15;106(6):1286–95. PMID:16470605
1890. Hino H, Nitadori JI, Ohno K, et al. An unusual invasive ectopic thymoma in the thyroid and anterior mediastinum. Ann Thorac Surg. 2018 Aug;106(2):e65–7. PMID:29626459
1891. Hino R, Motoi N, Toda K, et al. Stromal tiny black dots, like "sugar-coated", of von Kossa stain is a diagnostic clue to hyalinizing trabecular tumor of the thyroid gland. Pathol Int. 2018 Mar;68(3):176–82. PMID:29368414
1892. Hinton DR, Hahn JA, Weiss MH, et al. Loss of Rb expression in an ACTH-secreting pituitary carcinoma. Cancer Lett. 1998 Apr 24;126(2):209–14. PMID:9585068
1893. Hirasaki S, Kanzaki H, Okuda M, et al. Composite paraganglioma-ganglioneuroma in the retroperitoneum. World J Surg Oncol. 2009 Nov 5;7:81. PMID:19889235
1894. Hirokawa M, Carney JA. Cell membrane and cytoplasmic staining for MIB-1 in hyalinizing trabecular adenoma of the thyroid gland. Am J Surg Pathol. 2000 Apr;24(4):575–8. PMID:10757406
1895. Hirokawa M, Higuchi M, Suzuki A, et al. Noninvasive follicular thyroid neoplasm with papillary-like nuclear features: a single-institutional experience in Japan. Endocr J. 2017 Dec 28;64(12):1149–55. PMID:28904306
1896. Hirokawa M, Kuma S, Miyauchi A. Cytological findings of intrathyroidal epithelial thymoma/carcinoma showing thymus-like differentiation: a study of eight cases. Diagn Cytopathol. 2012 May;40 Suppl 1:E16–20. PMID:22619154
1897. Hirokawa M, Maekawa M, Kuma S, et al. Cribriform-morular variant of papillary thyroid carcinoma–cytological and immunocytochemical findings of 18 cases. Diagn Cytopathol. 2010 Dec;38(12):890–6. PMID:20091902
1898. Hirokawa M, Miyauchi A, Minato H, et al. Intrathyroidal epithelial thymoma/carcinoma showing thymus-like differentiation; comparison with thymic lymphoepithelioma-like carcinoma and a possibility of development from a multipotential stem cell. APMIS. 2013 Jun;121(6):523–30. PMID:23176314
1899. Hirokawa M, Suzuki A, Higuchi M, et al. Histological alterations following fine-needle aspiration for parathyroid adenoma: incidence and diagnostic problems. Pathol Int. 2021 Jun;71(6):400–5. PMID:33740321
1900. Hirokawa M, Takada N, Abe H, et al. Thyroid sclerosing mucoepidermoid carcinoma with eosinophilia distinct from the salivary type. Endocr J. 2018 Apr 26;65(4):427–36. PMID:29415898
1901. Hirsch MS, Faquin WC, Krane JF. Thyroid transcription factor-1, but not p53, is helpful in distinguishing moderately differentiated neuroendocrine carcinoma of the larynx from medullary carcinoma of the thyroid. Mod Pathol. 2004 Jun;17(6):631–6. PMID:15098009
1902. Hirshoren N, Neuman T, Udassin R, et al. The imperative of the Sistrunk operation: review of 160 thyroglossal tract remnant operations. Otolaryngol Head Neck Surg. 2009 Mar;140(3):338–42. PMID:19248939
1903. Hisama FM, Kubisch C, Martin GM, et al. Clinical utility gene card for: Werner syndrome–update 2014. Eur J Hum Genet. 2015 Jun;23(6):891. PMID:25182132
1904. Hishinuma A. [Genetics of thyroid diseases]. Nihon Rinsho. 2012 Nov;70(11):1885–91. Japanese. PMID:23214057
1905. Hjerpe SJ, Rahim U, Usman MS, et al. High-grade non-small cell neuroendocrine carcinoma of the esophagus. Cureus. 2018 Apr 3;10(4):e2416. PMID:29872597
1906. Hjorth L, Thomsen LB, Nielsen VT. Adenolipoma of the thyroid gland. Histopathology. 1986 Jan;10(1):91–6. PMID:3957249
1907. Ho AS, Luu M, Barrios L, et al. Incidence and mortality risk spectrum across aggressive variants of papillary thyroid carcinoma. JAMA Oncol. 2020 May 1;6(5):706–13. PMID:32134428
1908. Ho AS, Wang L, Palmer FL, et al. Postoperative nomogram for predicting cancer-specific mortality in medullary thyroid cancer. Ann Surg Oncol. 2015 Aug;22(8):2700–6. PMID:25366585
1909. Ho YH, Yap WM, Chuah KL. Solitary fibrous tumor of the adrenal gland with unusual immunophenotype: a potential diagnostic problem and a brief review of endocrine organ solitary fibrous tumor. Endocr Pathol. 2010 Jun;21(2):125–9. PMID:20191330
1910. Hoang JK, Middleton WD, Tessler FN. Update on ACR TI-RADS: successes, challenges, and future directions, from the AJR Special Series on radiology reporting and data systems. AJR Am J Roentgenol. 2021 Mar;216(3):570–8. PMID:33112199
1911. Hoang MP, Donizy P, Wu CL, et al. TdT expression is a marker of better survival in Merkel cell carcinoma, and expression of B-cell markers is associated with Merkel cell polyomavirus. Am J Clin Pathol. 2020 Jun 8;154(1):38–47. PMID:32134459
1912. Hoang MP, Hobbs CM, Sobin LH, et al. Carcinoid tumor of the esophagus: a clinicopathologic study of four cases. Am J Surg Pathol. 2002 Apr;26(4):517–22. PMID:11914632
1913. Hoang MP, Hruban RH, Albores-Saavedra J. Clear cell endocrine pancreatic tumor mimicking renal cell carcinoma: a distinctive neoplasm of von Hippel-Lindau disease. Am J Surg Pathol. 2001 May;25(5):602–9. PMID:11342771
1914. Hochwald SN, Zee S, Conlon KC, et al. Prognostic factors in pancreatic endocrine neoplasms: an analysis of 136 cases with a proposal for low-grade and intermediate-grade groups. J Clin Oncol. 2002 Jun 1;20(11):2633–42. PMID:12039924
1915. Hockman D, Adameyko I, Kaucka M, et al. Striking parallels between carotid body glomus cell and adrenal chromaffin cell development. Dev Biol. 2018 Dec 1;444 Suppl 1 (Suppl 1):S308–24. PMID:29807017
1916. Hodgson A, Pakbaz S, Mete O. A diagnostic approach to adrenocortical tumors. Surg Pathol Clin. 2019 Dec;12(4):967–95. PMID:31672302
1917. Hodgson A, Pakbaz S, Shenouda C, et al. Mixed sparsely granulated lactotroph and densely granulated somatotroph pituitary neuroendocrine tumor expands the spectrum of neuroendocrine neoplasms in ovarian teratomas: the role of pituitary neuroendocrine cell lineage biomarkers. Endocr Pathol. 2020 Sep;31(3):315–9. PMID:32632841
1918. Hodgson A, Pakbaz S, Tayyari F, et al. Diagnostic pitfall: parathyroid carcinoma expands the spectrum of calcitonin and calcitonin gene-related peptide expressing neuroendocrine neoplasms. Endocr Pathol. 2019 Jun;30(2):168–72. PMID:30903444
1919. Hodgson NC. Merkel cell carcinoma: changing incidence trends. J Surg Oncol. 2005 Jan 1;89(1):1–4. PMID:15611998
1920. Hoekstra AS, Devilee P, Bayley JP. Models of parent-of-origin tumorigenesis in hereditary paraganglioma. Semin Cell Dev Biol. 2015 Jul;43:117–24. PMID:26067997
1921. Hoffmann A, Boekhoff S, Gebhardt U, et al. History before diagnosis in childhood craniopharyngioma: associations with initial presentation and long-term prognosis. Eur J Endocrinol. 2015 Dec;173(6):853–62. PMID:26392473
1922. Hoffmann A, Brentrup A, Müller HL. First report on spinal metastasis in childhood-onset craniopharyngioma. J Neurooncol. 2016 Aug;129(1):193–4. PMID:27278607
1923. Hofland J, Herrera-Martínez AD, Zandee WT, et al. Management of carcinoid syndrome: a systematic review and meta-analysis. Endocr Relat Cancer. 2019 Mar;26(3):R145–56. PMID:30608900
1924. Hofland J, Kaltsas G, de Herder WW. Advances in the diagnosis and management of well-differentiated neuroendocrine neoplasms. Endocr Rev. 2020 Apr 1;41(2):371–403. PMID:31555796
1925. Hofman V, Lassalle S, Bonnetaud C, et al. Thyroid tumours of uncertain malignant potential: frequency and diagnostic reproducibility. Virchows Arch. 2009 Jul;455(1):21–33. PMID:19543912
1926. Hofstedter R, Sanabria-Salas MC, Di Jiang M, et al. FLCN-driven functional adrenal cortical carcinoma with high mitotic tumor grade: extending the endocrine manifestations of Birt-Hogg-Dubé syndrome. Endocr Pathol. 2023 Jun;34(2):257–64. PMID:36701047
1927. Hofstra RM, Landsvater RM, Ceccherini I, et al. A mutation in the RET proto-oncogene associated with multiple endocrine neoplasia type 2B and sporadic medullary thyroid carcinoma. Nature. 1994 Jan 27;367(6461):375–6. PMID:7906866
1928. Hofstra RM, Sijmons RH, Stelwagen T, et al. RET mutation screening in familial cutaneous lichen amyloidosis and in skin amyloidosis associated with multiple endocrine neoplasia. J Invest Dermatol. 1996 Aug;107(2):215–8. PMID:8757765
1929. Holm LE, Blomgren H, Löwhagen T.

Cancer risks in patients with chronic lymphocytic thyroiditis. N Engl J Med. 1985 Mar 7;312(10):601–4. PMID:3838363
1930. Holm R, Farrants GW, Nesland JM, et al. Ultrastructural and electron immunohistochemical features of medullary thyroid carcinoma. Virchows Arch A Pathol Anat Histopathol. 1989;414(5):375–84. PMID:2499093
1931. Holoubek SA, Yan H, Khokar AH, et al. Aggressive variants of papillary thyroid microcarcinoma are associated with high-risk features, but not decreased survival. Surgery. 2020 Jan;167(1):19–27. PMID:31627846
1932. Hölsken A, Kreutzer J, Hofmann BM, et al. Target gene activation of the Wnt signaling pathway in nuclear beta-catenin accumulating cells of adamantinomatous craniopharyngiomas. Brain Pathol. 2009 Jul;19(3):357–64. PMID:18540944
1933. Hölsken A, Sill M, Merkle J, et al. Adamantinomatous and papillary craniopharyngiomas are characterized by distinct epigenomic as well as mutational and transcriptomic profiles. Acta Neuropathol Commun. 2016 Feb 29;4:20. PMID:26927026
1934. Honeyman SI, Warr W, Curran OE, et al. Paraganglioma of the lumbar spine: a case report and literature review. Neurochirurgie. 2019 Dec;65(6):387–92. PMID:31247160
1935. Hong X, Qiao S, Li F, et al. Whole-genome sequencing reveals distinct genetic bases for insulinomas and non-functional pancreatic neuroendocrine tumours: leading to a new classification system. Gut. 2020 May;69(5):877–87. PMID:31462556
1936. Hong Y, Fang Y, Wu Q, et al. Ganglioglioma of the adenohypophysis mimicking pituitary adenoma: a case report and review of the literature. Medicine (Baltimore). 2018 Jul;97(30):e11583. PMID:30045287
1937. Hong Y, Hao Y, Hu J, et al. Adrenocortical oncocytoma: 11 case reports and review of the literature. Medicine (Baltimore). 2017 Dec;96(48):e8750. PMID:29310349
1938. Hong YA, Park KC, Kim BK, et al. Analyzing genetic differences between sporadic primary and secondary/tertiary hyperparathyroidism by targeted next-generation panel sequencing. Endocr Pathol. 2021 Dec;32(4):501–12. PMID:34215996
1939. Hori A. Suprasellar peri-infundibular ectopic adenohypophysis in fetal and adult brains. J Neurosurg. 1985 Jul;63(1):113–5. PMID:4009259
1940. Horn LC, Hentschel B, Bilek K, et al. Mixed small cell carcinomas of the uterine cervix: prognostic impact of focal neuroendocrine differentiation but not of Ki-67 labeling index. Ann Diagn Pathol. 2006 Jun;10(3):140–3. PMID:16730307
1941. Hornick JL, Fletcher CD. Sclerosing PEComa: clinicopathologic analysis of a distinctive variant with a predilection for the retroperitoneum. Am J Surg Pathol. 2008 Apr;32(4):493–501. PMID:18223480
1942. Horst W, Rösler H, Schneider C, et al. 306 cases of toxic adenoma: clinical aspects, findings in radioiodine diagnostics, radiochromatography and histology; results of 131-I and surgical treatment. J Nucl Med. 1967 Jul;8(7):515–28. PMID:4166326
1943. Horvath E, Chalvardjian A, Kovacs K, et al. Leydig-like cells in the adrenals of a woman with ectopic ACTH syndrome. Hum Pathol. 1980 May;11(3):284–7. PMID:7190543
1944. Horvath E, Kovacs K. Pathology of acromegaly. Neuroendocrinology. 2006;83(3-4):161–5. PMID:17047379
1945. Horvath E, Kovacs K, Killinger DW, et al. Mammosomatotroph cell adenoma of the human pituitary: a morphologic entity. Virchows Arch A Pathol Anat Histopathol. 1983;398(3):277–89. PMID:6402839
1946. Horvath E, Kovacs K, Killinger DW, et al. Silent corticotropic adenomas of the human pituitary gland: a histologic, immunocytologic, and ultrastructural study. Am J Pathol. 1980 Mar;98(3):617–38. PMID:6244736
1947. Horvath E, Kovacs K, Scheithauer BW, et al. Pituitary adenoma with neuronal choristoma (PANCH): composite lesion or lineage infidelity? Ultrastruct Pathol. 1994 Nov-Dec;18(6):565–74. PMID:7855931
1948. Horvath E, Kovacs K, Singer W, et al. Acidophil stem cell adenoma of the human pituitary. Arch Pathol Lab Med. 1977 Nov;101(11):594–9. PMID:199135
1949. Horvath E, Kovacs K, Singer W, et al. Acidophil stem cell adenoma of the human pituitary: clinicopathologic analysis of 15 cases. Cancer. 1981 Feb 15;47(4):761–71. PMID:6261917
1950. Horvath E, Kovacs K, Smyth HS, et al. A novel type of pituitary adenoma: morphological features and clinical correlations. J Clin Endocrinol Metab. 1988 Jun;66(6):1111–8. PMID:3372677
1951. Horvath E, Kovacs K, Smyth HS, et al. Silent adenoma subtype 3 of the pituitary–immunohistochemical and ultrastructural classification: a review of 29 cases. Ultrastruct Pathol. 2005 Nov-Dec;29(6):511–24. PMID:16316952
1952. Hosal SA, Apel RL, Freeman JL, et al. Immunohistochemical localization of p53 in human thyroid neoplasms: correlation with biological behavior. Endocr Pathol. 1997 Spring;8(1):21–8. PMID:12114668
1953. Hosny Mohammed K, Siddiqui MT, Willis BC, et al. Parafibromin, APC, and MIB-1 are useful markers for distinguishing parathyroid carcinomas from adenomas. Appl Immunohistochem Mol Morphol. 2017 Nov/Dec;25(10):731–5. PMID:27490759
1954. Hosoi H. Current status of treatment for pediatric rhabdomyosarcoma in the USA and Japan. Pediatr Int. 2016 Feb;58(2):81–7. PMID:26646016
1955. Hosoi H, Teramukai S, Matsumoto Y, et al. A review of 331 rhabdomyosarcoma cases in patients treated between 1991 and 2002 in Japan. Int J Clin Oncol. 2007 Apr;12(2):137–45. PMID:17443282
1956. Hou P, Liu D, Shan Y, et al. Genetic alterations and their relationship in the phosphatidylinositol 3-kinase/Akt pathway in thyroid cancer. Clin Cancer Res. 2007 Feb 15;13(4):1161–70. PMID:17317825
1957. Hou Y, He X, Chute DJ. Paraganglioma-like medullary thyroid carcinoma: a case report and literature review. Diagn Cytopathol. 2020 Jun;48(6):559–63. PMID:32125784
1958. Hough AJ, Hollifield JW, Page DL, et al. Prognostic factors in adrenal cortical tumors. A mathematical analysis of clinical and morphologic data. Am J Clin Pathol. 1979 Sep;72(3):390–9. PMID:474519
1959. Hovi SI, Kholová I. Vascular proliferation of the thyroid: potential histopathological pitfalls as a consequence of fine needle aspiration. Acta Cytol. 2017;61(3):179–86. PMID:28514786
1960. Howell VM, Gill A, Clarkson A, et al. Accuracy of combined protein gene product 9.5 and parafibromin markers for immunohistochemical diagnosis of parathyroid carcinoma. J Clin Endocrinol Metab. 2009 Feb;94(2):434–41. PMID:19017757
1961. Howell VM, Haven CJ, Kahnoski K, et al. HRPT2 mutations are associated with malignancy in sporadic parathyroid tumours. J Med Genet. 2003 Sep;40(9):657–63. PMID:12960210
1962. Howitt BE, Dong F, Vivero M, et al. Molecular characterization of neuroendocrine carcinomas of the endometrium: representation in all 4 TCGA groups. Am J Surg Pathol. 2020 Nov;44(11):1541–8. PMID:32773531
1963. Howitt BE, Kelly P, McCluggage WG. Pathology of neuroendocrine tumours of the female genital tract. Curr Oncol Rep. 2017 Sep;19(9):59. PMID:28735441
1964. Howitt BE, Paulson VA, Barletta JA. Absence of BRAF V600E in non-infiltrative, non-invasive follicular variant of papillary thyroid carcinoma. Histopathology. 2015 Oct;67(4):579–82. PMID:25736029
1966. Howlader N, Noone AM, Krapcho M, et al., editors. Surveillance, Epidemiology, and End Results (SEER) Program [Internet]. Bethesda (MD): National Cancer Institute; 2015. SEER Cancer Statistics Review, 1975-2012; based on November 2014 SEER data submission, posted to the SEER website in April 2015. Available from: https://seer.cancer.gov/archive/csr/1975_2012/.
1967. Howson P, Kruijff S, Aniss A, et al. Oxyphil cell parathyroid adenomas causing primary hyperparathyroidism: a clinico-pathological correlation. Endocr Pathol. 2015 Sep;26(3):250–4. PMID:26091632
1968. Hsiao HP, Chao MC, Lin CY, et al. Feminizing adrenocortical adenoma presenting as heterosexual precocious puberty: report of one case. Acta Paediatr Taiwan. 2005 Mar-Apr;46(2):97–100. PMID:16302588
1969. Hsiao HP, Kirschner LS, Bourdeau I, et al. Clinical and genetic heterogeneity, overlap with other tumor syndromes, and atypical glucocorticoid hormone secretion in adrenocorticotropin-independent macronodular adrenal hyperplasia compared with other adrenocortical tumors. J Clin Endocrinol Metab. 2009 Aug;94(8):2930–7. PMID:19509103
1970. Hsieh MH, Lin MC, Shun CT, et al. Fine needle aspiration cytology of mixed medullary-follicular thyroid carcinoma: a case report. Acta Cytol. 2008 May-Jun;52(3):361–5. PMID:18540307
1971. Hsieh MS, Chen JH, Lin LW. Myxoid adrenal cortical carcinoma presenting as primary hyperaldosteronism: case report and review of the literature. Int J Surg Pathol. 2011 Dec;19(6):803–7. PMID:20444728
1972. Hsing AW, Nam JM, Co Chien HT, et al. Risk factors for adrenal cancer: an exploratory study. Int J Cancer. 1996 Feb 8;65(4):432–6. PMID:8621222
1973. Hu J, Wu J, Cai L, et al. Retroperitoneal composite pheochromocytoma-ganglioneuroma : a case report and review of literature. Diagn Pathol. 2013 Apr 15;8:63. PMID:23587063
1974. Hu MI, Cote GJ. Medullary thyroid carcinoma: Who's on first? Thyroid. 2012 May;22(5):451–3. PMID:22545752
1975. Hu W, Huang J, Zhang Y, et al. A rare and easily misdiagnosed tumor of the urinary bladder: primary composite pheochromocytoma. Int J Clin Exp Pathol. 2017 Oct 1;10(10):10522–30. PMID:31966391
1976. Hu Y, Cui M, Xia Y, et al. The clinical features of cystic parathyroid adenoma in Chinese population: a single-center experience. Int J Endocrinol. 2018 Jul 15;2018:3745239. PMID:30123260
1977. Hu Y, Zhang X, Wang O, et al. The genomic profile of parathyroid carcinoma based on whole-genome sequencing. Int J Cancer. 2020 Nov 1;147(9):2446–57. PMID:32574388
1978. Huang C, Ezzat S, Asa SL, et al. Dopaminergic resistant prolactinomas in the peripubertal population. J Pediatr Endocrinol Metab. 2006 Jul;19(7):951–3. PMID:16995577
1979. Huang C, Wang L, Wang Y, et al. Carcinoma showing thymus-like differentiation of the thyroid (CASTLE). Pathol Res Pract. 2013 Oct;209(10):662–5. PMID:23920320
1980. Huang CC, Collins BT, Flint A, et al. Pulmonary neuroendocrine tumors: an entity in search of cytologic criteria. Diagn Cytopathol. 2013 Aug;41(8):689–96. PMID:23166111
1981. Huang CG, Li MZ, Wang SH, et al. The diagnosis of primary thyroid lymphoma by fine-needle aspiration, cell block, and immunohistochemistry technique. Diagn Cytopathol. 2020 Nov;48(11):1041–7. PMID:32609434
1982. Huang D, Peng Y, Xiong H, et al. Primary poorly differentiated neuroendocrine carcinoma of the oral cavity. Oral Dis. 2022 Oct;28(7):1811–5. PMID:33694290
1983. Huang Q, Wu H, Nie L, et al. Primary high-grade neuroendocrine carcinoma of the esophagus: a clinicopathologic and immunohistochemical study of 42 resection cases. Am J Surg Pathol. 2013 Apr;37(4):467–83. PMID:23426118
1984. Huang SF, Chuang WY, Cheng SD, et al. A colliding maxillary sinus cancer of adenosquamous carcinoma and small cell neuroendocrine carcinoma–a case report with EGFR copy number analysis. World J Surg Oncol. 2010 Oct 20;8:92. PMID:20961443
1985. Huang YC, Yang NN, Chen HC, et al. Clinicopathological features and prognostic factors associated with gastroenteropancreatic mixed neuroendocrine non-neuroendocrine neoplasms in Chinese patients. World J Gastroenterol. 2021 Feb 21;27(7):624–40. PMID:33642833
1986. Huei TJ, Lip HT, Rahman MS, et al. Large adrenal leiomyoma presented as adrenal incidentaloma in an AIDS patient: a rare entity. Med J Malaysia. 2017 Feb;72(1):65–7. PMID:28255146
1987. Hundahl SA, Cady B, Cunningham MP, et al. Initial results from a prospective cohort study of 5583 cases of thyroid carcinoma treated in the united states during 1996. U.S. and German Thyroid Cancer Study Group. An American College of Surgeons Commission on Cancer Patient Care Evaluation study. Cancer. 2000 Jul 1;89(1):202–17. PMID:10897019
1988. Hundahl SA, Fleming ID, Fremgen AM, et al. Two hundred eighty-six cases of parathyroid carcinoma treated in the U.S. between 1985-1995: a National Cancer Data Base report. Cancer. 1999 Aug 1;86(3):538–44. PMID:10430265
1989. Hung A, Ahmed S, Gupta A, et al. Performance of the aldosterone to renin ratio as a screening test for primary aldosteronism. J Clin Endocrinol Metab. 2021 Jul 13;106(8):2423–35. PMID:34008000
1990. Hung YP, Barletta JA. A user's guide to non-invasive follicular thyroid neoplasm with papillary-like nuclear features (NIFTP). Histopathology. 2018 Jan;72(1):53–69. PMID:29239036
1991. Hung YP, Diaz-Perez JA, Cote GM, et al. Dedifferentiated chordoma: clinicopathologic and molecular characteristics with integrative analysis. Am J Surg Pathol. 2020 Sep;44(9):1213–23. PMID:32427623
1992. Hung YP, Hornick JL. Immunohistochemical biomarkers of mesenchymal neoplasms in endocrine organs: diagnostic pitfalls and recent discoveries. Endocr Pathol. 2018 Jun;29(2):189–98. PMID:29340997
1993. Hunt JL, Barnes EL. Non-tumor-associated psammoma bodies in the thyroid. Am J Clin Pathol. 2003 Jan;119(1):90–4. PMID:12520702
1994. Hunt JL, Carty SE, Yim JH, et al. Allelic loss in parathyroid neoplasia can help characterize malignancy. Am J Surg Pathol. 2005 Aug;29(8):1049–55. PMID:16006799
1995. Hunt JL, LiVolsi VA, Barnes EL. p63 expression in sclerosing mucoepidermoid

carcinomas with eosinophilia arising in the thyroid. Mod Pathol. 2004 May;17(5):526–9. PMID:15001991
1997. Hunter JA, Skelly RH, Aylwin SJ, et al. The relationship between pituitary tumour transforming gene (PTTG) expression and in vitro hormone and vascular endothelial growth factor (VEGF) secretion from human pituitary adenomas. Eur J Endocrinol. 2003 Feb;148(2):203–11. PMID:12590639
1998. Huryn LA, Turriff A, Harney LA, et al. DICER1 syndrome: characterization of the ocular phenotype in a family-based cohort study. Ophthalmology. 2019 Feb;126(2):296–304. PMID:30339877
1999. Huson SM, Compston DA, Harper PS. A genetic study of von Recklinghausen neurofibromatosis in south east Wales. II. Guidelines for genetic counselling. J Med Genet. 1989 Nov;26(11):712–21. PMID:2511319
2000. Hussein MR. Central nervous system capillary haemangioblastoma: the pathologist's viewpoint. Int J Exp Pathol. 2007 Oct;88(5):311–24. PMID:17877533
2001. Hvilsom GB, Londero SC, Hahn CH, et al. Anaplastic thyroid carcinoma in Denmark 1996-2012: a national prospective study of 219 patients. Cancer Epidemiol. 2018 Apr;53:65–71. PMID:29414634
2002. Hwang JS, Beebe KS, Rojas J, et al. Malignant granular cell tumor of the thigh. Orthopedics. 2011 Aug 8;34(8):e428–31. PMID:21815590
2003. Hyjek E, Isaacson PG. Primary B cell lymphoma of the thyroid and its relationship to Hashimoto's thyroiditis. Hum Pathol. 1988 Nov;19(11):1315–26. PMID:3141260
2004. Hyrcza MD, Ezzat S, Mete O, et al. Pituitary adenomas presenting as sinonasal or nasopharyngeal masses: a case series illustrating potential diagnostic pitfalls. Am J Surg Pathol. 2017 Apr;41(4):525–34. PMID:28009611
2005. Hyrcza MD, Sargın P, Mete O. Parathyroid lipoadenoma: a clinicopathological diagnosis and possible trap for the unaware pathologist. Endocr Pathol. 2016 Mar;27(1):34–41. PMID:26585863
2006. Hyrcza MD, Winer D, Mete O. Images in endocrine pathology: papillary variant of medullary thyroid carcinoma with cystic change. Endocr Pathol. 2015 Mar;26(1):87–9. PMID:25246133
2007. Hyrcza MD, Winer DA, Shago M, et al. TFE3-expressing perivascular epithelioid cell neoplasm (PEComa) of the sella turcica. Endocr Pathol. 2017 Mar;28(1):22–6. PMID:27189222
2008. Hysek M, Jatta K, Stenman A, et al. Signet ring cell variant of follicular thyroid carcinoma: report of two cases with focus on morphological, expressional and genetic characteristics. Diagn Pathol. 2019 Nov 7;14(1):127. PMID:31699114
2009. Hysek M, Paulsson JO, Jatta K, et al. Clinical routine TERT promoter mutational screening of follicular thyroid tumors of uncertain malignant potential (FT-UMPs): a useful predictor of metastatic disease. Cancers (Basel). 2019 Sep 26;11(10):1443. PMID:31561592
2010. Iacobone M, Carnaille B, Palazzo FF, et al. Hereditary hyperparathyroidism–a consensus report of the European Society of Endocrine Surgeons (ESES). Langenbecks Arch Surg. 2015 Dec;400(8):867–86. PMID:26450137
2011. Iacobone M, Masi G, Barzon L, et al. Hyperparathyroidism-jaw tumor syndrome: a report of three large kindred. Langenbecks Arch Surg. 2009 Sep;394(5):817–25. PMID:19529956
2012. Iacobone M, Torresan F, Citton M, et al. Adrenal ganglioneuroma: the Padua Endocrine Surgery Unit experience. Int J Surg. 2017 May;41 Suppl 1:S103–8. PMID:28506406
2013. Iacocca MV, Abernethy JL, Stefanato CM, et al. Mixed Merkel cell carcinoma and squamous cell carcinoma of the skin. J Am Acad Dermatol. 1998 Nov;39(5 Pt 2):882–7. PMID:9810922
2014. Iacovazzo D, Carlsen E, Lugli F, et al. Factors predicting pasireotide responsiveness in somatotroph pituitary adenomas resistant to first-generation somatostatin analogues: an immunohistochemical study. Eur J Endocrinol. 2016 Feb;174(2):241–50. PMID:26586796
2015. Iacovazzo D, Caswell R, Bunce B, et al. Germline or somatic GPR101 duplication leads to X-linked acrogigantism: a clinico-pathological and genetic study. Acta Neuropathol Commun. 2016 Jun 1;4(1):56. PMID:27245663
2016. Iacovazzo D, Flanagan SE, Walker E, et al. MAFA missense mutation causes familial insulinomatosis and diabetes mellitus. Proc Natl Acad Sci U S A. 2018 Jan 30;115(5):1027–32. PMID:29339498
2017. Iakovou I, Konstantinidis I, Doumas A, et al. Squamous cell carcinoma in a thyroglossal duct cyst and 99mTc-MIBI findings. Hell J Nucl Med. 2011 Jan-Apr;14(1):62–4. PMID:21512669
2018. Iannalfi A, Fragkandrea I, Brock J, et al. Radiotherapy in craniopharyngiomas. Clin Oncol (R Coll Radiol). 2013 Nov;25(11):654–67. PMID:23910225
2019. Ibrahem HM. Ossifying fibroma of the jaw bones in hyperparathyroidism-jaw tumor syndrome: analysis of 24 cases retrieved from literatures. J Dent Sci. 2020 Dec;15(4):426–32. PMID:33505612
2020. Ibrahim NB, Milewski PJ, Gillett R, et al. Benign thyroid inclusions within cervical lymph nodes: an alarming incidental finding. Aust N Z J Surg. 1981 Apr;51(2):188–9. PMID:6940550
2021. Ibrahimpasic T, Ghossein R, Carlson DL, et al. Outcomes in patients with poorly differentiated thyroid carcinoma. J Clin Endocrinol Metab. 2014 Apr;99(4):1245–52. PMID:24512493
2022. Ichikawa S, Fukuhara N, Inoue A, et al. Clinicopathological analysis of primary adrenal diffuse large B-cell lymphoma: effectiveness of rituximab-containing chemotherapy including central nervous system prophylaxis. Exp Hematol Oncol. 2013 Aug 2;2(1):19. PMID:23915571
2023. Idowu BD, Al-Adnani M, O'Donnell P, et al. A sensitive mutation-specific screening technique for GNAS1 mutations in cases of fibrous dysplasia: the first report of a codon 227 mutation in bone. Histopathology. 2007 May;50(6):691–704. PMID:17493233
2024. Iesalnieks I, Winter H, Bareck E, et al. Thyroid metastases of renal cell carcinoma: clinical course in 45 patients undergoing surgery. Assessment of factors affecting patients' survival. Thyroid. 2008 Jun;18(6):615–24. PMID:18578610
2025. Iftikhar H, Awan MS, Ghaloo SK, et al. Sclerosing mucoepidermoid carcinoma with eosinophilia of thyroid. BMJ Case Rep. 2019 Aug 8;12(8):e225685. PMID:31399413
2026. Iglesias P, Díez JJ. Macroprolactinoma: a diagnostic and therapeutic update. QJM. 2013 Jun;106(6):495–504. PMID:23329574
2027. Iglesias P, Guerrero-Pérez F, Villabona C, et al. Adenohypophyseal hyperfunction syndromes and posterior pituitary tumors: prevalence, clinical characteristics, and pathophysiological mechanisms. Endocrine. 2020 Oct;70(1):15–23. PMID:32613546
2028. Igreja S, Chahal HS, King P, et al. Characterization of aryl hydrocarbon receptor interacting protein (AIP) mutations in familial isolated pituitary adenoma families. Hum Mutat. 2010 Aug;31(8):950–60. PMID:20506337
2029. Ikegaki N, Shimada H; International Neuroblastoma Pathology Committee. Subgrouping of unfavorable histology neuroblastomas with immunohistochemistry toward precision prognosis and therapy stratification. JCO Precis Oncol. 2019;3:PO.18.00312. PMID:31840131
2030. Ikota H, Tanimoto A, Komatsu H, et al. Ureteral leiomyoma causing hydronephrosis in type 1 multiple endocrine neoplasia. Pathol Int. 2004 Jun;54(6):457–9. PMID:15144407
2031. Ilie MD, Vasiljevic A, Louvet C, et al. Gonadotroph tumors show subtype differences that might have implications for therapy. Cancers (Basel). 2020 Apr 20;12(4):1012. PMID:32326042
2032. Imaizumi M, Ohishi W, Nakashima E, et al. Association of radiation dose with prevalence of thyroid nodules among atomic bomb survivors exposed in childhood (2007-2011). JAMA Intern Med. 2015 Feb;175(2):228–36. PMID:25545696
2033. Imanishi Y, Tahara H, Palanisamy N, et al. Clonal chromosomal defects in the molecular pathogenesis of refractory hyperparathyroidism of uremia. J Am Soc Nephrol. 2002 Jun;13(6):1490–8. PMID:12039978
2034. Inage T, Nakajima T, Fujiwara T, et al. Pathological diagnosis of pulmonary large cell neuroendocrine carcinoma by endobronchial ultrasound-guided transbronchial needle aspiration. Thorac Cancer. 2018 Feb;9(2):273–7. PMID:29271588
2035. Inoue K, Yamazaki Y, Tsurutani Y, et al. Evaluation of cortisol production in aldosterone-producing adenoma. Horm Metab Res. 2017 Nov;49(11):847–53. PMID:29069700
2036. International Association of Cancer Registries (IACR) [Internet]. Lyon (France): International Agency for Research on Cancer; 2021. International Classification of Diseases for Oncology (ICD-O) – ICD-O-3.2; updated 2021 Jan 25. Available from: http://www.iacr.com.fr/index.php?option=com_content&view=category&layout=blog&id=100&Itemid=577.
2037. Inzani F, Rindi G, Tamborrino E, et al. Extra-adrenal composite paraganglioma with ganglioneuroma component presenting as a pancreatic mass. Endocr Pathol. 2009 Fall;20(3):191–5. PMID:19598001
2038. Inzani F, Santoro A, Angelico G, et al. Neuroendocrine carcinoma of the uterine cervix: a clinicopathologic and immunohistochemical study with focus on novel markers (Sst2-Sst5). Cancers (Basel). 2020 May 12;12(5):1211. PMID:32408525
2039. Ioachimescu AG, Handa T, Goswami N, et al. Gender differences and temporal trends over two decades in acromegaly: a single center study in 112 patients. Endocrine. 2020 Feb;67(2):423–32. PMID:31677093
2040. Ippolito S, Bellevicine C, Arpaia D, et al. Spindle epithelial tumor with thymus-like differentiation (SETTLE): clinical-pathological features, differential pathological diagnosis and therapy. Endocrine. 2016 Mar;51(3):402–12. PMID:26289127
2041. Iqbal MS, Paleri V, Moor J, et al. Small cell neuroendocrine carcinoma of larynx: case series and literature review. J Laryngol Otol. 2015 Sep;129(9):910–5. PMID:26173932
2042. Irizarry-Villafañe G, Rivera-Santana N, Mangual-García M, et al. A rare case of uterine leiomyosarcoma with metastasis to the thyroid gland. Case Rep Endocrinol. 2020 Jun 29;2020:8889843. PMID:32665867
2043. Irwin MS, Naranjo A, Zhang FF, et al. Revised neuroblastoma risk classification system: a report from the Children's Oncology Group. J Clin Oncol. 2021 Oct 10;39(29):3229–41. PMID:34319759
2044. Ishida GM, Kato N, Hayasaka T, et al. Small cell neuroendocrine carcinomas of the uterine cervix: a histological, immunohistochemical, and molecular genetic study. Int J Gynecol Pathol. 2004 Oct;23(4):366–72. PMID:15381906
2045. Ishida M, Kashu I, Morisaki T, et al. Thyrolipomatosis: a case report with review of the literature. Mol Clin Oncol. 2017 Jun;6(6):893–5. PMID:28588784
2046. Ishida M, Sekine S, Fukagawa T, et al. Neuroendocrine carcinoma of the stomach: morphologic and immunohistochemical characteristics and prognosis. Am J Surg Pathol. 2013 Jul;37(7):949–59. PMID:23759931
2047. Ishida S, Akita M, Fujikura K, et al. Neuroendocrine carcinoma and mixed neuroendocrine–non-neuroendocrine neoplasm of the stomach: a clinicopathological and exome sequencing study. Hum Pathol. 2021 Apr;110:1–10. PMID:33359239
2048. Ishii H, Mihai R, Watkinson JC, et al. Systematic review of cure and recurrence rates following minimally invasive parathyroidectomy. BJS Open. 2018 May 28;2(6):364–70. PMID:30511037
2049. Ishikawa Y, Sugano H, Matsumoto T, et al. Unusual features of thyroid carcinomas in Japanese patients with Werner syndrome and possible genotype-phenotype relations to cell type and race. Cancer. 1999 Mar 15;85(6):1345–52. PMID:10189141
2050. Isidro ML, Iglesias Díaz P, Matías-Guiu X, et al. Acromegaly due to a growth hormone-releasing hormone-secreting intracranial gangliocytoma. J Endocrinol Invest. 2005 Feb;28(2):162–5. PMID:15887863
2051. Isotalo PA, Keeney GL, Sebo TJ, et al. Adenomatoid tumor of the adrenal gland: a clinicopathologic study of five cases and review of the literature. Am J Surg Pathol. 2003 Jul;27(7):969–77. PMID:12826889
2052. Itami H, Fujii T, Nakai T, et al. TRAF7 mutations and immunohistochemical study of uterine adenomatoid tumor compared with malignant mesothelioma. Hum Pathol. 2021 May;111:59–66. PMID:33667423
2053. Ito H, Kurokawa T, Yokoyama O. Composite paraganglioma with ganglioneuroma in the retroperitoneal space. Int J Urol. 2010 Apr;17(4):385–6. PMID:20409235
2054. Ito T, Igarashi H, Nakamura K, et al. Epidemiological trends of pancreatic and gastrointestinal neuroendocrine tumors in Japan: a nationwide survey analysis. J Gastroenterol. 2015 Jan;50(1):58–64. PMID:24499825
2055. Ito T, Igarashi H, Uehara H, et al. Causes of death and prognostic factors in multiple endocrine neoplasia type 1: a prospective study: comparison of 106 MEN1/Zollinger-Ellison syndrome patients with 1613 literature MEN1 patients with or without pancreatic endocrine tumors. Medicine (Baltimore). 2013 May;92(3):135–81. PMID:23645327
2056. Ito T, Lee L, Jensen RT. Treatment of symptomatic neuroendocrine tumor syndromes: recent advances and controversies. Expert Opin Pharmacother. 2016 Nov;17(16):2191–205. PMID:27635672
2057. Ito T, Takada R, Omoto S, et al. Analysis of prognostic factors in pancreatic metastases: a multicenter retrospective analysis. Pancreas. 2018 Sep;47(8):1033–9. PMID:30048381
2058. Ito Y, Hirokawa M, Hayashi T, et al. Case report: exceptionally rapid growth character of hobnail variant of papillary thyroid carcinoma: a report of four cases. Endocr J. 2020 Oct 28;67(10):1047–53. PMID:32554948
2059. Ito Y, Hirokawa M, Masuoka H, et al. Prognostic factors of minimally invasive follicular thyroid carcinoma: extensive vascular invasion significantly affects patient prognosis. Endocr J. 2013;60(5):637–42. PMID:23327839
2060. Ito Y, Hirokawa M, Miyauchi A, et al.

Prognostic significance of the proportion of tall cell components in papillary thyroid carcinoma. World J Surg. 2017 Mar;41(3):742–7. PMID:27807709

2061. Ito Y, Kakudo K, Hirokawa M, et al. Biological behavior and prognosis of familial papillary thyroid carcinoma. Surgery. 2009 Jan;145(1):100–5. PMID:19081481

2062. Ito Y, Miyauchi A, Arai K, et al. Usefulness of S100A9 for diagnosis of intrathyroid epithelial thymoma (ITET)/carcinoma showing thymus-like differentiation (CASTLE). Pathology. 2006 Dec;38(6):541–4. PMID:17393982

2063. Ito Y, Miyauchi A, Kihara M, et al. Static prognostic factors and appropriate surgical designs for patients with medullary thyroid carcinoma: the second report from a single-institution study in Japan. World J Surg. 2018 Dec;42(12):3954–66. PMID:30051240

2064. Ito Y, Miyauchi A, Nakamura Y, et al. Clinicopathologic significance of intrathyroidal epithelial thymoma/carcinoma showing thymus-like differentiation: a collaborative study with Member Institutes of The Japanese Society of Thyroid Surgery. Am J Clin Pathol. 2007 Feb;127(2):230–6. PMID:17210519

2065. Ito Y, Onoda N, Okamoto T. The revised clinical practice guidelines on the management of thyroid tumors by the Japan Associations of Endocrine Surgeons: core questions and recommendations for treatments of thyroid cancer. Endocr J. 2020 Jul 28;67(7):669–717. PMID:32269182

2066. Ivanova R, Soares P, Castro P, et al. Diffuse (or multinodular) follicular variant of papillary thyroid carcinoma: a clinicopathologic and immunohistochemical analysis of ten cases of an aggressive form of differentiated thyroid carcinoma. Virchows Arch. 2002 Apr;440(4):418–24. PMID:11956824

2067. Iwasa K, Imai MA, Noguchi M, et al. Spindle epithelial tumor with thymus-like differentiation (SETTLE) of the thyroid. Head Neck. 2002 Sep;24(9):888–93. PMID:12211053

2068. Iwasaki T, Matsushita M, Kuwamoto S, et al. Usefulness of significant morphologic characteristics in distinguishing between Merkel cell polyomavirus-positive and Merkel cell polyomavirus-negative Merkel cell carcinomas. Hum Pathol. 2013 Sep;44(9):1912–7. PMID:23664542

2069. Iwata E, Orosz Z, Teh J, et al. Neuroendocrine tumor arising in a tailgut cyst: a rare presacral tumor. Int J Surg Pathol. 2019 May;27(3):336–42. PMID:30176741

2070. Iyoda A, Hiroshima K, Nakatani Y, et al. Pulmonary large cell neuroendocrine carcinoma: its place in the spectrum of pulmonary carcinoma. Ann Thorac Surg. 2007 Aug;84(2):702–7. PMID:17643676

2071. Iype EM, Suresh S, Patil S, et al. Clinicopathological profile and treatment outcomes of sinonasal small cell neuroendocrine carcinoma: a rare case series. Indian J Otolaryngol Head Neck Surg. 2019 Nov;71(Suppl 3):2214–8. PMID:31763323

2072. Izraely S, Witz IP. Site-specific metastasis: a cooperation between cancer cells and the metastatic microenvironment. Int J Cancer. 2021 Mar 15;148(6):1308–22. PMID:32761606

2073. Jackson CE, Norum RA, Boyd SB, et al. Hereditary hyperparathyroidism and multiple ossifying jaw fibromas: a clinically and genetically distinct syndrome. Surgery. 1990 Dec;108(6):1006–12. PMID:2123361

2074. Jacobs IA, Kagan SA. Adrenal leiomyoma: a case report and review of the literature. J Surg Oncol. 1998 Oct;69(2):111–2. PMID:9808515

2075. Jacobsen E, Shanmugam V, Jagannathan J. Rosai-Dorfman disease with activating KRAS mutation - response to cobimetinib. N Engl J Med. 2017 Dec 14;377(24):2398–9. PMID:29236635

2076. Jacobson D, Nayan S, Macnay R, et al. Intra-thyroidal hemangioma–a rare congenital anomaly: case presentation and literature review. Int J Pediatr Otorhinolaryngol. 2014 Oct;78(10):1779–83. PMID:25130945

2077. Jacoby LB, MacCollin M, Barone R, et al. Frequency and distribution of NF2 mutations in schwannomas. Genes Chromosomes Cancer. 1996 Sep;17(1):45–55. PMID:8889506

2078. Jaffrain-Rea ML, Angelini M, Gargano D, et al. Expression of aryl hydrocarbon receptor (AHR) and AHR-interacting protein in pituitary adenomas: pathological and clinical implications. Endocr Relat Cancer. 2009 Sep;16(3):1029–43. PMID:19556287

2079. Jahangiri A, Wagner JR, Pekmezci M, et al. A comprehensive long-term retrospective analysis of silent corticotrophic adenomas vs hormone-negative adenomas. Neurosurgery. 2013 Jul;73(1):8–17. PMID:23685641

2080. Jain M, Khan A, Patwardhan N, et al. Follicular variant of papillary thyroid carcinoma: a comparative study of histopathologic features and cytology results in 141 patients. Endocr Pract. 2001 Mar-Apr;7(2):79–84. PMID:11421549

2081. Jain R, Gramigna V, Sanchez-Marull R, et al. Composite intestinal-type adenocarcinoma and small cell carcinoma of sinonasal tract. J Clin Pathol. 2009 Jul;62(7):634–7. PMID:19321468

2082. Jaiswal VR, Hoang MP. Primary combined squamous and small cell carcinoma of the larynx: a case report and review of the literature. Arch Pathol Lab Med. 2004 Nov;128(11):1279–82. PMID:15504064

2083. Jalaly JB, Baloch ZW. Hürthle-cell neoplasms of the thyroid: an algorithmic approach to pathologic diagnosis in light of molecular advances. Semin Diagn Pathol. 2020 Sep;37(5):234–42. PMID:32444244

2084. Jamilloux Y, Favier J, Pertuit M, et al. A MEN1 syndrome with a paraganglioma. Eur J Hum Genet. 2014 Feb;22(2):283–5. PMID:23778871

2085. Janeway KA, Kim SY, Lodish M, et al. Defects in succinate dehydrogenase in gastrointestinal stromal tumors lacking KIT and PDGFRA mutations. Proc Natl Acad Sci U S A. 2011 Jan 4;108(1):314–8. PMID:21173220

2086. Jang H, Park CK, Son EJ, et al. Hyalinizing trabecular tumor of the thyroid: diagnosis of a rare tumor using ultrasonography, cytology, and intraoperative frozen sections. Ultrasonography. 2016 Apr;35(2):131–9. PMID:26639939

2087. Jang JH, Kim KH, Lee YM, et al. Surgical results of pure endoscopic endonasal transsphenoidal surgery for 331 pituitary adenomas: a 15-year experience from a single institution. World Neurosurg. 2016 Dec;96:545–55. PMID:27663264

2088. Janoueix-Lerosey I, Lequin D, Brugières L, et al. Somatic and germline activating mutations of the ALK kinase receptor in neuroblastoma. Nature. 2008 Oct 16;455(7215):967–70. PMID:18923523

2089. Janoueix-Lerosey I, Lopez-Delisle L, Delattre O, et al. The ALK receptor in sympathetic neuron development and neuroblastoma. Cell Tissue Res. 2018 May;372(2):325–37. PMID:29374774

2090. Janovitz T, Williamson DFK, Wong KS, et al. Genomic profile of columnar cell variant of papillary thyroid carcinoma. Histopathology. 2021 Oct;79(4):491–8. PMID:33783022

2091. Janson ET, Knigge U, Dam G, et al. Nordic guidelines 2021 for diagnosis and treatment of gastroenteropancreatic neuroendocrine neoplasms. Acta Oncol. 2021 Jul;60(7):931–41. PMID:33999752

2092. Jarrell ST, Vortmeyer AO, Linehan WM, et al. Metastases to hemangioblastomas in von Hippel-Lindau disease. J Neurosurg. 2006 Aug;105(2):256–63. PMID:17219831

2093. Jastania RA, Alsaad KO, Al-Shraim M, et al. Double adenomas of the pituitary: transcription factors Pit-1, T-pit, and SF-1 identify cytogenesis and differentiation. Endocr Pathol. 2005 Fall;16(3):187–94. PMID:16299401

2094. Javaid MK, Boyce A, Appelman-Dijkstra N, et al. Best practice management guidelines for fibrous dysplasia/McCune-Albright syndrome: a consensus statement from the FD/MAS international consortium. Orphanet J Rare Dis. 2019 Jun 13;14(1):139. PMID:31196103

2095. Javanbakht A, D'Apuzzo M, Badie B, et al. Pituitary metastasis: a rare condition. Endocr Connect. 2018 Aug 23;7(10):1049–57. PMID:30139817

2096. Jayaram G, Hayati JN, Yip CH, et al. Cytologic, histologic and immunocytochemical features in fine needle aspiration of paraganglioma-like variant of medullary carcinoma. Acta Cytol. 2008 Jan-Feb;52(1):119–21. PMID:18323289

2097. Jensen K, Kohler S, Rouse RV. Cytokeratin staining in Merkel cell carcinoma: an immunohistochemical study of cytokeratins 5/6, 7, 17, and 20. Appl Immunohistochem Mol Morphol. 2000 Dec;8(4):310–5. PMID:11127923

2098. Jensen RT, Bodei L, Capdevila J, et al. Unmet needs in functional and nonfunctional pancreatic neuroendocrine neoplasms. Neuroendocrinology. 2019;108(1):26–36. PMID:30282083

2099. Jensen RT, Cadiot G, Brandi ML, et al. ENETS consensus guidelines for the management of patients with digestive neuroendocrine neoplasms: functional pancreatic endocrine tumor syndromes. Neuroendocrinology. 2012;95(2):98–119. PMID:22261919

2100. Jensen RT, Niederle B, Mitry E, et al. Gastrinoma (duodenal and pancreatic). Neuroendocrinology. 2006;84(3):173–82. PMID:17312377

2101. Jeon MJ, Kim WG, Chung KW, et al. Active surveillance of papillary thyroid microcarcinoma: Where do we stand? Eur Thyroid J. 2019 Dec;8(6):298–306. PMID:31934555

2102. Jeong SH, Hong HS, Kwak JJ, et al. Analysis of RAS mutation and PAX8/PPARγ rearrangements in follicular-derived thyroid neoplasms in a Korean population: frequency and ultrasound findings. J Endocrinol Invest. 2015 Aug;38(8):849–57. PMID:25999051

2103. Jeremie G, Lifante JC, Chazot FB, et al. [Myxoid variant of adrenocortical carcinoma]. Ann Pathol. 2021 Apr;41(2):186–91. French. PMID:33549334

2104. Jesinghaus M, Konukiewitz B, Keller G, et al. Colorectal mixed adenoneuroendocrine carcinomas and neuroendocrine carcinomas are genetically closely related to colorectal adenocarcinomas. Mod Pathol. 2017 Apr;30(4):610–9. PMID:28059096

2105. Jha S, El-Maouche D, Marko J, et al. Individualizing management of infertility in classic congenital adrenal hyperplasia and testicular adrenal rest tumors. J Endocr Soc. 2019 Oct 17;3(12):2290–4. PMID:31745525

2106. Jhala NC, Jhala D, Eloubeidi MA, et al. Endoscopic ultrasound-guided fine-needle aspiration biopsy of the adrenal glands: analysis of 24 patients. Cancer. 2004 Oct 25;102(5):308–14. PMID:15376200

2107. Ji JH, Oh YL, Hong M, et al. Identification of driving ALK fusion genes and genomic landscape of medullary thyroid cancer. PLoS Genet. 2015 Aug 21;11(8):e1005467. PMID:26295973

2108. Jiang J, Zhang J, Pang Y, et al. Sino-European differences in the genetic landscape and clinical presentation of pheochromocytoma and paraganglioma. J Clin Endocrinol Metab. 2020 Oct 1;105(10):dgaa502. PMID:32750708

2109. Jiang J, Zhang L, Wu Z, et al. A rare case of watery diarrhea, hypokalemia and achlorhydria syndrome caused by pheochromocytoma. BMC Cancer. 2014 Jul 31;14:553. PMID:25081061

2110. Jiao Y, Shi C, Edil BH, et al. DAXX/ATRX, MEN1, and mTOR pathway genes are frequently altered in pancreatic neuroendocrine tumors. Science. 2011 Mar 4;331(6021):1199–203. PMID:21252315

2111. Jimenez-Heffernan JA, Hardisson D, Palacios J, et al. Adrenal gland leiomyoma in a child with acquired immunodeficiency syndrome. Pediatr Pathol Lab Med. 1995 Nov-Dec;15(6):923–9. PMID:8705202

2112. Jimenez-Heffernan JA, Lopez-Ferrer P, Vicandi B, et al. Fine-needle aspiration cytology of large cell neuroendocrine carcinoma of the lung: a cytohistologic correlation study of 11 cases. Cancer. 2008 Jun 25;114(3):180–6. PMID:18433011

2113. Jiménez-Heffernan JA, Vicandi B, López-Ferrer P, et al. Cytologic features of pheochromocytoma and retroperitoneal paraganglioma: a morphologic and immunohistochemical study of 13 cases. Acta Cytol. 2006 Jul-Aug;50(4):372–8. PMID:16900997

2114. Jin L, Qian X, Kulig E, et al. Transforming growth factor-beta, transforming growth factor-beta receptor II, and p27Kip1 expression in nontumorous and neoplastic human pituitaries. Am J Pathol. 1997 Aug;151(2):509–19. PMID:9250163

2115. Jing X, Michael CW. Potential pitfalls for false suspicion of papillary thyroid carcinoma: a cytohistologic review of 22 cases. Diagn Cytopathol. 2012 May;40 Suppl 1:E74–9. PMID:21563322

2116. Jo JH, Chung TM, Youn H, et al. Cytoplasmic parafibromin/hCdc73 targets and destabilizes p53 mRNA to control p53-mediated apoptosis. Nat Commun. 2014 Nov 12;5:5433. PMID:25388829

2117. Jo VY, Fletcher CD. Epithelioid malignant peripheral nerve sheath tumor: clinicopathologic analysis of 63 cases. Am J Surg Pathol. 2015 May;39(5):673–82. PMID:25602794

2118. Jo VY, Krane JF, Pantanowitz L, et al. HPV-associated neuroendocrine carcinomas of the head and neck in FNA biopsies: clinicopathologic features of a rare entity. Cancer Cytopathol. 2019 Feb;127(1):26–34. PMID:30475447

2119. Job S, Draskovic I, Burnichon N, et al. Telomerase activation and ATRX mutations are independent risk factors for metastatic pheochromocytoma and paraganglioma. Clin Cancer Res. 2019 Jan 15;25(2):760–70. PMID:30301828

2120. Job S, Georges A, Burnichon N, et al. Transcriptome analysis of lncRNAs in pheochromocytomas and paragangliomas. J Clin Endocrinol Metab. 2020 Mar 1;105(3):dgz168. PMID:31678991

2121. Jochmanova I, Abcede AMT, Guerrero RJS, et al. Clinical characteristics and outcomes of SDHB-related pheochromocytoma and paraganglioma in children and adolescents. J Cancer Res Clin Oncol. 2020 Apr;146(4):1051–63. PMID:32062700

2122. Joehlin-Price AS, Hardesty DA, Arnold CA, et al. Case report: ACTH-secreting pituitary carcinoma metastatic to the liver in a patient with a history of atypical pituitary adenoma and Cushing's disease. Diagn Pathol. 2017 Apr 18;12(1):34. PMID:28420444

2123. Johannessen JV, Sobrinho-Simões M. The origin and significance of thyroid psammoma bodies. Lab Invest. 1980 Sep;43(3):287–96. PMID:7401638

2124. Johansen L, Haller W, Thyagarajan M, et al. Hepatic lesions associated with McCune Albright syndrome. J Pediatr Gastroenterol Nutr. 2019 Apr;68(4):e54–7. PMID:30628989
2125. Johnson KJ, Hussain I, Williams K, et al. Development of an international internet-based neurofibromatosis Type 1 patient registry. Contemp Clin Trials. 2013 Mar;34(2):305–11. PMID:23246715
2126. Johnson LN, Hepler RS, Yee RD, et al. Magnetic resonance imaging of craniopharyngioma. Am J Ophthalmol. 1986 Aug 15;102(2):242–4. PMID:3740186
2127. Johnson MD, Fan X, Bourne P, et al. Neuronal differentiation and expression of neural epitopes in pituitary adenomas. J Histochem Cytochem. 2007 Dec;55(12):1265–71. PMID:17875653
2128. Johnson RE, Scheithauer B. Massive hyperplasia of testicular adrenal rests in a patient with Nelson's syndrome. Am J Clin Pathol. 1982 Apr;77(4):501–7. PMID:7072659
2129. Johnson TL, Zarbo RJ, Lloyd RV, et al. Paragangliomas of the head and neck: immunohistochemical neuroendocrine and intermediate filament typing. Mod Pathol. 1988 May;1(3):216–23. PMID:2467285
2130. Johnston PC, Kennedy L, Weil RJ, et al. Ectopic ACTH-secreting pituitary adenomas within the sphenoid sinus. Endocrine. 2014 Dec;47(3):717–24. PMID:24927792
2131. Jokisch F, Kleinlein I, Haller B, et al. A small subgroup of Hashimoto's thyroiditis is associated with IgG4-related disease. Virchows Arch. 2016 Mar;468(3):321–7. PMID:26669779
2132. Jones RT, Abedalthagafi MS, Brahmandam M, et al. Cross-reactivity of the BRAF VE1 antibody with epitopes in axonemal dyneins leads to staining of cilia. Mod Pathol. 2015 Apr;28(4):596–606. PMID:25412847
2133. Joseph NM, Chen YY, Nasr A, et al. Genomic profiling of malignant peritoneal mesothelioma reveals recurrent alterations in epigenetic regulatory genes BAP1, SETD2, and DDX3X. Mod Pathol. 2017 Feb;30(2):246–54. PMID:27813512
2134. Jouinot A, Assie G, Libe R, et al. DNA methylation is an independent prognostic marker of survival in adrenocortical cancer. J Clin Endocrinol Metab. 2017 Mar 1;102(3):923–32. PMID:27967600
2135. Jovanovic L, Delahunt B, McIver B, et al. Thyroid gland clonality revisited: the embryonal patch size of the normal human thyroid gland is very large, suggesting X-chromosome inactivation tumor clonality studies of thyroid tumors have to be interpreted with caution. J Clin Endocrinol Metab. 2003 Jul;88(7):3284–91. PMID:12843177
2136. Juarez D, Brown RW, Ostrowski M, et al. Pheochromocytoma associated with neuroendocrine carcinoma. A new type of composite pheochromocytoma. Arch Pathol Lab Med. 1999 Dec;123(12):1274–9. PMID:10583935
2137. Jug R, Jiang X. Noninvasive follicular thyroid neoplasm with papillary-like nuclear features: an evidence-based nomenclature change. Patholog Res Int. 2017;2017:1057252. PMID:28280647
2138. Juhlin C, Larsson C, Yakoleva T, et al. Loss of parafibromin expression in a subset of parathyroid adenomas. Endocr Relat Cancer. 2006 Jun;13(2):509–23. PMID:16728578
2139. Juhlin CC. Challenges in paragangliomas and pheochromocytomas: from histology to molecular immunohistochemistry. Endocr Pathol. 2021 Jun;32(2):228–44. PMID:33768452
2140. Juhlin CC, Asa SL, Jatta K, et al. Perithyroidal salivary gland acinic cell carcinoma: morphological and molecular attributes of a unique lesion. Head Neck Pathol. 2021 Jun;15(2):628–37. PMID:32519264
2141. Juhlin CC, Bertherat J, Giordano TJ, et al. What did we learn from the molecular biology of adrenal cortical neoplasia? From histopathology to translational genomics. Endocr Pathol. 2021 Mar;32(1):102–33. PMID:33534120
2142. Juhlin CC, Bränström R, Shabo I, et al. Clear cell variant of a follicular thyroid tumor with uncertain malignant potential: a case report. Int J Surg Pathol. 2019 May;27(3):290–3. PMID:30370813
2143. Juhlin CC, Erickson LA. Genomics and epigenomics in parathyroid neoplasia: from bench to surgical pathology practice. Endocr Pathol. 2021 Mar;32(1):17–34. PMID:33269427
2144. Juhlin CC, Falhammar H, Zedenius J, et al. Lipoadenoma of the parathyroid gland: characterization of an institutional series spanning 28 years. Endocr Pathol. 2020 Jun;31(2):156–65. PMID:32193823
2145. Juhlin CC, Goh G, Healy JM, et al. Whole-exome sequencing characterizes the landscape of somatic mutations and copy number alterations in adrenocortical carcinoma. J Clin Endocrinol Metab. 2015 Mar;100(3):E493–502. PMID:25490274
2146. Juhlin CC, Haglund F, Obara T, et al. Absence of nucleolar parafibromin immunoreactivity in subsets of parathyroid malignant tumours. Virchows Arch. 2011 Jul;459(1):47–53. PMID:21221636
2147. Juhlin CC, Höög A. Clear cell variant of papillary thyroid carcinoma with associated anaplastic thyroid carcinoma: description of an extraordinary case. Int J Surg Pathol. 2019 Sep;27(6):658–63. PMID:30931661
2148. Juhlin CC, Kiss NB, Villablanca A, et al. Frequent promoter hypermethylation of the APC and RASSF1A tumour suppressors in parathyroid tumours. PLoS One. 2010 Mar 1;5(3):e9472. PMID:20208994
2149. Juhlin CC, Nilsson IL, Falhammar H, et al. Institutional characterisation of water clear cell parathyroid adenoma: a rare entity often unrecognised by TC-99m-sestamibi scintigraphy. Pathology. 2021 Dec;53(7):852–9. PMID:33994174
2150. Juhlin CC, Nilsson IL, Johansson K, et al. Parafibromin and APC as screening markers for malignant potential in atypical parathyroid adenomas. Endocr Pathol. 2010 Sep;21(3):166–77. PMID:20473645
2151. Juhlin CC, Nilsson IL, Lagerstedt-Robinson K, et al. Parafibromin immunostainings of parathyroid tumors in clinical routine: a near-decade experience from a tertiary center. Mod Pathol. 2019 Jul;32(8):1082–94. PMID:30923346
2152. Juhlin CC, Stenman A, Zedenius J. Macrofollicular variant follicular thyroid tumors are DICER1 mutated and exhibit distinct histological features. Histopathology. 2021 Oct;79(4):661–6. PMID:34008223
2153. Juhlin CC, Villablanca A, Sandelin K, et al. Parafibromin immunoreactivity: its use as an additional diagnostic marker for parathyroid tumor classification. Endocr Relat Cancer. 2007 Jun;14(2):501–12. PMID:17639063
2154. Juhlin CC, Zedenius J, Höög A. Clinical routine application of the second-generation neuroendocrine markers ISL1, INSM1, and secretagogin in neuroendocrine neoplasia: staining outcomes and potential clues for determining tumor origin. Endocr Pathol. 2020 Dec;31(4):401–10. PMID:32813226
2155. Jukes A, Allan R, Rawson R, et al. Growth hormone secreting pituitary adenoma with admixed gangliocytoma and ganglioglioma. J Clin Neurosci. 2016 Sep;31:202–4. PMID:27068013
2156. Jung CK, Choi YJ, Lee KY, et al. The cytological, clinical, and pathological features of the cribriform-morular variant of papillary thyroid carcinoma and mutation analysis of CTNNB1 and BRAF genes. Thyroid. 2009 Aug;19(8):905–13. PMID:19534622
2157. Kabara M, Nakagawa N, Chinda J, et al. Diagnosis of IgG4-related systemic disease by cytology of large pericardial effusion with fine needle aspiration. Int J Cardiol. 2011 May 5;148(3):392–3. PMID:21194763
2158. Kageji T, Miyamoto T, Kotani Y, et al. Congenital craniopharyngioma treated by radical surgery: case report and review of the literature. Childs Nerv Syst. 2017 Feb;33(2):357–62. PMID:27669698
2159. Kakkar A, Kaur K, Kumar T, et al. Pigmented pheochromocytoma: an unusual variant of a common tumor. Endocr Pathol. 2016 Mar;27(1):42–5. PMID:26578456
2160. Kakkar A, Purkait S, Agarwal S, et al. Primary thyroid lymphoma: a series from a tertiary care center in Northern India. J Cancer Res Ther. 2019 Jul-Sep;15(3):669–75. PMID:31169238
2161. Kakudo K, Bai Y, Liu Z, et al. Classification of thyroid follicular cell tumors: with special reference to borderline lesions. Endocr J. 2012;59(1):1–12. PMID:21908930
2162. Kakudo K, Bai Y, Liu Z, et al. Encapsulated papillary thyroid carcinoma, follicular variant: a misnomer. Pathol Int. 2012 Mar;62(3):155–60. PMID:22360502
2163. Kakudo K, Mori I, Tamaoki N, et al. Carcinoma of possible thymic origin presenting as a thyroid mass: a new subgroup of squamous cell carcinoma of the thyroid. J Surg Oncol. 1988 Jul;38(3):187–92. PMID:3260644
2164. Kakudo K, Wakasa T, Ohta Y, et al. Prognostic classification of thyroid follicular cell tumors using Ki-67 labeling index: risk stratification of thyroid follicular cell carcinomas. Endocr J. 2015;62(1):1–12. PMID:25195708
2165. Kalezic NK, Zivaljevic VR, Slijepcevic NA, et al. Risk factors for sporadic medullary thyroid carcinoma. Eur J Cancer Prev. 2013 May;22(3):262–7. PMID:22960778
2166. Kaltsas G, Caplin M, Davies P, et al. ENETS consensus guidelines for the standards of care in neuroendocrine tumors: pre- and perioperative therapy in patients with neuroendocrine tumors. Neuroendocrinology. 2017;105(3):245–54. PMID:28253514
2167. Kaltsas G, Kanakis G, Chrousos G. Carney complex. In: Feingold KR, Anawalt B, Blackman MR, et al., editors. Endotext. South Dartmouth (MA): MDText.com, Inc.; 2000 [updated 2023 Jul 13]. PMID:25905341
2168. Kamarashev J, French LE, Dummer R, et al. Symplastic glomus tumor - a rare but distinct benign histological variant with analogy to other 'ancient' benign skin neoplasms. J Cutan Pathol. 2009 Oct;36(10):1099–102. PMID:19602065
2169. Kamboj M, Gandhi JS, Gupta G, et al. Neuroendocrine carcinoma of gall bladder: a series of 19 cases with review of literature. J Gastrointest Cancer. 2015 Dec;46(4):356–64. PMID:26208508
2170. Kameneva P, Artemov AV, Kastriti ME, et al. Single-cell transcriptomics of human embryos identifies multiple sympathoblast lineages with potential implications for neuroblastoma origin. Nat Genet. 2021 May;53(5):694–706. PMID:33833454
2171. Kameyama K, Takami H. Proposal for the histological classification of parathyroid carcinoma. Endocr Pathol. 2005 Spring;16(1):49–52. PMID:16000846
2172. Kamihara J, Bourdeaut F, Foulkes WD, et al. Retinoblastoma and neuroblastoma predisposition and surveillance. Clin Cancer Res. 2017 Jul 1;23(13):e98–106. PMID:28674118
2173. Kamihara J, Paulson V, Breen MA, et al. DICER1-associated central nervous system sarcoma in children: comprehensive clinicopathologic and genetic analysis of a newly described rare tumor. Mod Pathol. 2020 Oct;33(10):1910–21. PMID:32291395
2174. Kamilaris CDC, Faucz FR, Voutetakis A, et al. Carney complex. Exp Clin Endocrinol Diabetes. 2019 Feb;127(2-03):156-164. PMID:30428497
2175. Kamilaris CDC, Stratakis CA, Hannah-Shmouni F. Molecular genetic and genomic alterations in Cushing's syndrome and primary aldosteronism. Front Endocrinol (Lausanne). 2021 Mar 12;12:632543. PMID:33776926
2176. Kaminskyi OV, Kopylova OV, Afanasyev DE, et al. [Hyperparathyroidism and parathyroid lesions in the ChNPP accident survivors]. Probl Radiac Med Radiobiol. 2019 Dec;24:380–94. Ukrainian. PMID:31841481
2177. Kaminuma Y, Tanahashi M, Yoshii N, et al. Bronchogenic gangliocytic paraganglioma. J Bronchology Interv Pulmonol. 2020 Jul;27(3):212–5. PMID:32205710
2178. Kamisawa T, Tu Y, Egawa N, et al. Ductal and acinar differentiation in pancreatic endocrine tumors. Dig Dis Sci. 2002 Oct;47(10):2254–61. PMID:12395898
2179. Kamiya-Matsuoka C, Cachia D, Waguespack SG, et al. Radiotherapy with concurrent temozolomide for the management of extraneural metastases in pituitary carcinoma. Pituitary. 2016 Aug;19(4):415–21. PMID:27106209
2180. Kamp K, Feelders RA, van Adrichem RC, et al. Parathyroid hormone-related peptide (PTHrP) secretion by gastroenteropancreatic neuroendocrine tumors (GEP-NETs): clinical features, diagnosis, management, and follow-up. J Clin Endocrinol Metab. 2014 Sep;99(9):3060–9. PMID:24905065
2181. Kanaji N, Watanabe N, Kita N, et al. Paraneoplastic syndromes associated with lung cancer. World J Clin Oncol. 2014 Aug 10;5(3):197–223. PMID:25114839
2182. Kanakis G, Kaltsas G, Granberg D, et al. Unusual complication of a pancreatic neuroendocrine tumor presenting with malignant hypercalcemia. J Clin Endocrinol Metab. 2012 Apr;97(4):E627–31. PMID:22319031
2183. Kanazawa S, Kammori M. Case report: 84-month disease-free survival after surgery for anaplastic thyroid carcinoma. J Nippon Med Sch. 2019;86(1):38–42. PMID:30918155
2184. Kanazawa T, Harris TS, Chikunguwo SM, et al. Larvicidal properties of macrophages induced by cloned murine schistosomal egg antigen-specific CD4 positive T-helper lymphocytes. Parasite Immunol. 1992 May;14(3):279–93. PMID:1385648
2185. Kanazawa T, Nokubi M, Takeoda K, et al. Atypical carcinoid of the larynx and expressions of proteins associated with molecular targeted therapy. Auris Nasus Larynx. 2011 Feb;38(1):123–6. PMID:20580173
2186. Kandil E, Abdel Khalek M, Abdullah O, et al. Primary peripheral nerve sheath tumors of the thyroid gland. Thyroid. 2010 Jun;20(6):583–6. PMID:20553194
2187. Kane AJ, Sughrue ME, Rutkowski MJ, et al. Atypia predicting prognosis for intracranial extraventricular neurocytomas. J Neurosurg. 2012 Feb;116(2):349–54. PMID:22054208
2188. Kaneko Y, Saito S, Takahashi K, et al. Neuroendocrine carcinoma of the esophagus with an adenocarcinoma component. Clin J Gastroenterol. 2019 Dec;12(6):534–8. PMID:31134449
2189. Kang H, Pettinga D, Schubert AD, et al. Genomic profiling of parathyroid carcinoma reveals genomic alterations suggesting benefit from therapy. Oncologist. 2019 Jun;24(6):791–7. PMID:30373905

2190. Kang Y, Pekmezci M, Folpe AL, et al. Diagnostic utility of SOX10 to distinguish malignant peripheral nerve sheath tumor from synovial sarcoma, including intraneural synovial sarcoma. Mod Pathol. 2014 Jan;27(1):55–61. PMID:23929265
2191. Kanitra JJ, Hardaway JC, Soleimani T, et al. Adrenocortical oncocytic neoplasm: a systematic review. Surgery. 2018 Dec;164(6):1351–9. PMID:30037428
2192. Kano Y, Kakinuma S, Goto F, et al. Primary hepatic neuroendocrine carcinoma with a cholangiocellular carcinoma component in one nodule. Clin J Gastroenterol. 2014 Oct;7(5):449–54. PMID:26184027
2193. Kansal A, Lahiri A, Nishikawa H. Sympathetic paraganglioma presenting with Horner's syndrome in a child. J Plast Reconstr Aesthet Surg. 2006;59(7):772–4. PMID:16782577
2194. Kao HL, Chang WC, Li WY, et al. Head and neck large cell neuroendocrine carcinoma should be separated from atypical carcinoid on the basis of different clinical features, overall survival, and pathogenesis. Am J Surg Pathol. 2012 Feb;36(2):185–92. PMID:22082601
2195. Kapran Y, Bauersfeld J, Anlauf M, et al. Multihormonality and entrapment of islets in pancreatic endocrine tumors. Virchows Arch. 2006 Apr;448(4):394–8. PMID:16418841
2196. Kapur A, Singh N, Mete O, et al. A young male with parafibromin-deficient parathyroid carcinoma due to a rare germline HRPT2/CDC73 mutation. Endocr Pathol. 2018 Dec;29(4):374–9. PMID:30361844
2197. Karageorgiadis AS, Papadakis GZ, Biro J, et al. Ectopic adrenocorticotropic hormone and corticotropin-releasing hormone co-secreting tumors in children and adolescents causing Cushing syndrome: a diagnostic dilemma and how to solve it. J Clin Endocrinol Metab. 2015 Jan;100(1):141–8. PMID:25291050
2198. Karaisli S, Haciyanli M, Gücek Haciyanli S, et al. Spindle epithelial tumour with thymus-like differentiation: report of two cases. Ann R Coll Surg Engl. 2020 Feb;102(2):e33–5. PMID:31530165
2199. Karak AK, Sahoo M, Bhatnagar D. Fine needle aspiration cytology, histology and MIB-1 proliferative index in a case of dyshormonogenetic goitre. Indian J Pathol Microbiol. 2001 Apr;44(2):169–72. PMID:11883139
2200. Karamchandani JR, Nielsen TO, van de Rijn M, et al. Sox10 and S100 in the diagnosis of soft-tissue neoplasms. Appl Immunohistochem Mol Morphol. 2012 Oct;20(5):445–50. PMID:22495377
2201. Karamzadeh Dashti N, Bahrami A, Lee SJ, et al. BRAF V600E mutations occur in a subset of glomus tumors, and are associated with malignant histologic characteristics. Am J Surg Pathol. 2017 Nov;41(11):1532–41. PMID:28834810
2202. Karavitaki N, Brufani C, Warner JT, et al. Craniopharyngiomas in children and adults: systematic analysis of 121 cases with long-term follow-up. Clin Endocrinol (Oxf). 2005 Apr;62(4):397–409. PMID:15807869
2203. Karim F, Loeffen J, Bramer W, et al. IgG4-related disease: a systematic review of this unrecognized disease in pediatrics. Pediatr Rheumatol Online J. 2016 Mar 25;14(1):18. PMID:27012661
2204. Karimi F. Primary adrenal lymphoma presenting with adrenal failure: a case report and review of the literature. Int J Endocrinol Metab. 2017 Oct 26;15(4):e12014. PMID:29344029
2205. Kariya S, Cureoglu S, Schachern PA, et al. Histopathological temporal bone study of the metastatic rhabdomyosarcoma. Auris Nasus Larynx. 2009 Apr;36(2):221–3. PMID:18606509
2206. Karl M, Lamberts SW, Koper JW, et al. Cushing's disease preceded by generalized glucocorticoid resistance: clinical consequences of a novel, dominant-negative glucocorticoid receptor mutation. Proc Assoc Am Physicians. 1996 Jul;108(4):296–307. PMID:8863343
2207. Karnezis AN, Wang Y, Keul J, et al. DICER1 and FOXL2 mutation status correlates with clinicopathologic features in ovarian Sertoli-Leydig cell tumors. Am J Surg Pathol. 2019 May;43(5):628–38. PMID:30986800
2208. Karpathiou G, Casteillo F, Dridi M, et al. L1CAM expression in cystic mesothelial lesions: a comparison with adenomatoid tumours, well-differentiated papillary mesothelial tumours and malignant mesotheliomas. Histopathology. 2021 Aug;79(2):272–4. PMID:33847416
2209. Karpathiou G, Hiroshima K, Peoc'h M. Adenomatoid tumor: a review of pathology with focus on unusual presentations and sites, histogenesis, differential diagnosis, and molecular and clinical aspects with a historic overview of its description. Adv Anat Pathol. 2020 Nov;27(6):394–407. PMID:32769378
2210. Karunamurthy A, Panebianco F, J Hsiao S, et al. Prevalence and phenotypic correlations of EIF1AX mutations in thyroid nodules. Endocr Relat Cancer. 2016 Apr;23(4):295–301. PMID:26911375
2211. Karvounaris DC, Symeonidis N, Triantafyllou A, et al. Ectopic parathyroid adenoma located inside the hypoglossal nerve. Head Neck. 2010 Sep;32(9):1273–6. PMID:19691113
2212. Kasaian K, Chindris AM, Wiseman SM, et al. MEN1 mutations in Hürthle cell (oncocytic) thyroid carcinoma. J Clin Endocrinol Metab. 2015 Apr;100(4):E611–5. PMID:25625803
2213. Kasajima A, Klöppel G. Neuroendocrine neoplasms of lung, pancreas and gut: a morphology-based comparison. Endocr Relat Cancer. 2020 Nov;27(11):R417–32. PMID:33032264
2214. Kasajima A, Konukiewitz B, Schlitter AM, et al. An analysis of 130 neuroendocrine tumors G3 regarding prevalence, origin, metastasis, and diagnostic features. Virchows Arch. 2022 Feb;480(2):359–68. PMID:34499237
2215. Kasajima A, Konukiewitz B, Schlitter AM, et al. Mesenchymal/non-epithelial mimickers of neuroendocrine neoplasms with a focus on fusion gene-associated and SWI/SNF-deficient tumors. Virchows Arch. 2021 Dec;479(6):1209–19. PMID:34350470
2216. Kasajima A, Nakamura Y, Adachi Y, et al. Oncocytic adrenocortical neoplasm arising from adrenal rest in the broad ligament of the uterus. Pathol Int. 2014 Apr;64(4):183–8. PMID:24750189
2217. Kasaliwal R, Goroshi M, Khadilkar K, et al. Primary adrenal lymphoma: a single-center experience. Endocr Pract. 2015 Jul;21(7):719–24. PMID:25716633
2218. Kasem K, Lam AK. Adrenal oncocytic phaeochromocytoma with putative adverse histologic features: a unique case report and review of the literature. Endocr Pathol. 2014 Dec;25(4):416–21. PMID:25252620
2219. Kaserer K, Scheuba C, Neuhold N, et al. C-cell hyperplasia and medullary thyroid carcinoma in patients routinely screened for serum calcitonin. Am J Surg Pathol. 1998 Jun;22(6):722–8. PMID:9630179
2220. Kaserer K, Scheuba C, Neuhold N, et al. Sporadic versus familial medullary thyroid microcarcinoma: a histopathologic study of 50 consecutive patients. Am J Surg Pathol. 2001 Oct;25(10):1245–51. PMID:11688458
2221. Kastriti ME, Kameneva P, Kamenev D, et al. Schwann cell precursors generate the majority of chromaffin cells in Zuckerkandl organ and some sympathetic neurons in paraganglia. Front Mol Neurosci. 2019 Jan 25;12:6. PMID:30740044
2222. Katabi N. Neuroendocrine neoplasms of the ear. Head Neck Pathol. 2018 Sep;12(3):362–6. PMID:30069842
2223. Kataoka K, Taguchi M, Takeshita A, et al. Recurrence of primary hyperparathyroidism following spontaneous remission with intracapsular hemorrhage of a parathyroid adenoma. J Bone Miner Metab. 2008;26(3):295–7. PMID:18470672
2224. Katayama A, Otsuka F, Takeda M, et al. Rhabdomyosarcoma discovered in the adrenal region of an elderly hypertensive patient. Hypertens Res. 2011 Jun;34(6):784–6. PMID:21412240
2225. Kato I, Tajima K, Suchi T, et al. Chronic thyroiditis as a risk factor of B-cell lymphoma in the thyroid gland. Jpn J Cancer Res. 1985 Nov;76(11):1085–90. PMID:3936828
2226. Kato K, Nakatani Y, Kanno H, et al. Possible linkage between specific histological structures and aberrant reactivation of the Wnt pathway in adamantinomatous craniopharyngioma. J Pathol. 2004 Jul;203(3):814–21. PMID:15221941
2227. Kato M, Inoshita N, Sugiyama T, et al. Differential expression of genes related to drug responsiveness between sparsely and densely granulated somatotroph adenomas. Endocr J. 2012;59(3):221–8. PMID:22200580
2228. Kato N, Kusumi T, Kamataki A, et al. DICER1 hotspot mutations in ovarian Sertoli-Leydig cell tumors: a potential association with androgenic effects. Hum Pathol. 2017 Jan;59:41–7. PMID:27664536
2229. Katz RL, Patel S, Mackay B, et al. Fine needle aspiration cytology of the adrenal gland. Acta Cytol. 1984 May-Jun;28(3):269–82. PMID:6587703
2230. Katznelson L, Laws ER Jr, Melmed S, et al. Acromegaly: an Endocrine Society clinical practice guideline. J Clin Endocrinol Metab. 2014 Nov;99(11):3933–51. PMID:25356808
2231. Kauffmann RM, Juhlin CC, Fohn LE, et al. Parathyroid carcinoma arising from four-gland hyperplasia. Endocr Pract. 2011 Mar-Apr;17(2):e37–42. PMID:21247853
2232. Kaufmann O, Dietel M. Expression of thyroid transcription factor-1 in pulmonary and extrapulmonary small cell carcinomas and other neuroendocrine carcinomas of various primary sites. Histopathology. 2000 May;36(5):415–20. PMID:10792482
2233. Kaur A, Jayaram G. Thyroid tumors: cytomorphology of medullary, clinically anaplastic, and miscellaneous thyroid neoplasms. Diagn Cytopathol. 1990;6(6):383–9. PMID:2292224
2234. Kaur J, Srinivasan R, Kakkar N. Fine needle aspiration cytology of a spindle epithelial tumour with thymus-like differentiation (SETTLE) occurring in the thyroid. Cytopathology. 2012 Dec;23(6):413–5. PMID:22136375
2235. Kaur R, Mehta J, Borges A. Extranodal follicular dendritic cell sarcoma-a review: "What the mind does not know the eye does not see". Adv Anat Pathol. 2021 Jan;28(1):21–9. PMID:32991350
2236. Kaur R, Mitra S, Rajwanshi A, et al. Fine needle aspiration cytology of IgG4-related disease: a potential diagnostic pitfall? Diagn Cytopathol. 2017 Jan;45(1):14–21. PMID:27666423
2237. Kawai K, Takahashi M. Intracellular RET signaling pathways activated by GDNF. Cell Tissue Res. 2020 Oct;382(1):113–23. PMID:32816064
2238. Kawaji H, Saito O, Amano S, et al. Extraventricular neurocytoma of the sellar region with spinal dissemination. Brain Tumor Pathol. 2014 Jan;31(1):51–6. PMID:23250388
2239. Kawakami K, Takeshita A, Furushima K, et al. Persistent fibroblast growth factor 23 signalling in the parathyroid glands for secondary hyperparathyroidism in mice with chronic kidney disease. Sci Rep. 2017 Jan 17;7:40534. PMID:28094278
2240. Kawamoto S, Shi C, Hruban RH, et al. Small serotonin-producing neuroendocrine tumor of the pancreas associated with pancreatic duct obstruction. AJR Am J Roentgenol. 2011 Sep;197(3):W482-8. PMID:21862776
2241. Kawanishi N, Norimatsu Y, Ohsaki H, et al. Diagnosis of pseudopapillary variant of medullary thyroid carcinoma by fine-needle aspiration cytology. Diagn Cytopathol. 2014 Sep;42(9):823–6. PMID:23894022
2242. Kawashima ST, Tagami T, Nakao K, et al. Serum levels of IgG and IgG4 in Hashimoto thyroiditis. Endocrine. 2014 Mar;45(2):236–43. PMID:23695895
2243. Kawashima ST, Usui T, Sano T, et al. P53 gene mutation in an atypical corticotroph adenoma with Cushing's disease. Clin Endocrinol (Oxf). 2009 Apr;70(4):656–7. PMID:18771563
2244. Kayakabe M, Takahashi K, Okamiya T, et al. Combined small cell carcinoma of the sinonasal tract associated with syndrome of inappropriate secretion of antidiuretic hormone: a case report. Oncol Lett. 2014 Apr;7(4):1253–6. PMID:24944702
2245. Kayani I, Conry BG, Groves AM, et al. A comparison of 68Ga-DOTATATE and 18F-FDG PET/CT in pulmonary neuroendocrine tumors. J Nucl Med. 2009 Dec;50(12):1927–32. PMID:19910422
2246. Kazaure HS, Roman SA, Sosa JA. Insular thyroid cancer: a population-level analysis of patient characteristics and predictors of survival. Cancer. 2012 Jul 1;118(13):3260–7. PMID:22252610
2247. Kazaure HS, Roman SA, Sosa JA. Medullary thyroid microcarcinoma: a population-level analysis of 310 patients. Cancer. 2012 Feb 1;118(3):620–7. PMID:21717441
2248. Kebebew E, Ituarte PH, Siperstein AE, et al. Medullary thyroid carcinoma: clinical characteristics, treatment, prognostic factors, and a comparison of staging systems. Cancer. 2000 Mar 1;88(5):1139–48. PMID:10699905
2249. Kefeli M, Mete O. An unusual malignant thyroid nodule: coexistence of epithelioid angiosarcoma and follicular variant papillary thyroid carcinoma. Endocr Pathol. 2014 Sep;25(3):350–2. PMID:23608996
2250. Kehrer-Sawatzki H, Farschtschi S, Mautner VF, et al. The molecular pathogenesis of schwannomatosis, a paradigm for the co-involvement of multiple tumour suppressor genes in tumorigenesis. Hum Genet. 2017 Feb;136(2):129–48. PMID:27921248
2251. Keitoku M, Konishi I, Nanbu K, et al. Extraovarian sex cord-stromal tumor: case report and review of the literature. Int J Gynecol Pathol. 1997 Apr;16(2):180–5. PMID:9100075
2252. Kelley MJ, Shi J, Ballew B, et al. Characterization of T gene sequence variants and germline duplications in familial and sporadic chordoma. Hum Genet. 2014 Oct;133(10):1289–97. PMID:24990759
2253. Kellie SJ, Hayes FA, Bowman L, et al. Primary extracranial neuroblastoma with central nervous system metastases characterization by clinicopathologic findings and neuroimaging. Cancer. 1991 Nov 1;68(9):1999–2006. PMID:1913549
2254. Kelly WF, Bradey N, Scoones D. Rosai-Dorfman disease presenting as a pituitary tumour. Clin Endocrinol (Oxf). 1999 Jan;50(1):133–7. PMID:10341867
2255. Kempermann G, Neumann HP, Volk B. Endolymphatic sac tumours. Histopathology. 1998 Jul;33(1):2–10. PMID:9726042
2256. Kempers RD, Dockerty MB, Hoffman DL, et al. Struma ovarii–ascitic, hyperthyroid, and asymptomatic syndromes. Ann Intern Med.

1970 Jun;72(6):883–93. PMID:5448747
2257. Kempná P, Flück CE. Adrenal gland development and defects. Best Pract Res Clin Endocrinol Metab. 2008 Feb;22(1):77–93. PMID:18279781
2258. Kennedy JM, Wang X, Plouffe KR, et al. Clinical and morphologic review of 60 hereditary renal tumors from 30 hereditary renal cell carcinoma syndrome patients: lessons from a contemporary single institution series. Med Oncol. 2019 Jul 22;36(9):74. PMID:31332543
2259. Kent RB 3rd, van Heerden JA, Weiland LH. Nonfunctioning islet cell tumors. Ann Surg. 1981 Feb;193(2):185–90. PMID:6258500
2260. Keraliya AR, Tirumani SH, Shinagare AB, et al. Solitary fibrous tumors: 2016 imaging update. Radiol Clin North Am. 2016 May;54(3):565–79. PMID:27153789
2261. Kervarrec T, Aljundi M, Appenzeller S, et al. Polyomavirus-positive Merkel cell carcinoma derived from a trichoblastoma suggests an epithelial origin of this Merkel cell carcinoma. J Invest Dermatol. 2020 May;140(5):976–85. PMID:31759946
2262. Kervarrec T, Appenzeller S, Samimi M, et al. Merkel cell polyomavirus–negative Merkel cell carcinoma originating from in situ squamous cell carcinoma: a keratinocytic tumor with neuroendocrine differentiation. J Invest Dermatol. 2022 Mar;142 3 Pt A:516–27. PMID:34480892
2263. Kervarrec T, Tallet A, Miquelestorena-Standley E, et al. Diagnostic accuracy of a panel of immunohistochemical and molecular markers to distinguish Merkel cell carcinoma from other neuroendocrine carcinomas. Mod Pathol. 2019 Apr;32(4):499–510. PMID:30349028
2264. Kervarrec T, Tallet A, Miquelestorena-Standley E, et al. Morphologic and immunophenotypical features distinguishing Merkel cell polyomavirus-positive and negative Merkel cell carcinoma. Mod Pathol. 2019 Nov;32(11):1605–16. PMID:31201352
2265. Ketata S, Ketata H, Sahnoun A, et al. Ectopic adrenal cortex tissue: an incidental finding during inguinoscrotal operations in pediatric patients. Urol Int. 2008;81(3):316–9. PMID:18931550
2266. Keutgen XM, Nilubol N, Kebebew E. Malignant-functioning neuroendocrine tumors of the pancreas: a survival analysis. Surgery. 2016 May;159(5):1382–9. PMID:26704781
2267. Khan MW, Worcester EM, Straus FH 2nd, et al. Parathyroid carcinoma in secondary and tertiary hyperparathyroidism. J Am Coll Surg. 2004 Aug;199(2):312–9. PMID:15275889
2268. Khan NE, Bauer AJ, Doros L, et al. Macrocephaly associated with the DICER1 syndrome. Genet Med. 2017 Feb;19(2):244–8. PMID:27441995
2269. Khan NE, Bauer AJ, Schultz KAP, et al. Quantification of thyroid cancer and multinodular goiter risk in the DICER1 syndrome: a family-based cohort study. J Clin Endocrinol Metab. 2017 May 1;102(5):1614–22. PMID:28323992
2270. Khan NE, Ling A, Raske ME, et al. Structural renal abnormalities in the DICER1 syndrome: a family-based cohort study. Pediatr Nephrol. 2018 Dec;33(12):2281–8. PMID:30178239
2271. Khandakar B, Dey S, Ray PS, et al. Ectopic paratubal adrenal cell rest associated with mucinous cystadenoma of ovary. J Clin Diagn Res. 2015 Oct;9(10):ED13–4. PMID:26557532
2272. Khayyata S, Barroeta JE, LiVolsi VA, et al. Papillary hyperplastic nodule: pitfall in the cytopathologic diagnosis of papillary thyroid carcinoma. Endocr Pract. 2008 Oct;14(7):863–8. PMID:18996814
2273. Khosroshahi A, Wallace ZS, Crowe JL, et al. International consensus guidance statement on the management and treatment of IgG4-related disease. Arthritis Rheumatol. 2015 Jul;67(7):1688–99. PMID:25809420
2274. Khunamornpong S, Settakorn J, Sukpan K, et al. Poorly differentiated thyroid carcinoma arising in struma ovarii. Case Rep Pathol. 2015;2015:826978. PMID:26185700
2275. Khurana R, Agarwal A, Bajpai VK, et al. Unraveling the amyloid associated with human medullary thyroid carcinoma. Endocrinology. 2004 Dec;145(12):5465–70. PMID:15459123
2276. Kikuchi K, Kowada M, Sasaki J, et al. Large pituitary adenoma of the sphenoid sinus and the nasopharynx: report of a case with ultrastructural evaluations. Surg Neurol. 1994 Oct;42(4):330–4. PMID:7974131
2277. Kikuchi Y, Wada R, Sakihara S, et al. Pheochromocytoma with histologic transformation to composite type, complicated by watery diarrhea, hypokalemia, and achlorhydria syndrome. Endocr Pract. 2012 Jul-Aug;18(4):e91–6. PMID:22440998
2278. Killian JK, Miettinen M, Walker RL, et al. Recurrent epimutation of SDHC in gastrointestinal stromal tumors. Sci Transl Med. 2014 Dec 24;6(268):268ra177. PMID:25540324
2279. Kim B, Kim HS, Moon KC. Primary renal well-differentiated neuroendocrine tumors: report of six cases with an emphasis on the Ki-67 index and mitosis. Diagn Pathol. 2019 Feb 7;14(1):12. PMID:30732641
2280. Kim BS, Ryu HS, Kang KH, et al. Parathyroid carcinoma in tertiary hyperparathyroidism. Asian J Surg. 2016 Oct;39(4):255–9. PMID:27664600
2281. Kim E, Wright MJ, Sioson L, et al. Utility of the succinate: fumarate ratio for assessing SDH dysfunction in different tumor types. Mol Genet Metab Rep. 2016 Dec 30;10:45–9. PMID:28070496
2282. Kim HJ, Lee HK, Seo JJ, et al. MR imaging of solitary fibrous tumors in the head and neck. Korean J Radiol. 2005 Jul-Sep;6(3):136–42. PMID:16145288
2283. Kim IE Jr, Amin A, Wang LJ, et al. Insulinoma-associated Protein 1 (INSM1) expression in small cell neuroendocrine carcinoma of the urinary tract. Appl Immunohistochem Mol Morphol. 2020 Oct;28(9):687–93. PMID:31876605
2284. Kim J, Field A, Schultz KAP, et al. The prevalence of DICER1 pathogenic variation in population databases. Int J Cancer. 2017 Nov 15;141(10):2030–6. PMID:28748527
2285. Kim J, Horowitz G, Hong M, et al. The dangers of parathyroid biopsy. J Otolaryngol Head Neck Surg. 2017 Jan 7;46(1):4. PMID:28061891
2286. Kim J, Schultz KAP, Hill DA, et al. The prevalence of germline DICER1 pathogenic variation in cancer populations. Mol Genet Genomic Med. 2019 Mar;7(3):e555. PMID:30672147
2287. Kim JH, Moon H, Noh J, et al. Epidemiology and prognosis of pheochromocytoma/paraganglioma in Korea: a nationwide study based on the National Health Insurance Service. Endocrinol Metab (Seoul). 2020 Mar;35(1):157–64. PMID:32207276
2288. Kim JH, Paulus W, Heim S. BRAF V600E mutation is a useful marker for differentiating Rathke's cleft cyst with squamous metaplasia from papillary craniopharyngioma. J Neurooncol. 2015 May;123(1):189–91. PMID:25820214
2289. Kim JM. The clinical importance of multifocality on tumor recurrence in papillary thyroid carcinoma. Gland Surg. 2021 Jan;10(1):273–8. PMID:33633983
2290. Kim JY, Brosnan-Cashman JA, An S, et al. Alternative lengthening of telomeres in primary pancreatic neuroendocrine tumors is associated with aggressive clinical behavior and poor survival. Clin Cancer Res. 2017 Mar 15;23(6):1598–606. PMID:27663587
2291. Kim JY, Brosnan-Cashman JA, Kim J, et al. Pancreatic acinar cell carcinomas and mixed acinar-neuroendocrine carcinomas are more clinically aggressive than grade 1 pancreatic neuroendocrine tumours. Pathology. 2020 Apr;52(3):336–47. PMID:32111396
2292. Kim JY, Kim MS, Kim KS, et al. Clinicopathologic and prognostic significance of multiple hormone expression in pancreatic neuroendocrine tumors. Am J Surg Pathol. 2015 May;39(5):592–601. PMID:25602797
2293. Kim K, Yamada S, Usui M, et al. Preoperative identification of clearly separated double pituitary adenomas. Clin Endocrinol (Oxf). 2004 Jul;61(1):26–30. PMID:15212641
2294. Kim KM, Kim MJ, Cho BK, et al. Genetic evidence for the multi-step progression of mixed glandular-neuroendocrine gastric carcinomas. Virchows Arch. 2002 Jan;440(1):85–93. PMID:11942581
2295. Kim MJ, Won JK, Jung KC, et al. Clinical characteristics of subtypes of follicular variant papillary thyroid carcinoma. Thyroid. 2018 Mar;28(3):311–8. PMID:29343212
2296. Kim SC, Sun HY, Kim HS, et al. Long-term ultrasound follow-up of incidentally detected thyroglossal duct cysts in adults. AJNR Am J Neuroradiol. 2018 Dec;39(12):2356–9. PMID:30467213
2297. Kim TH, Kim YE, Ahn S, et al. TERT promoter mutations and long-term survival in patients with thyroid cancer. Endocr Relat Cancer. 2016 Oct;23(10):813–23. PMID:27528624
2298. Kim TH, Lee M, Kwon AY, et al. Molecular genotyping of the non-invasive encapsulated follicular variant of papillary thyroid carcinoma. Histopathology. 2018 Mar;72(4):648–61. PMID:28940583
2299. Kim WY, Kim S, Hyun J, et al. Disseminated struma ovarii containing focal anaplastic carcinoma in peritoneal implants: a case report. Int J Gynecol Pathol. 2014 Nov;33(6):607–12. PMID:25272300
2300. Kim Y, Roh JL, Song D, et al. Predictors of recurrence after total thyroidectomy plus neck dissection and radioactive iodine ablation for high-risk papillary thyroid carcinoma. J Surg Oncol. 2020 Oct;122(5):906–13. PMID:32588461
2301. Kim YR, Kim JS, Min YH, et al. Prognostic factors in primary diffuse large B-cell lymphoma of adrenal gland treated with rituximab-CHOP chemotherapy from the Consortium for Improving Survival of Lymphoma (CISL). J Hematol Oncol. 2012 Aug 13;5:49. PMID:22889180
2302. Kim YS, Seo M, Park SH, et al. Should total thyroidectomy be recommended for patients with familial non-medullary thyroid cancer? World J Surg. 2020 Sep;44(9):3022–7. PMID:32556933
2303. Kimura N. Dopamine β-hydroxylase: an essential and optimal immunohistochemical marker for pheochromocytoma and sympathetic paraganglioma. Endocr Pathol. 2021 Jun;32(2):258–61. PMID:33405069
2304. Kimura N, Miura Y, Miura K, et al. Adrenal and retroperitoneal mixed neuroendocrine-neural tumors. Endocr Pathol. 1991 Sep;2(3):139–47. PMID:32357642
2305. Kimura N, Shiga K, Kaneko K, et al. The diagnostic dilemma of GATA3 immunohistochemistry in pheochromocytoma and paraganglioma. Endocr Pathol. 2020 Jun;31(2):95–100. PMID:32303954
2306. Kimura N, Takayanagi R, Takizawa N, et al. Pathological grading for predicting metastasis in phaeochromocytoma and paraganglioma. Endocr Relat Cancer. 2014 May 6;21(3):405–14. PMID:24521857
2307. Kimura N, Tateno H, Saijo S, et al. Familial cervical paragangliomas with lymph node metastasis expressing somatostatin receptor type 2A. Endocr Pathol. 2010 Jun;21(2):139–43. PMID:19936639
2308. Kimura N, Watanabe T, Fukase M, et al. Neurofibromin and NF1 gene analysis in composite pheochromocytoma and tumors associated with von Recklinghausen's disease. Mod Pathol. 2002 Mar;15(3):183–8. PMID:11904334
2309. Kimura T, Miyamoto H, Fukuya A, et al. Neuroendocrine carcinoma of the pancreas with similar genetic alterations to invasive ductal adenocarcinoma. Clin J Gastroenterol. 2016 Aug;9(4):261–5. PMID:27262570
2310. Kimura W, Kuroda A, Morioka Y. Clinical pathology of endocrine tumors of the pancreas. Analysis of autopsy cases. Dig Dis Sci. 1991 Jul;36(7):933–42. PMID:2070707
2311. Kindmark H, Sundin A, Granberg D, et al. Endocrine pancreatic tumors with glucagon hypersecretion: a retrospective study of 23 cases during 20 years. Med Oncol. 2007;24(3):330–7. PMID:17873310
2312. King KS, Prodanov T, Kantorovich V, et al. Metastatic pheochromocytoma/paraganglioma related to primary tumor development in childhood or adolescence: significant link to SDHB mutations. J Clin Oncol. 2011 Nov 1;29(31):4137–42. PMID:21969497
2313. Kinge NG, Paliwal VK, Neyaz Z, et al. Superficial siderosis in a patient with filum terminale paraganglioma. Neurol India. 2012 Nov-Dec;60(6):648–9. PMID:23287334
2314. Kini SR, Miller JM, Hamburger JI, et al. Cytopathology of papillary carcinoma of the thyroid by fine needle aspiration. Acta Cytol. 1980 Nov-Dec;24(6):511–21. PMID:6255716
2315. Kinjo T, al-Mefty O, Ciric I. Diaphragma sellae meningiomas. Neurosurgery. 1995 Jun;36(6):1082–92. PMID:7643985
2316. Kinoshita T, Yoshida J, Ishii G, et al. The differences of biological behavior based on the clinicopathological data between resectable large-cell neuroendocrine carcinoma and small-cell lung carcinoma. Clin Lung Cancer. 2013 Sep;14(5):535–40. PMID:23792008
2317. Kinslow CJ, May MS, Saqi A, et al. Large-cell neuroendocrine carcinoma of the lung: a population-based study. Clin Lung Cancer. 2020 Mar;21(2):e99–113. PMID:31601526
2318. Kirby PA, Ellison WA, Thomas PA. Spindle epithelial tumor with thymus-like differentiation (SETTLE) of the thyroid with prominent mitotic activity and focal necrosis. Am J Surg Pathol. 1999 Jun;23(6):712–6. PMID:10366154
2319. Kirkwood KS, Debas HT. Neuroendocrine tumors: common presentations of uncommon diseases. Compr Ther. 1995 Dec;21(12):719–25. PMID:8789136
2320. Kirschner LS. PRKAR1A and the evolution of pituitary tumors. Mol Cell Endocrinol. 2010 Sep 15;326(1-2):3–7. PMID:20451576
2321. Kiseljak-Vassiliades K, Bancos I, Hamrahian A, et al. American Association of Clinical Endocrinology Disease State Clinical Review on the evaluation and management of adrenocortical carcinoma in an adult: a practical approach. Endocr Pract. 2020 Nov;26(11):1366–83. PMID:33875173
2322. Kiseljak-Vassiliades K, Carlson NE, Borges MT, et al. Growth hormone tumor histological subtypes predict response to surgical and medical therapy. Endocrine. 2015 May;49(1):231–41. PMID:25129651
2323. Kitahara CM, Sosa JA. The changing incidence of thyroid cancer. Nat Rev Endocrinol. 2016 Nov;12(11):646–53. PMID:27418023
2324. Kitahara CM, Sosa JA. Understanding the ever-changing incidence of thyroid cancer. Nat Rev Endocrinol. 2020 Nov;16(11):617–8. PMID:32895503
2325. Kitawaki Y, Nakamura Y,

Kubota-Nakayama F, et al. Tumor microenvironment in functional adrenocortical adenomas: immune cell infiltration in cortisol-producing adrenocortical adenoma. Hum Pathol. 2018 Jul;77:88–97. PMID:29596893
2326. Kitazono I, Akahane T, Sakihama M, et al. Human papilloma virus 18-positive submucosal small cell neuroendocrine carcinoma of the vagina: an immunohistochemical and genomic study. Int J Surg Pathol. 2021 Dec;29(8):870–6. PMID:33792412
2327. Kittah NE, Gruber LM, Bancos I, et al. Bilateral pheochromocytoma: clinical characteristics, treatment and longitudinal follow-up. Clin Endocrinol (Oxf). 2020 Sep;93(3):288–95. PMID:32410303
2328. Kiyokawa H, Kineman RD, Manova-Todorova KO, et al. Enhanced growth of mice lacking the cyclin-dependent kinase inhibitor function of p27(Kip1). Cell. 1996 May 31;85(5):721–32. PMID:8646780
2329. Klein S, Lee H, Ghahremani S, et al. Expanding the phenotype of mutations in DICER1: mosaic missense mutations in the RNase IIIb domain of DICER1 cause GLOW syndrome. J Med Genet. 2014 May;51(5):294–302. PMID:24676357
2330. Kleinschmidt-DeMasters BK, Lillehei KO, Hankinson TC. Review of xanthomatous lesions of the sella. Brain Pathol. 2017 May;27(3):377–95. PMID:28236350
2331. Kleinschmidt-DeMasters BK, Lopes MB. Update on hypophysitis and TTF-1 expressing sellar region masses. Brain Pathol. 2013 Sep;23(5):495–514. PMID:23701182
2332. Kleinschmidt-DeMasters BK, Winston KR, Rubinstein D, et al. Ectopic pituitary adenoma of the third ventricle. Case report. J Neurosurg. 1990 Jan;72(1):139–42. PMID:2294174
2333. Klempner SJ, Gershenhorn B, Tran P, et al. BRAFV600E mutations in high-grade colorectal neuroendocrine tumors may predict responsiveness to BRAF-MEK combination therapy. Cancer Discov. 2016 Jun;6(6):594–600. PMID:27048246
2334. Klibanski A. Clinical practice. Prolactinomas. N Engl J Med. 2010 Apr 1;362(13):1219–26. PMID:20357284
2335. Kliewer KE, Cochran AJ. A review of the histology, ultrastructure, immunohistology, and molecular biology of extra-adrenal paragangliomas. Arch Pathol Lab Med. 1989 Nov;113(11):1209–18. PMID:2684087
2336. Klijanienko J, Caillaud JM, Orbach D, et al. Cyto-histological correlations in primary, recurrent and metastatic rhabdomyosarcoma: the Institut Curie's experience. Diagn Cytopathol. 2007 Aug;35(8):482–7. PMID:17636492
2337. Klimstra DS, Adsay V. Acinar neoplasms of the pancreas-a summary of 25 years of research. Semin Diagn Pathol. 2016 Sep;33(5):307–18. PMID:27320062
2338. Klimstra DS, Rosai J, Heffess CS. Mixed acinar-endocrine carcinomas of the pancreas. Am J Surg Pathol. 1994 Aug;18(8):765–78. PMID:8037290
2339. Klinck GH, Winship T. Psammoma bodies and thyroid cancer. Cancer. 1959 Jul-Aug;12(4):656–62. PMID:13663006
2340. Klöppel G. Mixed exocrine-endocrine tumors of the pancreas. Semin Diagn Pathol. 2000 May;17(2):104–8. PMID:10839610
2341. Klöppel G, Anlauf M. Gastrinoma–morphological aspects. Wien Klin Wochenschr. 2007;119(19-20):579–84. PMID:17985091
2342. Klöppel G, Anlauf M, Perren A, et al. Hyperplasia to neoplasia sequence of duodenal and pancreatic neuroendocrine diseases and pseudohyperplasia of the PP-cells in the pancreas. Endocr Pathol. 2014 Jun;25(2):181–5. PMID:24718881
2343. Klöppel G, Couvelard A, Perren A, et al. ENETS consensus guidelines for the standards of care in neuroendocrine tumors: towards a standardized approach to the diagnosis of gastroenteropancreatic neuroendocrine tumors and their prognostic stratification. Neuroendocrinology. 2009;90(2):162–6. PMID:19060454
2344. Klöppel G, Heitz PU. Morphology and functional activity of gastroenteropancreatic neuroendocrine tumours. Recent Results Cancer Res. 1990;118:27–36. PMID:1978380
2345. Klöppel G, Heitz PU. Pancreatic endocrine tumors. Pathol Res Pract. 1988 Apr;183(2):155–68. PMID:2898775
2346. Klöppel G, Willemer S, Stamm B, et al. Pancreatic lesions and hormonal profile of pancreatic tumors in multiple endocrine neoplasia type I. An immunocytochemical study of nine patients. Cancer. 1986 May 1;57(9):1824–32. PMID:2420439
2347. Kloub O, Perry A, Tu PH, et al. Spindle cell oncocytoma of the adenohypophysis: report of two recurrent cases. Am J Surg Pathol. 2005 Feb;29(2):247–53. PMID:15644783
2348. Klubo-Gwiezdzinska J, Yang L, Merkel R, et al. Results of screening in familial non-medullary thyroid cancer. Thyroid. 2017 Aug;27(8):1017–24. PMID:28657510
2349. Kluckova K, Tennant DA. Metabolic implications of hypoxia and pseudohypoxia in pheochromocytoma and paraganglioma. Cell Tissue Res. 2018 May;372(2):367–78. PMID:29450727
2350. Knepper TC, Montesion M, Russell JS, et al. The genomic landscape of Merkel cell carcinoma and clinicogenomic biomarkers of response to immune checkpoint inhibitor therapy. Clin Cancer Res. 2019 Oct 1;25(19):5961–71. PMID:31399473
2351. Knief J, Gebauer N, Bernard V, et al. Oncogenic mutations and chromosomal aberrations in primary extranodal diffuse large B-cell lymphomas of the thyroid–a study of 21 cases. J Clin Endocrinol Metab. 2015 Feb;100(2):754–62. PMID:25423572
2352. Kniseley RM, Baggenstoss AH. Primary melanoma of the adrenal gland. Arch Pathol (Chic). 1946 Sep;42:345–9. PMID:20999933
2353. Knobel M. Etiopathology, clinical features, and treatment of diffuse and multinodular nontoxic goiters. J Endocrinol Invest. 2016 Apr;39(4):357–73. PMID:26392367
2354. Knosp E, Steiner E, Kitz K, et al. Pituitary adenomas with invasion of the cavernous sinus space: a magnetic resonance imaging classification compared with surgical findings. Neurosurgery. 1993 Oct;33(4):610–7. PMID:8232800
2355. Ko JS, Prieto VG, Elson PJ, et al. Histological pattern of Merkel cell carcinoma sentinel lymph node metastasis improves stratification of Stage III patients. Mod Pathol. 2016 Feb;29(2):122–30. PMID:26541273
2356. Koay EJ, Teh BS, Paulino AC, et al. A Surveillance, Epidemiology, and End Results analysis of small cell carcinoma of the bladder: epidemiology, prognostic variables, and treatment trends. Cancer. 2011 Dec 1;117(23):5325–33. PMID:21567387
2357. Koba S, Nagase K, Ikeda S, et al. Merkel cell carcinoma with glandular differentiation admixed with sweat gland carcinoma and spindle cell carcinoma: histogenesis of Merkel cell carcinoma from hair follicle stem cells. Am J Dermatopathol. 2015 Mar;37(3):e31–6. PMID:25699980
2358. Kobayashi C, Monforte-Munoz HL, Gerbing RB, et al. Enlarged and prominent nucleoli may be indicative of MYCN amplification: a study of neuroblastoma (Schwannian stroma-poor), undifferentiated/poorly differentiated subtype with high mitosis-karyorrhexis index. Cancer. 2005 Jan 1;103(1):174–80. PMID:15549714
2359. Kober P, Boresowicz J, Rusetska N, et al. DNA methylation profiling in nonfunctioning pituitary adenomas. Mol Cell Endocrinol. 2018 Sep 15;473:194–204. PMID:29410024
2360. Kober P, Boresowicz J, Rusetska N, et al. The role of aberrant DNA methylation in misregulation of gene expression in gonadotroph nonfunctioning pituitary tumors. Cancers (Basel). 2019 Oct 25;11(11):1650. PMID:31731486
2361. Koch CA, Mauro D, Walther MM, et al. Pheochromocytoma in von Hippel-Lindau disease: distinct histopathologic phenotype compared to pheochromocytoma in multiple endocrine neoplasia type 2. Endocr Pathol. 2002 Spring;13(1):17–27. PMID:12114747
2362. Kocjan G, Cochand-Priollet B, de Agustin PP, et al. Diagnostic terminology for reporting thyroid fine needle aspiration cytology: European Federation of Cytology Societies thyroid working party symposium, Lisbon 2009. Cytopathology. 2010 Apr;21(2):86–92. PMID:21054822
2363. Koelsche C, Schrimpf D, Stichel D, et al. Sarcoma classification by DNA methylation profiling. Nat Commun. 2021 Jan 21;12(1):498. PMID:33479225
2364. Koelsche C, Schweizer L, Renner M, et al. Nuclear relocation of STAT6 reliably predicts NAB2-STAT6 fusion for the diagnosis of solitary fibrous tumour. Histopathology. 2014 Nov;65(5):613–22. PMID:24702701
2365. Koh CM, Khattar E, Leow SC, et al. Telomerase regulates MYC-driven oncogenesis independent of its reverse transcriptase activity. J Clin Invest. 2015 May;125(5):2109–22. PMID:25893605
2366. Koh J, Nam SK, Kwak Y, et al. Comprehensive genetic features of gastric mixed adenoneuroendocrine carcinomas and pure neuroendocrine carcinomas. J Pathol. 2021 Jan;253(1):94–105. PMID:32985687
2367. Koh JM, Ahn SH, Kim H, et al. Validation of pathological grading systems for predicting metastatic potential in pheochromocytoma and paraganglioma. PLoS One. 2017 Nov 8;12(11):e0187398. PMID:29117221
2368. Kohashi K, Kinoshita I, Oda Y. Soft tissue special issue: Skeletal muscle tumors: a clinicopathological review. Head Neck Pathol. 2020 Mar;14(1):12–20. PMID:31950473
2369. Kohl NE, Kanda N, Schreck RR, et al. Transposition and amplification of oncogene-related sequences in human neuroblastomas. Cell. 1983 Dec;35(2 Pt 1):359–67. PMID:6197179
2370. Kolli V, Kim H, Rao H, et al. Measurement of serum tenascin-X in patients with congenital adrenal hyperplasia at risk for Ehlers-Danlos contiguous gene deletion syndrome CAH-X. BMC Res Notes. 2019 Oct 30;12(1):711. PMID:31666125
2371. Kolson Kokohaare E, Riva FMG, Bernstein JM, et al. Malignant solitary fibrous tumor metastatic to widely invasive Hurthle cell thyroid carcinoma: a distinct tumor-to-tumor metastasis. Int J Surg Pathol. 2018 Sep;26(6):521–4. PMID:29616597
2372. Komatsubara K, Tahara S, Umeoka K, et al. Immunohistochemical analysis of p27 (Kip1) in human pituitary glands and in various types of pituitary adenomas. Endocr Pathol. 2001 Summer;12(2):181–8. PMID:11579684
2373. Komorowski RA, Hanson GA. Occult thyroid pathology in the young adult: an autopsy study of 138 patients without clinical thyroid disease. Hum Pathol. 1988 Jun;19(6):689–96. PMID:3378788
2374. Kon T, Wada R, Suzuki R, et al. VIP and calcitonin-producing pancreatic neuroendocrine tumor with watery diarrhea: clinicopathological features and the effect of somatostatin analogue. JOP. 2012 Mar 10;13(2):226–30. PMID:22406608
2375. Kondo T, Ezzat S, Asa SL. Pathogenetic mechanisms in thyroid follicular-cell neoplasia. Nat Rev Cancer. 2006 Apr;6(4):292–306. PMID:16557281
2376. Kondo T, Kato K, Nakazawa T, et al. Mucinous carcinoma (poorly differentiated carcinoma with extensive extracellular mucin deposition) of the thyroid: a case report with immunohistochemical studies. Hum Pathol. 2005 Jun;36(6):698–701. PMID:16021578
2377. Kondo T, Matsuyama R, Ashihara H, et al. A case of ectopic adrenocorticotropic hormone-producing pancreatic neuroendocrine tumor with multiple liver metastases. Endocr J. 2010;57(3):229–36. PMID:20032567
2378. Kong F, Ying H, Zhai R, et al. Clinical outcome of intensity modulated radiotherapy for carcinoma showing thymus-like differentiation. Oncotarget. 2016 Dec 6;7(49):81899–905. PMID:27626313
2379. Kong J, Wang O, Nie M, et al. Familial isolated primary hyperparathyroidism/hyperparathyroidism-jaw tumour syndrome caused by germline gross deletion or point mutations of CDC73 gene in Chinese. Clin Endocrinol (Oxf). 2014 Aug;81(2):222–30. PMID:24716902
2380. Kong SH, Kim JH, Park MY, et al. Epidemiology and prognosis of parathyroid carcinoma: real-world data using nationwide cohort. J Cancer Res Clin Oncol. 2021 Oct;147(10):3091–7. PMID:33738545
2381. Konomi K, Chijiiwa K, Katsuta T, et al. Pancreatic somatostatinoma: a case report and review of the literature. J Surg Oncol. 1990 Apr;43(4):259–65. PMID:1969977
2382. Kontogeorgos G, Asa SL, Kovacs K, et al. Production of alpha-subunit of glycoprotein hormones by pituitary somatotroph adenomas in vitro. Acta Endocrinol (Copenh). 1993 Dec;129(6):565–72. PMID:7509101
2383. Kontogeorgos G, Kapranos N, Orphanidis G, et al. Molecular cytogenetics of chromosome 11 in pituitary adenomas: a comparison of fluorescence in situ hybridization and DNA ploidy study. Hum Pathol. 1999 Nov;30(11):1377–82. PMID:10571521
2384. Kontogeorgos G, Kovacs K, Horvath E, et al. Multiple adenomas of the human pituitary. A retrospective autopsy study with clinical implications. J Neurosurg. 1991 Feb;74(2):243–7. PMID:1988594
2385. Kontogeorgos G, Kovacs K, Horvath E, et al. Null cell adenomas, oncocytomas, and gonadotroph adenomas of the human pituitary: an immunocytochemical and ultrastructural analysis of 300 cases. Endocr Pathol. 1993 Mar;4(1):20–7. PMID:32370437
2386. Kontogeorgos G, Mourouti G, Kyrodimou E, et al. Ganglion cell containing pituitary adenomas: signs of neuronal differentiation in adenoma cells. Acta Neuropathol. 2006 Jul;112(1):21–8. PMID:16699777
2387. Konukiewitz B, Enosawa T, Klöppel G. Glucagon expression in cystic pancreatic neuroendocrine neoplasms: an immunohistochemical analysis. Virchows Arch. 2011 Jan;458(1):47–53. PMID:20922407
2388. Konukiewitz B, Jesinghaus M, Steiger K, et al. Pancreatic neuroendocrine carcinomas reveal a closer relationship to ductal adenocarcinomas than to neuroendocrine tumors G3. Hum Pathol. 2018 Jul;77:70–9. PMID:29596894
2389. Konukiewitz B, Schlitter AM, Jesinghaus M, et al. Somatostatin receptor expression related to TP53 and RB1 alterations in pancreatic and extrapancreatic neuroendocrine neoplasms with a Ki67-index above 20. Mod Pathol. 2017 Apr;30(4):587–98. PMID:28059098
2390. Konukiewitz B, von Hornstein M, Jesinghaus M, et al. Pancreatic neuroendocrine

tumors with somatostatin expression and paraganglioma-like features. Hum Pathol. 2020 Aug;102:79–87. PMID:32668277
2391. Kooijman CD. Immature teratomas in children. Histopathology. 1988 May;12(5):491–502. PMID:3397045
2392. Koopmans KP, Jager PL, Kema IP, et al. 111In-octreotide is superior to 123I-metaiodobenzylguanidine for scintigraphic detection of head and neck paragangliomas. J Nucl Med. 2008 Aug;49(8):1232–7. PMID:18632829
2393. Kopp P. Perspective: genetic defects in the etiology of congenital hypothyroidism. Endocrinology. 2002 Jun;143(6):2019–24. PMID:12021164
2394. Korbonits M, Chahal HS, Kaltsas G, et al. Expression of phosphorylated p27(Kip1) protein and Jun activation domain-binding protein 1 in human pituitary tumors. J Clin Endocrinol Metab. 2002 Jun;87(6):2635–43. PMID:12050228
2395. Kordes U, Flitsch J, Hagel C, et al. Ectopic craniopharyngioma. Klin Padiatr. 2011 May;223(3):176–7. PMID:21462099
2396. Koren R, Bernheim J, Schachter P, et al. Black thyroid adenoma. Clinical, histochemical, and ultrastructural features. Appl Immunohistochem Mol Morphol. 2000 Mar;8(1):80–4. PMID:10937053
2397. Körner M, Waser B, Schonbrunn A, et al. Somatostatin receptor subtype 2A immunohistochemistry using a new monoclonal antibody selects tumors suitable for in vivo somatostatin receptor targeting. Am J Surg Pathol. 2012 Feb;36(2):242–52. PMID:22251942
2398. Korpershoek E, Favier J, Gaal J, et al. SDHA immunohistochemistry detects germline SDHA gene mutations in apparently sporadic paragangliomas and pheochromocytomas. J Clin Endocrinol Metab. 2011 Sep;96(9):E1472–6. PMID:21752896
2399. Korpershoek E, Koffy D, Eussen BH, et al. Complex MAX rearrangement in a family with malignant pheochromocytoma, renal oncocytoma, and erythrocytosis. J Clin Endocrinol Metab. 2016 Feb;101(2):453–60. PMID:26670126
2400. Korpershoek E, Petri BJ, Post E, et al. Adrenal medullary hyperplasia is a precursor lesion for pheochromocytoma in MEN2 syndrome. Neoplasia. 2014 Oct 23;16(10):868–73. PMID:25379023
2401. Korpi-Hyövälti E, Cranston T, Ryhänen E, et al. CDC73 intragenic deletion in familial primary hyperparathyroidism associated with parathyroid carcinoma. J Clin Endocrinol Metab. 2014 Sep;99(9):3044–8. PMID:24823466
2402. Korse CM, Taal BG, van Velthuysen ML, et al. Incidence and survival of neuroendocrine tumours in the Netherlands according to histological grade: experience of two decades of cancer registry. Eur J Cancer. 2013 May;49(8):1975–83. PMID:23352435
2403. Korytnaya E, Liu J, Camelo-Piragua S, et al. Ectopic prolactin secretion from a perivascular epithelioid cell tumor (PEComa). J Clin Endocrinol Metab. 2014 Nov;99(11):3960–4. PMID:25127092
2404. Kösem M, Kotan C, Algün E, et al. Simultaneous occurrence of papillary intrafollicular and microcarcinomas with bilateral medullary microcarcinoma of the thyroid in a patient with multiple endocrine neoplasia type 2A: report of a case. Surg Today. 2002;32(7):623–8. PMID:12111520
2405. Koshy A, Jain R, Srinivasan R, et al. Cytopathological spectrum of peripheral neuroblastic tumours in fine needle aspiration cytology and categorisation as per International Neuroblastoma Pathology Classification. Cytopathology. 2019 Nov;30(6):634–43. PMID:31231909
2406. Kostiainen I, Hakaste L, Kejo P, et al. Adrenocortical carcinoma: presentation and outcome of a contemporary patient series. Endocrine. 2019 Jul;65(1):166–74. PMID:30980285
2407. Kostoglou-Athanassiou I, Athanassiou P, Vecchini G, et al. Mixed medullary-follicular thyroid carcinoma. Report of a case and review of the literature. Horm Res. 2004;61(6):300–4. PMID:15153799
2408. Kotecha K, Paik J, Gill AJ, et al. Management of a rare cause of upper gastrointestinal bleed: the duodenal gangliocytic paraganglioma. ANZ J Surg. 2021 Nov;91(11):E724–6. PMID:33764657
2409. Kou HW, Yu MC, Chong SW, et al. Successful localization and resection of small pancreatic cystic insulinoma using intraoperative near-infrared fluorescence imaging: a case report and literature review. Pancreas. 2020 Nov/Dec;49(10):1388–92. PMID:33122530
2410. Kouba E, Cheng L. Neuroendocrine tumors of the urinary bladder according to the 2016 World Health Organization Classification: molecular and clinical characteristics. Endocr Pathol. 2016 Sep;27(3):188–99. PMID:27334654
2411. Kouhara H, Tatekawa T, Koga M, et al. Intracranial and intraspinal dissemination of an ACTH-secreting pituitary tumor. Endocrinol Jpn. 1992 Apr;39(2):177–84. PMID:1327728
2412. Koulouri O, Steuwe A, Gillett D, et al. A role for 11C-methionine PET imaging in ACTH-dependent Cushing's syndrome. Eur J Endocrinol. 2015 Oct;173(4):M107–20. PMID:26245763
2413. Kousta E, Konstantinidis K, Michalakis C, et al. Ectopic thyroid tissue in the lower neck with a coexisting normally located multinodular goiter and brief literature review. Hormones (Athens). 2005 Oct-Dec;4(4):231–4. PMID:16613822
2414. Kovács GL, Góth M, Rotondo F, et al. ACTH-secreting Crooke cell carcinoma of the pituitary. Eur J Clin Invest. 2013 Jan;43(1):20–6. PMID:23134557
2415. Kovacs K, Horvath E, Rewcastle NB, et al. Gonadotroph cell adenoma of the pituitary in a women with long-standing hypogonadism. Arch Gynecol. 1980 Jan;229(1):57–65. PMID:7362277
2416. Kovacs K, Horvath E, Ryan N, et al. Null cell adenoma of the human pituitary. Virchows Arch A Pathol Anat Histol. 1980;387(2):165–74. PMID:7456308
2417. Kovacs K, Horvath E, Thorner MO, et al. Mammosomatotroph hyperplasia associated with acromegaly and hyperprolactinemia in a patient with the McCune-Albright syndrome. A histologic, immunocytologic and ultrastructural study of the surgically-removed adenohypophysis. Virchows Arch A Pathol Anat Histopathol. 1984;403(1):77–86. PMID:6426154
2418. Kovacs K, Ryan N, Horvath E, et al. Pituitary adenomas in old age. J Gerontol. 1980 Jan;35(1):16–22. PMID:6243145
2419. Koyama T, Mikami Y, Saga T, et al. Secondary ovarian tumors: spectrum of CT and MR features with pathologic correlation. Abdom Imaging. 2007 Nov;32(6):784–95. PMID:17318680
2420. Kr A, Sebastian P, Somanathan T, et al. Significance of incidentally detected thyroid tissue in lymph nodes of neck dissections in patients with head and neck carcinoma. Int J Surg Pathol. 2012 Dec;20(6):564–9. PMID:22674918
2421. Kraft S, Faquin WC, Krane JF. HPV-associated neuroendocrine carcinoma of the oropharynx: a rare new entity with potentially aggressive clinical behavior. Am J Surg Pathol. 2012 Mar;36(3):321–30. PMID:22301491
2422. Kraimps JL, Canzian F, Jost C, et al. Mapping of a gene predisposing to familial thyroid tumors with cell oxyphilia to chromosome 19 and exclusion of JUN B as a candidate gene. Surgery. 1999 Dec;126(6):1188–94. PMID:10598206
2423. Krainev AA, Mathavan VK, Klink DF, et al. Pancreatic neuroendocrine microadenomatosis presenting as a functional VIPoma. J Surg Case Rep. 2019 Jun 28;2019(6):rjz196. PMID:31275551
2424. Krampitz GW, Norton JA. Current management of the Zollinger-Ellison syndrome. Adv Surg. 2013;47:59–79. PMID:24298844
2425. Krampitz GW, Norton JA. RET gene mutations (genotype and phenotype) of multiple endocrine neoplasia type 2 and familial medullary thyroid carcinoma. Cancer. 2014 Jul 1;120(13):1920–31. PMID:24699901
2426. Krane JF, Alexander EK, Cibas ES, et al. Coming to terms with NIFTP: a provisional approach for cytologists. Cancer Cytopathol. 2016 Nov;124(11):767–72. PMID:27564464
2427. Krause MW, Hedinger CE. Pathologic study of parathyroid glands in tertiary hyperparathyroidism. Hum Pathol. 1985 Aug;16(8):772–84. PMID:4018775
2428. Krauss T, Ferrara AM, Links TP, et al. Preventive medicine of von Hippel-Lindau disease-associated pancreatic neuroendocrine tumors. Endocr Relat Cancer. 2018 Sep;25(9):783–93. PMID:29748190
2429. Krausz Y, Freedman N, Rubinstein R, et al. 68Ga-DOTA-NOC PET/CT imaging of neuroendocrine tumors: comparison with ^{111}In-DTPA-octreotide (OctreoScan®). Mol Imaging Biol. 2011 Jun;13(3):583–93. PMID:20652423
2430. Krawitz PL. Topical glycerin as an adjunct treatment for flat anterior chamber. Ophthalmic Surg. 1994 May;25(5):330–1. PMID:8058267
2431. Krawitz R, Glover A, Koneru S, et al. The significance of histologically "large normal" parathyroid glands in primary hyperparathyroidism. World J Surg. 2020 Apr;44(4):1149–55. PMID:31773224
2432. Krejs GJ. VIPoma syndrome. Am J Med. 1987 May 29;82 5B:37–48. PMID:3035922
2433. Krenning EP, Kwekkeboom DJ, Oei HY, et al. Somatostatin receptor scintigraphy in carcinoids, gastrinomas and Cushing's syndrome. Digestion. 1994;55 Suppl 3:54–9. PMID:7698538
2434. Kreutzer J, Vance ML, Lopes MB, et al. Surgical management of GH-secreting pituitary adenomas: an outcome study using modern remission criteria. J Clin Endocrinol Metab. 2001 Sep;86(9):4072–7. PMID:11549628
2435. Kriegsmann K, Zgorzelski C, Kazdal D, et al. Insulinoma-associated protein 1 (INSM1) in thoracic tumors is less sensitive but more specific compared with synaptophysin, chromogranin A, and CD56. Appl Immunohistochem Mol Morphol. 2020 Mar;28(3):237–42. PMID:30358615
2436. Krohn K, Führer D, Bayer Y, et al. Molecular pathogenesis of euthyroid and toxic multinodular goiter. Endocr Rev. 2005 Jun;26(4):504–24. PMID:15615818
2437. Krokker L, Nyírő G, Reiniger L, et al. Differentially expressed miRNAs influence metabolic processes in pituitary oncocytoma. Neurochem Res. 2019 Oct;44(10):2360–71. PMID:30945144
2438. Kruijff S, Sidhu SB, Sywak MS, et al. Negative parafibromin staining predicts malignant behavior in atypical parathyroid adenomas. Ann Surg Oncol. 2014 Feb;21(2):426–33. PMID:24081804
2439. Kruljac I, Pavic I, Matesa N, et al. Intrathyroid parathyroid carcinoma with intrathyroidal metastasis to the contralateral lobe: source of diagnostic and treatment pitfalls. Jpn J Clin Oncol. 2011 Sep;41(9):1142–6. PMID:21742652
2440. Kuan EC, Alonso JE, Tajudeen BA, et al. Small cell carcinoma of the head and neck: a comparative study by primary site based on population data. Laryngoscope. 2017 Aug;127(8):1785–90. PMID:27859290
2441. Kuhel WI, Gonzales D, Hoda SA, et al. Synchronous water-clear cell double parathyroid adenomas a hitherto uncharacterized entity? Arch Pathol Lab Med. 2001 Feb;125(2):256–9. PMID:11175646
2442. Kuhn E, Ragazzi M, Ciarrocchi A, et al. Angiosarcoma and anaplastic carcinoma of the thyroid are two distinct entities: a morphologic, immunohistochemical, and genetic study. Mod Pathol. 2019 Jun;32(6):787–98. PMID:30723294
2443. Kuhn E, Teller L, Piana S, et al. Different clonal origin of bilateral papillary thyroid carcinoma, with a review of the literature. Endocr Pathol. 2012 Jun;23(2):101–7. PMID:22434481
2444. Kulaksiz H, Eissele R, Rössler D, et al. Identification of somatostatin receptor subtypes 1, 2A, 3, and 5 in neuroendocrine tumours with subtype specific antibodies. Gut. 2002 Jan;50(1):52–60. PMID:11772967
2445. Kulke MH, Anthony LB, Bushnell DL, et al. NANETS treatment guidelines: well-differentiated neuroendocrine tumors of the stomach and pancreas. Pancreas. 2010 Aug;39(6):735–52. PMID:20664472
2446. Kumar S, Nanjappa B. Giant benign adrenal adenoma. Urology. 2012 Sep;80(3):e25–6. PMID:22840871
2447. Kumar T, Nigam JS, Tewari P, et al. Warthin-like variant of papillary thyroid carcinoma: an uncommon variant. Cureus. 2020 Dec 28;12(12):e12350. PMID:33520545
2448. Kung AW, Pun KK, Lam K, et al. Addisonian crisis as presenting feature in malignancies. Cancer. 1990 Jan 1;65(1):177–9. PMID:2293863
2449. Kunstman JW, Juhlin CC, Goh G, et al. Characterization of the mutational landscape of anaplastic thyroid cancer via whole-exome sequencing. Hum Mol Genet. 2015 Apr 15;24(8):2318–29. PMID:25576899
2450. Kunwar S, Wilson CB. Pediatric pituitary adenomas. J Clin Endocrinol Metab. 1999 Dec;84(12):4385–9. PMID:10599692
2451. Kuo EJ, Sisk AE, Yang Z, et al. Adrenal teratoma: a case series and review of the literature. Endocr Pathol. 2017 Jun;28(2):152–8. PMID:28091891
2452. Kuo TC, Wu MH, Chen KY, et al. Ultrasonographic features for differentiating follicular thyroid carcinoma and follicular adenoma. Asian J Surg. 2020 Jan;43(1):339–46. PMID:31182260
2453. Kure S, Ohashi R. Thyroid Hürthle cell carcinoma: clinical, pathological, and molecular features. Cancers (Basel). 2020 Dec 23;13(1):26. PMID:33374707
2454. Kurihara K, Shimizu S, Chong J, et al. Nuclear localization of immunoreactive beta-catenin is specific to familial adenomatous polyposis in papillary thyroid carcinoma. Jpn J Cancer Res. 2000 Nov;91(11):1100–2. PMID:11092973
2455. Kurihara S, Hiyama E, Onitake Y, et al. Clinical features of ATRX or DAXX mutated neuroblastoma. J Pediatr Surg. 2014 Dec;49(12):1835–8. PMID:25487495
2456. Kurisaki-Arakawa A, Akaike K, Hara K, et al. A case of dedifferentiated solitary fibrous tumor in the pelvis with TP53 mutation. Virchows Arch. 2014 Nov;465(5):615–21. PMID:25015562
2457. Kuroki M, Tanaka R, Yokoyama M, et al. Subarachnoid dissemination of a pituitary adenoma. Surg Neurol. 1987 Jul;28(1):71–6.

PMID:3589946
2458. Kurosaki M, Saeger W, Lüdecke DK. Immunohistochemical localisation of cytokeratins in craniopharyngioma. Acta Neurochir (Wien). 2001;143(2):147–51. PMID:11459086
2459. Kusafuka K, Abe M, Iida Y, et al. Mucosal large cell neuroendocrine carcinoma of the head and neck regions in Japanese patients: a distinct clinicopathological entity. J Clin Pathol. 2012 Aug;65(8):704–9. PMID:22718848
2460. Kusafuka K, Ferlito A, Lewis JS Jr, et al. Large cell neuroendocrine carcinoma of the head and neck. Oral Oncol. 2012 Mar;48(3):211–5. PMID:22024350
2461. Kusaka A, Koie T, Yamamoto H, et al. Testicular metastasis of prostate cancer: a case report. Case Rep Oncol. 2014 Sep 18;7(3):643–7. PMID:25408658
2462. Kushchayev SV, Kushchayeva YS, Tella SH, et al. Medullary thyroid carcinoma: an update on imaging. J Thyroid Res. 2019 Jul 7;2019:1893047. PMID:31360432
2463. Kushchayeva YS, Kushchayev SV, Glushko TY, et al. Fibrous dysplasia for radiologists: beyond ground glass bone matrix. Insights Imaging. 2018 Dec;9(6):1035–56. PMID:30484079
2464. Kushner BH. Neuroblastoma: a disease requiring a multitude of imaging studies. J Nucl Med. 2004 Jul;45(7):1172–88. PMID:15235064
2465. Kutahyalioglu M, Nguyen HT, Kwatampora L, et al. Genetic profiling as a clinical tool in advanced parathyroid carcinoma. J Cancer Res Clin Oncol. 2019 Aug;145(8):1977–86. PMID:31309300
2466. Kwancharoen R, Blitz AM, Tavares F, et al. Clinical features of sellar and suprasellar meningiomas. Pituitary. 2014 Aug;17(4):342–8. PMID:23975080
2467. Kwiatkowski JL, Rutkowski JL, Yamashiro DJ, et al. Schwann cell-conditioned medium promotes neuroblastoma survival and differentiation. Cancer Res. 1998 Oct 15;58(20):4602–6. PMID:9788610
2468. Kwon H, Kim WG, Choi YM, et al. A cut-off value of basal serum calcitonin for detecting macroscopic medullary thyroid carcinoma. Clin Endocrinol (Oxf). 2015 Apr;82(4):598–603. PMID:25041034
2469. Kwon J, Kim BH, Jung HW, et al. The prognostic impacts of postoperative radiotherapy in the patients with resected anaplastic thyroid carcinoma: a systematic review and meta-analysis. Eur J Cancer. 2016 May;59:34–45. PMID:27014798
2470. Kwon JH, Kim HJ, Park DH, et al. Incidentally detected pancreatic neuroendocrine microadenoma with lymph node metastasis. Virchows Arch. 2018 Nov;473(5):649–53. PMID:30003325
2471. Kwon MJ, Rho YS, Jeong JC, et al. Cribriform-morular variant of papillary thyroid carcinoma: a study of 3 cases featuring the PIK3CA mutation. Hum Pathol. 2015 Aug;46(8):1180–8. PMID:26054797
2472. Kwon MJ, Suh YL. Pituicytoma with unusual histological features. Pathol Int. 2011 Oct;61(10):598–602. PMID:21951670
2473. Kwon MR, Shin JH, Hahn SY, et al. Histogram analysis of greyscale sonograms to differentiate between the subtypes of follicular variant of papillary thyroid cancer. Clin Radiol. 2018 Jun;73(6):591.e1–7. PMID:29317047
2474. Kwon T, Jeong IG, Pak S, et al. Renal tumor size is an independent prognostic factor for overall survival in von Hippel-Lindau disease. J Cancer Res Clin Oncol. 2014 Jul;140(7):1171–7. PMID:24671227
2475. Kwon Y, Hong EK, Koo HL, et al. Clinicopathological and immunohistochemical studies of thymic-related tumours in thyroid gland: report of five cases. Histopathology. 2006 Feb;48(3):312–5. PMID:16430482
2476. La Corte E, Younus I, Pivari F, et al. BRAF V600E mutant papillary craniopharyngiomas: a single-institutional case series. Pituitary. 2018 Dec;21(6):571–83. PMID:30187175
2477. La Rosa S, Adsay V, Albarello L, et al. Clinicopathologic study of 62 acinar cell carcinomas of the pancreas: insights into the morphology and immunophenotype and search for prognostic markers. Am J Surg Pathol. 2012 Dec;36(12):1782–95. PMID:23026929
2478. La Rosa S, Bernasconi B, Vanoli A, et al. c-MYC amplification and c-myc protein expression in pancreatic acinar cell carcinomas. New insights into the molecular signature of these rare cancers. Virchows Arch. 2018 Oct;473(4):435–41. PMID:29721608
2479. La Rosa S, Bonzini M, Sciarra A, et al. Exploring the prognostic role of Ki67 proliferative index in Merkel cell carcinoma of the skin: clinico-pathologic analysis of 84 cases and review of the literature. Endocr Pathol. 2020 Dec;31(4):392–400. PMID:32696301
2480. La Rosa S, Franzi F, Albarello L, et al. Serotonin-producing enterochromaffin cell tumors of the pancreas: clinicopathologic study of 15 cases and comparison with intestinal enterochromaffin cell tumors. Pancreas. 2011 Aug;40(6):883–95. PMID:21705949
2481. La Rosa S, Franzi F, Marchet S, et al. The monoclonal anti-BCL10 antibody (clone 331.1) is a sensitive and specific marker of pancreatic acinar cell carcinoma and pancreatic metaplasia. Virchows Arch. 2009 Feb;454(2):133–42. PMID:19066953
2482. La Rosa S, Furlan D, Franzi F, et al. Mixed exocrine-neuroendocrine carcinoma of the nasal cavity: clinico-pathologic and molecular study of a case and review of the literature. Head Neck Pathol. 2013 Mar;7(1):76–84. PMID:22740238
2483. La Rosa S, Inzani F, Vanoli A, et al. Histologic characterization and improved prognostic evaluation of 209 gastric neuroendocrine neoplasms. Hum Pathol. 2011 Oct;42(10):1373–84. PMID:21531442
2484. La Rosa S, Marando A, Furlan D, et al. Colorectal poorly differentiated neuroendocrine carcinomas and mixed adenoneuroendocrine carcinomas: insights into the diagnostic immunophenotype, assessment of methylation profile, and search for prognostic markers. Am J Surg Pathol. 2012 Apr;36(4):601–11. PMID:22314183
2485. La Rosa S, Marando A, Ghezzi F, et al. Cushing's syndrome due to a pancreatic neuroendocrine tumor metastatic to the ovaries: a clinicopathological description of a case. Endocr Pathol. 2011 Jun;22(2):118–24. PMID:21390554
2486. La Rosa S, Pariani D, Calandra C, et al. Ectopic duodenal insulinoma: a very rare and challenging tumor type. Description of a case and review of the literature. Endocr Pathol. 2013 Dec;24(4):213–9. PMID:24006218
2487. La Rosa S, Sahnane N, Cimetti L. Serotonin-producing tumor. In: La Rosa S, Sessa F, editors. Pancreatic neuroendocrine neoplasms: practical approach to diagnosis, classification, and therapy. Cham (Switzerland): Springer; 2015. pp. 117–24.
2488. La Rosa S, Sessa F, Capella C, et al. Prognostic criteria in nonfunctioning pancreatic endocrine tumours. Virchows Arch. 1996 Dec;429(6):323–33. PMID:8982376
2490. La Rosa S, Simbolo M, Franzi F, et al. Combined adenocarcinoma–atypical carcinoid of the lung. Targeted next-generation sequencing (NGS) suggests a monoclonal origin of the two components. Diagn Histopathol. 2018 Mar;24(3):120–3. doi:10.1016/j.mpdhp.2018.02.002.
2492. La Rosa S, Simbolo M, Luchini C, et al. MiNENs composed of adenocarcinoma and well differentiated neuroendocrine tumor have a monoclonal origin. Abstracts from USCAP 2020: Endocrine Pathology (565–611). Mod Pathol. 2020;33:720–63.
2493. La Rosa S, Simbolo M, Luchini C, et al. MiNENs composed of adenocarcinoma and well differentiated neuroendocrine tumor have a monoclonal origin. Abstracts from USCAP 2020: Endocrine Pathology (565–611). Mod Pathol. 2020;33:720–63.
2494. La Rosa S, Uccella S, Molinari F, et al. Mixed adenoma well-differentiated neuroendocrine tumor (MANET) of the digestive system: an indolent subtype of mixed neuroendocrine-nonneuroendocrine neoplasm (MiNEN). Am J Surg Pathol. 2018 Nov;42(11):1503–12. PMID:30001239
2495. Lacefield E, Raheem OA, Cox R, et al. Composite paraganglioma and neuroblastoma of the urinary bladder: a rare histopathological entity. Curr Urol. 2015 Dec;8(4):208–11. PMID:30263028
2496. Lack EE. Chapter 2: Congenital adrenal heterotopia, hyperplasia, and Beckwith-Wiedemann syndrome. In: Tumors of the adrenal glands and extraadrenal paraganglia. Washington, DC: American Registry of Pathology; 2007. (AFIP atlas of tumor pathology, series 4; fascicle 8).
2497. Lacroix A, Baldacchino V, Bourdeau I, et al. Cushing's syndrome variants secondary to aberrant hormone receptors. Trends Endocrinol Metab. 2004 Oct;15(8):375–82. PMID:15380809
2498. Lacroix A, Bourdeau I, Lampron A, et al. Aberrant G-protein coupled receptor expression in relation to adrenocortical overfunction. Clin Endocrinol (Oxf). 2010 Jul;73(1):1–15. PMID:19719763
2499. Lacroix A, N'Diaye N, Mircescu H, et al. Abnormal expression and function of hormone receptors in adrenal Cushing's syndrome. Endocr Res. 1998 Aug-Nov;24(3-4):835–43. PMID:9888584
2500. Lacy SE, Barrans SL, Beer PA, et al. Targeted sequencing in DLBCL, molecular subtypes, and outcomes: a Haematological Malignancy Research Network report. Blood. 2020 May 14;135(20):1759–71. PMID:32187361
2501. Laforga JB, Aranda FI. Pseudoangiosarcomatous features in medullary thyroid carcinoma spindle-cell variant. Report of a case studied by FNA and immunohistochemistry. Diagn Cytopathol. 2007 Jul;35(7):424–8. PMID:17580345
2502. LaGuette J, Matias-Guiu X, Rosai J. Thyroid paraganglioma: a clinicopathologic and immunohistochemical study of three cases. Am J Surg Pathol. 1997 Jul;21(7):748–53. PMID:9236830
2503. Lai JH, Fleming KE, Ly TY, et al. Pure versus combined Merkel cell carcinomas: immunohistochemical evaluation of cellular proteins (p53, Bcl-2, and c-kit) reveals significant overexpression of p53 in combined tumors. Hum Pathol. 2015 Sep;46(9):1290–6. PMID:26099430
2504. Lai WA, Hang JF, Liu CY, et al. PAX8 expression in anaplastic thyroid carcinoma is less than those reported in early studies: a multi-institutional study of 182 cases using the monoclonal antibody MRQ-50. Virchows Arch. 2020 Mar;476(3):431–7. PMID:31732814
2505. Lai WA, Liu CY, Lin SY, et al. Characterization of driver mutations in anaplastic thyroid carcinoma identifies RAS and PIK3CA mutations as negative survival predictors. Cancers (Basel). 2020 Jul 20;12(7):1973. PMID:32698386
2506. Lal P, Saleh MA, Khoudari G, et al. Epidemiology of large bowel carcinoid tumors in the USA: a population-based national study. Dig Dis Sci. 2020 Jan;65(1):269–75. PMID:31300994
2507. Lallier TE. Cell lineage and cell migration in the neural crest. Ann N Y Acad Sci. 1991;615:158–71. PMID:2039141
2508. Lam AK. Lipomatous tumours in adrenal gland: WHO updates and clinical implications. Endocr Relat Cancer. 2017 Mar;24(3):R65–79. PMID:28143811
2509. Lam AK. Squamous cell carcinoma of thyroid: a unique type of cancer in World Health Organization Classification. Endocr Relat Cancer. 2020 Jun;27(6):R177–92. PMID:32252028
2510. Lam AK, Fridman M. Characteristics of cribriform morular variant of papillary thyroid carcinoma in post-Chernobyl affected region. Hum Pathol. 2018 Apr;74:170–7. PMID:29320754
2511. Lam AK, Lo CY, Lam KS. Papillary carcinoma of thyroid: a 30-yr clinicopathological review of the histological variants. Endocr Pathol. 2005 Winter;16(4):323–30. PMID:16627919
2512. Lam KY, Lo CY. Adrenal lipomatous tumours: a 30 year clinicopathological experience at a single institution. J Clin Pathol. 2001 Sep;54(9):707–12. PMID:11533079
2513. Lam KY, Lo CY. Composite pheochromocytoma-ganglioneuroma of the adrenal gland: an uncommon entity with distinctive clinicopathologic features. Endocr Pathol. 1999 Winter;10(4):343–52. PMID:12114771
2514. Lam KY, Lo CY, Chan KW, et al. Insular and anaplastic carcinoma of the thyroid: a 45-year comparative study at a single institution and a review of the significance of p53 and p21. Ann Surg. 2000 Mar;231(3):329–38. PMID:10714625
2515. Lam KY, Loong F, Shek TW, et al. Composite paraganglioma-ganglioneuroma of the urinary bladder: a clinicopathologic, immunohistochemical, and ultrastructural study of a case and review of the literature. Endocr Pathol. 1998 Winter;9(1):353–61. PMID:12114785
2516. Lamlum H, Ilyas M, Rowan A, et al. The type of somatic mutation at APC in familial adenomatous polyposis is determined by the site of the germline mutation: a new facet to Knudson's 'two-hit' hypothesis. Nat Med. 1999 Sep;5(9):1071–5. PMID:10470088
2517. Lammy S, Brown J, Littlechild P. Cavernous sinus haemangioma masquerading as a pituitary macroadenoma: how the unexpected lurks in neurosurgery. Br J Neurosurg. 2023 Apr;37(2):234–6. PMID:33332201
2518. Lamolet B, Pulichino AM, Lamonerie T, et al. A pituitary cell-restricted T box factor, Tpit, activates POMC transcription in cooperation with Pitx homeoproteins. Cell. 2001 Mar 23;104(6):849–59. PMID:11290323
2519. Lancerotto L, Salmaso R, Sartore L, et al. Malignant glomus tumor of the leg developed in the context of a superficial typical glomus tumor. Int J Surg Pathol. 2012 Aug;20(4):420–4. PMID:22228777
2520. Landa I, Ibrahimpasic T, Boucai L, et al. Genomic and transcriptomic hallmarks of poorly differentiated and anaplastic thyroid cancers. J Clin Invest. 2016 Mar 1;126(3):1052–66. PMID:26878173
2521. Landau MS, Nikiforov YE, Ohori NP, et al. Impact of molecular testing on detecting mimics of oncocytic neoplasms in thyroid fine-needle aspirates diagnosed as follicular neoplasm of Hürthle cell (oncocytic) type. Cancer Cytopathol. 2021 Oct;129(10):788–97. PMID:33901345
2522. Landis CA, Masters SB, Spada A, et al. GTPase inhibiting mutations activate the alpha chain of Gs and stimulate adenylyl cyclase in

human pituitary tumours. Nature. 1989 Aug 31;340(6236):692–6. PMID:2549426
2523. Langer P, Cupisti K, Bartsch DK, et al. Adrenal involvement in multiple endocrine neoplasia type 1. World J Surg. 2002 Aug;26(8):891–6. PMID:12016472
2524. Langerman A, Athavale SM, Rangarajan SV, et al. Natural history of cervical paragangliomas: outcomes of observation of 43 patients. Arch Otolaryngol Head Neck Surg. 2012 Apr;138(4):341–5. PMID:22431860
2525. Lantuejoul S, Fernandez-Cuesta L, Damiola F, et al. New molecular classification of large cell neuroendocrine carcinoma and small cell lung carcinoma with potential therapeutic impacts. Transl Lung Cancer Res. 2020 Oct;9(5):2233–44. PMID:33209646
2526. Lanzafame S, Caltabiano R, Puzzo L, et al. Expression of thyroid transcription factor 1 (TTF-1) in extra thyroidal sites: papillary thyroid carcinoma of branchial cleft cysts and thyroglossal duct cysts and struma ovarii. Pathologica. 2006 Dec;98(6):640–4. PMID:17285841
2527. Lao Q, Mallappa A, Rueda Faucz F, et al. A TNXB splice donor site variant as a cause of hypermobility type Ehlers-Danlos syndrome in patients with congenital adrenal hyperplasia. Mol Genet Genomic Med. 2021 Feb;9(2):e1556. PMID:33332743
2528. Larger E, Wewer Albrechtsen NJ, Hansen LH, et al. Pancreatic α-cell hyperplasia and hyperglucagonemia due to a glucagon receptor splice mutation. Endocrinol Diabetes Metab Case Rep. 2016;2016:16-0081. PMID:27933176
2529. Larkin DF, Dervan PA, Munnelly J, et al. Sinus histiocytosis with massive lymphadenopathy simulating subacute thyroiditis. Hum Pathol. 1986 Mar;17(3):321–4. PMID:3512416
2530. Larkin S, Reddy R, Karavitaki N, et al. Granulation pattern, but not GSP or GHR mutation, is associated with clinical characteristics in somatostatin-naive patients with somatotroph adenomas. Eur J Endocrinol. 2013 Mar 15;168(4):491–9. PMID:23288882
2531. Larkin SJ, Preda V, Karavitaki N, et al. BRAF V600E mutations are characteristic for papillary craniopharyngioma and may coexist with CTNNB1-mutated adamantinomatous craniopharyngioma. Acta Neuropathol. 2014;127(6):927–9. PMID:24715106
2532. La Rosa S. Challenges in high-grade neuroendocrine neoplasms and mixed neuroendocrine/non-neuroendocrine neoplasms. Endocr Pathol. 2021 Jun;32(2):245–57. PMID:33786701
2533. La Rosa S, Sessa F, Uccella S. Mixed neuroendocrine-nonneuroendocrine neoplasms (MiNENs): unifying the concept of a heterogeneous group of neoplasms. Endocr Pathol. 2016 Dec;27(4):284–311. PMID:27169712
2534. La Rosa S, Solcia E. New insights into the classification of gastric neuroendocrine tumours, expanding the spectrum of ECL-cell tumours related to hypergastrinaemia. Histopathology. 2020 Dec;77(6):862–4. PMID:33190337
2535. La Rosa S, Vanoli A. Gastric neuroendocrine neoplasms and related precursor lesions. J Clin Pathol. 2014 Nov;67(11):938–48. PMID:25053544
2536. La Rosa S, Vanoli A. Republished: gastric neuroendocrine neoplasms and related precursor lesions. Postgrad Med J. 2015 Mar;91(1073):163–73. PMID:25740317
2537. Larose S, Bondaz L, Mermejo LM, et al. Coexistence of myelolipoma and primary bilateral macronodular adrenal hyperplasia with GIP-dependent Cushing's syndrome. Front Endocrinol (Lausanne). 2019 Sep 11;10:618. PMID:31572300
2538. Larouche V, Akirov A, Thomas CM, et al. A primer on the genetics of medullary thyroid cancer. Curr Oncol. 2019 Dec;26(6):389–94. PMID:31896937
2539. Larsson LI, Hirsch MA, Holst JJ, et al. Pancreatic somatostatinoma. Clinical features and physiological implications. Lancet. 1977 Mar 26;1(8013):666–8. PMID:66472
2540. Lassaletta L, Torres-Martín M, Peña-Granero C, et al. NF2 genetic alterations in sporadic vestibular schwannomas: clinical implications. Otol Neurotol. 2013 Sep;34(7):1355–61. PMID:23921927
2541. Lastoria S, Marciello F, Faggiano A, et al. Role of (68)Ga-DOTATATE PET/CT in patients with multiple endocrine neoplasia type 1 (MEN1). Endocrine. 2016 Jun;52(3):488–94. PMID:26242621
2542. Lau SK. Malignant PEComa of the adrenal gland. Pathol Res Pract. 2012 Feb 15;208(2):113–7. PMID:22154607
2543. Lauper JM, Krause A, Vaughan TL, et al. Spectrum and risk of neoplasia in Werner syndrome: a systematic review. PLoS One. 2013;8(4):e59709. PMID:23573208
2544. Laurberg P, Pedersen KM, Vestergaard H, et al. High incidence of multinodular toxic goitre in the elderly population in a low iodine intake area vs. high incidence of Graves' disease in the young in a high iodine intake area: comparative surveys of thyrotoxicosis epidemiology in East-Jutland Denmark and Iceland. J Intern Med. 1991 May;229(5):415–20. PMID:2040867
2545. Laury AR, Bongiovanni M, Tille JC, et al. Thyroid pathology in PTEN-hamartoma tumor syndrome: characteristic findings of a distinct entity. Thyroid. 2011 Feb;21(2):135–44. PMID:21190448
2546. Laury AR, Perets R, Piao H, et al. A comprehensive analysis of PAX8 expression in human epithelial tumors. Am J Surg Pathol. 2011 Jun;35(6):816–26. PMID:21552115
2547. Lawrence B, Gustafsson BI, Chan A, et al. The epidemiology of gastroenteropancreatic neuroendocrine tumors. Endocrinol Metab Clin North Am. 2011 Mar;40(1):1–18, vii. PMID:21349409
2548. Lawrence LEB, Saleem A, Sahoo MK, et al. Is Merkel cell carcinoma of lymph node actually metastatic cutaneous Merkel cell carcinoma? Am J Clin Pathol. 2020 Aug 5;154(3):369–80. PMID:32445471
2549. Lax SF, Beham A, Kronberger-Schönecker D, et al. Coexistence of papillary and medullary carcinoma of the thyroid gland-mixed or collision tumour? Clinicopathological analysis of three cases. Virchows Arch. 1994;424(4):441–7. PMID:8205357
2550. Layfield LJ, Glasgow BJ, Du Puis MH, et al. Aspiration cytology and immunohistochemistry of a pheochromocytoma-ganglioneuroma of the adrenal gland. Acta Cytol. 1987 Jan-Feb;31(1):33–9. PMID:3468715
2551. Le BH, Towfighi J, Kapadia SB, et al. Comparative immunohistochemical assessment of craniopharyngioma and related lesions. Endocr Pathol. 2007 Spring;18(1):23–30. PMID:17652797
2552. Le Bodic MF, Heymann MF, Lecomte M, et al. Immunohistochemical study of 100 pancreatic tumors in 28 patients with multiple endocrine neoplasia, type I. Am J Surg Pathol. 1996 Nov;20(11):1378–84. PMID:8898842
2553. Le Guellec S, Decouvelaere AV, Filleron T, et al. Malignant peripheral nerve sheath tumor is a challenging diagnosis: a systematic pathology review, immunohistochemistry, and molecular analysis in 160 patients from the French Sarcoma Group database. Am J Surg Pathol. 2016 Jul;40(7):896–908. PMID:27158754
2554. Le QV, Ngo DQ, Ngo QX. Primary mucoepidermoid carcinoma of the thyroid: a report of a rare case with bone metastasis and review of the literature. Case Rep Oncol. 2019 Mar 19;12(1):248–59. PMID:31011324
2555. Leath CA 3rd, Huh WK, Straughn JM Jr, et al. Uterine leiomyosarcoma metastatic to the thyroid. Obstet Gynecol. 2002 Nov;100(5 Pt 2):1122–4. PMID:12423830
2556. Lecomte P, Binquet C, Le Bras M, et al. Histologically proven bronchial neuroendocrine tumors in MEN1: a GTE 51-case cohort study. World J Surg. 2018 Jan;42(1):143–52. PMID:28785839
2557. Lecomte-Houcke M, Parent M, Carnaille B, et al. [Primary malignant teratoma of the thyroid. Two cases involving immunohistochemical and ultrastructural studies]. Ann Pathol. 1992;12(1):12–9. French. PMID:1580935
2558. Le Douarin NM, Ziller C. Plasticity in neural crest cell differentiation. Curr Opin Cell Biol. 1993 Dec;5(6):1036–43. PMID:8129941
2559. Lee BJ, Cho GJ, Norgren RB Jr, et al. TTF-1, a homeodomain gene required for diencephalic morphogenesis, is postnatally expressed in the neuroendocrine brain in a developmentally regulated and cell-specific fashion. Mol Cell Neurosci. 2001 Jan;17(1):107–26. PMID:11161473
2560. Lee CC, Harun F, Jalaludin MY, et al. A novel, homozygous c.1502T>G (p.Val501Gly) mutation in the thyroid peroxidase gene in Malaysian sisters with congenital hypothyroidism and multinodular goiter. Int J Endocrinol. 2013T;2013:987186. PMID:23737781
2561. Lee CC, Vance ML, Lopes MB, et al. Stereotactic radiosurgery for acromegaly: outcomes by adenoma subtype. Pituitary. 2015 Jun;18(3):326–34. PMID:24925503
2562. Lee CR, Park S, Kang SW, et al. Is familial papillary thyroid microcarcinoma more aggressive than sporadic form? Ann Surg Treat Res. 2017 Mar;92(3):129–35. PMID:28289666
2563. Lee DH, Cho HH, Cho YB. Typical carcinoid tumor of the nasal cavity. Auris Nasus Larynx. 2007 Dec;34(4):537–9. PMID:17481837
2564. Lee DH, Yoon TM, Lee JK, et al. Is fine needle aspiration cytology appropriate for preoperatively diagnosing thyroglossal duct cysts in children under the age of 10 years? Int J Pediatr Otorhinolaryngol. 2012 Apr;76(4):480–2. PMID:22277268
2565. Lee EB, Tihan T, Scheithauer BW, et al. Thyroid transcription factor 1 expression in sellar tumors: a histogenetic marker? J Neuropathol Exp Neurol. 2009 May;68(5):482–8. PMID:19525896
2566. Lee EJ, Park SM, Maeng L, et al. Composite glandular-endocrine cell carcinomas of the stomach: clinicopathologic and methylation study. APMIS. 2005 Sep;113(9):569–76. PMID:16218931
2567. Lee FY, Jan YJ, Chou G, et al. Thyroid involvement in Rosai-Dorfman disease. Thyroid. 2007 May;17(5):471–6. PMID:17542678
2568. Lee HE, Kim DH, Cho YH, et al. Tumor-to-tumor metastasis: hepatocellular carcinoma metastatic to parathyroid adenoma. Pathol Int. 2011 Oct;61(10):593–7. PMID:21951669
2569. Lee HJ, Wu CC, Wu HM, et al. Pretreatment diagnosis of suprasellar papillary craniopharyngioma and germ cell tumors of adult patients. AJNR Am J Neuroradiol. 2015 Mar;36(3):508–17. PMID:25339645
2570. Lee JH, Choi YD, Cho NH. An intrarenal adrenocortical carcinoma arising in an adrenal rest. J Pathol Transl Med. 2018 Nov;52(6):416–9. PMID:30269470
2571. Lee JH, Hwang Y, Song RY, et al. Relationship between iodine levels and papillary thyroid carcinoma: a systematic review and meta-analysis. Head Neck. 2017 Aug;39(8):1711–8. PMID:28513893
2572. Lee JH, Shin JH, Lee HW, et al. Sonographic and cytopathologic correlation of papillary thyroid carcinoma variants. J Ultrasound Med. 2015 Jan;34(1):1–15. PMID:25542934
2573. Lee JH, Song RY, Yi JW, et al. Case-control study of papillary thyroid carcinoma on urinary and dietary iodine status in South Korea. World J Surg. 2018 May;42(5):1424–31. PMID:29067516
2574. Lee JS, Cho KH, Hong EK, et al. Pituitary ependymoma, 10-year follow-up after partial resection and radiation therapy. Brain Tumor Res Treat. 2017 Oct;5(2):94–8. PMID:29188210
2575. Lee JY, Baek JH, Ha EJ, et al. 2020 Imaging guidelines for thyroid nodules and differentiated thyroid cancer: Korean Society of Thyroid Radiology. Korean J Radiol. 2021 May;22(5):840–60. PMID:33660459
2576. Lee M, Pellegata NS. Multiple endocrine neoplasia type 4. Front Horm Res. 2013;41:63–78. PMID:23652671
2577. Lee NC, Norton JA. Multiple endocrine neoplasia type 2B–genetic basis and clinical expression. Surg Oncol. 2000 Nov;9(3):111–8. PMID:11356339
2578. Lee PK, Jarosek SL, Virnig BA, et al. Trends in the incidence and treatment of parathyroid cancer in the United States. Cancer. 2007 May 1;109(9):1736–41. PMID:17372919
2579. Lee S, Borah S, Bahrami A. Detection of aberrant TERT promoter methylation by combined bisulfite restriction enzyme analysis for cancer diagnosis. J Mol Diagn. 2017 May;19(3):378–86. PMID:28284778
2580. Lee S, Han BK, Ko EY, et al. The ultrasonography features of hyalinizing trabecular tumor of the thyroid are more consistent with its benign behavior than cytology or frozen section readings. Thyroid. 2011 Mar;21(3):253–9. PMID:21190434
2581. Lee S, Kim YS, Lee JH, et al. Spindle epithelial tumor with thymus-like differentiation of the thyroid in a 70-year-old man. Ann Surg Treat Res. 2018 Jun;94(6):337–41. PMID:29854712
2582. Lee SE, Hwang TS, Choi YL, et al. Molecular profiling of papillary thyroid carcinoma in Korea with a high prevalence of BRAFV600E mutation. Thyroid. 2017 Jun;27(6):802–10. PMID:28293988
2583. Lee SE, Hwang TS, Choi YL, et al. Prognostic significance of TERT promoter mutations in papillary thyroid carcinomas in a BRAF(V600E) mutation-prevalent population. Thyroid. 2016 Jul;26(7):901–10. PMID:27184112
2584. Lee SM, Sung CO. Neuroendocrine carcinomas of the gallbladder: a clinicopathologic and immunohistochemical analysis of 34 resected cases. Am J Surg Pathol. 2020 Oct;44(10):1308–21. PMID:32739935
2585. Lee SW, Shin EA, Kwon KW, et al. Primary lymphangioma of the thyroid gland. Thyroid. 2009 Aug;19(8):915–6. PMID:19500020
2586. Lee SY, Thng CH, Chow PKh. Lipoma of the pancreas, a case report and a review of the literature. World J Radiol. 2011 Oct 28;3(10):246–8. PMID:22229078
2587. Lee TK, Myers RT, Marshall RB, et al. The significance of mitotic rate: a retrospective study of 127 thyroid carcinomas. Hum Pathol. 1985 Oct;16(10):1042–6. PMID:4043953
2588. Lee W, Teckie S, Wiesner T, et al. PRC2 is recurrently inactivated through EED or SUZ12 loss in malignant peripheral nerve sheath tumors. Nat Genet. 2014 Nov;46(11):1227–32. PMID:25240281
2589. Lee WS, Koh YS, Kim JC, et al. Zollinger-Ellison syndrome associated with neurofibromatosis type 1: a case report. BMC Cancer. 2005 Jul 21;5:85. PMID:16042772

2590. Lee YA, Im SW, Jung KC, et al. Predominant DICER1 pathogenic variants in pediatric follicular thyroid carcinomas. Thyroid. 2020 Aug;30(8):1120–31. PMID:32228164
2591. Lee YM, Yoon JH, Yi O, et al. Familial history of non-medullary thyroid cancer is an independent prognostic factor for tumor recurrence in younger patients with conventional papillary thyroid carcinoma. J Surg Oncol. 2014 Feb;109(2):168–73. PMID:24132694
2592. Lee YS, Kim Y, Jeon S, et al. Cytologic, clinicopathologic, and molecular features of papillary thyroid carcinoma with prominent hobnail features: 10 case reports and systematic literature review. Int J Clin Exp Pathol. 2015 Jul 1;8(7):7988–97. PMID:26339365
2593. Lee YY, Wang WC, Li CF. Aspiration cytology of an ectopic cervical thymoma misinterpreted as a lymphoproliferative lesion of the thyroid: a case report. Oncol Lett. 2015 Sep;10(3):1255–8. PMID:26622659
2594. Leeman-Neill RJ, Brenner AV, Little MP, et al. RET/PTC and PAX8/PPARγ chromosomal rearrangements in post-Chernobyl thyroid cancer and their association with iodine-131 radiation dose and other characteristics. Cancer. 2013 May 15;119(10):1792–9. PMID:23436219
2595. Leet AI, Chebli C, Kushner H, et al. Fracture incidence in polyostotic fibrous dysplasia and the McCune-Albright syndrome. J Bone Miner Res. 2004 Apr;19(4):571–7. PMID:15005844
2596. Lefebvre H, Duparc C, Chartrel N, et al. Intraadrenal adrenocorticotropin production in a case of bilateral macronodular adrenal hyperplasia causing Cushing's syndrome. J Clin Endocrinol Metab. 2003 Jul;88(7):3035–42. PMID:12843140
2597. Lei Y, Feng H, Qiang H, et al. Clinical characteristics and prognostic factors of surgically resected combined small cell lung cancer: a retrospective study. Lung Cancer. 2020 Aug;146:244–51. PMID:32592985
2598. Leibowitz-Amit R, Mete O, Asa SL, et al. Malignant pheochromocytoma secreting vasoactive intestinal peptide and response to sunitinib: a case report and literature review. Endocr Pract. 2014 Aug;20(8):e145–50. PMID:24936559
2599. Lelotte J, Mourin A, Fomekong E, et al. Both invasiveness and proliferation criteria predict recurrence of non-functioning pituitary macroadenomas after surgery: a retrospective analysis of a monocentric cohort of 120 patients. Eur J Endocrinol. 2018 Mar;178(3):237–46. PMID:29259039
2600. Lemmens I, Van de Ven WJ, Kas K, et al. Identification of the multiple endocrine neoplasia type 1 (MEN1) gene. The European Consortium on MEN1. Hum Mol Genet. 1997 Jul;6(7):1177–83. PMID:9215690
2601. Lemos MC, Thakker RV. Multiple endocrine neoplasia type 1 (MEN1): analysis of 1336 mutations reported in the first decade following identification of the gene. Hum Mutat. 2008 Jan;29(1):22–32. PMID:17879353
2602. Lenders JW, Eisenhofer G, Mannelli M, et al. Phaeochromocytoma. Lancet. 2005 Aug 20-26;366(9486):665–75. PMID:16112304
2603. Lenders JWM, Kerstens MN, Amar L, et al. Genetics, diagnosis, management and future directions of research of phaeochromocytoma and paraganglioma: a position statement and consensus of the Working Group on Endocrine Hypertension of the European Society of Hypertension. J Hypertens. 2020 Aug;38(8):1443–56. PMID:32412940
2604. Lenders N, McCormack A. Malignant transformation in non-functioning pituitary adenomas (pituitary carcinoma). Pituitary. 2018 Apr;21(2):217–29. PMID:29299820
2605. Lenders NF, Wilkinson AC, Wong SJ, et al. Transcription factor immunohistochemistry in the diagnosis of pituitary tumours. Eur J Endocrinol. 2021 May 10;184(6):891–901. PMID:33852418
2606. Lenzini L, Rossitto G, Maiolino G, et al. A meta-analysis of somatic KCNJ5 K(+) channel mutations in 1636 patients with an aldosterone-producing adenoma. J Clin Endocrinol Metab. 2015 Aug;100(8):E1089–95. PMID:26066531
2607. León X, Sancho FJ, García J, et al. Incidence and significance of clinically unsuspected thyroid tissue in lymph nodes found during neck dissection in head and neck carcinoma patients. Laryngoscope. 2005 Mar;115(3):470–4. PMID:15744160
2608. Leonardo E, Volante M, Barbareschi M, et al. Cell membrane reactivity of MIB-1 antibody to Ki67 in human tumors: fact or artifact? Appl Immunohistochem Mol Morphol. 2007 Jun;15(2):220–3. PMID:17525638
2609. Leoncini E, Carioli G, La Vecchia C, et al. Risk factors for neuroendocrine neoplasms: a systematic review and meta-analysis. Ann Oncol. 2016 Jan;27(1):68–81. PMID:26487581
2610. Leong AS, Chawla JC, Teh EC. Pituitary thyrotropic tumour secondary to long-standing primary hypothyroidism. Pathol Eur. 1976;11(1):49–55. PMID:934699
2611. Lepage C, Rachet B, Coleman MP. Survival from malignant digestive endocrine tumors in England and Wales: a population-based study. Gastroenterology. 2007 Mar;132(3):899–904. PMID:17383419
2612. Leporati P, Landek-Salgado MA, Lupi I, et al. IgG4-related hypophysitis: a new addition to the hypophysitis spectrum. J Clin Endocrinol Metab. 2011 Jul;96(7):1971–80. PMID:21593109
2613. Lerman RI, Kaplan ES, Daman L. Ganglioneuroma-paraganglioma of the intradural filum terminale. Case report. J Neurosurg. 1972 May;36(5):652–8. PMID:5026551
2614. Lerner J, Goldfarb M. Follicular variant papillary thyroid carcinoma in a pediatric population. Pediatr Blood Cancer. 2015 Nov;62(11):1942–6. PMID:26131690
2615. Leslie MD, Cheung KY. Malignant transformation of neurofibromas at multiple sites in a case of neurofibromatosis. Postgrad Med J. 1987 Feb;63(736):131–3. PMID:3118347
2616. Lesueur F, Stark M, Tocco T, et al. Genetic heterogeneity in familial nonmedullary thyroid carcinoma: exclusion of linkage to RET, MNG1, and TCO in 56 families. J Clin Endocrinol Metab. 1999 Jun;84(6):2157–62. PMID:10372725
2617. Levine SN, Ishaq S, Nanda A, et al. Occurrence of extensive spherical amyloid deposits in a prolactin-secreting pituitary macroadenoma: a radiologic-pathologic correlation. Ann Diagn Pathol. 2013 Aug;17(4):361–6. PMID:23602507
2618. Levy A, Hall L, Yeudall WA, et al. p53 gene mutations in pituitary adenomas: rare events. Clin Endocrinol (Oxf). 1994 Dec;41(6):809–14. PMID:7889618
2619. Levy MT, Braun JT, Pennant M, et al. Primary paraganglioma of the parathyroid: a case report and clinicopathologic review. Head Neck Pathol. 2010 Mar;4(1):37–43. PMID:20237987
2620. Levy RA. Paraganglioma of the filum terminale: MR findings. AJR Am J Roentgenol. 1993 Apr;160(4):851–2. PMID:8456679
2621. Lévy-Bohbot N, Merle C, Goudet P, et al. Prevalence, characteristics and prognosis of MEN 1-associated glucagonomas, VIPomas, and somatostatinomas: study from the GTE (Groupe des Tumeurs Endocrines) registry. Gastroenterol Clin Biol. 2004 Nov;28(11):1075–81. PMID:15657529
2622. Lewandowska-Graban K, Zdrojewska M, Jendrzejewski J, et al. A case report of melanoma metastasis to adrenal gland. Pol Arch Intern Med. 2019 Sep 30;129(9):636–7. PMID:31290484
2623. Lewis JE, Wick MR, Scheithauer BW, et al. Thymoma. A clinicopathologic review. Cancer. 1987 Dec 1;60(11):2727–43. PMID:3677008
2624. Lewis JS Jr, Spence DC, Chiosea S, et al. Large cell neuroendocrine carcinoma of the larynx: definition of an entity. Head Neck Pathol. 2010 Sep;4(3):198–207. PMID:20589486
2625. Li AF, Li AC, Hsu CY, et al. Small cell carcinomas in gastrointestinal tract: immunohistochemical and clinicopathological features. J Clin Pathol. 2010 Jul;63(7):620–5. PMID:20530158
2626. Li C, Lv L, Wang H, et al. Total parathyroidectomy versus total parathyroidectomy with autotransplantation for secondary hyperparathyroidism: systematic review and meta-analysis. Ren Fail. 2017 Nov;39(1):678–87. PMID:28853301
2627. Li C, Xie W, Rosenblum JS, et al. Somatic SF3B1 hotspot mutation in prolactinomas. Nat Commun. 2020 May 19;11(1):2506. PMID:32427851
2628. Li DH, Wang C, Chen HJ, et al. Clinical characteristics of the mixed form of neuroendocrine tumor in the lung: a retrospective study in 2501 lung cancer cases. Thorac Cancer. 2015 Jan;6(1):25–30. PMID:26273331
2629. Li H, Sisoudiya SD, Martin-Giacalone BA, et al. Germline cancer predisposition variants in pediatric rhabdomyosarcoma: a report from the Children's Oncology Group. J Natl Cancer Inst. 2021 Jul 1;113(7):875–83. PMID:33372952
2630. Li H, Zhao L, Singh R, et al. The first pediatric case of glucagon receptor defect due to biallelic mutations in GCGR is identified by newborn screening of elevated arginine. Mol Genet Metab Rep. 2018 Oct 2;17:46–52. PMID:30294546
2631. Li J, Li J, Xiong Y, et al. Atypical/malignant solitary fibrous tumor of the pancreas with spleen vein invasion: case report and literature review. Medicine (Baltimore). 2020 Apr;99(17):e19783. PMID:32332621
2632. Li JD, Zhuang Y, Li YF, et al. A clinicopathological aspect of primary small-cell carcinoma of the uterine cervix: a single-centre study of 25 cases. J Clin Pathol. 2011 Dec;64(12):1102–7. PMID:21965825
2633. Li JY, Racadot O, Kujas M, et al. Immunocytochemistry of four mixed pituitary adenomas and intrasellar gangliocytomas associated with different clinical syndromes: acromegaly, amenorrhea-galactorrhea, Cushing's disease and isolated tumoral syndrome. Acta Neuropathol. 1989;77(3):320–8. PMID:2922994
2634. Li M, Carcangiu ML, Rosai J. Abnormal intracellular and extracellular distribution of basement membrane material in papillary carcinoma and hyalinizing trabecular tumors of the thyroid: implication for deregulation of secretory pathways. Hum Pathol. 1997 Dec;28(12):1366–72. PMID:9416692
2635. Li M, Eastman CJ. The changing epidemiology of iodine deficiency. Nat Rev Endocrinol. 2012 Apr 3;8(7):434–40. PMID:22473332
2636. Li M, Liu F, Zhang Y, et al. Whole-genome sequencing reveals the mutational landscape of metastatic small-cell gallbladder neuroendocrine carcinoma (GB-SCNEC). Cancer Lett. 2017 Apr 10;391:20–7. PMID:28040546
2637. Li S, Yang T, Xiang Y, et al. Clinical characteristics and survival outcomes of malignant struma ovarii confined to the ovary. BMC Cancer. 2021 Apr 9;21(1):383. PMID:33836675
2638. Li X, Su J, Zhao L, et al. Familial Cushing syndrome due to thymic carcinoids in a multiple endocrine neoplasia type 1 kindred. Endocrine. 2014 Sep;47(1):183–90. PMID:24452869
2639. Li Y, Chen SH, Sheinberg D, et al. Imaging characteristics of a hypervascular pituitary spindle cell oncocytoma on magnetic resonance imaging and digital subtraction angiography. World Neurosurg. 2020 Jan;133:56–9. PMID:31568904
2640. Li Y, Gao H, Li Z, et al. Clinical characteristics of 76 patients with IgG4-related hypophysitis: a systematic literature review. Int J Endocrinol. 2019 Dec 18;2019:5382640. PMID:31929792
2641. Li Y, Zhang J, Adikaram PR, et al. Genotype of CDC73 germline mutation determines risk of parathyroid cancer. Endocr Relat Cancer. 2020 Sep;27(9):483–94. PMID:32590342
2642. Li Y, Zhou G, Ozaki T, et al. Distinct histopathological features of Hashimoto's thyroiditis with respect to IgG4-related disease. Mod Pathol. 2012 Aug;25(8):1086–97. PMID:22555173
2643. Li YR, Chen ST, Hseuh C, et al. Risk factors of distant metastasis in the follicular variant of papillary thyroid carcinoma. J Formos Med Assoc. 2016 Aug;115(8):665–71. PMID:26239193
2644. Li Z, Raynald, Wang Z, et al. Malignant transformation of craniofacial fibrous dysplasia: a systematic review of overall survival. Neurosurg Rev. 2020 Jun;43(3):911–21. PMID:30809751
2645. Li Z, Zhang J, Zhang L, et al. Natural history and growth kinetics of clear cell renal cell carcinoma in sporadic and von Hippel-Lindau disease. Transl Androl Urol. 2021 Mar;10(3):1064–70. PMID:33850741
2646. Liang Y, Yang Z, Qin B, et al. Primary Sjogren's syndrome and malignancy risk: a systematic review and meta-analysis. Ann Rheum Dis. 2014 Jun;73(6):1151–6. PMID:23687261
2647. Liao S, Song W, Liu Y, et al. Familial multinodular goiter syndrome with papillary thyroid carcinomas: mutational analysis of the associated genes in 5 cases from 1 Chinese family. BMC Endocr Disord. 2013 Oct 21;13:48. PMID:24144365
2648. Liapi-Avgeri G, Karabela-Bouropoulou V, Agnanti N. Glomus tumor. A histological, histochemical and immunohistochemical study of the various types. Pathol Res Pract. 1994 Jan;190(1):2–10. PMID:8065987
2649. Liatsikos EN, Papathanassiou Z, Voudoukis T, et al. Case report: laparoscopic adrenalectomy in a patient with primary adrenal malignant melanoma. J Endourol. 2006 Feb;20(2):123–6. PMID:16509796
2650. Libé R. Clinical and molecular prognostic factors in adrenocortical carcinoma. Minerva Endocrinol. 2019 Mar;44(1):58–69. PMID:30221891
2651. Libé R, Horvath A, Vezzosi D, et al. Frequent phosphodiesterase 11A gene (PDE11A) defects in patients with Carney complex (CNC) caused by PRKAR1A mutations: PDE11A may contribute to adrenal and testicular tumors in CNC as a modifier of the phenotype. J Clin Endocrinol Metab. 2011 Jan;96(1):E208–14. PMID:21047926
2652. Lichtenauer UD, Di Dalmazi G, Slater EP, et al. Frequency and clinical correlates of somatic Ying Yang 1 mutations in sporadic insulinomas. J Clin Endocrinol Metab. 2015 May;100(5):E776–82. PMID:25763608
2653. Liegl B, Hornick JL, Fletcher CD. Primary cutaneous PEComa: distinctive clear cell lesions of skin. Am J Surg Pathol. 2008 Apr;32(4):608–14. PMID:18277881
2654. Ligneau B, Lombard-Bohas C, Partensky C, et al. Cystic endocrine tumors of the pancreas: clinical, radiologic, and histopathologic features in 13 cases. Am J Surg Pathol. 2001 Jun;25(6):752–60. PMID:11395552

2655. Likhacheva A, Rosenthal DI, Hanna E, et al. Sinonasal neuroendocrine carcinoma: impact of differentiation status on response and outcome. Head Neck Oncol. 2011 Jul 27;3:32. PMID:21794118

2656. Lim H, Devesa SS, Sosa JA, et al. Trends in thyroid cancer incidence and mortality in the United States, 1974-2013. JAMA. 2017 Apr 4;317(13):1338–48. PMID:28362912

2657. Lim JS, Lee SE, Kim JH, et al. Characteristics of adrenocortical carcinoma in South Korea: a registry-based nationwide survey. Endocr Connect. 2020 Jun;9(6):519–29. PMID:32438344

2658. Lim S, Elston MS, Gill AJ, et al. Metastatic parathyroid carcinoma initially misdiagnosed as parathyroid adenoma: the role of parafibromin in increasing diagnostic accuracy. Intern Med J. 2011 Sep;41(9):695–9. PMID:21899683

2659. Lin AL, Jonsson P, Tabar V, et al. Marked response of a hypermutated ACTH-secreting pituitary carcinoma to ipilimumab and nivolumab. J Clin Endocrinol Metab. 2018 Oct 1;103(10):3925–30. PMID:30085142

2660. Lin B, Ma H, Ma M, et al. The incidence and survival analysis for anaplastic thyroid cancer: a SEER database analysis. Am J Transl Res. 2019 Sep 15;11(9):5888–96. PMID:31632557

2661. Lin CY, Huang WK, Chung FT, et al. Prognostic factors in cancer patients with symptomatic pituitary metastasis: a clinical case study. Anticancer Res. 2015 Feb;35(2):983–7. PMID:25667485

2662. Lin J, Wasco MJ, Korobkin M, et al. Leiomyoma of the adrenal gland presenting as a non-functioning adrenal incidentaloma: case report and review of the literature. Endocr Pathol. 2007 Winter;18(4):239–43. PMID:18197480

2663. Lin L, Zhang JH, Panicker LM, et al. The parafibromin tumor suppressor protein inhibits cell proliferation by repression of the c-myc proto-oncogene. Proc Natl Acad Sci U S A. 2008 Nov 11;105(45):17420–5. PMID:18987311

2664. Lin MW, Su KY, Su TJ, et al. Clinicopathological and genomic comparisons between different histologic components in combined small cell lung cancer and non-small cell lung cancer. Lung Cancer. 2018 Nov;125:282–90. PMID:30429033

2665. Lin ST, Tseng FY, Hsu CJ, et al. Thyroglossal duct cyst: a comparison between children and adults. Am J Otolaryngol. 2008 Mar-Apr;29(2):83–7. PMID:18314017

2666. Lin W, Watanabe H, Peng S, et al. Dynamic epigenetic regulation by menin during pancreatic islet tumor formation. Mol Cancer Res. 2015 Apr;13(4):689–98. PMID:25537453

2667. Lin X, Fan Y, Zhang Z, et al. Clinical characteristics of primary hyperparathyroidism: 15-year experience of 457 patients in a single center in China. Front Endocrinol (Lausanne). 2021 Feb 25;12:602221. PMID:33716964

2668. Lin X, Zhu B, Liu Y, et al. Follicular thyroid carcinoma invades venous rather than lymphatic vessels. Diagn Pathol. 2010 Jan 22;5:8. PMID:20205756

2669. Lin Y, Seger N, Tsagkozis P, et al. Telomerase promoter mutations and copy number alterations in solitary fibrous tumours. J Clin Pathol. 2018 Sep;71(9):832–9. PMID:29703757

2670. Lind P, Langsteger W, Molnar M, et al. Epidemiology of thyroid diseases in iodine sufficiency. Thyroid. 1998 Dec;8(12):1179–83. PMID:9920375

2671. Lindner S, Bachmann HS, Odersky A, et al. Absence of telomerase reverse transcriptase promoter mutations in neuroblastoma. Biomed Rep. 2015 Jul;3(4):443–6. PMID:26171145

2672. Lindsey JC, Schwalbe EC, Potluri S, et al. TERT promoter mutation and aberrant hypermethylation are associated with elevated expression in medulloblastoma and characterise the majority of non-infant SHH subgroup tumours. Acta Neuropathol. 2014 Feb;127(2):307–9. PMID:24337442

2673. Linos D, Kiriakopoulos AC, Tsakayannis DE, et al. Laparoscopic excision of bilateral primary adrenal leiomyosarcomas in a 14-year-old girl with acquired immunodeficiency syndrome (AIDS). Surgery. 2004 Nov;136(5):1098–100. PMID:15523410

2674. Lithgow K, Siqueira I, Senthil L, et al. Pituitary metastases: presentation and outcomes from a pituitary center over the last decade. Pituitary. 2020 Jun;23(3):258–65. PMID:32189207

2675. Liu AH, Juan LY, Yang AH, et al. Anaplastic thyroid cancer with uncommon long-term survival. J Chin Med Assoc. 2006 Oct;69(10):489–91. PMID:17098674

2676. Liu APY, Kelsey MM, Sabbaghian N, et al. Clinical outcomes and complications of pituitary blastoma. J Clin Endocrinol Metab. 2021 Jan 23;106(2):351–63. PMID:33236116

2677. Liu BJ, Zhang YF, Zhao CK, et al. Conventional ultrasound characteristics, TI-RADS category and shear wave speed measurement between follicular adenoma and follicular thyroid carcinoma. Clin Hemorheol Microcirc. 2020;75(3):291–301. PMID:32280082

2678. Liu C, Wu C, Wang F, et al. Mutations of GNAS and TSHR genes in subclinical toxic multinodular goiter. Ann Otol Rhinol Laryngol. 2010 Feb;119(2):118–24. PMID:20336923

2679. Liu C, Zhao Q, Li Z, et al. Mixed subtype thyroid cancer: a Surveillance, Epidemiology, and End results database analysis. Oncotarget. 2017 Sep 23;8(49):86556–65. PMID:29156816

2680. Liu CY, Bychkov A, Agarwal S, et al. Cytologic diagnosis of medullary thyroid carcinoma in the Asia-Pacific region. Diagn Cytopathol. 2021 Jan;49(1):60–9. PMID:32827355

2681. Liu G, Chen F, Li JN, et al. Carcinoid tumor of the middle ear: a case report and review of literature. Int J Clin Exp Pathol. 2014 Sep 15;7(10):7105–9. PMID:25400805

2682. Liu H, Yang D, Li L, et al. Appraisal of radioiodine refractory thyroid cancer: advances and challenges. Am J Cancer Res. 2020 Jul 1;10(7):1923–36. PMID:32774993

2683. Liu J, Cui N, Ding W, et al. Anaplastic thyroid carcinoma with chondrosarcomatous differentiation: a case report. Diagn Pathol. 2020 Jul 21;15(1):89. PMID:32693811

2684. Liu J, Guzman MA, Pezanowski D, et al. FOXO1-FGFR1 fusion and amplification in a solid variant of alveolar rhabdomyosarcoma. Mod Pathol. 2011 Oct;24(10):1327–35. PMID:21666686

2685. Liu J, Marcaccio MJ, Young JE, et al. Pancreatic struma with papillary thyroid carcinoma: a diagnostic dilemma. Endocr Pathol. 2017 Mar;28(1):91–4. PMID:28078619

2686. Liu J, Singh B, Tallini G, et al. Follicular variant of papillary thyroid carcinoma: a clinicopathologic study of a problematic entity. Cancer. 2006 Sep 15;107(6):1255–64. PMID:16900519

2687. Liu J, Wang Y, Da D, et al. Hyperfunctioning thyroid carcinoma: a systematic review. Mol Clin Oncol. 2019 Dec;11(6):535–50. PMID:31798874

2688. Liu JK, Couldwell WT. Contemporary management of prolactinomas. Neurosurg Focus. 2004 Apr 15;16(4):E2. PMID:15191331

2689. Liu L, Perry AM, Cao W, et al. Relationship between Rosai-Dorfman disease and IgG4-related disease: study of 32 cases. Am J Clin Pathol. 2013 Sep;140(3):395–402. PMID:23955459

2690. Liu R, Bishop J, Zhu G, et al. Mortality risk stratification by combining BRAF V600E and TERT promoter mutations in papillary thyroid cancer: genetic duet of BRAF and TERT promoter mutations in thyroid cancer mortality. JAMA Oncol. 2017 Feb 1;3(2):202–8. PMID:27581851

2691. Liu S, Tian Y, Chlenski A, et al. Cross-talk between Schwann cells and neuroblasts influences the biology of neuroblastoma xenografts. Am J Pathol. 2005 Mar;166(3):891–900. PMID:15743800

2692. Liu T, Brown TC, Juhlin CC, et al. The activating TERT promoter mutation C228T is recurrent in subsets of adrenal tumors. Endocr Relat Cancer. 2014 May 6;21(3):427–34. PMID:24803525

2693. Liu W, Asa SL, Ezzat S. Vitamin D and its analog EB1089 induce p27 accumulation and diminish association of p27 with Skp2 independent of PTEN in pituitary corticotroph cells. Brain Pathol. 2002 Oct;12(4):412–9. PMID:12408227

2694. Liu W, Zahr RS, McCartney S, et al. Clinical outcomes in male patients with lactotroph adenomas who required pituitary surgery: a retrospective single center study. Pituitary. 2018 Oct;21(5):454–62. PMID:29936681

2695. Liu X, Bishop J, Shan Y, et al. Highly prevalent TERT promoter mutations in aggressive thyroid cancers. Endocr Relat Cancer. 2013 Jul 12;20(4):603–10. PMID:23766237

2696. Liu Y, Chotai S, Ming C, et al. Characteristics of midline suprasellar meningiomas based on their origin and growth pattern. Clin Neurol Neurosurg. 2014 Oct;125:173–81. PMID:25171391

2697. Liu Y, Wu R, Yu T, et al. Malignant glomus tumor of the thyroid gland: a case report. J Int Med Res. 2019 Jun;47(6):2723–7. PMID:31039649

2698. Liu Y, Yao Y, Xing B, et al. Prolactinomas in children under 14. Clinical presentation and long-term follow-up. Childs Nerv Syst. 2015 Jun;31(6):909–16. PMID:25771923

2699. Liu Y, Yuan L, Yang D, et al. Serum calcitonin negative mixed medullary-follicular carcinoma initially diagnosed as medullary thyroid carcinoma by fine-needle aspiration cytology: a case report and review of the literatures. Diagn Cytopathol. 2018 Aug;46(8):690–3. PMID:29524315

2700. Liu Z, Li L, Yi Z, et al. Biological and clinical impact of central nervous system hemangioblastomas in Chinese patients with von Hippel-Lindau disease: implications for treatment. Hered Cancer Clin Pract. 2020 Oct 22;18:21. PMID:33110457

2701. Liu Z, Zeng W, Chen T, et al. A comparison of the clinicopathological features and prognoses of the classical and the tall cell variant of papillary thyroid cancer: a meta-analysis. Oncotarget. 2017 Jan 24;8(4):6222–32. PMID:28009980

2702. Liu Z, Zhou G, Nakamura M, et al. Encapsulated follicular thyroid tumor with equivocal nuclear changes, so-called well-differentiated tumor of uncertain malignant potential: a morphological, immunohistochemical, and molecular appraisal. Cancer Sci. 2011 Jan;102(1):288–94. PMID:21070478

2703. Livhits MJ, Zhu CY, Kuo EJ, et al. Effectiveness of molecular testing techniques for diagnosis of indeterminate thyroid nodules: a randomized clinical trial. JAMA Oncol. 2021 Jan 1;7(1):70–7. PMID:33300952

2704. LiVolsi VA. C cell hyperplasia/neoplasia. J Clin Endocrinol Metab. 1997 Jan;82(1):39–41. PMID:8989229

2705. Livolsi VA. Neuroendocrine tumors of the thyroid and their mimics. Endocr Pathol. 2021 Jun;32(2):211–21. PMID:33687689

2706. LiVolsi VA. Papillary thyroid carcinoma: an update. Mod Pathol. 2011 Apr;24 Suppl 2:S1–9. PMID:21455196

2707. LiVolsi VA, Abrosimov AA, Bogdanova T, et al. The Chernobyl thyroid cancer experience: pathology. Clin Oncol (R Coll Radiol). 2011 May;23(4):261–7. PMID:21333507

2708. LiVolsi VA, Asa SL. The demise of follicular carcinoma of the thyroid gland. Thyroid. 1994 Summer;4(2):233–6. PMID:7920009

2709. LiVolsi VA, Baloch ZW. The pathology of hyperthyroidism. Front Endocrinol (Lausanne). 2018 Dec 3;9:737. PMID:30559722

2710. LiVolsi VA, Merino MJ. Worrisome histologic alterations following fine-needle aspiration of the thyroid (WHAFFT). Pathol Annu. 1994:29 (Pt 2):99–120. PMID:7936753

2711. Llorens de Knecht E, Guadarrama Vega S, Donate G, et al. Robot-assisted radical prostatectomy due to a primary carcinoid prostatic tumor in a three-year-old child: a case report. Urology. 2019 Nov;133:216–8. PMID:31415779

2712. Lloyd RV, Carney JA, Ferreiro JA, et al. Immunohistochemical analysis of the cell cycle-associated antigens Ki-67 and retinoblastoma protein in parathyroid carcinomas and adenomas. Endocr Pathol. 1995 Winter;6(4):279–87. PMID:12114810

2713. Lloyd RV, Chandler WF, Kovacs K, et al. Ectopic pituitary adenomas with normal anterior pituitary glands. Am J Surg Pathol. 1986 Aug;10(8):546–52. PMID:3017137

2714. Lloyd RV, Osamura RY. Transcription factors in normal and neoplastic pituitary tissues. Microsc Res Tech. 1997 Oct 15;39(2):168–81. PMID:9361268

2716. Lloyd RV, Osamura RY, Klöppel G, et al., editors. WHO classification of tumours of endocrine organs. Lyon (France): International Agency for Research on Cancer; 2017. (WHO classification of tumours series, 4th ed.; vol. 10). https://publications.iarc.who.int/554.

2717. Lodewijk L, Bongers PJ, Kist JW, et al. Thyroid incidentalomas in patients with multiple endocrine neoplasia type 1. Eur J Endocrinol. 2015 Apr;172(4):337–42. PMID:25572387

2718. Lodish MB, Trivellin G, Stratakis CA. Pituitary gigantism: update on molecular biology and management. Curr Opin Endocrinol Diabetes Obes. 2016 Feb;23(1):72–80. PMID:26574647

2719. Loehry CA, Kingham JG, Whorwell PJ. Watery diarrhoea and hypokalaemia associated with a phaeochromocytoma. Postgrad Med J. 1975 Jun;51(596):416–9. PMID:175362

2720. Logani S, Gupta PK, LiVolsi VA, et al. Thyroid nodules with FNA cytology suspicious for follicular variant of papillary thyroid carcinoma: follow-up and management. Diagn Cytopathol. 2000 Dec;23(6):380–5. PMID:11074641

2721. Loh KC, Lo JC, Greenspan FS, et al. Familial papillary thyroid cancer: a case report. Ann Acad Med Singap. 1997 Jul;26(4):503–6. PMID:9395820

2722. Lohmann DR, Gillessen-Kaesbach G. Multiple subcutaneous granular-cell tumours in a patient with Noonan syndrome. Clin Dysmorphol. 2000 Oct;9(4):301–2. PMID:11045593

2723. Lolis E, Juhlin CC, Nordenström A, et al. Extensive bilateral adrenal rest testicular tumors in a patient with 3β-hydroxysteroid dehydrogenase type 2 deficiency. J Endocr Soc. 2018 May 1;2(6):513–7. PMID:29850650

2724. Lollar K, Farrag TY, Cao D, et al. Langerhans cell histiocytosis of the thyroid gland. Am J Otolaryngol. 2008 May-Jun;29(3):201–4. PMID:18439957

2725. Lomakina II, Skripnik SV. [Rhabdomyosarcoma mimicking anaplastic carcinoma of the thyroid gland]. Arkh Patol. 1983;45(4):71–4. Russian. PMID:6870584

2726. London F, Mulquin N, Fervaille C, et al. Radiologically atypical paraganglioma of the filum terminale as a rare cause of superficial siderosis of the central nervous system.

Acta Neurol Belg. 2020 Dec;120(6):1471–4. PMID:32152998
2727. Lonser RR, Kindzelski BA, Mehta GU, et al. Acromegaly without imaging evidence of pituitary adenoma. J Clin Endocrinol Metab. 2010 Sep;95(9):4192–6. PMID:20610592
2728. Lonser RR, Mehta GU, Kindzelski BA, et al. Surgical management of Carney complex-associated pituitary pathology. Neurosurgery. 2017 May 1;80(5):780–6. PMID:27509071
2729. Look AT, Hayes FA, Nitschke R, et al. Cellular DNA content as a predictor of response to chemotherapy in infants with unresectable neuroblastoma. N Engl J Med. 1984 Jul 26;311(4):231–5. PMID:6738617
2730. Lopes MB, Sloan E, Polder J. Mixed gangliocytoma-pituitary adenoma: insights on the pathogenesis of a rare sellar tumor. Am J Surg Pathol. 2017 May;41(5):586–95. PMID:28079576
2731. López F, Hunt JL, Nixon IJ, et al. How phenotype guides management of the neuroendocrine carcinomas of the larynx. J Laryngol Otol. 2018 Jul;132(7):568–74. PMID:29909787
2732. Lopez JA, Kleinschmidt-Demasters Bk Bk, Sze CI, et al. Silent corticotroph adenomas: further clinical and pathological observations. Hum Pathol. 2004 Sep;35(9):1137–47. PMID:15343517
2733. Lorenz L, von Rappard J, Arnold W, et al. Pembrolizumab in a patient with a metastatic CASTLE tumor of the parotid. Front Oncol. 2019 Aug 14;9:734. PMID:31475102
2734. Lorenzi L, Döring C, Rausch T, et al. Identification of novel follicular dendritic cell sarcoma markers, FDCSP and SRGN, by whole transcriptome sequencing. Oncotarget. 2017 Mar 7;8(10):16463–72. PMID:28145886
2735. Losa M, Mortini P, Barzaghi R, et al. Early results of surgery in patients with nonfunctioning pituitary adenoma and analysis of the risk of tumor recurrence. J Neurosurg. 2008 Mar;108(3):525–32. PMID:18312100
2736. Losa M, Mortini P, Pagnano A, et al. Clinical characteristics and surgical outcome in USP8-mutated human adrenocorticotropic hormone-secreting pituitary adenomas. Endocrine. 2019 Feb;63(2):240–6. PMID:30315484
2737. Losa M, Vimercati A, Acerno S, et al. Correlation between clinical characteristics and proliferative activity in patients with craniopharyngioma. J Neurol Neurosurg Psychiatry. 2004 Jun;75(6):889–92. PMID:15146007
2738. Lotan TL, Gupta NS, Wang W, et al. ERG gene rearrangements are common in prostatic small cell carcinomas. Mod Pathol. 2011 Jun;24(6):820–8. PMID:21336263
2739. Lott Limbach AA, Hoschar AP, Thompson LD, et al. Middle ear adenomas stain for two cell populations and lack myoepithelial cell differentiation. Head Neck Pathol. 2012 Sep;6(3):345–53. PMID:22623086
2740. Lottrup G, Nielsen JE, Skakkebæk NE, et al. Abundance of DLK1, differential expression of CYP11B1, CYP21A2 and MC2R, and lack of INSL3 distinguish testicular adrenal rest tumours from Leydig cell tumours. Eur J Endocrinol. 2015 Apr;172(4):491–9. PMID:25609776
2741. Louiset E, Duparc C, Young J, et al. Intraadrenal corticotropin in bilateral macronodular adrenal hyperplasia. N Engl J Med. 2013 Nov 28;369(22):2115–25. PMID:24283225
2742. Louiset E, Stratakis CA, Perraudin V, et al. The paradoxical increase in cortisol secretion induced by dexamethasone in primary pigmented nodular adrenocortical disease involves a glucocorticoid receptor-mediated effect of dexamethasone on protein kinase A catalytic subunits. J Clin Endocrinol Metab. 2009 Jul;94(7):2406–13. PMID:19383776
2743. Low G, Huang G, Fu W, et al. Review of renal cell carcinoma and its common subtypes in radiology. World J Radiol. 2016 May 28;8(5):484–500. PMID:27247714
2744. Lowe KM, Young WF Jr, Lyssikatos C, et al. Cushing syndrome in Carney complex: clinical, pathologic, and molecular genetic findings in the 17 affected Mayo Clinic patients. Am J Surg Pathol. 2017 Feb;41(2):171–81. PMID:27875378
2745. Lowery MA, Klimstra DS, Shia J, et al. Acinar cell carcinoma of the pancreas: new genetic and treatment insights into a rare malignancy. Oncologist. 2011;16(12):1714–20. PMID:22042785
2746. Lu H, Papathomas TG, van Zessen D, et al. Automated selection of hotspots (ASH): enhanced automated segmentation and adaptive step finding for Ki67 hotspot detection in adrenal cortical cancer. Diagn Pathol. 2014 Nov 25;9:216. PMID:25421287
2747. Lu HY, Sun WY, Chen B, et al. Epidermal growth factor receptor mutations in small cell lung cancer patients who received surgical resection in China. Neoplasma. 2012;59(1):100–4. PMID:22103903
2748. Lu Y, Liu QL, Lu T, et al. [Clinicopathological features of follicular dendritic cell sarcoma]. Zhongguo Yi Xue Ke Xue Yuan Xue Bao. 2020 Aug 30;42(4):504–12. Chinese. PMID:32895103
2749. Lu Z, Sheng J, Zhang Y, et al. Clonality analysis of multifocal papillary thyroid carcinoma by using genetic profiles. J Pathol. 2016 May;239(1):72–83. PMID:27071483
2750. Lubana SS, Singh N, Chan HC, et al. Primary neuroendocrine tumor (carcinoid tumor) of the testis: a case report with review of literature. Am J Case Rep. 2015 May 31;16:328–32. PMID:26027014
2751. Lubensky IA, Pack S, Ault D, et al. Multiple neuroendocrine tumors of the pancreas in von Hippel-Lindau disease patients: histopathological and molecular genetic analysis. Am J Pathol. 1998 Jul;153(1):223–31. PMID:9665483
2752. Lubitz CC, Economopoulos KP, Pawlak AC, et al. Hobnail variant of papillary thyroid carcinoma: an institutional case series and molecular profile. Thyroid. 2014 Jun;24(6):958–65. PMID:24417340
2753. Lubitz CC, Faquin WC, Yang J, et al. Clinical and cytological features predictive of malignancy in thyroid follicular neoplasms. Thyroid. 2010 Jan;20(1):25–31. PMID:20025540
2754. Luboshitzky R, Dharan M. Mixed follicular-medullary thyroid carcinoma: a case report. Diagn Cytopathol. 2004 Feb;30(2):122–4. PMID:14755766
2755. Luchini C, Lawlor RT, Bersani S, et al. Alternative lengthening of telomeres (ALT) in pancreatic neuroendocrine tumors: ready for prime-time in clinical practice? Curr Oncol Rep. 2021 Jul 16;23(9):106. PMID:34269919
2756. Luft FC. Toxic thyroid adenoma and toxic multinodular goiter. J Mol Med (Berl). 2001;78(12):657–60. PMID:11434717
2757. Lui WO, Zeng L, Rehrmann V, et al. CREB3L2-PPARgamma fusion mutation identifies a thyroid signaling pathway regulated by intramembrane proteolysis. Cancer Res. 2008 Sep 1;68(17):7156–64. PMID:18757431
2758. Luksch R, Castellani MR, Collini P, et al. Neuroblastoma (peripheral neuroblastic tumours). Crit Rev Oncol Hematol. 2016 Nov;107:163–81. PMID:27823645
2759. Lumbroso S, Paris F, Sultan C. Activating Gsalpha mutations: analysis of 113 patients with signs of McCune-Albright syndrome–a European Collaborative Study. J Clin Endocrinol Metab. 2004 May;89(5):2107–13. PMID:15126527
2760. Luna IE, Monrad N, Binderup T, et al. Somatostatin-immunoreactive pancreaticoduodenal neuroendocrine neoplasms: twenty-three cases evaluated according to the WHO 2010 classification. Neuroendocrinology. 2016;103(5). PMID:26505735
2761. Lundgren E, Hagström EG, Lundin J, et al. Primary hyperparathyroidism revisited in menopausal women with serum calcium in the upper normal range at population-based screening 8 years ago. World J Surg. 2002 Aug;26(8):931–6. PMID:12045863
2762. Luo M, Huang Y, Li Y, et al. Metastatic rectal cancer to papillary thyroid carcinoma: a case report and review of literature. BMC Gastroenterol. 2020 May 6;20(1):136. PMID:32375670
2763. Luo P, Zhang L, Yang L, et al. Progress in the pathogenesis, diagnosis, and treatment of TSH-secreting pituitary neuroendocrine tumor. Front Endocrinol (Lausanne). 2020 Nov 27;11:580264. PMID:33329389
2764. Luo Y, Jiang H, Xu W, et al. Clinical, pathological, and molecular characteristics correlating to the occurrence of radioiodine refractory differentiated thyroid carcinoma: a systematic review and meta-analysis. Front Oncol. 2020 Sep 30;10:549882. PMID:33117686
2765. Lupoli G, Vitale G, Caraglia M, et al. Familial papillary thyroid microcarcinoma: a new clinical entity. Lancet. 1999 Feb 20;353(9153):637–9. PMID:10030330
2766. Luzi E, Marini F, Giusti F, et al. The negative feedback-loop between the oncomir Mir-24-1 and menin modulates the Men1 tumorigenesis by mimicking the “Knudson's second hit”. PLoS One. 2012;7(6):e39767. PMID:22761894
2767. Luzi P, Miracco C, Lio R, et al. Endocrine inactive pituitary carcinoma metastasizing to cervical lymph nodes: a case report. Hum Pathol. 1987 Jan;18(1):90–2. PMID:3817801
2768. Lv L, Jiang Y, Yin S, et al. Mammosomatotroph and mixed somatotroph-lactotroph adenoma in acromegaly: a retrospective study with long-term follow-up. Endocrine. 2019 Nov;66(2):310–8. PMID:31368083
2769. Lynnhtun K, Achan A, Lam V. IgG4 related pseudotumour (calcifying fibrous tumour) of adrenal gland. Pathology. 2013 Aug;45(5):519–21. PMID:23842043
2770. Lyra J, Vinagre J, Batista R, et al. mTOR activation in medullary thyroid carcinoma with RAS mutation. Eur J Endocrinol. 2014 Nov;171(5):633–40. PMID:25163725
2771. Ma L, Xia Y, Wang L, et al. Sonographic features of the testicular adrenal rests tumors in patients with congenital adrenal hyperplasia: a single-center experience and literature review. Orphanet J Rare Dis. 2019 Nov 6;14(1):242. PMID:31694673
2772. Ma W, Ikeda H, Yoshimoto T. Clinicopathologic study of 123 cases of prolactin-secreting pituitary adenomas with special reference to multihormone production and clonality of the adenomas. Cancer. 2002 Jul 15;95(2):258–66. PMID:12124824
2773. Ma X, Xia C, Liu H, et al. Primary thyroid spindle cell tumors: spindle cell variant of papillary thyroid carcinoma? Int J Clin Exp Pathol. 2015 Oct 1;8(10):13528–31. PMID:26722568
2774. Ma YH, Gao HQ, Li WC. [Gangliocytic paragangliomas: a clinicopathologic study]. Zhonghua Bing Li Xue Za Zhi. 2018 Dec 8;47(12):941–4. Chinese. PMID:30522176
2775. Ma ZY, Song ZJ, Chen JH, et al. Recurrent gain-of-function USP8 mutations in Cushing's disease. Cell Res. 2015 Mar;25(3):306–17. PMID:25675982
2776. Maas M, Nassiri N, Bhanvadia S, et al. Discrepancies in the recommended management of adrenal incidentalomas by various guidelines. J Urol. 2021 Jan;205(1):52–9. PMID:32856984
2777. Macerola E, Poma AM, Vignali P, et al. Molecular genetics of follicular-derived thyroid cancer. Cancers (Basel). 2021 Mar 7;13(5):1139. PMID:33799953
2778. Machens A, Dralle H. Biological relevance of medullary thyroid microcarcinoma. J Clin Endocrinol Metab. 2012 May;97(5):1547–53. PMID:22399508
2779. Machens A, Dralle H. Familial prevalence and age of RET germline mutations: implications for screening. Clin Endocrinol (Oxf). 2008 Jul;69(1):81–7. PMID:18062802
2780. Machens A, Hauptmann S, Dralle H. Modification of multiple endocrine neoplasia 2A phenotype by cell membrane proximity of RET mutations in exon 10. Endocr Relat Cancer. 2009 Mar;16(1):171–7. PMID:18936155
2781. Maciel RMB, Maia AL. Global endocrinology: geographical variation in the profile of RET variants in patients with medullary thyroid cancer: a comprehensive review. Eur J Endocrinol. 2021 Dec 9;186(1):R15–30. PMID:34757920
2782. MacKay D, Nordenström A, Falhammar H. Bilateral adrenalectomy in congenital adrenal hyperplasia: a systematic review and meta-analysis. J Clin Endocrinol Metab. 2018 May 1;103(5):1767–78. PMID:29554355
2783. Mackenzie IS, Ashby MJ, Donovan T, et al. Bilateral adrenal masses: phaeochromocytoma or melanoma? J R Soc Med. 2006 Mar;99(3):153–5. PMID:16508056
2784. Maddock IR, Moran A, Maher ER, et al. A genetic register for von Hippel-Lindau disease. J Med Genet. 1996 Feb;33(2):120–7. PMID:8929948
2785. Maenhaut C, Detours V, Dom G, et al. Gene expression profiles for radiation-induced thyroid cancer. Clin Oncol (R Coll Radiol). 2011 May;23(4):282–8. PMID:21411301
2786. Maertens O, Prenen H, Debiec-Rychter M, et al. Molecular pathogenesis of multiple gastrointestinal stromal tumors in NF1 patients. Hum Mol Genet. 2006 Mar 15;15(6):1015–23. PMID:16461335
2787. Magalhàes MC. A new crystal-containing cell in human adrenal cortex. J Cell Biol. 1972 Oct;55(1):126–33. PMID:4347248
2788. Magiakou MA, Mastorakos G, Oldfield EH, et al. Cushing's syndrome in children and adolescents. Presentation, diagnosis, and therapy. N Engl J Med. 1994 Sep 8;331(10):629–36. PMID:8052272
2789. Magri F, Villa C, Locatelli D, et al. Prevalence of double pituitary adenomas in a surgical series: clinical, histological and genetic features. J Endocrinol Invest. 2010 May;33(5):325–31. PMID:19955848
2790. Magro G, Emmanuele C, Lopes M, et al. Solitary fibrous tumour of the kidney with sarcomatous overgrowth. Case report and review of the literature. APMIS. 2008 Nov;116(11):1020–5. PMID:19133003
2791. Magro G, Grasso S. Sustentacular cells in sporadic paraganglioma-like medullary thyroid carcinoma: report of a case with diagnostic and histogenetic considerations. Pathol Res Pract. 2000;196(1):55–9. PMID:10674273
2792. Maguire JA, Bilbao JM, Kovacs K, et al. Hypothalamic neurocytoma with vasopressin immunoreactivity: immunohistochemical and ultrastructural observations. Endocr Pathol. 1992 Jun;3(2):99–104. PMID:32138406
2793. Mahajan H, Lee D, Sharma R, et al. Composite phaeochromocytoma-ganglioneuroma, an uncommon entity: report of two cases. Pathology. 2010 Apr;42(3):295–8. PMID:20350228
2794. Mahalakshmi B, Baskaran R, Shanmugavadivu M, et al. Insulinoma-associated protein 1 (INSM1): a potential biomarker and therapeutic target for neuroendocrine tumors. Cell Oncol (Dordr). 2020 Jun;43(3):367–76. PMID:32219703

2795. Maher ER, Yates JR, Harries R, et al. Clinical features and natural history of von Hippel-Lindau disease. Q J Med. 1990 Nov;77(283):1151–63. PMID:2274658
2796. Mai KT, Khanna P, Yazdi HM, et al. Differentiated thyroid carcinomas with vascular invasion: a comparative study of follicular, Hürthle cell and papillary thyroid carcinoma. Pathology. 2002 Jun;34(3):239–44. PMID:12109784
2797. Maillet M, Bourdeau I, Lacroix A. Update on primary micronodular bilateral adrenocortical diseases. Curr Opin Endocrinol Diabetes Obes. 2020 Jun;27(3):132–9. PMID:32209819
2798. Maiorana A, Collina G, Cesinaro AM, et al. Epithelioid angiosarcoma of the thyroid. Clinicopathological analysis of seven cases from non-Alpine areas. Virchows Arch. 1996 Oct;429(2-3):131–7. PMID:8917714
2799. Maiter D, Delgrange E. Therapy of endocrine disease: the challenges in managing giant prolactinomas. Eur J Endocrinol. 2014 Jun;170(6):R213–27. PMID:24536090
2800. Majd N, Waguespack SG, Janku F, et al. Efficacy of pembrolizumab in patients with pituitary carcinoma: report of four cases from a phase II study. J Immunother Cancer. 2020 Dec;8(2):e001532. PMID:33427689
2801. Majoor BC, Boyce AM, Bovée JV, et al. Increased risk of breast cancer at a young age in women with fibrous dysplasia. J Bone Miner Res. 2018 Jan;33(1):84–90. PMID:28856726
2802. Majumder S, Chakraborty PP, Ghosh PC, et al. Cushing's syndrome in early infancy due to isolated sporadic bilateral micronodular adrenocortical disease associated with myosin heavy chain 8 mutation: diagnostic challenges, too many! BMJ Case Rep. 2020 Oct 27;13(10):e236850. PMID:33109698
2803. Majumder S, Grabska J, Trikudanathan G, et al. Functional 'composite' pheochromocytoma-ganglioneuroma presenting as a pancreatic mass. Pancreatology. 2012 May-Jun;12(3):211–4. PMID:22687375
2804. Mak JK, Kay M. Carotid body tumour associated with cyanotic heart disease. BMJ Case Rep. 2016 Mar 9;2016:bcr2016214728. PMID:26961564
2805. Makhlouf HR, Ishak KG, Shekar R, et al. Melanoma markers in angiomyolipoma of the liver and kidney: a comparative study. Arch Pathol Lab Med. 2002 Jan;126(1):49–55. PMID:11800647
2806. Maki M, Kaneko Y, Ohta Y, et al. Somatostatinoma of the pancreas associated with von Hippel-Lindau disease. Intern Med. 1995 Jul;34(7):661–5. PMID:7496080
2807. Makino K, Kojima R, Nakamura H, et al. Ectopic adrenal cortical adenoma in the spinal region: case report and review of the literature. Brain Tumor Pathol. 2010 Oct;27(2):121–5. PMID:21046315
2808. Makuuchi R, Terashima M, Kusuhara M, et al. Comprehensive analysis of gene mutation and expression profiles in neuroendocrine carcinomas of the stomach. Biomed Res. 2017;38(1):19–27. PMID:28239029
2809. Malandrino P, Russo M, Regalbuto C, et al. Outcome of the diffuse sclerosing variant of papillary thyroid cancer: a meta-analysis. Thyroid. 2016 Sep;26(9):1285–92. PMID:27349273
2810. Malandrino P, Russo M, Ronchi A, et al. Increased thyroid cancer incidence in a basaltic volcanic area is associated with non-anthropogenic pollution and biocontamination. Endocrine. 2016 Aug;53(2):471–9. PMID:26438396
2811. Malanga D, De Gisi S, Riccardi M, et al. Functional characterization of a rare germline mutation in the gene encoding the cyclin-dependent kinase inhibitor p27Kip1 (CDKN1B) in a Spanish patient with multiple endocrine neoplasia-like phenotype. Eur J Endocrinol. 2012 Mar;166(3):551–60. PMID:22129891
2812. Malchoff CD, Sarfarazi M, Tendler B, et al. Papillary thyroid carcinoma associated with papillary renal neoplasia: genetic linkage analysis of a distinct heritable tumor syndrome. J Clin Endocrinol Metab. 2000 May;85(5):1758–64. PMID:10843148
2813. Malempati S, Hawkins DS. Rhabdomyosarcoma: review of the Children's Oncology Group (COG) Soft-Tissue Sarcoma Committee experience and rationale for current COG studies. Pediatr Blood Cancer. 2012 Jul 15;59(1):5–10. PMID:22378628
2814. Maleszewski JJ, Larsen BT, Kip NS, et al. PRKAR1A in the development of cardiac myxoma: a study of 110 cases including isolated and syndromic tumors. Am J Surg Pathol. 2014 Aug;38(8):1079–87. PMID:24618615
2815. Malgulwar PB, Nambirajan A, Pathak P, et al. Study of β-catenin and BRAF alterations in adamantinomatous and papillary craniopharyngiomas: mutation analysis with immunohistochemical correlation in 54 cases. J Neurooncol. 2017 Jul;133(3):487–95. PMID:28500561
2816. Malinowska I, Kwiatkowski DJ, Weiss S, et al. Perivascular epithelioid cell tumors (PEComas) harboring TFE3 gene rearrangements lack the TSC2 alterations characteristic of conventional PEComas: further evidence for a biological distinction. Am J Surg Pathol. 2012 May;36(5):783–4. PMID:22456611
2817. Mamilla D, Manukyan I, Fetsch PA, et al. Immunohistochemical distinction of paragangliomas from epithelial neuroendocrine tumors-gangliocytic duodenal and cauda equina paragangliomas align with epithelial neuroendocrine tumors. Hum Pathol. 2020 Sep;103:72–82. PMID:32668278
2818. Mancikova V, Cruz R, Inglada-Pérez L, et al. Thyroid cancer GWAS identifies 10q26.12 and 6q14.1 as novel susceptibility loci and reveals genetic heterogeneity among populations. Int J Cancer. 2015 Oct 15;137(8):1870–8. PMID:25855579
2819. Mandish SF, Gaskins JT, Yusuf MB, et al. Extrapulmonary small cell carcinoma: prognostic factors, patterns of care, and overall survival. Eur J Surg Oncol. 2020 Sep;46(9):1596–604. PMID:32336623
2820. Mangum MD, Greco FA, Hainsworth JD, et al. Combined small-cell and non-small-cell lung cancer. J Clin Oncol. 1989 May;7(5):607–12. PMID:2540288
2821. Maniam P, Zhou K, Lonergan M, et al. Pathogenicity and penetrance of germline SDHA variants in pheochromocytoma and paraganglioma (PPGL). J Endocr Soc. 2018 Jun 18;2(7):806–16. PMID:29978154
2822. Manivel C, Wick MR, Sibley RK. Neuroendocrine differentiation in müllerian neoplasms. An immunohistochemical study of a "pure" endometrial small-cell carcinoma and a mixed müllerian tumor containing small-cell carcinoma. Am J Clin Pathol. 1986 Oct;86(4):438–43. PMID:3020961
2823. Manjila S, Asmar NE, Vidalis BM, et al. Intratumoral Rathke's cleft cyst remnants within craniopharyngioma, pituitary adenoma, suprasellar dermoid, and epidermoid cysts: a ubiquitous signature of ectodermal lineage or a transitional entity? Neurosurgery. 2019 Aug 1;85(2):180–8. PMID:30010935
2824. Mann CM, Bramhall SR, Buckels JA, et al. An unusual case of duodenal obstruction-gangliocytic paraganglioma. J Hepatobiliary Pancreat Surg. 2009;16(4):562–5. PMID:19517054
2825. Manning MA, Paal EE, Srivastava A, et al. Nonepithelial neoplasms of the pancreas, part 2: malignant tumors and tumors of uncertain malignant potential from the radiologic pathology archives. Radiographics. 2018 Jul-Aug;38(4):1047–72. PMID:29787363
2826. Manoharan J, Albers MB, Bartsch DK. The future: diagnostic and imaging advances in MEN1 therapeutic approaches and management strategies. Endocr Relat Cancer. 2017 Oct;24(10):T209–25. PMID:28790162
2827. Manojlovic-Gacic E, Bollerslev J, Casar-Borota O. Invited review: Pathology of pituitary neuroendocrine tumours: present status, modern diagnostic approach, controversies and future perspectives from a neuropathological and clinical standpoint. Neuropathol Appl Neurobiol. 2020 Feb;46(2):89–110. PMID:31112312
2828. Manoranjan B, Koziarz A, Kameda-Smith MM, et al. Multiple recurrences require long-term follow-up in patients diagnosed with spindle cell oncocytoma of the sella turcica. J Clin Neurosci. 2017 Sep;43:134–46. PMID:28668473
2829. Manski TJ, Heffner DK, Glenn GM, et al. Endolymphatic sac tumors. A source of morbid hearing loss in von Hippel-Lindau disease. JAMA. 1997 May 14;277(18):1461–6. PMID:9145719
2830. Mansouri H, Gaye M, Errihani H, et al. Leiomyosarcoma of the thyroid gland. Acta Otolaryngol. 2008 Mar;128(3):335–6. PMID:18274920
2831. Mantzoros I, Bitsianis S, Loutzidou L, et al. Giant adrenocortical carcinoma: a case report and review of the relevant literature. Am J Case Rep. 2021 Apr 4;22:e928875. PMID:33813589
2832. Mantzoros I, Kyriakidou D, Galanos-Demiris K, et al. A rare case of primary hyperparathyroidism caused by a giant solitary parathyroid adenoma. Am J Case Rep. 2018 Nov 8;19:1334–7. PMID:30405093
2833. Mao C, Shah A, Hanson DJ, et al. Von Recklinghausen's disease associated with duodenal somatostatinoma: contrast of duodenal versus pancreatic somatostatinomas. J Surg Oncol. 1995 May;59(1):67–73. PMID:7745981
2834. Mao R, Shi L, Yan W, et al. Anaplastic thyroid carcinoma combined with sclerosing mucoepidermoid carcinoma with eosinophilia: a case report. Medicine (Baltimore). 2020 Oct 16;99(42):e22783. PMID:33080749
2835. Mao X, Wu Y, Yu S, et al. Genetic alteration profiles and clinicopathological associations in atypical parathyroid adenoma. Int J Genomics. 2021 Mar 9;2021:6666257. PMID:33778063
2836. Maragliano R, Vanoli A, Albarello L, et al. ACTH-secreting pancreatic neoplasms associated with Cushing syndrome: clinicopathologic study of 11 cases and review of the literature. Am J Surg Pathol. 2015 Mar;39(3):374–82. PMID:25353285
2837. Marangoni R, Mauramati S, Bertino G, et al. Hypopharyngeal squamous cell carcinoma and laryngeal neuroendocrine carcinoma colliding in the aryepiglottic fold: a case report. Tumori. 2017 Nov 15;103(Suppl. 1):e1–4. PMID:28430347
2838. Marcadis AR, Valderrabano P, Ho AS, et al. Interinstitutional variation in predictive value of the ThyroSeq v2 genomic classifier for cytologically indeterminate thyroid nodules. Surgery. 2019 Jan;165(1):17–24. PMID:30360906
2839. Marchand-Crety C, Pascard M, Debreuve-Theresette A, et al. Prognostic factors and survival score for patients with anaplastic thyroid carcinoma: a retrospective study from a regional registry. Anticancer Res. 2021 Mar;41(3):1555–61. PMID:33788749
2840. Marchesa P, Fazio VW, Church JM, et al. Adrenal masses in patients with familial adenomatous polyposis. Dis Colon Rectum. 1997 Sep;40(9):1023–8. PMID:9293929
2841. Marchevsky AM. Lung tumors derived from ectopic tissues. Semin Diagn Pathol. 1995 May;12(2):172–84. PMID:7638449
2842. Marchiò C, Da Cruz Paula A, Gularte-Merida R, et al. PAX8-GLIS3 gene fusion is a pathognomonic genetic alteration of hyalinizing trabecular tumors of the thyroid. Mod Pathol. 2019 Dec;32(12):1734–43. PMID:31273314
2843. Marcocci C, Cetani F. Clinical practice. Primary hyperparathyroidism. N Engl J Med. 2011 Dec 22;365(25):2389–97. PMID:22187986
2844. Margraf RL, Crockett DK, Krautscheid PM, et al. Multiple endocrine neoplasia type 2 RET protooncogene database: repository of MEN2-associated RET sequence variation and reference for genotype/phenotype correlations. Hum Mutat. 2009 Apr;30(4):548–56. PMID:19177457
2845. Marincola Smith P, Kiernan CM, Tran TB, et al. Role of additional organ resection in adrenocortical carcinoma: analysis of 167 patients from the U.S. adrenocortical carcinoma database. Ann Surg Oncol. 2018 Aug;25(8):2308–15. PMID:29868977
2846. Marinelli JP, Cass SP, Mann SE, et al. Adenomatous neuroendocrine tumors of the middle ear: a multi-institutional investigation of 32 cases and development of a staging system. Otol Neurotol. 2018 Sep;39(8):e712–21. PMID:30001283
2847. Marini A, Kanakis M, Valakis K, et al. Thyroid carcinoma showing thymic-like differentiation causing fracture of the trachea. Case Rep Med. 2016;2016:7962385. PMID:27110248
2848. Marinoni I, Kurrer AS, Vassella E, et al. Loss of DAXX and ATRX are associated with chromosome instability and reduced survival of patients with pancreatic neuroendocrine tumors. Gastroenterology. 2014 Feb;146(2):453–60.e5. PMID:24148618
2849. Maris JM. Recent advances in neuroblastoma. N Engl J Med. 2010 Jun 10;362(23):2202–11. PMID:20558371
2850. Mark J, Bush S, Glazer E, et al. Metastatic VIPoma presenting as an ovarian mass. Int J Surg Case Rep. 2015;17:167–9. PMID:26657531
2851. Marmor S, Koren R, Halpern M, et al. Transthoracic needle biopsy in the diagnosis of large-cell neuroendocrine carcinoma of the lung. Diagn Cytopathol. 2005 Oct;33(4):238–43. PMID:16138368
2852. Marques AR, Espadinha C, Catarino AL, et al. Expression of PAX8-PPAR gamma 1 rearrangements in both follicular thyroid carcinomas and adenomas. J Clin Endocrinol Metab. 2002 Aug;87(8):3947–52. PMID:12161538
2853. Marques B, Monteiro AR, Martins RG, et al. Metastatic VIPoma, cosecreting insulin, with complete response to lanreotide, capecitabine, and temozolomide. Pancreas. 2020 Mar;49(3):e19–20. PMID:32168252
2854. Marques NV, Kasuki L, Coelho MC, et al. Frequency of familial pituitary adenoma syndromes among patients with functioning pituitary adenomas in a reference outpatient clinic. J Endocrinol Invest. 2017 Dec;40(12):1381–7. PMID:28689311
2855. Marques P, Caimari F, Hernández-Ramírez LC, et al. Significant benefits of AIP testing and clinical screening in familial isolated and young-onset pituitary tumors. J Clin Endocrinol Metab. 2020 Jun 1;105(6):e2247–60. PMID:31996917
2856. Marsh DJ, Hahn MA, Howell VM, et al. Molecular diagnosis of primary hyperparathyroidism in familial cancer syndromes. Expert Opin Med Diagn. 2007 Nov;1(3):377–92. PMID:23489357
2857. Martin B, Poblet E, Rios JJ, et al. Merkel cell carcinoma with divergent differentiation: histopathological and immunohistochemical study of 15 cases with PCR analysis for Merkel cell polyomavirus. Histopathology. 2013

Apr;62(5):711–22. PMID:23530585
2858. Martin JT, Alkhoury F, Helton S, et al. Metastatic adenocarcinoma within a functioning adrenal adenoma: a case report. Cases J. 2009 Jul 2;2:7965. PMID:19830028
2859. Martínez de LaPiscina I, Hernández-Ramírez LC, Portillo N, et al. Rare germline DICER1 variants in pediatric patients with Cushing's disease: What is their role? Front Endocrinol (Lausanne). 2020 Jul 3;11:433. PMID:32714280
2860. Martins CS, Camargo RC, Coeli-Lacchini FB, et al. USP8 mutations and cell cycle regulation in corticotroph adenomas. Horm Metab Res. 2020 Feb;52(2):117–23. PMID:32053843
2861. Martins-Filho SN, Almeida MQ, Soares I, et al. Clinical impact of pathological features including the Ki-67 labeling index on diagnosis and prognosis of adult and pediatric adrenocortical tumors. Endocr Pathol. 2021 Jun;32(2):288–300. PMID:33443677
2862. Maru DM, Khurana H, Rashid A, et al. Retrospective study of clinicopathologic features and prognosis of high-grade neuroendocrine carcinoma of the esophagus. Am J Surg Pathol. 2008 Sep;32(9):1404–11. PMID:18670347
2863. Masi G, Barzon L, Iacobone M, et al. Clinical, genetic, and histopathologic investigation of CDC73-related familial hyperparathyroidism. Endocr Relat Cancer. 2008 Dec;15(4):1115–26. PMID:18755853
2864. Masi G, Iacobone M, Sinigaglia A, et al. Characterization of a new CDC73 missense mutation that impairs parafibromin expression and nucleolar localization. PLoS One. 2014 May 19;9(5):e97994. PMID:24842573
2865. Massaro F, Dolcino M, Degrandi R, et al. Calcitonin assay in wash-out fluid after fine-needle aspiration biopsy in patients with a thyroid nodule and border-line value of the hormone. J Endocrinol Invest. 2009 Apr;32(4):308–12. PMID:19636196
2866. Massironi S, Rossi RE, Ferrero S, et al. An esophageal gastrointestinal stromal tumor in a patient with MEN1-related pancreatic gastrinoma: an unusual association and review of the literature. J Cancer Res Ther. 2014 Apr-Jun;10(2):443–5. PMID:25022420
2867. Massironi S, Zilli A, Rossi RE, et al. Gastrinoma and neurofibromatosis type 2: the first case report and review of the literature. BMC Gastroenterol. 2014 Jun 24;14:110. PMID:24961548
2868. Massoth LR, Hung YP, Ferry JA, et al. Histiocytic and dendritic cell sarcomas of hematopoietic origin share targetable genomic alterations distinct from follicular dendritic cell sarcoma. Oncologist. 2021 Jul;26(7):e1263–72. PMID:33904632
2869. Mastracci L, Rindi G, Grillo F, et al. Neuroendocrine neoplasms of the esophagus and stomach. Pathologica. 2021 Feb;113(1):5–11. PMID:33686305
2870. Masuda Y, Kurisaki-Arakawa A, Hara K, et al. A case of dedifferentiated solitary fibrous tumor of the thoracic cavity. Int J Clin Exp Pathol. 2013 Dec 15;7(1):386–93. PMID:24427361
2871. Masui T, Ito T, Komoto I, et al. Recent epidemiology of patients with gastro-entero-pancreatic neuroendocrine neoplasms (GEP-NEN) in Japan: a population-based study. BMC Cancer. 2020 Nov 14;20(1):1104. PMID:33189127
2872. Matarazzo P, Lala R, Andreo M, et al. McCune-Albright syndrome: persistence of autonomous ovarian hyperfunction during adolescence and early adult age. J Pediatr Endocrinol Metab. 2006 May;19 Suppl 2:607–17. PMID:16789624
2873. Matheson CL, Blair GK, Bush J. Spindle epithelial tumor with thymus-like differentiation (SETTLE): a case report. Fetal Pediatr Pathol. 2019 Oct;38(5):399–405. PMID:30998418
2874. Mathiasen RA, Jarrahy R, Cha ST, et al. Pituitary lymphoma: a case report and literature review. Pituitary. 2000 May;2(4):283–7. PMID:11081150
2875. Mathiesen JS, Kroustrup JP, Vestergaard P, et al. Distribution of RET mutations in multiple endocrine neoplasia 2 in Denmark 1994-2014: a nationwide study. Thyroid. 2017 Feb;27(2):215–23. PMID:27809725
2876. Mathiesen JS, Kroustrup JP, Vestergaard P, et al. Survival and long-term biochemical cure in medullary thyroid carcinoma in Denmark 1997-2014: a nationwide study. Thyroid. 2019 Mar;29(3):368–77. PMID:30618340
2877. Mathon B, Carpentier A, Clemenceau S, et al. [Paraganglioma of the cauda equina region: report of six cases and review of the literature]. Neurochirurgie. 2012 Dec;58(6):341–5. French. PMID:22770767
2878. Mathur A, Olson MT, Zeiger MA. Follicular lesions of the thyroid. Surg Clin North Am. 2014 Jun;94(3):499–513. PMID:24857573
2879. Matias-Guiu X, De Lellis R. Medullary thyroid carcinoma: a 25-year perspective. Endocr Pathol. 2014 Mar;25(1):21–9. PMID:24343523
2880. Matias-Guiu X, Garrastazu MT. Composite phaeochromocytoma-ganglioneuroblastoma in a patient with multiple endocrine neoplasia type IIA. Histopathology. 1998 Mar;32(3):281–2. PMID:9568520
2881. Matias-Guiu X, LaGuette J, Puras-Gil AM, et al. Metastatic neuroendocrine tumors to the thyroid gland mimicking medullary carcinoma: a pathologic and immunohistochemical study of six cases. Am J Surg Pathol. 1997 Jul;21(7):754–62. PMID:9236831
2882. Matkar S, Thiel A, Hua X. Menin: a scaffold protein that controls gene expression and cell signaling. Trends Biochem Sci. 2013 Aug;38(8):394–402. PMID:23850066
2883. Maton PN, Gardner JD, Jensen RT. Cushing's syndrome in patients with the Zollinger-Ellison syndrome. N Engl J Med. 1986 Jul 3;315(1):1–5. PMID:2872593
2884. Matos LPL, Penha RCC, Cardoso-Weide LC, et al. Regulation of thyroid sodium-iodide symporter in different stages of goiter: possible involvement of reactive oxygen species. Clin Exp Pharmacol Physiol. 2018 Apr;45(4):326–34. PMID:29112772
2885. Matoso A, Easley SE, Mangray S, et al. Spindle cell foci in the thyroid gland: an immunohistochemical analysis. Appl Immunohistochem Mol Morphol. 2011 Oct;19(5):400–7. PMID:21297445
2886. Matsui K, Jin XM, Kitagawa M, et al. Clinicopathologic features of neuroendocrine carcinomas of the stomach: appraisal of small cell and large cell variants. Arch Pathol Lab Med. 1998 Nov;122(11):1010–7. PMID:9822131
2887. Matsumoto H, Shimokawa M, Nasu K, et al. Clinicopathologic features, treatment, prognosis and prognostic factors of neuroendocrine carcinoma of the endometrium: a retrospective analysis of 42 cases from the Kansai Clinical Oncology Group/Intergroup study in Japan. J Gynecol Oncol. 2019 Nov;30(6):e103. PMID:31576694
2888. Matsumoto S, Hosoya Y, Lefor AK, et al. A black adrenal adenoma with high FDG uptake on PET/CT scan in a patient with esophageal carcinoma: a case report. Int J Surg Case Rep. 2018;44:118–21. PMID:29499515
2889. Matsumura A, Meguro K, Doi M, et al. Suprasellar ectopic pituitary adenoma: case report and review of the literature. Neurosurgery. 1990 Apr;26(4):681–5. PMID:2184378
2890. Matsuno R, Gifford AJ, Fang J, et al. Rare MYC-amplified neuroblastoma with large cell histology. Pediatr Dev Pathol. 2018 Sep-Oct;21(5):461–6. PMID:29426276
2891. Matter MS, Bihl M, Juskevicius D, et al. Is Rosai-Dorfman disease a reactve process? Detection of a MAP2K1 L115V mutation in a case of Rosai-Dorfman disease. Virchows Arch. 2017 Oct;471(4):545–7. PMID:28597077
2892. Matyakhina L, Freedman RJ, Bourdeau I, et al. Hereditary leiomyomatosis associated with bilateral, massive, macronodular adrenocortical disease and atypical Cushing syndrome: a clinical and molecular genetic investigation. J Clin Endocrinol Metab. 2005 Jun;90(6):3773–9. PMID:15741255
2893. Matyakhina L, Pack S, Kirschner LS, et al. Chromosome 2 (2p16) abnormalities in Carney complex tumours. J Med Genet. 2003 Apr;40(4):268–77. PMID:12676898
2894. Mauclet C, Duplaquet F, Pirard L, et al. Complete tumor response of a locally advanced lung large-cell neuroendocrine carcinoma after palliative thoracic radiotherapy and immunotherapy with nivolumab. Lung Cancer. 2019 Feb;128:53–6. PMID:30642453
2895. Maurer CA, Baer HU, Dyong TH, et al. Carcinoid of the pancreas: clinical characteristics and morphological features. Eur J Cancer. 1996 Jun;32A(7):1109–16. PMID:8758239
2896. Máximo V, Botelho T, Capela J, et al. Somatic and germline mutation in GRIM-19, a dual function gene involved in mitochondrial metabolism and cell death, is linked to mitochondrion-rich (Hurthle cell) tumours of the thyroid. Br J Cancer. 2005 May 23;92(10):1892–8. PMID:15841082
2897. Máximo V, Lima J, Prazeres H, et al. The biology and the genetics of Hurthle cell tumors of the thyroid. Endocr Relat Cancer. 2012 Jul 18;19(4):R131–47. PMID:22514109
2898. Máximo V, Rios E, Sobrinho-Simões M. Oncocytic lesions of the thyroid, kidney, salivary glands, adrenal cortex, and parathyroid glands. Int J Surg Pathol. 2014 Feb;22(1):33–6. PMID:24406625
2899. Maxwell EL, Hall FT, Freeman JL. Familial non-medullary thyroid cancer: a matched-case control study. Laryngoscope. 2004 Dec;114(12):2182–6. PMID:15564841
2900. Mayr B, Buslei R, Theodoropoulou M, et al. Molecular and functional properties of densely and sparsely granulated GH-producing pituitary adenomas. Eur J Endocrinol. 2013 Sep 12;169(4):391–400. PMID:23847328
2901. Mazeh H, Benavidez J, Poehls JL, et al. In patients with thyroid cancer of follicular cell origin, a family history of nonmedullary thyroid cancer in one first-degree relative is associated with more aggressive disease. Thyroid. 2012 Jan;22(1):3–8. PMID:22136209
2902. Mazeh H, Sippel RS. Familial nonmedullary thyroid carcinoma. Thyroid. 2013 Sep;23(9):1049–56. PMID:23734600
2903. Mazzucchelli L, Burckhardt E, Hirsiger H, et al. Interphase cytogenetics in oncocytic adenomas and carcinomas of the thyroid gland. Hum Pathol. 2000 Jul;31(7):854–9. PMID:10923924
2904. Mazzuco TL, Thomas M, Martinie M, et al. Cellular and molecular abnormalities of a macronodular adrenal hyperplasia causing beta-blocker-sensitive Cushing's syndrome. Arq Bras Endocrinol Metabol. 2007 Dec;51(9):1452–62. PMID:18209887
2905. McCall CM, Shi C, Cornish TC, et al. Grading of well-differentiated pancreatic neuroendocrine tumors is improved by the inclusion of both Ki67 proliferative index and mitotic rate. Am J Surg Pathol. 2013 Nov;37(11):1671–7. PMID:24121170
2906. McCall CM, Shi C, Klein AP, et al. Serotonin expression in pancreatic neuroendocrine tumors correlates with a trabecular histologic pattern and large duct involvement. Hum Pathol. 2012 Aug;43(8):1169–76. PMID:22221702
2907. McClain KL, Leach CT, Jenson HB, et al. Association of Epstein-Barr virus with leiomyosarcomas in young people with AIDS. N Engl J Med. 1995 Jan 5;332(1):12–8. PMID:7990860
2908. McCluggage WG, Chong AL, de Kock L, et al. Somatic tumour testing establishes that bilateral DICER1-associated ovarian Sertoli-Leydig cell tumours represent independent primary neoplasms. Histopathology. 2020 Aug;77(2):223–30. PMID:32333409
2909. McCluggage WG, Foulkes WD. DICER1-associated sarcomas at different sites exhibit morphological overlap arguing for a unified nomenclature. Virchows Arch. 2021 Aug;479(2):431–3. PMID:33825038
2910. McCluggage WG, Foulkes WD. DICER1-associated sarcomas: towards a unified nomenclature. Mod Pathol. 2021 Jun;34(6):1226–8. PMID:32572152
2911. McCluggage WG, Kennedy K, Busam KJ. An immunohistochemical study of cervical neuroendocrine carcinomas: neoplasms that are commonly TTF1 positive and which may express CK20 and P63. Am J Surg Pathol. 2010 Apr;34(4):525–32. PMID:20182342
2912. McCluggage WG, Sloan JM. Hyalinizing trabecular carcinoma of thyroid gland. Histopathology. 1996 Apr;28(4):357–62. PMID:8732345
2913. McCluggage WG, Young RH. Immunohistochemistry as a diagnostic aid in the evaluation of ovarian tumors. Semin Diagn Pathol. 2005 Feb;22(1):3–32. PMID:16512597
2914. McCormack A, Dekkers OM, Petersenn S, et al. Treatment of aggressive pituitary tumours and carcinomas: results of a European Society of Endocrinology (ESE) survey 2016. Eur J Endocrinol. 2018 Mar;178(3):265–76. PMID:29330228
2915. McCoy KL, Seethala RR, Armstrong MJ, et al. The clinical importance of parathyroid atypia: Is long-term surveillance necessary? Surgery. 2015 Oct;158(4):929–35. PMID:26210223
2916. McCrary HC, Babajanian E, Calquin M, et al. Characterization of malignant head and neck paragangliomas at a single institution across multiple decades. JAMA Otolaryngol Head Neck Surg. 2019 Jul 1;145(7):641–6. PMID:31194233
2917. McDonald TJ, Driedger AA, Garcia BM, et al. Familial papillary thyroid carcinoma: a retrospective analysis. J Oncol. 2011;2011:948786. PMID:22131992
2918. McGaughran JM, Harris DI, Donnai D, et al. A clinical study of type 1 neurofibromatosis in north west England. J Med Genet. 1999 Mar;36(3):197–203. PMID:10204844
2919. McKay JD, Lesueur F, Jonard L, et al. Localization of a susceptibility gene for familial nonmedullary thyroid carcinoma to chromosome 2q21. Am J Hum Genet. 2001 Aug;69(2):440–6. PMID:11438887
2920. McKay JD, Thompson D, Lesueur F, et al. Evidence for interaction between the TCO and NMTC1 loci in familial non-medullary thyroid cancer. J Med Genet. 2004 Jun;41(6):407–12. PMID:15173224
2921. McKeeby JL, Li X, Zhuang Z, et al. Multiple leiomyomas of the esophagus, lung, and uterus in multiple endocrine neoplasia type 1. Am J Pathol. 2001 Sep;159(3):1121–7. PMID:11549605
2922. McMaster MJ, Soule EH, Ivins JC. Hemangiopericytoma. A clinicopathologic study and long-term followup of 60 patients. Cancer. 1975 Dec;36(6):2232–44. PMID:1203874
2923. Meacham R, Matrka L, Ozer E, et al. Neuroendocrine carcinoma of the head and neck: a 20-year case series. Ear Nose Throat J. 2012 Mar;91(3):E20–4. PMID:22430343

2924. Medina-Arana V, Delgado L, González L, et al. Adrenocortical carcinoma, an unusual extracolonic tumor associated with Lynch II syndrome. Fam Cancer. 2011 Jun;10(2):265–71. PMID:21225464
2925. Meeks M, Grace S, Veerapong J, et al. Primary angiosarcoma of the pancreas. J Gastrointest Cancer. 2017 Dec;48(4):369–72. PMID:27228987
2926. Mehdi G, Maheshwari V, Ansari HA, et al. FNAC diagnosis of medullary carcinoma thyroid: a report of three cases with review of literature. J Cytol. 2010 Apr;27(2):66–8. PMID:21157553
2927. Mehrabi A, Fischer L, Hafezi M, et al. A systematic review of localization, surgical treatment options, and outcome of insulinoma. Pancreas. 2014 Jul;43(5):675–86. PMID:24921202
2928. Mehta A, Patel D, Rosenberg A, et al. Hyperparathyroidism-jaw tumor syndrome: results of operative management. Surgery. 2014 Dec;156(6):1315–24. PMID:25444225
2929. Mehta R, Lam-Chung CE, Hinojosa-Amaya JM, et al. High molecular weight ACTH-precursor presence in a metastatic pancreatic neuroendocrine tumor causing severe ectopic Cushing's syndrome: a case report. Front Endocrinol (Lausanne). 2020 Aug 13;11:557. PMID:32903471
2930. Meij BP, Lopes MB, Vance ML, et al. Double pituitary lesions in three patients with Cushing's disease. Pituitary. 2000 Nov;3(3):159–68. PMID:11383480
2931. Meijs AC, Schroijen MA, Snel M, et al. Interleukin-6 producing pheochromocytoma/paraganglioma: case series from a tertiary referral centre for pheochromocytomas and paragangliomas. J Endocrinol Invest. 2021 Oct;44(10):2253–9. PMID:33715142
2932. Melmed S, Casanueva FF, Klibanski A, et al. A consensus on the diagnosis and treatment of acromegaly complications. Pituitary. 2013 Sep;16(3):294–302. PMID:22903574
2933. Melmed S, Ezrin C, Kovacs K, et al. Acromegaly due to secretion of growth hormone by an ectopic pancreatic islet-cell tumor. N Engl J Med. 1985 Jan 3;312(1):9–17. PMID:2981107
2934. Melo M, da Rocha AG, Vinagre J, et al. TERT promoter mutations are a major indicator of poor outcome in differentiated thyroid carcinomas. J Clin Endocrinol Metab. 2014 May;99(5):E754–65. PMID:24476079
2935. Meltzer CJ, Irish J, Angelos P, et al. American Head and Neck Society Endocrine Section clinical consensus statement: North American quality statements and evidence-based multidisciplinary workflow algorithms for the evaluation and management of thyroid nodules. Head Neck. 2019 Apr;41(4):843–56. PMID:30561068
2936. Mendelsohn G, Baylin SB, Bigner SH, et al. Anaplastic variants of medullary thyroid carcinoma: a light-microscopic and immunohistochemical study. Am J Surg Pathol. 1980 Aug;4(4):333–41. PMID:6999920
2937. Mendenhall WM, Suárez C, Skálová A, et al. Current treatment of endolymphatic sac tumor of the temporal bone. Adv Ther. 2018 Jul;35(7):887–98. PMID:29923043
2938. Méndez JC, Carrasco R, Prieto MA, et al. Paraganglioma of the cauda equina: MR and angiographic findings. Radiol Case Rep. 2019 Jul 25;14(10):1185–7. PMID:31379984
2939. Mendola M, Dolci A, Piscopello L, et al. Rare case of Cushing's disease due to double ACTH-producing adenomas, one located in the pituitary gland and one into the stalk. Hormones (Athens). 2014 Oct-Dec;13(4):574–8. PMID:25402386
2940. Meng K, Chen W, Tian W, et al. Medullary thyroid carcinoma with breast metastasis: two case reports. Medicine (Baltimore). 2018 Nov;97(47):e13193. PMID:30461619
2941. Menke JR, Raleigh DR, Gown AM, et al. Somatostatin receptor 2a is a more sensitive diagnostic marker of meningioma than epithelial membrane antigen. Acta Neuropathol. 2015 Sep;130(3):441–3. PMID:26195322
2942. Menon MP, Evbuomwan MO, Rosai J, et al. A subset of Rosai-Dorfman disease cases show increased IgG4-positive plasma cells: another red herring or a true association with IgG4-related disease? Histopathology. 2014 Feb;64(3):455–9. PMID:24215263
2943. Menon RK, Ferrau F, Kurzawinski TR, et al. Adrenal cancer in neurofibromatosis type 1: case report and DNA analysis. Endocrinol Diabetes Metab Case Rep. 2014;2014:140074. PMID:25520849
2944. Mentzel T, Reisshauer S, Rütten A, et al. Cutaneous clear cell myomelanocytic tumour: a new member of the growing family of perivascular epithelioid cell tumours (PEComas). Clinicopathological and immunohistochemical analysis of seven cases. Histopathology. 2005 May;46(5):498–504. PMID:15842631
2945. Merino MJ, Chuaqui R, Fernandez P. Parathyroid hemangioma: a report of two cases. Endocr Pathol. 1996 Winter;7(4):319–22. PMID:12114803
2946. Merke DP, Auchus RJ. Congenital adrenal hyperplasia due to 21-hydroxylase deficiency. N Engl J Med. 2020 Sep 24;383(13):1248–61. PMID:32966723
2947. Mesolella M, Allosso S, Varricchio S, et al. Small-cell carcinoma of nasopharynx: a case report of unusual localization. Ear Nose Throat J. 2023 Jan;102(1):NP13–8. PMID:33371727
2948. Messiaen LM, Callens T, Mortier G, et al. Exhaustive mutation analysis of the NF1 gene allows identification of 95% of mutations and reveals a high frequency of unusual splicing defects. Hum Mutat. 2000;15(6):541–55. PMID:10862084
2949. Messinger YH, Stewart DR, Priest JR, et al. Pleuropulmonary blastoma: a report on 350 central pathology-confirmed pleuropulmonary blastoma cases by the International Pleuropulmonary Blastoma Registry. Cancer. 2015 Jan 15;121(2):276–85. PMID:25209242
2950. Mete O, Alshaikh OM, Cintosun A, et al. Synchronous multiple pituitary neuroendocrine tumors of different cell lineages. Endocr Pathol. 2018 Dec;29(4):332–8. PMID:30215160
2951. Mete O, Asa SL. Aldosterone-producing adrenal cortical adenoma with oncocytic change and cytoplasmic eosinophilic globular inclusions. Endocr Pathol. 2009 Fall;20(3):182–5. PMID:19462261
2952. Mete O, Asa SL. Clinicopathological correlations in pituitary adenomas. Brain Pathol. 2012 Jul;22(4):443–53. PMID:22697380
2953. Mete O, Asa SL. Morphological distinction of cortisol-producing and aldosterone-producing adrenal cortical adenomas: not only possible but a critical clinical responsibility. Histopathology. 2012 May;60(6):1015–6. PMID:22320848
2954. Mete O, Asa SL. Oncocytes, oxyphils, Hürthle, and Askanazy cells: morphological and molecular features of oncocytic thyroid nodules. Endocr Pathol. 2010 Mar;21(1):16–24. PMID:20013317
2955. Mete O, Asa SL. Pathological definition and clinical significance of vascular invasion in thyroid carcinomas of follicular epithelial derivation. Mod Pathol. 2011 Dec;24(12):1545–52. PMID:21804527
2956. Mete O, Asa SL. Precursor lesions of endocrine system neoplasms. Pathology. 2013 Apr;45(3):316–30. PMID:23478233
2957. Mete O, Asa SL. Structure, function, and morphology in the classification of pituitary neuroendocrine tumors: the importance of routine analysis of pituitary transcription factors. Endocr Pathol. 2020 Dec;31(4):330–6. PMID:32813227
2958. Mete O, Asa SL. Therapeutic implications of accurate classification of pituitary adenomas. Semin Diagn Pathol. 2013 Aug;30(3):158–64. PMID:24144285
2959. Mete O, Asa SL, Giordano TJ, et al. Immunohistochemical biomarkers of adrenal cortical neoplasms. Endocr Pathol. 2018 Jun;29(2):137–49. PMID:29542002
2960. Mete O, Chetty R. Pancreatic endocrine neoplasia: familial syndromes. Diagn Histopathol. 2017;23(8):378–85.
2961. Mete O, Cintosun A, Pressman I, et al. Epidemiology and biomarker profile of pituitary adenohypophysial tumors. Mod Pathol. 2018 Jun;31(6):900–9. PMID:29434339
2962. Mete O, Davis JL, Rudzinski ER, et al. Protocol for the examination of specimens from patients with carcinoma of the adrenal gland. Version: Adrenal Gland 4.1.0.0. Northfield (IL): College of American Pathologists; 2020 Feb. Available from: https://www.cap.org/protocols-and-guidelines/cancer-reporting-tools/cancer-protocol-templates.
2963. Mete O, Duan K. The many faces of primary aldosteronism and Cushing syndrome: a reflection of adrenocortical tumor heterogeneity. Front Med (Lausanne). 2018 Mar 12;5:54. PMID:29594118
2964. Mete O, Essa A, Bramdev A, et al. MEN2 syndrome-related medullary thyroid carcinoma with focal tyrosine hydroxylase expression: Does it represent a hybrid cellular phenotype or functional state of tumor cells? Endocr Pathol. 2017 Dec;28(4):362–6. PMID:28493102
2965. Mete O, Ezzat S, Asa SL. Biomarkers of aggressive pituitary adenomas. J Mol Endocrinol. 2012 Aug 30;49(2):R69–78. PMID:22822048
2966. Mete O, Gomez-Hernandez K, Kucharczyk W, et al. Silent subtype 3 pituitary adenomas are not always silent and represent poorly differentiated monomorphous plurihormonal Pit-1 lineage adenomas. Mod Pathol. 2016 Feb;29(2):131–42. PMID:26743473
2967. Mete O, Gucer H, Kefeli M, et al. Diagnostic and prognostic biomarkers of adrenal cortical carcinoma. Am J Surg Pathol. 2018 Feb;42(2):201–13. PMID:28877067
2968. Mete O, Hannah-Shmouni F, Kim R, et al. Inherited neuroendocrine neoplasms. In: Asa SL, La Rosa S, Mete O, editors. The spectrum of neuroendocrine neoplasia: a practical approach to diagnosis, classification and therapy. Cham (Switzerland): Springer; 2021. pp. 409–59.
2969. Mete O, Hayhurst C, Alahmadi H, et al. The role of mediators of cell invasiveness, motility, and migration in the pathogenesis of silent corticotroph adenomas. Endocr Pathol. 2013 Dec;24(4):191–8. PMID:24091601
2970. Mete O, Kapran Y, Güllüoğlu MG, et al. Anti-CD10 (56C6) is expressed variably in adrenocortical tumors and cannot be used to discriminate clear cell renal cell carcinomas. Virchows Arch. 2010 May;456(5):515–21. PMID:20390424
2971. Mete O, Kefeli M, Çalışkan S, et al. GATA3 immunoreactivity expands the transcription factor profile of pituitary neuroendocrine tumors. Mod Pathol. 2019 Apr;32(4):484–9. PMID:30390035
2972. Mete O, Lopes MB. Overview of the 2017 WHO classification of pituitary tumors. Endocr Pathol. 2017 Sep;28(3):228–43. PMID:28766057
2973. Mete O, Lopes MB, Asa SL. Spindle cell oncocytomas and granular cell tumors of the pituitary are variants of pituicytoma. Am J Surg Pathol. 2013 Nov;37(11):1694–9. PMID:23887161
2974. Mete O, Ng T, Christie-David D, et al. Silent corticotroph adenoma with adrenal cortical choristoma: a rare but distinct morphological entity. Endocr Pathol. 2013 Sep;24(3):162–6. PMID:23872913
2975. Mete O, Pakbaz S, Lerario AM, et al. Significance of alpha-inhibin expression in pheochromocytomas and paragangliomas. Am J Surg Pathol. 2021 Sep 1;45(9):1264–73. PMID:33826547
2976. Mete O, Raphael S, Pirzada A, et al. Is adrenal ovarian thecal metaplasia a misnomer? Report of three cases of radial scar-like spindle cell myofibroblastic nodule of the adrenal gland. Endocr Pathol. 2011 Dec;22(4):222–5. PMID:21858518
2977. Mete O, Tischler AS, de Krijger R, et al. Protocol for the examination of specimens from patients with pheochromocytomas and extra-adrenal paragangliomas. Arch Pathol Lab Med. 2014 Feb;138(2):182–8. PMID:24476517
2978. Mete O, van der Kwast TH. Epithelioid angiomyolipoma: a morphologically distinct variant that mimics a variety of intra-abdominal neoplasms. Arch Pathol Lab Med. 2011 May;135(5):665–70. PMID:21526965
2979. Meyer JS, Steinberg LS. Microscopically benign thyroid follicles in cervical lymph nodes. Serial section study of lymph node inclusions and entire thyroid gland in 5 cases. Cancer. 1969 Aug;24(2):302–11. PMID:5796776
2980. Meyer PN, Fu K, Greiner TC, et al. Immunohistochemical methods for predicting cell of origin and survival in patients with diffuse large B-cell lymphoma treated with rituximab. J Clin Oncol. 2011 Jan 10;29(2):200–7. PMID:21135273
2981. Meyer-Rochow GY, Alvarado R, Sywak MS, et al. Letter 2: Intraoperative diagnosis and treatment of parathyroid cancer and atypical parathyroid adenoma (Br J Surg 2007; 94: 566-570). Br J Surg. 2007 Aug;94(8):1043. PMID:17636522
2982. Mezmezian MB, Fernandez Ugazio G, Paparella ML. Histopathological features of malignant craniopharyngioma: case report and literature review. Clin Neuropathol. 2020 Jan/Feb;39(1):25–31. PMID:31661068
2983. Mhawej R, Farah C, Haddad A, et al. Primary neuroendocrine tumors of the ear, nose and throat: a report of three cases and a review of the literature. Oncol Lett. 2015 Oct;10(4):2533–6. PMID:26622884
2984. Mian C, Pennelli G, Barollo S, et al. Combined RET and Ki-67 assessment in sporadic medullary thyroid carcinoma: a useful tool for patient risk stratification. Eur J Endocrinol. 2011 Jun;164(6):971–6. PMID:21422198
2985. Mian M, Gaidano G, Conconi A, et al. High response rate and improvement of long-term survival with combined treatment modalities in patients with poor-risk primary thyroid diffuse large B-cell lymphoma: an International Extranodal Lymphoma Study Group and Intergruppo Italiano Linfomi study. Leuk Lymphoma. 2011 May;52(5):823–32. PMID:21338283
2986. Miao J, Chen S, Li Y, et al. A primary cavernous hemangioma of the thyroid gland: a case report and literature review. Medicine (Baltimore). 2017 Dec;96(49):e8651. PMID:29245224
2987. Miao R, Wang H, Jacobson A, et al. Radiation-induced and neurofibromatosis-associated malignant peripheral nerve sheath tumors (MPNST) have worse outcomes than sporadic MPNST. Radiother Oncol. 2019 Aug;137:61–70. PMID:31078939
2988. Miccoli P, Bakkar S. Surgical management of papillary thyroid carcinoma: an overview. Updates Surg. 2017 Jun;69(2):145–50. PMID:28405952
2989. Michalski K, Kurz P, Fuellgraf H, et al.

TTF-1 positive atypical carcinoid of the epiglottis mimicking medullary thyroid carcinoma. Nuklearmedizin. 2019 Jun;58(3):279–81. PMID:30974468
2990. Michelow PM, Leiman G. Metastases to the thyroid gland: diagnosis by aspiration cytology. Diagn Cytopathol. 1995 Oct;13(3):209–13. PMID:8575279
2991. Miettinen M, Chatten J, Paetau A, et al. Monoclonal antibody NB84 in the differential diagnosis of neuroblastoma and other small round cell tumors. Am J Surg Pathol. 1998 Mar;22(3):327–32. PMID:9500774
2992. Miettinen M, McCue PA, Sarlomo-Rikala M, et al. GATA3: a multispecific but potentially useful marker in surgical pathology: a systematic analysis of 2500 epithelial and nonepithelial tumors. Am J Surg Pathol. 2014 Jan;38(1):13–22. PMID:24145643
2993. Miettinen M, Paal E, Lasota J, et al. Gastrointestinal glomus tumors: a clinicopathologic, immunohistochemical, and molecular genetic study of 32 cases. Am J Surg Pathol. 2002 Mar;26(3):301–11. PMID:11859201
2994. Miettinen M, Saari A. Pheochromocytoma combined with malignant schwannoma: unusual neoplasm of the adrenal medulla. Ultrastruct Pathol. 1988 Sep-Oct;12(5):513–27. PMID:3194994
2995. Miettinen M, Wang Z, Lasota J, et al. Nuclear brachyury expression is consistent in chordoma, common in germ cell tumors and small cell carcinomas, and rare in other carcinomas and sarcomas: an immunohistochemical study of 5229 cases. Am J Surg Pathol. 2015 Oct;39(10):1305–12. PMID:26099010
2996. Miettinen M, Wang ZF, Sarlomo-Rikala M, et al. Succinate dehydrogenase-deficient GISTs: a clinicopathologic, immunohistochemical, and molecular genetic study of 66 gastric GISTs with predilection to young age. Am J Surg Pathol. 2011 Nov;35(11):1712–21. PMID:21997692
2997. Miki H, Sumitomo M, Inoue H, et al. Parathyroid carcinoma in patients with chronic renal failure on maintenance hemodialysis. Surgery. 1996 Nov;120(5):897–901. PMID:8909528
2998. Mikić A, Zvrko E, Trivić A, et al. Small cell neuroendocrine tumor of the larynx–a small case series. Coll Antropol. 2012 Nov;36 Suppl 2:201–4. PMID:23397787
2999. Milanesi A, Yu R, Geller SA, et al. Concurrent primary hyperparathyroidism and humoral hypercalcemia of malignancy in a patient with multiple endocrine neoplasia type 1. Pancreas. 2011 May;40(4):634–7. PMID:21483254
3000. Milanetto AC, Fassan M, David A, et al. Serotonin-secreting neuroendocrine tumours of the pancreas. J Clin Med. 2020 May 6;9(5):1363. PMID:32384679
3001. Milano AF. Thyroid cancer: 20-year comparative mortality and survival analysis of six thyroid cancer histologic subtypes by age, sex, race, stage, cohort entry time-period and disease duration (SEER*Stat 8.3.2) A systematic review of 145,457 cases for diagnosis years 1993-2013. J Insur Med. 2018 Jan;47(3):143–58. PMID:30192723
3002. Milas M, Mester J, Metzger R, et al. Should patients with Cowden syndrome undergo prophylactic thyroidectomy? Surgery. 2012 Dec;152(6):1201–10. PMID:23158187
3003. Milas M, Wagner K, Easley KA, et al. Double adenomas revisited: nonuniform distribution favors enlarged superior parathyroids (fourth pouch disease). Surgery. 2003 Dec;134(6):995–1003. PMID:14668733
3004. Milde P, Sidawy MK. Thymoma presenting as a palpable thyroid nodule: a pitfall in fine needle aspiration (FNA) of the neck. Cytopathology. 1999 Dec;10(6):415–9. PMID:10607013
3005. Milias S, Hytiroglou P, Kourtis D, et al. Granular cell tumour of the thyroid gland. Histopathology. 2004 Feb;44(2):190–1. PMID:14764065
3006. Miliauskas JR, Worthley C, Allen PW. Glomangiomyoma (glomus tumour) of the pancreas: a case report. Pathology. 2002 Apr;34(2):193–5. PMID:12009105
3007. Milione M, Maisonneuve P, Grillo F, et al. Ki-67 index of 55% distinguishes two groups of bronchopulmonary pure and composite large cell neuroendocrine carcinomas with distinct prognosis. Neuroendocrinology. 2021;111(5):475–89. PMID:32365350
3008. Milione M, Maisonneuve P, Pellegrinelli A, et al. Ki67 proliferative index of the neuroendocrine component drives MANEC prognosis. Endocr Relat Cancer. 2018 May;25(5):583–93. PMID:29592868
3009. Milione M, Maisonneuve P, Spada F, et al. The clinicopathologic heterogeneity of grade 3 gastroenteropancreatic neuroendocrine neoplasms: morphological differentiation and proliferation identify different prognostic categories. Neuroendocrinology. 2017;104(1):85–93. PMID:26943788
3010. Milione M, Parente P, Grillo F, et al. Neuroendocrine neoplasms of the duodenum, ampullary region, jejunum and ileum. Pathologica. 2021 Feb;113(1):12–8. PMID:33686306
3011. Miller BS, Rusinko RY, Fowler L. Synchronous thymoma and thymic carcinoid in a woman with multiple endocrine neoplasia type 1: case report and review. Endocr Pract. 2008 Sep;14(6):713–6. PMID:18996790
3012. Miller DL, Thompson LDR, Bishop JA, et al. Malignant teratomas of the thyroid gland: clinico-radiologic and cytomorphologic features of a rare entity. J Am Soc Cytopathol. 2020 Jul-Aug;9(4):221–31. PMID:32448730
3013. Miller HC, Kidd M, Modlin IM, et al. Glucagon receptor gene mutations with hyperglucagonemia but without the glucagonoma syndrome. World J Gastrointest Surg. 2015 Apr 27;7(4):60–6. PMID:25914784
3014. Miller MB, Bi WL, Ramkissoon LA, et al. MAPK activation and HRAS mutation identified in pituitary spindle cell oncocytoma. Oncotarget. 2016 Jun 14;7(24):37054–63. PMID:27175596
3015. Miller WL, Merke DP. Tenascin-X, congenital adrenal hyperplasia, and the CAH-X syndrome. Horm Res Paediatr. 2018;89(5):352–61. PMID:29734195
3016. Miller WT Jr, Gefter WB, Miller WT. Thymoma mimicking a thyroid mass. Radiology. 1992 Jul;184(1):75–6. PMID:1609105
3017. Mills SE, Cooper PH, Garland TA, et al. Small cell undifferentiated carcinoma of the larynx. Report of two patients and review of 13 additional cases. Cancer. 1983 Jan 1;51(1):116–20. PMID:6295589
3018. Min KW, Clemens A, Bell J, et al. Malignant peripheral nerve sheath tumor and pheochromocytoma. A composite tumor of the adrenal. Arch Pathol Lab Med. 1988 Mar;112(3):266–70. PMID:2894207
3019. Mindermann T, Wilson CB. Age-related and gender-related occurrence of pituitary adenomas. Clin Endocrinol (Oxf). 1994 Sep;41(3):359–64. PMID:7893282
3020. Mindermann T, Wilson CB. Pediatric pituitary adenomas. Neurosurgery. 1995 Feb;36(2):259–68. PMID:7731505
3021. Miner AG, Patel RM, Wilson DA, et al. Cytokeratin 20-negative Merkel cell carcinoma is infrequently associated with the Merkel cell polyomavirus. Mod Pathol. 2015 Apr;28(4):498–504. PMID:25394777
3022. Minkov M, Grois N, Heitger A, et al. Response to initial treatment of multisystem Langerhans cell histiocytosis: an important prognostic indicator. Med Pediatr Oncol. 2002 Dec;39(6):581–5. PMID:12376981
3023. Mir SA, Masoodi SR, Bashir MI, et al. Dissociated hypopituitarism after spontaneous pituitary apoplexy in acromegaly. Indian J Endocrinol Metab. 2013 Oct;17(Suppl 1):S102–4. PMID:24251123
3024. Mirabile A, Biafora M, Giordano L, et al. Uncommon site of metastasis and prolonged survival in patients with anaplastic thyroid carcinoma: a systematic review of the literature. Cancers (Basel). 2020 Sep 10;12(9):2585. PMID:32927794
3025. Miranda-Filho A, Lortet-Tieulent J, Bray F, et al. Thyroid cancer incidence trends by histology in 25 countries: a population-based study. Lancet Diabetes Endocrinol. 2021 Apr;9(4):225–34. PMID:33662333
3026. Miras AD, Mogford JT, Wright J, et al. Ovarian hyperstimulation from ectopic hypersecretion of follicle stimulating hormone. Lancet. 2015 Jan 24;385(9965):392. PMID:25706853
3027. Miret M, Horváth-Puhó E, Déruaz-Luyet A, et al. Potential paraneoplastic syndromes and selected autoimmune conditions in patients with non-small cell lung cancer and small cell lung cancer: a population-based cohort study. PLoS One. 2017 Aug 2;12(8):e0181564. PMID:28767671
3028. Mirshahi UL, Kim J, Best AF, et al. A genome-first approach to characterize DICER1 pathogenic variant prevalence, penetrance, and phenotype. JAMA Netw Open. 2021 Feb 1;4(2):e210112. PMID:33630087
3029. Mirsharifi A, Vasei M, Sadeghian E, et al. Extra-adrenal, non-functional adrenocortical carcinoma presenting with acute abdomen: a case report. J Med Case Rep. 2020 Jul 8;14(1):107. PMID:32635927
3030. Misawa K, Kawasaki H, Matsuo R, et al. Human papillomavirus-associated small cell carcinoma/neuroendocrine carcinoma of the oropharynx: a report of two cases. Springerplus. 1847;20165(1). PMID:27818885
3031. Misgar RA, Sahu D, Purra S, et al. Multiple uterine leiomyomas in multiple endocrine neoplasia type 1 with a novel MEN1 gene mutation. J Hum Reprod Sci. 2020 Jan-Mar;13(1):75–7. PMID:32577074
3032. Mishra T, Goel NA, Goel AH. Primary paraganglioma of the spine: a clinicopathological study of eight cases. J Craniovertebr Junction Spine. 2014 Jan;5(1):20–4. PMID:25013343
3033. Misra RK, Mitra S, Yadav R, et al. Spindle epithelial tumor with thymus-like differentiation: a case report and review of literature. Acta Cytol. 2013;57(3):303–8. PMID:23635450
3034. Missiaglia E, Williamson D, Chisholm J, et al. PAX3/FOXO1 fusion gene status is the key prognostic molecular marker in rhabdomyosarcoma and significantly improves current risk stratification. J Clin Oncol. 2012 May 10;30(14):1670–7. PMID:22454413
3035. Mistry R, Hillyar C, Nibber A, et al. Ultrasound classification of thyroid nodules: a systematic review. Cureus. 2020 Mar 11;12(3):e7239. PMID:32190531
3036. Mitchell A, Scheithauer BW, Sasano H, et al. Symptomatic intradural adrenal adenoma of the spinal nerve root: report of two cases. Neurosurgery. 1993 Apr;32(4):658–61. PMID:8474656
3037. Mitsutake N, Saenko V. Molecular pathogenesis of pediatric thyroid carcinoma. J Radiat Res. 2021 May 5;62(Supplement_1):i71–7. PMID:33978172
3038. Mitsuya K, Nakasu Y, Nioka H, et al. Ectopic growth hormone-releasing adenoma in the cavernous sinus–case report. Neurol Med Chir (Tokyo). 2004 Jul;44(7):380–5. PMID:15347217
3039. Mixson AJ, Friedman TC, Katz DA, et al. Thyrotropin-secreting pituitary carcinoma. J Clin Endocrinol Metab. 1993 Feb;76(2):529–33. PMID:8432799
3040. Miyakawa M, Sato K, Hasegawa M, et al. Severe thyrotoxicosis induced by thyroid metastasis of lung adenocarcinoma: a case report and review of the literature. Thyroid. 2001 Sep;11(9):883–8. PMID:11575859
3041. Miyaki M, Iijima T, Ishii R, et al. Molecular evidence for multicentric development of thyroid carcinomas in patients with familial adenomatous polyposis. Am J Pathol. 2000 Dec;157(6):1825–7. PMID:11106555
3042. Miyauchi A, Kuma K, Matsuzuka F, et al. Intrathyroidal epithelial thymoma: an entity distinct from squamous cell carcinoma of the thyroid. World J Surg. 1985 Feb;9(1):128–35. PMID:3984364
3043. Miyoshi T, Umemura S, Matsumura Y, et al. Genomic profiling of large-cell neuroendocrine carcinoma of the lung. Clin Cancer Res. 2017 Feb 1;23(3):757–65. PMID:27507618
3044. Mizukami Y, Matsubara F, Hashimoto T, et al. Primary mucoepidermoid carcinoma in the thyroid gland. A case report including an ultrastructural and biochemical study. Cancer. 1984 Apr 15;53(8):1741–5. PMID:6697313
3045. Mizukami Y, Michigishi T, Nonomura A, et al. Autonomously functioning (hot) nodule of the thyroid gland. A clinical and histopathologic study of 17 cases. Am J Clin Pathol. 1994 Jan;101(1):29–35. PMID:8279452
3046. Mizukami Y, Michigishi T, Nonomura A, et al. Mixed medullary-follicular carcinoma of the thyroid occurring in familial form. Histopathology. 1993 Mar;22(3):284–7. PMID:8495962
3047. Mizukami Y, Nonomura A, Michigishi T, et al. Diffuse follicular variant of papillary carcinoma of the thyroid. Histopathology. 1995 Dec;27(6):575–7. PMID:8838340
3048. Mizukami Y, Nonomura A, Michigishi T, et al. Mixed medullary-follicular carcinoma of the thyroid gland: a clinicopathologic variant of medullary thyroid carcinoma. Mod Pathol. 1996 Jun;9(6):631–5. PMID:8782199
3049. Mizuno T, Masaoka A, Hashimoto T, et al. Coexisting thymic carcinoid tumor and thymoma. Ann Thorac Surg. 1990 Oct;50(4):650–2. PMID:2222057
3050. Mizuuchi Y, Yamamoto H, Nakamura K, et al. Solitary fibrous tumor of the thyroid gland. Med Mol Morphol. 2014 Jun;47(2):117–22. PMID:24013381
3051. Mnif Feki M, Mnif F, Kamoun M, et al. Ectopic secretion of GHRH by a pancreatic neuroendocrine tumor associated with an empty sella. Ann Endocrinol (Paris). 2011 Dec;72(6):522–5. PMID:21963237
3052. Mochizuki K, Kondo T, Oishi N, et al. Low frequency of PAX8-PPARγ rearrangement in follicular thyroid carcinomas in Japanese patients. Pathol Int. 2015 May;65(5):250–3. PMID:25708358
3053. Modigliani E, Cohen R, Campos JM, et al. Prognostic factors for survival and for biochemical cure in medullary thyroid carcinoma: results in 899 patients. The GETC Study Group. Groupe d'étude des tumeurs à calcitonine. Clin Endocrinol (Oxf). 1998 Mar;48(3):265–73. PMID:9578814
3054. Modigliani E, Vasen HM, Raue K, et al. Pheochromocytoma in multiple endocrine neoplasia type 2: European study. J Intern Med. 1995 Oct;238(4):363–7. PMID:7595173
3055. Modlin IM, Lye KD, Kidd M. A 5-decade analysis of 13,715 carcinoid tumors. Cancer. 2003 Feb 15;97(4):934–59. PMID:12569593
3056. Modlin IM, Shapiro MD, Kidd M. An analysis of rare carcinoid tumors: clarifying these clinical conundrums. World J Surg. 2005 Jan;29(1):92–101. PMID:15599742
3057. Mohajeri A, Tayebwa J, Collin A, et al.

Comprehensive genetic analysis identifies a pathognomonic NAB2/STAT6 fusion gene, nonrandom secondary genomic imbalances, and a characteristic gene expression profile in solitary fibrous tumor. Genes Chromosomes Cancer. 2013 Oct;52(10):873–86. PMID:23761323
3058. Mohammed AZ, Edino ST, Umar AB. Leiomyoma of the thyroid gland with psammoma bodies. Niger Med J. 2015 Jan-Feb;56(1):71–3. PMID:25657499
3059. Mohan DR, Lerario AM, Else T, et al. Targeted assessment of G0S2 methylation identifies a rapidly recurrent, routinely fatal molecular subtype of adrenocortical carcinoma. Clin Cancer Res. 2019 Jun 1;25(11):3276–88. PMID:30770352
3060. Mohanty SK, Tiwari A, Bhardwaj N, et al. Positivity for SATB2 distinguishes Islet1 positive rectal neuroendocrine tumours from pancreaticoduodenal neuroendocrine tumours. J Clin Pathol. 2021 Sep;74(9):582–8. PMID:32934105
3061. Mohindroo C, McAllister F, De Jesus-Acosta A. Genetics of pancreatic neuroendocrine tumors. Hematol Oncol Clin North Am. 2022 Oct;36(5):1033–51. PMID:36154786
3062. Mohr VH, Vortmeyer AO, Zhuang Z, et al. Histopathology and molecular genetics of multiple cysts and microcystic (serous) adenomas of the pancreas in von Hippel-Lindau patients. Am J Pathol. 2000 Nov;157(5):1615–21. PMID:11073821
3063. Moke DJ, Thomas SM, Hiemenz MC, et al. Three synchronous malignancies in a patient with DICER1 syndrome. Eur J Cancer. 2018 Apr;93:140–3. PMID:29395683
3064. Molatore S, Marinoni I, Lee M, et al. A novel germline CDKN1B mutation causing multiple endocrine tumors: clinical, genetic and functional characterization. Hum Mutat. 2010 Nov;31(11):E1825–35. PMID:20824794
3065. Molberg K, Albores-Saavedra J. Hyalinizing trabecular carcinoma of the thyroid gland. Hum Pathol. 1994 Feb;25(2):192–7. PMID:8119720
3066. Moley JF. Medullary thyroid carcinoma: management of lymph node metastases. J Natl Compr Canc Netw. 2010 May;8(5):549–56. PMID:20495084
3067. Molinaro AM, Pearson BJ. Myths vs. FACS: What do we know about planarian stem cell lineages? Int J Dev Biol.201862. PMID:29938764
3068. Moline J, Eng C. Multiple endocrine neoplasia type 2: an overview. Genet Med. 2011 Sep;13(9):755–64. PMID:21552134
3069. Momota H, Ichimiya S, Ikeda T, et al. Immunohistochemical analysis of the p53 family members in human craniopharyngiomas. Brain Tumor Pathol. 2003;20(2):73–7. PMID:14756444
3070. Mon SY, Riedlinger G, Abbott CE, et al. Cancer risk and clinicopathological characteristics of thyroid nodules harboring thyroid-stimulating hormone receptor gene mutations. Diagn Cytopathol. 2018 May;46(5):369–77. PMID:29516685
3071. Monaghan TF, Michelson KP, Suss NR, et al. Primary small cell carcinoma of the kidney: disease characteristics and treatment outcomes. Medicines (Basel). 2021 Jan 18;8(1):6. PMID:33477429
3072. Monclair T, Brodeur GM, Ambros PF, et al. The International Neuroblastoma Risk Group (INRG) staging system: an INRG Task Force report. J Clin Oncol. 2009 Jan 10;27(2):298–303. PMID:19047290
3073. Monclair T, Ruud E, Holmstrøm H, et al. Extra-adrenal composite phaeochromocytoma/neuroblastoma in a 15-month-old child. J Pediatr Surg Case Rep. 2015 Aug;3(8):348–50. doi:10.1016/j.epsc.2015.06.014.
3074. Mondin V, Ferlito A, Muzzi E, et al. Thyroglossal duct cyst: personal experience and literature review. Auris Nasus Larynx. 2008 Mar;35(1):11–25. PMID:17720342
3075. Monfared A, Gorti G, Kim D. Microsurgical anatomy of the laryngeal nerves as related to thyroid surgery. Laryngoscope. 2002 Feb;112(2):386–92. PMID:11889402
3076. Monsalves E, Larjani S, Loyola Godoy B, et al. Growth patterns of pituitary adenomas and histopathological correlates. J Clin Endocrinol Metab. 2014 Apr;99(4):1330–8. PMID:24423330
3077. Monsefi N, Dehghani M, Nowshadi PA, et al. Leiomyoma of the adrenal gland presenting as an incidentaloma. Arch Iran Med. 2011 Nov;14(6):419–22. PMID:22039848
3078. Montani M, Heinimann K, von Teichman A, et al. VHL-gene deletion in single renal tubular epithelial cells and renal tubular cysts: further evidence for a cyst-dependent progression pathway of clear cell renal carcinoma in von Hippel-Lindau disease. Am J Surg Pathol. 2010 Jun;34(6):806–15. PMID:20431476
3079. Montefusco L, Harari S, Elia D, et al. Endocrine and metabolic assessment in adults with Langerhans cell histiocytosis. Eur J Intern Med. 2018 May;51:61–7. PMID:29198444
3080. Montone KT, Baloch ZW, LiVolsi VA. The thyroid Hürthle (oncocytic) cell and its associated pathologic conditions: a surgical pathology and cytopathology review. Arch Pathol Lab Med. 2008 Aug;132(8):1241–50. PMID:18684023
3081. Monzani A, Prodam F, Rapa A, et al. Endocrine disorders in childhood and adolescence. Natural history of subclinical hypothyroidism in children and adolescents and potential effects of replacement therapy: a review. Eur J Endocrinol. 2012 Dec 10;168(1):R1–11. PMID:22989466
3082. Moody S, Thompson JS, Chuang SS, et al. Novel GPR34 and CCR6 mutation and distinct genetic profiles in MALT lymphomas of different sites. Haematologica. 2018 Aug;103(8):1329–36. PMID:29674500
3084. Moo-Young TA, Traugott AL, Moley JF. Sporadic and familial medullary thyroid carcinoma: state of the art. Surg Clin North Am. 2009 Oct;89(5):1193–204. PMID:19836492
3085. Mora-Guzmán I, Alonso-Casado A, Rodríguez Sánchez A, et al. Neuroendocrine tumour arising inside a tailgut cyst. Ann R Coll Surg Engl. 2017 Feb;99(2):e91–3. PMID:27917670
3086. Moran CA, Rush W, Mena H. Primary spinal paragangliomas: a clinicopathological and immunohistochemical study of 30 cases. Histopathology. 1997 Aug;31(2):167–73. PMID:9279569
3087. Morandi L, Righi A, Maletta F, et al. Somatic mutation profiling of hobnail variant of papillary thyroid carcinoma. Endocr Relat Cancer. 2017 Feb;24(2):107–17. PMID:28062544
3088. Morariu EM, McCoy KL, Chiosea SI, et al. Clinicopathologic characteristics of thyroid nodules positive for the THADA-IGF2BP3 fusion on preoperative molecular analysis. Thyroid. 2021 Aug;31(8):1212–8. PMID:33487086
3089. Moreland DB. Intrasellar pituitary schwannoma. J Clin Neurosci. 2006 Aug;13(7):771–4. PMID:16860986
3090. Moreno S, Guillermo M, Decoulx M, et al. Feminizing adreno-cortical carcinomas in male adults. A dire prognosis. Three cases in a series of 801 adrenalectomies and review of the literature. Ann Endocrinol (Paris). 2006 Mar;67(1):32–8. PMID:16596055
3091. Mori Y, Sato N, Taniguchi R, et al. Pancreatic somatostatinoma diagnosed preoperatively: report of a case. JOP. 2014 Jan 10;15(1):66–71. PMID:24413789
3092. Morimoto R, Satoh F, Murakami O, et al. Immunohistochemistry of a proliferation marker Ki67/MIB1 in adrenocortical carcinomas: Ki67/MIB1 labeling index is a predictor for recurrence of adrenocortical carcinomas. Endocr J. 2008 Mar;55(1):49–55. PMID:18187873
3093. Morin A, Goncalves J, Moog S, et al. TET-mediated hypermethylation primes SDH-deficient cells for HIF2α-driven mesenchymal transition. Cell Rep. 2020 Mar 31;30(13):4551–4566.e7. PMID:32234487
3094. Morin E, Mete O, Wasserman JD, et al. Carney complex with adrenal cortical carcinoma. J Clin Endocrinol Metab. 2012 Feb;97(2):E202–6. PMID:22112809
3095. Morioka M, Furukawa Y, Kobayashi T, et al. Aldosterone-producing adrenal cortical cancer: a case report and analysis of steroidogenic enzymes in the tumor. Endocr J. 1997 Aug;44(4):547–52. PMID:9447288
3096. Morita M, Taguchi K, Kagawa M, et al. Treatment strategies for neuroendocrine carcinoma of the upper digestive tract. Int J Clin Oncol. 2020 May;25(5):842–50. PMID:32036480
3097. Morotti RA, Nicol KK, Parham DM, et al. An immunohistochemical algorithm to facilitate diagnosis and subtyping of rhabdomyosarcoma: the Children's Oncology Group experience. Am J Surg Pathol. 2006 Aug;30(8):962–8. PMID:16861966
3098. Morrison PJ, Nevin NC. Multiple endocrine neoplasia type 2B (mucosal neuroma syndrome, Wagenmann-Froboese syndrome). J Med Genet. 1996 Sep;33(9):779–82. PMID:8880581
3099. Mortini P, Barzaghi LR, Albano L, et al. Microsurgical therapy of pituitary adenomas. Endocrine. 2018 Jan;59(1):72–81. PMID:29067608
3100. Morton LM, Karyadi DM, Stewart C, et al. Radiation-related genomic profile of papillary thyroid carcinoma after the Chernobyl accident. Science. 2021 May 14;372(6543):eabg2538. PMID:33888599
3101. Moses W, Weng J, Kebebew E. Prevalence, clinicopathologic features, and somatic genetic mutation profile in familial versus sporadic nonmedullary thyroid cancer. Thyroid. 2011 Apr;21(4):367–71. PMID:21190444
3102. Moshiri AS, Doumani R, Yelistratova L, et al. Polyomavirus-negative Merkel cell carcinoma: a more aggressive subtype based on analysis of 282 cases using multimodal tumor virus detection. J Invest Dermatol. 2017 Apr;137(4):819–27. PMID:27815175
3103. Moshynska OV, Saxena A. Clonal relationship between Hashimoto thyroiditis and thyroid lymphoma. J Clin Pathol. 2008 Apr;61(4):438–44. PMID:18006670
3104. Mosimann C, Hausmann G, Basler K. Parafibromin/Hyrax activates Wnt/Wg target gene transcription by direct association with beta-catenin/Armadillo. Cell. 2006 Apr 21;125(2):327–41. PMID:16630820
3105. Moslehi M, Shahi Z, Badihian S, et al. Differentiated thyroid cancer in Iran - initial observations, histological features, management of the disease, and tumor recurrence: a review of 1689 cases. Indian J Cancer. 2016 Apr-Jun;53(2):261–4. PMID:28071623
3106. Mosquera JM, Fletcher CD. Expanding the spectrum of malignant progression in solitary fibrous tumors: a study of 8 cases with a discrete anaplastic component–is this dedifferentiated SFT? Am J Surg Pathol. 2009 Sep;33(9):1314–21. PMID:19718788
3107. Mosquera JM, Sboner A, Zhang L, et al. Novel MIR143-NOTCH fusions in benign and malignant glomus tumors. Genes Chromosomes Cancer. 2013 Nov;52(11):1075–87. PMID:23999936
3108. Mosquera JM, Sboner A, Zhang L, et al. Recurrent NCOA2 gene rearrangements in congenital/infantile spindle cell rhabdomyosarcoma. Genes Chromosomes Cancer. 2013 Jun;52(6):538–50. PMID:23463663
3109. Mossé YP. Anaplastic lymphoma kinase as a cancer target in pediatric malignancies. Clin Cancer Res. 2016 Feb 1;22(3):546–52. PMID:26503946
3110. Mossé YP, Laudenslager M, Longo L, et al. Identification of ALK as a major familial neuroblastoma predisposition gene. Nature. 2008 Oct 16;455(7215):930–5. PMID:18724359
3111. Mostoufi-Moab S, Labourier E, Sullivan L, et al. Molecular testing for oncogenic gene alterations in pediatric thyroid lesions. Thyroid. 2018 Jan;28(1):60–7. PMID:29108474
3112. Mouaqit O, Belkacem Z, Ifrine L, et al. A rare tumor of the thyroid gland: report on one case of leiomyosarcoma and review of literature. Updates Surg. 2014 Jun;66(2):165–7. PMID:23335096
3113. Mouat IC, Omata K, McDaniel AS, et al. Somatic mutations in adrenocortical carcinoma with primary aldosteronism or hyperreninemic hyperaldosteronism. Endocr Relat Cancer. 2019 Feb;26(2):217–25. PMID:30475217
3114. Moura MM, Cabrera RA, Esteves S, et al. Correlation of molecular data with histopathological and clinical features in a series of 66 patients with medullary thyroid carcinoma. J Endocrinol Invest. 2021 Sep;44(9):1837–46. PMID:33575974
3115. Moura MM, Cavaco BM, Pinto AE, et al. Correlation of RET somatic mutations with clinicopathological features in sporadic medullary thyroid carcinomas. Br J Cancer. 2009 Jun 2;100(11):1777–83. PMID:19401695
3116. Moura MM, Cavaco BM, Pinto AE, et al. High prevalence of RAS mutations in RET-negative sporadic medullary thyroid carcinomas. J Clin Endocrinol Metab. 2011 May;96(5):E863–8. PMID:21325462
3117. Movahedi-Lankarani S, Hruban RH, Westra WH, et al. Primitive neuroectodermal tumors of the pancreas: a report of seven cases of a rare neoplasm. Am J Surg Pathol. 2002 Aug;26(8):1040–7. PMID:12170091
3118. Mow C, Edwards A, Hayman JA. Ectopic pituitary with pregnancy changes in a benign cystic teratoma of the ovary. Pathology. 1999 Nov;31(4):431–3. PMID:10643021
3119. Mozos A, Ye H, Chuang WY, et al. Most primary adrenal lymphomas are diffuse large B-cell lymphomas with non-germinal center B-cell phenotype, BCL6 gene rearrangement and poor prognosis. Mod Pathol. 2009 Sep;22(9):1210–7. PMID:19525926
3120. Mrad K, Charfi L, Dhouib R, et al. [Extranodal Rosai-Dorfman disease: a case report with thyroid involvement]. Ann Pathol. 2004 Oct;24(5):446–9. French. PMID:15738872
3121. Mravic M, LaChaud G, Nguyen A, et al. Clinical and histopathological diagnosis of glomus tumor: an institutional experience of 138 cases. Int J Surg Pathol. 2015 May;23(3):181–8. PMID:25614464
3122. Mu Q, Yu J, Qu L, et al. Spindle cell oncocytoma of the adenohypophysis: two case reports and a review of the literature. Mol Med Rep. 2015 Jul;12(1):871–6. PMID:25777996
3123. Muderris T, Bercin S, Sevil E, et al. Transoral robotic surgery for atypical carcinoid tumor of the larynx. J Craniofac Surg. 2013 Nov;24(6):1996–9. PMID:24220389
3124. Muhammad A, Coopmans EC, Gatto F, et al. Pasireotide responsiveness in acromegaly is mainly driven by somatostatin receptor subtype 2 expression. J Clin Endocrinol Metab. 2019 Mar 1;104(3):915–24. PMID:30346538
3125. Mukhida K, Asa S, Gentili F, et al. Ependymoma of the pituitary fossa. Case report and

review of the literature. J Neurosurg. 2006 Oct;105(4):616–20. PMID:17044567
3126. Mulatero P, Schiavi F, Williams TA, et al. ARMC5 mutation analysis in patients with primary aldosteronism and bilateral adrenal lesions. J Hum Hypertens. 2016 Jun;30(6):374–8. PMID:26446392
3127. Müller HL. Craniopharyngioma: long-term consequences of a chronic disease. Expert Rev Neurother. 2015;15(11):1241–4. PMID:26523617
3128. Müller HL, Bueb K, Bartels U, et al. Obesity after childhood craniopharyngioma–German multicenter study on pre-operative risk factors and quality of life. Klin Padiatr. 2001 Jul-Aug;213(4):244–9. PMID:11528558
3129. Müller HL, Emser A, Faldum A, et al. Longitudinal study on growth and body mass index before and after diagnosis of childhood craniopharyngioma. J Clin Endocrinol Metab. 2004 Jul;89(7):3298–305. PMID:15240606
3130. Müller HL, Gebhardt U, Teske C, et al. Post-operative hypothalamic lesions and obesity in childhood craniopharyngioma: results of the multinational prospective trial KRANIOPHARYNGEOM 2000 after 3-year follow-up. Eur J Endocrinol. 2011 Jul;165(1):17–24. PMID:21490122
3131. Müller HL, Merchant TE, Warmuth-Metz M, et al. Craniopharyngioma. Nat Rev Dis Primers. 2019 Nov 7;5(1):75. PMID:31699993
3132. Muller KE, Tafe LJ, Gonzalez JL, et al. Ovarian strumal carcinoid producing peptide YY associated with severe constipation: a case report and review of the literature. Int J Gynecol Pathol. 2015 Jan;34(1):30–5. PMID:25473750
3133. Müller-Scholden J, Lehrnbecher T, Müller HL, et al. Radical surgery in a neonate with craniopharyngioma. report of a case. Pediatr Neurosurg. 2000 Nov;33(5):265–9. PMID:11155065
3134. Mulligan LM. RET revisited: expanding the oncogenic portfolio. Nat Rev Cancer. 2014 Mar;14(3):173–86. PMID:24561444
3135. Mulligan LM, Eng C, Healey CS, et al. Specific mutations of the RET proto-oncogene are related to disease phenotype in MEN 2A and FMTC. Nat Genet. 1994 Jan;6(1):70–4. PMID:7907913
3136. Mulligan LM, Kwok JB, Healey CS, et al. Germ-line mutations of the RET proto-oncogene in multiple endocrine neoplasia type 2A. Nature. 1993 Jun 3;363(6428):458–60. PMID:8099202
3137. Munakata S, Murai Y, Koizumi A, et al. Mixed neuroendocrine carcinoma and squamous cell carcinoma of the colon: case report and literature review. Case Rep Gastroenterol. 2018 Jun 5;12(2):240–6. PMID:30022911
3138. Murahashi N, Abe T, Matsumoto R, et al. [A case of WDHA water diarrhea hypokalemia achlorhydria syndrome that developed after multimodal therapy for retroperitoneal paraganglioma]. Hinyokika Kiyo. 2019 Jul;65(7):277–82. Japanese. PMID:31501391
3139. Murakami I, Matsushita M, Iwasaki T, et al. Interleukin-1 loop model for pathogenesis of Langerhans cell histiocytosis. Cell Commun Signal. 2015 Feb 22;13:13. PMID:25889448
3140. Murakami I, Matsushita M, Iwasaki T, et al. Merkel cell polyomavirus DNA sequences in peripheral blood and tissues from patients with Langerhans cell histiocytosis. Hum Pathol. 2014 Jan;45(1):119–26. PMID:24321520
3141. Murakami M, Kamiya Y, Yanagita Y, et al. Gs alpha mutations in hyperfunctioning thyroid adenomas. Arch Med Res. 1999 Nov-Dec;30(6):514–21. PMID:10714366
3142. Murakami M, Katayama K, Kato S, et al. Large-cell neuroendocrine carcinoma of the common bile duct: a case report and a review of literature. Surg Case Rep. 2016 Dec;2(1):141. PMID:27888490
3143. Murase T, Takino H, Shimizu S, et al. Clonality analysis of different histological components in combined small cell and non-small cell carcinoma of the lung. Hum Pathol. 2003 Nov;34(11):1178–84. PMID:14652820
3144. Murphy E, Smith R, Lindesay J, et al. Increased mortality rates in late-life depression. Br J Psychiatry. 1988 Mar;152:347–53. PMID:3167369
3145. Musat M, Korbonits M, Pyle M, et al. The expression of the F-box protein Skp2 is negatively associated with p27 expression in human pituitary tumors. Pituitary. 2002;5(4):235–42. PMID:14558671
3146. Musholt TJ, Musholt PB, Petrich T, et al. Familial papillary thyroid carcinoma: genetics, criteria for diagnosis, clinical features, and surgical treatment. World J Surg. 2000 Nov;24(11):1409–17. PMID:11038215
3147. Müssnich P, Raverot G, Jaffrain-Rea ML, et al. Downregulation of miR-410 targeting the cyclin B1 gene plays a role in pituitary gonadotroph tumors. Cell Cycle. 2015;14(16):2590–7. PMID:26125663
3148. Muth A, Hammarstedt L, Hellström M, et al. Cohort study of patients with adrenal lesions discovered incidentally. Br J Surg. 2011 Oct;98(10):1383–91. PMID:21618498
3149. Muzza M. The clonal origin of multifocal papillary thyroid cancer: intrathyroidal spread or independent tumors? Minerva Endocrinol (Torino). 2021 Mar;46(1):35–44. PMID:33045819
3150. Nabhan F, Ringel MD. Thyroid nodules and cancer management guidelines: comparisons and controversies. Endocr Relat Cancer. 2017 Feb;24(2):R13–26. PMID:27965276
3151. Nadaf J, de Kock L, Chong AS, et al. Molecular characterization of DICER1-mutated pituitary blastoma. Acta Neuropathol. 2021 Jun;141(6):929–44. PMID:33644822
3152. Nadas AS, Alimurung MM, Sieracki LA. Cardiac manifestations of Friedreich's ataxia. N Engl J Med. 1951 Feb 15;244(7):239–44. PMID:14796821
3153. Nagasaki K, Shibata N, Nyuzuki H, et al. A Japanese family with DICER1 syndrome found in childhood-onset multinodular goitre. Horm Res Paediatr. 2020;93(7-8):477–82. PMID:33080613
3154. Nagata Y, Inoshita N, Fukuhara N, et al. Growth hormone-producing pituitary adenomas in childhood and young adulthood: clinical features and outcomes. Pituitary. 2018 Feb;21(1):1–9. PMID:28849339
3155. Nagiredla P, Tummidi S, Patro MK. Carotid body tumor diagnosed by on-site FNA: a case report. Indian J Surg Oncol. 2019 Jun;10(2):396–9. PMID:31168271
3156. Naidoo J, Santos-Zabala ML, Iyriboz T, et al. Large cell neuroendocrine carcinoma of the lung: clinico-pathologic features, treatment, and outcomes. Clin Lung Cancer. 2016 Sep;17(5):e121–9. PMID:26898325
3157. Nair SK, Burley SK. X-ray structures of Myc-Max and Mad-Max recognizing DNA. Molecular bases of regulation by proto-oncogenic transcription factors. Cell. 2003 Jan 24;112(2):193–205. PMID:12553908
3158. Najdawi F, Ahmadi S, Capelletti M, et al. Evaluation of grade in a genotyped cohort of sporadic medullary thyroid carcinomas. Histopathology. 2021 Sep;79(3):427–36. PMID:33763905
3159. Nakagawara A, Ikeda K, Tsuneyoshi M, et al. Malignant pheochromocytoma with ganglioneuroblastoma elements in a patient with von Recklinghausen's disease. Cancer. 1985 Jun 15;55(12):2794–8. PMID:3922614
3160. Nakagawara A, Li Y, Izumi H, et al. Neuroblastoma. Jpn J Clin Oncol. 2018 Mar 1;48(3):214–41. PMID:29378002
3161. Nakajo M, Jinguji M, Tani A, et al. Application of adrenal maximum standardized uptake value to 131I-6β-iodomethyl-19-norcholesterol SPECT/CT for characterizing unilateral hyperfunctioning adrenocortical masses. Eur J Radiol. 2020 Dec;133:109397. PMID:33190101
3162. Nakamura K, Kimura S, Yamazaki M, et al. Immunohistochemical analyses of thyroid-specific enhancer-binding protein in the fetal and adult rat hypothalami and pituitary glands. Brain Res Dev Brain Res. 2001 Oct 24;130(2):159–66. PMID:11675118
3163. Nakamura N, Erickson LA, Jin L, et al. Immunohistochemical separation of follicular variant of papillary thyroid carcinoma from follicular adenoma. Endocr Pathol. 2006 Fall;17(3):213–23. PMID:17308358
3164. Nakamura S, Shiota M, Nakagawa A, et al. Anaplastic large cell lymphoma: a distinct molecular pathologic entity: a reappraisal with special reference to p80(NPM/ALK) expression. Am J Surg Pathol. 1997 Dec;21(12):1420–32. PMID:9414185
3165. Nakamura Y, Maekawa T, Felizola SJ, et al. Adrenal CYP11B1/2 expression in primary aldosteronism: immunohistochemical analysis using novel monoclonal antibodies. Mol Cell Endocrinol. 2014 Jul 5;392(1-2):73–9. PMID:24837548
3166. Nakano A, Hirabayashi K, Yamamuro H, et al. Combined primary hepatic neuroendocrine carcinoma and hepatocellular carcinoma: case report and literature review. World J Surg Oncol. 2021 Mar 16;19(1):78. PMID:33726764
3167. Nakano T, Motoshita J, Tanaka R, et al. Primary combined small cell carcinoma and squamous cell carcinoma of the oropharynx with special reference to EGFR status of small cell carcinoma component: case report and review of the literature. Auris Nasus Larynx. 2017 Aug;44(4):472–8. PMID:27496009
3168. Nakano-Tateno T, Tateno T, Hlaing MM, et al. FGFR4 polymorphic variants modulate phenotypic features of Cushing disease. Mol Endocrinol. 2014 Apr;28(4):525–33. PMID:24625004
3169. Nakata K, Ito Y, Magadi W, et al. Childhood cancer incidence and survival in Japan and England: a population-based study (1993-2010). Cancer Sci. 2018 Feb;109(2):422–34. PMID:29178401
3170. Nakayama K, Ishida N, Shirane M, et al. Mice lacking p27(Kip1) display increased body size, multiple organ hyperplasia, retinal dysplasia, and pituitary tumors. Cell. 1996 May 31;85(5):707–20. PMID:8646779
3171. Nakazawa T, Cameselle-Teijeiro J, Vinagre J, et al. C-cell-derived calcitonin-free neuroendocrine carcinoma of the thyroid: the diagnostic importance of CGRP immunoreactivity. Int J Surg Pathol. 2014 Sep;22(6):530–5. PMID:24599901
3172. Nakazawa T, Celestino R, Machado JC, et al. Cribriform-morular variant of papillary thyroid carcinoma displaying poorly differentiated features. Int J Surg Pathol. 2013 Aug;21(4):379–89. PMID:23349472
3173. Nam JH, Han CW, Kim NI, et al. The cytological features of sclerosing mucoepidermoid carcinoma with eosinophilia of the thyroid gland: a case report. Cytopathology. 2020 Nov;31(6):593–7. PMID:32671907
3174. Namba H, Matsuo K, Fagin JA. Clonal composition of benign and malignant human thyroid tumors. J Clin Invest. 1990 Jul;86(1):120–5. PMID:1973172
3175. Nambirajan A, Singh V, Irugu DVK, et al. Spindle epithelial tumour with thymus-like elements presenting with lymph node metastasis: an illustrative case report with review of literature. Cytopathology. 2019 Nov;30(6):657–61. PMID:31209931
3176. Nambron R, Rosenthal R, Bahl D. Diagnosis and evaluation of thyroid nodules-the clinician's perspective. Radiol Clin North Am. 2020 Nov;58(6):1009–18. PMID:33040844
3177. Namekawa T, Utsumi T, Imamoto T, et al. Composite pheochromocytoma with a malignant peripheral nerve sheath tumor: case report and review of the literature. Asian J Surg. 2016 Jul;39(3):187–90. PMID:27338175
3178. Nanarng V, Jacob S, Mahapatra D, et al. Intraoperative diagnosis of central nervous system lesions: comparison of squash smear, touch imprint, and frozen section. J Cytol. 2015 Jul-Sep;32(3):153–8. PMID:26729974
3179. Nanba K, Blinder AR, Rege J, et al. Somatic CACNA1H mutation as a cause of aldosterone-producing adenoma. Hypertension. 2020 Mar;75(3):645–9. PMID:31983310
3180. Nanba K, Omata K, Else T, et al. Targeted molecular characterization of aldosterone-producing adenomas in White Americans. J Clin Endocrinol Metab. 2018 Oct 1;103(10):3869–76. PMID:30085035
3181. Nanba K, Omata K, Gomez-Sanchez CE, et al. Genetic characteristics of aldosterone-producing adenomas in Blacks. Hypertension. 2019 Apr;73(4):885–92. PMID:30739536
3182. Nanba K, Tsuiki M, Sawai K, et al. Histopathological diagnosis of primary aldosteronism using CYP11B2 immunohistochemistry. J Clin Endocrinol Metab. 2013 Apr;98(4):1567–74. PMID:23443813
3183. Nanba K, Yamazaki Y, Bick N, et al. Prevalence of somatic mutations in aldosterone-producing adenomas in Japanese patients. J Clin Endocrinol Metab. 2020 Nov 1;105(11):e4066–73. PMID:32844168
3184. Nandagopal R, Vortmeyer A, Oldfield EH, et al. Cushing's syndrome due to a pituitary corticotropinoma in a child with tuberous sclerosis: an association or a coincidence? Clin Endocrinol (Oxf). 2007 Oct;67(4):639–41. PMID:17596199
3185. Nandini H, Shetty V, Lakshmikantha A, et al. SETTLE tumor of thyroid: oldest case in literature. Indian J Pathol Microbiol. 2019 Jan-Mar;62(1):175–7. PMID:30706893
3186. Nangue C, Bron L, Portmann L, et al. Mixed medullary-papillary carcinoma of the thyroid: report of a case and review of the literature. Head Neck. 2009 Jul;31(7):968–74. PMID:19260112
3187. Naniwadekar MR, Jagtap SV, Kshirsagar AY, et al. Fine needle aspiration diagnosis of carotid body tumor in a case of multiple paragangliomas presenting with facial palsy: a case report. Acta Cytol. 2010 Jul-Aug;54(4):635–9. PMID:20715670
3188. Narayanan D, Mandal R, Hardin H, et al. Long non-coding RNAs in pulmonary neuroendocrine neoplasms. Endocr Pathol. 2020 Sep;31(3):254–63. PMID:32388776
3189. Nardi V, Song Y, Santamaria-Barria JA, et al. Activation of PI3K signaling in Merkel cell carcinoma. Clin Cancer Res. 2012 Mar 1;18(5):1227–36. PMID:22261808
3190. Narisawa Y, Koba S, Inoue T, et al. Histogenesis of pure and combined Merkel cell carcinomas: an immunohistochemical study of 14 cases. J Dermatol. 2015 May;42(5):445–52. PMID:25720654
3191. Narla S, Govindraj J, Chandrasekar K, et al. Craniopharyngioma with malignant transformation: review of literature. Neurol India. 2017 Mar-Apr;65(2):418–20. PMID:28290422
3192. Nascimento AF, Fletcher CD. Spindle cell rhabdomyosarcoma in adults. Am J Surg Pathol. 2005 Aug;29(8):1106–13. PMID:16006807
3193. Nasioudis D, Chapman-Davis E, Frey MK, et al. Small cell carcinoma of the ovary: a rare tumor with a poor prognosis. Int J

Gynecol Cancer. 2018 Jun;28(5):932–8. PMID:29621125
3194. Nasioudis D, Frey MK, Chapman-Davis E, et al. Primary malignant ovarian carcinoid; management and outcomes. Gynecol Oncol. 2020 Apr;157(1):101–5. PMID:31959493
3195. Nasr C, Mason A, Mayberg M, et al. Acromegaly and somatotroph hyperplasia with adenomatous transformation due to pituitary metastasis of a growth hormone-releasing hormone-secreting pulmonary endocrine carcinoma. J Clin Endocrinol Metab. 2006 Dec;91(12):4776–80. PMID:16968791
3196. Nassar H, Albores-Saavedra J, Klimstra DS. High-grade neuroendocrine carcinoma of the ampulla of vater: a clinicopathologic and immunohistochemical analysis of 14 cases. Am J Surg Pathol. 2005 May;29(5):588–94. PMID:15832081
3197. Nath MC, Erickson LA. Aggressive variants of papillary thyroid carcinoma: hobnail, tall cell, columnar, and solid. Adv Anat Pathol. 2018 May;25(3):172–9. PMID:29351089
3198. Nath V, Parks GE, Baliga M, et al. Mucoepidermoid carcinoma of the thyroid with concomitant papillary carcinoma: comparison of findings on fine-needle aspiration biopsy and histology. Endocr Pathol. 2014 Dec;25(4):427–32. PMID:25307114
3199. National Institutes of Health Consensus Development Conference. Neurofibromatosis. Conference statement. Arch Neurol. 1988 May;45(5):575–8. PMID:3128965
3200. Navone F, Jahn R, Di Gioia G, et al. Protein p38: an integral membrane protein specific for small vesicles of neurons and neuroendocrine cells. J Cell Biol. 1986 Dec;103(6 Pt 1):2511–27. PMID:3097029
3201. Naziat A, Karavitaki N, Thakker R, et al. Confusing genes: a patient with MEN2A and Cushing's disease. Clin Endocrinol (Oxf). 2013 Jun;78(6):966–8. PMID:23072303
3202. Neely D, Gray S. Primary carcinoid tumour of the testis. Ulster Med J. 2011 May;80(2):79–81. PMID:22347748
3203. Negri E, Ron E, Franceschi S, et al. Risk factors for medullary thyroid carcinoma: a pooled analysis. Cancer Causes Control. 2002 May;13(4):365–72. PMID:12074506
3204. Nelson DS, Quispel W, Badalian-Very G, et al. Somatic activating ARAF mutations in Langerhans cell histiocytosis. Blood. 2014 May 15;123(20):3152–5. PMID:24652991
3205. Nelson DS, van Halteren A, Quispel WT, et al. MAP2K1 and MAP3K1 mutations in Langerhans cell histiocytosis. Genes Chromosomes Cancer. 2015 Jun;54(6):361–8. PMID:25899310
3206. Nemenqani D, Yaqoob N, Khoja H. Leiomyosarcoma metastatic to the thyroid diagnosed by fine needle aspiration cytology. J Pak Med Assoc. 2010 Apr;60(4):307–9. PMID:20419977
3207. Nemir J, Štenger M, Jakovčević A, et al. Adrenal cortical adenoma in the spinal canal: a case report and review of the literature. J Neurol Surg A Cent Eur Neurosurg. 2020 Jan;81(1):71–4. PMID:31127594
3208. Neou M, Villa C, Armignacco R, et al. Pangenomic classification of pituitary neuroendocrine tumors. Cancer Cell. 2020 Jan 13;37(1):123–134.e5. PMID:31883967
3209. Nermoen I, Falhammar H. Prevalence and characteristics of adrenal tumors and myelolipomas in congenital adrenal hyperplasia: a systematic review and meta-analysis. Endocr Pract. 2020 Nov;26(11):1351–65. PMID:33471666
3210. Nermoen I, Falhammar H. Prevalence and characteristics of adrenal tumors and myelolipomas in congenital adrenal hyperplasia: a systematic review and meta-analysis. Endocr Pract. 2020 Nov;26(11):1351–65. PMID:33471666
3211. Nermoen I, Rørvik J, Holmedal SH, et al. High frequency of adrenal myelolipomas and testicular adrenal rest tumours in adult Norwegian patients with classical congenital adrenal hyperplasia because of 21-hydroxylase deficiency. Clin Endocrinol (Oxf). 2011 Dec;75(6):753–9. PMID:21689130
3212. Nery B, Bernardes Filho F, Costa RAF, et al. Neurocytoma mimicking macroadenoma. Surg Neurol Int. 2019 Jan 21;10:8. PMID:30775062
3213. Nesi G, Marcucci T, Rubio CA, et al. Somatostatinoma: clinico-pathological features of three cases and literature reviewed. J Gastroenterol Hepatol. 2008 Apr;23(4):521–6. PMID:17645474
3214. Nettore IC, Colao A, Macchia PE. Nutritional and environmental factors in thyroid carcinogenesis. Int J Environ Res Public Health. 2018 Aug 13;15(8):1735. PMID:30104523
3215. Neumann HPH, Tsoy U, Bancos I, et al. Comparison of pheochromocytoma-specific morbidity and mortality among adults with bilateral pheochromocytomas undergoing total adrenalectomy vs cortical-sparing adrenalectomy. JAMA Netw Open. 2019 Aug 2;2(8):e198898. PMID:31397861
3216. Neumann S, Bayer Y, Reske A, et al. Further indications for genetic heterogeneity of euthyroid familial goiter. J Mol Med (Berl). 2003 Nov;81(11):736–45. PMID:14564411
3217. National Institutes of Health Consensus Development Conference. Neurofibromatosis. Conference statement. Arch Neurol. 1988 May;45(5):575–8. PMID:3128965
3218. Newey PJ, Bowl MR, Cranston T, et al. Cell division cycle protein 73 homolog (CDC73) mutations in the hyperparathyroidism-jaw tumor syndrome (HPT-JT) and parathyroid tumors. Hum Mutat. 2010 Mar;31(3):295–307. PMID:20052758
3219. Newey PJ, Nesbit MA, Rimmer AJ, et al. Whole-exome sequencing studies of nonfunctioning pituitary adenomas. J Clin Endocrinol Metab. 2013 Apr;98(4):E796–800. PMID:23450047
3220. Newman E, Shaha AR. Substernal goiter. J Surg Oncol. 1995 Nov;60(3):207–12. PMID:7475073
3221. Ng HK, Poon WS. Sinus histiocytosis with massive lymphadenopathy localized to the sella. Br J Neurosurg. 1995;9(4):551–5. PMID:7576285
3222. Ng WK, Collins RJ, Shek WH, et al. Cytologic Diagnosis of "CASTLE" of thyroid gland: report of a case with histologic correlation. Diagn Cytopathol. 1996 Sep;15(3):224–7. PMID:8955605
3223. Ngan ES, Lang BH, Liu T, et al. A germline mutation (A339V) in thyroid transcription factor-1 (TITF-1/NKX2.1) in patients with multinodular goiter and papillary thyroid carcinoma. J Natl Cancer Inst. 2009 Feb 4;101(3):162–75. PMID:19176457
3224. Ngeow J, Mester J, Rybicki LA, et al. Incidence and clinical characteristics of thyroid cancer in prospective series of individuals with Cowden and Cowden-like syndrome characterized by germline PTEN, SDH, or KLLN alterations. J Clin Endocrinol Metab. 2011 Dec;96(12):E2063–71. PMID:21956414
3225. Ngeow J, Ni Y, Tohme R, et al. Germline alterations in RASAL1 in Cowden syndrome patients presenting with follicular thyroid cancer and in individuals with apparently sporadic epithelial thyroid cancer. J Clin Endocrinol Metab. 2014 Jul;99(7):E1316–21. PMID:24712574
3226. Toledo RA, Burnichon N, Cascon A, et al. Consensus statement on next-generation-sequencing-based diagnostic testing of hereditary phaeochromocytomas and paragangliomas. Nat Rev Endocrinol. 2017 Apr;13(4):233–47. PMID:27857127
3227. Nguyen AH, O'Leary MP, De Andrade JP, et al. Natural history of renal neuroendocrine neoplasms: A NET by any other name? Front Endocrinol (Lausanne). 2021 Feb 5;11:624251. PMID:33613455
3228. Nguyen KD, Waitt T, Alleyne CH Jr. Sellar/suprasellar ganglioglioma: clinical image. World Neurosurg. 2019 Dec;132:1–3. PMID:31442637
3229. Nguyen MT, Lavi E. Pituitary adenoma-neuronal choristoma is a pituitary adenoma with ganglionic differentiation. Exp Mol Pathol. 2015 Dec;99(3):628–31. PMID:26551086
3230. Nguyen PL, Poetker DM, Zambrano E. Parathyroid hemangioma: a case report in proof of its existence. Endocr Pathol. 2011 Mar;22(1):53–6. PMID:21286857
3231. Nguyen TH, Barr FG. Therapeutic approaches targeting PAX3-FOXO1 and its regulatory and transcriptional pathways in rhabdomyosarcoma. Molecules. 2018 Oct 28;23(11):2798. PMID:30373318
3232. Ni Y, He X, Chen J, et al. Germline SDHx variants modify breast and thyroid cancer risks in Cowden and Cowden-like syndrome via FAD/NAD-dependant destabilization of p53. Hum Mol Genet. 2012 Jan 15;21(2):300–10. PMID:21979946
3233. Nicholson SA, Beasley MB, Brambilla E, et al. Small cell lung carcinoma (SCLC): a clinicopathologic study of 100 cases with surgical specimens. Am J Surg Pathol. 2002 Sep;26(9):1184–97. PMID:12218575
3234. Nicolis G, Shimshi M, Allen C, et al. Gonadotropin-producing pituitary adenoma in a man with long-standing primary hypogonadism. J Clin Endocrinol Metab. 1988 Jan;66(1):237–41. PMID:2447114
3235. Nicolson NG, Murtha TD, Dong W, et al. Comprehensive genetic analysis of follicular thyroid carcinoma predicts prognosis independent of histology. J Clin Endocrinol Metab. 2018 Jul 1;103(7):2640–50. PMID:29726952
3236. Niederle B, Selberherr A, Bartsch DK, et al. Multiple endocrine neoplasia type 1 and the pancreas: diagnosis and treatment of functioning and non-functioning pancreatic and duodenal neuroendocrine neoplasia within the men1 syndrome - an international consensus statement. Neuroendocrinology. 2021;111(7):609–30. PMID:32971521
3237. Niederle MB, Hackl M, Kaserer K, et al. Gastroenteropancreatic neuroendocrine tumours: the current incidence and staging based on the WHO and European Neuroendocrine Tumour Society classification: an analysis based on prospectively collected parameters. Endocr Relat Cancer. 2010 Oct 5;17(4):909–18. PMID:20702725
3238. Nielsen EH, Feldt-Rasmussen U, Poulsgaard L, et al. Incidence of craniopharyngioma in Denmark (n = 189) and estimated world incidence of craniopharyngioma in children and adults. J Neurooncol. 2011 Sep;104(3):755–63. PMID:21336771
3239. Nielsen GP, Dickersin GR, Provenzal JM, et al. Lipomatous hemangiopericytoma. A histologic, ultrastructural and immunohistochemical study of a unique variant of hemangiopericytoma. Am J Surg Pathol. 1995 Jul;19(7):748–56. PMID:7793472
3240. Nieman LK. Cushing's syndrome: update on signs, symptoms and biochemical screening. Eur J Endocrinol. 2015 Oct;173(4):M33–8. PMID:26156970
3241. Niemas-Teshiba R, Matsuno R, Wang LL, et al. MYC-family protein overexpression and prominent nucleolar formation represent prognostic indicators and potential therapeutic targets for aggressive high-MKI neuroblastomas: a report from the Children's Oncology Group. Oncotarget. 2017 Dec 15;9(5):6416–32. PMID:29464082
3242. Nieminen TT, Walker CJ, Olkinuora A, et al. Thyroid carcinomas that occur in familial adenomatous polyposis patients recurrently harbor somatic variants in APC, BRAF, and KTM2D. Thyroid. 2020 Mar;30(3):380–8. PMID:32024448
3243. Nießen A, Schimmack S, Weber TF, et al. Presentation and outcome of mixed neuroendocrine non-neuroendocrine neoplasms of the pancreas. Pancreatology. 2021 Jan;21(1):224–35. PMID:33309225
3244. Nigawara K, Suzuki T, Tazawa H, et al. A case of recurrent malignant pheochromocytoma complicated by watery diarrhea, hypokalemia, achlorhydria syndrome. J Clin Endocrinol Metab. 1987 Nov;65(5):1053–6. PMID:3667875
3245. Niitsu N, Okamoto M, Nakamura N, et al. Clinicopathologic correlations of stage IE/IIE primary thyroid diffuse large B-cell lymphoma. Ann Oncol. 2007 Jul;18(7):1203–8. PMID:17429099
3246. Niiya F, Takano Y, Azami T, et al. A case of pancreatic mixed acinar-neuroendocrine carcinoma successfully diagnosed with endoscopic ultrasound-guided fine needle aspiration. Clin J Gastroenterol. 2020 Oct;13(5):951–8. PMID:32529486
3247. Nijhoff MF, Dekkers OM, Vleming LJ, et al. ACTH-producing pheochromocytoma: clinical considerations and concise review of the literature. Eur J Intern Med. 2009 Nov;20(7):682–5. PMID:19818286
3248. Nikfarjam M, Warshaw AL, Axelrod L, et al. Improved contemporary surgical management of insulinomas: a 25-year experience at the Massachusetts General Hospital. Ann Surg. 2008 Jan;247(1):165–72. PMID:18156937
3249. Nikiforov YE. Role of molecular markers in thyroid nodule management: then and now. Endocr Pract. 2017 Aug;23(8):979–88. PMID:28534687
3250. Nikiforov YE. Thyroid cancer in 2015: molecular landscape of thyroid cancer continues to be deciphered. Nat Rev Endocrinol. 2016 Feb;12(2):67–8. PMID:26668120
3251. Nikiforov YE, Baloch ZW. Clinical validation of the ThyroSeq v3 genomic classifier in thyroid nodules with indeterminate FNA cytology. Cancer Cytopathol. 2019 Apr;127(4):225–30. PMID:30811896
3252. Nikiforov YE, Baloch ZW, Hodak SP, et al. Change in diagnostic criteria for noninvasive follicular thyroid neoplasm with papillary-like nuclear features. JAMA Oncol. 2018 Aug 1;4(8):1125–6. PMID:29902314
3253. Nikiforov YE, Carty SE, Chiosea SI, et al. Highly accurate diagnosis of cancer in thyroid nodules with follicular neoplasm/suspicious for a follicular neoplasm cytology by ThyroSeq v2 next-generation sequencing assay. Cancer. 2014 Dec 1;120(23):3627–34. PMID:25209362
3254. Nikiforov YE, Erickson LA, Nikiforova MN, et al. Solid variant of papillary thyroid carcinoma: incidence, clinical-pathologic characteristics, molecular analysis, and biologic behavior. Am J Surg Pathol. 2001 Dec;25(12):1478–84. PMID:11717536
3255. Nikiforov YE, Seethala RR, Tallini G, et al. Nomenclature revision for encapsulated follicular variant of papillary thyroid carcinoma: a paradigm shift to reduce overtreatment of indolent tumors. JAMA Oncol. 2016 Aug 1;2(8):1023–9. PMID:27078145
3256. Nikiforova MN, Biddinger PW, Caudill CM, et al. PAX8-PPARgamma rearrangement in thyroid tumors: RT-PCR and immunohistochemical analyses. Am J Surg Pathol. 2002

Aug;26(8):1016–23. PMID:12170088
3257. Nikiforova MN, Lynch RA, Biddinger PW, et al. RAS point mutations and PAX8-PPAR gamma rearrangement in thyroid tumors: evidence for distinct molecular pathways in thyroid follicular carcinoma. J Clin Endocrinol Metab. 2003 May;88(5):2318–26. PMID:12727991
3258. Nikiforova MN, Mercurio S, Wald AI, et al. Analytical performance of the ThyroSeq v3 genomic classifier for cancer diagnosis in thyroid nodules. Cancer. 2018 Apr 15;124(8):1682–90. PMID:29345728
3259. Nikiforova MN, Nikiforov YE, Ohori NP. GLIS rearrangements in thyroid nodules: a key to preoperative diagnosis of hyalinizing trabecular tumor. Cancer Cytopathol. 2019 Sep;127(9):560–6. PMID:31373774
3260. Nikiforova MN, Nikitski AV, Panebianco F, et al. GLIS rearrangement is a genomic hallmark of hyalinizing trabecular tumor of the thyroid gland. Thyroid. 2019 Feb;29(2):161–73. PMID:30648929
3261. Nikiforova MN, Wald AI, Roy S, et al. Targeted next-generation sequencing panel (ThyroSeq) for detection of mutations in thyroid cancer. J Clin Endocrinol Metab. 2013 Nov;98(11):E1852–60. PMID:23979959
3262. Nilsson M, Williams D. On the origin of cells and derivation of thyroid cancer: C cell story revisited. Eur Thyroid J. 2016 Jul;5(2):79–93. PMID:27493881
3263. Nishi T, Kawabata Y, Hari Y, et al. A case of pancreatic neuroendocrine tumor in a patient with neurofibromatosis-1. World J Surg Oncol. 2012 Jul 23;10:153. PMID:22824559
3264. Nishigami K, Liu Z, Taniguchi E, et al. Cytological features of well-differentiated tumors of uncertain malignant potential: indeterminate cytology and WDT-UMP. Endocr J. 2012;59(6):483–7. PMID:22484994
3265. Nishino M, Mateo R, Kilim H, et al. Repeat fine needle aspiration cytology refines the selection of thyroid nodules for afirma gene expression classifier testing. Thyroid. 2021 Aug;31(8):1253–63. PMID:33813868
3266. Nishino M, Nikiforova M. Update on molecular testing for cytologically indeterminate thyroid nodules. Arch Pathol Lab Med. 2018 Apr;142(4):446–57. PMID:29336606
3267. Nishioka H, Fukuhara N, Horiguchi K, et al. Aggressive transsphenoidal resection of tumors invading the cavernous sinus in patients with acromegaly: predictive factors, strategies, and outcomes. J Neurosurg. 2014 Sep;121(3):505–10. PMID:25014437
3268. Nishioka H, Haraoka J, Akada K, et al. Gender-related differences in prolactin secretion in pituitary prolactinomas. Neuroradiology. 2002 May;44(5):407–10. PMID:12012125
3269. Nishioka H, Inoshita N, Mete O, et al. The complementary role of transcription factors in the accurate diagnosis of clinically nonfunctioning pituitary adenomas. Endocr Pathol. 2015 Dec;26(4):349–55. PMID:26481628
3270. Nishioka H, Inoshita N, Sano T, et al. Correlation between histological subtypes and MRI findings in clinically nonfunctioning pituitary adenomas. Endocr Pathol. 2012 Sep;23(3):151–6. PMID:22569896
3271. Nishioka H, Shibuya M, Izawa H, et al. Primary suprasellar malignant tumor with odontogenic features: case report. Neurosurgery. 2009 Aug;65(2):E380–2. PMID:19625894
3272. Nishishinya MB, Pereda CA, Muñoz-Fernández S, et al. Identification of lymphoma predictors in patients with primary Sjögren's syndrome: a systematic literature review and meta-analysis. Rheumatol Int. 2015 Jan;35(1):17–26. PMID:24899571
3273. Nishizawa H, Fukuoka H, Iguchi G, et al. AIP mutation identified in a patient with acromegaly caused by pituitary somatotroph adenoma with neuronal choristoma. Exp Clin Endocrinol Diabetes. 2013 May;121(5):295–9. PMID:23674160
3274. Niu M, Liu A, Zhao Y, et al. Malignant transformation of a mature teratoma of the adrenal gland: a rare case report and literature review. Medicine (Baltimore). 2017 Nov;96(45):e8333. PMID:29137015
3275. Nixon IJ, Coca-Pelaz A, Kaleva AI, et al. Metastasis to the thyroid gland: a critical review. Ann Surg Oncol. 2017 Jun;24(6):1533–9. PMID:27873099
3276. Nixon IJ, Suárez C, Simo R, et al. The impact of family history on non-medullary thyroid cancer. Eur J Surg Oncol. 2016 Oct;42(10):1455–63. PMID:27561845
3277. Noctor E, Gupta S, Brown T, et al. Paediatric cyclical Cushing's disease due to corticotroph cell hyperplasia. BMC Endocr Disord. 2015 Jun 12;15:27. PMID:26063496
3278. Noel M, Delehaye MC, Segond N, et al. Study of calcitonin and thyroglobulin gene expression in human mixed follicular and medullary thyroid carcinoma. Thyroid. 1991 Summer;1(3):249–56. PMID:1824340
3279. Nogales FF, Goyenaga P, Preda O, et al. An analysis of five clear cell papillary cystadenomas of mesosalpinx and broad ligament: four associated with von Hippel-Lindau disease and one aggressive sporadic type. Histopathology. 2012 Apr;60(5):748–57. PMID:22296276
3280. Noh JM, Ha SY, Ahn YC, et al. Potential role of adjuvant radiation therapy in cervical thymic neoplasm involving thyroid gland or neck. Cancer Res Treat. 2015 Jul;47(3):436–40. PMID:25648096
3281. Nölting S, Grossman AB. Signaling pathways in pheochromocytomas and paragangliomas: prospects for future therapies. Endocr Pathol. 2012 Mar;23(1):21–33. PMID:22391976
3282. Nomura Y, Nakashima O, Akiba J, et al. Clinicopathological features of neoplasms with neuroendocrine differentiation occurring in the liver. J Clin Pathol. 2017 Jul;70(7):563–70. PMID:27881473
3283. Nonaka D. Study of parathyroid transcription factor Gcm2 expression in parathyroid lesions. Am J Surg Pathol. 2011 Jan;35(1):145–51. PMID:21164298
3284. Nonaka D, Chiriboga L, Rubin BP. Sox10: a pan-schwannian and melanocytic marker. Am J Surg Pathol. 2008 Sep;32(9):1291–8. PMID:18636017
3285. Nonaka D, Rodriguez J, Rosai J. Extraneural hemangioblastoma: a report of 5 cases. Am J Surg Pathol. 2007 Oct;31(10):1545–51. PMID:17895756
3286. Nonaka D, Tang Y, Chiriboga L, et al. Diagnostic utility of thyroid transcription factors Pax8 and TTF-2 (FoxE1) in thyroid epithelial neoplasms. Mod Pathol. 2008 Feb;21(2):192–200. PMID:18084247
3287. Nonaka K, Matsuda Y, Okaniwa A, et al. Pancreatic gangliocytic paraganglioma harboring lymph node metastasis: a case report and literature review. Diagn Pathol. 2017 Aug 2;12(1):57. PMID:28764742
3288. Noor M, Russell DK, Israel AK, et al. Thyroid sclerosing mucoepidermoid carcinoma with eosinophilia in conjunction with parotid basal cell adenoma: cytologic, histologic, and molecular features. Diagn Cytopathol. 2021 Jul;49(7):E262–8. PMID:33484239
3289. Norman J, Politz D, Browarsky I. Diagnostic aspiration of parathyroid adenomas causes severe fibrosis complicating surgery and final histologic diagnosis. Thyroid. 2007 Dec;17(12):1251–5. PMID:17887929
3290. Norris HJ, Zirkin HJ, Benson WL. Immature (malignant) teratoma of the ovary: a clinical and pathologic study of 58 cases. Cancer. 1976 May;37(5):2359–72. PMID:1260722
3291. North JH Jr, Foley AM, Hamill RL. Intrathyroid cysts of thyroglossal duct origin. Am Surg. 1998 Sep;64(9):886–8. PMID:9731820
3293. Nosé V, Paner GP, Greenson JK, et al., editors. Diagnostic pathology: familial cancer syndromes. Salt Lake City (UT): Amirsys Publishing; 2013.
3294. Nosé V. DICER1 gene alterations in thyroid diseases. Cancer Cytopathol. 2020 Oct;128(10):688–9. PMID:32897630
3295. Nosé V. Familial follicular cell tumors: classification and morphological characteristics. Endocr Pathol. 2010 Dec;21(4):219–26. PMID:20878367
3296. Nosé V. Familial non-medullary thyroid carcinoma: an update. Endocr Pathol. 2008 Winter;19(4):226–40. PMID:18931957
3297. Nosé V. Familial thyroid cancer: a review. Mod Pathol. 2011 Apr;24 Suppl 2:S19–33. PMID:21455198
3298. Nosé V. Genodermatosis affecting the skin and mucosa of the head and neck: clinicopathologic, genetic, and molecular aspect–PTEN-hamartoma tumor syndrome/ Cowden syndrome. Head Neck Pathol. 2016 Jun;10(2):131–8. PMID:26975628
3299. Nosé V. Thyroid cancer of follicular cell origin in inherited tumor syndromes. Adv Anat Pathol. 2010 Nov;17(6):428–36. PMID:20966648
3300. Nosé V, Ezzat S, Horvath E, et al. Protocol for the examination of specimens from patients with primary pituitary tumors. Arch Pathol Lab Med. 2011 May;135(5):640–6. PMID:21526962
3301. Nose-Alberti V, Mesquita MI, Martin LC, et al. Adrenocorticotropin-producing pituitary carcinoma with expression of c-erbB-2 and high PCNA index: a comparative study with pituitary adenomas and normal pituitary tissues. Endocr Pathol. 1998 Spring;9(1):53–62. PMID:12114662
3302. Novotný F, Konopík J. [Report on the resuming of cooperation between the Czechoslovak Dermato-Venereological Society and the Allunion Scientific Society of Dermatologists and Venereologists of the USSR]. Cesk Dermatol. 1978 Feb;53(2):141–2. Czech. PMID:657301
3303. Nozaki Y, Yamamoto H, Iwasaki T, et al. Clinicopathological features and immunohistochemical utility of NTRK-, ALK-, and ROS1-rearranged papillary thyroid carcinomas and anaplastic thyroid carcinomas. Hum Pathol. 2020 Dec;106:82–92. PMID:32980422
3304. Nozières C, Chardon L, Goichot B, et al. Neuroendocrine tumors producing calcitonin: characteristics, prognosis and potential interest of calcitonin monitoring during follow-up. Eur J Endocrinol. 2016 Mar;174(3):335–41. PMID:26671974
3305. Ntali G, Capatina C, Grossman A, et al. Clinical review: functioning gonadotroph adenomas. J Clin Endocrinol Metab. 2014 Dec;99(12):4423–33. PMID:25166722
3306. Nunez AL, Elgin JN, Fatima H. Fine-needle aspiration biopsy of alveolar rhabdomyosarcoma of Stensen's duct: a case report and review of the literature. Diagn Cytopathol. 2014 Dec;42(12):1069–74. PMID:24599626
3307. Nwokoro NA, Korytkowski MT, Rose S, et al. Spectrum of malignancy and premalignancy in Carney syndrome. Am J Med Genet. 1997 Dec 31;73(4):369–77. PMID:9415461
3308. Oak CY, Kim HK, Yoon TM, et al. Benign teratoma of the thyroid gland. Endocrinol Metab (Seoul). 2013 Jun;28(2):144–8. PMID:24396669
3309. Obari A, Sano T, Ohyama K, et al. Clinicopathological features of growth hormone-producing pituitary adenomas: difference among various types defined by cytokeratin distribution pattern including a transitional form. Endocr Pathol. 2008 Summer;19(2):82–91. PMID:18629656
3310. Oberg K, Modlin IM, De Herder W, et al. Consensus on biomarkers for neuroendocrine tumour disease. Lancet Oncol. 2015 Sep;16(9):e435–46. PMID:26370353
3311. O'Brien T, Young WF Jr, Davila DG, et al. Cushing's syndrome associated with ectopic production of corticotrophin-releasing hormone, corticotrophin and vasopressin by a phaeochromocytoma. Clin Endocrinol (Oxf). 1992 Nov;37(5):460–7. PMID:1283118
3312. Occhi G, Regazzo D, Trivellin G, et al. A novel mutation in the upstream open reading frame of the CDKN1B gene causes a MEN4 phenotype. PLoS Genet. 2013 Mar;9(3):e1003350. PMID:23555276
3313. Odate T, Oishi N, Kawai M, et al. Progression of papillary thyroid carcinoma to anaplastic carcinoma in metastatic lymph nodes: solid/insular growth and hobnail cell change in lymph nodes are predictors of subsequent anaplastic transformation. Endocr Pathol. 2021 Sep;32(3):347–56. PMID:33761111
3314. Odate T, Oishi N, Vuong HG, et al. Genetic differences in follicular thyroid carcinoma between Asian and Western countries: a systematic review. Gland Surg. 2020 Oct;9(5):1813–26. PMID:33224857
3315. Odrzywolski KJ, Mukhopadhyay S. Papillary cystadenoma of the epididymis. Arch Pathol Lab Med. 2010 Apr;134(4):630–3. PMID:20367315
3316. Offergeld C, Brase C, Yaremchuk S, et al. Head and neck paragangliomas: clinical and molecular genetic classification. Clinics (Sao Paulo). 2012 Suppl 1(Suppl 1):19-28. PMID:22584701
3317. O'Gorman CS, Hamilton J, Rachmiel M, et al. Thyroid cancer in childhood: a retrospective review of childhood course. Thyroid. 2010 Apr;20(4):375–80. PMID:20373982
3318. Ogundoyin OO, Ogun G, Oluwasola A, et al. Spindle epithelial tumor of thymus-like differentiation (SETTLE) in a 3-year-old African girl. Clin Case Rep. 2019 Apr 25;7(6):1119–22. PMID:31183079
3319. Oh CM, Jung KW, Won YJ, et al. Age-period-cohort analysis of thyroid cancer incidence in Korea. Cancer Res Treat. 2015 Jul;47(3):362–9. PMID:25672579
3320. Oh EJ, Lee S, Bae JS, et al. TERT promoter mutation in an aggressive cribriform morular variant of papillary thyroid carcinoma. Endocr Pathol. 2017 Mar;28(1):49–53. PMID:27688081
3321. Oh JE, Ohta T, Satomi K, et al. Alterations in the NF2/LATS1/LATS2/YAP pathway in schwannomas. J Neuropathol Exp Neurol. 2015 Oct;74(10):952–9. PMID:26360373
3322. Oh JS, Kim HJ, Hann HJ, et al. Incidence, mortality, and cardiovascular diseases in pituitary adenoma in Korea: a nationwide population-based study. Pituitary. 2021 Feb;24(1):38–47. PMID:32949324
3323. Oh YL, Ko YH, Ree HJ. Aspiration cytology of ectopic cervical thymoma mimicking a thyroid mass. A case report. Acta Cytol. 1998 Sep-Oct;42(5):1167–71. PMID:9755676
3324. Ohara Y, Oda T, Hashimoto S, et al. Pancreatic neuroendocrine tumor and solid-pseudopapillary neoplasm: key immunohistochemical profiles for differential diagnosis. World J Gastroenterol. 2016 Oct 14;22(38):8596–604. PMID:27784972
3325. Ohashi R. Solid variant of papillary thyroid carcinoma: an under-recognized entity. Endocr J. 2020 Mar 28;67(3):241–8. PMID:31983699
3326. Ohashi R, Kawahara K, Namimatsu S, et al. Clinicopathological significance of a solid component in papillary thyroid carcinoma.

Histopathology. 2017 Apr;70(5):775–81. PMID:27882585
3327. Ohashi R, Murase Y, Matsubara M, et al. Fine needle aspiration cytology of the papillary thyroid carcinoma with a solid component: a cytological and clinical correlation. Diagn Cytopathol. 2017 May;45(5):391–8. PMID:28224716
3328. Ohike N, Jürgensen A, Pipeleers-Marichal M, et al. Mixed ductal-endocrine carcinomas of the pancreas and ductal adenocarcinomas with scattered endocrine cells: characterization of the endocrine cells. Virchows Arch. 2003 Mar;442(3):258–65. PMID:12647216
3329. Ohike N, Kosmahl M, Klöppel G. Mixed acinar-endocrine carcinoma of the pancreas. A clinicopathological study and comparison with acinar-cell carcinoma. Virchows Arch. 2004 Sep;445(3):231–5. PMID:15517367
3330. Ohike N, Morohoshi T. Exocrine pancreatic neoplasms of nonductal origin: acinar cell carcinoma, pancreatoblastoma, and solid-pseudopapillary neoplasm. Surg Pathol Clin. 2011 Jun;4(2):579–88. PMID:26837489
3331. Ohsugi H, Takizawa N, Kinoshita H, et al. Pheochromocytoma arising from an ectopic adrenal tissue in multiple endocrine neoplasia type 2A. Endocrinol Diabetes Metab Case Rep. 2019 Oct 12;2019:19-0073. PMID:31610522
3332. Ohtake H, Yamakawa M. Interdigitating dendritic cell sarcoma and follicular dendritic cell sarcoma: histopathological findings for differential diagnosis. J Clin Exp Hematop. 2013;53(3):179–84. PMID:24369219
3333. Ohtsuki Y, Watanabe R, Okada Y, et al. Composite paraganglioma and ganglioneuroma in the retroperitoneum: a case report. Med Mol Morphol. 2012 Jun;45(3):168–72. PMID:23001299
3334. Oka H, Kameya T, Sasano H, et al. Pituitary choristoma composed of corticotrophs and adrenocortical cells in the sella turcica. Virchows Arch. 1996 Mar;427(6):613–7. PMID:8605573
3335. Okada Y, Matsushita S, Yamaguchi K. Investigation of Cushing's and subclinical Cushing's syndromes using adrenocortical scintigraphy. Nucl Med Commun. 2021 Jun 1;42(6):619–24. PMID:33596032
3336. Okamatsu C, London WB, Naranjo A, et al. Clinicopathological characteristics of ganglioneuroma and ganglioneuroblastoma: a report from the CCG and COG. Pediatr Blood Cancer. 2009 Oct;53(4):563–9. PMID:19530234
3337. O'Kane AM, O'Donnell ME, Shah R, et al. Small cell carcinoma of the appendix. World J Surg Oncol. 2008 Jan 15;6:4. PMID:18197972
3338. Okazaki M, Sano Y, Soga Y, et al. Combined atypical carcinoid tumour and squamous cell carcinoma of the lung. Intern Med. 2015;54(11):1385–8. PMID:26027992
3339. Okubo Y. Gangliocytic paraganglioma: an overview and future perspective. World J Clin Oncol. 2019 Sep 24;10(9):300–2. PMID:31572665
3340. Okubo Y, Nemoto T, Wakayama M, et al. Gangliocytic paraganglioma: a multi-institutional retrospective study in Japan. BMC Cancer. 2015 Apr 12;15:269. PMID:25886293
3341. Okubo Y, Sakai M, Yamazaki H, et al. Histopathological study of carcinoma showing thymus-like differentiation (CASTLE). Malays J Pathol. 2020 Aug;42(2):259–65. PMID:32860379
3342. Okubo Y, Wakayama M, Nemoto T, et al. Literature survey on epidemiology and pathology of gangliocytic paraganglioma. BMC Cancer. 2011 May 20;11:187. PMID:21599949
3343. Okubo Y, Yokose T, Motohashi O, et al. Duodenal rare neuroendocrine tumor: clinicopathological characteristics of patients with gangliocytic paraganglioma. Gastroenterol Res Pract. 2016;2016:5257312. PMID:28096810
3344. Okubo Y, Yoshioka E, Suzuki M, et al. Diagnosis, pathological findings, and clinical management of gangliocytic paraganglioma: a systematic review. Front Oncol. 2018 Jul 27;8:291. PMID:30101131
3345. Okuyucu K, Alagoz E, Arslan N, et al. Clinicopathologic features and prognostic factors of tall cell variant of papillary thyroid carcinoma: comparison with classic variant of papillary thyroid carcinoma. Nucl Med Commun. 2015 Oct;36(10):1021–5. PMID:26225942
3346. Oldfield EH, Vance ML, Louis RG, et al. Crooke's changes in Cushing's syndrome depends on degree of hypercortisolism and individual susceptibility. J Clin Endocrinol Metab. 2015 Aug;100(8):3165–71. PMID:26147609
3347. Oliver RL, Davis JR, White A. Characterisation of ACTH related peptides in ectopic Cushing's syndrome. Pituitary. 2003;6(3):119–26. PMID:14971736
3348. Olmedilla Y, Khan S, Young V, et al. Plurihormonal Pit-1 lineage adenoma presenting as meningitis with recurrence after somatostatin analogue. Endocrinol Diabetes Metab Case Rep. 2019 Mar 21;2019:18-0130. PMID:30897548
3349. Olofson AM, Tafe LJ. A case of a primary lung cancer comprised of adenocarcinoma and atypical carcinoid tumor with both components harboring BRAF p.V600E mutation. Exp Mol Pathol. 2018 Feb;104(1):26–8. PMID:29248665
3350. Olsen CM, Pandeya N, Whiteman DC. International increases in Merkel cell carcinoma incidence rates between 1997 and 2016. J Invest Dermatol. 2021 Nov;141(11):2596–2601.e1. PMID:33932460
3351. Olsson DS, Andersson E, Bryngelsson IL, et al. Excess mortality and morbidity in patients with craniopharyngioma, especially in patients with childhood onset: a population-based study in Sweden. J Clin Endocrinol Metab. 2015 Feb;100(2):467–74. PMID:25375987
3352. Omofoye OA, Lechpammer M, Steele TO, et al. Pituitary stalk gangliogliomas: case report and literature review. Clin Neurol Neurosurg. 2021 Feb;201:106405. PMID:33340839
3353. Oneal PA, Kwitkowski V, Luo L, et al. FDA approval summary: vemurafenib for the treatment of patients with Erdheim-Chester disease with the BRAFV600 mutation. Oncologist. 2018 Dec;23(12):1520–4. PMID:30120160
3354. O'Neill CJ, Vaughan L, Learoyd DL, et al. Management of follicular thyroid carcinoma should be individualised based on degree of capsular and vascular invasion. Eur J Surg Oncol. 2011 Feb;37(2):181–5. PMID:21144693
3355. Onozawa M, Fukuhara T, Minoguchi M, et al. Hypokalemic rhabdomyolysis due to WDHA syndrome caused by VIP-producing composite pheochromocytoma: a case in neurofibromatosis type 1. Jpn J Clin Oncol. 2005 Sep;35(9):559–63. PMID:16027147
3356. Opsahl EM, Akslen LA, Schlichting E, et al. Trends in diagnostics, surgical treatment, and prognostic factors for outcomes in medullary thyroid carcinoma in Norway: a nationwide population-based study. Eur Thyroid J. 2019 Jan;8(1):31–40. PMID:30800639
3357. Ordóñez NG. Value of GATA3 immunostaining in the diagnosis of parathyroid tumors. Appl Immunohistochem Mol Morphol. 2014 Nov-Dec;22(10):756–61. PMID:25046229
3358. Ordóñez NG. Value of GATA3 immunostaining in tumor diagnosis: a review. Adv Anat Pathol. 2013 Sep;20(5):352–60. PMID:23939152
3359. Orgiazzi J. [Multinodular goiter: natural history]. Ann Chir. 1999;53(3):233–6. French. PMID:10339866
3360. Orois A, Gara SK, Mora M, et al. NOP53 as a candidate modifier locus for familial non-medullary thyroid cancer. Genes (Basel). 2019 Nov 7;10(11):899. PMID:31703244
3361. Orrell JM, Hales SA. Paragangliomas of the cauda equina have a distinctive cytokeratin immunophenotype. Histopathology. 1992 Nov;21(5):479–81. PMID:1280616
3362. Orselli RC, Bassler TJ. Theca granuloma cell tumor arising in adrenal. Cancer. 1973 Feb;31(2):474–7. PMID:4687888
3363. Ortiz E, Peldoza M, Monnier E, et al. Ectopic pituitary adenoma of the TSH-secreting sphenoidal sinus with excellent response to somatostatin analogs. Theory of the embryogenesis and literature review from a clinical case. Steroids. 2020 Feb;154:108535. PMID:31704334
3364. Osawa N, Onoda N, Kawajiri H, et al. Diagnosis of parathyroid carcinoma using immunohistochemical staining against hTERT. Int J Mol Med. 2009 Dec;24(6):733–41. PMID:19885612
3365. Oshima J, Martin GM, Hisama FM. Werner syndrome. In: Adam MP, Feldman J, Mirzaa GM, et al., editors. GeneReviews. Seattle (WA): University of Washington, Seattle; 2002 Dec 2 [updated 2021 May 13]. PMID:20301687
3366. Oshima J, Sidorova JM, Monnat RJ Jr. Werner syndrome: clinical features, pathogenesis and potential therapeutic interventions. Ageing Res Rev. 2017 Jan;33:105–14. PMID:26993153
3367. Osinga TE, Korpershoek E, de Krijger RR, et al. Catecholamine-synthesizing enzymes are expressed in parasympathetic head and neck paraganglioma tissue. Neuroendocrinology. 2015;101(4):289–95. PMID:25677368
3368. O'steen L, Indelicato DJ. Advances in the management of craniopharyngioma. F1000Res. 20187
3369. Ostrom QT, Gittleman H, Liao P, et al. CBTRUS statistical report: primary brain and central nervous system tumors diagnosed in the United States in 2007-2011. Neuro Oncol. 2014 Oct;16 Suppl 4(Suppl 4):iv1-63. PMID:25304271
3370. Ostrom QT, Gittleman H, Truitt G, et al. CBTRUS statistical report: primary brain and other central nervous system tumors diagnosed in the United States in 2011-2015. Neuro Oncol. 2018 Oct 1;20(suppl_4):iv1–86. PMID:30445539
3371. Osuga T, Hayashi T, Ishiwatari H, et al. Pancreatic metastasis from a solitary fibrous tumor of the central nervous system. JOP. 2014 Jan 10;15(1):58–62. PMID:24413787
3372. O'Toole K, Fenoglio-Preiser C, Pushparaj N. Endocrine changes associated with the human aging process: III. Effect of age on the number of calcitonin immunoreactive cells in the thyroid gland. Hum Pathol. 1985 Oct;16(10):991–1000. PMID:3899904
3373. Otsuka H, Kohashi K, Yoshimoto M, et al. Immunohistochemical evaluation of H3K27 trimethylation in malignant peripheral nerve sheath tumors. Pathol Res Pract. 2018 Mar;214(3):417–25. PMID:29482987
3374. Otto AI, Marschalko M, Zalatnai A, et al. Glucagon cell adenomatosis: a new entity associated with necrolytic migratory erythema and glucagonoma syndrome. J Am Acad Dermatol. 2011 Aug;65(2):458–9. PMID:21763589
3375. Oudijk L, Gaal J, de Krijger RR. The role of immunohistochemistry and molecular analysis of succinate dehydrogenase in the diagnosis of endocrine and non-endocrine tumors and related syndromes. Endocr Pathol. 2019 Mar;30(1):64–73. PMID:30421319
3376. Owens CL, Fraire AE. Combined carcinoid tumor and squamous cell carcinoma of lung: expanding the spectrum of combined tumors of lung. Int J Surg Pathol. 2011 Apr;19(2):273–5. PMID:21427100
3377. Oyama K, Sanno N, Teramoto A, et al. Expression of neuro D1 in human normal pituitaries and pituitary adenomas. Mod Pathol. 2001 Sep;14(9):892–9. PMID:11557786
3378. Oyewumi M, Inarejos E, Greer ML, et al. Ultrasound to differentiate thyroglossal duct cysts and dermoid cysts in children. Laryngoscope. 2015 Apr;125(4):998–1003. PMID:25234770
3379. Øystese KA, Casar-Borota O, Normann KR, et al. Estrogen receptor α, a sex-dependent predictor of aggressiveness in nonfunctioning pituitary adenomas: SSTR and sex hormone receptor distribution in NFPA. J Clin Endocrinol Metab. 2017 Sep 1;102(9):3581–90. PMID:28911153
3380. Ozkara SK, Gürbüz Y, Müezzinoğlu B, et al. Encapsulated cystic papillary variant of medullary carcinoma of thyroid gland. Endocr Pathol. 2002 Summer;13(2):167–71. PMID:12165666
3381. Ozolek JA. Selected topics in the pathology of the thyroid and parathyroid glands in children and adolescents. Head Neck Pathol. 2021 Mar;15(1):85–106. PMID:33723755
3382. Oztürk O, Demirci L, Egeli E, et al. Papillary carcinoma of the thyroglossal duct cyst in childhood. Eur Arch Otorhinolaryngol. 2003 Nov;260(10):541–3. PMID:12764621
3383. Ozturk Sari S, Taskin OC, Gundogdu G, et al. The impact of phosphohistone-H3-assisted mitotic count and Ki67 score in the determination of tumor grade and prediction of distant metastasis in well-differentiated pancreatic neuroendocrine tumors. Endocr Pathol. 2016 Jun;27(2):162–70. PMID:26936845
3384. Özyurt J, Müller HL, Thiel CM. A systematic review of cognitive performance in patients with childhood craniopharyngioma. J Neurooncol. 2015 Oct;125(1):9–21. PMID:26369768
3385. Pacini F, Castagna MG, Cipri C, et al. Medullary thyroid carcinoma. Clin Oncol (R Coll Radiol). 2010 Aug;22(6):475–85. PMID:20627492
3386. Pacini F, Elisei R, Romei C, et al. RET proto-oncogene mutations in thyroid carcinomas: clinical relevance. J Endocrinol Invest. 2000 May;23(5):328–38. PMID:10882153
3387. Paik JY, Hall G, Clarkson A, et al. Immunohistochemistry for Merkel cell polyomavirus is highly specific but not sensitive for the diagnosis of Merkel cell carcinoma in the Australian population. Hum Pathol. 2011 Oct;42(10):1385–90. PMID:21453956
3388. Paja M, Zafón C, Iglesias C, et al. Rate of non-invasive follicular thyroid neoplasms with papillary-like nuclear features depends on pathologist's criteria: a multicentre retrospective Southern European study with prolonged follow-up. Endocrine. 2021 Jul;73(1):131–40. PMID:33484411
3389. Pak K, Suh S, Goh TS, et al. BRAF-positive multifocal and unifocal papillary thyroid cancer show different messenger RNA expressions. Clin Endocrinol (Oxf). 2019 Apr;90(4):601–7. PMID:30592330
3390. Pakbaz S, Mete O. Adrenal cortical neoplasia: from histology to molecular biology. Diagn Histopathol. 2019 May;25(5):178–89. doi:10.1016/j.mpdhp.2019.02.004.
3391. Paker I, Kokenek TD, Yılmazer D, et al. Oncocytic variant of papillary thyroid carcinoma with lymphocytic stroma (Warthin-like variant): report of a case with fine needle aspiration cytology and review of the literature. Cytopathology. 2012 Dec;23(6):408–10. PMID:21645139
3392. Pal T, Vogl FD, Chappuis PO, et al. Increased risk for nonmedullary thyroid cancer in the first degree relatives of prevalent cases of nonmedullary thyroid cancer: a hospital-based study. J Clin Endocrinol Metab. 2001

Nov;86(11):5307–12. PMID:11701697
3393. Pallares J, Perez-Ruiz L, Ros S, et al. Malignant peripheral nerve sheath tumor of the thyroid: a clinicopathological and ultrastructural study of one case. Endocr Pathol. 2004 Summer;15(2):167–74. PMID:15299203
3394. Palos-Paz F, Perez-Guerra O, Cameselle-Teijeiro J, et al. Prevalence of mutations in TSHR, GNAS, PRKAR1A and RAS genes in a large series of toxic thyroid adenomas from Galicia, an iodine-deficient area in NW Spain. Eur J Endocrinol. 2008 Nov;159(5):623–31. PMID:18694911
3395. Pamporaki C, Hamplova B, Peitzsch M, et al. Characteristics of pediatric vs adult pheochromocytomas and paragangliomas. J Clin Endocrinol Metab. 2017 Apr 1;102(4):1122–32. PMID:28324046
3396. Pan CC, Chung MY, Ng KF, et al. Constant allelic alteration on chromosome 16p (TSC2 gene) in perivascular epithelioid cell tumour (PEComa): genetic evidence for the relationship of PEComa with angiomyolipoma. J Pathol. 2008 Feb;214(3):387–93. PMID:18085521
3397. Pan J, Qi S, Liu Y, et al. Growth patterns of craniopharyngiomas: clinical analysis of 226 patients. J Neurosurg Pediatr. 2016 Apr;17(4):418–33. PMID:26636252
3398. Pan KS, Heiss JD, Brown SM, et al. Chiari I malformation and basilar invagination in fibrous dysplasia: prevalence, mechanisms, and clinical implications. J Bone Miner Res. 2018 Nov;33(11):1990–8. PMID:29924878
3399. Pan Z, Kleinschmidt-DeMasters BK. CNS Erdheim-Chester disease: a challenge to diagnose. J Neuropathol Exp Neurol. 2017 Dec 1;76(12):986–96. PMID:29096034
3400. Pandey P, Ojha BK, Mahapatra AK. Pediatric pituitary adenoma: a series of 42 patients. J Clin Neurosci. 2005 Feb;12(2):124–7. PMID:15749410
3401. Pandeya N, McLeod DS, Balasubramaniam K, et al. Increasing thyroid cancer incidence in Queensland, Australia 1982-2008 - true increase or overdiagnosis? Clin Endocrinol (Oxf). 2016 Feb;84(2):257–64. PMID:25597380
3402. Pandya C, Uzilov AV, Bellizzi J, et al. Genomic profiling reveals mutational landscape in parathyroid carcinomas. JCI Insight. 2017 Mar 23;2(6):e92061. PMID:28352668
3403. Panebianco F, Nikitski AV, Nikiforova MN, et al. Characterization of thyroid cancer driven by known and novel ALK fusions. Endocr Relat Cancer. 2019 Nov;26(11):803–14. PMID:31539879
3404. Panebianco F, Nikitski AV, Nikiforova MN, et al. Spectrum of TERT promoter mutations and mechanisms of activation in thyroid cancer. Cancer Med. 2019 Oct;8(13):5831–9. PMID:31408918
3405. Panicker LM, Zhang JH, Dagur PK, et al. Defective nucleolar localization and dominant interfering properties of a parafibromin L95P missense mutant causing the hyperparathyroidism-jaw tumor syndrome. Endocr Relat Cancer. 2010 May 18;17(2):513–24. PMID:20304979
3406. Paniza ACJ, Mendes TB, Viana MDB, et al. Revised criteria for diagnosis of NIFTP reveals a better correlation with tumor biological behavior. Endocr Connect. 2019 Nov;8(11):1529–38. PMID:31671409
3407. Papaconstantinou D, Machairas N, Damaskou V, et al. Duodenal gangliocytic paraganglioma, successfully treated by local surgical excision-a case report. Int J Surg Case Rep. 2017;32:5–8. PMID:28213067
3408. Papanikolaou A, Michala L. Autonomous ovarian cysts in prepubertal girls. How aggressive should we be? A review of the literature. J Pediatr Adolesc Gynecol. 2015 Oct;28(5):292–6. PMID:26228588
3409. Papathomas TG, Duregon E, Korpershoek E, et al. Sarcomatoid adrenocortical carcinoma: a comprehensive pathological, immunohistochemical, and targeted next-generation sequencing analysis. Hum Pathol. 2016 Dec;58:113–22. PMID:27589897
3410. Papathomas TG, Gaal J, Corssmit EP, et al. Non-pheochromocytoma (PCC)/paraganglioma (PGL) tumors in patients with succinate dehydrogenase-related PCC-PGL syndromes: a clinicopathological and molecular analysis. Eur J Endocrinol. 2013 Nov 22;170(1):1–12. PMID:24096523
3411. Papathomas TG, Nosé V. New and emerging biomarkers in endocrine pathology. Adv Anat Pathol. 2019 May;26(3):198–209. PMID:30730313
3412. Papathomas TG, Oudijk L, Persu A, et al. SDHB/SDHA immunohistochemistry in pheochromocytomas and paragangliomas: a multicenter interobserver variation analysis using virtual microscopy: a Multinational Study of the European Network for the Study of Adrenal Tumors (ENS@T). Mod Pathol. 2015 Jun;28(6):807–21. PMID:25720320
3413. Papathomas TG, Oudijk L, Zwarthoff EC, et al. Telomerase reverse transcriptase promoter mutations in tumors originating from the adrenal gland and extra-adrenal paraganglia. Endocr Relat Cancer. 2014 Aug;21(4):653–61. PMID:24951106
3414. Papathomas TG, Pucci E, Giordano TJ, et al. An international Ki67 reproducibility study in adrenal cortical carcinoma. Am J Surg Pathol. 2016 Apr;40(4):569–76. PMID:26685085
3415. Papathomas TG, Suurd DPD, Pacak K, et al. What have we learned from molecular biology̌ of paragangliomas and pheochromocytomas? Endocr Pathol. 2021 Mar;32(1):134–53. PMID:33433885
3416. Papi G, Corrado S, LiVolsi VA. Primary spindle cell lesions of the thyroid gland; an overview. Am J Clin Pathol. 2006 Jun;125 Suppl:S95–123. PMID:16830961
3417. Papi G, Fadda G, Corsello SM, et al. Metastases to the thyroid gland: prevalence, clinicopathological aspects and prognosis: a 10-year experience. Clin Endocrinol (Oxf). 2007 Apr;66(4):565–71. PMID:17371476
3418. Papo M, Emile JF, Maciel TT, et al. Erdheim-Chester disease: a concise review. Curr Rheumatol Rep. 2019 Dec 5;21(12):66. PMID:31807955
3419. Papotti M, Arrondini M, Tavaglione V, et al. Diagnostic controversies in vascular proliferations of the thyroid gland. Endocr Pathol. 2008 Fall;19(3):175–83. PMID:18766472
3420. Papotti M, Duregon E, Volante M, et al. Pathology of the adrenal cortex: a reappraisal of the past 25 years focusing on adrenal cortical tumors. Endocr Pathol. 2014 Mar;25(1):35–48. PMID:24382573
3421. Papotti M, Manazza AD, Chiarle R, et al. Confocal microscope analysis and tridimensional reconstruction of papillary thyroid carcinoma nuclei. Virchows Arch. 2004 Apr;444(4):350–5. PMID:14758551
3422. Papotti M, Negro F, Carney JA, et al. Mixed medullary-follicular carcinoma of the thyroid. A morphological, immunohistochemical and in situ hybridization analysis of 11 cases. Virchows Arch. 1997 May;430(5):397–405. PMID:9174630
3423. Papotti M, Sambataro D, Pecchioni C, et al. The pathology of medullary carcinoma of the thyroid: review of the literature and personal experience on 62 cases. Endocr Pathol. 1996 Spring;7(1):1–20. PMID:12114676
3424. Papotti M, Volante M, Duregon E, et al. Adrenocortical tumors with myxoid features: a distinct morphologic and phenotypical variant exhibiting malignant behavior. Am J Surg Pathol. 2010 Jul;34(7):973–83. PMID:20534995
3425. Papotti M, Volante M, Giuliano A, et al. RET/PTC activation in hyalinizing trabecular tumors of the thyroid. Am J Surg Pathol. 2000 Dec;24(12):1615–21. PMID:11117781
3426. Papotti M, Volante M, Komminoth P, et al. Thyroid carcinomas with mixed follicular and C-cell differentiation patterns. Semin Diagn Pathol. 2000 May;17(2):109–19. PMID:10839611
3427. Pareja F, Brandes AH, Basili T, et al. Loss-of-function mutations in ATP6AP1 and ATP6AP2 in granular cell tumors. Nat Commun. 2018 Aug 30;9(1):3533. PMID:30166553
3428. Parelkar SV, Sampat NP, Sanghvi BV, et al. Case report of bilateral adrenal leiomyoma with review of literature. Pediatr Surg Int. 2013 Jun;29(6):655–8. PMID:23354505
3429. Parente DN, Kluijfhout WP, Bongers PJ, et al. Clinical safety of renaming encapsulated follicular variant of papillary thyroid carcinoma: Is NIFTP truly benign? World J Surg. 2018 Feb;42(2):321–6. PMID:28828746
3430. Parfitt AM, Wang Q, Palnitkar S. Rates of cell proliferation in adenomatous, suppressed, and normal parathyroid tissue: implications for pathogenesis. J Clin Endocrinol Metab. 1998 Mar;83(3):863–9. PMID:9506741
3431. Parfitt JR, McLean CA, Joseph MG, et al. Granular cell tumours of the gastrointestinal tract: expression of nestin and clinicopathological evaluation of 11 patients. Histopathology. 2006 Mar;48(4):424–30. PMID:16487364
3432. Parham DM, Barr FG. Classification of rhabdomyosarcoma and its molecular basis. Adv Anat Pathol. 2013 Nov;20(6):387–97. PMID:24113309
3433. Park DH, Park YK, Oh JI, et al. Oncocytic paraganglioma of the cauda equina in a child. Case report and review of the literature. Pediatr Neurosurg. 2002 May;36(5):260–5. PMID:12053045
3434. Park HK, Han HS. Duodenal gangliocytic paraganglioma with lymph node metastasis. Arch Pathol Lab Med. 2016 Jan;140(1):94–8. PMID:26717062
3435. Park J, Kim JW, Park H, et al. Multifocality in a patient with cribriform-morular variant of papillary thyroid carcinoma is an important clue for the diagnosis of familial adenomatous polyposis. Thyroid. 2019 Nov;29(11):1606–14. PMID:31469036
3436. Park J, Lee S, Kim K, et al. TERT promoter mutations and the 8th edition TNM classification in predicting the survival of thyroid cancer patients. Cancers (Basel). 2021 Feb;13(4):648. PMID:33562809
3437. Park JK, Paik WH, Lee K, et al. DAXX/ATRX and MEN1 genes are strong prognostic markers in pancreatic neuroendocrine tumors. Oncotarget. 2017 Jul 25;8(30):49796–806. PMID:28591701
3438. Park JR, Bagatell R, London WB, et al. Children's Oncology Group's 2013 blueprint for research: neuroblastoma. Pediatr Blood Cancer. 2013 Jun;60(6):985–93. PMID:23255319
3439. Park P, Chandler WF, Barkan AL, et al. The role of radiation therapy after surgical resection of nonfunctional pituitary macroadenomas. Neurosurgery. 2004 Jul;55(1):100–6. PMID:15214978
3440. Park S, Kim HS, Park KS, et al. A case of coincidental intrasellar chordoma and pituitary adenoma. Brain Tumor Res Treat. 2017 Apr;5(1):49–52. PMID:28516081
3441. Park SH, Suh EH, Chi JG. A histopathologic study on 1,095 surgically resected thyroid specimens. Jpn J Clin Oncol. 1988 Dec;18(4):297–302. PMID:3204680
3442. Park SY, Rhee Y, Youn JC, et al. Ectopic Cushing's syndrome due to concurrent corticotropin-releasing hormone (CRH) and adrenocorticotropic hormone (ACTH) secreted by malignant gastrinoma. Exp Clin Endocrinol Diabetes. 2007 Jan;115(1):13–6. PMID:17286228
3443. Park YJ, Ahn HY, Choi HS, et al. The long-term outcomes of the second generation of familial nonmedullary thyroid carcinoma are more aggressive than sporadic cases. Thyroid. 2012 Apr;22(4):356–62. PMID:22280228
3444. Park YJ, Kim YA, Lee YJ, et al. Papillary microcarcinoma in comparison with larger papillary thyroid carcinoma in BRAF(V600E) mutation, clinicopathological features, and immunohistochemical findings. Head Neck. 2010 Jan;32(1):38–45. PMID:19475551
3445. Parker KG, White MG, Cipriani NA. Comparison of molecular methods and BRAF immunohistochemistry (VE1 clone) for the detection of BRAF V600E mutation in papillary thyroid carcinoma: a meta-analysis. Head Neck Pathol. 2020 Dec;14(4):1067–79. PMID:32358715
3446. Parker LA, Vincent LM. Detection of adrenal melanoma with computed tomography. Urol Radiol. 1986;8(4):209–10. PMID:3798606
3447. Parker LN, Kollin J, Wu SY, et al. Carcinoma of the thyroid with a mixed medullary, papillary, follicular, and undifferentiated pattern. Arch Intern Med. 1985 Aug;145(8):1507–9. PMID:3896182
3448. Parma J, Duprez L, Van Sande J, et al. Somatic mutations in the thyrotropin receptor gene cause hyperfunctioning thyroid adenomas. Nature. 1993 Oct 14;365(6447):649–51. PMID:8413627
3449. Partelli S, Ramage JK, Massironi S, et al. Management of asymptomatic sporadic nonfunctioning pancreatic neuroendocrine neoplasms (ASPEN) ≤2 cm: study protocol for a prospective observational study. Front Med (Lausanne). 2020 Dec 23;7:598438. PMID:33425946
3450. Partington MD, Davis DH, Laws ER Jr, et al. Pituitary adenomas in childhood and adolescence. Results of transsphenoidal surgery. J Neurosurg. 1994 Feb;80(2):209–16. PMID:8283258
3451. Parvanescu A, Cros J, Ronot M, et al. Lessons from McCune-Albright syndrome-associated intraductal papillary mucinous neoplasms: GNAS-activating mutations in pancreatic carcinogenesis. JAMA Surg. 2014 Aug;149(8):858–62. PMID:24898823
3452. Parwani AV, Galindo R, Steinberg DM, et al. Solitary fibrous tumor of the thyroid: cytopathologic findings and differential diagnosis. Diagn Cytopathol. 2003 Apr;28(4):213–6. PMID:12672098
3453. Pascual JM, Prieto R, Castro-Dufourny I, et al. Craniopharyngiomas primarily involving the hypothalamus: a model of neurosurgical lesions to elucidate the neurobiological basis of psychiatric disorders. World Neurosurg. 2018 Dec;120:e1245–78. PMID:30240857
3454. Pascual JM, Prieto R, Castro-Dufourny I, et al. Topographic diagnosis of papillary craniopharyngiomas: the need for an accurate MRI-surgical correlation. AJNR Am J Neuroradiol. 2015 Aug;36(8):E55–6. PMID:26113067
3455. Pasquali D, Torella A, Accardo G, et al. BROX haploinsufficiency in familial nonmedullary thyroid cancer. J Endocrinol Invest. 2021 Jan;44(1):165–71. PMID:32385852
3456. Pasquali S, Gronchi A, Strauss D, et al. Resectable extra-pleural and extra-meningeal solitary fibrous tumours: a multi-centre prognostic study. Eur J Surg Oncol. 2016 Jul;42(7):1064–70. PMID:26924782
3457. Pasternak S, Carter MD, Ly TY, et al. Immunohistochemical profiles of different subsets of Merkel cell carcinoma. Hum Pathol. 2018 Dec;82:232–8. PMID:30067951

3458. Patchefsky AS, Hoch WS. Psammoma bodies in diffuse toxic goiter. Am J Clin Pathol. 1972 May;57(5):551–6. PMID:4337189
3459. Patel K, Allen J, Zagzag D, et al. Radiologic response to MEK inhibition in a patient with a WNT-activated craniopharyngioma. Pediatr Blood Cancer. 2021 Mar;68(3):e28753. PMID:33073916
3460. Patel KJ, Chandana SR, Wiese DA, et al. Unusual presentation of large-cell poorly differentiated neuroendocrine carcinoma of the epiglottis. J Clin Oncol. 2010 Sep 20;28(27):e461–3. PMID:20679623
3461. Patel S, Bhatt AA. Thyroglossal duct pathology and mimics. Insights Imaging. 2019 Feb 6;10(1):12. PMID:30725193
3462. Patel S, Jinjuvadia R, Devara A, et al. Performance characteristics of EUS-FNA biopsy for adrenal lesions: a meta-analysis. Endosc Ultrasound. 2019 May-Jun;8(3):180–7. PMID:30880721
3463. Patel TD, Vazquez A, Dubal PM, et al. Sinonasal neuroendocrine carcinoma: a population-based analysis of incidence and survival. Int Forum Allergy Rhinol. 2015 May;5(5):448–53. PMID:25727332
3464. Patel YA, Dhalla S, Olson MT, et al. Pancreatic metastasis from a solitary fibrous tumor of the kidney: a rare cause of acute recurrent pancreatitis. Pancreatology. 2013 Nov-Dec;13(6):631–3. PMID:24280583
3465. Pathak KA, Klonisch T, Nason RW, et al. FDG-PET characteristics of Hürthle cell and follicular adenomas. Ann Nucl Med. 2016 Aug;30(7):506–9. PMID:27221817
3466. Pathmanathan N, Murali R. Composite phaeochromocytoma with intratumoural metastatic squamous cell carcinoma. Pathology. 2003 Jun;35(3):263–5. PMID:14506975
3467. Patrova J, Jarocka I, Wahrenberg H, et al. Clinical outcomes in adrenal incidentaloma: experience from one center. Endocr Pract. 2015 Aug;21(8):870–7. PMID:26121453
3468. Patten DK, Wani Z, Tolley N. Solitary langerhans histiocytosis of the thyroid gland: a case report and literature review. Head Neck Pathol. 2012 Jun;6(2):279–89. PMID:22198822
3469. Paulson KG, Iyer JG, Blom A, et al. Systemic immune suppression predicts diminished Merkel cell carcinoma-specific survival independent of stage. J Invest Dermatol. 2013 Mar;133(3):642–6. PMID:23190897
3470. Paulson KG, Iyer JG, Tegeder AR, et al. Transcriptome-wide studies of Merkel cell carcinoma and validation of intratumoral CD8+ lymphocyte invasion as an independent predictor of survival. J Clin Oncol. 2011 Apr 20;29(12):1539–46. PMID:21422430
3471. Paulson KG, Park SY, Vandeven NA, et al. Merkel cell carcinoma: current US incidence and projected increases based on changing demographics. J Am Acad Dermatol. 2018 Mar;78(3):457–463.e2. PMID:29102486
3472. Paulsson JO, Mu N, Shabo I, et al. TERT aberrancies: a screening tool for malignancy in follicular thyroid tumours. Endocr Relat Cancer. 2018 Jul;25(7):723–33. PMID:29692346
3473. Paulus W, Honegger J, Keyvani K, et al. Xanthogranuloma of the sellar region: a clinicopathological entity different from adamantinomatous craniopharyngioma. Acta Neuropathol. 1999 Apr;97(4):377–82. PMID:10208277
3474. Paulus W, Stöckel C, Krauss J, et al. Odontogenic classification of craniopharyngiomas: a clinicopathological study of 54 cases. Histopathology. 1997 Feb;30(2):172–6. PMID:9067743
3475. Pavlus JD, Carter BW, Tolley MD, et al. Imaging of thoracic neurogenic tumors. AJR Am J Roentgenol. 2016 Sep;207(3):552–61. PMID:27340927
3476. Pazienza V, la Torre A, Baorda F, et al. Identification and functional characterization of three NoLS (nucleolar localisation signals) mutations of the CDC73 gene. PLoS One. 2013 Dec 5;8(12):e82292. PMID:24340015
3477. Pea A, Hruban RH, Wood LD. Genetics of pancreatic neuroendocrine tumors: implications for the clinic. Expert Rev Gastroenterol Hepatol. 2015;9(11):1407–19. PMID:26413978
3478. Peard L, Cost NG, Saltzman AF. Pediatric pheochromocytoma: current status of diagnostic imaging and treatment procedures. Curr Opin Urol. 2019 Sep;29(5):493–9. PMID:31246590
3479. Pease M, Ling C, Mack WJ, et al. The role of epigenetic modification in tumorigenesis and progression of pituitary adenomas: a systematic review of the literature. PLoS One. 2013 Dec 18;8(12):e82619. PMID:24367530
3480. Pecce V, Verrienti A, Abballe L, et al. Loss of function SETD2 mutations in poorly differentiated metastases from two Hürthle cell carcinomas of the thyroid. Cancers (Basel). 2020 Jul 14;12(7):1892. PMID:32674319
3481. Pęczkowska M, Kowalska A, Sygut J, et al. Testing new susceptibility genes in the cohort of apparently sporadic phaeochromocytoma/paraganglioma patients with clinical characteristics of hereditary syndromes. Clin Endocrinol (Oxf). 2013 Dec;79(6):817–23. PMID:23551045
3482. Pedersen RK, Pedersen NT. Primary non-Hodgkin's lymphoma of the thyroid gland: a population based study. Histopathology. 1996 Jan;28(1):25–32. PMID:8838117
3483. Pedrazzini L, Baroli A, Marzoli L, et al. Cancer recurrence in papillary thyroid microcarcinoma: a multivariate analysis on 231 patients with a 12-year follow-up. Minerva Endocrinol. 2013 Sep;38(3):269–79. PMID:24126547
3484. Pei L, Melmed S. Isolation and characterization of a pituitary tumor-transforming gene (PTTG). Mol Endocrinol. 1997 Apr;11(4):433–41. PMID:9092795
3485. Pei L, Melmed S, Scheithauer B, et al. H-ras mutations in human pituitary carcinoma metastases. J Clin Endocrinol Metab. 1994 Apr;78(4):842–6. PMID:8157709
3486. Pei X, Xiang L, Chen W, et al. The next generation sequencing of cancer-related genes in small cell neuroendocrine carcinoma of the cervix. Gynecol Oncol. 2021 Jun;161(3):779–86. PMID:33888337
3487. Peifer M, Hertwig F, Roels F, et al. Telomerase activation by genomic rearrangements in high-risk neuroblastoma. Nature. 2015 Oct 29;526(7575):700–4. PMID:26466568
3488. Peiling Yang S, Ngeow J. Familial non-medullary thyroid cancer: unraveling the genetic maze. Endocr Relat Cancer. 2016 Dec;23(12):R577–95. PMID:27807061
3489. Peiretti V, Mussa A, Feyles F, et al. Thyroid involvement in two patients with Bannayan-Riley-Ruvalcaba syndrome. J Clin Res Pediatr Endocrinol. 2013;5(4):261–5. PMID:24379037
3490. Pekmezci M, Cuevas-Ocampo AK, Perry A, et al. Significance of H3K27me3 loss in the diagnosis of malignant peripheral nerve sheath tumors. Mod Pathol. 2017 Dec;30(12):1710–9. PMID:28776579
3491. Pekmezci M, Louie J, Gupta N, et al. Clinicopathological characteristics of adamantinomatous and papillary craniopharyngiomas: University of California, San Francisco experience 1985-2005. Neurosurgery. 2010 Nov;67(5):1341–9. PMID:20871436
3492. Pekova B, Sykorova V, Mastnikova K, et al. NTRK fusion genes in thyroid carcinomas: clinicopathological characteristics and their impacts on prognosis. Cancers (Basel). 2021 Apr 16;13(8):1932. PMID:33923728
3493. Pelizzo MR, Piotto A, Bergamasco A, et al. [Parathyroid carcinoma. Therapeutic strategies derived from 20 years of experience]. Minerva Endocrinol. 2001 Mar;26(1):23–9. Italian. PMID:11323564
3494. Pellegata NS, Quintanilla-Martinez L, Siggelkow H, et al. Germ-line mutations in p27Kip1 cause a multiple endocrine neoplasia syndrome in rats and humans. Proc Natl Acad Sci U S A. 2006 Oct 17;103(42):15558–63. PMID:17030811
3495. Pelletier G, Cortot A, Launay JM, et al. Serotonin-secreting and insulin-secreting ileal carcinoid tumor and the use of in vitro culture of tumoral cells. Cancer. 1984 Jul 15;54(2):319–22. PMID:6372987
3496. Pellini R, Ruggieri M, Pichi B, et al. A case of cervical metastases from temporal bone carcinoid. Head Neck. 2005 Jul;27(7):644–7. PMID:15825200
3497. Pelosi G, Bresaola E, Bogina G, et al. Endocrine tumors of the pancreas: Ki-67 immunoreactivity on paraffin sections is an independent predictor for malignancy: a comparative study with proliferating-cell nuclear antigen and progesterone receptor protein immunostaining, mitotic index, and other clinicopathologic variables. Hum Pathol. 1996 Nov;27(11):1124–34. PMID:8912819
3498. Pelosi G, Sonzogni A, Galetta D, et al. Combined small-cell carcinoma of the lung with quadripartite differentiation of epithelial, neuroendocrine, skeletal muscle, and myofibroblastic type. Virchows Arch. 2011 Apr;458(4):497–503. PMID:21210145
3499. Pemayun TG. Current diagnosis and management of thyroid nodules. Acta Med Indones. 2016 Jul;48(3):247–57. PMID:27840362
3500. Pemberton LS, Dougal M, Magee B, et al. Experience of external beam radiotherapy given adjuvantly or at relapse following surgery for craniopharyngioma. Radiother Oncol. 2005 Oct;77(1):99–104. PMID:16216361
3501. Pemov A, Hansen NF, Sindiri S, et al. Low mutation burden and frequent loss of CDKN2A/B and SMARCA2, but not PRC2, define premalignant neurofibromatosis type 1-associated atypical neurofibromas. Neuro Oncol. 2019 Aug 5;21(8):981–92. PMID:30722027
3502. Pemov A, Li H, Patidar R, et al. The primacy of NF1 loss as the driver of tumorigenesis in neurofibromatosis type 1-associated plexiform neurofibromas. Oncogene. 2017 Jun 1;36(22):3168–77. PMID:28068329
3503. Pemov A, Sung H, Hyland PL, et al. Genetic modifiers of neurofibromatosis type 1-associated café-au-lait macule count identified using multi-platform analysis. PLoS Genet. 2014 Oct 16;10(10):e1004575. PMID:25329635
3504. Penel N, Lebellec L, Blay JY, et al. Overview of « druggable » alterations by histological subtypes of sarcomas and connective tissue intermediate malignancies. Crit Rev Oncol Hematol. 2020 Jun;150:102960. PMID:32320927
3505. Peng P, Chen F, Zhou D, et al. Neurocytoma of the pituitary gland: a case report and literature review. Biomed Rep. 2015 May;3(3):301–3. PMID:26137226
3506. Peng S, Shepard MJ, Wang J, et al. Genotype-phenotype correlations in Chinese von Hippel-Lindau disease patients. Oncotarget. 2017 Jun 13;8(24):38456–65. PMID:28388566
3507. Peng X, Chen J, Wang J, et al. Natural history of renal tumours in von Hippel-Lindau disease: a large retrospective study of Chinese patients. J Med Genet. 2019 Jun;56(6):380–7. PMID:30745424
3508. Penn I, First MR. Merkel's cell carcinoma in organ recipients: report of 41 cases. Transplantation. 1999 Dec 15;68(11):1717–21. PMID:10609948
3509. Penna GC, Vaisman F, Vaisman M, et al. Molecular markers involved in tumorigenesis of thyroid carcinoma: focus on aggressive histotypes. Cytogenet Genome Res. 2016;150(3-4):194–207. PMID:28231576
3510. Pennanen M, Heiskanen I, Sane T, et al. Helsinki score-a novel model for prediction of metastases in adrenocortical carcinomas. Hum Pathol. 2015 Mar;46(3):404–10. PMID:25582500
3511. Perakakis N, Flohr F, Kayser G, et al. Multiple endocrine neoplasia type 1 associated with a new germline Men1 mutation in a family with atypical tumor phenotype. Hormones (Athens). 2016 Jan-Mar;15(1):113–7. PMID:26732163
3512. Pereira AM, Schmid EM, Schutte PJ, et al. High prevalence of long-term cardiovascular, neurological and psychosocial morbidity after treatment for craniopharyngioma. Clin Endocrinol (Oxf). 2005 Feb;62(2):197–204. PMID:15670196
3513. Pereira BD, Raimundo L, Mete O, et al. Monomorphous plurihormonal pituitary adenoma of Pit-1 lineage in a giant adolescent with central hyperthyroidism. Endocr Pathol. 2016 Mar;27(1):25–33. PMID:26330191
3514. Pereira JS, da Silva JG, Tomaz RA, et al. Identification of a novel germline FOXE1 variant in patients with familial non-medullary thyroid carcinoma (FNMTC). Endocrine. 2015 May;49(1):204–14. PMID:25381600
3515. Pereira M, Williams VL, Hallanger Johnson J, et al. Thyroid cancer incidence trends in the United States: association with changes in professional guideline recommendations. Thyroid. 2020 Aug;30(8):1132–40. PMID:32098591
3516. Perera MT, McKiernan PJ, Brundler MA, et al. Embryonal rhabdomyosarcoma of the ampulla of Vater in early childhood: report of a case and review of literature. J Pediatr Surg. 2009 Feb;44(2):e9–11. PMID:19231522
3517. Perez-Montiel MD, Frankel WL, Suster S. Neuroendocrine carcinomas of the pancreas with 'Rhabdoid' features. Am J Surg Pathol. 2003 May;27(5):642–9. PMID:12717248
3518. Perez-Ordoñez B. Neuroendocrine carcinomas of the larynx and head and neck: challenges in classification and grading. Head Neck Pathol. 2018 Mar;12(1):1–8. PMID:29557536
3519. Perez-Ordonez B, Caruana SM, Huvos AG, et al. Small cell neuroendocrine carcinoma of the nasal cavity and paranasal sinuses. Hum Pathol. 1998 Aug;29(8):826–32. PMID:9712424
3520. Perez-Rivas LG, Theodoropoulou M, Ferraù F, et al. The gene of the ubiquitin-specific protease 8 is frequently mutated in adenomas causing Cushing's disease. J Clin Endocrinol Metab. 2015 Jul;100(7):E997–1004. PMID:25942478
3521. Pergolizzi S, Ascenti G, Settineri N, et al. Primitive sinonasal malignant mucosal melanoma: description of a case treated with radiotherapy (0-7-21 regimen). Anticancer Res. 1999 Jan-Feb;19 1B:657–60. PMID:10216472
3522. Périgny M, Hammel P, Corcos O, et al. Pancreatic endocrine microadenomatosis in patients with von Hippel-Lindau disease: characterization by VHL/HIF pathway proteins expression. Am J Surg Pathol. 2009 May;33(5):739–48. PMID:19238077
3523. Perkins JA, Inglis AF, Sie KC, et al. Recurrent thyroglossal duct cysts: a 23-year experience and a new method for management. Ann Otol Rhinol Laryngol. 2006 Nov;115(11):850–6. PMID:17165669
3524. Permana H, Darmawan G, Ritonga E, et al. An interesting case of hepatic adrenocortical carcinoma. Acta Med Indones. 2018 Jul;50(3):257–9. PMID:30333277
3525. Pernicone PJ, Scheithauer BW, Sebo TJ, et al. Pituitary carcinoma: a clinicopathologic

study of 15 cases. Cancer. 1997 Feb 15;79(4):804–12. PMID:9024719
3526. Perren A, Anlauf M, Henopp T, et al. Multiple endocrine neoplasia type 1 (MEN1): loss of one MEN1 allele in tumors and monohormonal endocrine cell clusters but not in islet hyperplasia of the pancreas. J Clin Endocrinol Metab. 2007 Mar;92(3):1118–28. PMID:17179192
3527. Perren A, Wiesli P, Schmid S, et al. Pancreatic endocrine tumors are a rare manifestation of the neurofibromatosis type 1 phenotype: molecular analysis of a malignant insulinoma in a NF-1 patient. Am J Surg Pathol. 2006 Aug;30(8):1047–51. PMID:16861979
3528. Perrone T, Sibley RK, Rosai J. Duodenal gangliocytic paraganglioma. An immunohistochemical and ultrastructural study and a hypothesis concerning its origin. Am J Surg Pathol. 1985 Jan;9(1):31–41. PMID:2578747
3529. Perry A, Graffeo CS, Marcellino C, et al. Pediatric pituitary adenoma: case series, review of the literature, and a skull base treatment paradigm. J Neurol Surg B Skull Base. 2018 Feb;79(1):91–114. PMID:29404245
3530. Perry A, Molberg K, Albores-Saavedra J. Physiologic versus neoplastic C-cell hyperplasia of the thyroid: separation of distinct histologic and biologic entities. Cancer. 1996 Feb 15;77(4):750–6. PMID:8616768
3531. Perry A, Roth KA, Banerjee R, et al. NF1 deletions in S-100 protein-positive and negative cells of sporadic and neurofibromatosis 1 (NF1)-associated plexiform neurofibromas and malignant peripheral nerve sheath tumors. Am J Pathol. 2001 Jul;159(1):57–61. PMID:11438454
3532. Perry A, Stafford SL, Scheithauer BW, et al. Meningioma grading: an analysis of histologic parameters. Am J Surg Pathol. 1997 Dec;21(12):1455–65. PMID:9414189
3533. Perry AM, Nelson M, Sanger WG, et al. Cytogenetic abnormalities in follicular dendritic cell sarcoma: report of two cases and literature review. In Vivo. 2013 Mar-Apr;27(2):211–4. PMID:23422480
3534. Persani L, Rurale G, de Filippis T, et al. Genetics and management of congenital hypothyroidism. Best Pract Res Clin Endocrinol Metab. 2018 Aug;32(4):387–96. PMID:30086865
3535. Pery C Jr, Avallone S, Regenet N, et al. Intraductal papillary mucinous tumor of the pancreas in 2 twin brothers diagnosed as having the Carney complex. Pancreas. 2009 Mar;38(2):237–9. PMID:19238031
3536. Peters C, van Trotsenburg ASP, Schoenmakers N. Diagnosis of endocrine disease: congenital hypothyroidism: update and perspectives. Eur J Endocrinol. 2018 Dec 1;179(6):R297–317. PMID:30324792
3537. Petignot S, Daly AF, Castermans E, et al. Pancreatic neuroendocrine neoplasm associated with a familial MAX deletion. Horm Metab Res. 2020 Nov;52(11):784–7. PMID:32521546
3538. Petrone G, Santoro A, Angrisani B, et al. Neuroendocrine tumors of the submandibular gland: literature review and report of a case. Int J Surg Pathol. 2013 Feb;21(1):85–8. PMID:22614165
3539. Petrossians P, Daly AF, Natchev E, et al. Acromegaly at diagnosis in 3173 patients from the Liège Acromegaly Survey (LAS) Database. Endocr Relat Cancer. 2017 Oct;24(10):505–18. PMID:28733467
3540. Petterson T, MacFarlane IA, MacKenzie JM, et al. Prolactin secreting pituitary carcinoma. J Neurol Neurosurg Psychiatry. 1992 Dec;55(12):1205–6. PMID:1479402
3541. Peuchmaur M, d'Amore ES, Joshi VV, et al. Revision of the International Neuroblastoma Pathology Classification: confirmation of favorable and unfavorable prognostic subsets in ganglioneuroblastoma, nodular. Cancer. 2003 Nov 15;98(10):2274–81. PMID:14601099
3542. Pezzolo A, Rossi E, Gimelli S, et al. Presence of 1q gain and absence of 7p gain are new predictors of local or metastatic relapse in localized resectable neuroblastoma. Neuro Oncol. 2009 Apr;11(2):192–200. PMID:18923191
3543. Pfaltz M, Hedinger CE, Mühlethaler JP. Mixed medullary and follicular carcinoma of the thyroid. Virchows Arch A Pathol Anat Histopathol. 1983;400(1):53–9. PMID:6407193
3544. Phillips JJ, Misra A, Feuerstein BG, et al. Pituicytoma: characterization of a unique neoplasm by histology, immunohistochemistry, ultrastructure, and array-based comparative genomic hybridization. Arch Pathol Lab Med. 2010 Jul;134(7):1063–9. PMID:20586639
3545. Piaditis G, Angellou A, Kontogeorgos G, et al. Ectopic bioactive luteinizing hormone secretion by a pancreatic endocrine tumor, manifested as luteinized granulosa-thecal cell tumor of the ovaries. J Clin Endocrinol Metab. 2005 Apr;90(4):2097–103. PMID:15687346
3546. Piana S, Frasoldati A, Di Felice E, et al. Encapsulated well-differentiated follicular-patterned thyroid carcinomas do not play a significant role in the fatality rates from thyroid carcinoma. Am J Surg Pathol. 2010 Jun;34(6):868–72. PMID:20463572
3547. Piana S, Ragazzi M, Tallini G, et al. Papillary thyroid microcarcinoma with fatal outcome: evidence of tumor progression in lymph node metastases: report of 3 cases, with morphological and molecular analysis. Hum Pathol. 2013 Apr;44(4):556–65. PMID:23079204
3548. Picard C, Orbach D, Carton M, et al. Revisiting the role of the pathological grading in pediatric adrenal cortical tumors: results from a national cohort study with pathological review. Mod Pathol. 2019 Apr;32(4):546–59. PMID:30401946
3549. Pichard DC, Boyce AM, Collins MT, et al. Oral pigmentation in McCune-Albright syndrome. JAMA Dermatol. 2014 Jul;150(7):760–3. PMID:24671640
3550. Pickleman JR, Lee JF, Straus FH 2nd, et al. Thyroid hemangioma. Am J Surg. 1975 Mar;129(3):331–3. PMID:1119698
3551. Pierre C, Agopiantz M, Brunaud L, et al. COPPS, a composite score integrating pathological features, PS100 and SDHB losses, predicts the risk of metastasis and progression-free survival in pheochromocytomas/paragangliomas. Virchows Arch. 2019 Jun;474(6):721–34. PMID:30868297
3552. Piersigilli F, Auriti C, Mondì V, et al. Decreased CDKN1C expression in congenital alveolar rhabdomyosarcoma associated with Beckwith-Wiedemann syndrome. Indian J Pediatr. 2016 Nov;83(12-13):1476–8. PMID:27345568
3553. Pieterman CR, Conemans EB, Dreijerink KM, et al. Thoracic and duodenopancreatic neuroendocrine tumors in multiple endocrine neoplasia type 1: natural history and function of menin in tumorigenesis. Endocr Relat Cancer. 2014 May 6;21(3):R121–42. PMID:24389729
3554. Pieterman CR, van Hulsteijn LT, den Heijer M, et al. Primary hyperparathyroidism in MEN1 patients: a cohort study with longterm follow-up on preferred surgical procedure and the relation with genotype. Ann Surg. 2012 Jun;255(6):1171–8. PMID:22470073
3555. Pieterman CRC, de Laat JM, Twisk JWR, et al. Long-term natural course of small nonfunctional pancreatic neuroendocrine tumors in MEN1-results from the Dutch MEN1 Study Group. J Clin Endocrinol Metab. 2017 Oct 1;102(10):3795–805. PMID:28938468
3556. Pieterman CRC, Hyde SM, Wu SY, et al. Understanding the clinical course of genotype-negative MEN1 patients can inform management strategies. Surgery. 2021 Jan;169(1):175–84. PMID:32703679
3557. Pignatelli D, Carvalho BL, Palmeiro A, et al. The complexities in genotyping of congenital adrenal hyperplasia: 21-hydroxylase deficiency. Front Endocrinol (Lausanne). 2019 Jul 4;10:432. PMID:31333583
3558. Pilati C, Shinde J, Alexandrov LB, et al. Mutational signature analysis identifies MUTYH deficiency in colorectal cancers and adrenocortical carcinomas. J Pathol. 2017 May;242(1):10–5. PMID:28127763
3559. Pileri SA, Grogan TM, Harris NL, et al. Tumours of histiocytes and accessory dendritic cells: an immunohistochemical approach to classification from the International Lymphoma Study Group based on 61 cases. Histopathology. 2002 Jul;41(1):1–29. PMID:12121233
3560. Pillai S, Gopalan V, Smith RA, et al. Diffuse sclerosing variant of papillary thyroid carcinoma–an update of its clinicopathological features and molecular biology. Crit Rev Oncol Hematol. 2015 Apr;94(1):64–73. PMID:25577570
3561. Pillarisetty VG, Katz SC, Ghossein RA, et al. Micromedullary thyroid cancer: how micro is truly micro? Ann Surg Oncol. 2009 Oct;16(10):2875–81. PMID:19568813
3562. Pimenta FJ, Gontijo Silveira LF, Tavares GC, et al. HRPT2 gene alterations in ossifying fibroma of the jaws. Oral Oncol. 2006 Aug;42(7):735–9. PMID:16458039
3563. Pinato DJ, Ramachandran R, Toussi ST, et al. Immunohistochemical markers of the hypoxic response can identify malignancy in phaeochromocytomas and paragangliomas and optimize the detection of tumours with VHL germline mutations. Br J Cancer. 2013 Feb 5;108(2):429–37. PMID:23257898
3564. Pinchot SN, Sippel R, Chen H. ACTH-producing carcinoma of the pituitary with refractory Cushing's disease and hepatic metastases: a case report and review of the literature. World J Surg Oncol. 2009 Apr 8;7:39. PMID:19356251
3565. Pini GM, Uccella S, Corinti M, et al. Primary MiNEN of the urinary bladder: an hitherto undescribed entity composed of large cell neuroendocrine carcinoma and adenocarcinoma with a distinct clinical behavior : description of a case and review of the pertinent literature. Virchows Arch. 2021 Jul;479(1):69–78. PMID:33454836
3566. Pinto K, Chetty R. Gene of the month: GLIS1-3. J Clin Pathol. 2020 Sep;73(9):527–30. PMID:32699115
3567. Pipeleers-Marichal M, Somers G, Willems G, et al. Gastrinomas in the duodenums of patients with multiple endocrine neoplasia type 1 and the Zollinger-Ellison syndrome. N Engl J Med. 1990 Mar 15;322(11):723–7. PMID:1968616
3568. Pires C, Marques IJ, Dias D, et al. A pathogenic variant in CHEK2 shows a founder effect in Portuguese Roma patients with thyroid cancer. Endocrine. 2021 Sep;73(3):588–97. PMID:33683595
3569. Pisapia P, Pepe F, Iaccarino A, et al. BRAF: a two-faced Janus. Cells. 2020 Nov 27;9(12):2549. PMID:33260892
3570. Pitner H, Elmaraghy C, Fischer B, et al. Diagnostic accuracy of midline pediatric neck masses. Otolaryngol Head Neck Surg. 2019 Jun;160(6):1111–7. PMID:30717638
3571. Pitsava G, Zhu C, Sundaram R, et al. Predicting the risk of cardiac myxoma in Carney complex. Genet Med. 2021 Jan;23(1):80–5. PMID:32893266
3572. Pitt SC, Sippel RS, Chen H. Secondary and tertiary hyperparathyroidism, state of the art surgical management. Surg Clin North Am. 2009 Oct;89(5):1227–39. PMID:19836494
3573. Pivonello R, De Leo M, Cozzolino A, et al. The treatment of Cushing's disease. Endocr Rev. 2015 Aug;36(4):385–486. PMID:26067718
3574. Pivovarova AI, Patrick S, Reddy PJ. Sporadic medullary thyroid carcinoma with paraneoplastic Cushing syndrome. Case Rep Endocrinol. 2019 Dec 8;2019:6414921. PMID:31885947
3575. Pluta RM, Wait SD, Butman JA, et al. Sacral hemangioblastoma in a patient with von Hippel-Lindau disease. Case report and review of the literature. Neurosurg Focus. 2003 Aug 15;15(2):E11. PMID:15350042
3576. Pocrnich CE, Ramalingam P, Euscher ED, et al. Neuroendocrine carcinoma of the endometrium: a clinicopathologic study of 25 cases. Am J Surg Pathol. 2016 May;40(5):577–86. PMID:26945341
3577. Podda M, Saba A, Porru F, et al. Follicular thyroid carcinoma: differences in clinical relevance between minimally invasive and widely invasive tumors. World J Surg Oncol. 2015 Jun 4;13:193. PMID:26041024
3578. Point du Jour KS, Alwelaie Y, Coleman A, et al. Adrenal gland fine needle aspiration: a multi-institutional analysis of 139 cases. J Am Soc Cytopathol. 2021 Mar-Apr;10(2):168–74. PMID:32988789
3579. Pointer KB, Ko HC, Brower JV, et al. Small cell carcinoma of the head and neck: an analysis of the National Cancer Database. Oral Oncol. 2017 Jun;69:92–8. PMID:28559027
3580. Polak M. Hyperfunctioning thyroid adenoma and activating mutations in the TSH receptor gene. Arch Med Res. 1999 Nov-Dec;30(6):510–3. PMID:10714365
3581. Polat SB, Cakir B, Evranos B, et al. Preoperative predictors and prognosis of bilateral multifocal papillary thyroid carcinomas. Surg Oncol. 2019 Mar;28:145–9. PMID:30851890
3582. Poli R, Scatolini M, Grosso E, et al. Malignant struma ovarii: next-generation sequencing of six cases revealed Nras, Braf, and Jak3 mutations. Endocrine. 2021 Jan;71(1):216–24. PMID:32743766
3583. Policarpio-Nicolas ML, Le BH, Mandell JW, et al. Granular cell tumor of the neurohypophysis: report of a case with intraoperative cytologic diagnosis. Diagn Cytopathol. 2008 Jan;36(1):58–63. PMID:18064694
3584. Pollak N, Renner GJ, Miick R, et al. Endometrioid adenocarcinoma metastatic to the thyroid, presenting like anaplastic thyroid cancer. Case Rep Endocrinol. 2011;2011:246872. PMID:22937279
3585. Pollard PJ, Brière JJ, Alam NA, et al. Accumulation of Krebs cycle intermediates and over-expression of HIF1alpha in tumours which result from germline FH and SDH mutations. Hum Mol Genet. 2005 Aug 1;14(15):2231–9. PMID:15987702
3586. Pollock WJ, McConnell CF, Hilton C, et al. Virilizing Leydig cell adenoma of adrenal gland. Am J Surg Pathol. 1986 Nov;10(11):816–22. PMID:3022613
3587. Polyak K. The p27Kip1 tumor suppressor gene: still a suspect or proven guilty? Cancer Cell. 2006 Nov;10(5):352–4. PMID:17097557
3588. Poma AM, Condello V, Denaro M, et al. DICER1 somatic mutations strongly impair miRNA processing even in benign thyroid lesions. Oncotarget. 2019 Mar 5;10(19):1785–97. PMID:30956758
3589. Ponder TB, Collins BT, Bee CS, et al. Diagnosis of cervical thymoma by fine needle aspiration biopsy with flow cytometry. A case report. Acta Cytol. 2002 Nov-Dec;46(6):1129–32. PMID:12462094
3590. Ponnudurai T, Lensen AH, van Gemert GJ, et al. Sporozoite load of mosquitoes infected with Plasmodium falciparum. Trans R Soc Trop Med Hyg. 1989 Jan-Feb;83(1):67–70. PMID:2690418

3591. Pontén E, Frisk S, Taylan F, et al. A complex DICER1 syndrome phenotype associated with a germline pathogenic variant affecting the RNase IIIa domain of DICER1. J Med Genet. 2022 Feb;59(2):141–6. PMID:33208384
3592. Porcellini A, Fenzi G, Avvedimento EV. Mutations of thyrotropin receptor gene. J Mol Med (Berl). 1997 Aug;75(8):567–75. PMID:9297624
3593. Poretti A, Grotzer MA, Ribi K, et al. Outcome of craniopharyngioma in children: long-term complications and quality of life. Dev Med Child Neurol. 2004 Apr;46(4):220–9. PMID:15077699
3594. Pósfai B, Kuthi L, Varga L, et al. The colorful palette of neuroendocrine neoplasms in the genitourinary tract. Anticancer Res. 2018 Jun;38(6):3243–54. PMID:29848671
3595. Potorac I, Petrossians P, Daly AF, et al. Pituitary MRI characteristics in 297 acromegaly patients based on T2-weighted sequences. Endocr Relat Cancer. 2015 Apr;22(2):169–77. PMID:25556181
3596. Potrony M, Puig-Butille JA, Ribera-Sola M, et al. POT1 germline mutations but not TERT promoter mutations are implicated in melanoma susceptibility in a large cohort of Spanish melanoma families. Br J Dermatol. 2019 Jul;181(1):105–13. PMID:30451293
3597. Póvoa AA, Teixeira E, Bella-Cueto MR, et al. Clinicopathological features as prognostic predictors of poor outcome in papillary thyroid carcinoma. Cancers (Basel). 2020 Oct 29;12(11):3186. PMID:33138175
3598. Powell JG, Goellner JR, Nowak LE, et al. Rosai-Dorfman disease of the thyroid masquerading as anaplastic carcinoma. Thyroid. 2003 Feb;13(2):217–21. PMID:12699598
3599. Poyhonen M, Kytölä S, Leisti J. Epidemiology of neurofibromatosis type 1 (NF1) in northern Finland. J Med Genet. 2000 Aug;37(8):632–6. PMID:10991696
3600. Pozdeyev N, Gay LM, Sokol ES, et al. Genetic analysis of 779 advanced differentiated and anaplastic thyroid cancers. Clin Cancer Res. 2018 Jul 1;24(13):3059–68. PMID:29615459
3601. Pozza C, Sesti F, Di Dato C, et al. A novel MAX gene mutation variant in a patient with multiple and "composite" neuroendocrine-neuroblastic tumors. Front Endocrinol (Lausanne). 2020 May 19;11:234. PMID:32508744
3602. Pradeep PV, Jayashree B. Thyroglossal cysts in a pediatric population: apparent differences from adult thyroglossal cysts. Ann Saudi Med. 2013 Jan-Feb;33(1):45–8. PMID:23458940
3603. Pradella LM, Zuntini R, Magini P, et al. Two distinct thyroid tumours in a patient with Cowden syndrome carrying both a 10q23 and a mitochondrial DNA germline deletion. J Med Genet. 2011 Nov;48(11):779–82. PMID:21926107
3604. Prall OWJ, Nastevski V, Xu H, et al. RAF1 rearrangements are common in pancreatic acinar cell carcinomas. Mod Pathol. 2020 Sep;33(9):1811–21. PMID:32358589
3605. Prasad ML, Vyas M, Horne MJ, et al. NTRK fusion oncogenes in pediatric papillary thyroid carcinoma in northeast United States. Cancer. 2016 Apr 1;122(7):1097–107. PMID:26784937
3606. Prat-Acín R, Galeano-Senabre I, García-Sánchez D, et al. Superficial siderosis of the central nervous system in a patient with asymptomatic sacral paraganglioma as source of chronic bleeding. Rev Neurol. 2020 Oct 1;71(7):253–6. PMID:32959357
3607. Prazeres HJ, Rodrigues F, Soares P, et al. Loss of heterozygosity at 19p13.2 and 2q21 in tumours from familial clusters of non-medullary thyroid carcinoma. Fam Cancer. 2008;7(2):141–9. PMID:17823852
3608. Preda V, Korbonits M, Cudlip S, et al. Low rate of germline AIP mutations in patients with apparently sporadic pituitary adenomas before the age of 40: a single-centre adult cohort. Eur J Endocrinol. 2014 Nov;171(5):659–66. PMID:25184284
3609. Preda V, Sywak M, Learoyd D. A new association - multiple endocrine neoplasia type 1 and malignant peripheral nerve sheath tumor. Clin Case Rep. 2015 Jan;3(1):29–31. PMID:25678969
3610. Preston DL, Ron E, Yonehara S, et al. Tumors of the nervous system and pituitary gland associated with atomic bomb radiation exposure. J Natl Cancer Inst. 2002 Oct 16;94(20):1555–63. PMID:12381708
3611. Prete A, Borges de Souza P, Censi S, et al. Update on fundamental mechanisms of thyroid cancer. Front Endocrinol (Lausanne). 2020 Mar 13;11:102. PMID:32231639
3612. Prévot S, Penna C, Imbert JC, et al. Solitary fibrous tumor of the adrenal gland. Mod Pathol. 1996 Dec;9(12):1170–4. PMID:8972477
3613. Prichard RS, Lee JC, Gill AJ, et al. Mucoepidermoid carcinoma of the thyroid: a report of three cases and postulated histogenesis. Thyroid. 2012 Feb;22(2):205–9. PMID:22224821
3614. Priemer DS, Montironi R, Wang L, et al. Neuroendocrine tumors of the prostate: emerging insights from molecular data and updates to the 2016 World Health Organization Classification. Endocr Pathol. 2016 Jun;27(2):123–35. PMID:26885643
3615. Priemer DS, Trevino K, Chen S, et al. Paratesticular soft-tissue masses in orchiectomy specimens: a 17-year survey of primary and incidental cases from one institution. Int J Surg Pathol. 2017 Sep;25(6):480–7. PMID:28459169
3616. Prieto R, Pascual JM, Barrios L. Letter: A clinical rule for preoperative prediction of BRAF mutation status in craniopharyngiomas. Neurosurgery. 2019 Nov 1;85(5):E962–5. PMID:31435663
3617. Prieto R, Pascual JM, Barrios L. Optic chiasm distortions in craniopharyngiomas: a sign of hypothalamic involvement. Acta Neurochir (Wien). 2017 Aug;159(8):1533–5. PMID:28660394
3618. Prieto R, Pascual JM, Rosdolsky M, et al. Craniopharyngioma adherence: a comprehensive topographical categorization and outcome-related risk stratification model based on the methodical examination of 500 tumors. Neurosurg Focus. 2016 Dec;41(6):E13. PMID:27903121
3619. Prieto-Granada CN, Wiesner T, Messina JL, et al. Loss of H3K27me3 expression is a highly sensitive marker for sporadic and radiation-induced MPNST. Am J Surg Pathol. 2016 Apr;40(4):479–89. PMID:26645727
3620. Pringle DR, Yin Z, Lee AA, et al. Thyroid-specific ablation of the Carney complex gene, PRKAR1A, results in hyperthyroidism and follicular thyroid cancer. Endocr Relat Cancer. 2012 May 24;19(3):435–46. PMID:22514108
3621. Proboka G, Tilgase A, Isajevs S, et al. Adrenal gland and gastric malignant melanoma without evidence of skin lesion treated with the oncolytic virus Rigvir. Case Rep Oncol. 2020 Apr 17;13(1):424–30. PMID:32399011
3622. Proietti A, Sartori C, Macerola E, et al. Low frequency of TERT promoter mutations in a series of well-differentiated follicular-patterned thyroid neoplasms. Virchows Arch. 2017 Dec;471(6):769–73. PMID:28975450
3623. Pu RT, Yang J, Wasserman PG, et al. Does Hurthle cell lesion/neoplasm predict malignancy more than follicular lesion/neoplasm on thyroid fine-needle aspiration? Diagn Cytopathol. 2006 May;34(5):330–4. PMID:16604553
3624. Puar T, Engels M, van Herwaarden AE, et al. Bilateral testicular tumors resulting in recurrent Cushing disease after bilateral adrenalectomy. J Clin Endocrinol Metab. 2017 Feb 1;102(2):339–44. PMID:27901643
3625. Puchner MJ, Lüdecke DK, Saeger W, et al. Gangliocytomas of the sellar region–a review. Exp Clin Endocrinol Diabetes. 1995;103(3):129–49. PMID:7584515
3626. Puchner MJ, Lüdecke DK, Valdueza JM, et al. Cushing's disease in a child caused by a corticotropin-releasing hormone-secreting intrasellar gangliocytoma associated with an adrenocorticotropic hormone-secreting pituitary adenoma. Neurosurgery. 1993 Nov;33(5):920–4. PMID:8264895
3627. Puente S, Velasco A, Gallel P, et al. Metastatic small cell carcinoma to the thyroid gland: a pathologic and molecular study demonstrating the origin in the urinary bladder. Endocr Pathol. 2008 Fall;19(3):190–6. PMID:18446450
3628. Pugh TJ, Yu W, Yang J, et al. Exome sequencing of pleuropulmonary blastoma reveals frequent biallelic loss of TP53 and two hits in DICER1 resulting in retention of 5p-derived miRNA hairpin loop sequences. Oncogene. 2014 Nov 6;33(45):5295–302. PMID:24909177
3629. Pugnale N, Waridel F, Bouzourène H, et al. Pharyngeal pituitary non-functioning adenoma with normal intra-sellar gland: massive tumor shrinkage on octreotide therapy. Eur J Endocrinol. 2003 Mar;148(3):357–64. PMID:12611618
3630. Pulitzer DR, Martin PC, Reed RJ. Epithelioid glomus tumor. Hum Pathol. 1995 Sep;26(9):1022–7. PMID:7672784
3631. Pulitzer MP, Amin BD, Busam KJ. Merkel cell carcinoma: review. Adv Anat Pathol. 2009 May;16(3):135–44. PMID:19395876
3632. Pulitzer MP, Brannon AR, Berger MF, et al. Cutaneous squamous and neuroendocrine carcinoma: genetically and immunohistochemically different from Merkel cell carcinoma. Mod Pathol. 2015 Aug;28(8):1023–32. PMID:26022453
3633. Pulvirenti A, Raj N, Cingarlini S, et al. Platinum-based treatment for well- and poorly differentiated pancreatic neuroendocrine neoplasms. Pancreas. 2021 Feb 1;50(2):138–46. PMID:33565789
3634. Pusztaszeri M, Wang H, Cibas ES, et al. Fine-needle aspiration biopsy of secondary neoplasms of the thyroid gland: a multi-institutional study of 62 cases. Cancer Cytopathol. 2015 Jan;123(1):19–29. PMID:25369542
3635. Pusztaszeri MP, Bongiovanni M, Faquin WC. Update on the cytologic and molecular features of medullary thyroid carcinoma. Adv Anat Pathol. 2014 Jan;21(1):26–35. PMID:24316908
3636. Pusztaszeri MP, Krane JF, Cibas ES, et al. FNAB of benign thyroid nodules with papillary hyperplasia: a cytological and histological evaluation. Cancer Cytopathol. 2014 Sep;122(9):666–77. PMID:24891128
3637. Pusztaszeri MP, Sauder KJ, Cibas ES, et al. Fine-needle aspiration of primary Langerhans cell histiocytosis of the thyroid gland, a potential mimic of papillary thyroid carcinoma. Acta Cytol. 2013;57(4):406–12. PMID:23860349
3638. Pytel P, Krausz T, Wollmann R, et al. Ganglioneuromatous paraganglioma of the cauda equina–a pathological case study. Hum Pathol. 2005 Apr;36(4):444–6. PMID:15892009
3639. Qi XP, Lin GB, Chen B, et al. Multiple endocrine neoplasia type 2B associated mixed medullary and follicular thyroid carcinoma in a Chinese patient with RET M918T germline mutation. Endocr Metab Immune Disord Drug Targets. 2021;21(3):554–60. PMID:32660411
3640. Qi XP, Zhao JQ, Cao ZL, et al. The clinical spectrum of multiple endocrine neoplasia type 2A with cutaneous lichen amyloidosis in ethnic Han Chinese. Cancer Invest. 2018 Feb 7;36(2):141–51. PMID:29420094
3641. Qian ZR, Sano T, Yoshimoto K, et al. Tumor-specific downregulation and methylation of the CDH13 (H-cadherin) and CDH1 (E-cadherin) genes correlate with aggressiveness of human pituitary adenomas. Mod Pathol. 2007 Dec;20(12):1269–77. PMID:17873891
3642. Qiao N, Ye Z, Wang Y, et al. Gangliocytomas in the sellar region. Clin Neurol Neurosurg. 2014 Nov;126:156–61. PMID:25259876
3643. Qie S, Wang XF, Ran YG, et al. Nomogram for predicting the survival of patients with small cell carcinoma of the esophagus: a population study based on the Surveillance, Epidemiology, and End Results database. Medicine (Baltimore). 2021 Apr 16;100(15):e25427. PMID:33847642
3644. Qin N, de Cubas AA, Garcia-Martin R, et al. Opposing effects of HIF1α and HIF2α on chromaffin cell phenotypic features and tumor cell proliferation: insights from MYC-associated factor X. Int J Cancer. 2014 Nov 1;135(9):2054–64. PMID:24676840
3645. Qiu ZL, Shen CT, Sun ZK, et al. Distant metastases from pathologically proven benign follicular nodules of the thyroid: clinicopathological features and predictors of long-term survival. Endocrine. 2020 Jul;69(1):113–25. PMID:32189188
3646. Qu R, Wang C, Dong Z, et al. Another strategy for the treatment of thyroglossal duct cyst: totally endoscopic surgery by breast approach. Surg Laparosc Endosc Percutan Tech. 2018 Apr;28(2):118–22. PMID:29521676
3647. Quah BL, Donofrio CA, La Rosa S, et al. Primary glomus tumour of the pituitary gland: diagnostic challenges of a rare and potentially aggressive neoplasm. Virchows Arch. 2021 May;478(5):977–84. PMID:32918169
3648. Qualman S, Lynch J, Bridge J, et al. Prevalence and clinical impact of anaplasia in childhood rhabdomyosarcoma : a report from the Soft Tissue Sarcoma Committee of the Children's Oncology Group. Cancer. 2008 Dec 1;113(11):3242–7. PMID:18985676
3649. Qualman SJ, Coffin CM, Newton WA, et al. Intergroup Rhabdomyosarcoma Study: update for pathologists. Pediatr Dev Pathol. 1998 Nov-Dec;1(6):550–61. PMID:9724344
3650. Quidde J, Alsdorf WH, von Amsberg G, et al. Treatment of metastatic spindle epithelial tumor with thymus-like differentiation (SETTLE) - long-term disease control by multimodal therapy. Oncol Res Treat. 2018;41(1-2):58–60. PMID:29402817
3651. Quiroga-Garza G, Lee JH, El-Naggar A, et al. Sclerosing mucoepidermoid carcinoma with eosinophilia of the thyroid: more aggressive than previously reported. Hum Pathol. 2015 May;46(5):725–31. PMID:25754017
3652. Raaf HN, Grant LD, Santoscoy C, et al. Adenomatoid tumor of the adrenal gland: a report of four new cases and a review of the literature. Mod Pathol. 1996 Nov;9(11):1046–51. PMID:8933514
3653. Rabban JT, Lerwill MF, McCluggage WG, et al. Primary ovarian carcinoid tumors may express CDX-2: a potential pitfall in distinction from metastatic intestinal carcinoid tumors involving the ovary. Int J Gynecol Pathol. 2009 Jan;28(1):41–8. PMID:19047909
3654. Rabban JT, Zaloudek CJ. A practical approach to immunohistochemical diagnosis of ovarian germ cell tumours and sex cord-stromal tumours. Histopathology. 2013 Jan;62(1):71–88. PMID:23240671

3655. Rabinowits G, Barletta J, Sholl LM, et al. Successful management of a patient with malignant thyroid teratoma. Thyroid. 2017 Jan;27(1):125–8. PMID:27784193
3656. Raco A, Bristot R, Domenicucci M, et al. Meningiomas of the tuberculum sellae. Our experience in 69 cases surgically treated between 1973 and 1993. J Neurosurg Sci. 1999 Dec;43(4):253–60. PMID:10864387
3657. Raddatz D, Horstmann O, Basenau D, et al. Cushing's syndrome due to ectopic adrenocorticotropic hormone production by a non-metastatic gastrinoma after long-term conservative treatment of Zollinger-Ellison syndrome. Ital J Gastroenterol Hepatol. 1998 Dec;30(6):636–40. PMID:10076790
3658. Radice PA, Matthews MJ, Ihde DC, et al. The clinical behavior of "mixed" small cell/large cell bronchogenic carcinoma compared to "pure" small cell subtypes. Cancer. 1982 Dec 15;50(12):2894–902. PMID:6291745
3659. Raess PW, Habashi A, El Rassi E, et al. Overlapping morphologic and immunohistochemical features of Hashimoto thyroiditis and IgG4-related thyroid disease. Endocr Pathol. 2015 May;26(2):170–7. PMID:25898816
3660. Ragazzi M, Torricelli F, Donati B, et al. Coexisting well-differentiated and anaplastic thyroid carcinoma in the same primary resection specimen: immunophenotypic and genetic comparison of the two components in a consecutive series of 13 cases and a review of the literature. Virchows Arch. 2021 Feb;478(2):265–81. PMID:32683537
3661. Raghavan R, Dickey WT Jr, Margraf LR, et al. Proliferative activity in craniopharyngiomas: clinicopathological correlations in adults and children. Surg Neurol. 2000 Sep;54(3):241–7. PMID:11118571
3662. Ragni A, Nervo A, Papotti M, et al. Pituitary metastases from neuroendocrine neoplasms: case report and narrative review. Pituitary. 2021 Oct;24(5):828–37. PMID:34342837
3663. Rahimi A, Shahbazi R, Nikuei P, et al. A pediatric parathyroid carcinoma: an unusual clinical presentation and mini-review. Int J Endocrinol Metab. 2021 Jan 25;19(1):e110234. PMID:33815520
3664. Raj N, Valentino E, Capanu M, et al. Treatment response and outcomes of grade 3 pancreatic neuroendocrine neoplasms based on morphology: well differentiated versus poorly differentiated. Pancreas. 2017 Mar;46(3):296–301. PMID:27759713
3665. Rajaratnam A, Waugh J. Adrenal metastases of malignant melanoma: characteristic computed tomography appearances. Australas Radiol. 2005 Aug;49(4):325–9. PMID:16026441
3666. Rajeshwari M, Sakthivel P, Yogal R, et al. Composite tumor of the larynx: a case report. JNMA J Nepal Med Assoc. 2020 Jan;58(221):52–5. PMID:32335641
3667. Rajeshwari M, Singh V, Nambirajan A, et al. Carcinoma showing thymus like elements: report of a case with EGFR T790M mutation. Diagn Cytopathol. 2018 May;46(5):413–8. PMID:29115061
3668. Rak B, Maksymowicz M, Grzywa TM, et al. Pituitary tumours - a large retrospective single-centre study of over 2300 cases. Experience of a tertiary reference centre. Endokrynol Pol. 2020;71(2):116–25. PMID:32154573
3669. Rak B, Maksymowicz M, Pękul M, et al. Clinical, biological, radiological pathological and immediate post-operative remission of sparsely and densely granulated corticotroph pituitary tumors: a retrospective study of a cohort of 277 patients with Cushing's disease. Front Endocrinol (Lausanne). 2021 May 31;12:672178. PMID:34135861
3670. Ramani B, Gupta R, Wu J, et al. The immunohistochemical, DNA methylation, and chromosomal copy number profile of cauda equina paraganglioma is distinct from extra-spinal paraganglioma. Acta Neuropathol. 2020 Dec;140(6):907–17. PMID:32892244
3671. Ramaswamy PV, Storm CA, Filiano JJ, et al. Multiple granular cell tumors in a child with Noonan syndrome. Pediatr Dermatol. 2010 Mar-Apr;27(2):209–11. PMID:20537083
3672. Ramesh BG, Bhargav PR, Rajesh BG, et al. Genotype-phenotype correlations of dyshormonogenetic goiter in children and adolescents from South India. Indian J Endocrinol Metab. 2016 Nov-Dec;20(6):816–24. PMID:27867886
3673. Ramírez C, Cheng S, Vargas G, et al. Expression of Ki-67, PTTG1, FGFR4, and SSTR 2, 3, and 5 in nonfunctioning pituitary adenomas: a high throughput TMA, immunohistochemical study. J Clin Endocrinol Metab. 2012 May;97(5):1745–51. PMID:22419713
3674. Ramírez C, Hernández-Ramirez LC, Espinosa-de-los-Monteros AL, et al. Ectopic acromegaly due to a GH-secreting pituitary adenoma in the sphenoid sinus: a case report and review of the literature. BMC Res Notes. 2013 Oct 12;6:411. PMID:24119925
3675. Ramlagun D, Shadhu K, Sang M, et al. Simultaneous occurrence of primary aldosteronism due to aldosteronoma and ectopic meningioma in the adrenal gland: a case report. Medicine (Baltimore). 2018 Dec;97(50):e13591. PMID:30558028
3676. Ramsay JA, Asa SL, van Nostrand AW, et al. Lipid degeneration in pheochromocytomas mimicking adrenal cortical tumors. Am J Surg Pathol. 1987 Jun;11(6):480–6. PMID:3592062
3677. Ramsey MJ, Nadol JB Jr, Pilch BZ, et al. Carcinoid tumor of the middle ear: clinical features, recurrences, and metastases. Laryngoscope. 2005 Sep;115(9):1660–6. PMID:16148713
3678. Rao Q, Shen Q, Xia QY, et al. PSF/SFPQ is a very common gene fusion partner in TFE3 rearrangement-associated perivascular epithelioid cell tumors (PEComas) and melanotic Xp11 translocation renal cancers: clinicopathologic, immunohistochemical, and molecular characteristics suggesting classification as a distinct entity. Am J Surg Pathol. 2015 Sep;39(9):1181–96. PMID:26274027
3679. Rao SN, Zafereo M, Dadu R, et al. Patterns of treatment failure in anaplastic thyroid carcinoma. Thyroid. 2017 May;27(5):672–81. PMID:28068873
3680. Raphael SJ. The meanings of markers: ancillary techniques in diagnosis of thyroid neoplasia. Endocr Pathol. 2002 Winter;13(4):301–11. PMID:12665648
3681. Rashid FA, Munkhdelger J, Fukuoka J, et al. Prevalence of BRAFV600E mutation in Asian series of papillary thyroid carcinoma-a contemporary systematic review. Gland Surg. 2020 Oct;9(5):1878–900. PMID:33224863
3682. Rashidi A, Fisher SI. Primary adrenal lymphoma: a systematic review. Ann Hematol. 2013 Dec;92(12):1583–93. PMID:23771429
3683. Rasmussen P, Lindholm J. Ectopic pituitary adenomas. Clin Endocrinol (Oxf). 1979 Jul;11(1):69–74. PMID:519872
3684. Rasmussen SA, Friedman JM. NF1 gene and neurofibromatosis 1. Am J Epidemiol. 2000 Jan 1;151(1):33–40. PMID:10625171
3685. Rassi-Cruz M, Maria AG, Faucz FR, et al. Phosphodiesterase 2A and 3B variants are associated with primary aldosteronism. Endocr Relat Cancer. 2021 Jan;28(1):1–13. PMID:33112806
3686. Ratliff JK, Oldfield EH. Multiple pituitary adenomas in Cushing's disease. J Neurosurg. 2000 Nov;93(5):753–61. PMID:11059654
3687. Ratner N, Miller SJ. A RASopathy gene commonly mutated in cancer: the neurofibromatosis type 1 tumour suppressor. Nat Rev Cancer. 2015 May;15(5):290–301. PMID:25877329
3688. Raue F, Frank-Raue K. Epidemiology and clinical presentation of medullary thyroid carcinoma. Recent Results Cancer Res. 2015;204:61–90. PMID:26494384
3689. Raveendran Nair AKA, George NA, Kumar R, et al. Sclerosing mucoepidermoid carcinoma with eosinophilia of thyroid gland: Not so indolent a neoplasm? Indian J Pathol Microbiol. 2018 Apr-Jun;61(2):242–4. PMID:29676367
3690. Ravella L, Lopez J, Descotes F, et al. [DICER1 mutated, solid/trabecular thyroid papillary carcinoma in an 11-year-old child]. Ann Pathol. 2018 Oct;38(5):316–20. French. PMID:29884466
3691. Raverot G, Dantony E, Beauvy J, et al. Risk of recurrence in pituitary neuroendocrine tumors: a prospective study using a five-tiered classification. J Clin Endocrinol Metab. 2017 Sep 1;102(9):3368–74. PMID:28651368
3692. Raverot G, Jouanneau E, Trouillas J. Management of endocrine disease: clinicopathological classification and molecular markers of pituitary tumours for personalized therapeutic strategies. Eur J Endocrinol. 2014 Mar 13;170(4):R121–32. PMID:24431196
3693. Raverot G, Vasiljevic A, Jouanneau E. Prognostic factors of regrowth in nonfunctioning pituitary tumors. Pituitary. 2018 Apr;21(2):176–82. PMID:29288467
3694. Raverot G, Vasiljevic A, Jouanneau E, et al. A prognostic clinicopathologic classification of pituitary endocrine tumors. Endocrinol Metab Clin North Am. 2015 Mar;44(1):11–8. PMID:25732637
3695. Ravindran A, Goyal G, Go RS, et al. Rosai-Dorfman disease displays a unique monocyte-macrophage phenotype characterized by expression of OCT2. Am J Surg Pathol. 2021 Jan;45(1):35–44. PMID:33177341
3696. Rayess HM, Monk I, Svider PF, et al. Thyroglossal duct cyst carcinoma: a systematic review of clinical features and outcomes. Otolaryngol Head Neck Surg. 2017 May;156(5):794–802. PMID:28322121
3697. Raygada M, Raffeld M, Bernstein A, et al. Case report of adrenocortical carcinoma associated with double germline mutations in MSH2 and RET. Am J Med Genet A. 2021 Apr;185(4):1282–7. PMID:33615670
3698. Rayhan N, Sano T, Qian ZR, et al. Histological and immunohistochemical study of composite neuroendocrine-exocrine carcinomas of the stomach. J Med Invest. 2005 Aug;52(3-4):191–202. PMID:16167538
3699. Raymond VM, Everett JN, Furtado LV, et al. Adrenocortical carcinoma is a lynch syndrome-associated cancer. J Clin Oncol. 2013 Aug 20;31(24):3012–8. PMID:23752102
3700. Reagh J, Bullock M, Andrici J, et al. NRASQ61R mutation-specific immunohistochemistry also identifies the HRASQ61R mutation in medullary thyroid cancer and may have a role in triaging genetic testing for MEN2. Am J Surg Pathol. 2017 Jan;41(1):75–81. PMID:27635947
3701. Rebecchini C, Nobile A, Piana S, et al. Papillary thyroid carcinoma with nodular fasciitis-like stroma and β-catenin mutations should be renamed papillary thyroid carcinoma with desmoid-type fibromatosis. Mod Pathol. 2017 Feb;30(2):236–45. PMID:27713418
3702. Recondo G Jr, Busaidy N, Erasmus J, et al. Spindle epithelial tumor with thymus-like differentiation: a case report and comprehensive review of the literature and treatment options. Head Neck. 2015 May;37(5):746–54. PMID:24677409
3703. Reddy B, Aggarwal V, Ajmani AK, et al. Primary leiomyosarcoma of the thyroid gland - a rare malignancy. Eur Endocrinol. 2019 Apr;15(1):44–6. PMID:31244910
3704. Reddy R, Cudlip S, Byrne JV, et al. Can we ever stop imaging in surgically treated and radiotherapy-naive patients with non-functioning pituitary adenoma? Eur J Endocrinol. 2011 Nov;165(5):739–44. PMID:21900406
3705. Redlich A, Pamporaki C, Lessel L, et al. Pseudohypoxic pheochromocytomas and paragangliomas dominate in children. Pediatr Blood Cancer. 2021 Jul;68(7):e28981. PMID:33682326
3706. Redman BG, Pazdur R, Zingas AP, et al. Prospective evaluation of adrenal insufficiency in patients with adrenal metastasis. Cancer. 1987 Jul 1;60(1):103–7. PMID:3581024
3706A. Rednam SP, Erez A, Druker H, et al. Von Hippel-Lindau and hereditary pheochromocytoma/paraganglioma syndromes: clinical features, genetics, and surveillance recommendations in childhood. Clin Cancer Res. 2017 Jun;23(12):e68–75. PMID:28620007
3707. Regairaz M, Munier F, Sartelet H, et al. Mutation-independent activation of the anaplastic lymphoma kinase in neuroblastoma. Am J Pathol. 2016 Feb;186(2):435–45. PMID:26687816
3708. Rege J, Nanba K, Blinder AR, et al. Identification of somatic mutations in CLCN2 in aldosterone-producing adenomas. J Endocr Soc. 2020 Oct 1;4(10):bvaa123. PMID:33033789
3709. Rehfeld JF, Federspiel B, Agersnap M, et al. The uncovering and characterization of a CCKoma syndrome in enteropancreatic neuroendocrine tumor patients. Scand J Gastroenterol. 2016 Oct;51(10):1172–8. PMID:27191542
3710. Rehfeld JF, Federspiel B, Bardram L. A neuroendocrine tumor syndrome from cholecystokinin secretion. N Engl J Med. 2013 Mar 21;368(12):1165–6. PMID:23514309
3711. Reich M, Jaegle S, Neumann-Haefelin E, et al. Genotype-phenotype correlation in von Hippel-Lindau disease. Acta Ophthalmol. 2021 Dec;99(8):e1492–500. PMID:33720516
3712. Reid M. Cytology of the pancreas: a practical review for cytopathologists. Surg Pathol Clin. 2011 Jun;4(2):651–91. PMID:26837492
3713. Reid MD, Bagci P, Ohike N, et al. Calculation of the Ki67 index in pancreatic neuroendocrine tumors: a comparative analysis of four counting methodologies. Mod Pathol. 2015 May;28(5):686–94. PMID:25412850
3714. Reid MD, Balci S, Saka B, et al. Neuroendocrine tumors of the pancreas: current concepts and controversies. Endocr Pathol. 2014 Mar;25(1):65–79. PMID:24430597
3715. Reimann JD, Dorfman DM, Nosé V. Carcinoma showing thymus-like differentiation of the thyroid (CASTLE): a comparative study: evidence of thymic differentiation and solid cell nest origin. Am J Surg Pathol. 2006 Aug;30(8):994–1001. PMID:16861971
3716. Reincke M, Sbiera S, Hayakawa A, et al. Mutations in the deubiquitinase gene USP8 cause Cushing's disease. Nat Genet. 2015 Jan;47(1):31–8. PMID:25485838
3717. Reisenauer JS, Mneimneh W, Jenkins S, et al. Comparison of risk stratification models to predict recurrence and survival in pleuropulmonary solitary fibrous tumor. J Thorac Oncol. 2018 Sep;13(9):1349–62. PMID:29935303
3718. Rekhi B, Patil B, Deodhar KK, et al. Spectrum of neuroendocrine carcinomas of the uterine cervix, including histopathologic features, terminology, immunohistochemical profile, and clinical outcomes in a series of 50 cases from a single institution in India. Ann Diagn Pathol. 2013 Feb;17(1):1–9. PMID:22534245
3719. Rekhtman N, Pietanza CM, Sabari J, et al. Pulmonary large cell neuroendocrine carcinoma with adenocarcinoma-like

features: napsin A expression and genomic alterations. Mod Pathol. 2018 Jan;31(1):111–21. PMID:28884744
3720. Rekhtman N, Pietanza MC, Hellmann MD, et al. Next-generation sequencing of pulmonary large cell neuroendocrine carcinoma reveals small cell carcinoma-like and non-small cell carcinoma-like subsets. Clin Cancer Res. 2016 Jul 15;22(14):3618–29. PMID:26960398
3721. Relles D, Baek J, Witkiewicz A, et al. Periampullary and duodenal neoplasms in neurofibromatosis type 1: two cases and an updated 20-year review of the literature yielding 76 cases. J Gastrointest Surg. 2010 Jun;14(6):1052–61. PMID:20300877
3722. Remstein ED, Dogan A, Einerson RR, et al. The incidence and anatomic site specificity of chromosomal translocations in primary extranodal marginal zone B-cell lymphoma of mucosa-associated lymphoid tissue (MALT lymphoma) in North America. Am J Surg Pathol. 2006 Dec;30(12):1546–53. PMID:17122510
3723. Ren R, Guo M, Sneige N, et al. Fine-needle aspiration of adrenal cortical carcinoma: cytologic spectrum and diagnostic challenges. Am J Clin Pathol. 2006 Sep;126(3):389–98. PMID:16880150
3724. Ren W, Zhi K, Zhao L, et al. Presentations and management of thyroglossal duct cyst in children versus adults: a review of 106 cases. Oral Surg Oral Med Oral Pathol Oral Radiol Endod. 2011 Feb;111(2):e1–6. PMID:21237423
3725. Ren WH, Dong K, Huang XZ, et al. Intrathyroidal thymic carcinoma exhibiting neuroendocrine differentiation: case report with cytomorphology, immunocytochemistry, and review of the literature focusing on cytology. Diagn Cytopathol. 2019 Nov;47(11):1197–202. PMID:31318494
3726. Ren Y, Kyriazidis N, Faquin WC, et al. The presence of Hürthle cells does not increase the risk of malignancy in most Bethesda categories in thyroid fine-needle aspirates. Thyroid. 2020 Mar;30(3):425–31. PMID:32013786
3727. Renaudin K, Smati S, Wargny M, et al. Clinicopathological description of 43 oncocytic adrenocortical tumors: importance of Ki-67 in histoprognostic evaluation. Mod Pathol. 2018 Nov;31(11):1708–16. PMID:29921900
3728. Rendl G, Manzl M, Hitzl W, et al. Long-term prognosis of medullary thyroid carcinoma. Clin Endocrinol (Oxf). 2008 Sep;69(3):497–505. PMID:18331612
3729. Renshaw AA. Hürthle cell carcinoma is a better gold standard than Hürthle cell neoplasm for fine-needle aspiration of the thyroid: defining more consistent and specific cytologic criteria. Cancer. 2002 Oct 25;96(5):261–6. PMID:12378592
3730. Resende de Paiva C, Grønhøj C, Feldt-Rasmussen U, et al. Association between Hashimoto's thyroiditis and thyroid cancer in 64,628 patients. Front Oncol. 2017 Apr 10;7:53. PMID:28443243
3731. Reyes CV, Wang T. Undifferentiated small cell carcinoma of the pancreas: a report of five cases. Cancer. 1981 May 15;47(10):2500–2. PMID:6268272
3732. Reyes-Vivas H, Diaz A, Peon J, et al. Disulfide bridges in the mesophilic triosephosphate isomerase from Giardia lamblia are related to oligomerization and activity. J Mol Biol. 2007 Jan 19;365(3):752–63. PMID:17095008
3733. Ribon V, Leff T, Saltiel AR. c-Myc does not require max for transcriptional activity in PC-12 cells. Mol Cell Neurosci. 1994 Jun;5(3):277–82. PMID:8087425
3734. Ricci C, Morandi L, Ambrosi F, et al. Intron 4-5 hTERT DNA hypermethylation in Merkel cell carcinoma: frequency, association with other clinico-pathological features and prognostic relevance. Endocr Pathol. 2021 Sep;32(3):385–95. PMID:33909215
3735. Ricci C, Partelli S, Landoni L, et al. Sporadic non-functioning pancreatic neuroendocrine tumours: multicentre analysis. Br J Surg. 2021 Jul 23;108(7):811–6. PMID:33724300
3736. Riccio L, Donofrio CA, Tomacelli G, et al. Ectopic GH-secreting pituitary adenoma of the clivus: systematic literature review of a challenging tumour. Pituitary. 2020 Aug;23(4):457–66. PMID:32504302
3737. Richard C, Debreuve-Theresette A, Patey M, et al. Long-term progression of non-invasive follicular thyroid neoplasm with papillary-like nuclear features: a single-center retrospective study of the French Marne-Ardennes thyroid cancer registry. Ann Endocrinol (Paris). 2020 Feb;81(1):34–8. PMID:32057425
3738. Richard MA, Lupo PJ, Morton LM, et al. Genetic variation in POT1 and risk of thyroid subsequent malignant neoplasm: a report from the Childhood Cancer Survivor Study. PLoS One. 2020 Feb 10;15(2):e0228887. PMID:32040538
3739. Richard S, Gardie B, Couvé S, et al. Von Hippel-Lindau: how a rare disease illuminates cancer biology. Semin Cancer Biol. 2013 Feb;23(1):26–37. PMID:22659535
3740. Rickert CH, Hasselblatt M, Jeibmann A, et al. Cellular and reticular variants of hemangioblastoma differ in their cytogenetic profiles. Hum Pathol. 2006 Nov;37(11):1452–7. PMID:16949923
3741. Rickert CH, Paulus W. Lack of chromosomal imbalances in adamantinomatous and papillary craniopharyngiomas. J Neurol Neurosurg Psychiatry. 2003 Feb;74(2):260–1. PMID:12531965
3742. Ricklefs FL, Fita KD, Rotermund R, et al. Genome-wide DNA methylation profiles distinguish silent from non-silent ACTH adenomas. Acta Neuropathol. 2020 Jul;140(1):95–7. PMID:32185515
3743. Riedlinger WF, Lack EE, Robson CD, et al. Primary thyroid teratomas in children: a report of 11 cases with a proposal of criteria for their diagnosis. Am J Surg Pathol. 2005 May;29(5):700–6. PMID:15832097
3744. Rigaud C, Barkaoui MA, Thomas C, et al. Langerhans cell histiocytosis: therapeutic strategy and outcome in a 30-year nationwide cohort of 1478 patients under 18 years of age. Br J Haematol. 2016 Sep;174(6):887–98. PMID:27273725
3745. Righi A, Morandi L, Leonardi E, et al. Galectin-3 expression in pituitary adenomas as a marker of aggressive behavior. Hum Pathol. 2013 Nov;44(11):2400–9. PMID:24007691
3746. Riminucci M, Collins MT, Fedarko NS, et al. FGF-23 in fibrous dysplasia of bone and its relationship to renal phosphate wasting. J Clin Invest. 2003 Sep;112(5):683–92. PMID:12952917
3747. Rindi G, Falconi M, Klersy C, et al. TNM staging of neoplasms of the endocrine pancreas: results from a large international cohort study. J Natl Cancer Inst. 2012 May 16;104(10):764–77. PMID:22525418
3748. Rindi G, Klersy C, Albarello L, et al. Competitive testing of the WHO 2010 versus the WHO 2017 grading of pancreatic neuroendocrine neoplasms: data from a large international cohort study. Neuroendocrinology. 2018;107(4):375–86. PMID:30300897
3749. Rindi G, Klimstra DS, Abedi-Ardekani B, et al. A common classification framework for neuroendocrine neoplasms: an International Agency for Research on Cancer (IARC) and World Health Organization (WHO) expert consensus proposal. Mod Pathol. 2018 Dec;31(12):1770–86. PMID:30140036
3750. Rindi G, Klöppel G, Alhman H, et al. TNM staging of foregut (neuro)endocrine tumors: a consensus proposal including a grading system. Virchows Arch. 2006 Oct;449(4):395–401. PMID:16967267
3751. Rindi G, Wiedenmann B. Neuroendocrine neoplasia of the gastrointestinal tract revisited: towards precision medicine. Nat Rev Endocrinol. 2020 Oct;16(10):590–607. PMID:32839579
3752. Rindi G, Wiedenmann B. Neuroendocrine neoplasms of the gut and pancreas: new insights. Nat Rev Endocrinol. 2011 Aug 2;8(1):54–64. PMID:21808296
3753. Rinke A, Müller HH, Schade-Brittinger C, et al. Placebo-controlled, double-blind, prospective, randomized study on the effect of octreotide LAR in the control of tumor growth in patients with metastatic neuroendocrine midgut tumors: a report from the PROMID Study Group. J Clin Oncol. 2009 Oct 1;27(28):4656–63. PMID:19704057
3754. Ríos A, Rodríguez JM, Martínez E, et al. Cavernous hemangioma of the thyroid. Thyroid. 2001 Mar;11(3):279–80. PMID:11327620
3755. Rivera M, Ghossein RA, Schoder H, et al. Histopathologic characterization of radioactive iodine-refractory fluorodeoxyglucose-positron emission tomography-positive thyroid carcinoma. Cancer. 2008 Jul 1;113(1):48–56. PMID:18484584
3756. Rivera M, Ricarte-Filho J, Knauf J, et al. Molecular genotyping of papillary thyroid carcinoma follicular variant according to its histological subtypes (encapsulated vs infiltrative) reveals distinct BRAF and RAS mutation patterns. Mod Pathol. 2010 Sep;23(9):1191–200. PMID:20526288
3757. Rivera M, Ricarte-Filho J, Patel S, et al. Encapsulated thyroid tumors of follicular cell origin with high grade features (high mitotic rate/tumor necrosis): a clinicopathologic and molecular study. Hum Pathol. 2010 Feb;41(2):172–80. PMID:19913280
3758. Rivera M, Tuttle RM, Patel S, et al. Encapsulated papillary thyroid carcinoma: a clinico-pathologic study of 106 cases with emphasis on its morphologic subtypes (histologic growth pattern). Thyroid. 2009 Feb;19(2):119–27. PMID:19191744
3759. Rivero A, Liang J. Sinonasal small cell neuroendocrine carcinoma: a systematic review of 80 patients. Int Forum Allergy Rhinol. 2016 Jul;6(7):744–51. PMID:26880574
3760. Roake CM, Artandi SE. DNA repair: telomere-lengthening mechanism revealed. Nature. 2016 Nov 3;539(7627):35–6. PMID:27760112
3761. Robberecht P, Conlon TP, Gardner JD. Interaction of porcine vasoactive intestinal peptide with dispersed pancreatic acinar cells from the guinea pig. Structural requirements for effects of vasoactive intestinal peptide and secretin on cellular adenosine 3':5'-monophosphate. J Biol Chem. 1976 Aug 10;251(15):4635–9. PMID:181379
3762. Robboy SJ, Norris HJ, Scully RE. Insular carcinoid primary in the ovary. A clinicopathologic analysis of 48 cases. Cancer. 1975 Aug;36(2):404–18. PMID:1157010
3763. Robboy SJ, Scully RE. Ovarian teratoma with glial implants on the peritoneum. An analysis of 12 cases. Hum Pathol. 1970 Dec;1(4):643–53. PMID:5521737
3764. Robboy SJ, Scully RE. Strumal carcinoid of the ovary: an analysis of 50 cases of a distinctive tumor composed of thyroid tissue and carcinoid. Cancer. 1980 Nov 1;46(9):2019–34. PMID:7427909
3765. Robboy SJ, Scully RE, Norris HJ. Primary trabecular carcinoid of the ovary. Obstet Gynecol. 1977 Feb;49(2):202–7. PMID:834404
3766. Robboy SJ, Shaco-Levy R, Peng RY, et al. Malignant struma ovarii: an analysis of 88 cases, including 27 with extraovarian spread. Int J Gynecol Pathol. 2009 Sep;28(5):405–22. PMID:19696610
3767. Robenshtok E, Tzvetov G, Grozinsky-Glasberg S, et al. Clinical characteristics and outcome of familial nonmedullary thyroid cancer: a retrospective controlled study. Thyroid. 2011 Jan;21(1):43–8. PMID:20954815
3768. Roberts JA, Gonzalez RS, Das S, et al. Expression of PD-1 and PD-L1 in poorly differentiated neuroendocrine carcinomas of the digestive system: a potential target for anti-PD-1/PD-L1 therapy. Hum Pathol. 2017 Dec;70:49–54. PMID:29037958
3769. Roberts S, Borges MT, Lillehei KO, et al. Double separate versus contiguous pituitary adenomas: MRI features and endocrinological follow up. Pituitary. 2016 Oct;19(5):472–81. PMID:27209585
3770. Robinson C, Estrada A, Zaheer A, et al. Clinical and radiographic gastrointestinal abnormalities in McCune-Albright syndrome. J Clin Endocrinol Metab. 2018 Nov 1;103(11):4293–303. PMID:30124968
3771. Robinson DR, Wu YM, Kalyana-Sundaram S, et al. Identification of recurrent NAB2-STAT6 gene fusions in solitary fibrous tumor by integrative sequencing. Nat Genet. 2013 Feb;45(2):180–5. PMID:23313952
3772. Robinson JB, Im DD, Logan L, et al. Extraovarian granulosa cell tumor. Gynecol Oncol. 1999 Jul;74(1):123–7. PMID:10385563
3773. Robinson L, Schouwstra CM, van Heerden WFP. Oropharyngeal mixed neuroendocrine-nonneuroendocrine neoplasm (MiNEN): a case report and literature review. Head Neck Pathol. 2021 Dec;15(4):1415–20. PMID:33709305
3774. Roche AM, Fedewa SA, Shi LL, et al. Treatment and survival vary by race/ethnicity in patients with anaplastic thyroid cancer. Cancer. 2018 Apr 15;124(8):1780–90. PMID:29409119
3775. Roche PH, Figarella-Branger D, Regis J, et al. Cauda equina paraganglioma with subsequent intracranial and intraspinal metastases. Acta Neurochir (Wien). 1996;138(4):475–9. PMID:8738400
3776. Rockall AG, Babar SA, Sohaib SA, et al. CT and MR imaging of the adrenal glands in ACTH-independent Cushing syndrome. Radiographics. 2004 Mar-Apr;24(2):435–52. PMID:15026592
3777. Roden AC, Hu X, Kip S, et al. BRAF V600E expression in Langerhans cell histiocytosis: clinical and immunohistochemical study on 25 pulmonary and 54 extrapulmonary cases. Am J Surg Pathol. 2014 Apr;38(4):548–51. PMID:24625419
3778. Rodriguez FJ, Aubry MC, Tazelaar HD, et al. Pulmonary chondroma: a tumor associated with Carney triad and different from pulmonary hamartoma. Am J Surg Pathol. 2007 Dec;31(12):1844–53. PMID:18043038
3779. Rodriguez FJ, Folpe AL, Giannini C, et al. Pathology of peripheral nerve sheath tumors: diagnostic overview and update on selected diagnostic problems. Acta Neuropathol. 2012 Mar;123(3):295–319. PMID:22327363
3780. Rodriguez FJ, Scheithauer BW, Tsunoda S, et al. The spectrum of malignancy in craniopharyngioma. Am J Surg Pathol. 2007 Jul;31(7):1020–8. PMID:17592268
3781. Rodriguez M, Martin-Malo A, Martinez ME, et al. Calcemic response to parathyroid hormone in renal failure: role of phosphorus and its effect on calcitriol. Kidney Int. 1991 Dec;40(6):1055–62. PMID:1762306
3782. Rodriguez Pena MDC, Salles DC, Epstein JI, et al. Well-differentiated neuroendocrine tumors of the lower urinary tract: biologic behavior of a rare entity. Hum Pathol. 2021

Mar;109:53–8. PMID:33301750
3783. Rodriguez-Galindo C, Allen CE. Langerhans cell histiocytosis. Blood. 2020 Apr 16;135(16):1319–31. PMID:32106306
3784. Rodríguez-Ortiz ME, Rodríguez M. Recent advances in understanding and managing secondary hyperparathyroidism in chronic kidney disease. F1000Res. 2020 Sep 1;9:F1000 Faculty Rev-1077. PMID:32913635
3785. Roethlisberger M, Jayapalan RR, Hostettler IC, et al. Evolving strategies for resection of sellar/parasellar synchronous tumors via endoscopic endonasal approach: a technical case report and systematic review of the literature. World Neurosurg. 2020 Jan;133:381–391.e2. PMID:31476461
3786. Roh MH, Jo VY, Stelow EB, et al. The predictive value of the fine-needle aspiration diagnosis "suspicious for a follicular neoplasm, Hurthle cell type" in patients with Hashimoto thyroiditis. Am J Clin Pathol. 2011 Jan;135(1):139–45. PMID:21173136
3787. Rohayem J, Bäumer LM, Zitzmann M, et al. Semen quality and testicular adrenal rest tumour development in 46,XY congenital adrenal hyperplasia: the importance of optimal hormonal replacement. Eur J Endocrinol. 2021 Apr;184(4):487–501. PMID:33524003
3788. Rojiani AM, Owen DA, Berry K, et al. Hepatic hemangioblastoma. An unusual presentation in a patient with von Hippel-Lindau disease. Am J Surg Pathol. 1991 Jan;15(1):81–6. PMID:1898683
3789. Roman S, Lin R, Sosa JA. Prognosis of medullary thyroid carcinoma: demographic, clinical, and pathologic predictors of survival in 1252 cases. Cancer. 2006 Nov 1;107(9):2134–42. PMID:17019736
3790. Romanet P, Guerin C, Pedini P, et al. Pathological and genetic characterization of bilateral adrenomedullary hyperplasia in a patient with germline MAX mutation. Endocr Pathol. 2017 Dec;28(4):302–7. PMID:27838885
3791. Romanet P, Mohamed A, Giraud S, et al. UMD-MEN1 database: an overview of the 370 MEN1 variants present in 1676 patients from the French population. J Clin Endocrinol Metab. 2019 Mar 1;104(3):753–64. PMID:30339208
3792. Roman-Gonzalez A, Jimenez C. Malignant pheochromocytoma-paraganglioma: pathogenesis, TNM staging, and current clinical trials. Curr Opin Endocrinol Diabetes Obes. 2017 Jun;24(3):174–83. PMID:28234804
3793. Romei C, Casella F, Tacito A, et al. New insights in the molecular signature of advanced medullary thyroid cancer: evidence of a bad outcome of cases with double RET mutations. J Med Genet. 2016 Nov;53(11):729–34. PMID:27468888
3794. Romei C, Ciampi R, Elisei R. A comprehensive overview of the role of the RET proto-oncogene in thyroid carcinoma. Nat Rev Endocrinol. 2016 Apr;12(4):192–202. PMID:26868437
3795. Romei C, Elisei R. A narrative review of genetic alterations in primary thyroid epithelial cancer. Int J Mol Sci. 2021 Feb 9;22(4):1726. PMID:33572167
3796. Romei C, Mariotti S, Fugazzola L, et al. Multiple endocrine neoplasia type 2 syndromes (MEN 2): results from the ItaMEN network analysis on the prevalence of different genotypes and phenotypes. Eur J Endocrinol. 2010 Aug;163(2):301–8. PMID:20516206
3797. Romei C, Ugolini C, Cosci B, et al. Low prevalence of the somatic M918T RET mutation in micro-medullary thyroid cancer. Thyroid. 2012 May;22(5):476–81. PMID:22404432
3798. Romero OA, Torres-Diz M, Pros E, et al. MAX inactivation in small cell lung cancer disrupts MYC-SWI/SNF programs and is synthetic lethal with BRG1. Cancer Discov. 2014 Mar;4(3):292–303. PMID:24362264
3799. Romero-Rojas A, Bella-Cueto MR, Meza-Cabrera IA, et al. Ectopic thyroid tissue in the adrenal gland: a report of two cases with pathogenetic implications. Thyroid. 2013 Dec;23(12):1644–50. PMID:23510370
3800. Romero-Rojas AE, Diaz-Perez JA, Mastrodimos M, et al. Follicular thyroid carcinoma with signet ring cell morphology: fine-needle aspiration cytology, histopathology, and immunohistochemistry. Endocr Pathol. 2013 Dec;24(4):239–45. PMID:24068558
3801. Romero-Rojas AE, Melo-Uribe MA, Barajas-Solano PA, et al. Spindle cell oncocytoma of the adenohypophysis. Brain Tumor Pathol. 2011 Oct;28(4):359–64. PMID:21833579
3802. Ron E, Modan B, Boice JD Jr, et al. Tumors of the brain and nervous system after radiotherapy in childhood. N Engl J Med. 1988 Oct 20;319(16):1033–9. PMID:3173432
3803. Ron E, Modan B, Preston D, et al. Thyroid neoplasia following low-dose radiation in childhood. Radiat Res. 1989 Dec;120(3):516–31. PMID:2594972
3804. Roncaroli F, Faustini-Fustini M, Mauri F, et al. Crooke's hyalinization in silent corticotroph adenoma: report of two cases. Endocr Pathol. 2002 Fall;13(3):245–9. PMID:12446925
3805. Roncaroli F, Scheithauer BW, Cenacchi G, et al. 'Spindle cell oncocytoma' of the adenohypophysis: a tumor of folliculostellate cells? Am J Surg Pathol. 2002 Aug;26(8):1048–55. PMID:12170092
3806. Roncaroli F, Scheithauer BW, Horvath E, et al. Silent subtype 3 carcinoma of the pituitary: a case report. Neuropathol Appl Neurobiol. 2010 Feb;36(1):90–4. PMID:19811617
3807. Ronchi CL, Sbiera S, Volante M, et al. CYP2W1 is highly expressed in adrenal glands and is positively associated with the response to mitotane in adrenocortical carcinoma. PLoS One. 2014 Aug 21;9(8):e105855. PMID:25144458
3808. Rooper LM, Bishop JA, Westra WH. INSM1 is a sensitive and specific marker of neuroendocrine differentiation in head and neck tumors. Am J Surg Pathol. 2018 May;42(5):665–71. PMID:29438167
3809. Rooper LM, Bynum JP, Miller KP, et al. Recurrent DICER1 hotspot mutations in malignant thyroid gland teratomas: molecular characterization and proposal for a separate classification. Am J Surg Pathol. 2020 Jun;44(6):826–33. PMID:31917706
3810. Rooper LM, Sharma R, Li QK, et al. INSM1 demonstrates superior performance to the individual and combined use of synaptophysin, chromogranin and CD56 for diagnosing neuroendocrine tumors of the thoracic cavity. Am J Surg Pathol. 2017 Nov;41(11):1561–9. PMID:28719469
3811. Roque L, Nunes VM, Ribeiro C, et al. Karyotypic characterization of papillary thyroid carcinomas. Cancer. 2001 Nov 15;92(10):2529–38. PMID:11745186
3812. Rosa M. Cytological features of medullary thyroid carcinoma in ascitic effusion. Diagn Cytopathol. 2017 Nov;45(11):1030–2. PMID:28643384
3813. Rosai J. Immunohistochemical markers of thyroid tumors: significance and diagnostic applications. Tumori. 2003 Sep-Oct;89(5):517–9. PMID:14870775
3814. Rosai J. The encapsulated follicular variant of papillary thyroid carcinoma: back to the drawing board. Endocr Pathol. 2010 Mar;21(1):7–11. PMID:20066572
3815. Rosai J, Kuhn E, Carcangiu ML. Pitfalls in thyroid tumour pathology. Histopathology. 2006 Aug;49(2):107–20. PMID:16879388
3816. Rosai J, LiVolsi VA, Sobrinho-Simoes M, et al. Renaming papillary microcarcinoma of the thyroid gland: the Porto proposal. Int J Surg Pathol. 2003 Oct;11(4):249–51. PMID:14615819
3817. Rosario PW, Mourão GF. Noninvasive follicular thyroid neoplasm with papillary-like nuclear features (NIFTP): a review for clinicians. Endocr Relat Cancer. 2019 May 1;26(5):R259–66. PMID:30913533
3818. Rosario PW, Mourão GF, Nunes MB, et al. Noninvasive follicular thyroid neoplasm with papillary-like nuclear features. Endocr Relat Cancer. 2016 Dec;23(12):893–7. PMID:27660403
3819. Rosell A, Muñoz de Nova JL, Lahera M, et al. Clear cell thyroid carcinoma in a patient with clear cell renal cell carcinoma: not as clear as it seems. Cytopathology. 2021 Jul;32(4):541–4. PMID:33848035
3820. Rosemberg S, Fujiwara D. Epidemiology of pediatric tumors of the nervous system according to the WHO 2000 classification: a report of 1,195 cases from a single institution. Childs Nerv Syst. 2005 Nov;21(11):940–4. PMID:16044344
3821. Rosen RD, Bordoni B. Embryology, parathyroid. 2023 May 1. In: StatPearls. Treasure Island (FL): StatPearls Publishing; 2024 Jan–. PMID:32119467
3822. Rosen RD, Sapra A. Embryology, thyroid. 2023 May 1. In: StatPearls. Treasure Island (FL): StatPearls Publishing; 2024 Jan–. PMID:31869075
3823. Rosenbaum JN, Guo Z, Baus RM, et al. INSM1: a novel immunohistochemical and molecular marker for neuroendocrine and neuroepithelial neoplasms. Am J Clin Pathol. 2015 Oct;144(4):579–91. PMID:26386079
3824. Ross DS, Burch HB, Cooper DS, et al. 2016 American Thyroid Association guidelines for diagnosis and management of hyperthyroidism and other causes of thyrotoxicosis. Thyroid. 2016 Oct;26(10):1343–421. PMID:27521067
3825. Rosset A, Greenman Y, Osher E, et al. Revisiting Cushing syndrome, milder forms are now a common occurrence: a single-center cohort of 76 subjects. Endocr Pract. 2021 Sep;27(9):859–65. PMID:33652108
3826. Rossi D. Thyroid lymphoma: beyond antigen stimulation. Leuk Res. 2009 May;33(5):607–9. PMID:19128828
3827. Rossi ED, Faquin WC. NIFTP revised: chronicle of a change foretold. Cancer Cytopathol. 2018 Nov;126(11):897–901. PMID:30339322
3828. Rossi ED, Faquin WC, Pantanowitz L. Cytologic features of aggressive variants of follicular-derived thyroid carcinoma. Cancer Cytopathol. 2019 Jul;127(7):432–46. PMID:31150164
3829. Rossi ED, Pantanowitz L, Hornick JL. A worldwide journey of thyroid cancer incidence centred on tumour histology. Lancet Diabetes Endocrinol. 2021 Apr;9(4):193–4. PMID:33662332
3830. Rossi ED, Pantanowitz L, Hornick JL. Cytologic and histological features of rare nonepithelial and nonlymphoid tumors of the thyroid. Cancer Cytopathol. 2021 Aug;129(8):583–602. PMID:33493367
3831. Rossi ED, Papotti M, Faquin W, et al. The diagnosis of hyalinizing trabecular tumor: a difficult and controversial thyroid entity. Head Neck Pathol. 2020 Sep;14(3):778–84. PMID:31571046
3832. Rossi ED, Raffaelli M, Mule' A, et al. Simultaneous immunohistochemical expression of HBME-1 and galectin-3 differentiates papillary carcinomas from hyperfunctioning lesions of the thyroid. Histopathology. 2006 Jun;48(7):795–800. PMID:16722927
3833. Rossi ED, Straccia P, Martini M, et al. The role of thyroid fine-needle aspiration cytology in the pediatric population: an institutional experience. Cancer Cytopathol. 2014 May;122(5):359–67. PMID:24474727
3834. Rossi G, Cavazza A, Marchioni A, et al. Role of chemotherapy and the receptor tyrosine kinases KIT, PDGFRalpha, PDGFR-beta, and Met in large-cell neuroendocrine carcinoma of the lung. J Clin Oncol. 2005 Dec 1;23(34):8774–85. PMID:16314638
3835. Rostomyan L, Daly AF, Petrossians P, et al. Clinical and genetic characterization of pituitary gigantism: an international collaborative study in 208 patients. Endocr Relat Cancer. 2015 Oct;22(5):745–57. PMID:26187128
3836. Roszko KL, Blouch E, Blake M, et al. Case report of a prolactinoma in a patient with a novel MAX mutation and bilateral pheochromocytomas. J Endocr Soc. 2017 Oct 23;1(11):1401–7. PMID:29264463
3837. Roth LM, Karseladze AI. Highly differentiated follicular carcinoma arising from struma ovarii: a report of 3 cases, a review of the literature, and a reassessment of so-called peritoneal strumosis. Int J Gynecol Pathol. 2008 Apr;27(2):213–22. PMID:18317221
3838. Roth LM, Miller AW 3rd, Talerman A. Typical thyroid-type carcinoma arising in struma ovarii: a report of 4 cases and review of the literature. Int J Gynecol Pathol. 2008 Oct;27(4):496–506. PMID:18753973
3839. Roth LM, Talerman A. Recent advances in the pathology and classification of ovarian germ cell tumors. Int J Gynecol Pathol. 2006 Oct;25(4):305–20. PMID:16990705
3840. Roth LM, Talerman A. The enigma of struma ovarii. Pathology. 2007 Feb;39(1):139–46. PMID:17365830
3841. Roth SI, Marshall RB. Pathology and ultrastructure of the human parathyroid glands in chronic renal failure. Arch Intern Med. 1969 Oct;124(4):397–407. PMID:5823010
3842. Rothenberg AB, Berdon WE, D'Angio GJ, et al. The association between neuroblastoma and opsoclonus-myoclonus syndrome: a historical review. Pediatr Radiol. 2009 Jul;39(7):723–6. PMID:19430769
3843. Rothenberg HJ, Goellner JR, Carney JA. Hyalinizing trabecular adenoma of the thyroid gland: recognition and characterization of its cytoplasmic yellow body. Am J Surg Pathol. 1999 Jan;23(1):118–25. PMID:9888712
3844. Rothenberg HJ, Goellner JR, Carney JA. Prevalence and incidence of cytoplasmic yellow bodies in thyroid neoplasms. Arch Pathol Lab Med. 2003 Jun;127(6):715–7. PMID:12741896
3845. Rotman JA, Kucharczyk W, Zadeh G, et al. Spindle cell oncocytoma of the adenohypophysis: a case report illustrating its natural history with 8-year observation and a review of the literature. Clin Imaging. 2014 Jul-Aug;38(4):499–504. PMID:24721021
3846. Rotman LE, Vaughan TB, Hackney JR, et al. Long-term survival after transformation of an adrenocorticotropic hormone-secreting pituitary macroadenoma to a silent corticotroph pituitary carcinoma. World Neurosurg. 2019 Feb;122:417–23. PMID:30447452
3847. Rotondi M, Carbone A, Coperchini F, et al. Diagnosis of endocrine disease: IgG4-related thyroid autoimmune disease. Eur J Endocrinol. 2019 May 1;180(5):R175–83. PMID:30889549
3848. Rotondo F, Munoz DG, Hegele RG, et al. Rosai-Dorfman disease involving the neurohypophysis. Pituitary. 2010 Sep;13(3):256–9. PMID:20405324
3849. Rottenburger C, Papantoniou D, Mandair D, et al. A case series of molecular imaging of glucagonoma after initial therapy-68Ga-DOTATATE PET/CT reveals similar results as in neuroendocrine tumors of other origin in follow-up and re-evaluation. Clin Nucl Med. 2018

Apr;43(4):252–5. PMID:29432346
3851. Rowland KJ, Moley JF. Hereditary thyroid cancer syndromes and genetic testing. J Surg Oncol. 2015 Jan;111(1):51–60. PMID:25351655
3852. Roy M, Chen H, Sippel RS. Current understanding and management of medullary thyroid cancer. Oncologist. 2013;18(10):1093–100. PMID:24037980
3853. Roy S, LaFramboise WA, Liu TC, et al. Loss of chromatin-remodeling proteins and/or CDKN2A associates with metastasis of pancreatic neuroendocrine tumors and reduced patient survival times. Gastroenterology. 2018 Jun;154(8):2060–2063.e8. PMID:29486199
3854. Rozenblatt-Rosen O, Hughes CM, Nannepaga SJ, et al. The parafibromin tumor suppressor protein is part of a human Paf1 complex. Mol Cell Biol. 2005 Jan;25(2):612–20. PMID:15632063
3855. Rudzinski ER, Anderson JR, Chi YY, et al. Histology, fusion status, and outcome in metastatic rhabdomyosarcoma: a report from the Children's Oncology Group. Pediatr Blood Cancer. 2017 Dec;64(12). PMID:28521080
3856. Ruggieri P, Sim FH, Bond JR, et al. Malignancies in fibrous dysplasia. Cancer. 1994 Mar 1;73(5):1411–24. PMID:8111708
3857. Rumeh ASAL, Bafaqeeh M, Khairan SJA, et al. Pituicytoma associated with Cushing's disease: a case report and literature review. J Surg Case Rep. 2020 Jun 15;2020(6):rjaa104. PMID:32577204
3858. Rupp AP, Bocklage TJ. Mammary analog secretory carcinoma of thyroid: a case report. Diagn Cytopathol. 2017 Jan;45(1):45–50. PMID:27633961
3859. Russo M, Malandrino P, Moleti M, et al. Tall cell and diffuse sclerosing variants of papillary thyroid cancer: outcome and predicting value of risk stratification methods. J Endocrinol Invest. 2017 Nov;40(11):1235–41. PMID:28528434
3860. Rüter A, Dreifus J, Jones M, et al. Overexpression of p53 in tall cell variants of papillary thyroid carcinoma. Surgery. 1996 Dec;120(6):1046–50. PMID:8957493
3861. Rutter MM, Jha P, Schultz KA, et al. DICER1 mutations and differentiated thyroid carcinoma: evidence of a direct association. J Clin Endocrinol Metab. 2016 Jan;101(1):1–5. PMID:26555935
3862. Ruzevick J, Koh EK, Gonzalez-Cuyar LF, et al. Clival paragangliomas: a report of two cases involving the midline skull base and review of the literature. J Neurooncol. 2017 May;132(3):473–8. PMID:28299533
3863. Ryhänen EM, Leijon H, Metso S, et al. A nationwide study on parathyroid carcinoma. Acta Oncol. 2017 Jul;56(7):991–1003. PMID:28362521
3864. Ryska A, Cap J, Vaclavikova E, et al. Paraganglioma-like medullary thyroid carcinoma: fine needle aspiration cytology features with histological correlation. Cytopathology. 2009 Jun;20(3):188–94. PMID:18631354
3865. Rzepecka A, Babińska A, Sworczak K. IgG4-related disease in endocrine practice. Arch Med Sci. 2019 Jan;15(1):55–64. PMID:30697253
3866. Saavedra A, Lima J, Castro L, et al. Malignant paraganglioma and somatotropinoma in a patient with germline SDHB mutation-genetic and clinical features. Endocrine. 2019 Jan;63(1):182–7. PMID:30155846
3867. Sadanandam A, Wullschleger S, Lyssiotis CA, et al. A cross-species analysis in pancreatic neuroendocrine tumors reveals molecular subtypes with distinctive clinical, metastatic, developmental, and metabolic characteristics. Cancer Discov. 2015 Dec;5(12):1296–313. PMID:26446169
3868. Sadashivam S, Menon G, Abraham M, et al. Adult craniopharyngioma: the role of extent of resection in tumor recurrence and long-term functional outcome. Clin Neurol Neurosurg. 2020 May;192:105711. PMID:32036264
3869. Sadler C, Gow KW, Beierle EA, et al. Parathyroid carcinoma in more than 1,000 patients: a population-level analysis. Surgery. 2014 Dec;156(6):1622–9. PMID:25456964
3870. Sadow PM, Hartford NM, Nosé V. Familial endocrine syndromes. Surg Pathol Clin. 2014 Dec;7(4):577–98. PMID:26837556
3871. Sadow PM, Hunt JL. Mixed medullary-follicular-derived carcinomas of the thyroid gland. Adv Anat Pathol. 2010 Jul;17(4):282–5. PMID:20574174
3872. Saeed Kamil Z, Sinson G, Gucer H, et al. TTF-1 expressing sellar neoplasm with ependymal rosettes and oncocytic change: mixed ependymal and oncocytic variant pituicytoma. Endocr Pathol. 2014 Dec;25(4):436–8. PMID:24242699
3873. Saeger W, Ebrahimi A, Beschorner R, et al. Teratoma of the sellar region: a case report. Endocr Pathol. 2017 Dec;28(4):315–9. PMID:28102527
3874. Saeger W, Koch A. Clinical implications of the new WHO classification 2017 for pituitary tumors. Exp Clin Endocrinol Diabetes. 2021 Mar;129(3):146–56. PMID:33690870
3875. Saeger W, Lohe B, Engels CL, et al. IgG4-associated adrenalitis-a case report. Endocr Pathol. 2018 Sep;29(3):294–8. PMID:29766416
3876. Saeger W, Lubke D. Pituitary carcinomas. Endocr Pathol. 1996 Spring;7(1):21–35. PMID:12114677
3877. Saeger W, Lüdecke DK, Buchfelder M, et al. Pathohistological classification of pituitary tumors: 10 years of experience with the German Pituitary Tumor Registry. Eur J Endocrinol. 2007 Feb;156(2):203–16. PMID:17287410
3878. Saeger W, Petersenn S, Schöfl C, et al. Emerging histopathological and genetic parameters of pituitary adenomas: clinical impact and recommendation for future WHO classification. Endocr Pathol. 2016 Jun;27(2):115–22. PMID:26874696
3879. Saeger W, Puchner MJ, Lüdecke DK. Combined sellar gangliocytoma and pituitary adenoma in acromegaly or Cushing's disease. A report of 3 cases. Virchows Arch. 1994;425(1):93–9. PMID:7921420
3880. Saeger W, von Schöning J, Flitsch J, et al. Co-occurrence of pituitary neuroendocrine tumors (PitNETs) and tumors of the neurohypophysis. Endocr Pathol. 2021 Dec;32(4):473–9. PMID:34129177
3881. Sağlıcan Y, Kurtulmus N, Tunca F, et al. Mesothelial derived adenomatoid tumour in a location devoid of mesothelium: adrenal adenomatoid tumour. BMJ Case Rep. 2015 Aug 4;2015:bcr2015211147. PMID:26243749
3882. Saglietti C, Onenerk AM, Faquin WC, et al. FNA diagnosis of poorly differentiated thyroid carcinoma. A review of the recent literature. Cytopathology. 2017 Dec;28(6):467–74. PMID:29094425
3883. Saglietti C, Piana S, La Rosa S, et al. Hyalinizing trabecular tumour of the thyroid: fine-needle aspiration cytological diagnosis and correlation with histology. J Clin Pathol. 2017 Aug;70(8):641–7. PMID:28424236
3884. Sagna Y, Courtillot C, Drabo JY, et al. Endocrine manifestations in a cohort of 63 adulthood and childhood onset patients with Langerhans cell histiocytosis. Eur J Endocrinol. 2019 Sep;181(3):275–85. PMID:31269469
3885. Sahakitrungruang T, Srichomthong C, Pornkunwilai S, et al. Germline and somatic DICER1 mutations in a pituitary blastoma causing infantile-onset Cushing's disease. J Clin Endocrinol Metab. 2014 Aug;99(8):E1487–92. PMID:24823459
3886. Sahin A, Robinson RA. Papillae formation in parathyroid adenoma. A source of possible diagnostic error. Arch Pathol Lab Med. 1988 Jan;112(1):99–100. PMID:3337625
3887. Şahin Mİ, Vural A, Yüce İ, et al. Thyroid leiomyosarcoma: presentation of two cases and review of the literature. Braz J Otorhinolaryngol. 2016 Nov-Dec;82(6):715–21. PMID:27080750
3888. Sahm F, Toprak UH, Hübschmann D, et al. Meningiomas induced by low-dose radiation carry structural variants of NF2 and a distinct mutational signature. Acta Neuropathol. 2017 Jul;134(1):155–8. PMID:28474103
3889. Sahnane N, Furlan D, Monti M, et al. Microsatellite unstable gastrointestinal neuroendocrine carcinomas: a new clinicopathologic entity. Endocr Relat Cancer. 2015 Feb;22(1):35–45. PMID:25465415
3890. Said SI. Evidence for secretion of vasoactive intestinal peptide by tumours of pancreas, adrenal medulla, thyroid and lung: support for the unifying APUD concept. Clin Endocrinol (Oxf). 1976;5 Suppl:201S–4S. PMID:29733
3891. Said SI, Faloona GR. Elevated plasma and tissue levels of vasoactive intestinal polypeptide in the watery-diarrhea syndrome due to pancreatic, bronchogenic and other tumors. N Engl J Med. 1975 Jul 24;293(4):155–60. PMID:166313
3892. Said-Al-Naief N, Sciandra K, Gnepp DR. Moderately differentiated neuroendocrine carcinoma (atypical carcinoid) of the parotid gland: report of three cases with contemporary review of salivary neuroendocrine carcinomas. Head Neck Pathol. 2013 Sep;7(3):295–303. PMID:23456649
3893. Sakaguchi N, Sano K, Ito M, et al. A case of von Recklinghausen's disease with bilateral pheochromocytoma-malignant peripheral nerve sheath tumors of the adrenal and gastrointestinal autonomic nerve tumors. Am J Surg Pathol. 1996 Jul;20(7):889–97. PMID:8669538
3894. Sakaki S, Yokoyama S, Mamitsuka K, et al. A case of pituitary adenoma associated with McCune-Albright syndrome. Pituitary. 1999 May;1(3-4):297–302. PMID:11081212
3895. Sakata K, Fujimori K, Komaki S, et al. Pituitary gangliocytoma producing TSH and TRH: a review of "Gangliocytomas of the sellar region". J Clin Endocrinol Metab. 2020 Oct 1;105(10):3109–21. PMID:32706866
3896. Sakellariou M, Dellaportas D, Peppa M, et al. Review of the literature on leiomyoma and leiomyosarcoma of the adrenal gland: a systematic analysis of case reports. In Vivo. 2020 Sep-Oct;34(5):2233–48. PMID:32871746
3897. Sakorafas GH, Giannopoulos GA, Parasi A, et al. Large somatostatin-producing endocrine carcinoma of the ampulla of vater in association with GIST in a patient with von Recklinghausen's disease. Case report and review of the literature. JOP. 2008 Sep 2;9(5):633–9. PMID:18762695
3898. Sakorafas GH, Giotakis J, Stafyla V. Papillary thyroid microcarcinoma: a surgical perspective. Cancer Treat Rev. 2005 Oct;31(6):423–38. PMID:16005155
3899. Sakurai A, Suzuki S, Kosugi S, et al. Multiple endocrine neoplasia type 1 in Japan: establishment and analysis of a multicentre database. Clin Endocrinol (Oxf). 2012 Apr;76(4):533–9. PMID:21950691
3900. Sakurai K, Onouchi T, Yamada S, et al. Cytohistology of morule in cribriform-morular variant of papillary thyroid carcinoma. Malays J Pathol. 2019 Dec;41(3):339–43. PMID:31901919
3901. Sala E, Ferrante E, Verrua E, et al. Growth hormone-releasing hormone-producing pancreatic neuroendocrine tumor in a multiple endocrine neoplasia type 1 family with an uncommon phenotype. Eur J Gastroenterol Hepatol. 2013 Jul;25(7):858–62. PMID:23542451
3902. Sala TD, Mureşan S, Roman R, et al. Hypercalcaemic crisis due to primary hyperparathyroidism: report of two cases. J Crit Care Med (Targu Mures). 2019 Feb 4;5(1):34–9. PMID:30766921
3903. Salama Y, Albanyan S, Szybowska M, et al. Comprehensive characterization of a Canadian cohort of von Hippel-Lindau disease patients. Clin Genet. 2019 Nov;96(5):461–7. PMID:31368132
3904. Salas S, Resseguier N, Blay JY, et al. Prediction of local and metastatic recurrence in solitary fibrous tumor: construction of a risk calculator in a multicenter cohort from the French Sarcoma Group (FSG) database. Ann Oncol. 2017 Aug 1;28(8):1979–87. PMID:28838212
3905. Saleh HA, Jin B, Barnwell J, et al. Utility of immunohistochemical markers in differentiating benign from malignant follicular-derived thyroid nodules. Diagn Pathol. 2010 Jan 26;5:9. PMID:20181018
3906. Salehi F, Agur A, Scheithauer BW, et al. Ki-67 in pituitary neoplasms: a review–part I. Neurosurgery. 2009 Sep;65(3):429–37. PMID:19687686
3907. Salehi F, Scheithauer BW, Kovacs K, et al. O-6-methylguanine-DNA methyltransferase (MGMT) immunohistochemical expression in pituitary corticotroph adenomas. Neurosurgery. 2012 Feb;70(2):491–6. PMID:21822153
3908. Salehi F, Scheithauer BW, Moyes VJ, et al. Low immunohistochemical expression of MGMT in ACTH secreting pituitary tumors of patients with Nelson syndrome. Endocr Pathol. 2010 Dec;21(4):227–9. PMID:21061089
3909. Salenave S, Ancelle D, Bahougne T, et al. Macroprolactinomas in children and adolescents: factors associated with the response to treatment in 77 patients. J Clin Endocrinol Metab. 2015 Mar;100(3):1177–86. PMID:25532043
3910. Salenave S, Boyce AM, Collins MT, et al. Acromegaly and McCune-Albright syndrome. J Clin Endocrinol Metab. 2014 Jun;99(6):1955–69. PMID:24517150
3911. Salge-Arrieta FJ, Carrasco-Moro R, Rodríguez-Berrocal V, et al. Clinical features, diagnosis and therapy of pituicytoma: an update. J Endocrinol Invest. 2019 Apr;42(4):371–84. PMID:30030746
3912. Salgues B, Guerin C, Amodru V, et al. Risk stratification of adrenal masses by [18 F] FDG PET/CT: changing tactics. Clin Endocrinol (Oxf). 2021 Feb;94(2):133–40. PMID:32978795
3913. Saliba I, Evrard AS. Middle ear glandular neoplasms: adenoma, carcinoma or adenoma with neuroendocrine differentiation: a case series. Cases J. 2009 Mar 13;2:6508. PMID:20111612
3914. Saliba M, Katabi N, Dogan S, et al. NRAS Q61R immunohistochemical staining in thyroid pathology: sensitivity, specificity and utility. Histopathology. 2021 Oct;79(4):650–60. PMID:33960437
3915. Saliba M, Mohanty AS, Ho AL, et al. Secretory carcinoma of the thyroid in a 49-year-old man treated with larotrectinib: protracted clinical course of disease despite the high-grade histologic features. Head Neck Pathol. 2022 Jun;16(2):612–20. PMID:34655408
3916. Salle L, Mas R, Teissier-Clément MP. Ectopic adrenocortical carcinoma of the ovary: an unexpected outcome. Ann Endocrinol (Paris). 2020 Oct;81(5):516–8. PMID:32822651
3917. Salpea P, Stratakis CA. Carney complex and McCune Albright syndrome: an overview of clinical manifestations and human molecular genetics. Mol Cell Endocrinol. 2014 Apr

5;386(1-2):85–91. PMID:24012779
3918. Saltman B, Singh B, Hedvat CV, et al. Patterns of expression of cell cycle/apoptosis genes along the spectrum of thyroid carcinoma progression. Surgery. 2006 Dec;140(6):899–905. PMID:17188136
3919. Salvatore G, Chiappetta G, Nikiforov YE, et al. Molecular profile of hyalinizing trabecular tumours of the thyroid: high prevalence of RET/PTC rearrangements and absence of B-raf and N-ras point mutations. Eur J Cancer. 2005 Mar;41(5):816–21. PMID:15763659
3920. Salvatori M, Perotti G, Rufini V, et al. Solitary liver metastasis from Hürthle cell thyroid cancer: a case report and review of the literature. J Endocrinol Invest. 2004 Jan;27(1):52–6. PMID:15053244
3921. Salzman R, Stárek I, Tichá V, et al. Metastasizing middle ear carcinoid: an unusual case report, with focus on ultrastructural and immunohistochemical findings. Otol Neurotol. 2012 Oct;33(8):1418–21. PMID:22935814
3922. Samarasinghe S, Yuksel S, Mehrotra S. Intermixed medullary and papillary thyroid cancer in a patient with renal cell carcinoma. Endocrinol Diabetes Metab Case Rep. 2020 Jun 4;2020:20-0025. PMID:32538376
3923. Sambade C, Baldaque-Faria A, Cardoso-Oliveira M, et al. Follicular and papillary variants of medullary carcinoma of the thyroid. Pathol Res Pract. 1988 Dec;184(1):98–107. PMID:3068650
3924. Sambade C, Franssila K, Cameselle-Teijeiro J, et al. Hyalinizing trabecular adenoma: a misnomer for a peculiar tumor of the thyroid gland. Endocr Pathol. 1991 Jun;2(2):83–91. PMID:32138392
3925. Sambugaro S, Di Ruvo M, Ambrosio MR, et al. Early onset acromegaly associated with a novel deletion in CDKN1B 5'UTR region. Endocrine. 2015 May;49(1):58–64. PMID:25645465
3926. Sameer KS, Mohanty S, Correa MM, et al. Lingual thyroglossal duct cysts–a review. Int J Pediatr Otorhinolaryngol. 2012 Feb;76(2):165–8. PMID:22192899
3927. Sams SB, Tompkins KD, Mayson S, et al. Oncocytic variant of medullary thyroid carcinoma; a rare tumor with numerous diagnostic mimics by fine needle aspiration. Diagn Cytopathol. 2017 Dec;45(12):1148–52. PMID:28802094
3928. Samuels SL, Surrey LF, Hawkes CP, et al. Characteristics of Follicular variant papillary thyroid carcinoma in a pediatric cohort. J Clin Endocrinol Metab. 2018 Apr 1;103(4):1639–48. PMID:29438531
3929. Samulski TD, Bai S, LiVolsi VA, et al. Malignant potential of small oncocytic follicular carcinoma/Hürthle cell carcinoma: an institutional experience. Histopathology. 2013 Oct;63(4):568–73. PMID:23952654
3930. Samyn I, Fontaine C, Van Tussenbroek F, et al. Paraneoplastic syndromes in cancer: Case 1. Polycythemia as a result of ectopic erythropoietin production in metastatic pancreatic carcinoid tumor. J Clin Oncol. 2004 Jun 1;22(11):2240–2. PMID:15169813
3931. Sancak S, Jaeschke H, Eren F, et al. High prevalence of TSHR/Gsα mutation-negative clonal hot thyroid nodules (HNs) in a Turkish cohort. Horm Metab Res. 2011 Jul;43(8):562–8. PMID:21773967
3932. Sancho JJ, Triponez F, Montet X, et al. Surgical management of adrenal metastases. Langenbecks Arch Surg. 2012 Feb;397(2):179–94. PMID:22205385
3933. Sandoval M, Carrasco-Zuber J, Gonzalez S. Extradigital symplastic glomus tumor of the hand: report of 2 cases and literature review. Am J Dermatopathol. 2015 Jul;37(7):560–2. PMID:25051107
3934. Sanghvi S, Misra P, Patel NR, et al. Incidence trends and long-term survival analysis of sinonasal rhabdomyosarcoma. Am J Otolaryngol. 2013 Nov-Dec;34(6):682–9. PMID:23743294
3935. Sanguedolce F, Calò B, Chirico M, et al. Urinary tract large cell neuroendocrine carcinoma: diagnostic, prognostic and therapeutic issues. Anticancer Res. 2020 May;40(5):2439–47. PMID:32366387
3936. Sankhla S, Khan GM. Cauda equina paraganglioma presenting with intracranial hypertension: case report and review of the literature. Neurol India. 2004 Jun;52(2):243–4. PMID:15269482
3937. Sanno N, Teramoto A, Osamura RY, et al. A growth hormone-releasing hormone-producing pancreatic islet cell tumor metastasized to the pituitary is associated with pituitary somatotroph hyperplasia and acromegaly. J Clin Endocrinol Metab. 1997 Aug;82(8):2731–7. PMID:9253362
3938. Sano T, Asa SL, Kovacs K. Growth hormone-releasing hormone-producing tumors: clinical, biochemical, and morphological manifestations. Endocr Rev. 1988 Aug;9(3):357–73. PMID:3145190
3939. Sano T, Horiguchi H, Xu B, et al. Double pituitary adenomas: six surgical cases. Pituitary. 1999 May;1(3-4):243–50. PMID:11081204
3940. Sano T, Rong QZ, Kagawa N, et al. Down-regulation of E-cadherin and catenins in human pituitary growth hormone-producing adenomas. Front Horm Res. 2004;32:127–32. PMID:15281343
3941. Sansone ME, Liwnicz BH, Mandybur TI. Giant pituitary cavernous hemangioma: case report. J Neurosurg. 1980 Jul;53(1):124–6. PMID:7411202
3942. Santana NO, Freitas RMC, Marcos VN, et al. Diagnostic performance of thyroid ultrasound in Hürthle cell carcinomas. Arch Endocrinol Metab. 2019 May-Jun;63(3):300–5. PMID:31038598
3943. Santoro A, Minniti G, Ruggeri A, et al. Biochemical remission and recurrence rate of secreting pituitary adenomas after transsphenoidal adenomectomy: long-term endocrinologic follow-up results. Surg Neurol. 2007 Nov;68(5):513–8. PMID:17961741
3944. Santoro C, Perrotta S, Picariello S, et al. Pretreatment endocrine disorders due to optic pathway gliomas in pediatric neurofibromatosis type 1: multicenter study. J Clin Endocrinol Metab. 2020 Jun 1;105(6):dgaa138. PMID:32294191
3945. Santoro M, Carlomagno F, Romano A, et al. Activation of RET as a dominant transforming gene by germline mutations of MEN2A and MEN2B. Science. 1995 Jan 20;267(5196):381–3. PMID:7824936
3946. Santos-Pinheiro F, Penas-Prado M, Kamiya-Matsuoka C, et al. Treatment and long-term outcomes in pituitary carcinoma: a cohort study. Eur J Endocrinol. 2019 Oct;181(4):397–407. PMID:31349217
3947. Santucci N, Gaujoux S, Binquet C, et al. Pancreatoduodenectomy for neuroendocrine tumors in patients with multiple endocrine neoplasia type 1: an AFCE (Association Francophone de Chirurgie Endocrinienne) and GTE (Groupe d'étude des Tumeurs Endocrines) study. World J Surg. 2021 Jun;45(6):1794–802. PMID:33649917
3948. Saqcena M, Leandro-Garcia LJ, Maag JLV, et al. SWI/SNF complex mutations promote thyroid tumor progression and insensitivity to redifferentiation therapies. Cancer Discov. 2021 May;11(5):1158–75. PMID:33318036
3949. Saqi A, Kuker AP, Ebner SA, et al. Langerhans cell histiocytosis: diagnosis on thyroid aspirate and review of the literature. Head Neck Pathol. 2015 Dec;9(4):496–502. PMID:25596951
3950. Sarioglu S, Akturk G, Aslier NG, et al. Atypical carcinoid tumor and chondroid and glandular hamartoma of the arythenoid region. J Craniofac Surg. 2016 Mar;27(2):e175–6. PMID:26854777
3951. Sarkar S, Sahoo PK, Mahata S, et al. Mitotic checkpoint defects: en route to cancer and drug resistance. Chromosome Res. 2021 Jun;29(2):131–44. PMID:33409811
3952. Sarkaria IS, Iyoda A, Roh MS, et al. Neoadjuvant and adjuvant chemotherapy in resected pulmonary large cell neuroendocrine carcinomas: a single institution experience. Ann Thorac Surg. 2011 Oct;92(4):1180–6. PMID:21867986
3953. Sarkis LM, Clifton-Bligh R, Veivers D, et al. SDH deficiency is very common in carotid body paragangliomas: genetic counseling and testing should be offered to all patients. Head Neck. 2023 Jun;45(6):1497–502. PMID:37010365
3954. Sarkisian SS, Schultz AL. Pituitary ependymoma. U S Armed Forces Med J. 1956 Dec;7(12):1813–6. PMID:13392185
3955. Sarquis M, Moraes DC, Bastos-Rodrigues L, et al. Germline mutations in familial papillary thyroid cancer. Endocr Pathol. 2020 Mar;31(1):14–20. PMID:32034658
3956. Sarquis MS, Silveira LG, Pimenta FJ, et al. Familial hyperparathyroidism: surgical outcome after 30 years of follow-up in three families with germline HRPT2 mutations. Surgery. 2008 May;143(5):630–40. PMID:18436011
3957. Sartoretti-Schefer S, Wichmann W, Aguzzi A, et al. MR differentiation of adamantinous and squamous-papillary craniopharyngiomas. AJNR Am J Neuroradiol. 1997 Jan;18(1):77–87. PMID:9010523
3958. Sasaki Y, Shiozawa E, Watanabe N, et al. t(3;14)(p14.1;q32)/FOXP1-IGH translocation in thyroid extranodal marginal zone lymphoma of mucosa-associated lymphoid tissue (MALT lymphoma). Leuk Res. 2020 Aug;95:106399. PMID:32534365
3959. Sasano H, Miyazaki S, Sawai T, et al. Primary pigmented nodular adrenocortical disease (PPNAD): immunohistochemical and in situ hybridization analysis of steroidogenic enzymes in eight cases. Mod Pathol. 1992 Jan;5(1):23–9. PMID:1542635
3960. Sasano H, Sato S, Yajima A, et al. Adrenal rest tumor of the broad ligament: case report with immunohistochemical study of steroidogenic enzymes. Pathol Int. 1997 Jul;47(7):493–6. PMID:9234389
3961. Sasano H, Suzuki T, Nagura H. ACTH-independent macronodular adrenocortical hyperplasia: immunohistochemical and in situ hybridization studies of steroidogenic enzymes. Mod Pathol. 1994 Feb;7(2):215–9. PMID:8008746
3962. Sasidharan K, Babu AS, Pandey AP, et al. Primary melanoma of the adrenal gland: a case report. J Urol. 1977 May;117(5):663–4. PMID:859207
3963. Satake H, Inoue K, Kamada M, et al. Malignant composite pheochromocytoma of the adrenal gland in a patient with von Recklinghausen's disease. J Urol. 2001 Apr;165(4):1199–200. PMID:11257670
3964. Satapathy S, Mittal BR, Bhansali A. 'Peptide receptor radionuclide therapy in the management of advanced pheochromocytoma and paraganglioma: a systematic review and meta-analysis'. Clin Endocrinol (Oxf). 2019 Dec;91(6):718–27. PMID:31569282
3965. Sathananthan M, Sathananthan A, Scheithauer BW, et al. Sellar meningiomas: an endocrinologic perspective. Pituitary. 2013 Jun;16(2):182–8. PMID:22644157
3966. Sathe PA, Shah HU, Kothari KS, et al. Bilateral Epstein-Barr virus-associated adrenal leiomyomas in a child without an established immunodeficiency. Pediatr Dev Pathol. 2012 Jul-Aug;15(4):329–32. PMID:22483165
3967. Sato H, Imamura Y, Sakamoto S, et al. Adrenalectomy in Japanese patients with subclinical Cushing syndrome: 1-mg dexamethasone suppression test to predict the surgical benefit. Int J Urol. 2021 Mar;28(3):273–9. PMID:33258172
3968. Sato K, Oka H, Utsuki S, et al. Ciliated craniopharyngioma may arise from Rathke cleft cyst. Clin Neuropathol. 2006 Jan-Feb;25(1):25–8. PMID:16465771
3969. Sato Y, Maekawa S, Ishii R, et al. Recurrent somatic mutations underlie corticotropin-independent Cushing's syndrome. Science. 2014 May 23;344(6186):917–20. PMID:24855271
3970. Sato Y, Nakamura N, Nakamura S, et al. Deviated VH4 immunoglobulin gene usage is found among thyroid mucosa-associated lymphoid tissue lymphomas, similar to the usage at other sites, but is not found in thyroid diffuse large B-cell lymphomas. Mod Pathol. 2006 Dec;19(12):1578–84. PMID:16980947
3971. Sauer CM, Haugg AM, Chteinberg E, et al. Reviewing the current evidence supporting early B-cells as the cellular origin of Merkel cell carcinoma. Crit Rev Oncol Hematol. 2017 Aug;116:99–105. PMID:28693804
3972. Saygin C, Uzunaslan D, Ozguroglu M, et al. Dendritic cell sarcoma: a pooled analysis including 462 cases with presentation of our case series. Crit Rev Oncol Hematol. 2013 Nov;88(2):253–71. PMID:23755890
3973. Sbiera S, Kunz M, Weigand I, et al. The new genetic landscape of Cushing's disease: deubiquitinases in the spotlight. Cancers (Basel). 2019 Nov 8;11(11):1761. PMID:31717455
3974. Sbiera S, Perez-Rivas LG, Taranets L, et al. Driver mutations in USP8 wild-type Cushing's disease. Neuro Oncol. 2019 Oct 9;21(10):1273–83. PMID:31222332
3975. Sbiera S, Schmull S, Assie G, et al. High diagnostic and prognostic value of steroidogenic factor-1 expression in adrenal tumors. J Clin Endocrinol Metab. 2010 Oct;95(10):E161–71. PMID:20660055
3976. Scardoni M, Vittoria E, Volante M, et al. Mixed adenoneuroendocrine carcinomas of the gastrointestinal tract: targeted next-generation sequencing suggests a monoclonal origin of the two components. Neuroendocrinology. 2014;100(4):310–6. PMID:25342539
3977. Scarpa A, Chang DK, Nones K, et al. Whole-genome landscape of pancreatic neuroendocrine tumours. Nature. 2017 Mar 2;543(7643):65–71. PMID:28199314
3978. Scarpa A, Mantovani W, Capelli P, et al. Pancreatic endocrine tumors: improved TNM staging and histopathological grading permit a clinically efficient prognostic stratification of patients. Mod Pathol. 2010 Jun;23(6):824–33. PMID:20305616
3979. Scarsbrook AF, Thakker RV, Wass JA, et al. Multiple endocrine neoplasia: spectrum of radiologic appearances and discussion of a multitechnique imaging approach. Radiographics. 2006 Mar-Apr;26(2):433–51. PMID:16549608
3980. Schaapveld M, Jorna FH, Aben KK, et al. Incidence and prognosis of parathyroid gland carcinoma: a population-based study in The Netherlands estimating the preoperative diagnosis. Am J Surg. 2011 Nov;202(5):590–7. PMID:21861982
3981. Schaefer IM, Dong F, Garcia EP, et al. Recurrent SMARCB1 inactivation in epithelioid malignant peripheral nerve sheath tumors. Am J Surg Pathol. 2019 Jun;43(6):835–43. PMID:30864974
3982. Schaefer IM, Fletcher CD, Hornick JL.

Loss of H3K27 trimethylation distinguishes malignant peripheral nerve sheath tumors from histologic mimics. Mod Pathol. 2016 Jan;29(1):4–13. PMID:26585554
3983. Schaefer S, Shipotko M, Meyer S, et al. Natural course of small adrenal lesions in multiple endocrine neoplasia type 1: an endoscopic ultrasound imaging study. Eur J Endocrinol. 2008 May;158(5):699–704. PMID:18426829
3984. Schalin-Jäntti C, Asa SL, Arola J, et al. Recurrent acute-onset Cushing's syndrome 6 years after removal of a thymic neuroendocrine carcinoma: from ectopic ACTH to CRH. Endocr Pathol. 2013 Mar;24(1):25–9. PMID:23233312
3985. Schantz A, Castleman B. Parathyroid carcinoma. A study of 70 cases. Cancer. 1973 Mar;31(3):600–5. PMID:4693587
3986. Scharpf J, Kamani D, Sadow PM, et al. The follicular variant of papillary thyroid cancer and noninvasive follicular thyroid neoplasm with papillary-like nuclear features (NIFTP). Curr Opin Oncol. 2017 Jan;29(1):20–4. PMID:27845971
3987. Schatz-Siemers N, Brandler TC, Oweity T, et al. Hürthle cell lesions on thyroid fine needle aspiration cytology: molecular and histologic correlation. Diagn Cytopathol. 2019 Oct;47(10):977–85. PMID:31293091
3988. Schaumann N, Hussein K. Hepatic and adrenocortical choristomas in the placenta. Fetal Pediatr Pathol. 2022 Apr;41(2):320–9. PMID:32696693
3989. Scheithauer BW, Horvath E, Abel TW, et al. Pituitary blastoma: a unique embryonal tumor. Pituitary. 2012 Sep;15(3):365–73. PMID:21805093
3990. Scheithauer BW, Horvath E, Kovacs K. Ultrastructure of the neurohypophysis. Microsc Res Tech. 1992 Jan 15;20(2):177–86. PMID:1547358
3991. Scheithauer BW, Horvath E, Kovacs K, et al. Prolactin-producing pituitary adenoma and carcinoma with neuronal components–a metaplastic lesion. Pituitary. 1999 May;1(3-4):197–205. PMID:11081198
3992. Scheithauer BW, Jaap AJ, Horvath E, et al. Clinically silent corticotroph tumors of the pituitary gland. Neurosurgery. 2000 Sep;47(3):723–9. PMID:10981760
3993. Scheithauer BW, Kovacs K, Horvath E, et al. Pituitary blastoma. Acta Neuropathol. 2008 Dec;116(6):657–66. PMID:18551299
3994. Scheithauer BW, Nora FE, LeChago J, et al. Duodenal gangliocytic paraganglioma. Clinicopathologic and immunocytochemical study of 11 cases. Am J Clin Pathol. 1986 Nov;86(5):559–65. PMID:2877566
3995. Scheithauer BW, Swearingen B, Whyte ET, et al. Ependymoma of the sella turcica: a variant of pituicytoma. Hum Pathol. 2009 Mar;40(3):435–40. PMID:18992914
3996. Schernthaner-Reiter MH, Trivellin G, Stratakis CA. MEN1, MEN4, and Carney complex: pathology and molecular genetics. Neuroendocrinology. 2016;103(1):18–31. PMID:25592387
3997. Schilling T, Bürck J, Sinn HP, et al. Prognostic value of codon 918 (ATG-->ACG) RET proto-oncogene mutations in sporadic medullary thyroid carcinoma. Int J Cancer. 2001 Jan 20;95(1):62–6. PMID:11241313
3998. Schittenhelm J, Psaras T, Meyermann R, et al. Pituitary adenomas and craniopharyngiomas are CDX2 negative neoplasms. Folia Neuropathol. 2010;48(2):75–80. PMID:20602288
3999. Schlaffer SM, Buchfelder M, Stoehr R, et al. Rathke's cleft cyst as origin of a pediatric papillary craniopharyngioma. Front Genet. 2018 Feb 22;9:49. PMID:29520296
4000. Schleiermacher G, Delattre O, Peter M, et al. Clinical relevance of loss heterozygosity of the short arm of chromosome 1 in neuroblastoma: a single-institution study. Int J Cancer. 1996 Apr 22;69(2):73–8. PMID:8608986
4001. Schleiermacher G, Mosseri V, London WB, et al. Segmental chromosomal alterations have prognostic impact in neuroblastoma: a report from the INRG project. Br J Cancer. 2012 Oct 9;107(8):1418–22. PMID:22976801
4002. Schlumberger M, Chevillard S, Ory K, et al. [Thyroid cancer following exposure to ionising radiation]. Cancer Radiother. 2011 Aug;15(5):394–9. French. PMID:21723770
4003. Schmalisch K, Beschorner R, Psaras T, et al. Postoperative intracranial seeding of craniopharyngiomas–report of three cases and review of the literature. Acta Neurochir (Wien). 2010 Feb;152(2):313–9. PMID:19859655
4004. Schmid S, Solomon DA, Perez E, et al. Genetic and epigenetic characterization of posterior pituitary tumors. Acta Neuropathol. 2021 Dec;142(6):1025–43. PMID:34661724
4005. Schmidt J, Derr V, Heinrich MC, et al. BRAF in papillary thyroid carcinoma of ovary (struma ovarii). Am J Surg Pathol. 2007 Sep;31(9):1337–43. PMID:17721188
4006. Schmitt A, Saremaslani P, Schmid S, et al. IGFII and MIB1 immunohistochemistry is helpful for the differentiation of benign from malignant adrenocortical tumours. Histopathology. 2006 Sep;49(3):298–307. PMID:16918977
4007. Schmitt AM, Anlauf M, Rousson V, et al. WHO 2004 criteria and CK19 are reliable prognostic markers in pancreatic endocrine tumors. Am J Surg Pathol. 2007 Nov;31(11):1677–82. PMID:18059224
4008. Schmitt AM, Blank A, Perren A. Gastrinoma. In: La Rosa S, Sessa F, editors. Pancreatic neuroendocrine neoplasms: practical approach to diagnosis, classification, and therapy. Cham (Switzerland): Springer; 2015. pp. 105–8.
4009. Schmitt AM, Schmid S, Rudolph T, et al. VHL inactivation is an important pathway for the development of malignant sporadic pancreatic endocrine tumors. Endocr Relat Cancer. 2009 Dec;16(4):1219–27. PMID:19690016
4010. Schmitt HP, Wurster K, Bauer M, et al. Mixed chemodectoma-ganglioneuroma of the conus medullaris region. Acta Neuropathol. 1982;57(4):275–81. PMID:6291307
4011. Schmitz BA, Singh C, Gulbahce HE, et al. Florid capsular and pericapsular papillary endothelial proliferation associated with poorly differentiated thyroid carcinoma. Int J Surg Pathol. 2011 Feb;19(1):110–2. PMID:20042405
4012. Schmitz R, Wright GW, Huang DW, et al. Genetics and pathogenesis of diffuse large B-cell lymphoma. N Engl J Med. 2018 Apr 12;378(15):1396–407. PMID:29641966
4013. Schneider N, Hallin M, Thway K. STAT6 loss in dedifferentiated solitary fibrous tumor. Int J Surg Pathol. 2017 Feb;25(1):58–60. PMID:27189111
4014. Schneider R, Bartsch-Herzog S, Ramaswamy A, et al. Immunohistochemical expression of E-cadherin in atypical parathyroid adenoma. World J Surg. 2015 Oct;39(10):2477–83. PMID:26154578
4015. Schneider R, Waldmann J, Swaid Z, et al. Calcitonin-secreting pancreatic endocrine tumors: systematic analysis of a rare tumor entity. Pancreas. 2011 Mar;40(2):213–21. PMID:21178652
4016. Scholfield DW, Fitzgerald CWR, Boe LA, et al. Defining the genomic landscape of diffuse sclerosing papillary thyroid carcinoma: prognostic implications of RET fusions. Ann Surg Oncol. 2024 Sep;31(9):5525–36. PMID:38847983
4017. Scholl UI, Goh G, Stölting G, et al. Somatic and germline CACNA1D calcium channel mutations in aldosterone-producing adenomas and primary aldosteronism. Nat Genet. 2013 Sep;45(9):1050–4. PMID:23913001
4018. Scholl UI, Stölting G, Nelson-Williams C, et al. Recurrent gain of function mutation in calcium channel CACNA1H causes early-onset hypertension with primary aldosteronism. Elife. 2015 Apr 24;4:e06315. PMID:25907736
4019. Scholl UI, Stölting G, Schewe J, et al. CLCN2 chloride channel mutations in familial hyperaldosteronism type II. Nat Genet. 2018 Mar;50(3):349–54. PMID:29403011
4020. Schoonhoven LM, Sparnaay T, van Wissen W, et al. Seven-week persistence of an oviposition-deterrent pheromone. J Chem Ecol. 1981 May;7(3):583–8. PMID:24420597
4021. Schrader KA, Nelson TN, De Luca A, et al. Multiple granular cell tumors are an associated feature of LEOPARD syndrome caused by mutation in PTPN11. Clin Genet. 2009 Feb;75(2):185–9. PMID:19054014
4022. Schreinemakers JM, Pieterman CR, Scholten A, et al. The optimal surgical treatment for primary hyperparathyroidism in MEN1 patients: a systematic review. World J Surg. 2011 Sep;35(9):1993–2005. PMID:21713580
4023. Schröder S, Böcker W. Clear-cell carcinomas of thyroid gland: a clinicopathological study of 13 cases. Histopathology. 1986 Jan;10(1):75–89. PMID:3957248
4024. Schröder S, Böcker W. Signet-ring-cell thyroid tumors. Follicle cell tumors with arrest of folliculogenesis. Am J Surg Pathol. 1985 Sep;9(9):619–29. PMID:2996373
4025. Schröder S, Böcker W, Hüsselmann H, et al. Adenolipoma (thyrolipoma) of the thyroid gland report of two cases and review of literature. Virchows Arch A Pathol Anat Histopathol. 1984;404(1):99–103. PMID:6433552
4026. Schulte JH, Schulte S, Heukamp LC, et al. Targeted therapy for neuroblastoma: ALK inhibitors. Klin Padiatr. 2013 Nov;225(6):303–8. PMID:24166094
4027. Schulte JJ, Pease G, Taxy JB, et al. Distinguishing parathyromatosis, atypical parathyroid adenomas, and parathyroid carcinomas utilizing histologic and clinical features. Head Neck Pathol. 2021 Sep;15(3):727–36. PMID:33394375
4028. Schulte KM, Gill AJ, Barczynski M, et al. Classification of parathyroid cancer. Ann Surg Oncol. 2012 Aug;19(8):2620–8. PMID:22434247
4029. Schultheis AM, de Bruijn I, Selenica P, et al. Genomic characterization of small cell carcinomas of the uterine cervix. Mol Oncol. 2022 Feb;16(4):833–45. PMID:33830625
4030. Schultz KAP, Stewart DR, Kamihara J, et al. DICER1 tumor predisposition. In: Adam MP, Feldman J, Mirzaa GM, et al., editors. GeneReviews. Seattle (WA): University of Washington, Seattle; 2014 Apr 24 [updated 2020 Apr 30]. PMID:24761742
4031. Schultz KAP, Williams GM, Kamihara J, et al. DICER1 and associated conditions: identification of at-risk individuals and recommended surveillance strategies. Clin Cancer Res. 2018 May 15;24(10):2251–61. PMID:29343557
4032. Schulz B, Altendorf-Hofmann A, Kirchner T, et al. Loss of CD34 and high IGF2 are associated with malignant transformation in solitary fibrous tumors. Pathol Res Pract. 2014 Feb;210(2):92–7. PMID:24360568
4033. Schulz T, Hartschuh W. Merkel cells are absent in basal cell carcinomas but frequently found in trichoblastomas. An immunohistochemical study. J Cutan Pathol. 1997 Jan;24(1):14–24. PMID:9027628
4034. Schwarzkopf G, Pfisterer J. [Metastasizing gastrinoma and tuberous sclerosis complex. Association or coincidence?]. Zentralbl Pathol. 1994 Feb;139(6):477–81. German. PMID:8161496
4035. Schweizer L, Capper D, Hölsken A, et al. BRAF V600E analysis for the differentiation of papillary craniopharyngiomas and Rathke's cleft cysts. Neuropathol Appl Neurobiol. 2015 Oct;41(6):733–42. PMID:25442675
4036. Schweizer L, Koelsche C, Sahm F, et al. Meningeal hemangiopericytoma and solitary fibrous tumors carry the NAB2-STAT6 fusion and can be diagnosed by nuclear expression of STAT6 protein. Acta Neuropathol. 2013 May;125(5):651–8. PMID:23575898
4037. Schweizer L, Thierfelder F, Thomas C, et al. Molecular characterization of CNS paragangliomas identifies cauda equina paragangliomas as a distinct tumor entity. Acta Neuropathol. 2020 Dec;140(6):893–906. PMID:32926213
4038. Sciarra A, Missiaglia E, Trimech M, et al. Gallbladder mixed neuroendocrine-non-neuroendocrine neoplasm (MiNEN) arising in intracholecystic papillary neoplasm: clinicopathologic and molecular analysis of a case and review of the literature. Endocr Pathol. 2020 Mar;31(1):84–93. PMID:31981075
4039. Scognamiglio T, Hyjek E, Kao J, et al. Diagnostic usefulness of HBME1, galectin-3, CK19, and CITED1 and evaluation of their expression in encapsulated lesions with questionable features of papillary thyroid carcinoma. Am J Clin Pathol. 2006 Nov;126(5):700–8. PMID:17050067
4040. Scollo C, Baudin E, Travagli JP, et al. Rationale for central and bilateral lymph node dissection in sporadic and hereditary medullary thyroid cancer. J Clin Endocrinol Metab. 2003 May;88(5):2070–5. PMID:12727956
4041. Scott DW, Wright GW, Williams PM, et al. Determining cell-of-origin subtypes of diffuse large B-cell lymphoma using gene expression in formalin-fixed paraffin-embedded tissue. Blood. 2014 Feb 20;123(8):1214–7. PMID:24398326
4042. Scott MP, Helm KF. Cytokeratin 20: a marker for diagnosing Merkel cell carcinoma. Am J Dermatopathol. 1999 Feb;21(1):16–20. PMID:10027519
4043. Scully KM, Gleiberman AS, Lindzey J, et al. Role of estrogen receptor-alpha in the anterior pituitary gland. Mol Endocrinol. 1997 Jun;11(6):674–81. PMID:9171231
4044. Scully KM, Rosenfeld MG. Pituitary development: regulatory codes in mammalian organogenesis. Science. 2002 Mar 22;295(5563):2231–5. PMID:11910101
4045. Scully RE, Cohen RB. Ganglioneuroma of adrenal medulla containing cells morphologically identical to hilus cells (extraparenchymal Leydig cells). Cancer. 1961 Mar-Apr;14:421–5. PMID:13749451
4046. Scurry J, Brand A, Planner R, et al. Vulvar Merkel cell tumor with glandular and squamous differentiation. Gynecol Oncol. 1996 Aug;62(2):292–7. PMID:8751563
4047. Seabrook AJ, Harris JE, Velosa SB, et al. Multiple endocrine tumors associated with germline MAX mutations: Multiple endocrine neoplasia type 5? J Clin Endocrinol Metab. 2021 Mar 25;106(4):1163–82. PMID:33367756
4048. Sebastiano C, Zhao X, Deng FM, et al. Cystic lesions of the adrenal gland: our experience over the last 20 years. Hum Pathol. 2013 Sep;44(9):1797–803. PMID:23618356
4049. Sebro R, DeLaney T, Hornicek F, et al. Differences in sex distribution, anatomic location and MR imaging appearance of pediatric compared to adult chordomas. BMC Med Imaging. 2016 Sep 8;16(1):53. PMID:27609115
4050. Seefelder C, Sparks JW, Chirnomas D, et al. Perioperative management of a child with severe hypertension from a catecholamine secreting neuroblastoma. Paediatr Anaesth. 2005 Jul;15(7):606–10. PMID:15960647
4051. Seeger RC, Brodeur GM, Sather H,

et al. Association of multiple copies of the N-myc oncogene with rapid progression of neuroblastomas. N Engl J Med. 1985 Oct 31;313(18):1111–6. PMID:4047115
4052. Seethala RR, Baloch ZW, Barletta JA, et al. Noninvasive follicular thyroid neoplasm with papillary-like nuclear features: a review for pathologists. Mod Pathol. 2018 Jan;31(1):39–55. PMID:29052599
4053. Seethala RR, Chiosea SI. Solid cell nests, papillary thyroid microcarcinoma, and HBME1. Am J Clin Pathol. 2010 Jul;134(1):169–70. PMID:20551283
4054. Seethala RR, Ogilvie JB, Carty SE, et al. Parathyroid lipoadenomas and lipohyperplasias: clinicopathologic correlations. Am J Surg Pathol. 2008 Dec;32(12):1854–67. PMID:18813123
4055. Segkos K, Schmidt C, Nabhan F. Isolated liver metastasis in Hürthle cell thyroid cancer treated with microwave ablation. Case Rep Endocrinol. 2017;2017:2790741. PMID:28163939
4056. Sehested M, Hirsch FR, Osterlind K, et al. Morphologic variations of small cell lung cancer. A histopathologic study of pretreatment and posttreatment specimens in 104 patients. Cancer. 1986 Feb 15;57(4):804–7. PMID:3002587
4057. Sekimizu M, Yoshida A, Mitani S, et al. Frequent mutations of genes encoding vacuolar H+ -ATPase components in granular cell tumors. Genes Chromosomes Cancer. 2019 Jun;58(6):373–80. PMID:30597645
4058. Sekine S, Shibata T, Kokubu A, et al. Craniopharyngiomas of adamantinomatous type harbor beta-catenin gene mutations. Am J Pathol. 2002 Dec;161(6):1997–2001. PMID:12466115
4059. Selfe J, Olmos D, Al-Saadi R, et al. Impact of fusion gene status versus histology on risk-stratification for rhabdomyosarcoma: retrospective analyses of patients on UK trials. Pediatr Blood Cancer. 2017 Jul;64(7). PMID:28035744
4060. Seltzer J, Ashton CE, Scotton TC, et al. Gene and protein expression in pituitary corticotroph adenomas: a systematic review of the literature. Neurosurg Focus. 2015 Feb;38(2):E17. PMID:25639319
4061. Seltzer J, Lucas J, Commins D, et al. Ectopic ACTH-secreting pituitary adenoma of the sphenoid sinus: case report of endoscopic endonasal resection and systematic review of the literature. Neurosurg Focus. 2015 Feb;38(2):E10. PMID:25639312
4062. Semple PL, De Villiers JC, Bowen RM, et al. Pituitary apoplexy: do histological features influence the clinical presentation and outcome? J Neurosurg. 2006 Jun;104(6):931–7. PMID:16776337
4063. Sen F, Borczuk AC. Combined carcinoid tumor of the lung: a combination of carcinoid and adenocarcinoma. Lung Cancer. 1998 Jul;21(1):53–8. PMID:9792054
4064. Senescende L, Bitolog PL, Auberger E, et al. Adrenal ectopy of adult groin region: a systematic review of an unexpected anatomopathologic diagnosis. Hernia. 2016 Dec;20(6):879–85. PMID:27601037
4065. Sensaki K, Aida S, Takagi K, et al. Coexisting undifferentiated thymic carcinoma and thymic carcinoid tumor. Respiration. 1993;60(4):247–9. PMID:8265883
4066. Seo HS, Lee DH, Park SH, et al. Thyroid follicular neoplasms: can sonography distinguish between adenomas and carcinomas? J Clin Ultrasound. 2009 Nov-Dec;37(9):493–500. PMID:19746451
4067. Sergeant C, Jublanc C, Leclercq D, et al. Transdifferentiation of neuroendocrine cells: gangliocytoma associated with two pituitary adenomas of different lineage in MEN1. Am J Surg Pathol. 2017 Jun;41(6):849–53. PMID:28079577
4068. Service FJ, McMahon MM, O'Brien PC, et al. Functioning insulinoma–incidence, recurrence, and long-term survival of patients: a 60-year study. Mayo Clin Proc. 1991 Jul;66(7):711–9. PMID:1677058
4069. Seshamani M, Einhorn E, Mirza N. Atypical carcinoid of the larynx and potential complications of the carcinoid syndrome: a case report. Ear Nose Throat J. 2009 Jan;88(1):E1. PMID:19172557
4070. Seth AK, Argani P, Campbell KA. Angiosarcoma of the pancreas: discussion of a rare epithelioid neoplasm. Pancreas. 2008 Aug;37(2):230–1. PMID:18665093
4071. Seth R, Ahmed M, Hoschar AP, et al. Cervical sympathetic chain paraganglioma: a report of 2 cases and a literature review. Ear Nose Throat J. 2014 Mar;93(3):E22–7. PMID:24652566
4072. Sethi K, Sarkar S, Das S, et al. Biomarkers for the diagnosis of thyroid cancer. J Exp Ther Oncol. 2010;8(4):341–52. PMID:21222366
4073. Settakorn J, Sirivanichai C, Rangdaeng S, et al. Fine-needle aspiration cytology of adrenal myelolipoma: case report and review of the literature. Diagn Cytopathol. 1999 Dec;21(6):409–12. PMID:10572274
4074. Settas N, Faucz FR, Stratakis CA. Succinate dehydrogenase (SDH) deficiency, Carney triad and the epigenome. Mol Cell Endocrinol. 2018 Jul 5;469:107–11. PMID:28739378
4075. Shaco-Levy R, Peng RY, Snyder MJ, et al. Malignant struma ovarii: a blinded study of 86 cases assessing which histologic features correlate with aggressive clinical behavior. Arch Pathol Lab Med. 2012 Feb;136(2):172–8. PMID:22288964
4076. Shaffer MM, Oertel YC, Oertel JE. Thyroglossal duct cysts: diagnostic criteria by fine-needle aspiration. Arch Pathol Lab Med. 1996 Nov;120(11):1039–43. PMID:12049106
4077. Shafqat H, Ali S, Salhab M, et al. Survival of patients with neuroendocrine carcinoma of the colon and rectum: a population-based analysis. Dis Colon Rectum. 2015 Mar;58(3):294–303. PMID:25664707
4078. Shah AA, La Fortune K, Miller C, et al. Thyroid sclerosing mucoepidermoid carcinoma with eosinophilia: a clinicopathologic and molecular analysis of a distinct entity. Mod Pathol. 2017 Mar;30(3):329–39. PMID:27910944
4079. Shah K, Perez-Ordóñez B. Neuroendocrine neoplasms of the sinonasal tract: neuroendocrine carcinomas and olfactory neuroblastoma. Head Neck Pathol. 2016 Mar;10(1):85–94. PMID:26830400
4080. Shah R, Schniederjan M, DelGaudio JM, et al. Visual vignette. Ectopic ACTH-secreting pituitary adenoma. Endocr Pract. 2011 Nov-Dec;17(6):966. PMID:21803709
4081. Shah S, Gosain R, Groman A, et al. Incidence and survival outcomes in patients with lung neuroendocrine neoplasms in the United States. Cancers (Basel). 2021 Apr 7;13(8):1753. PMID:33916960
4082. Shaha AR, Shah JP. Parathyroid carcinoma: a diagnostic and therapeutic challenge. Cancer. 1999 Aug 1;86(3):378–80. PMID:10430243
4083. Shames JM, Dhurandhar NR, Blackard WG. Insulin-secreting bronchial carcinoid tumor with widespread metastases. Am J Med. 1968 Apr;44(4):632–7. PMID:4296076
4084. Shamir ER, Devine WP, Pekmezci M, et al. Identification of high-risk human papillomavirus and Rb/E2F pathway genomic alterations in mutually exclusive subsets of colorectal neuroendocrine carcinoma. Mod Pathol. 2019 Feb;32(2):290–305. PMID:30237525
4085. Shankar GM, Chen L, Kim AH, et al. Composite ganglioneuroma-paraganglioma of the filum terminale. J Neurosurg Spine. 2010 Jun;12(6):709–13. PMID:20515359
4086. Shankar SK, Tandon PN, Roy S. Third ventricular chromophobe adenoma with normal adenohypophysis. Acta Neuropathol. 1976 Aug 16;35(4):353–6. PMID:961385
4087. Shanmugam V, Margolskee E, Kluk M, et al. Rosai-Dorfman disease harboring an activating KRAS K117N missense mutation. Head Neck Pathol. 2016 Sep;10(3):394–9. PMID:26922062
4088. Shao N, Wang HK, Zhu Y, et al. Modification of American Joint Committee on cancer prognostic groups for renal cell carcinoma. Cancer Med. 2018 Nov;7(11):5431–8. PMID:30306741
4089. Shao QQ, Zhao BB, Dong LB, et al. Surgical management of Zollinger-Ellison syndrome: classical considerations and current controversies. World J Gastroenterol. 2019 Aug 28;25(32):4673–81. PMID:31528093
4090. Sharma A, Gaikwad SB, Goyal M, et al. Calcified filum terminale paraganglioma causing superficial siderosis. AJR Am J Roentgenol. 1998 Jun;170(6):1650–2. PMID:9609190
4091. Sharma A, Mukewar S, Vege SS. Clinical profile of pancreatic cystic lesions in von Hippel-Lindau disease: a series of 48 patients seen at a tertiary institution. Pancreas. 2017 Aug;46(7):948–52. PMID:28697137
4092. Sharma A, Sharma S, Patnaik N, et al. Cytomorphologic and immunophenotypic profile of a cohort of small cell carcinoma of the urinary bladder. Acta Cytol. 2016;60(5):475–80. PMID:27698324
4093. Sharretts JM, Kebebew E, Simonds WF. Parathyroid cancer. Semin Oncol. 2010 Dec;37(6):580–90. PMID:21167377
4094. Shattuck TM, Välimäki S, Obara T, et al. Somatic and germ-line mutations of the HRPT2 gene in sporadic parathyroid carcinoma. N Engl J Med. 2003 Oct 30;349(18):1722–9. PMID:14585940
4095. Shawa H, Elsayes KM, Javadi S, et al. Clinical and radiologic features of pheochromocytoma/ganglioneuroma composite tumors: a case series with comparative analysis. Endocr Pract. 2014 Sep;20(9):864–9. PMID:24641930
4096. Shawky M, Proctor I, Kurzawinski T, et al. Papillary thyroid microcarcinoma presenting as a metastasis to the brain. Ann R Coll Surg Engl. 2020 May;102(5):e107–10. PMID:32233872
4097. Shehadeh NJ, Vernick J, Lonardo F, et al. Sclerosing mucoepidermoid carcinoma with eosinophilia of the thyroid: a case report and review of the literature. Am J Otolaryngol. 2004 Jan-Feb;25(1):48–53. PMID:15011206
4098. Shekhar S, Sinaii N, Irizarry-Caro JA, et al. Prevalence of hypothyroidism in patients with Erdheim-Chester disease. JAMA Netw Open. 2020 Oct 1;3(10):e2019169. PMID:33119105
4099. Shen P, Jing Y, Zhang R, et al. Comprehensive genomic profiling of neuroendocrine bladder cancer pinpoints molecular origin and potential therapeutics. Oncogene. 2018 May;37(22):3039–44. PMID:29535424
4100. Shenker Y, LLoyd RV, Weatherbee L, et al. Ectopic prolactinoma in a patient with hyperparathyroidism and abnormal sellar radiography. J Clin Endocrinol Metab. 1986 May;62(5):1065–9. PMID:3958123
4101. Shenoy BV, Carpenter PC, Carney JA. Bilateral primary pigmented nodular adrenocortical disease. Rare cause of the Cushing syndrome. Am J Surg Pathol. 1984 May;8(5):335–44. PMID:6329005
4102. Shenoy VG, Thota A, Shankar R, et al. Adrenal myelolipoma: controversies in its management. Indian J Urol. 2015 Apr-Jun;31(2):94–101. PMID:25878407
4103. Shern JF, Chen L, Chmielecki J, et al. Comprehensive genomic analysis of rhabdomyosarcoma reveals a landscape of alterations affecting a common genetic axis in fusion-positive and fusion-negative tumors. Cancer Discov. 2014 Feb;4(2):216–31. PMID:24436047
4104. Shetty S, Varghese RT, Shanthly N, et al. Toxic thyroid adenoma in McCune-Albright syndrome. J Clin Diagn Res. 2014 Feb;8(2):281–2. PMID:24701557
4105. Shetty T, Chase TN. Central monoamines and hyperkinase of childhood. Neurology. 1976 Oct;26(10):1000–2. PMID:986582
4106. Sheu SY, Schwertheim S, Worm K, et al. Diffuse sclerosing variant of papillary thyroid carcinoma: lack of BRAF mutation but occurrence of RET/PTC rearrangements. Mod Pathol. 2007 Jul;20(7):779–87. PMID:17464312
4107. Sheu SY, Vogel E, Worm K, et al. Hyalinizing trabecular tumour of the thyroid-differential expression of distinct miRNAs compared with papillary thyroid carcinoma. Histopathology. 2010 Apr;56(5):632–40. PMID:20459574
4108. Sheu SY, Wenzel RR, Kersting C, et al. Erdheim-Chester disease: case report with multisystemic manifestations including testes, thyroid, and lymph nodes, and a review of literature. J Clin Pathol. 2004 Nov;57(11):1225–8. PMID:15509691
4109. Shi C, Klimstra DS. Pancreatic neuroendocrine tumors: pathologic and molecular characteristics. Semin Diagn Pathol. 2014 Nov;31(6):498–511. PMID:25441311
4110. Shi H, Qi C, Meng L, et al. Do neuroendocrine carcinomas and mixed neuroendocrine-non-neuroendocrine neoplasm of the gastrointestinal tract have the same prognosis? A SEER database analysis of 12,878 cases. Ther Adv Endocrinol Metab. 2020 Jul 6;11:2042018820938304. PMID:32670540
4111. Shia J, Tang LH, Weiser MR, et al. Is nonsmall cell type high-grade neuroendocrine carcinoma of the tubular gastrointestinal tract a distinct disease entity? Am J Surg Pathol. 2008 May;32(5):719–31. PMID:18360283
4112. Shibata M, Inaishi T, Miyajima N, et al. Synchronous bilateral pheochromocytomas and paraganglioma with novel germline mutation in MAX: a case report. Surg Case Rep. 2017 Dec 28;3(1):131. PMID:29282558
4113. Shibata Y, Yamazaki M, Takei M, et al. Early-onset, severe, and recurrent primary hyperparathyroidism associated with a novel CDC73 mutation. Endocr J. 2015;62(7):627–32. PMID:25959515
4114. Shibuya M. Welcoming the new WHO classification of pituitary tumors 2017: revolution in TTF-1-positive posterior pituitary tumors. Brain Tumor Pathol. 2018 Apr;35(2):62–70. PMID:29500747
4115. Shield PW, Crous H. Fine-needle aspiration cytology of Merkel cell carcinoma-a review of 69 cases. Diagn Cytopathol. 2014 Nov;42(11):924–8. PMID:24678011
4116. Shih AR, Cote GM, Chebib I, et al. Clinicopathologic characteristics of poorly differentiated chordoma. Mod Pathol. 2018 Aug;31(8):1237–45. PMID:29483606
4117. Shimada H. In situ neuroblastoma: an important concept related to the natural history of neural crest tumors. Pediatr Dev Pathol. 2005 May-Jun;8(3):305–6. PMID:16010489
4118. Shimada H, Ambros IM, Dehner LP, et al. Terminology and morphologic criteria of neuroblastic tumors: recommendations by the International Neuroblastoma Pathology Committee. Cancer. 1999 Jul 15;86(2):349–63. PMID:10421272
4119. Shimada H, Ambros IM, Dehner LP, et al. The International Neuroblastoma Pathology Classification (the Shimada system). Cancer.

1999 Jul 15;86(2):364–72. PMID:10421273
4120. Shimada H, Aoyama C, Chiba T, et al. Prognostic subgroups for undifferentiated neuroblastoma: immunohistochemical study with anti-S-100 protein antibody. Hum Pathol. 1985 May;16(5):471–6. PMID:3886523
4121. Shimada H, Chatten J, Newton WA Jr, et al. Histopathologic prognostic factors in neuroblastic tumors: definition of subtypes of ganglioneuroblastoma and an age-linked classification of neuroblastomas. J Natl Cancer Inst. 1984 Aug;73(2):405–16. PMID:6589432
4122. Shimada H, Umehara S, Monobe Y, et al. International neuroblastoma pathology classification for prognostic evaluation of patients with peripheral neuroblastic tumors: a report from the Children's Cancer Group. Cancer. 2001 Nov 1;92(9):2451–61. PMID:11745303
4123. Shimojo N, Hirokawa YS, Kanayama K, et al. Cytological features of adenocarcinoma admixed with small cell neuroendocrine carcinoma of the uterine cervix. Cytojournal. 2017 May 26;14:12. PMID:28603541
4124. Shimon I, Sosa E, Mendoza V, et al. Giant prolactinomas larger than 60 mm in size: a cohort of massive and aggressive prolactin-secreting pituitary adenomas. Pituitary. 2016 Aug;19(4):429–36. PMID:27138902
4125. Shin TJ, Rabbani CC, Murthy HD, et al. Hürthle cell neoplasms of the thyroid: pathologic outcomes and ultrasonographic analysis. Laryngoscope Investig Otolaryngol. 2020 Oct 7;5(6):1254–9. PMID:33364419
4126. Shindo K, Aishima S, Okido M, et al. A poor prognostic case of mucoepidermoid carcinoma of the thyroid: a case report. Case Rep Endocrinol. 2012;2012:862545. PMID:22970393
4127. Shinohara M, Shitara T, Hatakeyama SI, et al. An infant with systemic hypertension, renal artery stenosis, and neuroblastoma. J Pediatr Surg. 2004 Jan;39(1):103–6. PMID:14694383
4128. Shinozaki H, Sasakura Y, Shinozaki S, et al. Cystic pancreatic neuroendocrine tumor in a patient with neurofibromatosis type 1. Case Rep Gastroenterol. 2021 Feb 1;15(1):108–14. PMID:33708057
4129. Shirafkan Md A, Boroumand Md N, Komak Md S, et al. Pancreatic pleomorphic rhabdomyosarcoma. Int J Surg Case Rep. 2015;13:33–6. PMID:26092712
4130. Shiroko T, Yokoo N, Okamoto K, et al. Mixed medullary-papillary carcinoma of the thyroid with lymph node metastases: report of a case. Surg Today. 2001;31(4):317–21. PMID:11321340
4131. Shojaei-Brosseau T, Chompret A, Abel A, et al. Genetic epidemiology of neuroblastoma: a study of 426 cases at the Institut Gustave-Roussy in France. Pediatr Blood Cancer. 2004 Jan;42(1):99–105. PMID:14752801
4132. Shore RE, Hildreth N, Dvoretsky P, et al. Benign thyroid adenomas among persons X-irradiated in infancy for enlarged thymus glands. Radiat Res. 1993 May;134(2):217–23. PMID:8488255
4133. Shorter NA, Glick RD, Klimstra DS, et al. Malignant pancreatic tumors in childhood and adolescence: the Memorial Sloan-Kettering experience, 1967 to present. J Pediatr Surg. 2002 Jun;37(6):887–92. PMID:12037756
4134. Shugart RR, Soule EH, Johnson EW Jr. Glomus tumor. Surg Gynecol Obstet. 1963 Sep;117:334–40. PMID:14080348
4135. Siddappa PK, Vege SS. Vasoactive intestinal peptide-secreting tumors: a review. Pancreas. 2019 Oct;48(9):1119–25. PMID:31609932
4136. Sidwell RU, Rouse P, Owen RA, et al. Granular cell tumor of the scrotum in a child with Noonan syndrome. Pediatr Dermatol. 2008 May-Jun;25(3):341–3. PMID:18577039
4137. Sievers P, Stichel D, Schrimpf D, et al. FGFR1:TACC1 fusion is a frequent event in molecularly defined extraventricular neurocytoma. Acta Neuropathol. 2018 Aug;136(2):293–302. PMID:29978331
4138. Sigel CS, Klimstra DS. Cytomorphologic and immunophenotypical features of acinar cell neoplasms of the pancreas. Cancer Cytopathol. 2013 Aug;121(8):459–70. PMID:23408736
4139. Sigel CS, Krauss Silva VW, Reid MD, et al. Assessment of cytologic differentiation in high-grade pancreatic neuroendocrine neoplasms: a multi-institutional study. Cancer Cytopathol. 2018 Jan;126(1):44–53. PMID:29044913
4140. Sigel CS, Krauss Silva VW, Reid MD, et al. Well differentiated grade 3 pancreatic neuroendocrine tumors compared with related neoplasms: a morphologic study. Cancer Cytopathol. 2018 May;126(5):326–35. PMID:29451738
4141. Sihto H, Böhling T, Kavola H, et al. Tumor infiltrating immune cells and outcome of Merkel cell carcinoma: a population-based study. Clin Cancer Res. 2012 May 15;18(10):2872–81. PMID:22467679
4142. Sihto H, Kukko H, Koljonen V, et al. Clinical factors associated with Merkel cell polyomavirus infection in Merkel cell carcinoma. J Natl Cancer Inst. 2009 Jul 1;101(13):938–45. PMID:19535775
4143. Sihto H, Kukko H, Koljonen V, et al. Merkel cell polyomavirus infection, large T antigen, retinoblastoma protein and outcome in Merkel cell carcinoma. Clin Cancer Res. 2011 Jul 15;17(14):4806–13. PMID:21642382
4144. Silva-Figueroa AM, Bassett R Jr, Christakis I, et al. Using a novel diagnostic nomogram to differentiate malignant from benign parathyroid neoplasms. Endocr Pathol. 2019 Dec;30(4):285–96. PMID:31734935
4145. Silveira LG, Dias EP, Marinho BC, et al. HRPT2-related familial isolated hyperparathyroidism: could molecular studies direct the surgical approach? Arq Bras Endocrinol Metabol. 2008 Nov;52(8):1211–20. PMID:19169472
4146. Silverberg SG, Vidone RA. Carcinoma of the thyroid in surgical and postmortem material. Analysis of 300 cases at autopsy and literature review. Ann Surg. 1966 Aug;164(2):291–9. PMID:5915940
4147. Silverstein GE, Burke G, Cogan R. The natural history of the autonomous hyperfunctioning thyroid nodule. Ann Intern Med. 1967 Sep;67(3):539–48. PMID:4167139
4148. Simanshu DK, Nissley DV, McCormick F. RAS proteins and their regulators in human disease. Cell. 2017 Jun 29;170(1):17–33. PMID:28666118
4149. Simbolo M, Bilotta M, Mafficini A, et al. Gene expression profiling of pancreas neuroendocrine tumors with different Ki67-based grades. Cancers (Basel). 2021 Apr 23;13(9):2054. PMID:33922803
4150. Simbolo M, Mafficini A, Sikora KO, et al. Lung neuroendocrine tumours: deep sequencing of the four World Health Organization histotypes reveals chromatin-remodelling genes as major players and a prognostic role for TERT, RB1, MEN1 and KMT2D. J Pathol. 2017 Mar;241(4):488–500. PMID:27873319
4151. Simbolo M, Mian C, Barollo S, et al. High-throughput mutation profiling improves diagnostic stratification of sporadic medullary thyroid carcinomas. Virchows Arch. 2014 Jul;465(1):73–8. PMID:24828033
4152. Simões-Pereira J, Bugalho MJ, Limbert E, et al. Retrospective analysis of 140 cases of medullary thyroid carcinoma followed-up in a single institution. Oncol Lett. 2016 Jun;11(6):3870–4. PMID:27313709
4153. Simon LM, Magit AE. Impact of incision and drainage of infected thyroglossal duct cyst on recurrence after Sistrunk procedure. Arch Otolaryngol Head Neck Surg. 2012 Jan;138(1):20–4. PMID:22249624
4154. Simonds WF, Robbins CM, Agarwal SK, et al. Familial isolated hyperparathyroidism is rarely caused by germline mutation in HRPT2, the gene for the hyperparathyroidism-jaw tumor syndrome. J Clin Endocrinol Metab. 2004 Jan;89(1):96–102. PMID:14715834
4155. Simonds WF, Varghese S, Marx SJ, et al. Cushing's syndrome in multiple endocrine neoplasia type 1. Clin Endocrinol (Oxf). 2012 Mar;76(3):379–86. PMID:21916912
4156. Singarayer R, Mete O, Perrier L, et al. A systematic review and meta-analysis of the diagnostic performance of BRAF V600E immunohistochemistry in thyroid histopathology. Endocr Pathol. 2019 Sep;30(3):201–18. PMID:31300997
4157. Singh BK, Arumugaswamy PR, Chumber S, et al. Giant secretory multifocal adrenal myelolipoma: a diagnostic dilemma. BMJ Case Rep. 2021 Jan 29;14(1):e239441. PMID:33514622
4158. Singh HK, Kilpatrick SE, Silverman JF. Fine needle aspiration biopsy of soft tissue sarcomas: utility and diagnostic challenges. Adv Anat Pathol. 2004 Jan;11(1):24–37. PMID:14676638
4159. Singh Ospina N, Sebo TJ, Thompson GB, et al. Prevalence of parathyroid carcinoma in 348 patients with multiple endocrine neoplasia type 1 - case report and review of the literature. Clin Endocrinol (Oxf). 2016 Feb;84(2):244–9. PMID:25557532
4160. Singh Ospina N, Thompson GB, C Nichols F 3rd, et al. Thymic and bronchial carcinoid tumors in multiple endocrine neoplasia type 1: the Mayo Clinic experience from 1977 to 2013. Horm Cancer. 2015 Dec;6(5-6):247–53. PMID:26070346
4161. Singh R, Basturk O, Klimstra DS, et al. Lipid-rich variant of pancreatic endocrine neoplasms. Am J Surg Pathol. 2006 Feb;30(2):194–200. PMID:16434893
4162. Singhi AD, Chu LC, Tatsas AD, et al. Cystic pancreatic neuroendocrine tumors: a clinicopathologic study. Am J Surg Pathol. 2012 Nov;36(11):1666–73. PMID:23073325
4163. Singhi AD, Liu TC, Roncaioli JL, et al. Alternative lengthening of telomeres and loss of DAXX/ATRX expression predicts metastatic disease and poor survival in patients with pancreatic neuroendocrine tumors. Clin Cancer Res. 2017 Jan 15;23(2):600–9. PMID:27407094
4164. Singhi AD, Nikiforova MN, Fasanella KE, et al. Preoperative GNAS and KRAS testing in the diagnosis of pancreatic mucinous cysts. Clin Cancer Res. 2014 Aug 15;20(16):4381–9. PMID:24938521
4165. Sinha S, Sharma MC, Sharma BS. Malignant paraganglioma of the sellar region mimicking a pituitary macroadenoma. J Clin Neurosci. 2008 Aug;15(8):937–9. PMID:18482839
4166. Sinkre PA, Murakata L, Rabin L, et al. Clear cell carcinoid tumor of the gallbladder: another distinctive manifestation of von Hippel-Lindau disease. Am J Surg Pathol. 2001 Oct;25(10):1334–9. PMID:11688471
4167. Sinno S, Assaad AM, Salem Shabb N. Human papillomavirus-associated oropharyngeal high-grade neuroendocrine carcinoma in an adolescent: case report and review of literature. Clin Med Insights Pediatr. 2019 Sep 9;13:1179556519870520. PMID:31523135
4168. Siołek M, Cybulski C, Gąsior-Perczak D, et al. CHEK2 mutations and the risk of papillary thyroid cancer. Int J Cancer. 2015 Aug 1;137(3):548–52. PMID:25583358
4169. Sipos B, Sperveslage J, Anlauf M, et al. Glucagon cell hyperplasia and neoplasia with and without glucagon receptor mutations. J Clin Endocrinol Metab. 2015 May;100(5):E783–8. PMID:25695890
4170. Sippel RS, Caron NR, Clark OH. An evidence-based approach to familial nonmedullary thyroid cancer: screening, clinical management, and follow-up. World J Surg. 2007 May;31(5):924–33. PMID:17429563
4171. Sirikanjanapong S, Melamed J, Patel RR. Intraepidermal and dermal Merkel cell carcinoma with squamous cell carcinoma in situ: a case report with review of literature. J Cutan Pathol. 2010 Aug;37(8):881–5. PMID:19702685
4172. Sirvent N, Coindre JM, Maire G, et al. Detection of MDM2-CDK4 amplification by fluorescence in situ hybridization in 200 paraffin-embedded tumor samples: utility in diagnosing adipocytic lesions and comparison with immunohistochemistry and real-time PCR. Am J Surg Pathol. 2007 Oct;31(10):1476–89. PMID:17895748
4173. Sisto JM, Liu FW, Geffner ME, et al. Para-ovarian adrenal rest tumors: gynecologic manifestations of untreated congenital adrenal hyperplasia. Gynecol Endocrinol. 2018 Aug;34(8):644–6. PMID:29460643
4174. Sjöstedt E, Bollerslev J, Mulder J, et al. A specific antibody to detect transcription factor T-Pit: a reliable marker of corticotroph cell differentiation and a tool to improve the classification of pituitary neuroendocrine tumours. Acta Neuropathol. 2017 Oct;134(4):675–7. PMID:28823042
4175. Sjöstedt E, Kolnes AJ, Olarescu NC, et al. TGFBR3L-an uncharacterised pituitary specific membrane protein detected in the gonadotroph cells in non-neoplastic and tumour tissue. Cancers (Basel). 2020 Dec 31;13(1):114. PMID:33396509
4176. Skacel M, Ross CW, Hsi ED. A reassessment of primary thyroid lymphoma: high-grade MALT-type lymphoma as a distinct subtype of diffuse large B-cell lymphoma. Histopathology. 2000 Jul;37(1):10–8. PMID:10931213
4177. Skala SL, Dhanasekaran SM, Mehra R. Hereditary leiomyomatosis and renal cell carcinoma syndrome (HLRCC): a contemporary review and practical discussion of the differential diagnosis for HLRCC-associated renal cell carcinoma. Arch Pathol Lab Med. 2018 Oct;142(10):1202–15. PMID:30281371
4178. Skapek SX, Anderson J, Barr FG, et al. PAX-FOXO1 fusion status drives unfavorable outcome for children with rhabdomyosarcoma: a children's oncology group report. Pediatr Blood Cancer. 2013 Sep;60(9):1411–7. PMID:23526739
4179. Skapek SX, Ferrari A, Gupta AA, et al. Rhabdomyosarcoma. Nat Rev Dis Primers. 2019 Jan 7;5(1):1. PMID:30617281
4180. Skogseid B, Larsson C, Lindgren PG, et al. Clinical and genetic features of adrenocortical lesions in multiple endocrine neoplasia type 1. J Clin Endocrinol Metab. 1992 Jul;75(1):76–81. PMID:1352309
4181. Skogseid B, Rastad J, Gobl A, et al. Adrenal lesion in multiple endocrine neoplasia type 1. Surgery. 1995 Dec;118(6):1077–82. PMID:7491526
4182. Slater DN, Cotton DW, Azzopardi JG. Oncocytic glomus tumour: a new variant. Histopathology. 1987 May;11(5):523–31. PMID:3038728
4183. Slingerland J, Pagano M. Regulation of the CDK inhibitor p27 and its deregulation in cancer. J Cell Physiol. 2000 Apr;183(1):10–7. PMID:10699961
4184. Smedby KE, Baecklund E, Askling J. Malignant lymphomas in autoimmunity and inflammation: a review of risks, risk factors, and lymphoma characteristics. Cancer Epidemiol

Biomarkers Prev. 2006 Nov;15(11):2069–77. PMID:17119030
4185. Smeets EE, Span PN, van Herwaarden AE, et al. Molecular characterization of testicular adrenal rest tumors in congenital adrenal hyperplasia: lesions with both adrenocortical and Leydig cell features. J Clin Endocrinol Metab. 2015 Mar;100(3):E524–30. PMID:25485724
4186. Smith A, Galli M, Piga I, et al. Molecular signatures of medullary thyroid carcinoma by matrix-assisted laser desorption/ionisation mass spectrometry imaging. J Proteomics. 2019 Jan 16;191:114–23. PMID:29581064
4187. Smith J, Kulkarni A, Birkeland AC, et al. Whole-exome sequencing of sinonasal small cell carcinoma arising within a papillary Schneiderian carcinoma in situ. Otolaryngol Head Neck Surg. 2018 Nov;159(5):859–65. PMID:29734873
4188. Smith JD, Harvey RN, Darr OA, et al. Head and neck paragangliomas: a two-decade institutional experience and algorithm for management. Laryngoscope Investig Otolaryngol. 2017 Nov 11;2(6):380–9. PMID:29299512
4189. Smith JD, Reidy DL, Goodman KA, et al. A retrospective review of 126 high-grade neuroendocrine carcinomas of the colon and rectum. Ann Surg Oncol. 2014 Sep;21(9):2956–62. PMID:24763982
4190. Smith JR, Marqusee E, Webb S, et al. Thyroid nodules and cancer in children with PTEN hamartoma tumor syndrome. J Clin Endocrinol Metab. 2011 Jan;96(1):34–7. PMID:20962022
4191. Smith NJ, Mukherjee D, Wang Y, et al. Epidemiology and outcomes of primary pediatric lung malignancies: updates from the SEER database. Am J Surg. 2021 Oct;222(4):861–6. PMID:33549297
4192. Smith SL, Branton SA, Avino AJ, et al. Vasoactive intestinal polypeptide secreting islet cell tumors: a 15-year experience and review of the literature. Surgery. 1998 Dec;124(6):1050–5. PMID:9854582
4193. Smith TG, Clark SK, Katz DE, et al. Adrenal masses are associated with familial adenomatous polyposis. Dis Colon Rectum. 2000 Dec;43(12):1739–42. PMID:11156460
4194. Smith TR, Hulou MM, Huang KT, et al. Current indications for the surgical treatment of prolactinomas. J Clin Neurosci. 2015 Nov;22(11):1785–91. PMID:26277642
4195. Snaith JR, McLeod D, Richardson A, et al. Multifocal insulinoma secondary to insulinomatosis: persistent hypoglycaemia despite total pancreatectomy. Endocrinol Diabetes Metab Case Rep. 2020 Dec 24;2020:20-0091. PMID:33434149
4196. Snover DC, Foucar K. Mitotic activity in benign parathyroid disease. Am J Clin Pathol. 1981 Mar;75(3):345–7. PMID:7211756
4197. Snyder PJ. Gonadotroph cell adenomas of the pituitary. Endocr Rev. 1985 Fall;6(4):552–63. PMID:2416559
4198. Snyder V, Bayrak S, Woodroof J, et al. A parathyroid hemangioma of the retropharynx. JAMA Otolaryngol Head Neck Surg. 2018 Dec 1;144(12):1181–3. PMID:30242327
4199. So JS, Epstein JI. GATA3 expression in paragangliomas: a pitfall potentially leading to misdiagnosis of urothelial carcinoma. Mod Pathol. 2013 Oct;26(10):1365–70. PMID:23599157
4200. So YK, Kim MJ, Kim S, et al. Lateral lymph node metastasis in papillary thyroid carcinoma: a systematic review and meta-analysis for prevalence, risk factors, and location. Int J Surg. 2018 Feb;50:94–103. PMID:29329789
4201. Soares P, Póvoa AA, Melo M, et al. Molecular pathology of non-familial follicular epithelial-derived thyroid cancer in adults: from RAS/BRAF-like tumor designations to molecular risk stratification. Endocr Pathol. 2021 Mar;32(1):44–62. PMID:33651322
4202. Sobrinho-Simões M, Eloy C, Magalhães J, et al. Follicular thyroid carcinoma. Mod Pathol. 2011 Apr;24 Suppl 2:S10–8. PMID:21455197
4203. Sobrinho-Simões M, Nesland JM, Johannessen JV. Columnar-cell carcinoma. Another variant of poorly differentiated carcinoma of the thyroid. Am J Clin Pathol. 1988 Feb;89(2):264–7. PMID:3341287
4204. Sofela AA, Hettige S, Curran O, et al. Malignant transformation in craniopharyngiomas. Neurosurgery. 2014 Sep;75(3):306–14. PMID:24978859
4205. Soffer D, Pittaluga S, Caine Y, et al. Paraganglioma of cauda equina. A report of a case and review of the literature. Cancer. 1983 May 15;51(10):1907–10. PMID:6831356
4206. Soga J. Carcinoids and their variant endocrinomas. An analysis of 11842 reported cases. J Exp Clin Cancer Res. 2003 Dec;22(4):517–30. PMID:15053292
4207. Soga J. Carcinoids of the pancreas: an analysis of 156 cases. Cancer. 2005 Sep 15;104(6):1180–7. PMID:16104045
4208. Soga J, Osaka M, Yakuwa Y. Laryngeal endocrinomas (carcinoids and relevant neoplasms): analysis of 278 reported cases. J Exp Clin Cancer Res. 2002 Mar;21(1):5–13. PMID:12071530
4209. Soga J, Tazawa K. Pathologic analysis of carcinoids. Histologic reevaluation of 62 cases. Cancer. 1971 Oct;28(4):990–8. PMID:4106849
4210. Soga J, Yakuwa Y. Glucagonomas/diabetico-dermatogenic syndrome (DDS): a statistical evaluation of 407 reported cases. J Hepatobiliary Pancreat Surg. 1998;5(3):312–9. PMID:9880781
4211. Soga J, Yakuwa Y. Somatostatinoma/inhibitory syndrome: a statistical evaluation of 173 reported cases as compared to other pancreatic endocrinomas. J Exp Clin Cancer Res. 1999 Mar;18(1):13–22. PMID:10374671
4212. Soga J, Yakuwa Y. The gastrinoma/Zollinger-Ellison syndrome: statistical evaluation of a Japanese series of 359 cases. J Hepatobiliary Pancreat Surg. 1998;5(1):77–85. PMID:9683758
4213. Soga J, Yakuwa Y. Vipoma/diarrheogenic syndrome: a statistical evaluation of 241 reported cases. J Exp Clin Cancer Res. 1998 Dec;17(4):389–400. PMID:10089056
4214. Sohn SY, Lee JJ, Lee JH. Molecular profile and clinicopathologic features of follicular variant papillary thyroid carcinoma. Pathol Oncol Res. 2020 Apr;26(2):927–36. PMID:30900082
4215. Sohn SY, Park WY, Shin HT, et al. Highly concordant key genetic alterations in primary tumors and matched distant metastases in differentiated thyroid cancer. Thyroid. 2016 May;26(5):672–82. PMID:26971368
4216. Solcia E, Capella C, Riva C, et al. The morphology and neuroendocrine profile of pancreatic epithelial VIPomas and extrapancreatic, VIP-producing, neurogenic tumors. Ann N Y Acad Sci. 1988;527:508–17. PMID:2839087
4217. Soldozy S, Yeghyayan M, Yağmurlu K, et al. Endoscopic endonasal surgery outcomes for pediatric craniopharyngioma: a systematic review. Neurosurg Focus. 2020 Jan 1;48(1):E6. PMID:31896083
4218. Sollfrank L, Lettmaier S, Erdmann M, et al. Panniculitis under successful targeted inhibition of the MAPK/ERK signaling pathway in a patient with BRAF V600E-mutated spindle cell oncocytoma of the pituitary gland. Anticancer Res. 2019 Jul;39(7):3955–9. PMID:31262927
4219. Solomon A, Gupta PK, LiVolsi VA, et al. Distinguishing tall cell variant of papillary thyroid carcinoma from usual variant of papillary thyroid carcinoma in cytologic specimens. Diagn Cytopathol. 2002 Sep;27(3):143–8. PMID:12203860
4220. Solomon AC, Baloch ZW, Salhany KE, et al. Thyroid sclerosing mucoepidermoid carcinoma with eosinophilia: mimic of Hodgkin disease in nodal metastases. Arch Pathol Lab Med. 2000 Mar;124(3):446–9. PMID:10705405
4221. Solomon D, Schwartz A. Renal pathology in von Hippel-Lindau disease. Hum Pathol. 1988 Sep;19(9):1072–9. PMID:3417291
4222. Song E, Jeon MJ, Oh HS, et al. Do aggressive variants of papillary thyroid carcinoma have worse clinical outcome than classic papillary thyroid carcinoma? Eur J Endocrinol. 2018 Sep;179(3):135–42. PMID:29875289
4223. Song IH, Lee YS, Sun DI, et al. Metachronous double primary neuroendocrine tumors in larynx and lung: a case report. J Int Med Res. 2020 Nov;48(11):300060520962928. PMID:33167723
4224. Song M, Wang H, Song L, et al. Ectopic TSH-secreting pituitary tumor: a case report and review of prior cases. BMC Cancer. 2014 Jul 28;14:544. PMID:25069990
4225. Song T, Chen L, Zhang H, et al. Multimodal treatment based on thyroidectomy improves survival in patients with metastatic anaplastic thyroid carcinoma: a SEER analysis from 1998 to 2015. Gland Surg. 2020 Oct;9(5):1205–13. PMID:33224795
4226. Song X, Zheng S, Yang G, et al. Glucagonoma and the glucagonoma syndrome. Oncol Lett. 2018 Mar;15(3):2749–55. PMID:29435000
4227. Song YL, Xu J, Zhao DC, et al. Mutation and expression of gene YY1 in pancreatic neuroendocrine tumors and its clinical significance. Endocr Pract. 2021 Sep;27(9):874–80. PMID:33705973
4228. Song Z, Liu Y, Cheng G, et al. Distinct mutational backgrounds and clonal architectures implicated prognostic discrepancies in small-cell carcinomas of the esophagus and lung. Cell Death Dis. 2021 May 12;12(5):472. PMID:33980813
4229. Sonneland PR, Scheithauer BW, LeChago J, et al. Paraganglioma of the cauda equina region. Clinicopathologic study of 31 cases with special reference to immunocytology and ultrastructure. Cancer. 1986 Oct 15;58(8):1720–35. PMID:2875784
4230. Soon PS, Gill AJ, Benn DE, et al. Microarray gene expression and immunohistochemistry analyses of adrenocortical tumors identify IGF2 and Ki-67 as useful in differentiating carcinomas from adenomas. Endocr Relat Cancer. 2009 Jun;16(2):573–83. PMID:19218281
4231. Soon PS, Tacon LJ, Gill AJ, et al. miR-195 and miR-483-5p identified as predictors of poor prognosis in adrenocortical cancer. Clin Cancer Res. 2009 Dec 15;15(24):7684–92. PMID:19996210
4232. Soong CP, Arnold A. Recurrent ZFX mutations in human sporadic parathyroid adenomas. Oncoscience. 2014 May 6;1(5):360–6. PMID:25594030
4233. Soravia C, Sugg SL, Berk T, et al. Familial adenomatous polyposis-associated thyroid cancer: a clinical, pathological, and molecular genetics study. Am J Pathol. 1999 Jan;154(1):127–35. PMID:9916927
4234. Sorbye H, Strosberg J, Baudin E, et al. Gastroenteropancreatic high-grade neuroendocrine carcinoma. Cancer. 2014 Sep 15;120(18):2814–23. PMID:24771552
4235. Sorbye H, Welin S, Langer SW, et al. Predictive and prognostic factors for treatment and survival in 305 patients with advanced gastrointestinal neuroendocrine carcinoma (WHO G3): the NORDIC NEC study. Ann Oncol. 2013 Jan;24(1):152–60. PMID:22967994
4236. Sorrenti S, Carbotta G, Di Matteo FM, et al. Evaluation of clinicopathological and molecular parameters on disease recurrence of papillary thyroid cancer patient: a retrospective observational study. Cancers (Basel). 2020 Dec 4;12(12):3637. PMID:33291668
4237. Sorrenti S, Trimboli P, Catania A, et al. Comparison of malignancy rate in thyroid nodules with cytology of indeterminate follicular or indeterminate Hürthle cell neoplasm. Thyroid. 2009 Apr;19(4):355–60. PMID:19355826
4238. Soukup J, Česák T, Hornychová H, et al. Stem cell transcription factor Sox2 is expressed in a subset of folliculo-stellate cells of growth hormone-producing pituitary neuroendocrine tumours and its expression shows no association with tumour size or IGF1 levels: a clinicopathological study of 109 cases. Endocr Pathol. 2020 Dec;31(4):337–47. PMID:32632839
4239. Soukup J, Kasparova P, Kohout A, et al. Evaluation of expression of somatostatin receptor 1, 2, 3, 5 and dopamine D2 receptor in spindle cell oncocytomas of posterior pituitary. Pituitary. 2019 Feb;22(1):70–8. PMID:30607746
4240. Sousa J, O'Brien D, Crooks D. Paraganglioma of the filum terminale. J Clin Neurosci. 2005 Jun;12(5):584–5. PMID:15921911
4241. Souteiro P, Donato S, Costa C, et al. Diagnosis, treatment, and survival analysis of adrenocortical carcinomas: a multicentric study. Hormones (Athens). 2020 Jun;19(2):197–203. PMID:31823340
4242. Sovinz P, Urban C, Uhrig S, et al. Pheochromocytoma in a 2.75-year-old-girl with a germline von Hippel-Lindau mutation Q164R. Am J Med Genet A. 2010 Jul;152A(7):1752–5. PMID:20583150
4243. Spada A, Mantovani G, Lania AG, et al. Pituitary tumors: genetic and molecular factors underlying pathogenesis and clinical behavior. Neuroendocrinology. 2022;112(1):15–33. PMID:33524974
4244. Spadigam A, Dhupar A, Syed S, et al. Small cell neuroendocrine carcinoma of the paranasal sinus with intraoral involvement: report of a rare case and review of the literature. J Oral Maxillofac Pathol. 2017 May-Aug;21(2):286–95. PMID:28932042
4245. Spaulding SL, Ho R, Everest S, et al. The role of molecular testing in the diagnosis of medullary thyroid cancer: a case report of oncocytic medullary thyroid carcinoma and review of the literature. Am J Otolaryngol. 2020 Jan-Feb;41(1):102312. PMID:31727331
4246. Speel EJ, Richter J, Moch H, et al. Genetic differences in endocrine pancreatic tumor subtypes detected by comparative genomic hybridization. Am J Pathol. 1999 Dec;155(6):1787–94. PMID:10595906
4247. Speiser PW, Arlt W, Auchus RJ, et al. Congenital adrenal hyperplasia due to steroid 21-hydroxylase deficiency: an Endocrine Society Clinical Practice Guideline. J Clin Endocrinol Metab. 2018 Nov 1;103(11):4043–88. PMID:30272171
4248. Speiser PW, Azziz R, Baskin LS, et al. A summary of the Endocrine Society clinical practice guidelines on congenital adrenal hyperplasia due to steroid 21-hydroxylase deficiency. Int J Pediatr Endocrinol. 2010;2010:494173. PMID:20981249
4249. Speisky D, Duces A, Bièche I, et al. Molecular profiling of pancreatic neuroendocrine tumors in sporadic and Von Hippel-Lindau patients. Clin Cancer Res. 2012 May 15;18(10):2838–49. PMID:22461457
4250. Spinelli C, Rossi L, Barbetta A, et al. Incidental ganglioneuromas: a presentation of 14 surgical cases and literature review. J Endocrinol Invest. 2015 May;38(5):547–54. PMID:25501841

4251. Spinelli C, Strambi S, Bakkar S, et al. Surgical management of diffuse sclerosing variant of papillary thyroid carcinoma. Experience in 25 patients. World J Surg. 2020 Jan;44(1):155–62. PMID:31605177

4252. Šplíchalová E, Holý R, Traboulsi E, et al. Nonfunctional parathyroid cancer a case report. Rozhl Chir. 2021 Spring;100(3):133–7. PMID:33910359

4253. Sponziello M, Benvenuti S, Gentile A, et al. Whole exome sequencing identifies a germline MET mutation in two siblings with hereditary wild-type RET medullary thyroid cancer. Hum Mutat. 2018 Mar;39(3):371–7. PMID:29219214

4254. Sponziello M, Durante C, Boichard A, et al. Epigenetic-related gene expression profile in medullary thyroid cancer revealed the overexpression of the histone methyltransferases EZH2 and SMYD3 in aggressive tumours. Mol Cell Endocrinol. 2014 Jul 5;392(1-2):8–13. PMID:24813658

4255. Spurbeck JL, Carlson RO, Allen JE, et al. Culturing and robotic harvesting of bone marrow, lymph nodes, peripheral blood, fibroblasts, and solid tumors with in situ techniques. Cancer Genet Cytogenet. 1988 May;32(1):59–66. PMID:3281746

4256. Squires MH 3rd, Volkan Adsay N, Schuster DM, et al. Octreoscan versus FDG-PET for neuroendocrine tumor staging: a biological approach. Ann Surg Oncol. 2015 Jul;22(7):2295–301. PMID:25786743

4257. Srirangam Nadhamuni V, Iacovazzo D, Evanson J, et al. GHRH secretion from a pancreatic neuroendocrine tumor causing gigantism in a patient with MEN1. Endocrinol Diabetes Metab Case Rep. 2021 Jun 1;2021:20-0208. PMID:34156350

4258. Srivastava A, Giangiobbe S, Skopelitou D, et al. Whole genome sequencing prioritizes CHEK2, EWSR1, and TIAM1 as possible predisposition genes for familial non-medullary thyroid cancer. Front Endocrinol (Lausanne). 2021 Feb 22;12:600682. PMID:33692755

4259. Srivastava A, Hornick JL. Immunohistochemical staining for CDX-2, PDX-1, NESP-55, and TTF-1 can help distinguish gastrointestinal carcinoid tumors from pancreatic endocrine and pulmonary carcinoid tumors. Am J Surg Pathol. 2009 Apr;33(4):626–32. PMID:19065104

4260. Srivastava A, Kumar A, Giangiobbe S, et al. Whole genome sequencing of familial non-medullary thyroid cancer identifies germline alterations in MAPK/ERK and PI3K/AKT signaling pathways. Biomolecules. 2019 Oct 13;9(10):605. PMID:31614935

4261. Srivastava A, Miao B, Skopelitou D, et al. A germline mutation in the POT1 gene is a candidate for familial non-medullary thyroid cancer. Cancers (Basel). 2020 Jun 1;12(6):1441. PMID:32492864

4262. Sroussi M, Elaidi R, Fléchon A, et al. Neuroendocrine carcinoma of the urinary bladder: a large, retrospective study from the French Genito-Urinary Tumor Group. Clin Genitourin Cancer. 2020 Aug;18(4):295–303.e3. PMID:31882335

4263. Stack BC Jr, Tolley NS, Bartel TB, et al. AHNS Series: Do you know your guidelines? Optimizing outcomes in reoperative parathyroid surgery: definitive multidisciplinary joint consensus guidelines of the American Head and Neck Society and the British Association of Endocrine and Thyroid Surgeons. Head Neck. 2018 Aug;40(8):1617–29. PMID:30070413

4264. Stack BC Jr, Twining C, Rastatter J, et al. Consensus statement by the American Association of Clinical Endocrinology (AACE) and the American Head and Neck Society Endocrine Surgery Section (AHNS) on pediatric benign and malignant thyroid surgery. Endocr Pract. 2021 Mar;27(3):174–84. PMID:33779552

4265. Stacpoole PW. The glucagonoma syndrome: clinical features, diagnosis, and treatment. Endocr Rev. 1981 Summer;2(3):347–61. PMID:6268399

4266. Stahnke MJ, Dickel C, Schröder S, et al. Inhibition of human insulin gene transcription and MafA transcriptional activity by the dual leucine zipper kinase. Cell Signal. 2014 Sep;26(9):1792–9. PMID:24726898

4267. Stanek J, Busseniers AE. Fine-needle aspiration diagnosis of ectopic thyroid: report of one case. Diagn Cytopathol. 1993;9(1):59–62. PMID:8458284

4268. Stang A, Becker JC, Nghiem P, et al. The association between geographic location and incidence of Merkel cell carcinoma in comparison to melanoma: an international assessment. Eur J Cancer. 2018 May;94:47–60. PMID:29533867

4269. Starker LF, Svedlund J, Udelsman R, et al. The DNA methylome of benign and malignant parathyroid tumors. Genes Chromosomes Cancer. 2011 Sep;50(9):735–45. PMID:21638518

4270. Starling CE, Sabra J, Brady B, et al. Malignant teratoma of the thyroid: a difficult diagnosis by fine-needle aspiration. Diagn Cytopathol. 2019 Sep;47(9):930–4. PMID:31120625

4271. Starr JS, Attia S, Joseph RW, et al. Follicular dendritic cell sarcoma presenting as a thyroid mass. J Clin Oncol. 2015 Jun 10;33(17):e74–6. PMID:24663046

4272. Stefaneanu L, Kovacs K, Scheithauer BW, et al. Effect of dopamine agonists on lactotroph adenomas of the human pituitary. Endocr Pathol. 2000 Winter;11(4):341–52. PMID:12114758

4273. Stein T, Murugan P, Li F, et al. Can medullary thyroid carcinoma arise in thyroglossal duct cysts? A search for parafollicular C-cells in 41 resected cases. Head Neck Pathol. 2018 Mar;12(1):71–4. PMID:28536894

4274. Stelow EB, Moskaluk CA, Mills SE. The mismatch repair protein status of colorectal small cell neuroendocrine carcinomas. Am J Surg Pathol. 2006 Nov;30(11):1401–4. PMID:17063080

4275. Stemmer-Rachamimov AO, Xu L, Gonzalez-Agosti C, et al. Universal absence of merlin, but not other ERM family members, in schwannomas. Am J Pathol. 1997 Dec;151(6):1649–54. PMID:9403715

4276. Stenman A, Zedenius J, Juhlin CC. Over-diagnosis of potential malignant behavior in MEN 2A-associated pheochromocytomas using the PASS and GAPP algorithms. Langenbecks Arch Surg. 2018 Sep;403(6):785–90. PMID:29779047

4277. Stenman A, Zedenius J, Juhlin CC. The value of histological algorithms to predict the malignancy potential of pheochromocytomas and abdominal paragangliomas-a meta-analysis and systematic review of the literature. Cancers (Basel). 2019 Feb 15;11(2):225. PMID:30769931

4278. Stephen AE, Chen KT, Milas M, et al. The coming of age of radiation-induced hyperparathyroidism: evolving patterns of thyroid and parathyroid disease after head and neck irradiation. Surgery. 2004 Dec;136(6):1143–53. PMID:15657569

4279. Stephens M, Williams GT, Jasani B, et al. Synchronous duodenal neuroendocrine tumours in von Recklinghausen's disease–a case report of co-existing gangliocytic paraganglioma and somatostatin-rich glandular carcinoid. Histopathology. 1987 Dec;11(12):1331–40. PMID:2894342

4280. Sterkenburg AS, Hoffmann A, Gebhardt U, et al. Survival, hypothalamic obesity, and neuropsychological/psychosocial status after childhood-onset craniopharyngioma: newly reported long-term outcomes. Neuro Oncol. 2015 Jul;17(7):1029–38. PMID:25838139

4281. Sterrer E, Windisch F, Frey K, et al. Middle ear adenoma with neuroendocrine differentiation : a pediatric case report. Wien Klin Wochenschr. 2017 Mar;129(5-6):208–11. PMID:27761737

4282. Stetsenko GY, Malekirad J, Paulson KG, et al. p63 expression in Merkel cell carcinoma predicts poorer survival yet may have limited clinical utility. Am J Clin Pathol. 2013 Dec;140(6):838–44. PMID:24225752

4283. Stevens TM, Morlote D, Swensen J, et al. Spindle epithelial tumor with thymus-like differentiation (SETTLE): a next-generation sequencing study. Head Neck Pathol. 2019 Jun;13(2):162–8. PMID:29736783

4284. Stewart DR, Best AF, Williams GM, et al. Neoplasm risk among individuals with a pathogenic germline variant in DICER1. J Clin Oncol. 2019 Mar 10;37(8):668–76. PMID:30715996

4285. Stewart DR, Sloan JL, Yao L, et al. Diagnosis, management, and complications of glomus tumours of the digits in neurofibromatosis type 1. J Med Genet. 2010 Aug;47(8):525–32. PMID:20530151

4286. Stewart PM, Carey MP, Graham CT, et al. Growth hormone secreting pituitary carcinoma: a case report and literature review. Clin Endocrinol (Oxf). 1992 Aug;37(2):189–94. PMID:1395070

4287. Carreira AL, Korbonits M. Familial isolated pituitary adenoma. In: Feingold KR, Anawalt B, Blackman MR, et al., editors. Endotext. South Dartmouth (MA): MDText.com, Inc.; 2000 [updated 2024 Mar 7]. PMID:25905184

4288. Stojadinovic A, Brennan MF, Hoos A, et al. Adrenocortical adenoma and carcinoma: histopathological and molecular comparative analysis. Mod Pathol. 2003 Aug;16(8):742–51. PMID:12920217

4289. Stojadinovic A, Hoos A, Nissan A, et al. Parathyroid neoplasms: clinical, histopathological, and tissue microarray-based molecular analysis. Hum Pathol. 2003 Jan;34(1):54–64. PMID:12605367

4290. Stoll K, Tomkovich A, Howells J. Small cell carcinoma of the bladder presenting with paraneoplastic syndrome of inappropriate antidiuretic hormone. BMJ Case Rep. 2019 Dec 29;12(12):e232128. PMID:31888898

4291. Storr HL, Isidori AM, Monson JP, et al. Prepubertal Cushing's disease is more common in males, but there is no increase in severity at diagnosis. J Clin Endocrinol Metab. 2004 Aug;89(8):3818–20. PMID:15292311

4292. Storr HL, Savage MO. Management of endocrine disease: paediatric Cushing's disease. Eur J Endocrinol. 2015 Jul;173(1):R35–45. PMID:26036813

4293. Stoupa A, Kariyawasam D, Muzza M, et al. New genetics in congenital hypothyroidism. Endocrine. 2021 Mar;71(3):696–705. PMID:33650047

4294. Strait AM, Sharma N, Tsapakos MJ, et al. Pancreatic mixed acinar-neuroendocrine carcinoma, a unique diagnostic challenge on FNA cytology: a small series of two cases with literature review. Diagn Cytopathol. 2018 Nov;46(11):971–6. PMID:30284406

4295. Stratakis CA. Carney complex. In: Adam MP, Feldman J, Mirzaa GM, et al., editors. GeneReviews. Seattle (WA): University of Washington, Seattle; 2003 Feb 5 [updated 2023 Sep 21]. PMID:20301463

4296. Stratakis CA. Carney complex: a familial lentiginosis predisposing to a variety of tumors. Rev Endocr Metab Disord. 2016 Sep;17(3):367–71. PMID:27943004

4297. Stratakis CA, Boikos SA. Genetics of adrenal tumors associated with Cushing's syndrome: a new classification for bilateral adrenocortical hyperplasias. Nat Clin Pract Endocrinol Metab. 2007 Nov;3(11):748–57. PMID:17955016

4298. Stratakis CA, Courcoutsakis NA, Abati A, et al. Thyroid gland abnormalities in patients with the syndrome of spotty skin pigmentation, myxomas, endocrine overactivity, and schwannomas (Carney complex). J Clin Endocrinol Metab. 1997 Jul;82(7):2037–43. PMID:9215269

4299. Stratakis CA, Kirschner LS, Carney JA. Clinical and molecular features of the Carney complex: diagnostic criteria and recommendations for patient evaluation. J Clin Endocrinol Metab. 2001 Sep;86(9):4041–6. PMID:11549623

4300. Stratakis CA, Papageorgiou T, Premkumar A, et al. Ovarian lesions in Carney complex: clinical genetics and possible predisposition to malignancy. J Clin Endocrinol Metab. 2000 Nov;85(11):4359–66. PMID:11095480

4301. Stratakis CA, Tichomirowa MA, Boikos S, et al. The role of germline AIP, MEN1, PRKAR1A, CDKN1B and CDKN2C mutations in causing pituitary adenomas in a large cohort of children, adolescents, and patients with genetic syndromes. Clin Genet. 2010 Nov;78(5):457–63. PMID:20507346

4302. Straus FH 2nd, Kaplan EL, Nishiyama RH, et al. Five cases of parathyroid lipohyperplasia. Surgery. 1983 Dec;94(6):901–5. PMID:6648802

4303. Streubel B, Huber D, Wöhrer S, et al. Frequency of chromosomal aberrations involving MALT1 in mucosa-associated lymphoid tissue lymphoma in patients with Sjögren's syndrome. Clin Cancer Res. 2004 Jan 15;10(2):476–80. PMID:14760068

4304. Streubel B, Vinatzer U, Lamprecht A, et al. T(3;14)(p14.1;q32) involving IGH and FOXP1 is a novel recurrent chromosomal aberration in MALT lymphoma. Leukemia. 2005 Apr;19(4):652–8. PMID:15703784

4305. Strojan P, Hernandez-Prera JC, Beitler JJ, et al. Small cell and large cell neuroendocrine carcinoma of the larynx: a comparative analysis. Cancer Treat Rev. 2019 Aug;78:42–51. PMID:31437725

4306. Strommer KN, Brandner S, Sarioglu AC, et al. Symptomatic cerebellar metastasis and late local recurrence of a cauda equina paraganglioma. Case report. J Neurosurg. 1995 Jul;83(1):166–9. PMID:7782837

4307. Strong VE, Kennedy T, Al-Ahmadie H, et al. Prognostic indicators of malignancy in adrenal pheochromocytomas: clinical, histopathologic, and cell cycle/apoptosis gene expression analysis. Surgery. 2008 Jun;143(6):759–68. PMID:18549892

4308. Strosberg JR, Coppola D, Klimstra DS, et al. The NANETS consensus guidelines for the diagnosis and management of poorly differentiated (high-grade) extrapulmonary neuroendocrine carcinomas. Pancreas. 2010 Aug;39(6):799–800. PMID:20664477

4309. Sturgeon C, Clark OH. Familial nonmedullary thyroid cancer. Thyroid. 2005 Jun;15(6):588–93. PMID:16029126

4310. Sturiale A, Giudici F, Alemanno G, et al. Massive intrathoracic lipoma in MEN1 syndrome. Int J Surg Case Rep. 2015;6C:247–50. PMID:25545711

4311. Styne DM, Isaac R, Miller WL, et al. Endocrine, histological, and biochemical studies of adrenocorticotropin-producing islet cell carcinoma of the pancreas in childhood with characterization of proopiomelanocortin. J Clin Endocrinol Metab. 1983 Oct;57(4):723–31. PMID:6309881

4312. Su L, Beals T, Bernacki EG, et al. Spindle epithelial tumor with thymus-like differentiation:

a case report with cytologic, histologic, immunohistologic, and ultrastructural findings. Mod Pathol. 1997 May;10(5):510–4. PMID:9160319
4313. Suárez AL, Louis P, Kitts J, et al. Clinical and dermoscopic features of combined cutaneous squamous cell carcinoma (SCC)/ neuroendocrine [Merkel cell] carcinoma (MCC). J Am Acad Dermatol. 2015 Dec;73(6):968–75. PMID:26433246
4314. Subramaniam MM, Lim XY, Venkateswaran K, et al. Dedifferentiated solitary fibrous tumour of the nasal cavity: the first case reported with molecular characterization of a TP53 mutation. Histopathology. 2011 Dec;59(6):1269–74. PMID:22026427
4315. Suenaga S, Ichiyanagi O, Ito H, et al. Expression of extracellular signal-regulated kinase 5 and ankyrin repeat domain 1 in composite pheochromocytoma and ganglioneuroblastoma detected incidentally in the adult adrenal gland. Intern Med. 2016;55(24):3611–21. PMID:27980262
4316. Suganuma N, Iwasaki H, Shimizu S, et al. Non-functioning parathyroid carcinoma: a case report. Surg Case Rep. 2017 Dec;3(1):81. PMID:28726134
4317. Suganuma R, Wang LL, Sano H, et al. Peripheral neuroblastic tumors with genotype-phenotype discordance: a report from the Children's Oncology Group and the International Neuroblastoma Pathology Committee. Pediatr Blood Cancer. 2013 Mar;60(3):363–70. PMID:22744966
4318. Sugino K, Ito K Jr, Ozaki O, et al. Papillary microcarcinoma of the thyroid. J Endocrinol Invest. 1998 Jul-Aug;21(7):445–8. PMID:9766259
4319. Sugino K, Kameyama K, Ito K, et al. Does Hürthle cell carcinoma of the thyroid have a poorer prognosis than ordinary follicular thyroid carcinoma? Ann Surg Oncol. 2013 Sep;20(9):2944–50. PMID:23616135
4320. Sugino K, Kameyama K, Nagahama M, et al. Follicular thyroid carcinoma with distant metastasis: outcome and prognostic factor. Endocr J. 2014;61(3):273–9. PMID:24420337
4321. Sugitani I, Fujimoto Y. Symptomatic versus asymptomatic papillary thyroid microcarcinoma: a retrospective analysis of surgical outcome and prognostic factors. Endocr J. 1999 Feb;46(1):209–16. PMID:10426589
4322. Sugitani I, Miyauchi A, Sugino K, et al. Prognostic factors and treatment outcomes for anaplastic thyroid carcinoma: ATC Research Consortium of Japan cohort study of 677 patients. World J Surg. 2012 Jun;36(6):1247–54. PMID:22311136
4323. Sugiyama T, Tajiri T, Hiraiwa S, et al. Hepatic adrenal rest tumor: diagnostic pitfall and proposed algorithms to prevent misdiagnosis as lipid-rich hepatocellular carcinoma. Pathol Int. 2015 Feb;65(2):95–9. PMID:25572108
4324. Suh I, Filetti S, Vriens MR, et al. Distinct loci on chromosome 1q21 and 6q22 predispose to familial nonmedullary thyroid cancer: a SNP array-based linkage analysis of 38 families. Surgery. 2009 Dec;146(6):1073–80. PMID:19958934
4325. Suh J, Heimann A, Cohen H. True adrenal mesothelial cyst in a patient with flank pain and hematuria: a case report. Endocr Pathol. 2008 Fall;19(3):203–5. PMID:18446449
4326. Suh YJ, Park JH, Jeon JH, et al. Extrapleural solitary fibrous tumor of the thyroid gland: a case report and review of literature. World J Clin Cases. 2020 Feb 26;8(4):782–9. PMID:32149061
4327. Sujoy V, Pinto A, Nosé V. Columnar cell variant of papillary thyroid carcinoma: a study of 10 cases with emphasis on CDX2 expression. Thyroid. 2013 Jun;23(6):714–9. PMID:23488912
4328. Sukumar JS, Sukumar S, Purohit D, et al. Activating BRAF mutation in sclerosing mucoepidermoid carcinoma with eosinophilia of the thyroid gland: two case reports and review of the literature. J Med Case Rep. 2019 Dec 28;13(1):385. PMID:31882020
4329. Sulaiman L, Haglund F, Hashemi J, et al. Genome-wide and locus specific alterations in CDC73/HRPT2-mutated parathyroid tumors. PLoS One. 2012;7(9):e46325. PMID:23029479
4330. Sulaiman L, Juhlin CC, Nilsson IL, et al. Global and gene-specific promoter methylation analysis in primary hyperparathyroidism. Epigenetics. 2013 Jun;8(6):646–55. PMID:23764768
4331. Sumegi J, Streblow R, Frayer RW, et al. Recurrent t(2;2) and t(2;8) translocations in rhabdomyosarcoma without the canonical PAX-FOXO1 fuse PAX3 to members of the nuclear receptor transcriptional coactivator family. Genes Chromosomes Cancer. 2010 Mar;49(3):224–36. PMID:19953635
4332. Summaria V, Rufini V, Mirk P, et al. Diagnostic imaging of differentiated thyroid carcinoma. Rays. 2000 Apr-Jun;25(2):177–90. PMID:11370536
4333. Sun L, Cliften PF, Duncavage EJ, et al. UV Signature mutations reclassify salivary high-grade neuroendocrine carcinomas as occult metastatic cutaneous Merkel cell carcinomas. Am J Surg Pathol. 2019 May;43(5):682–7. PMID:30986802
4334. Sun T, Wang Z, Wang J, et al. Outcome of radical resection and postoperative radiotherapy for thyroid carcinoma showing thymus-like differentiation. World J Surg. 2011 Aug;35(8):1840–6. PMID:21597887
4335. Sun W, Kuang XL, Liu YP, et al. Crystal structure of the N-terminal domain of human CDC73 and its implications for the hyperparathyroidism-jaw tumor (HPT-JT) syndrome. Sci Rep. 2017 Nov 15;7(1):15638. PMID:29142233
4336. Sun Y, Sun Q, Shen J, et al. Cauda equina hemangioblastoma at L5 vertebral level related to von Hippel-Lindau disease. Br J Neurosurg. 2012 Aug;26(4):576–7. PMID:22133049
4337. Sundaram V, Schuster DP, Falko JM. Unusual manifestations of Cushing's syndrome in a multiple endocrine neoplasia type I kindred. Endocr Pract. 1998 Jul-Aug;4(4):190–4. PMID:15251731
4338. Sundararajan V, Robinson-Smith TM, Lowy AM. Duodenal gangliocytic paraganglioma with lymph node metastasis: a case report and review of the literature. Arch Pathol Lab Med. 2003 Mar;127(3):e139–41. PMID:12653602
4339. Sundin A, Vullierme MP, Kaltsas G, et al. ENETS consensus guidelines for the standards of care in neuroendocrine tumors: radiological examinations. Neuroendocrinology. 2009;90(2):167–83. PMID:19077417
4340. Sung S, Saqi A, Margolskee EM, et al. Cytomorphologic features distinguishing Bethesda category IV thyroid lesions from parathyroid. Cytojournal. 2017 Apr 28;14:10. PMID:28567111
4341. Sung TY, Lee YM, Yoon JH, et al. Surgical management of familial papillary thyroid microcarcinoma: a single institution study of 94 cases. World J Surg. 2015 Aug;39(8):1930–5. PMID:25894401
4342. Surov A, Gottschling S, Wienke A, et al. Primary thyroid sarcoma: a systematic review. Anticancer Res. 2015 Oct;35(10):5185–91. PMID:26408676
4343. Surov A, Machens A, Holzhausen HJ, et al. Radiological features of metastases to the thyroid. Acta Radiol. 2016 Apr;57(4):444–50. PMID:25907117
4344. Suster D, Michal M, Nishino M, et al. Papillary thyroid carcinoma with prominent myofibroblastic stromal component: clinicopathologic, immunohistochemical and next-generation sequencing study of seven cases. Mod Pathol. 2020 Sep;33(9):1702–11. PMID:32291398
4345. Suzuki A, Hirokawa M, Kanematsu R, et al. Fine-needle aspiration of parathyroid adenomas: indications as a diagnostic approach. Diagn Cytopathol. 2021 Jan;49(1):70–6. PMID:32833315
4346. Suzuki A, Hirokawa M, Takada N, et al. Diagnostic significance of PAX8 in thyroid squamous cell carcinoma. Endocr J. 2015;62(11):991–5. PMID:26354716
4347. Suzuki A, Hirokawa M, Takada N, et al. Utility of monoclonal PAX8 antibody for distinguishing intrathyroid thymic carcinoma from follicular cell-derived thyroid carcinoma. Endocr J. 2018 Dec 28;65(12):1171–5. PMID:30210064
4348. Suzuki K, Saenko V, Yamashita S, et al. Radiation-induced thyroid cancers: overview of molecular signatures. Cancers (Basel). 2019 Sep 2;11(9):1290. PMID:31480712
4349. Suzuki M, Egashira N, Kajiya H, et al. ACTH and alpha-subunit are co-expressed in rare human pituitary corticotroph cell adenomas proposed to originate from ACTH-committed early pituitary progenitor cells. Endocr Pathol. 2008 Spring;19(1):17–26. PMID:18228160
4350. Svahn F, Paulsson JO, Stenman A, et al. TERT promoter hypermethylation is associated with poor prognosis in adrenocortical carcinoma. Int J Mol Med. 2018 Sep;42(3):1675–83. PMID:29956721
4351. Svec A, Bury Y. Haemangioma of the parathyroid gland. Does it really exist? Pathol Oncol Res. 2010 Sep;16(3):443–6. PMID:20063187
4352. Svedlund J, Aurén M, Sundström M, et al. Aberrant WNT/β-catenin signaling in parathyroid carcinoma. Mol Cancer. 2010 Nov 15;9:294. PMID:21078161
4353. Swaak-Kragten AT, de Wilt JH, Schmitz PI, et al. Multimodality treatment for anaplastic thyroid carcinoma–treatment outcome in 75 patients. Radiother Oncol. 2009 Jul;92(1):100–4. PMID:19328572
4354. Swaby R. Lingual thyroid: ectopic gland in the tongue base. Arch Dis Child. 2020;105:586. doi:10.1136/archdischild-2018-316508.
4355. Swanson AA, Erickson D, Donegan DM, et al. Clinical, biological, radiological, and pathological comparison of sparsely and densely granulated somatotroph adenomas: a single center experience from a cohort of 131 patients with acromegaly. Pituitary. 2021 Apr;24(2):192–206. PMID:33074402
4356. Sy J, Ang LC. Cytomorphologic spectrum of mixed pituitary adenoma-gangliocytomas: a report of two cases. Acta Cytol. 2010 Sep-Oct;54(5 Suppl):981–4. PMID:21053582
4357. Sykorova V, Dvorakova S, Vcelak J, et al. Search for new genetic biomarkers in poorly differentiated and anaplastic thyroid carcinomas using next generation sequencing. Anticancer Res. 2015 Apr;35(4):2029–36. PMID:25862857
4358. Syro LV, Horvath E, Kovacs K. Double adenoma of the pituitary: a somatotroph adenoma colliding with a gonadotroph adenoma. J Endocrinol Invest. 2000 Jan;23(1):37–41. PMID:10698050
4359. Szablewski V, Neuville A, Terrier P, et al. Adult sinonasal soft tissue sarcoma: analysis of 48 cases from the French Sarcoma Group database. Laryngoscope. 2015 Mar;125(3):615–23. PMID:25186315
4360. Szabó J, Heath B, Hill VM, et al. Hereditary hyperparathyroidism-jaw tumor syndrome: the endocrine tumor gene HRPT2 maps to chromosome 1q21-q31. Am J Hum Genet. 1995 Apr;56(4):944–50. PMID:7717405
4361. Szabo Yamashita T, Baky FJ, McKenzie TJ, et al. Occurrence and natural history of thyroid cancer in patients with Cowden syndrome. Eur Thyroid J. 2020 Sep;9(5):243–6. PMID:33088792
4362. Szalat A, Mazeh H, Freund HR. Lithium-associated hyperparathyroidism: report of four cases and review of the literature. Eur J Endocrinol. 2009 Feb;160(2):317–23. PMID:19001061
4363. Szczepanek-Parulska E, Hernik A, Ruchała M. Thyroid ectopy - diagnostic and therapeutic challenges before and in the era of TSH neonatal screening. Endokrynol Pol. 2017;68(6):708–21. PMID:29238947
4364. Szeifert GT, Pásztor E. Could craniopharyngiomas produce pituitary hormones? Neurol Res. 1993 Feb;15(1):68–9. PMID:8098858
4365. Szeliga A, Pralat A, Witczak W, et al. CHEK2 mutation in patient with multiple endocrine glands tumors. Case Report. Int J Environ Res Public Health. 2020 Jun 18;17(12):4397. PMID:32570972
4366. Szporn AH, Yuan S, Wu M, et al. Cellular swirls in fine needle aspirates of papillary thyroid carcinoma: a new diagnostic criterion. Mod Pathol. 2006 Nov;19(11):1470–3. PMID:16951672
4367. Szyfelbein WM, Young RH, Scully RE. Cystic struma ovarii: a frequently unrecognized tumor. A report of 20 cases. Am J Surg Pathol. 1994 Aug;18(8):785–8. PMID:8037292
4368. Tachibana O, Yamashima T, Yamashita J, et al. Immunohistochemical expression of human chorionic gonadotropin and P-glycoprotein in human pituitary glands and craniopharyngiomas. J Neurosurg. 1994 Jan;80(1):79–84. PMID:7903692
4369. Tadokoro R, Sato S, Otsuka F, et al. Metastatic pancreatic neuroendocrine tumor that progressed to ectopic adrenocorticotropic hormone (ACTH) syndrome with growth hormone-releasing hormone (GHRH) production. Intern Med. 2016;55(20):2979–83. PMID:27746436
4370. Taggart JL, Summerlin DJ, Moore MG. Parathyroid carcinosarcoma: a rare form of parathyroid carcinoma with normal parathyroid hormone levels. Int J Surg Pathol. 2013 Aug;21(4):394–8. PMID:23493876
4371. Tahara E, Ito H, Nakagami K, et al. Scirrhous argyrophil cell carcinoma of the stomach with multiple production of polypeptide hormones, amine, CEA, lysozyme, and HCG. Cancer. 1982 May 1;49(9):1904–15. PMID:6176315
4372. Tahara I, Oishi N, Mochizuki K, et al. Identification of recurrent TERT promoter mutations in intrathyroid thymic carcinomas. Endocr Pathol. 2020 Sep;31(3):274–82. PMID:32594366
4373. Taïeb D, Jha A, Guerin C, et al. 18F-FDOPA PET/CT imaging of MAX-related pheochromocytoma. J Clin Endocrinol Metab. 2018 Apr 1;103(4):1574–82. PMID:29534198
4374. Taïeb D, Pacak K. Molecular imaging and theranostic approaches in pheochromocytoma and paraganglioma. Cell Tissue Res. 2018 May;372(2):393–401. PMID:29450723
4375. Takada N, Hirokawa M, Ito M, et al. Papillary thyroid carcinoma with desmoid-type fibromatosis: a clinical, pathological, and immunohistochemical study of 14 cases. Endocr J. 2017 Oct 28;64(10):1017–23. PMID:28794344
4376. Takada N, Hirokawa M, Ohbayashi C, et al. Re-evaluation of MIB-1 immunostaining for diagnosing hyalinizing trabecular tumour of the thyroid: semi-automated techniques with manual antigen retrieval are more accurate than fully automated techniques. Endocr J. 2018 Feb 26;65(2):239–44. PMID:29199205
4377. Takada N, Mussazhanova Z, Hirokawa M, et al. Immunohistochemical and molecular

analyses focusing on mesenchymal cells in papillary thyroid carcinoma with desmoid-type fibromatosis. Pathobiology. 2018;85(5-6):300–3. PMID:30223266

4378. Takagi N, Hirokawa M, Nobuoka Y, et al. Diffuse sclerosing variant of papillary thyroid carcinoma: a study of fine needle aspiration cytology in 20 patients. Cytopathology. 2014 Jun;25(3):199–204. PMID:23781895

4379. Takahashi K, Mikata R, Tsuyuguchi T, et al. Granular cell tumor of the pancreas diagnosed by endoscopic ultrasound-guided fine-needle aspiration. Clin J Gastroenterol. 2018 Jun;11(3):193–9. PMID:29380119

4380. Takahashi M, Ritz J, Cooper GM. Activation of a novel human transforming gene, ret, by DNA rearrangement. Cell. 1985 Sep;42(2):581–8. PMID:2992805

4381. Takasugi J, Shimamura M, Koda T, et al. Paraneoplastic cerebellar degeneration and Lambert-Eaton myasthenic syndrome associated with neuroendocrine carcinoma of the oropharynx. Intern Med. 2018 Feb 15;57(4):587–90. PMID:29093415

4382. Takayama F, Takashima S, Matsuba H, et al. MR imaging of primary leiomyosarcoma of the thyroid gland. Eur J Radiol. 2001 Jan;37(1):36–41. PMID:11274837

4383. Takeda M, Kasai T, Enomoto Y, et al. 9p21 deletion in the diagnosis of malignant mesothelioma, using fluorescence in situ hybridization analysis. Pathol Int. 2010 May;60(5):395–9. PMID:20518890

4384. Takei Y, Seyama S, Pearl GS, et al. Ultrastructural study of the human neurohypophysis. II. Cellular elements of neural parenchyma, the pituicytes. Cell Tissue Res. 1980;205(2):273–87. PMID:7188885

4385. Takeshima K, Ariyasu H, Uraki S, et al. False-positive staining of thyroglobulin distinguished from mixed medullary and follicular thyroid carcinoma by duplex in situ hybridization. Endocr J. 2020 Oct 28;67(10):1007–17. PMID:32522910

4386. Takeshima K, Li Y, Kakudo K, et al. Proposal of diagnostic criteria for IgG4-related thyroid disease. Endocr J. 2021 Jan 28;68(1):1–6. PMID:33311000

4387. Takimoto Sato M, Ikezawa Y, Sato M, et al. Large cell neuroendocrine carcinoma of the lung that responded to nivolumab: a case report. Mol Clin Oncol. 2020 Jul;13(1):43–7. PMID:32499913

4388. Talat N, Schulte KM. Clinical presentation, staging and long-term evolution of parathyroid cancer. Ann Surg Oncol. 2010 Aug;17(8):2156–74. PMID:20221704

4389. Talerman A. Carcinoid tumors of the ovary. J Cancer Res Clin Oncol. 1984;107(2):125–35. PMID:6715397

4390. Talerman A, Evans MI. Primary trabecular carcinoid tumor of the ovary. Cancer. 1982 Oct 1;50(7):1403–7. PMID:7104979

4391. Tallini G. Poorly differentiated thyroid carcinoma. Are we there yet? Endocr Pathol. 2011 Dec;22(4):190–4. PMID:21969055

4392. Tallini G, Carcangiu ML, Rosai J. Oncocytic neoplasms of the thyroid gland. Acta Pathol Jpn. 1992 May;42(5):305–15. PMID:1636432

4393. Tallini G, De Leo A, Repaci A, et al. Does the site of origin of the microcarcinoma with respect to the thyroid surface matter? A multicenter pathologic and clinical study for risk stratification. Cancers (Basel). 2020 Jan 19;12(1):246. PMID:31963890

4394. Tallini G, Garcia-Rostan G, Herrero A, et al. Downregulation of p27KIP1 and Ki67/Mib1 labeling index support the classification of thyroid carcinoma into prognostically relevant categories. Am J Surg Pathol. 1999 Jun;23(6):678–85. PMID:10366150

4395. Tallini G, Tuttle RM, Ghossein RA. The history of the follicular variant of papillary thyroid carcinoma. J Clin Endocrinol Metab. 2017 Jan 1;102(1):15–22. PMID:27732333

4396. Tamaki I, Hosoda Y, Sasano H, et al. Primary pancreatic glomus tumor invading into the superior mesenteric vein: a case report. Surg Case Rep. 2020 Nov 3;6(1):279. PMID:33141292

4397. Tamburrino A, Molinolo AA, Salerno P, et al. Activation of the mTOR pathway in primary medullary thyroid carcinoma and lymph node metastases. Clin Cancer Res. 2012 Jul 1;18(13):3532–40. PMID:22753663

4398. Tamiya H, Miyakawa M, Suzuki H, et al. A large functioning parathyroid cyst in a patient with multiple endocrine neoplasia type 1. Endocr J. 2013;60(6):709–14. PMID:23386389

4399. Tamouridis N, Deladetsima JK, Kastanias I, et al. Cold thyroid nodule as the sole manifestation of Rosai-Dorfman disease with mild lymphadenopathy, coexisting with chronic autoimmune thyroiditis. J Endocrinol Invest. 1999 Dec;22(11):866–70. PMID:10710276

4400. Tampourlou M, Ntali G, Ahmed S, et al. Outcome of nonfunctioning pituitary adenomas that regrow after primary treatment: a study from two large UK centers. J Clin Endocrinol Metab. 2017 Jun 1;102(6):1889–97. PMID:28323946

4401. Tamura A, Ogasawara T, Fujii Y, et al. Glucagonoma with necrolytic migratory erythema: metabolic profile and detection of biallelic inactivation of DAXX gene. J Clin Endocrinol Metab. 2018 Jul 1;103(7):2417–23. PMID:29688432

4402. Tan A, Stewart CJ, Garrett KL, et al. Novel BRAF and KRAS mutations in papillary thyroid carcinoma arising in struma ovarii. Endocr Pathol. 2015 Dec;26(4):296–301. PMID:26362194

4403. Tan CL, Pang YH, Lim KHC, et al. Two extraordinary sellar neuronal tumors: literature review and comparison of clinicopathologic features. Am J Clin Pathol. 2019 Feb 4;151(3):241–54. PMID:30551183

4404. Tan HL, Sood A, Rahimi HA, et al. Rb loss is characteristic of prostatic small cell neuroendocrine carcinoma. Clin Cancer Res. 2014 Feb 15;20(4):890–903. PMID:24323898

4405. Tan MH, Mester J, Peterson C, et al. A clinical scoring system for selection of patients for PTEN mutation testing is proposed on the basis of a prospective study of 3042 probands. Am J Hum Genet. 2011 Jan 7;88(1):42–56. PMID:21194675

4406. Tan MH, Morrison C, Wang P, et al. Loss of parafibromin immunoreactivity is a distinguishing feature of parathyroid carcinoma. Clin Cancer Res. 2004 Oct 1;10(19):6629–37. PMID:15475453

4407. Tan W, Tao L, Zhou Z, et al. Tumor-to-tumor metastasis: a rare case of breast carcinoma metastasizing to a pheochromocytoma, and a literature review. Diagn Pathol. 2019 May 20;14(1):46. PMID:31109373

4408. Tanaka A, Hirokawa M, Higuchi M, et al. Diagnostic clues indicating tall cell variants of papillary thyroid carcinoma in fine needle aspiration. Diagn Cytopathol. 2019 May;47(5):452–7. PMID:30582297

4409. Tanaka M, Kato K, Gomi K, et al. Perivascular epithelioid cell tumor with SFPQ/PSF-TFE3 gene fusion in a patient with advanced neuroblastoma. Am J Surg Pathol. 2009 Sep;33(9):1416–20. PMID:19606011

4410. Tanaka T, Yoshimi N, Iwata H, et al. Fine-needle aspiration cytology of pheochromocytoma-ganglioneuroma of the organ of Zuckerkandl. Diagn Cytopathol. 1989;5(1):64–8. PMID:2721353

4411. Tang L, Li X, Wang B, et al. Clinical characteristics of aldosterone- and cortisol-coproducing adrenal adenoma in primary aldosteronism. Int J Endocrinol. 2018 Mar 25;2018:4920841. PMID:29770148

4412. Tang LH. Pancreatic neuroendocrine neoplasms: landscape and horizon. Arch Pathol Lab Med. 2020 Jul 1;144(7):816–28. PMID:32298138

4413. Tang LH, Basturk O, Sue JJ, et al. A practical approach to the classification of WHO grade 3 (G3) well-differentiated neuroendocrine tumor (WD-NET) and poorly differentiated neuroendocrine carcinoma (PD-NEC) of the pancreas. Am J Surg Pathol. 2016 Sep;40(9):1192–202. PMID:27259015

4414. Tang LH, Untch BR, Reidy DL, et al. Well-differentiated neuroendocrine tumors with a morphologically apparent high-grade component: a pathway distinct from poorly differentiated neuroendocrine carcinomas. Clin Cancer Res. 2016 Feb 15;22(4):1011–7. PMID:26482044

4415. Tang W, Robles AI, Beyer RP, et al. The Werner syndrome RECQ helicase targets G4 DNA in human cells to modulate transcription. Hum Mol Genet. 2016 May 15;25(10):2060–9. PMID:26984941

4416. Tang Z, Zhang H, Ma C, et al. Colorimetric determination of the activity of alkaline phosphatase based on the use of Cu(II)-modulated G-quadruplex-based DNAzymes. Mikrochim Acta. 2018 Jan 10;185(2):109. PMID:29594418

4417. Tani E, Wejde J, Åström K, et al. FNA cytology of solitary fibrous tumors and the diagnostic value of STAT6 immunocytochemistry. Cancer Cytopathol. 2018 Jan;126(1):36–43. PMID:28914981

4418. Tanigawa M, Nakayama M, Taira T, et al. Insulinoma-associated protein 1 (INSM1) is a useful marker for pancreatic neuroendocrine tumor. Med Mol Morphol. 2018 Mar;51(1):32–40. PMID:28849340

4419. Tanizaki Y, Jin L, Scheithauer BW, et al. P53 gene mutations in pituitary carcinomas. Endocr Pathol. 2007 Winter;18(4):217–22. PMID:18026859

4420. Tarabay A, Cossu G, Berhouma M, et al. Primary pituitary lymphoma: an update of the literature. J Neurooncol. 2016 Dec;130(3):383–95. PMID:27581598

4421. Tarantola TI, Vallow LA, Halyard MY, et al. Unknown primary Merkel cell carcinoma: 23 new cases and a review. J Am Acad Dermatol. 2013 Mar;68(3):433–40. PMID:23182060

4422. Tardío JC, Machado I, Alemany I, et al. Solitary fibrous tumor of the vulva: report of 2 cases, including a de novo dedifferentiated solitary fibrous tumor diagnosed after molecular demonstration of NAB2-STAT6 gene fusion. Int J Gynecol Pathol. 2018 Nov;37(6):547–53. PMID:28968297

4423. Tarpey PS, Behjati S, Young MD, et al. The driver landscape of sporadic chordoma. Nat Commun. 2017 Oct 12;8(1):890. PMID:29026114

4424. Tas F, Keskin S, Karadeniz A, et al. Noncutaneous melanoma have distinct features from each other and cutaneous melanoma. Oncology. 2011;81(5-6):353–8. PMID:22248874

4425. Taskin OC, Gucer H, Mete O. An unusual adrenal cortical nodule: composite adrenal cortical adenoma and adenomatoid tumor. Endocr Pathol. 2015 Dec;26(4):370–3. PMID:25861051

4426. Tatematsu A, Shimizu J, Murakami Y, et al. Epidermal growth factor receptor mutations in small cell lung cancer. Clin Cancer Res. 2008 Oct 1;14(19):6092–6. PMID:18829487

4427. Tateno T, Asa SL, Zheng L, et al. The FGFR4-G388R polymorphism promotes mitochondrial STAT3 serine phosphorylation to facilitate pituitary growth hormone cell tumorigenesis. PLoS Genet. 2011 Dec;7(12):e1002400. PMID:22174695

4428. Tateyama H, Tada T, Okabe M, et al. Different keratin profiles in craniopharyngioma subtypes and ameloblastomas. Pathol Res Pract. 2001;197(11):735–42. PMID:11770017

4429. Tatsi C, Stratakis CA. The genetics of pituitary adenomas. J Clin Med. 2019 Dec 21;9(1):30. PMID:31877737

4430. Tavarelli M, Russo M, Terranova R, et al. Familial non-medullary thyroid cancer represents an independent risk factor for increased cancer aggressiveness: a retrospective analysis of 74 families. Front Endocrinol (Lausanne). 2015 Aug 3;6:117. PMID:26284028

4431. Taweevisit M, Sampatanukul P, Thorner PS. Ectopic thymoma can mimic benign and malignant thyroid lesions on fine needle aspiration cytology: a case report and literature review. Acta Cytol. 2013;57(2):213–20. PMID:23406665

4432. Taylor SL, Barakos JA, Harsh GR 4th, et al. Magnetic resonance imaging of tuberculum sellae meningiomas: preventing preoperative misdiagnosis as pituitary macroadenoma. Neurosurgery. 1992 Oct;31(4):621–7. PMID:1407446

4433. Tempfer CB, Tischoff I, Dogan A, et al. Neuroendocrine carcinoma of the cervix: a systematic review of the literature. BMC Cancer. 2018 May 4;18(1):530. PMID:29728073

4434. Teng L, Deng W, Lu J, et al. Hobnail variant of papillary thyroid carcinoma: molecular profiling and comparison to classical papillary thyroid carcinoma, poorly differentiated thyroid carcinoma and anaplastic thyroid carcinoma. Oncotarget. 2017 Mar 28;8(13):22023–33. PMID:28423545

4435. Terada T, Kovacs K, Stefaneanu L, et al. Incidence, pathology, and recurrence of pituitary adenomas: study of 647 unselected surgical cases. Endocr Pathol. 1995 Winter;6(4):301–10. PMID:12114812

4436. Terada T, Matsunaga Y, Maeta H, et al. Mixed ductal-endocrine carcinoma of the pancreas presenting as gastrinoma with Zollinger-Ellison syndrome: an autopsy case with a 24-year survival period. Virchows Arch. 1999 Dec;435(6):606–11. PMID:10628803

4437. Termote B, Verswijvel G, Palmers Y. Fat containing adrenal cavernous haemangioma: CT and MRI findings. JBR-BTR. 2007 Nov-Dec;90(6):516–8. PMID:18376767

4438. Tessaris D, Boyce AM, Zacharin M, et al. Growth hormone-Insulin-like growth factor 1 axis hyperactivity on bone fibrous dysplasia in McCune-Albright syndrome. Clin Endocrinol (Oxf). 2018 Jul;89(1):56–64. PMID:29672904

4439. Tessaris D, Corrias A, Matarazzo P, et al. Thyroid abnormalities in children and adolescents with McCune-Albright syndrome. Horm Res Paediatr. 2012;78(3):151–7. PMID:23006743

4440. Tetzlaff MT, Nagarajan P. Update on Merkel cell carcinoma. Head Neck Pathol. 2018 Mar;12(1):31–43. PMID:29556962

4441. Tezelman S, Borucu I, Senyurek Giles Y, et al. The change in surgical practice from subtotal to near-total or total thyroidectomy in the treatment of patients with benign multinodular goiter. World J Surg. 2009 Mar;33(3):400–5. PMID:18958517

4442. Thakkar K, Ramteke-Jadhav S, Kasaliwal R, et al. Sellar surprises: a single-centre experience of unusual sellar masses. Endocr Connect. 2020 Feb;9(2):111–21. PMID:31910151

4443. Thakker RV. Genetics of parathyroid tumours. J Intern Med. 2016 Dec;280(6):574–83. PMID:27306766

4444. Thakker RV. Multiple endocrine neoplasia type 1 (MEN1) and type 4 (MEN4). Mol

Cell Endocrinol. 2014 Apr 5;386(1-2):2–15. PMID:23933118
4445. Thakker RV, Newey PJ, Walls GV, et al. Clinical practice guidelines for multiple endocrine neoplasia type 1 (MEN1). J Clin Endocrinol Metab. 2012 Sep;97(9):2990–3011. PMID:22723327
4446. Thakral B, Zhou J, Medeiros LJ. Extranodal hematopoietic neoplasms and mimics in the head and neck: an update. Hum Pathol. 2015 Aug;46(8):1079–100. PMID:26118762
4447. Thakur A, Sebag F, Micco CD, et al. Ectopic cervical thymoma mimicking as papillary thyroid carcinoma: a diagnostic dilemma. Indian J Pathol Microbiol. 2010 Apr-Jun;53(2):305–7. PMID:20551539
4448. Thakur JS, Verma N, Singh R. Hürthle cell carcinoma in a lingual thyroid. Med Princ Pract. 2018;27(5):489–92. PMID:29898455
4449. Thapar K, Kovacs K, Scheithauer BW, et al. Proliferative activity and invasiveness among pituitary adenomas and carcinomas: an analysis using the MIB-1 antibody. Neurosurgery. 1996 Jan;38(1):99–106. PMID:8747957
4450. Thapar K, Scheithauer BW, Kovacs K, et al. p53 expression in pituitary adenomas and carcinomas: correlation with invasiveness and tumor growth fractions. Neurosurgery. 1996 Apr;38(4):765–70. PMID:8692397
4451. Thar YY, Patel P, Huang T, et al. An extremely rare case of advanced metastatic small cell neuroendocrine carcinoma of sinonasal tract. Case Rep Oncol Med. 2016;2016:1496916. PMID:27529044
4452. The I, Hannigan GE, Cowley GS, et al. Rescue of a Drosophila NF1 mutant phenotype by protein kinase A. Science. 1997 May 2;276(5313):791–4. PMID:9115203
4453. Theodoropoulou M, Reincke M, Fassnacht M, et al. Decoding the genetic basis of Cushing's disease: USP8 in the spotlight. Eur J Endocrinol. 2015 Oct;173(4):M73–83. PMID:26012588
4454. Therrell BL Jr, Berenbaum SA, Manter-Kapanke V, et al. Results of screening 1.9 million Texas newborns for 21-hydroxylase-deficient congenital adrenal hyperplasia. Pediatrics. 1998 Apr;101(4 Pt 1):583–90. PMID:9521938
4455. Theurer S, Siebolts U, Lorenz K, et al. [Ectopic tissue of the thyroid gland and the parathyroid glands]. Pathologe. 2018 Sep;39(5):379–89. German. PMID:30105609
4456. Thevenon J, Bourredjem A, Faivre L, et al. Higher risk of death among MEN1 patients with mutations in the JunD interacting domain: a Groupe d'etude des Tumeurs Endocrines (GTE) cohort study. Hum Mol Genet. 2013 May 15;22(10):1940–8. PMID:23376981
4457. Thewjitcharoen Y, Chatchomchuan W, Karndumri K, et al. Impacts of the American Joint Committee on Cancer (AJCC) 8th edition tumor, node, metastasis (TNM) staging system on outcomes of differentiated thyroid cancer in Thai patients. Heliyon. 2021 Mar 30;7(3):e06624. PMID:33869853
4458. Thieblemont C, Bastion Y, Berger F, et al. Mucosa-associated lymphoid tissue gastrointestinal and nongastrointestinal lymphoma behavior: analysis of 108 patients. J Clin Oncol. 1997 Apr;15(4):1624–30. PMID:9193362
4459. Thieblemont C, Cascione L, Conconi A, et al. A MALT lymphoma prognostic index. Blood. 2017 Sep 21;130(12):1409–17. PMID:28720586
4460. Thieblemont C, Mayer A, Dumontet C, et al. Primary thyroid lymphoma is a heterogeneous disease. J Clin Endocrinol Metab. 2002 Jan;87(1):105–11. PMID:11788631
4461. Thiel A, Reis AC, Haase M, et al. PRKACA mutations in cortisol-producing adenomas and adrenal hyperplasia: a single-center study of 60 cases. Eur J Endocrinol. 2015 Jun;172(6):677–85. PMID:25750087
4462. Thiel AT, Huang J, Lei M, et al. Menin as a hub controlling mixed lineage leukemia. Bioessays. 2012 Sep;34(9):771–80. PMID:22829075
4463. Thimsen V, John N, Buchfelder M, et al. Expression of SRY-related HMG box transcription factors (Sox) 2 and 9 in craniopharyngioma subtypes and surrounding brain tissue. Sci Rep. 2017 Nov 20;7(1):15856. PMID:29158570
4464. Thines L, Lejeune JP, Ruchoux MM, et al. Management of delayed intracranial and intraspinal metastases of intradural spinal paragangliomas. Acta Neurochir (Wien). 2006 Jan;148(1):63–6. PMID:16283104
4465. Thodou E, Kontogeorgos G. Somatostatin receptor profile in pituitary thyrotroph adenomas. Clin Neurol Neurosurg. 2020 Aug;195:105865. PMID:32416325
4466. Thomas CM, Asa SL, Ezzat S, et al. Diagnosis and pathologic characteristics of medullary thyroid carcinoma-review of current guidelines. Curr Oncol. 2019 Oct;26(5):338–44. PMID:31708652
4467. Thompson CF, Kim BJ, Lai C, et al. Sinonasal rhabdomyosarcoma: prognostic factors and treatment outcomes. Int Forum Allergy Rhinol. 2013 Aug;3(8):678–83. PMID:23424037
4468. Thompson ED, Stelow EB, Mills SE, et al. Large cell neuroendocrine carcinoma of the head and neck: a clinicopathologic series of 10 cases with an emphasis on HPV status. Am J Surg Pathol. 2016 Apr;40(4):471–8. PMID:26735857
4469. Thompson ED, Wood LD. Pancreatic neoplasms with acinar differentiation: a review of pathologic and molecular features. Arch Pathol Lab Med. 2020 Jul 1;144(7):808–15. PMID:31869246
4470. Thompson L. Dyshormonogenetic goiter of the thyroid gland. Ear Nose Throat J. 2005 Apr;84(4):200. PMID:15929313
4471. Thompson LD. Ninety-four cases of encapsulated follicular variant of papillary thyroid carcinoma: a name change to noninvasive follicular thyroid neoplasm with papillary-like nuclear features would help prevent overtreatment. Mod Pathol. 2016 Jul;29(7):698–707. PMID:27102347
4472. Thompson LD. Pheochromocytoma of the Adrenal gland Scaled Score (PASS) to separate benign from malignant neoplasms: a clinicopathologic and immunophenotypic study of 100 cases. Am J Surg Pathol. 2002 May;26(5):551–66. PMID:11979086
4473. Thompson LD, Herrera HB, Lau SK. A clinicopathologic series of 685 thyroglossal duct remnant cysts. Head Neck Pathol. 2016 Dec;10(4):465–74. PMID:27161104
4474. Thompson LD, Rosai J, Heffess CS. Primary thyroid teratomas: a clinicopathologic study of 30 cases. Cancer. 2000 Mar 1;88(5):1149–58. PMID:10699906
4475. Thompson LD, Seethala RR, Müller S. Ectopic sphenoid sinus pituitary adenoma (ESSPA) with normal anterior pituitary gland: a clinicopathologic and immunophenotypic study of 32 cases with a comprehensive review of the english literature. Head Neck Pathol. 2012 Mar;6(1):75–100. PMID:22430769
4476. Thompson LD, Wenig BM, Adair CF, et al. Langerhans cell histiocytosis of the thyroid: a series of seven cases and a review of the literature. Mod Pathol. 1996 Feb;9(2):145–9. PMID:8657721
4477. Thompson LD, Wenig BM, Adair CF, et al. Peripheral nerve sheath tumors of the thyroid gland: a series of four cases and a review of the literature. Endocr Pathol. 1996 Winter;7(4):309–18. PMID:12114802
4478. Thompson LD, Wenig BM, Adair CF, et al. Primary smooth muscle tumors of the thyroid gland. Cancer. 1997 Feb 1;79(3):579–87. PMID:9028371
4479. Thompson LD, Wieneke JA, Paal E, et al. A clinicopathologic study of minimally invasive follicular carcinoma of the thyroid gland with a review of the English literature. Cancer. 2001 Feb 1;91(3):505–24. PMID:11169933
4480. Thompson LDR. High grade differentiated follicular cell-derived thyroid carcinoma versus poorly differentiated thyroid carcinoma: a clinicopathologic analysis of 41 cases. Endocr Pathol. 2023 Jun;34(2):234–46. PMID:37195480
4481. Thompson LDR, Gagan J, Washington A, et al. Biphenotypic branchioma: a better name than ectopic hamartomatous thymoma for a neoplasm with HRAS mutation. Head Neck Pathol. 2020 Dec;14(4):884–8. PMID:32026292
4482. Thompson LDR, Gill AJ, Asa SL, et al. Data set for the reporting of pheochromocytoma and paraganglioma: explanations and recommendations of the guidelines from the International Collaboration on Cancer Reporting. Hum Pathol. 2021 Apr;110:83–97. PMID:32407815
4483. Thompson LDR, Herrera HB, Lau SK. Thyroglossal duct cyst carcinomas in pediatric patients: report of two cases with a comprehensive literature review. Head Neck Pathol. 2017 Dec;11(4):442–9. PMID:28293858
4484. Thompson LDR, Herrera HB, Lau SK. Thyroglossal duct cyst carcinomas: a clinicopathologic series of 22 cases with staging recommendations. Head Neck Pathol. 2017 Jun;11(2):175–85. PMID:27704385
4485. Thompson LDR, Jo VY, Agaimy A, et al. Sinonasal tract alveolar rhabdomyosarcoma in adults: a clinicopathologic and immunophenotypic study of fifty-two cases with emphasis on epithelial immunoreactivity. Head Neck Pathol. 2018 Jun;12(2):181–92. PMID:28875443
4486. Thompson LDR, Magliocca KR, Andreasen S, et al. CAIX and pax-8 commonly immunoreactive in endolymphatic sac tumors: a clinicopathologic study of 26 cases with differential considerations for metastatic renal cell carcinoma in von Hippel-Lindau patients. Head Neck Pathol. 2019 Sep;13(3):355–63. PMID:30291511
4487. Thompson LDR, Poller DN, Kakudo K, et al. An international interobserver variability reporting of the nuclear scoring criteria to diagnose noninvasive follicular thyroid neoplasm with papillary-like nuclear features: a validation study. Endocr Pathol. 2018 Sep;29(3):242–9. PMID:29508145
4488. Thompson LDR, Wei C, Rooper LM, et al. Thyroid gland solitary fibrous tumor: report of 3 cases and a comprehensive review of the literature. Head Neck Pathol. 2019 Dec;13(4):597–605. PMID:30758754
4490. Thompson NW, Eckhauser FE, Harness JK. The anatomy of primary hyperparathyroidism. Surgery. 1982 Nov;92(5):814–21. PMID:7135202
4491. Thomson N, Pacak K, Schmidt MH, et al. Leptomeningeal dissemination of a low-grade lumbar paraganglioma: case report. J Neurosurg Spine. 2017 Apr;26(4):501–6. PMID:28128698
4492. Thosani S, Ayala-Ramirez M, Román-González A, et al. Constipation: an overlooked, unmanaged symptom of patients with pheochromocytoma and sympathetic paraganglioma. Eur J Endocrinol. 2015 Sep;173(3):377–87. PMID:26060051
4493. Thway K, Hayes A, Ieremia E, et al. Heterologous osteosarcomatous and rhabdomyosarcomatous elements in dedifferentiated solitary fibrous tumor: further support for the concept of dedifferentiation in solitary fibrous tumor. Ann Diagn Pathol. 2013 Oct;17(5):457–63. PMID:23040384
4494. Thway K, Olmos D, Shah C, et al. Oncocytic adrenal cortical carcinosarcoma with pleomorphic rhabdomyosarcomatous metastases. Am J Surg Pathol. 2012 Mar;36(3):470–7. PMID:22343339
4495. Tichomirowa MA, Barlier A, Daly AF, et al. High prevalence of AIP gene mutations following focused screening in young patients with sporadic pituitary macroadenomas. Eur J Endocrinol. 2011 Oct;165(4):509–15. PMID:21753072
4496. Tichomirowa MA, Lee M, Barlier A, et al. Cyclin-dependent kinase inhibitor 1B (CDKN1B) gene variants in AIP mutation-negative familial isolated pituitary adenoma kindreds. Endocr Relat Cancer. 2012 May 3;19(3):233–41. PMID:22291433
4497. Tigas S, Carroll PV, Jones R, et al. Simultaneous Cushing's disease and tuberous sclerosis; a potential role for TSC in pituitary ontogeny. Clin Endocrinol (Oxf). 2005 Dec;63(6):694–5. PMID:16343106
4498. Timerbulatov VM, Lopatin VM. Giniiatulin ShKh. [Liver abscess after surgery of hemorrhoids]. Vestn Khir Im I I Grek. 1988 Sep;141(9):135–6. Russian. PMID:3238850
4499. Timmers HJ, Pacak K, Huynh TT, et al. Biochemically silent abdominal paragangliomas in patients with mutations in the succinate dehydrogenase subunit B gene. J Clin Endocrinol Metab. 2008 Dec;93(12):4826–32. PMID:18840642
4500. Timmers HJ, Taieb D, Pacak K. Current and future anatomical and functional imaging approaches to pheochromocytoma and paraganglioma. Horm Metab Res. 2012 May;44(5):367–72. PMID:22399235
4501. Timonera ER, Paiva ME, Lopes JM, et al. Composite adenomatoid tumor and myelolipoma of adrenal gland: report of 2 cases. Arch Pathol Lab Med. 2008 Feb;132(2):265–7. PMID:18251587
4502. Ting J, Bell D, Ahmed S, et al. Primary malignant thyroid teratoma: an institutional experience. Thyroid. 2019 Feb;29(2):229–36. PMID:30759052
4503. Tingi E, Ogah J. Ectopic adrenal rest cells of the fallopian tube: a case report and review of the literature. J Obstet Gynaecol. 2018 May;38(4):578–9. PMID:29385841
4504. Tiosano D, Vlodavsky E, Filmar S, et al. Ovarian adrenal rest tumor in a congenital adrenal hyperplasia patient with adrenocorticotropin hypersecretion following adrenalectomy. Horm Res Paediatr. 2010;74(3):223–8. PMID:20431278
4505. Tirabosco R, Mangham DC, Rosenberg AE, et al. Brachyury expression in extra-axial skeletal and soft tissue chordomas: a marker that distinguishes chordoma from mixed tumor/myoepithelioma/parachordoma in soft tissue. Am J Surg Pathol. 2008 Apr;32(4):572–80. PMID:18301055
4506. Tirado Y, Williams MD, Hanna EY, et al. CRTC1/MAML2 fusion transcript in high grade mucoepidermoid carcinomas of salivary and thyroid glands and Warthin's tumors: implications for histogenesis and biologic behavior. Genes Chromosomes Cancer. 2007 Jul;46(7):708–15. PMID:17437281
4507. Tischler AS, Dayal Y, Balogh K, et al. The distribution of immunoreactive chromogranins, S-100 protein, and vasoactive intestinal peptide in compound tumors of the adrenal medulla. Hum Pathol. 1987 Sep;18(9):909–17. PMID:3623551
4508. Tish S, Habboub G, Jones J, et al. The epidemiology of central and extraventricular neurocytoma in the United States between 2006 and 2014. J Neurooncol. 2019

May;143(1):123–7. PMID:30859483
4509. Tish S, Habboub G, Prayson RA, et al. Extraventricular neurocytoma with ganglioid differentiation of the sellar and parasellar regions in an elderly patient: a case report. Surg Neurol Int. 2019 May 10;10:82. PMID:31528420
4510. Tissier F, Cavard C, Groussin L, et al. Mutations of beta-catenin in adrenocortical tumors: activation of the Wnt signaling pathway is a frequent event in both benign and malignant adrenocortical tumors. Cancer Res. 2005 Sep 1;65(17):7622–7. PMID:16140927
4511. Titgemeyer C, Grois N, Minkov M, et al. Pattern and course of single-system disease in Langerhans cell histiocytosis data from the DAL-HX 83- and 90-study. Med Pediatr Oncol. 2001 Aug;37(2):108–14. PMID:11496348
4512. Tjörnstrand A, Gunnarsson K, Evert M, et al. The incidence rate of pituitary adenomas in western Sweden for the period 2001-2011. Eur J Endocrinol. 2014 Oct;171(4):519–26. PMID:25084775
4513. Tjörnstrand A, Nyström HF. Diagnosis of endocrine disease: diagnostic approach to TSH-producing pituitary adenoma. Eur J Endocrinol. 2017 Oct;177(4):R183–97. PMID:28566440
4514. Tohme CA, Mattar WE, Ghorra CS. Extra-adrenal composite pheochromocytoma-ganglioneuroma. Saudi Med J. 2006 Oct;27(10):1594–7. PMID:17013491
4515. Tolbert VP, Coggins GE, Maris JM. Genetic susceptibility to neuroblastoma. Curr Opin Genet Dev. 2017 Feb;42:81–90. PMID:28458126
4516. Tomic S, Warner T. Pancreatic somatostatin-secreting gangliocytic paraganglioma with lymph node metastases. Am J Gastroenterol. 1996 Mar;91(3):607–8. PMID:8633524
4517. Tominaga Y, Numano M, Uchida K, et al. Lung metastasis from parathyroid carcinoma causing recurrent renal hyperparathyroidism in a hemodialysis patient: report of a case. Surg Today. 1995;25(11):984–6. PMID:8640028
4518. Tomsic J, He H, Akagi K, et al. A germline mutation in SRRM2, a splicing factor gene, is implicated in papillary thyroid carcinoma predisposition. Sci Rep. 2015 Jul 2;5:10566. PMID:26135620
4519. Tonacchera M, Chiovato L, Pinchera A, et al. Hyperfunctioning thyroid nodules in toxic multinodular goiter share activating thyrotropin receptor mutations with solitary toxic adenoma. J Clin Endocrinol Metab. 1998 Feb;83(2):492–8. PMID:9467563
4520. Tonacchera M, Pinchera A, Vitti P. Assessment of nodular goitre. Best Pract Res Clin Endocrinol Metab. 2010 Feb;24(1):51–61. PMID:20172470
4521. Tonelli F, Giudici F, Giusti F, et al. A heterozygous frameshift mutation in exon 1 of CDKN1B gene in a patient affected by MEN4 syndrome. Eur J Endocrinol. 2014 Aug;171(2):K7–17. PMID:24819502
4522. Tong GX, Hamele-Bena D, Wei XJ, et al. Fine-needle aspiration biopsy of monophasic variant of spindle epithelial tumor with thymus-like differentiation of the thyroid: report of one case and review of the literature. Diagn Cytopathol. 2007 Feb;35(2):113–9. PMID:17230570
4523. Tonomura S, Kitaichi T, Onishi R, et al. A dural metastatic small cell carcinoma of the gallbladder as the first manifestation: a case report. World J Surg Oncol. 2018 Mar 16;16(1):57. PMID:29548338
4524. Tordjman KM, Greenman Y, Ram Z, et al. Plurihormonal pituitary tumor of Pit-1 and SF-1 lineages, with synchronous collision corticotroph tumor: a possible stem cell phenomenon. Endocr Pathol. 2019 Mar;30(1):74–80. PMID:30610567
4525. Tornóczky T, Kálmán E, Kajtár PG, et al. Large cell neuroblastoma: a distinct phenotype of neuroblastoma with aggressive clinical behavior. Cancer. 2004 Jan 15;100(2):390–7. PMID:14716776
4526. Tornóczky T, Semjén D, Shimada H, et al. Pathology of peripheral neuroblastic tumors: significance of prominent nucleoli in undifferentiated/poorly differentiated neuroblastoma. Pathol Oncol Res. 2007;13(4):269–75. PMID:18158560
4527. Torpy DJ. Screening for ACTH-dependent hypercortisolism in patients with pituitary incidentaloma. Eur J Endocrinol. 2015 Apr;172(4):C1–4. PMID:25609777
4528. Torres Luna N, Mosquera JE, Comba IY, et al. A primary adrenal epithelioid angiomyolipoma (PEComa) in a patient with tuberous sclerosis complex: report of a case and review of the literature. Case Rep Med. 2020 Mar 17;2020:5131736. PMID:32256603
4529. Torres MB, Diggs LP, Wei JS, et al. Ataxia telangiectasia mutated germline pathogenic variant in adrenocortical carcinoma. Cancer Genet. 2021 Aug;256-257:21–5. PMID:33836455
4530. Torresan F, Iacobone M. Clinical features, treatment, and surveillance of hyperparathyroidism-jaw tumor syndrome: an up-to-date and review of the literature. Int J Endocrinol. 2019 Dec 18;2019:1761030. PMID:31929790
4531. Torske KR, Thompson LD. Adenoma versus carcinoid tumor of the middle ear: a study of 48 cases and review of the literature. Mod Pathol. 2002 May;15(5):543–55. PMID:12011260
4532. Tosios KI, Papanikolaou V, Vlachodimitropoulos D, et al. Primary large cell neuroendocrine carcinoma of the parotid gland. report of a rare case. Head Neck Pathol. 2021 Dec;15(4):1377–84. PMID:33544384
4533. Tovi F, Fliss DM, Inbar-Yanai I. Hurthle cell adenoma of the thyroglossal duct. Head Neck Surg. 1988 May-Jun;10(5):346–9. PMID:3220776
4534. Trabelsi A, Ben Abdelkarim S, Hadfi M, et al. Primary mesenteric Sertoli-Leydig cell tumor: a case report and review of the literature. J Oncol. 2008;2008:619637. PMID:19266086
4535. Trabzonlu L, Paksoy N. Cytomorphological analysis of thyroid nodules diagnosed as follicular variant of papillary thyroid carcinoma: a fine needle aspiration study of diagnostic clues in 42 cases and the impact of using Bethesda system in reporting-an institutional experience. Endocr Pathol. 2018 Dec;29(4):351–6. PMID:30315491
4536. Tran L, Fitzpatrick C, Cohn SL, et al. Composite tumor with pheochromocytoma and immature neuroblastoma: report of two cases with cytogenetic analysis and discussion of current terminology. Virchows Arch. 2017 Oct;471(4):553–7. PMID:28864906
4537. Trastour C, Rahili A, Chevallier A, et al. Isolated bilateral adrenal choriocarcinoma. Lancet Oncol. 2005 Nov;6(11):905–7. PMID:16257799
4538. Travis WD. Pathology and diagnosis of neuroendocrine tumors: lung neuroendocrine. Thorac Surg Clin. 2014 Aug;24(3):257–66. PMID:25065926
4540. Travis WD, Brambilla E, Burke AP, et al., editors. WHO classification of tumours of the lung, pleura, thymus and heart. Lyon (France): International Agency for Research on Cancer; 2015. (WHO classification of tumours series, 4th ed.; vol. 7). https://publications.iarc.who.int/17.
4541. Travis WD, Linnoila RI, Tsokos MG, et al. Neuroendocrine tumors of the lung with proposed criteria for large-cell neuroendocrine carcinoma. An ultrastructural, immunohistochemical, and flow cytometric study of 35 cases. Am J Surg Pathol. 1991 Jun;15(6):529–53. PMID:1709558
4542. Travis WD, Rush W, Flieder DB, et al. Survival analysis of 200 pulmonary neuroendocrine tumors with clarification of criteria for atypical carcinoid and its separation from typical carcinoid. Am J Surg Pathol. 1998 Aug;22(8):934–44. PMID:9706973
4543. Traylor KS. Computed tomography and MR imaging of thyroid disease. Radiol Clin North Am. 2020 Nov;58(6):1059–70. PMID:33040848
4544. Treglia G, Annunziata S, Muoio B, et al. The role of fluorine-18-fluorodeoxyglucose positron emission tomography in aggressive histological subtypes of thyroid cancer: an overview. Int J Endocrinol. 2013;2013:856189. PMID:23653645
4545. Treglia G, Castaldi P, Villani MF, et al. Comparison of 18F-DOPA, 18F-FDG and 68Ga-somatostatin analogue PET/CT in patients with recurrent medullary thyroid carcinoma. Eur J Nucl Med Mol Imaging. 2012 Apr;39(4):569–80. PMID:22223169
4546. Triantafyllou A, Williams MD, Angelos P, et al. Incidental findings of thyroid tissue in cervical lymph nodes: old controversy not yet resolved? Eur Arch Otorhinolaryngol. 2016 Oct;273(10):2867–75. PMID:26459007
4547. Trimboli P, Cremonini N, Ceriani L, et al. Calcitonin measurement in aspiration needle washout fluids has higher sensitivity than cytology in detecting medullary thyroid cancer: a retrospective multicentre study. Clin Endocrinol (Oxf). 2014 Jan;80(1):135–40. PMID:23627255
4548. Trimboli P, Giovanella L, Valabrega S, et al. Ultrasound features of medullary thyroid carcinoma correlate with cancer aggressiveness: a retrospective multicenter study. J Exp Clin Cancer Res. 2014 Oct 25;33(1):87. PMID:25344474
4549. Trimboli P, Treglia G, Guidobaldi L, et al. Detection rate of FNA cytology in medullary thyroid carcinoma: a meta-analysis. Clin Endocrinol (Oxf). 2015 Feb;82(2):280–5. PMID:25047365
4550. Trindade F, Tellechea O, Torrelo A, et al. Wilms tumor 1 expression in vascular neoplasms and vascular malformations. Am J Dermatopathol. 2011 Aug;33(6):569–72. PMID:21697701
4551. Tripathi M, Maskara P, Deora H, et al. Role of stereotactic radiosurgery in intracranial histiocytosis: a systematic review of literature of an emerging modality for localized disease. World Neurosurg. 2021 Jun;150:64–70. PMID:33744421
4552. Triponez F, Sadowski SM, Pattou F, et al. Long-term follow-up of MEN1 patients who do not have initial surgery for small ≤2 cm nonfunctioning pancreatic neuroendocrine tumors, an AFCE and GTE study: Association Francophone de Chirurgie Endocrinienne & Groupe d'Etude des Tumeurs Endocrines. Ann Surg. 2018 Jul;268(1):158–64. PMID:28263205
4553. Triponez F, Wong M, Sturgeon C, et al. Does familial non-medullary thyroid cancer adversely affect survival? World J Surg. 2006 May;30(5):787–93. PMID:16479341
4554. Tritos NA, Eppakayala S, Swearingen B, et al. Pathologic and clinical features of pituitary adenomas showing TSH immunoreactivity. Pituitary. 2013 Sep;16(3):287–93. PMID:22869255
4555. Trivellin G, Daly AF, Faucz FR, et al. Gigantism and acromegaly due to Xq26 microduplications and GPR101 mutation. N Engl J Med. 2014 Dec 18;371(25):2363–74. PMID:25470569
4556. Trost BN, Koenig MP, Zimmermann A, et al. Virilization of a post-menopausal woman by a testosterone-secreting Leydig cell type adrenal adenoma. Acta Endocrinol (Copenh). 1981 Oct;98(2):274–82. PMID:6270941
4557. Trouillas J, Delgrange E, Jouanneau E, et al. [Prolactinoma in man: clinical and histological characteristics]. Ann Endocrinol (Paris). 2000 Sep;61(3):253–7. French. PMID:10970951
4558. Trouillas J, Jaffrain-Rea ML, Vasiljevic A, et al. How to classify the pituitary neuroendocrine tumors (PitNET)s in 2020. Cancers (Basel). 2020 Feb 22;12(2):514. PMID:32098443
4559. Trouillas J, Labat-Moleur F, Sturm N, et al. Pituitary tumors and hyperplasia in multiple endocrine neoplasia type 1 syndrome (MEN1): a case-control study in a series of 77 patients versus 2509 non-MEN1 patients. Am J Surg Pathol. 2008 Apr;32(4):534–43. PMID:18300794
4560. Trouillas J, Roy P, Sturm N, et al. A new prognostic clinicopathological classification of pituitary adenomas: a multicentric case-control study of 410 patients with 8 years post-operative follow-up. Acta Neuropathol. 2013 Jul;126(1):123–35. PMID:23400299
4561. Trovisco V, Soares P, Preto A, et al. Type and prevalence of BRAF mutations are closely associated with papillary thyroid carcinoma histotype and patients' age but not with tumour aggressiveness. Virchows Arch. 2005 Jun;446(6):589–95. PMID:15902486
4562. Trovisco V, Soares P, Soares R, et al. A new BRAF gene mutation detected in a case of a solid variant of papillary thyroid carcinoma. Hum Pathol. 2005 Jun;36(6):694–7. PMID:16021577
4563. Trovisco V, Vieira de Castro I, Soares P, et al. BRAF mutations are associated with some histological types of papillary thyroid carcinoma. J Pathol. 2004 Feb;202(2):247–51. PMID:14743508
4564. Trpkov K, Hes O, Williamson SR, et al. New developments in existing WHO entities and evolving molecular concepts: the Genitourinary Pathology Society (GUPS) update on renal neoplasia. Mod Pathol. 2021 Jul;34(7):1392–424. PMID:33664427
4565. Trpkov K, Williamson SR, Gill AJ, et al. Novel, emerging and provisional renal entities: the Genitourinary Pathology Society (GUPS) update on renal neoplasia. Mod Pathol. 2021 Jun;34(6):1167–84. PMID:33526874
4566. Trülzsch B, Krohn K, Wonerow P, et al. Detection of thyroid-stimulating hormone receptor and Gsalpha mutations: in 75 toxic thyroid nodules by denaturing gradient gel electrophoresis. J Mol Med (Berl). 2001;78(12):684–91. PMID:11434721
4567. Truran PP, Johnson SJ, Bliss RD, et al. Parafibromin, galectin-3, PGP9.5, Ki67, and cyclin D1: using an immunohistochemical panel to aid in the diagnosis of parathyroid cancer. World J Surg. 2014 Nov;38(11):2845–54. PMID:25002250
4568. Tsai HK, Hornick JL, Vivero M. INSM1 expression in a subset of thoracic malignancies and small round cell tumors: rare potential pitfalls for small cell carcinoma. Mod Pathol. 2020 Aug;33(8):1571–80. PMID:32203089
4569. Tsai PJ, Liu KY, Wang SE, et al. Solitary neurofibroma of the pancreas body not associated with type 1 neurofibromatosis. J Chin Med Assoc. 2012 Mar;75(3):132–5. PMID:22440272
4570. Tsai WH, Chen TC, Dai SH, et al. Case report: ectopic adrenocortical carcinoma in the ovary. Front Endocrinol (Lausanne). 2021 Mar 19;12:662377. PMID:33815299
4571. Tsang JCH, Ng CS, Fung CF, et al. Glomus tumor of sella turcica with synaptophysin expression mimicking pituitary adenoma. Int J Surg Pathol. 2020 Jun;28(4):401–5.

PMID:31948309
4572. Tsang K, Duggan MA. Vascular proliferation of the thyroid. A complication of fine-needle aspiration. Arch Pathol Lab Med. 1992 Oct;116(10):1040–2. PMID:1417444
4573. Tsang VH, Dwight T, Benn DE, et al. Overexpression of miR-210 is associated with SDH-related pheochromocytomas, paragangliomas, and gastrointestinal stromal tumours. Endocr Relat Cancer. 2014 May 6;21(3):415–26. PMID:24623741
4574. Tsang VH, Tacon LJ, Learoyd DL, et al. Pheochromocytomas in multiple endocrine neoplasia type 2. Recent Results Cancer Res. 2015;204:157–78. PMID:26494388
4575. Tsilou ET, Chan CC, Sandrini F, et al. Eyelid myxoma in Carney complex without PRKAR1A allelic loss. Am J Med Genet A. 2004 Nov 1;130A(4):395–7. PMID:15368482
4576. Tsuji H, Yasuoka H, Nakamura Y, et al. Aggressive cribriform-morular variant of papillary thyroid carcinoma: report of an unusual case with pulmonary metastasis displaying poorly differentiated features. Pathol Int. 2018 Dec;68(12):700–5. PMID:30376202
4577. Tsukada T, Yoshida H, Ishikawa M, et al. Malignant struma ovarii presenting with follicular carcinoma: a case report with molecular analysis. Gynecol Oncol Rep. 2019 Sep 9;30:100498. PMID:31538107
4578. Tsuruoka K, Horinouchi H, Goto Y, et al. PD-L1 expression in neuroendocrine tumors of the lung. Lung Cancer. 2017 Jun;108:115–20. PMID:28625622
4579. Tsutsui H, Hoshi M, Kubota M, et al. Management of thyroid carcinoma showing thymus-like differentiation (CASTLE) invading the trachea. Surg Today. 2013 Nov;43(11):1261–8. PMID:23543082
4580. Tsybrovskyy O, Rössmann-Tsybrovskyy M. Oncocytic versus mitochondrion-rich follicular thyroid tumours: should we make a difference? Histopathology. 2009 Dec;55(6):665–82. PMID:20002768
4581. Tu X, Chang T, Nie L, et al. Large cell neuroendocrine carcinoma of the prostate: a systematic review and pooled analysis. Urol Int. 2019;103(4):383–90. PMID:30965328
4582. Tufton N, Roncaroli F, Hadjidemetriou I, et al. Pituitary carcinoma in a patient with an SDHB mutation. Endocr Pathol. 2017 Dec;28(4):320–5. PMID:28284009
4583. Tufton N, Shapiro L, Srirangalingam U, et al. Outcomes of annual surveillance imaging in an adult and paediatric cohort of succinate dehydrogenase B mutation carriers. Clin Endocrinol (Oxf). 2017 Feb;86(2):286–96. PMID:27678251
4584. Tulbah A, Al-Dayel F, Fawaz I, et al. Epstein-Barr virus-associated leiomyosarcoma of the thyroid in a child with congenital immunodeficiency: a case report. Am J Surg Pathol. 1999 Apr;23(4):473–6. PMID:10199478
4585. Tunca F, Sormaz IC, Iscan Y, et al. Comparison of histopathological features and prognosis of classical and follicular variant papillary thyroid carcinoma. J Endocrinol Invest. 2015 Dec;38(12):1327–34. PMID:26280320
4586. Turan H, Tarçın G, Mete Ö, et al. Silent corticotroph tumor with adrenocortical choristoma in an eleven-year-old boy. J Clin Res Pediatr Endocrinol. 2022 Mar 3;14(1):126–30. PMID:33586921
4587. Turchini J, Cheung VKY, Tischler AS, et al. Pathology and genetics of phaeochromocytoma and paraganglioma. Histopathology. 2018 Jan;72(1):97–105. PMID:29239044
4588. Turchini J, Fuchs TL, Chou A, et al. A critical assessment of diagnostic criteria for the tall cell subtype of papillary thyroid carcinoma-How much? How tall? And when is it relevant? Endocr Pathol. 2023 Dec;34(4):461–70. PMID:37864666
4589. Turchini J, Gill AJ. Hereditary parathyroid disease: sometimes pathologists do not know what they are missing. Endocr Pathol. 2020 Sep;31(3):218–30. PMID:32468209
4590. Turchini J, Gill AJ. Morphologic clues to succinate dehydrogenase (SDH) deficiency in pheochromocytomas and paragangliomas. Am J Surg Pathol. 2020 Mar;44(3):422–4. PMID:31789631
4591. Turchini J, Sioson L, Clarkson A, et al. The presence of typical "BRAFV600E-like" atypia in papillary thyroid carcinoma is highly specific for the presence of the BRAFV600E mutation. Endocr Pathol. 2023 Mar;34(1):112–8. PMID:36709221
4592. Turchini J, Sioson L, Clarkson A, et al. Utility of GATA-3 expression in the analysis of pituitary neuroendocrine tumour (PitNET) transcription factors. Endocr Pathol. 2020 Jun;31(2):150–5. PMID:32193825
4593. Turkdogan S, Forest VI, Hier MP, et al. Carcinoembryonic antigen levels correlated with advanced disease in medullary thyroid cancer. J Otolaryngol Head Neck Surg. 2018 Sep 17;47(1):55. PMID:30223887
4594. Türkmen E, Erdoğan B, Kodaz H, et al. A small cell carcinoma in the testis associated with testicular teratoma. Balkan Med J. 2014 Jun;31(2):191–2. PMID:25207197
4595. Turri-Zanoni M, Maragliano R, Battaglia P, et al. The clinicopathological spectrum of olfactory neuroblastoma and sinonasal neuroendocrine neoplasms: refinements in diagnostic criteria and impact of multimodal treatments on survival. Oral Oncol. 2017 Nov;74:21–9. PMID:29103747
4596. Tusié-Luna MT, White PC. Gene conversions and unequal crossovers between CYP21 (steroid 21-hydroxylase gene) and CYP21P involve different mechanisms. Proc Natl Acad Sci U S A. 1995 Nov 7;92(23):10796–800. PMID:7479886
4597. Tuttle RM, Lemar H, Burch HB. Clinical features associated with an increased risk of thyroid malignancy in patients with follicular neoplasia by fine-needle aspiration. Thyroid. 1998 May;8(5):377–83. PMID:9623727
4598. Tzigkalidis T, Skandalou E, Manthou ME, et al. Adrenal cortical rests in the fallopian tube: report of a case and review of the literature. Medicines (Basel). 2021 Mar 12;8(3):14. PMID:33809106
4599. Ubayasiri KM, Brocklehurst J, Judd O, et al. A decade of experience of thyroglossal cyst excision. Ann R Coll Surg Engl. 2013 May;95(4):263–5. PMID:23676810
4600. Uccella S. Molecular classification of gastrointestinal and pancreatic neuroendocrine neoplasms: Are we ready for that? Endocr Pathol. 2024 Jun;35(2):91–106. PMID:38470548
4601. Uccella S, Blank A, Maragliano R, et al. Calcitonin-producing neuroendocrine neoplasms of the pancreas: clinicopathological study of 25 cases and review of the literature. Endocr Pathol. 2017 Dec;28(4):351–61. PMID:29063495
4602. Uccella S, Finzi G, Sessa F, et al. On the endless dilemma of neuroendocrine neoplasms of the breast: a journey through concepts and entities. Endocr Pathol. 2020 Dec;31(4):321–9. PMID:32613538
4603. Uccella S, La Rosa S, Metovic J, et al. Genomics of high-grade neuroendocrine neoplasms: well-differentiated neuroendocrine tumor with high-grade features (G3 NET) and neuroendocrine carcinomas (NEC) of various anatomic sites. Endocr Pathol. 2021 Mar;32(1):192–210. PMID:33433884
4604. Uccella S, La Rosa S, Volante M, et al. Immunohistochemical biomarkers of gastrointestinal, pancreatic, pulmonary, and thymic neuroendocrine neoplasms. Endocr Pathol. 2018 Jun;29(2):150–68. PMID:29520563
4605. Uccella S, La Rosa S. Looking into digestive mixed neuroendocrine - nonneuroendocrine neoplasms: subtypes, prognosis, and predictive factors. Histopathology. 2020 Nov;77(5):700–17. PMID:32538468
4606. Uccella S, Ottini G, Facco C, et al. Neuroendocrine neoplasms of the head and neck and olfactory neuroblastoma. Diagnosis and classification. Pathologica. 2017 Mar;109(1):14–30. PMID:28635990
4607. Uchida K, Masamune A, Shimosegawa T, et al. Prevalence of IgG4-related disease in Japan based on nationwide survey in 2009. Int J Rheumatol. 2012;2012:358371. PMID:22899936
4608. Uchino S, Ishikawa H, Miyauchi A, et al. Age- and gender-specific risk of thyroid cancer in patients with familial adenomatous polyposis. J Clin Endocrinol Metab. 2016 Dec;101(12):4611–7. PMID:27623068
4609. Uchino S, Noguchi S, Kawamoto H, et al. Familial nonmedullary thyroid carcinoma characterized by multifocality and a high recurrence rate in a large study population. World J Surg. 2002 Aug;26(8):897–902. PMID:11965446
4610. Uchino S, Noguchi S, Yamashita H, et al. Mutational analysis of the APC gene in cribriform-morula variant of papillary thyroid carcinoma. World J Surg. 2006 May;30(5):775–9. PMID:16680592
4611. Udager AM, Magers MJ, Goerke DM, et al. The utility of SDHB and FH immunohistochemistry in patients evaluated for hereditary paraganglioma-pheochromocytoma syndromes. Hum Pathol. 2018 Jan;71:47–54. PMID:29079178
4612. Udelsman R, Chen H. The current management of thyroid cancer. Adv Surg. 1999;33:1–27. PMID:10572560
4613. Ueki I, Ando T, Haraguchi A, et al. A case of mixed medullary and follicular cell carcinoma of the thyroid. Intern Med. 2011;50(12):1313–6. PMID:21673468
4614. Uğurlu MÜ, Seven İE, Eren F, et al. Minimally invasive thyroid anaplastic carcinoma with long survival. Turk J Surg. 2018 Dec 1;34(4):319–22. PMID:30664432
4615. UICC [Internet]. Geneva (Switzerland): Union for International Cancer Control; 2020. TNM Publications and Resources – Errata; updated 2020 Oct 6. Available from: https://www.uicc.org/resources/tnm/publications-resources.
4616. UICC [Internet]. Geneva (Switzerland): Union for International Cancer Control; 2022. TNM Publications and Resources – Errata; updated 2022 Jan 25. Available from: https://www.uicc.org/resources/tnm/publications-resources.
4617. Ulbright TM. Germ cell tumors of the gonads: a selective review emphasizing problems in differential diagnosis, newly appreciated, and controversial issues. Mod Pathol. 2005 Feb;18 Suppl 2:S61–79. PMID:15761467
4618. Ulrich JD, Specht K, Schlitter AM, et al. A rare case of perivascular epithelioid cell tumor (PEComa) of the pancreas diagnosed by endoscopic ultrasound. Endosc Int Open. 2020 Jan;8(1):E25–8. PMID:31921981
4619. Uludağ M, Tanal M, İşgör A. Standards and definitions in neck dissections of differentiated thyroid cancer. Sisli Etfal Hastan Tip Bul. 2018 Oct 1;52(3):149–63. PMID:32595391
4620. Umehara S, Nakagawa A, Matthay KK, et al. Histopathology defines prognostic subsets of ganglioneuroblastoma, nodular. Cancer. 2000 Sep 1;89(5):1150–61. PMID:10964346
4621. Umeoka K, Sanno N, Osamura RY, et al. Expression of GATA-2 in human pituitary adenomas. Mod Pathol. 2002 Jan;15(1):11–7. PMID:11796836
4622. Unger P, Hoffman K, Pertsemlidis D, et al. S100 protein-positive sustentacular cells in malignant and locally aggressive adrenal pheochromocytomas. Arch Pathol Lab Med. 1991 May;115(5):484–7. PMID:1673596
4623. Urakawa I, Yamazaki Y, Shimada T, et al. Klotho converts canonical FGF receptor into a specific receptor for FGF23. Nature. 2006 Dec 7;444(7120):770–4. PMID:17086194
4624. Uraki S, Ariyasu H, Doi A, et al. Atypical pituitary adenoma with MEN1 somatic mutation associated with abnormalities of DNA mismatch repair genes; MLH1 germline mutation and MSH6 somatic mutation. Endocr J. 2017 Sep 30;64(9):895–906. PMID:28701629
4625. Urano M, Kiriyama Y, Takakuwa Y, et al. Tall cell variant of papillary thyroid carcinoma: its characteristic features demonstrated by fine-needle aspiration cytology and immunohistochemical study. Diagn Cytopathol. 2009 Oct;37(10):732–7. PMID:19373912
4626. Urbini M, Nannini M, Astolfi A, et al. Whole exome sequencing uncovers germline variants of cancer-related genes in sporadic pheochromocytoma. Int J Genomics. 2018 Aug 19;2018:6582014. PMID:30211214
4627. Usher I, Flanagan AM, Choi D. Systematic review of clinical, radiologic, and histologic features of benign notochordal cell tumors: implications for patient management. World Neurosurg. 2019 Oct;130:13–23. PMID:31421435
4628. Us-Krasovec M, Golouh R. Papillary thyroid carcinoma with exuberant nodular fasciitis-like stroma in a fine needle aspirate. A case report. Acta Cytol. 1999 Nov-Dec;43(6):1101–4. PMID:10578985
4629. Usuda H, Emura I. Composite paraganglioma-ganglioneuroma of the urinary bladder. Pathol Int. 2005 Sep;55(9):596–601. PMID:16143037
4630. Uusitalo E, Rantanen M, Kallionpää RA, et al. Distinctive cancer associations in patients with neurofibromatosis type 1. J Clin Oncol. 2016 Jun 10;34(17):1978–86. PMID:26926675
4631. Uyanıkoglu H, Ozer G, Kahraman S. A spontaneous pregnancy and live birth in a woman with primary infertility following the excision of an ovarian adrenal rest tumor: a rare case. Clin Exp Reprod Med. 2020 Dec;47(4):319–22. PMID:33105528
4632. Uzilov AV, Taik P, Cheesman KC, et al. USP8 and TP53 drivers are associated with CNV in a corticotroph adenoma cohort enriched for aggressive tumors. J Clin Endocrinol Metab. 2021 Mar 8;106(3):826–42. PMID:33221858
4633. Vaduva P, Bonnet F, Bertherat J. Molecular basis of primary aldosteronism and adrenal Cushing syndrome. J Endocr Soc. 2020 Jun 29;4(9):bvaa075. PMID:32783015
4634. Vaidya A, Nehs M, Kilbridge K. Treatment of adrenocortical carcinoma. Surg Pathol Clin. 2019 Dec;12(4):997–1006. PMID:31672303
4635. Vajtai I, Beck J, Kappeler A, et al. Spindle cell oncocytoma of the pituitary gland with follicle-like component: organotypic differentiation to support its origin from folliculo-stellate cells. Acta Neuropathol. 2011 Aug;122(2):253–8. PMID:21590491
4636. Valassi E, Biller BM, Klibanski A, et al. Clinical features of nonpituitary sellar lesions in a large surgical series. Clin Endocrinol (Oxf). 2010 Dec;73(6):798–807. PMID:20874772
4637. Valdiserri RO, Yunis EJ. Sacrococcygeal teratomas: a review of 68 cases. Cancer. 1981 Jul 1;48(1):217–21. PMID:6165455
4638. Valentijn LJ, Koster J, Zwijnenburg DA, et al. TERT rearrangements are frequent in neuroblastoma and identify aggressive

tumors. Nat Genet. 2015 Dec;47(12):1411–4. PMID:26523776
4639. Välimäki N, Demir H, Pitkänen E, et al. Whole-genome sequencing of growth hormone (GH)-secreting pituitary adenomas. J Clin Endocrinol Metab. 2015 Oct;100(10):3918–27. PMID:26280510
4640. Vallat-Decouvelaere AV, Dry SM, Fletcher CD. Atypical and malignant solitary fibrous tumors in extrathoracic locations: evidence of their comparability to intra-thoracic tumors. Am J Surg Pathol. 1998 Dec;22(12):1501–11. PMID:9850176
4641. van Beek DJ, Nell S, Pieterman CRC, et al. Prognostic factors and survival in MEN1 patients with gastrinomas: results from the DutchMEN Study Group (DMSG). J Surg Oncol. 2019 Nov;120(6):966–75. PMID:31401809
4642. van den Broek MFM, de Laat JM, van Leeuwaarde RS, et al. The management of neuroendocrine tumors of the lung in MEN1: results from the Dutch MEN1 Study Group. J Clin Endocrinol Metab. 2021 Jan 23;106(2):e1014–27. PMID:33135721
4643. Van den Eynden GG, Neyret A, Fumey G, et al. PTHrP, calcitonin and calcitriol in a case of severe, protracted and refractory hypercalcemia due to a pancreatic neuroendocrine tumor. Bone. 2007 Apr;40(4):1166–71. PMID:17188588
4644. van der Laan TP, Bij HP, van Hemel BM, et al. The importance of multimodality therapy in the treatment of sinonasal neuroendocrine carcinoma. Eur Arch Otorhinolaryngol. 2013 Sep;270(9):2565–8. PMID:23740425
4645. van der Laan TP, Iepsma R, Witjes MJ, et al. Meta-analysis of 701 published cases of sinonasal neuroendocrine carcinoma: the importance of differentiation grade in determining treatment strategy. Oral Oncol. 2016 Dec;63:1–9. PMID:27938993
4646. van der Laan TP, Plaat BE, van der Laan BF, et al. Clinical recommendations on the treatment of neuroendocrine carcinoma of the larynx: a meta-analysis of 436 reported cases. Head Neck. 2015 May;37(5):707–15. PMID:24596175
4647. van der Laan TP, van der Laan BF, Plaat BE, et al. Neuroendocrine carcinoma of the larynx - an extraordinary malignancy with high recurrence rates and long survival: our experience in 11 patients. Clin Otolaryngol. 2012 Feb;37(1):63–6. PMID:22433139
4648. van der Tuin K, Tops CMJ, Adank MA, et al. CDC73-related disorders: clinical manifestations and case detection in primary hyperparathyroidism. J Clin Endocrinol Metab. 2017 Dec 1;102(12):4534–40. PMID:29040582
4649. van Eeden S, de Leng WW, Offerhaus GJ, et al. Ductuloinsular tumors of the pancreas: endocrine tumors with entrapped nonneoplastic ductules. Am J Surg Pathol. 2004 Jun;28(6):813–20. PMID:15166675
4650. van Heerden JA, Hay ID, Goellner JR, et al. Follicular thyroid carcinoma with capsular invasion alone: a nonthreatening malignancy. Surgery. 1992 Dec;112(6):1130–6. PMID:1455315
4651. van Hoeven KH, Hudock JA, Woodruff JM, et al. Small cell neuroendocrine carcinoma of the endometrium. Int J Gynecol Pathol. 1995 Jan;14(1):21–9. PMID:7883422
4652. van Houdt WJ, Westerveld CM, Vrijenhoek JE, et al. Prognosis of solitary fibrous tumors: a multicenter study. Ann Surg Oncol. 2013 Dec;20(13):4090–5. PMID:24052313
4653. van Keimpema M, Grüneberg LJ, Mokry M, et al. FOXP1 directly represses transcription of proapoptotic genes and cooperates with NF-κB to promote survival of human B cells. Blood. 2014 Nov 27;124(23):3431–40. PMID:25267198
4654. van Nederveen FH, Gaal J, Favier J, et al. An immunohistochemical procedure to detect patients with paraganglioma and phaeochromocytoma with germline SDHB, SDHC, or SDHD gene mutations: a retrospective and prospective analysis. Lancet Oncol. 2009 Aug;10(8):764–71. PMID:19576851
4655. van Nederveen FH, Korpershoek E, Lenders JW, et al. Somatic SDHB mutation in an extraadrenal pheochromocytoma. N Engl J Med. 2007 Jul 19;357(3):306–8. PMID:17634472
4656. van Slooten H, Schaberg A, Smeenk D, et al. Morphologic characteristics of benign and malignant adrenocortical tumors. Cancer. 1985 Feb 15;55(4):766–73. PMID:3967172
4657. van Treijen MJC, van Beek DJ, van Leeuwaarde RS, et al. Diagnosing nonfunctional pancreatic NETs in MEN1: the evidence base. J Endocr Soc. 2018 Jul 31;2(9):1067–88. PMID:30202829
4658. van Trotsenburg P, Stoupa A, Léger J, et al. Congenital hypothyroidism: a 2020-2021 consensus guidelines update-an ENDO-European reference network initiative endorsed by the European Society for Pediatric Endocrinology and the European Society for Endocrinology. Thyroid. 2021 Mar;31(3):387–419. PMID:33272083
4659. Vance ML. Nonfunctioning pituitary adenoma. Curr Ther Endocrinol Metab. 1997;6:33–5. PMID:9174695
4660. VandenBussche CJ, Allison DB, Graham MK, et al. Alternative lengthening of telomeres and ATRX/DAXX loss can be reliably detected in FNAs of pancreatic neuroendocrine tumors. Cancer Cytopathol. 2017 Jul;125(7):544–51. PMID:28371511
4661. Vanderveen KA, Thompson SM, Callstrom MR, et al. Biopsy of pheochromocytomas and paragangliomas: potential for disaster. Surgery. 2009 Dec;146(6):1158–66. PMID:19958944
4662. Van Leeuwen BJ, Bavitz MM, Boyle S. Primary extragonadal yolk sac tumor originating from adrenal gland. Can J Urol. 2019 Dec;26(6):10064–6. PMID:31860425
4663. van Nederveen FH, de Krijger RR. Precursor lesions of the adrenal gland. Pathobiology. 2007;74(5):285–90. PMID:17890895
4664. Vannucci L, Marini F, Giusti F, et al. MEN1 in children and adolescents: data from patients of a regional referral center for hereditary endocrine tumors. Endocrine. 2018 Feb;59(2):438–48. PMID:28530019
4665. Vanoli A, La Rosa S, Klersy C, et al. Four neuroendocrine tumor types and neuroendocrine carcinoma of the duodenum: analysis of 203 cases. Neuroendocrinology. 2017;104(2):112–25. PMID:26910321
4666. Vanoli A, La Rosa S, Miceli E, et al. Prognostic evaluations tailored to specific gastric neuroendocrine neoplasms: analysis of 200 cases with extended follow-up. Neuroendocrinology. 2018;107(2):114–26. PMID:29895024
4667. van Treijen MJC, de Vries LH, Hertog D, et al. Multiple endocrine neoplasia type 2. In: Feingold KR, Anawalt B, Blackman MR, et al., editors. Endotext. South Dartmouth (MA): MDText.com, Inc.; 2000 [updated 2022 Jan 2]. PMID:29465928
4668. Vanzati A, Mercalli F, Rosai J. The "sprinkling" sign in the follicular variant of papillary thyroid carcinoma: a clue to the recognition of this entity. Arch Pathol Lab Med. 2013 Dec;137(12):1707–9. PMID:24283853
4669. Variakojis D, Getz ML, Paloyan E, et al. Papillary clear cell carcinoma of the thyroid gland. Hum Pathol. 1975 May;6(3):384–90. PMID:1132876
4670. Varlamov EV, Wood MD, Netto JP, et al. Cystic appearance on magnetic resonance imaging in bihormonal growth hormone and prolactin tumors in acromegaly. Pituitary. 2020 Dec;23(6):672–80. PMID:32870441
4671. Varoquaux A, Kebebew E, Sebag F, et al. Endocrine tumors associated with the vagus nerve. Endocr Relat Cancer. 2016 Sep;23(9):R371–9. PMID:27406876
4672. Vasei M, Kumar PV, Malekhoseini SA, et al. Papillary Hürthle cell carcinoma (Warthin-like tumor) of the thyroid. Report of a case with fine needle aspiration findings. Acta Cytol. 1998 Nov-Dec;42(6):1437–40. PMID:9850656
4673. Vasen HF, Möslein G, Alonso A, et al. Guidelines for the clinical management of familial adenomatous polyposis (FAP). Gut. 2008 May;57(5):704–13. PMID:18194984
4674. Vasiloff J, Chideckel EW, Boyd CB, et al. Testosterone-secreting adrenal adenoma containing crystalloids characteristic of Leydig cells. Am J Med. 1985 Dec;79(6):772–6. PMID:3000178
4675. Vasko V, Ferrand M, Di Cristofaro J, et al. Specific pattern of RAS oncogene mutations in follicular thyroid tumors. J Clin Endocrinol Metab. 2003 Jun;88(6):2745–52. PMID:12788883
4676. Vázquez Ramírez F, Otal Salaverri C, Argueta Manzano O, et al. Fine needle aspiration cytology of high grade mucoepidermoid carcinoma of the thyroid. A case report. Acta Cytol. 2000 Mar-Apr;44(2):259–64. PMID:10740618
4677. Vázquez-Benítez G, Pérez-Campos A, Masgrau NA, et al. Unexpected tumor: primary asymptomatic schwannoma in thyroid gland. Endocr Pathol. 2016 Mar;27(1):46–9. PMID:26615394
4678. Veiga LH, Neta G, Aschebrook-Kilfoy B, et al. Thyroid cancer incidence patterns in Sao Paulo, Brazil, and the U.S. SEER program, 1997-2008. Thyroid. 2013 Jun;23(6):748–57. PMID:23410185
4679. Veits L, Mechtersheimer G, Steger C, et al. Chromosomal imbalances in carcinoma showing thymus-like elements (CASTLE). Virchows Arch. 2011 Aug;459(2):221–6. PMID:21735166
4680. Veits L, Schupfner R, Hufnagel P, et al. KRAS, EGFR, PDGFR-α, KIT and COX-2 status in carcinoma showing thymus-like elements (CASTLE). Diagn Pathol. 2014 Jun 16;9:116. PMID:24934485
4681. Vengrove MA, Schimmel M, Atkinson BF, et al. Invasive cervical thymoma masquerading as a solitary thyroid nodule. Report of a case studied by fine needle aspiration. Acta Cytol. 1991 Jul-Aug;35(4):431–3. PMID:1927177
4682. Venkatesh S, Ordonez NG, Ajani J, et al. Islet cell carcinoma of the pancreas. A study of 98 patients. Cancer. 1990 Jan 15;65(2):354–7. PMID:2153046
4683. Ventura M, Melo M, Carrilho F. Outcome and long-term follow-up of adrenal lesions in multiple endocrine neoplasia type 1. Arch Endocrinol Metab. 2019 Sep 2;63(5):516–23. PMID:31482957
4684. Veras E, Deavers MT, Silva EG, et al. Ovarian nonsmall cell neuroendocrine carcinoma: a clinicopathologic and immunohistochemical study of 11 cases. Am J Surg Pathol. 2007 May;31(5):774–82. PMID:17460463
4685. Verdonk C, Guerin C, Lufkin E, et al. Activation of virilizing adrenal rest tissues by excessive ACTH production. An unusual presentation of Nelson's syndrome. Am J Med. 1982 Sep;73(3):455–9. PMID:7124773
4686. Verga U, Fugazzola L, Cambiaghi S, et al. Frequent association between MEN 2A and cutaneous lichen amyloidosis. Clin Endocrinol (Oxf). 2003 Aug;59(2):156–61. PMID:12864791
4687. Vergès B, Boureille F, Goudet P, et al. Pituitary disease in MEN type 1 (MEN1): data from the France-Belgium MEN1 multicenter study. J Clin Endocrinol Metab. 2002 Feb;87(2):457–65. PMID:11836268
4688. Vergez S, Rouquette I, Ancey M, et al. Langerhans cell histiocytosis of the thyroid is a rare entity, but an association with a papillary thyroid carcinoma is often described. Endocr Pathol. 2010 Dec;21(4):274–6. PMID:20848238
4689. Vergilio J, Baloch ZW, LiVolsi VA. Spindle cell metaplasia of the thyroid arising in association with papillary carcinoma and follicular adenoma. Am J Clin Pathol. 2002 Feb;117(2):199–204. PMID:11863215
4690. Verloes A, Stevenaert A, Teh BT, et al. Familial acromegaly: case report and review of the literature. Pituitary. 1999 May;1(3-4):273–7. PMID:11081208
4691. Verma A, Kane S, Vinarkar S, et al. Small cell medullary thyroid carcinoma: a diagnostic dilemma. Indian J Pathol Microbiol. 2017 Oct-Dec;60(4):562–4. PMID:29323074
4692. Vermi W, Lonardi S, Bosisio D, et al. Identification of CXCL13 as a new marker for follicular dendritic cell sarcoma. J Pathol. 2008 Nov;216(3):356–64. PMID:18792075
4693. Verset L, Arvanitakis M, Loi P, et al. TTF-1 positive small cell cancers: Don't think they're always primary pulmonary! World J Gastrointest Oncol. 2011 Oct 15;3(10):144–7. PMID:22046491
4694. Vetrivel S, Zhang R, Engel M, et al. Circulating microRNA expression in Cushing's syndrome. Front Endocrinol (Lausanne). 2021 Feb 22;12:620012. PMID:33692756
4695. Vezzosi D, Tenenbaum F, Cazabat L, et al. Hormonal, radiological, NP-59 scintigraphy, and pathological correlations in patients with Cushing's syndrome due to primary pigmented nodular adrenocortical disease (PPNAD). J Clin Endocrinol Metab. 2015 Nov;100(11):4332–8. PMID:26390100
4696. Viaene AN, Lee EB, Nasrallah MP. Intraoperative cytology of pituicytomas. Diagn Cytopathol. 2020 Apr;48(4):342–9. PMID:31883319
4697. Viaene AN, Lee EB, Rosenbaum JN, et al. Histologic, immunohistochemical, and molecular features of pituicytomas and atypical pituicytomas. Acta Neuropathol Commun. 2019 May 2;7(1):69. PMID:31046843
4698. Vickery AL Jr. The diagnosis of malignancy in dyshormonogenetic goitre. Clin Endocrinol Metab. 1981 Jul;10(2):317–35. PMID:7285382
4699. Vickery AL Jr. Thyroid papillary carcinoma. Pathological and philosophical controversies. Am J Surg Pathol. 1983 Dec;7(8):797–807. PMID:6660352
4700. Vickery AL Jr, Carcangiu ML, Johannessen JV, et al. Papillary carcinoma. Semin Diagn Pathol. 1985 May;2(2):90–100. PMID:3843693
4701. Vidal S, Kovacs K, Horvath E, et al. Microvessel density in pituitary adenomas and carcinomas. Virchows Arch. 2001 Jun;438(6):595–602. PMID:11469692
4702. Vidal S, Kovacs K, Horvath E, et al. Topoisomerase IIalpha expression in pituitary adenomas and carcinomas: relationship to tumor behavior. Mod Pathol. 2002 Nov;15(11):1205–12. PMID:12429800
4703. Vigovich FA, Hurt MA, Santa Cruz DJ. Sclerotic glomus tumor. Am J Dermatopathol. 2010 Feb;32(1):76–8. PMID:19940754
4704. Vijayvergia N, Boland PM, Handorf E, et al. Molecular profiling of neuroendocrine malignancies to identify prognostic and therapeutic markers: a Fox Chase Cancer Center pilot study. Br J Cancer. 2016 Aug 23;115(5):564–70. PMID:27482646
4705. Vilallonga R, Zafon C, Ruiz-Marcellan C, et al. Malignant thyroid teratoma: report of an aggressive tumor in a 64-year-old man. Endocr Pathol. 2013 Sep;24(3):132–5.

PMID:23702575
4706. Villa C, Lagonigro MS, Magri F, et al. Hyperplasia-adenoma sequence in pituitary tumorigenesis related to aryl hydrocarbon receptor interacting protein gene mutation. Endocr Relat Cancer. 2011 Jun 8;18(3):347–56. PMID:21450940
4707. Villa C, Vasiljevic A, Jaffrain-Rea ML, et al. A standardised diagnostic approach to pituitary neuroendocrine tumours (PitNETs): a European Pituitary Pathology Group (EPPG) proposal. Virchows Arch. 2019 Dec;475(6):687–92. PMID:31578606
4708. Villagelin DG, Santos RB, Romaldini JH. Is diffuse and peritumoral lymphocyte infiltration in papillary thyroid cancer a marker of good prognosis? J Endocrinol Invest. 2011 Dec;34(11):e403–8. PMID:21765238
4709. Villar-del-Moral J, Jiménez-García A, Salvador-Egea P, et al. Prognostic factors and staging systems in parathyroid cancer: a multicenter cohort study. Surgery. 2014 Nov;156(5):1132–44. PMID:25444314
4710. Villares Fragoso MC, Wanichi IQ, Cavalcante IP, et al. The role of gsp mutations on the development of adrenocortical tumors and adrenal hyperplasia. Front Endocrinol (Lausanne). 2016 Jul 27;7:104. PMID:27512387
4711. Villar-Taibo R, Peteiro-González D, Cabezas-Agrícola JM, et al. Aggressiveness of the tall cell variant of papillary thyroid carcinoma is independent of the tumor size and patient age. Oncol Lett. 2017 May;13(5):3501–7. PMID:28529577
4712. Vinayek R, Capurso G, Larghi A. Grading of EUS-FNA cytologic specimens from patients with pancreatic neuroendocrine neoplasms: it is time move to tissue core biopsy? Gland Surg. 2014 Nov;3(4):222–5. PMID:25493252
4713. Vinik A. Neurotensinomas. In: Feingold KR, Anawalt B, Blackman MR, et al., editors. Endotext. South Dartmouth (MA): MDText.com, Inc.; 2000 [updated 2017 Jun 5]. PMID:25905306
4714. Vinik AI, Strodel WE, Eckhauser FE, et al. Somatostatinomas, PPomas, neurotensinomas. Semin Oncol. 1987 Sep;14(3):263–81. PMID:2820062
4715. Virgone C, Andreetta M, Avanzini S, et al. Pheochromocytomas and paragangliomas in children: data from the Italian Cooperative Study (TREP). Pediatr Blood Cancer. 2020 Aug;67(8):e28332. PMID:32491270
4716. Visser J, Hukin J, Sargent M, et al. Late mortality in pediatric patients with craniopharyngioma. J Neurooncol. 2010 Oct;100(1):105–11. PMID:20204458
4717. Vivero M, Kraft S, Barletta JA. Risk stratification of follicular variant of papillary thyroid carcinoma. Thyroid. 2013 Mar;23(3):273–9. PMID:23025507
4718. Vlaemynck K, De Man M, De Man K, et al. Neuroendocrine tumor with diarrhea: not always the usual suspects - a case report of metastatic calcitoninoma with literature review. Acta Clin Belg. 2021 Jun;76(3):239–43. PMID:31900071
4719. Vo KT, Matthay KK, Neuhaus J, et al. Clinical, biologic, and prognostic differences on the basis of primary tumor site in neuroblastoma: a report from the international neuroblastoma risk group project. J Clin Oncol. 2014 Oct 1;32(28):3169–76. PMID:25154816
4720. Vocke CD, Ricketts CJ, Ball MW, et al. CDC73 germline mutation in a family with mixed epithelial and stromal tumors. Urology. 2019 Feb;124:91–7. PMID:30452964
4721. Vogelstein B, Kinzler KW. The path to cancer –three strikes and you're out. N Engl J Med. 2015 Nov 12;373(20):1895–8. PMID:26559569
4722. Voit D, Saeger W, Lüdecke DK. Pituitary adenomas in acromegaly: comparison of different adenoma types with clinical data. Endocr Pathol. 1999 Jun;10(2):123–35. PMID:27519216
4723. Volante M, Birocco N, Gatti G, et al. Extrapulmonary neuroendocrine small and large cell carcinomas: a review of controversial diagnostic and therapeutic issues. Hum Pathol. 2014 Apr;45(4):665–73. PMID:23806528
4724. Volante M, Bollito E, Sperone P, et al. Clinicopathological study of a series of 92 adrenocortical carcinomas: from a proposal of simplified diagnostic algorithm to prognostic stratification. Histopathology. 2009 Nov;55(5):535–43. PMID:19912359
4725. Volante M, Brizzi MP, Faggiano A, et al. Somatostatin receptor type 2A immunohistochemistry in neuroendocrine tumors: a proposal of scoring system correlated with somatostatin receptor scintigraphy. Mod Pathol. 2007 Nov;20(11):1172–82. PMID:17873898
4726. Volante M, Collini P, Nikiforov YE, et al. Poorly differentiated thyroid carcinoma: the Turin proposal for the use of uniform diagnostic criteria and an algorithmic diagnostic approach. Am J Surg Pathol. 2007 Aug;31(8):1256–64. PMID:17667551
4727. Volante M, Grillo F, Massa F, et al. Neuroendocrine neoplasms of the appendix, colon and rectum. Pathologica. 2021 Feb;113(1):19–27. PMID:33686307
4728. Volante M, La Rosa S, Castellano I, et al. Clinico-pathological features of a series of 11 oncocytic endocrine tumours of the pancreas. Virchows Arch. 2006 May;448(5):545–51. PMID:16491376
4729. Volante M, Lam AK, Papotti M, et al. Molecular pathology of poorly differentiated and anaplastic thyroid cancer: What do pathologists need to know? Endocr Pathol. 2021 Mar;32(1):63–76. PMID:33543394
4730. Volante M, Landolfi S, Chiusa L, et al. Poorly differentiated carcinomas of the thyroid with trabecular, insular, and solid patterns: a clinicopathologic study of 183 patients. Cancer. 2004 Mar 1;100(5):950–7. PMID:14983490
4731. Volante M, Mete O, Pelosi G, et al. Molecular pathology of well-differentiated pulmonary and thymic neuroendocrine tumors: What do pathologists need to know? Endocr Pathol. 2021 Mar;32(1):154–68. PMID:33641055
4732. Volante M, Monica V, Birocco N, et al. Expression analysis of genes involved in DNA repair or synthesis in mixed neuroendocrine/nonneuroendocrine carcinomas. Neuroendocrinology. 2015;101(2):151–60. PMID:25633872
4733. Volante M, Papotti M. A practical diagnostic approach to solid/trabecular nodules in the thyroid. Endocr Pathol. 2008 Summer;19(2):75–81. PMID:18409025
4734. Volante M, Papotti M, Roth J, et al. Mixed medullary-follicular thyroid carcinoma. Molecular evidence for a dual origin of tumor components. Am J Pathol. 1999 Nov;155(5):1499–509. PMID:10550306
4735. Volante M, Terzolo M, Fassnacht M, et al. Ribonucleotide reductase large subunit (RRM1) gene expression may predict efficacy of adjuvant mitotane in adrenocortical cancer. Clin Cancer Res. 2012 Jun 15;18(12):3452–61. PMID:22547773
4736. Volpe C, Hamberger B, Zedenius J, et al. Impact of immunohistochemistry on the diagnosis and management of primary aldosteronism: an important tool for improved patient follow-up. Scand J Surg. 2020 Jun;109(2):133–42. PMID:30654730
4737. Volpe C, Höög A, Ogishima T, et al. Immunohistochemistry improves histopathologic diagnosis in primary aldosteronism. J Clin Pathol. 2013 Apr;66(4):351–4. PMID:23436930
4738. Volta AD, Cosentini D, Antonelli A, et al. Transformation of prostate adenocarcinoma into small-cell neuroendocrine cancer under androgen deprivation therapy: much is achieved but more information is needed. J Clin Oncol. 2019 Feb 1;37(4):350–1. PMID:30557524
4739. Vortmeyer AO, Falke EA, Gläsker S, et al. Nervous system involvement in von Hippel-Lindau disease: pathology and mechanisms. Acta Neuropathol. 2013 Mar;125(3):333–50. PMID:23400300
4740. Vortmeyer AO, Gläsker S, Mehta GU, et al. Somatic GNAS mutation causes widespread and diffuse pituitary disease in acromegalic patients with McCune-Albright syndrome. J Clin Endocrinol Metab. 2012 Jul;97(7):2404–13. PMID:22564667
4741. Vortmeyer AO, Gnarra JR, Emmert-Buck MR, et al. Von Hippel-Lindau gene deletion detected in the stromal cell component of a cerebellar hemangioblastoma associated with von Hippel-Lindau disease. Hum Pathol. 1997 May;28(5):540–3. PMID:9158701
4742. Vos EL, Grewal RK, Russo AE, et al. Predicting malignancy in patients with adrenal tumors using 18 F-FDG-PET/CT SUVmax. J Surg Oncol. 2020 Dec;122(8):1821–6. PMID:32914407
4743. Voss RK, Feng L, Lee JE, et al. Medullary thyroid carcinoma in MEN2A: ATA moderate- or high-risk RET mutations do not predict disease aggressiveness. J Clin Endocrinol Metab. 2017 Aug 1;102(8):2807–13. PMID:28609830
4744. Vujanić GM, Harach HR, Minić P, et al. Thyroid/cervical teratomas in children: immunohistochemical studies for specific thyroid epithelial cell markers. Pediatr Pathol. 1994 Mar-Apr;14(2):369–75. PMID:8008695
4745. Vujanić GM, Kelsey A, Perlman EJ, et al. Anaplastic sarcoma of the kidney: a clinicopathologic study of 20 cases of a new entity with polyphenotypic features. Am J Surg Pathol. 2007 Oct;31(10):1459–68. PMID:17895746
4746. Vujhini SK, Kolte SS, Satarkar RN, et al. Fine needle aspiration diagnosis of Rosai-Dorfman disease involving thyroid. J Cytol. 2012 Jan;29(1):83–5. PMID:22438629
4747. Vujovic S, Henderson S, Presneau N, et al. Brachyury, a crucial regulator of notochordal development, is a novel biomarker for chordomas. J Pathol. 2006 Jun;209(2):157–65. PMID:16538613
4748. Vuong HG, Kondo T, Pham TQ, et al. Prognostic significance of diffuse sclerosing variant papillary thyroid carcinoma: a systematic review and meta-analysis. Eur J Endocrinol. 2017 Apr;176(4):433–41. PMID:28183787
4749. Vuong HG, Long NP, Anh NH, et al. Papillary thyroid carcinoma with tall cell features is as aggressive as tall cell variant: a meta-analysis. Endocr Connect. 2018 Dec 1;7(12):R286–93. PMID:30352403
4750. Vuong HG, Ngo TNM, Dunn IF. Consolidating the Hyams grading system in esthesioneuroblastoma - an individual participant data meta-analysis. J Neurooncol. 2021 May;153(1):15–22. PMID:33770323
4751. Vuong HG, Odate T, Duong UNP, et al. Prognostic importance of solid variant papillary thyroid carcinoma: a systematic review and meta-analysis. Head Neck. 2018 Jul;40(7):1588–97. PMID:29509280
4752. Vuong HG, Odate T, Ngo HTT, et al. Clinical significance of RET and RAS mutations in sporadic medullary thyroid carcinoma: a meta-analysis. Endocr Relat Cancer. 2018 Jun;25(6):633–41. PMID:29615431
4753. Vural Ç, Kiraz U, Turan G, et al. Solid variant of papillary thyroid carcinoma: an analysis of 28 cases with current literature. Ann Diagn Pathol. 2021 Jun;52:151737. PMID:33838489
4754. Vyas M, Tang LH, Rekhtman N, et al. Alterations in Ki67 labeling following treatment of poorly differentiated neuroendocrine carcinomas: a potential diagnostic pitfall. Am J Surg Pathol. 2021 Jan;45(1):25–34. PMID:33177340
4755. Wachenfeld C, Beuschlein F, Zwermann O, et al. Discerning malignancy in adrenocortical tumors: Are molecular markers useful? Eur J Endocrinol. 2001 Sep;145(3):335–41. PMID:11517015
4756. Wachtel H, Hutchens T, Baraban E, et al. Predicting metastatic potential in pheochromocytoma and paraganglioma: a comparison of PASS and GAPP scoring systems. J Clin Endocrinol Metab. 2020 Dec 1;105(12):e4661–70. PMID:32877928
4757. Wagner AS, Fleitz JM, Kleinschmidt-Demasters BK. Pediatric adrenal cortical carcinoma: brain metastases and relationship to NF-1, case reports and review of the literature. J Neurooncol. 2005 Nov;75(2):127–33. PMID:16132517
4758. Wagner J, Portwine C, Rabin K, et al. High frequency of germline p53 mutations in childhood adrenocortical cancer. J Natl Cancer Inst. 1994 Nov 16;86(22):1707–10. PMID:7966399
4759. Wakasaki T, Yasumatsu R, Masuda M, et al. Small cell carcinoma in the head and neck. Ann Otol Rhinol Laryngol. 2019 Nov;128(11):1006–12. PMID:31161776
4760. Waldmann J, Bartsch DK, Kann PH, et al. Adrenal involvement in multiple endocrine neoplasia type 1: results of 7 years prospective screening. Langenbecks Arch Surg. 2007 Jul;392(4):437–43. PMID:17235589
4761. Walia R, Gupta R, Bhansali A, et al. Molecular imaging targeting corticotropin-releasing hormone receptor for corticotropinoma: a changing paradigm. J Clin Endocrinol Metab. 2021 Mar 25;106(4):e1816–26. PMID:33079979
4762. Waligórska-Stachura J, Gut P, Sawicka-Gutaj N, et al. Growth hormone-secreting macroadenoma of the pituitary gland successfully treated with the radiolabeled somatostatin analog (90)Y-DOTATATE: case report. J Neurosurg. 2016 Aug;125(2):346–9. PMID:26636388
4763. Walker CJ, Rush CM, Dama P, et al. MAX mutations in endometrial cancer: clinicopathologic associations and recurrent MAX p.His28Arg functional characterization. J Natl Cancer Inst. 2018 May 1;110(5):517–26. PMID:29155953
4764. Walker JD, Grossman A, Anderson JV, et al. Malignant prolactinoma with extracranial metastases: a report of three cases. Clin Endocrinol (Oxf). 1993 Apr;38(4):411–9. PMID:8319373
4765. Wallace ZS, Deshpande V, Mattoo H, et al. IgG4-related disease: clinical and laboratory features in one hundred twenty-five patients. Arthritis Rheumatol. 2015 Sep;67(9):2466–75. PMID:25988916
4766. Walls GV, Stevenson M, Lines KE, et al. Mice deleted for cell division cycle 73 gene develop parathyroid and uterine tumours: model for the hyperparathyroidism-jaw tumour syndrome. Oncogene. 2017 Jul 13;36(28):4025–36. PMID:28288139
4767. Walsh NM. Primary neuroendocrine (Merkel cell) carcinoma of the skin: morphologic diversity and implications thereof. Hum Pathol. 2001 Jul;32(7):680–9. PMID:11486166
4768. Walter T, Hervieu V, Adham M, et al. Primary neuroendocrine tumors of the main pancreatic duct: a rare entity. Virchows Arch. 2011 May;458(5):537–46. PMID:21431402
4769. Walther MM, Herring J, Enquist E, et al. Von Recklinghausen's disease and pheochromocytomas. J Urol. 1999 Nov;162(5):1582–6. PMID:10524872
4770. Walther MM, Reiter R, Keiser HR, et al. Clinical and genetic characterization of

pheochromocytoma in von Hippel-Lindau families: comparison with sporadic pheochromocytoma gives insight into natural history of pheochromocytoma. J Urol. 1999 Sep;162(3 Pt 1):659–64. PMID:10458336
4771. Walts AE, Mirocha JM, Marchevsky AM. Challenges in Ki-67 assessments in pulmonary large-cell neuroendocrine carcinomas. Histopathology. 2021 Apr;78(5):699–709. PMID:33025627
4772. Wan SK, Chan JK, Tang SK. Paucicellular variant of anaplastic thyroid carcinoma. A mimic of Reidel's thyroiditis. Am J Clin Pathol. 1996 Apr;105(4):388–93. PMID:8604680
4773. Wanebo JE, Lonser RR, Glenn GM, et al. The natural history of hemangioblastomas of the central nervous system in patients with von Hippel-Lindau disease. J Neurosurg. 2003 Jan;98(1):82–94. PMID:12546356
4774. Wang C, Yun T, Wang Z, et al. Pathological characteristics and genetic features of melanin-producing medullary thyroid carcinoma. Diagn Pathol. 2018 Nov 13;13(1):86. PMID:30424779
4775. Wang CJ, Li J, Qin J. Primary pleomorphic rhabdomyosarcoma of the adrenal gland in an adult: a case report. Oncol Lett. 2014 Jan;7(1):137–9. PMID:24348835
4776. Wang CY, Chang TC. Preoperative thyroid ultrasonography and fine-needle aspiration cytology in ectopic thyroid. Am Surg. 1995 Dec;61(12):1029–31. PMID:7486437
4777. Wang DZ, Liu P, Yao L, et al. Aberrant expression of thyroid transcription factor-1 in schwannomas. Hum Pathol. 2018 Jan;71:84–90. PMID:29104109
4778. Wang F, He Y, Li C, et al. Malignant craniopharyngioma: a report of seven cases and review of the literature. World Neurosurg. 2020 Mar;135:e194–201. PMID:31785438
4779. Wang G, Xiao L, Zhang M, et al. Small cell carcinoma of the urinary bladder: a clinicopathological and immunohistochemical analysis of 81 cases. Hum Pathol. 2018 Sep;79:57–65. PMID:29763719
4780. Wang H, Correa H, Sanders M, et al. Noninvasive follicular thyroid neoplasm with papillary-like nuclear features in children: an institutional experience and literature review. Pediatr Dev Pathol. 2020 Mar-Apr;23(2):121–6. PMID:31483741
4781. Wang H, Mehrad M, Ely KA, et al. Incidence and malignancy rates of indeterminate pediatric thyroid nodules. Cancer Cytopathol. 2019 Apr;127(4):231–9. PMID:30768868
4782. Wang H, Wang R, Hu T, et al. Nonfunctioning pituitary adenomas in pediatric and adolescent patients: a clinical analysis of a series of 14 patients. J Neurooncol. 2020 May;148(1):179–86. PMID:32333187
4783. Wang HH, Chen YL, Kao HL, et al. Extra-adrenal paraganglioma of the prostate. Can Urol Assoc J. 2013 May-Jun;7(5-6):E370–2. PMID:23766843
4784. Wang HY, Zou J, Zhou GY, et al. Primary small cell neuroendocrine carcinoma of the tonsil: a case report and review of the literature. Int J Clin Exp Pathol. 2014 Apr 15;7(5):2678–82. PMID:24966986
4785. Wang J, Liu D, Meng Y, et al. Extrapulmonary small cell carcinoma of the external auditory canal: a case report and review of the literature. J Int Med Res. 2020 Aug;48(8):300060520946517. PMID:32851892
4786. Wang J, Song DL, Deng L, et al. Extraventricular neurocytoma of the sellar region: case report and literature review. Springerplus. 2016 Jul 7;5(1):987. PMID:27398267
4787. Wang J, Ye L, Cai H, et al. Comparative study of large cell neuroendocrine carcinoma and small cell lung carcinoma in high-grade neuroendocrine tumors of the lung: a large population-based study. J Cancer. 2019 Jul 10;10(18):4226–36. PMID:31413741
4788. Wang J, Zhu XZ, Zhang RY. [Malignant granular cell tumor: a clinicopathologic analysis of 10 cases with review of literature]. Zhonghua Bing Li Xue Za Zhi. 2004 Dec;33(6):497–502. Chinese. PMID:15634442
4789. Wang JY, Peng SH, Li T, et al. Risk factors for survival in patients with von Hippel-Lindau disease. J Med Genet. 2018 May;55(5):322–8. PMID:29330336
4790. Wang KR, Jia YJ, Zhou SH, et al. Cutaneous and subcutaneous metastases from atypical laryngeal carcinoids: case report and review of the literature. Medicine (Baltimore). 2016 Feb;95(7):e2796. PMID:26886629
4791. Wang L, Ouyang N, Guo HX, et al. Middle ear adenoma with uncommon presentation and literature review. BMJ Case Rep. 2017 Jun 13;2017:bcr2016216694. PMID:28611057
4792. Wang L, Yang M, Zhang Y, et al. Prognostic validation of the WHO 2010 grading system in pancreatic insulinoma patients. Neoplasma. 2015;62(3):484–90. PMID:25866230
4793. Wang LE, Zhang DX, Li YJ, et al. Neuroendocrine carcinoma in the auditory canal and middle ear. Chin Med J (Engl). 2012 Sep;125(18):3357–8. PMID:22964339
4794. Wang LL, Suganuma R, Ikegaki N, et al. Neuroblastoma of undifferentiated subtype, prognostic significance of prominent nucleolar formation, and MYC/MYCN protein expression: a report from the Children's Oncology Group. Cancer. 2013 Oct 15;119(20):3718–26. PMID:23901000
4795. Wang LL, Teshiba R, Ikegaki N, et al. Augmented expression of MYC and/or MYCN protein defines highly aggressive MYC-driven neuroblastoma: a Children's Oncology Group study. Br J Cancer. 2015 Jun 30;113(1):57–63. PMID:26035700
4796. Wang LY, Ganly I. Post-treatment surveillance of thyroid cancer. Eur J Surg Oncol. 2018 Mar;44(3):357–66. PMID:28754228
4797. Wang N, Kjellin H, Sofiadis A, et al. Genetic and epigenetic background and protein expression profiles in relation to telomerase activation in medullary thyroid carcinoma. Oncotarget. 2016 Apr 19;7(16):21332–46. PMID:26870890
4798. Wang O, Wang C, Nie M, et al. Novel HRPT2/CDC73 gene mutations and loss of expression of parafibromin in Chinese patients with clinically sporadic parathyroid carcinomas. PLoS One. 2012;7(9):e45567. PMID:23029104
4799. Wang P, Xue S, Wang S, et al. Clinical characteristics and treatment outcomes of parathyroid carcinoma: a retrospective review of 234 cases. Oncol Lett. 2017 Dec;14(6):7276–82. PMID:29344163
4800. Wang S, Li MY, Liu Y, et al. The role of microRNA in cisplatin resistance or sensitivity. Expert Opin Ther Targets. 2020 Sep;24(9):885–97. PMID:32559147
4801. Wang S, Zong W, Li Y, et al. Pituitary ependymoma: a case report and review of the literature. World Neurosurg. 2018 Feb;110:43–54. PMID:29102750
4802. Wang TS, Ocal IT, Salem RR, et al. Leiomyosarcoma of the adrenal vein: a novel approach to surgical resection. World J Surg Oncol. 2007 Oct 3;5:109. PMID:17910774
4803. Wang TT, Zhang R, Wang L, et al. Two cases of multiple ossifying fibromas in the jaws. Diagn Pathol. 2014 Mar 28;9:75. PMID:24678936
4804. Wang TY, Lee CH, Yang AH, et al. Metastatic leiomyosarcoma of the thyroid: a case report. Zhonghua Yi Xue Za Zhi (Taipei). 1998 Jun;61(6):353–7. PMID:9684512
4805. Wang VE, Urisman A, Albacker L, et al. Checkpoint inhibitor is active against large cell neuroendocrine carcinoma with high tumor mutation burden. J Immunother Cancer. 2017 Sep 19;5(1):75. PMID:28923100
4806. Wang W, Epstein JI. Small cell carcinoma of the prostate. A morphologic and immunohistochemical study of 95 cases. Am J Surg Pathol. 2008 Jan;32(1):65–71. PMID:18162772
4807. Wang W, Xu C, Chen H, et al. Genomic alterations and clinical outcomes in patients with lung adenocarcinoma with transformation to small cell lung cancer after treatment with EGFR tyrosine kinase inhibitors: a multicenter retrospective study. Lung Cancer. 2021 May;155:20–7. PMID:33714778
4808. Wang X, Cheng W, Li J, et al. Endocrine tumours: familial nonmedullary thyroid carcinoma is a more aggressive disease: a systematic review and meta-analysis. Eur J Endocrinol. 2015 Jun;172(6):R253–62. PMID:25637073
4809. Wang X, Cheng W, Liu C, et al. Tall cell variant of papillary thyroid carcinoma: current evidence on clinicopathologic features and molecular biology. Oncotarget. 2016 Jun 28;7(26):40792–9. PMID:27008708
4810. Wang Y, Hou P, Yu H, et al. High prevalence and mutual exclusivity of genetic alterations in the phosphatidylinositol-3-kinase/AKT pathway in thyroid tumors. J Clin Endocrinol Metab. 2007 Jun;92(6):2387–90. PMID:17426084
4811. Wang Y, Karnezis AN, Magrill J, et al. DICER1 hot-spot mutations in ovarian gynandroblastoma. Histopathology. 2018 Aug;73(2):306–13. PMID:29660837
4812. Wang Y, Li Q, Wang J, et al. Small cell carcinoma of the bladder: the characteristics of molecular alterations, treatment, and follow-up. Med Oncol. 2019 Oct 29;36(12):98. PMID:31664527
4813. Wang Y, Ren Y, Ma L, et al. Clinical features of 50 patients with primary adrenal lymphoma. Front Endocrinol (Lausanne). 2020 Sep 24;11:595. PMID:33071959
4814. Wang YY, Kearney T, du Plessis D, et al. Extraventricular neurocytoma of the sellar region. Br J Neurosurg. 2012 Jun;26(3):420–2. PMID:22122710
4815. Wang Z, Yang Z, Wang W, et al. Diagnosis of testicular adrenal rest tumors on ultrasound: a retrospective study of 15 cases report. Medicine (Baltimore). 2015 Sep;94(36):e1471. PMID:26356704
4816. Wanichi IQ, de Paula Mariani BM, Frassetto FP, et al. Cushing's disease due to somatic USP8 mutations: a systematic review and meta-analysis. Pituitary. 2019 Aug;22(4):435–42. PMID:31273566
4817. Wannachalee T, Zhao L, Nanba K, et al. Three discrete patterns of primary aldosteronism lateralization in response to cosyntropin during adrenal vein sampling. J Clin Endocrinol Metab. 2019 Dec 1;104(12):5867–76. PMID:31408156
4818. Warmuth-Metz M, Gnekow AK, Müller H, et al. Differential diagnosis of suprasellar tumors in children. Klin Padiatr. 2004 Nov-Dec;216(6):323–30. PMID:15565547
4819. Warnakulasuriya S, Markwell BD, Williams DM. Familial hyperparathyroidism associated with cementifying fibromas of the jaws in two siblings. Oral Surg Oral Med Oral Pathol. 1985 Mar;59(3):269–74. PMID:3856818
4820. Warner E, Ofo E, Connor S, et al. Mucoepidermoid carcinoma in a thyroglossal duct remnant. Int J Surg Case Rep. 2015;13:43–7. PMID:26101054
4821. Warren M, Matsuno R, Tran H, et al. Utility of Phox2b immunohistochemical stain in neural crest tumours and non-neural crest tumours in paediatric patients. Histopathology. 2018 Mar;72(4):685–96. PMID:28986989
4822. Washecka R, Dresner MI, Honda SA. Testicular tumors in Carney's complex. J Urol. 2002 Mar;167(3):1299–302. PMID:11832717
4823. Wass JA, Reddy R, Karavitaki N. The postoperative monitoring of nonfunctioning pituitary adenomas. Nat Rev Endocrinol. 2011 Apr 5;7(7):431–4. PMID:21467969
4824. Wasserman JD, Novokmet A, Eichler-Jonsson C, et al. Prevalence and functional consequence of TP53 mutations in pediatric adrenocortical carcinoma: a children's oncology group study. J Clin Oncol. 2015 Feb 20;33(6):602–9. PMID:25584008
4825. Wasserman JD, Sabbaghian N, Fahiminiya S, et al. DICER1 mutations are frequent in adolescent-onset papillary thyroid carcinoma. J Clin Endocrinol Metab. 2018 May 1;103(5):2009–15. PMID:29474644
4826. Wasserman JD, Tomlinson GE, Druker H, et al. Multiple endocrine neoplasia and hyperparathyroid-jaw tumor syndromes: clinical features, genetics, and surveillance recommendations in childhood. Clin Cancer Res. 2017 Jul 1;23(13):e123–32. PMID:28674121
4827. Watanabe N, Noh JY, Narimatsu H, et al. Clinicopathological features of 171 cases of primary thyroid lymphoma: a long-term study involving 24553 patients with Hashimoto's disease. Br J Haematol. 2011 Apr;153(2):236–43. PMID:21371004
4828. Watanabe T, Araki K, Ishii N, et al. A surgically resected pancreatic schwannoma with obstructive jaundice with special reference to differential diagnosis from other cystic lesions in the pancreas. Case Rep Gastroenterol. 2018 Feb 21;12(1):85–91. PMID:29606941
4829. Watutantrige-Fernando S, Vianello F, Barollo S, et al. The hobnail variant of papillary thyroid carcinoma: clinical/molecular characteristics of a large monocentric series and comparison with conventional histotypes. Thyroid. 2018 Jan;28(1):96–103. PMID:29179638
4830. Wcislak SM, King WS, Waller BR 3rd, et al. Multifocal pheochromocytoma-paraganglioma in a 29-year-old woman with cyanotic congenital heart disease. Surgery. 2019 Jan;165(1):228–31. PMID:30340856
4831. Weaver J, Downs-Kelly E, Goldblum JR, et al. Fluorescence in situ hybridization for MDM2 gene amplification as a diagnostic tool in lipomatous neoplasms. Mod Pathol. 2008 Aug;21(8):943–9. PMID:18500263
4832. Wei J, Song X, Liu X, et al. Glucagonoma and glucagonoma syndrome: one center's experience of six cases. J Pancreat Cancer. 2018 May 1;4(1):11–6. PMID:30631852
4833. Wei S, Baloch ZW, LiVolsi VA. Pathology of struma ovarii: a report of 96 cases. Endocr Pathol. 2015 Dec;26(4):342–8. PMID:26374222
4834. Wei S, LiVolsi VA, Baloch ZW. Pathology of thyroglossal duct: an institutional experience. Endocr Pathol. 2015 Mar;26(1):75–9. PMID:25577275
4835. Wei S, LiVolsi VA, Montone KT, et al. PTEN and TP53 mutations in oncocytic follicular carcinoma. Endocr Pathol. 2015 Dec;26(4):365–9. PMID:26530486
4836. Wei SJ, Nguyen TH, Yang IH, et al. MYC transcription activation mediated by OCT4 as a mechanism of resistance to 13-cisRA-mediated differentiation in neuroblastoma. Cell Death Dis. 2020 May 14;11(5):368. PMID:32409685
4837. Wei Z, Sun B, Wang ZP, et al. Whole-exome sequencing identifies novel recurrent somatic mutations in sporadic parathyroid adenomas. Endocrinology. 2018 Aug 1;159(8):3061–8. PMID:29982334
4838. Weinhäusel A, Behmel A, Ponder BA, et al. Long-term follow up of a "sporadic" unilateral pheochromocytoma revealing multiple endocrine neoplasia MEN2A-2 in an elderly woman. Endocr Pathol. 2003 Winter;14(4):375–82. PMID:14739494

4839. Weinstein JL, Katzenstein HM, Cohn SL. Advances in the diagnosis and treatment of neuroblastoma. Oncologist. 2003;8(3):278–92. PMID:12773750
4840. Weinstein LS, Shenker A, Gejman PV, et al. Activating mutations of the stimulatory G protein in the McCune-Albright syndrome. N Engl J Med. 1991 Dec 12;325(24):1688–95. PMID:1944469
4841. Weisbrod AB, Zhang L, Jain M, et al. Altered PTEN, ATRX, CHGA, CHGB, and TP53 expression are associated with aggressive VHL-associated pancreatic neuroendocrine tumors. Horm Cancer. 2013 Jun;4(3):165–75. PMID:23361940
4842. Weiss DE, Vogel H, Lopes MB, et al. Ectopic acromegaly due to a pancreatic neuroendocrine tumor producing growth hormone-releasing hormone. Endocr Pract. 2011 Jan-Feb;17(1):79–84. PMID:20713338
4843. Weiss LM. Comparative histologic study of 43 metastasizing and nonmetastasizing adrenocortical tumors. Am J Surg Pathol. 1984 Mar;8(3):163–9. PMID:6703192
4844. Weiss LM, Medeiros LJ, Vickery AL Jr. Pathologic features of prognostic significance in adrenocortical carcinoma. Am J Surg Pathol. 1989 Mar;13(3):202–6. PMID:2919718
4845. Weissferdt A, Moran CA. Ectopic primary intrathyroidal thymoma: a clinicopathological and immunohistochemical analysis of 3 cases. Hum Pathol. 2016 Mar;49:71–6. PMID:26826412
4846. Welander J, Söderkvist P, Gimm O. The NF1 gene: a frequent mutational target in sporadic pheochromocytomas and beyond. Endocr Relat Cancer. 2013 Jul 4;20(4):C13–7. PMID:23756430
4847. Wells SA Jr. Advances in the management of MEN2: from improved surgical and medical treatment to novel kinase inhibitors. Endocr Relat Cancer. 2018 Feb;25(2):T1–13. PMID:29142004
4848. Wells SA Jr, Asa SL, Dralle H, et al. Revised American Thyroid Association guidelines for the management of medullary thyroid carcinoma. Thyroid. 2015 Jun;25(6):567–610. PMID:25810047
4849. Wells SA Jr, Pacini F, Robinson BG, et al. Multiple endocrine neoplasia type 2 and familial medullary thyroid carcinoma: an update. J Clin Endocrinol Metab. 2013 Aug;98(8):3149–64. PMID:23744408
4850. Wendzicki JA, Moore PS, Chang Y. Large T and small T antigens of Merkel cell polyomavirus. Curr Opin Virol. 2015 Apr;11:38–43. PMID:25681708
4851. Wenig BM, Abbondanzo SL, Heffess CS. Epithelioid angiosarcoma of the adrenal glands. A clinicopathologic study of nine cases with a discussion of the implications of finding "epithelial-specific" markers. Am J Surg Pathol. 1994 Jan;18(1):62–73. PMID:8279629
4852. Wenig BM, Adair CF, Heffess CS. Primary mucoepidermoid carcinoma of the thyroid gland: a report of six cases and a review of the literature of a follicular epithelial-derived tumor. Hum Pathol. 1995 Oct;26(10):1099–108. PMID:7557943
4853. Wenig BM, Thompson LD, Adair CF, et al. Thyroid papillary carcinoma of columnar cell type: a clinicopathologic study of 16 cases. Cancer. 1998 Feb 15;82(4):740–53. PMID:9477108
4854. Wenter V, Albert NL, Unterrainer M, et al. Clinical impact of follicular oncocytic (Hürthle cell) carcinoma in comparison with corresponding classical follicular thyroid carcinoma. Eur J Nucl Med Mol Imaging. 2021 Feb;48(2):449–60. PMID:32683470
4855. Wenter V, Jellinek A, Unterrainer M, et al. Long-term outcome of rare oncocytic papillary (Hürthle cell) thyroid carcinoma following (adjuvant) initial radioiodine therapy. Eur J Nucl Med Mol Imaging. 2019 Nov;46(12):2526–35. PMID:31410542
4856. Wermers RA, Fatourechi V, Wynne AG, et al. The glucagonoma syndrome. Clinical and pathologic features in 21 patients. Medicine (Baltimore). 1996 Mar;75(2):53–63. PMID:8606627
4857. Werner S, Zottola C, Steinberg J, et al. Ovarian teratoma with pituitary tissue: a case report. Case Rep Womens Health. 2020 Dec 10;29:e00279. PMID:33364180
4858. Westra WH. Human papillomavirus-related neuroendocrine carcinomas of the head and neck. Head Neck Pathol. 2018 Mar;12(1):9–12. PMID:29556964
4859. Whaley RD, Thompson LDR. Primary thyroid gland alveolar soft part sarcoma. Head Neck Pathol. 2020 Sep;14(3):701–6. PMID:31782115
4860. Wheeler YY, Stoll LM, Sheth S, et al. Metastatic signet ring cell carcinoma presenting as a thyroid nodule: report of a case with fine-needle aspiration cytology. Diagn Cytopathol. 2010 Aug;38(8):597–602. PMID:20014306
4861. White PC. Update on diagnosis and management of congenital adrenal hyperplasia due to 21-hydroxylase deficiency. Curr Opin Endocrinol Diabetes Obes. 2018 Jun;25(3):178–84. PMID:29718004
4862. White PC, Curnow KM, Pascoe L. Disorders of steroid 11 beta-hydroxylase isozymes. Endocr Rev. 1994 Aug;15(4):421–38. PMID:7988480
4863. Whitehair R, Stelow EB. The cytologic and immunohistochemical findings of pancreatic mixed acinar-endocrine carcinoma. Diagn Cytopathol. 2021 Feb;49(2):287–94. PMID:33128511
4864. WHO Classification of Tumours Editorial Board. Breast tumours. Lyon (France): International Agency for Research on Cancer; 2019. (WHO classification of tumours series, 5th ed.; vol. 2). https://publications.iarc.who.int/581.
4865. WHO Classification of Tumours Editorial Board. Central nervous system tumours. Lyon (France): International Agency for Research on Cancer; 2021. (WHO classification of tumours series, 5th ed.; vol. 6). https://publications.iarc.who.int/601.
4866. WHO Classification of Tumours Editorial Board. Digestive system tumours. Lyon (France): International Agency for Research on Cancer; 2019. (WHO classification of tumours series, 5th ed.; vol. 1). https://publications.iarc.who.int/579.
4867. WHO Classification of Tumours Editorial Board. Female genital tumours. Lyon (France): International Agency for Research on Cancer; 2020. (WHO classification of tumours series, 5th ed.; vol. 4). https://publications.iarc.who.int/592.
4868. WHO Classification of Tumours Editorial Board. Head and neck tumours. Lyon (France): International Agency for Research on Cancer; 2024. (WHO classification of tumours series, 5th ed.; vol. 9). https://publications.iarc.who.int/629.
4869. WHO Classification of Tumours Editorial Board. Skin tumours [Internet; beta version ahead of print]. Lyon (France): International Agency for Research on Cancer; 2023. (WHO classification of tumours series, 5th ed.; vol. 12). https://tumourclassification.iarc.who.int/chapters/64.
4870. WHO Classification of Tumours Editorial Board. Soft tissue and bone tumours. Lyon (France): International Agency for Research on Cancer; 2020. (WHO classification of tumours series, 5th ed.; vol. 3). https://publications.iarc.who.int/588.
4871. WHO Classification of Tumours Editorial Board. Thoracic tumours. Lyon (France): International Agency for Research on Cancer; 2021. (WHO classification of tumours series, 5th ed.; vol. 5). https://publications.iarc.who.int/595.
4872. WHO Classification of Tumours Editorial Board. Urinary and male genital tumours. Lyon (France): International Agency for Research on Cancer; 2022. (WHO classification of tumours series, 5th ed.; vol. 8). https://publications.iarc.who.int/610.
4873. Wiatrowska BA, Krol J, Zakowski MF. Large-cell neuroendocrine carcinoma of the lung: proposed criteria for cytologic diagnosis. Diagn Cytopathol. 2001 Jan;24(1):58–64. PMID:11135471
4874. Widder S, Guggisberg K, Khalil M, et al. A pathologic re-review of follicular thyroid neoplasms: the impact of changing the threshold for the diagnosis of the follicular variant of papillary thyroid carcinoma. Surgery. 2008 Jul;144(1):80–5. PMID:18571588
4875. Wiemels J, Wrensch M, Claus EB. Epidemiology and etiology of meningioma. J Neurooncol. 2010 Sep;99(3):307–14. PMID:20821343
4876. Wieneke JA, Thompson LD, Heffess CS. Adrenal cortical neoplasms in the pediatric population: a clinicopathologic and immunophenotypic analysis of 83 patients. Am J Surg Pathol. 2003 Jul;27(7):867–81. PMID:12826878
4877. Wierinckx A, Delgrange E, Bertolino P, et al. Sex-related differences in lactotroph tumor aggressiveness are associated with a specific gene-expression signature and genome instability. Front Endocrinol (Lausanne). 2018 Nov 30;9:706. PMID:30555413
4878. Wierinckx A, Roche M, Raverot G, et al. Integrated genomic profiling identifies loss of chromosome 11p impacting transcriptomic activity in aggressive pituitary PRL tumors. Brain Pathol. 2011 Sep;21(5):533–43. PMID:21251114
4879. Wierzchowski W, Szybiński P, Nowak W, et al. [Poorly differentiated carcinoma of the thyroid--immunohistochemical evaluation of p53 and p27 protein expression]. Wiad Lek. 2001;54 Suppl 1:79–87. Polish. PMID:12182066
4880. Wiles AB, Kraft AO, Mueller SM, et al. Sclerosing mucoepidermoid carcinoma with eosinophilia of the thyroid: case report of a rare lesion with novel genetic mutation. Diagn Cytopathol. 2019 Jun;47(6):589–93. PMID:30677251
4881. Willén H, Akerman M, Dal Cin P, et al. Comparison of chromosomal patterns with clinical features in 165 lipomas: a report of the CHAMP study group. Cancer Genet Cytogenet. 1998 Apr 1;102(1):46–9. PMID:9530339
4882. Williams D. Inherited thyroid tumours. Endocrine. 2020 May;68(2):271–3. PMID:32189189
4883. Williams ED. Guest editorial: two proposals regarding the terminology of thyroid tumors. Int J Surg Pathol. 2000 Jul;8(3):181–3. PMID:11493987
4884. Williams ED, Pollock DJ. Multiple mucosal neuromata with endocrine tumours: a syndrome allied to von Recklinghausen's disease. J Pathol Bacteriol. 1966 Jan;91(1):71–80. PMID:4957444
4885. Williams MD. Paragangliomas of the head and neck: an overview from diagnosis to genetics. Head Neck Pathol. 2017 Sep;11(3):278–87. PMID:28321772
4886. Williams MD, DeLellis RA, Erickson LA, et al. Pathology data set for reporting parathyroid carcinoma and atypical parathyroid neoplasm: recommendations from the International Collaboration on Cancer Reporting. Hum Pathol. 2021 Apr;110:73–82. PMID:32687943
4887. Williams TA, Gomez-Sanchez CE, Rainey WE, et al. International histopathology consensus for unilateral primary aldosteronism. J Clin Endocrinol Metab. 2021 Jan 1;106(1):42–54. PMID:32717746
4888. Williams TA, Monticone S, Schack VR, et al. Somatic ATP1A1, ATP2B3, and KCNJ5 mutations in aldosterone-producing adenomas. Hypertension. 2014 Jan;63(1):188–95. PMID:24082052
4889. Williams VC, Lucas J, Babcock MA, et al. Neurofibromatosis type 1 revisited. Pediatrics. 2009 Jan;123(1):124–33. PMID:19117870
4890. Williamson D, Missiaglia E, de Reyniès A, et al. Fusion gene-negative alveolar rhabdomyosarcoma is clinically and molecularly indistinguishable from embryonal rhabdomyosarcoma. J Clin Oncol. 2010 May 1;28(13):2151–8. PMID:20351326
4891. Williamson SR, Eble JN, Amin MB, et al. Succinate dehydrogenase-deficient renal cell carcinoma: detailed characterization of 11 tumors defining a unique subtype of renal cell carcinoma. Mod Pathol. 2015 Jan;28(1):80–94. PMID:25034258
4892. Williamson SR, Gill AJ, Argani P, et al. Report from the International Society of Urological Pathology (ISUP) consultation conference on molecular pathology of urogenital cancers: III: molecular pathology of kidney cancer. Am J Surg Pathol. 2020 Jul;44(7):e47–65. PMID:32251007
4893. Williamson SR, Hornick JL, Eble JN, et al. Renal cell carcinoma with angioleiomyoma-like stroma and clear cell papillary renal cell carcinoma: exploring SDHB protein immunohistochemistry and the relationship to tuberous sclerosis complex. Hum Pathol. 2018 May;75:10–5. PMID:29180251
4894. Wilson JB, Zopey M, Augustine J, et al. High prevalence of adrenal remnant tissue in patients undergoing bilateral adrenalectomy for Cushing's disease. Horm Metab Res. 2021 Mar;53(3):161–8. PMID:33091942
4895. Wilson NW, Pambakian H, Richardson TC, et al. Epithelial markers in thyroid carcinoma: an immunoperoxidase study. Histopathology. 1986 Aug;10(8):815–29. PMID:2428725
4896. Wilson TL, Hattangady N, Lerario AM, et al. A new POT1 germline mutation-expanding the spectrum of POT1-associated cancers. Fam Cancer. 2017 Oct;16(4):561–6. PMID:28389767
4897. Wiltshire JJ, Drake TM, Uttley L, et al. Systematic review of trends in the incidence rates of thyroid cancer. Thyroid. 2016 Nov;26(11):1541–52. PMID:27571228
4898. Winer DA, Winer S, Rotstein L, et al. Villous papillary thyroid carcinoma: a variant associated with marfan syndrome. Endocr Pathol. 2012 Dec;23(4):254–9. PMID:22847364
4899. Winters SJ, Vitaz T, Nowacki MR, et al. Addison's disease and pituitary enlargement. Am J Med Sci. 2015 Jun;349(6):526–9. PMID:25004119
4900. Winther KH, Rayman MP, Bonnema SJ, et al. Selenium in thyroid disorders - essential knowledge for clinicians. Nat Rev Endocrinol. 2020 Mar;16(3):165–76. PMID:32001830
4901. Wirth LJ, Sherman E, Robinson B, et al. Efficacy of selpercatinib in RET-altered thyroid cancers. N Engl J Med. 2020 Aug 27;383(9):825–35. PMID:32846061
4902. Witek P, Maksymowicz M, Szamotulska K, et al. MGMT expression in pituitary corticotroph adenomas and its relationship to clinical, pathological, and ultrastructural parameters in patients with Cushing's disease. Folia Neuropathol. 2020;58(4):357–64. PMID:33480240
4903. Witkiewicz A, Galler A, Yeo CJ, et al. Gangliocytic paraganglioma: case report and review of the literature. J Gastrointest Surg.

2007 Oct;11(10):1351–4. PMID:17653595
4904. Witteveen JE, Hamdy NA, Dekkers OM, et al. Downregulation of CASR expression and global loss of parafibromin staining are strong negative determinants of prognosis in parathyroid carcinoma. Mod Pathol. 2011 May;24(5):688–97. PMID:21240254
4905. Witzigmann H, Loracher C, Geissler F, et al. Neuroendocrine tumours of the duodenum. Clinical aspects, pathomorphology and therapy. Langenbecks Arch Surg. 2002 Jan;386(7):525–33. PMID:11819111
4906. Woischke C, Jung P, Jung A, et al. Mixed large cell neuroendocrine carcinoma and squamous cell carcinoma of the colon: detailed molecular characterisation of two cases indicates a distinct colorectal cancer entity. J Pathol Clin Res. 2021 Jan;7(1):75–85. PMID:33197299
4907. Woischke C, Schaaf CW, Yang HM, et al. In-depth mutational analyses of colorectal neuroendocrine carcinomas with adenoma or adenocarcinoma components. Mod Pathol. 2017 Jan;30(1):95–103. PMID:27586204
4908. Wolf KI, Jacobs MF, Mehra R, et al. A family with a carotid body paraganglioma and thyroid neoplasias with a new SDHAF2 germline variant. J Endocr Soc. 2019 Sep 5;3(11):2151–7. PMID:31687641
4909. Wolfe HJ, Delellis RA. Familial medullary thyroid carcinoma and C cell hyperplasia. Clin Endocrinol Metab. 1981 Jul;10(2):351–65. PMID:7285384
4910. Wolfe SQ, Heros RC. A Rathke cleft cyst to craniopharyngioma: Is there a spectrum? J Neurosurg. 2010 Jun;112(6):1322–3. PMID:19961318
4911. Wolff M, Goodman EN. Functioning lipoadenoma of a supernumerary parathyroid gland in the mediastinum. Head Neck Surg. 1980 Mar-Apr;2(4):302–7. PMID:7364585
4912. Wong CW, Schumm MA, Zhu CY, et al. Quality of life following molecular marker testing for indeterminate thyroid nodules. Endocr Pract. 2020 Sep;26(9):960–6. PMID:33471700
4913. Wong KS, Angell TE, Barletta JA, et al. Hürthle cell lesions of the thyroid: progress made and challenges remaining. Cancer Cytopathol. 2021 May;129(5):347–62. PMID:33108684
4914. Wong KS, Chen TY, Higgins SE, et al. A potential diagnostic pitfall for hobnail variant of papillary thyroid carcinoma. Histopathology. 2020 Apr;76(5):707–13. PMID:31811787
4915. Wong KS, Dong F, Telatar M, et al. Papillary thyroid carcinoma with high-grade features versus poorly differentiated thyroid carcinoma: an analysis of clinicopathologic and molecular features and outcome. Thyroid. 2021 Jun;31(6):933–40. PMID:33143568
4916. Wong KS, Higgins SE, Marqusee E, et al. Tall cell variant of papillary thyroid carcinoma: impact of change in WHO definition and molecular analysis. Endocr Pathol. 2019 Mar;30(1):43–8. PMID:30565013
4917. Wong KS, Jo VY, Lowe AC, et al. Malignancy risk for solitary and multiple nodules in Hürthle cell-predominant thyroid fine-needle aspirations: a multi-institutional study. Cancer Cytopathol. 2020 Jan;128(1):68–75. PMID:31751003
4918. Wong KS, Lorch JH, Alexander EK, et al. Histopathologic features and clinical outcome of anaplastic thyroid carcinoma with a minor anaplastic component. Endocr Pathol. 2020 Sep;31(3):283–90. PMID:32445173
4919. Wong KS, Lorch JH, Alexander EK, et al. Prognostic significance of extent of invasion in poorly differentiated thyroid carcinoma. Thyroid. 2019 Sep;29(9):1255–61. PMID:31397224
4920. Wong KT, Ahuja AT. Ultrasound of thyroid cancer. Cancer Imaging. 2005 Dec 9;5(1):157–66. PMID:16361145
4921. Wong MY, Andrews KA, Challis BG, et al. Clinical practice guidance: surveillance for phaeochromocytoma and paraganglioma in paediatric succinate dehydrogenase gene mutation carriers. Clin Endocrinol (Oxf). 2019 Apr;90(4):499–505. PMID:30589099
4922. Wong R, Farrell SG, Grossmann M. Thyroid nodules: diagnosis and management. Med J Aust. 2018 Jul 16;209(2):92–8. PMID:29996756
4923. Wong SBJ, Nga ME, Michal M, et al. SOX11 expression in a case of papillary thyroid carcinoma with fibromatosis/fasciitis-like stroma containing BRAF c.1799_1801delTGA and CTNNB1 c.133T>C mutations. Virchows Arch. 2019 Oct;475(4):519–25. PMID:31327063
4924. Wong SQ, Waldeck K, Vergara IA, et al. UV-associated mutations underlie the etiology of MCV-negative Merkel cell carcinomas. Cancer Res. 2015 Dec 15;75(24):5228–34. PMID:26627015
4925. Wong YN, Jack RH, Mak V, et al. The epidemiology and survival of extrapulmonary small cell carcinoma in South East England, 1970-2004. BMC Cancer. 2009 Jun 29;9:209. PMID:19563623
4926. Wongthim S, Hemachudha T, Punthumchinda K. Respiratory insufficiency associated with acute hepatic porphyria. J Med Assoc Thai. 1989 Nov;72(11):655–9. PMID:2635211
4927. Wont TW, Warner NE. Ovarian thecal metaplasia in the adrenal gland. Arch Pathol. 1971 Nov;92(5):319–28. PMID:5110570
4928. Woo Young K, Young Ran K, Sang Uk W, et al. Pulmonary leiomyosarcoma metastatic to the thyroid gland: case report and review of the literature. Ann Endocrinol (Paris). 2011 Sep;72(4):314–6. PMID:21784409
4929. Woo YS, Isidori AM, Wat WZ, et al. Clinical and biochemical characteristics of adrenocorticotropin-secreting macroadenomas. J Clin Endocrinol Metab. 2005 Aug;90(8):4963–9. PMID:15886242
4930. Wood CB, Bigcas JL, Alava I, et al. Papillary-type carcinoma of the thyroglossal duct cyst: the case for conservative management. Ann Otol Rhinol Laryngol. 2018 Oct;127(10):710–6. PMID:30091370
4931. Wood K, Vini L, Harmer C. Metastases to the thyroid gland: the Royal Marsden experience. Eur J Surg Oncol. 2004 Aug;30(6):583–8. PMID:15256229
4932. Wood LD, Klimstra DS. Pathology and genetics of pancreatic neoplasms with acinar differentiation. Semin Diagn Pathol. 2014 Nov;31(6):491–7. PMID:25441307
4933. Wood LD, Noë M, Hackeng W, et al. Patients with McCune-Albright syndrome have a broad spectrum of abnormalities in the gastrointestinal tract and pancreas. Virchows Arch. 2017 Apr;470(4):391–400. PMID:28188442
4934. Woodford RL, Nikiforov YE, Hunt JL, et al. Encapsulated papillary oncocytic neoplasms of the thyroid: morphologic, immunohistochemical, and molecular analysis of 18 cases. Am J Surg Pathol. 2010 Nov;34(11):1582–90. PMID:20924280
4935. Woodruff JD, Rauh JT, Markley RL. Ovarian struma. Obstet Gynecol. 1966 Feb;27(2):194–201. PMID:5909538
4936. Wooten MD, King DK. Adrenal cortical carcinoma. Epidemiology and treatment with mitotane and a review of the literature. Cancer. 1993 Dec 1;72(11):3145–55. PMID:8242539
4937. Workman AD, Soylu S, Kamani D, et al. Limitations of preoperative cytology for medullary thyroid cancer: proposal for improved preoperative diagnosis for optimal initial medullary thyroid carcinoma specific surgery. Head Neck. 2021 Mar;43(3):920–7. PMID:33269526
4938. Worth PJ, Turner M, Hammill CW. Incidental angiosarcoma of the pancreas: a case report of a rare, asymptomatic tumor. J Pancreat Cancer. 2017 May 1;3(1):24–7. PMID:30631836
4939. Wright JP, Montgomery KW, Tierney J, et al. Ectopic, retroperitoneal adrenocortical carcinoma in the setting of Lynch syndrome. Fam Cancer. 2018 Jul;17(3):381–5. PMID:28940135
4940. Wu AW, Bhuta S, Salamon N, et al. Chondroid chordoma of the sella turcica mimicking a pituitary adenoma. Ear Nose Throat J. 2015 Oct-Nov;94(10-11):E47–9. PMID:26535833
4941. Wu AW, Suh JD, Metson R, et al. Prognostic factors in sinonasal sarcomas: analysis of the Surveillance, Epidemiology and End Result Database. Laryngoscope. 2012 Oct;122(10):2137–42. PMID:22777866
4942. Wu B, Sun T, Gu Y, et al. CT and MR imaging of thyroid carcinoma showing thymus-like differentiation (CASTLE): a report of ten cases. Br J Radiol. 2016;89(1060):20150726. PMID:26954328
4943. Wu CS, Wang XW, Qin T, et al. Primary intraosseous ganglioneuromatous paraganglioma of the sacrum with immunopositivity for cytokeratin. Eur Rev Med Pharmacol Sci. 2015;19(6):931–5. PMID:25855915
4944. Wu EY, Lebastchi J, Marqusee E, et al. A case of primary secretory carcinoma of the thyroid with high-grade features. Histopathology. 2017 Oct;71(4):665–9. PMID:28556362
4945. Wu F, Watanabe N, Tzioni MM, et al. Thyroid MALT lymphoma: self-harm to gain potential T-cell help. Leukemia. 2021 Dec;35(12):3497–508. PMID:34021249
4946. Wu HH, Clouse J, Ren R. Fine-needle aspiration cytology of Hürthle cell carcinoma of the thyroid. Diagn Cytopathol. 2008 Mar;36(3):149–54. PMID:18232004
4947. Wu L, Xie J, Jiang L, et al. Feminizing adrenocortical carcinoma: the source of estrogen production and the role of adrenal-gonadal dedifferentiation. J Clin Endocrinol Metab. 2018 Oct 1;103(10):3706–13. PMID:30053001
4948. Wu VC, Wang SM, Chueh SJ, et al. The prevalence of CTNNB1 mutations in primary aldosteronism and consequences for clinical outcomes. Sci Rep. 2017 Jan 19;7:39121. PMID:28102204
4949. Wu Y, Gao L, Guo X, et al. Pituitary adenomas in patients with multiple endocrine neoplasia type 1: a single-center experience in China. Pituitary. 2019 Apr;22(2):113–23. PMID:30637623
4950. Wurm J, Constantinidis J, Grabenbauer GG, et al. Rhabdomyosarcomas of the nose and paranasal sinuses: treatment results in 15 cases. Otolaryngol Head Neck Surg. 2005 Jul;133(1):42–50. PMID:16025051
4951. Wynne AG, van Heerden J, Carney JA, et al. Parathyroid carcinoma: clinical and pathologic features in 43 patients. Medicine (Baltimore). 1992 Jul;71(4):197–205. PMID:1518393
4952. Xavier-Júnior JCC, Camilo-Júnior DJ, D'Ávilla SCGP, et al. Fine-needle aspiration of the Warthin-like variant of papillary thyroid carcinoma: a report of three cases. Diagn Cytopathol. 2019 Dec;47(12):1293–6. PMID:31513354
4953. Xekouki P, Azevedo M, Stratakis CA. Anterior pituitary adenomas: inherited syndromes, novel genes and molecular pathways. Expert Rev Endocrinol Metab. 2010 Sep 1;5(5):697–709. PMID:21264206
4954. Xekouki P, Brennand A, Whitelaw B, et al. The 3PAs: an update on the association of pheochromocytomas, paragangliomas, and pituitary tumors. Horm Metab Res. 2019 Jul;51(7):419–36. PMID:30273935
4955. Xekouki P, Pacak K, Almeida M, et al. Succinate dehydrogenase (SDH) D subunit (SDHD) inactivation in a growth-hormone-producing pituitary tumor: a new association for SDH? J Clin Endocrinol Metab. 2012 Mar;97(3):E357–66. PMID:22170724
4956. Xekouki P, Szarek E, Bullova P, et al. Pituitary adenoma with paraganglioma/pheochromocytoma (3PAs) and succinate dehydrogenase defects in humans and mice. J Clin Endocrinol Metab. 2015 May;100(5):E710–9. PMID:25695889
4957. Xia CX, Li R, Wang ZH, et al. A rare cause of goiter: Langerhans cell histiocytosis of the thyroid. Endocr J. 2012;59(1):47–54. PMID:22019948
4958. Xia Q, Wang W, Xu J, et al. Evidence from an updated meta-analysis of the prognostic impacts of postoperative radiotherapy and chemotherapy in patients with anaplastic thyroid carcinoma. Onco Targets Ther. 2018 Apr 19;11:2251–7. PMID:29719407
4959. Xia QY, Wang XT, Zhan XM, et al. Xp11 translocation renal cell carcinomas (RCCs) with RBM10-TFE3 gene fusion demonstrating melanotic features and overlapping morphology with t(6;11) RCC: interest and diagnostic pitfall in detecting a paracentric inversion of TFE3. Am J Surg Pathol. 2017 May;41(5):663–76. PMID:28288037
4960. Xiang N, Dong F, Zhan X, et al. Incidence and prognostic factors of primary thyroid lymphoma and construction of prognostic models for post-chemotherapy and post-operative patients: a population-based study. BMC Endocr Disord. 2021 Apr 13;21(1):68. PMID:33849490
4961. Xiao RY, Yao X, Wang WL. A huge pancreatic lipoma mimicking a well-differentiated liposarcoma: a case report and systematic literature review. World J Clin Cases. 2019 Aug 26;7(16):2352–9. PMID:31531331
4962. Xie C, Tanakchi S, Raygada M, et al. Case report of an adrenocortical carcinoma associated with germline CHEK2 mutation. J Endocr Soc. 2018 Dec 12;3(1):284–90. PMID:30623166
4963. Xin W, Rubin MA, McKeever PE. Differential expression of cytokeratins 8 and 20 distinguishes craniopharyngioma from Rathke cleft cyst. Arch Pathol Lab Med. 2002 Oct;126(10):1174–8. PMID:12296753
4964. Xin Y, Zhao T, Wei B, et al. Intrapericardial parathyroid carcinoma: a case report. Endocrine. 2020 Aug;69(2):456–60. PMID:32248393
4965. Xing M, Liu R, Liu X, et al. BRAF V600E and TERT promoter mutations cooperatively identify the most aggressive papillary thyroid cancer with highest recurrence. J Clin Oncol. 2014 Sep 1;32(25):2718–26. PMID:25024077
4966. Xing Y, Lerario AM, Rainey W, et al. Development of adrenal cortex zonation. Endocrinol Metab Clin North Am. 2015 Jun;44(2):243–74. PMID:26038200
4967. Xiu Q, Wang XJ, Zhu DD, et al. Diagnosis and comprehensive therapy for cutaneous neuroendocrine carcinoma of the external auditory canal: a case report and literature review. Braz J Otorhinolaryngol. 2018 Nov-Dec;84(6):799–801. PMID:27166275
4968. Xu B, David J, Dogan S, et al. Primary high-grade non-anaplastic thyroid carcinoma: a retrospective study of 364 cases. Histopathology. 2022 Jan;80(2):322–37. PMID:34449926
4969. Xu B, Farhat N, Barletta JA, et al. Should subcentimeter non-invasive encapsulated, follicular variant of papillary thyroid carcinoma be included in the noninvasive follicular thyroid neoplasm with papillary-like nuclear features category? Endocrine. 2018 Jan;59(1):143–50. PMID:29204912
4970. Xu B, Fuchs T, Dogan S, et al. Dissecting anaplastic thyroid carcinoma: a comprehensive clinical, histologic, immunophenotypic, and

molecular study of 360 cases. Thyroid. 2020 Oct;30(10):1505–17. PMID:32284020
4971. Xu B, Fuchs TL, Ahmadi S, et al. International medullary thyroid carcinoma grading system: a validated grading system for medullary thyroid carcinoma. J Clin Oncol. 2022 Jan 1;40(1):96–104. PMID:34731032
4972. Xu B, Ghossein R. Encapsulated thyroid carcinoma of follicular cell origin. Endocr Pathol. 2015 Sep;26(3):191–9. PMID:26003547
4973. Xu B, Ghossein R. Evolution of the histologic classification of thyroid neoplasms and its impact on clinical management. Eur J Surg Oncol. 2018 Mar;44(3):338–47. PMID:28554832
4974. Xu B, Ghossein R. Genomic landscape of poorly differentiated and anaplastic thyroid carcinoma. Endocr Pathol. 2016 Sep;27(3):205–12. PMID:27372303
4975. Xu B, Ghossein RA. Crucial parameters in thyroid carcinoma reporting - challenges, controversies and clinical implications. Histopathology. 2018 Jan;72(1):32–9. PMID:28782127
4976. Xu B, Ghossein RA. Noninvasive follicular thyroid neoplasm with papillary-like nuclear features (NIFTP): an update. Head Neck Pathol. 2020 Jun;14(2):303–10. PMID:32124418
4977. Xu B, Hirokawa M, Yoshimoto K, et al. Spindle epithelial tumor with thymus-like differentiation of the thyroid: a case report with pathological and molecular genetics study. Hum Pathol. 2003 Feb;34(2):190–3. PMID:12612889
4978. Xu B, Hong Y, Jin M, et al. Primary adrenal malignant melanoma: a case report and review of literature. Medicine (Baltimore). 2017 Dec;96(51):e8956. PMID:29390427
4979. Xu B, Ibrahimpasic T, Wang L, et al. Clinicopathologic features of fatal non-anaplastic follicular cell-derived thyroid carcinomas. Thyroid. 2016 Nov;26(11):1588–97. PMID:27480016
4980. Xu B, Reznik E, Tuttle RM, et al. Outcome and molecular characteristics of non-invasive encapsulated follicular variant of papillary thyroid carcinoma with oncocytic features. Endocrine. 2019 Apr;64(1):97–108. PMID:30689169
4981. Xu B, Sano T, Yoshimoto K, et al. Downregulation of E-cadherin and its undercoat proteins in pituitary growth hormone cell adenomas with prominent fibrous bodies. Endocr Pathol. 2002 Winter;13(4):341–51. PMID:12665652
4982. Xu B, Serrette R, Tuttle RM, et al. How many papillae in conventional papillary carcinoma? A clinical evidence-based pathology study of 235 unifocal encapsulated papillary thyroid carcinomas, with emphasis on the diagnosis of noninvasive follicular thyroid neoplasm with papillary-like nuclear features. Thyroid. 2019 Dec;29(12):1792–803. PMID:31452453
4983. Xu B, Suurmeijer AJH, Agaram NP, et al. Head and neck rhabdomyosarcoma with TFCP2 fusions and ALK overexpression: a clinicopathological and molecular analysis of 11 cases. Histopathology. 2021 Sep;79(3):347–57. PMID:33382123
4984. Xu B, Tallini G, Scognamiglio T, et al. Outcome of large noninvasive follicular thyroid neoplasm with papillary-like nuclear features. Thyroid. 2017 Apr;27(4):512–7. PMID:28136139
4985. Xu B, Viswanathan K, Ahadi MS, et al. Association of the genomic profile of medullary thyroid carcinoma with tumor characteristics and clinical outcomes in an international multicenter study. Thyroid. 2024 Feb;34(2):167–76. PMID:37842841
4986. Xu B, Wang L, Tuttle RM, et al. Prognostic impact of extent of vascular invasion in low-grade encapsulated follicular cell-derived thyroid carcinomas: a clinicopathologic study of 276 cases. Hum Pathol. 2015 Dec;46(12):1789–98. PMID:26482605
4987. Xu B, Yoshimoto K, Miyauchi A, et al. Cribriform-morular variant of papillary thyroid carcinoma: a pathological and molecular genetic study with evidence of frequent somatic mutations in exon 3 of the beta-catenin gene. J Pathol. 2003 Jan;199(1):58–67. PMID:12474227
4988. Xu F, Ma J, Yi H, et al. Clinicopathological aspects of small cell neuroendocrine carcinoma of the uterine cervix: a multicenter retrospective study and meta-analysis. Cell Physiol Biochem. 2018;50(3):1113–22. PMID:30355937
4989. Xu JL, Guo Y. Clinical characteristics and survival of extrapulmonary small cell carcinoma in 11 different primary tumor sites in the United States, 1975-2016. Curr Med Res Opin. 2021 Jan;37(1):71–81. PMID:33135938
4990. Xu KM, Liu Y, Gillespie TW, et al. Small-cell carcinoma of the prostate: report of outcomes of localized disease using the National Cancer Database. Clin Genitourin Cancer. 2021 Aug;19(4):e193–9. PMID:33582100
4991. Xu Z, Ellis S, Lee CC, et al. Silent corticotroph adenomas after stereotactic radiosurgery: a case-control study. Int J Radiat Oncol Biol Phys. 2014 Nov 15;90(4):903–10. PMID:25216855
4992. Yachida S, Vakiani E, White CM, et al. Small cell and large cell neuroendocrine carcinomas of the pancreas are genetically similar and distinct from well-differentiated pancreatic neuroendocrine tumors. Am J Surg Pathol. 2012 Feb;36(2):173–84. PMID:22251937
4993. Yakushina VD, Lerner LV, Lavrov AV. Gene fusions in thyroid cancer. Thyroid. 2018 Feb;28(2):158–67. PMID:29281951
4994. Yamada H, Haratake J, Narasaki T, et al. Embryonal craniopharyngioma. Case report of the morphogenesis of a craniopharyngioma. Cancer. 1995 Jun 15;75(12):2971–7. PMID:7773950
4995. Yamada M, Nakajima Y, Taguchi R, et al. KCNJ5 mutations in aldosterone- and cortisol-co-secreting adrenal adenomas. Endocr J. 2012;59(8):735–41. PMID:22863749
4996. Yamada S, Fukuhara N, Horiguchi K, et al. Clinicopathological characteristics and therapeutic outcomes in thyrotropin-secreting pituitary adenomas: a single-center study of 90 cases. J Neurosurg. 2014 Dec;121(6):1462–73. PMID:25237847
4997. Yamada S, Inoshita N, Fukuhara N, et al. Therapeutic outcomes in patients undergoing surgery after diagnosis of Cushing's disease: a single-center study. Endocr J. 2015;62(12):1115–25. PMID:26477323
4998. Yamada S, Ohyama K, Taguchi M, et al. A study of the correlation between morphological findings and biological activities in clinically nonfunctioning pituitary adenomas. Neurosurgery. 2007 Sep;61(3):580–4. PMID:17881972
4999. Yamagata K, Ohki K, Uchida F, et al. A rare primary neuroendocrine tumor (typical carcinoid) of the sublingual gland. Case Rep Dent. 2016;2016:7462690. PMID:27840746
5000. Yamagata K, Terada K, Uchida F, et al. A case of primary combined squamous cell carcinoma with neuroendocrine (atypical carcinoid) tumor in the floor of the mouth. Case Rep Dent. 2016;2016:7532805. PMID:28116178
5001. Yamagishi S, Yokoyama-Ohta M. A rare case of pituitary hyperplasia with suprasellar extension due to primary myxoedema: case report. J Int Med Res. 1999 Jan-Feb;27(1):49–52. PMID:10417962
5002. Yamamoto N, Minami S, Kidoguchi M, et al. Large cell neuroendocrine carcinoma of the submandibular gland: case report and literature review. Auris Nasus Larynx. 2014 Feb;41(1):105–8. PMID:23953500
5003. Yaman H, Durmaz A, Arslan HH, et al. Thyroglossal duct cysts: evaluation and treatment of 49 cases. B-ENT. 2011;7(4):267–71. PMID:22338239
5004. Yamasaki M, Sato Y, Nomura T, et al. Composite paraganglioma-ganglioneuroma concomitant with adrenal metastasis of medullary thyroid carcinoma in a patient with multiple endocrine neoplasia type 2B: a case report. Asian J Endosc Surg. 2017 Feb;10(1):66–9. PMID:27704704
5005. Yamashina M. Follicular neoplasms of the thyroid. Total circumferential evaluation of the fibrous capsule. Am J Surg Pathol. 1992 Apr;16(4):392–400. PMID:1373582
5006. Yamashita H, Murakami N, Noguchi S, et al. Cervical thymoma and incidence of cervical thymus. Acta Pathol Jpn. 1983 Jan;33(1):189–94. PMID:6687653
5007. Yamashita K, Fletcher CD. PEComa presenting in bone: clinicopathologic analysis of 6 cases and literature review. Am J Surg Pathol. 2010 Nov;34(11):1622–9. PMID:20975340
5008. Yamazaki H, Sugino K, Katoh R, et al. Outcomes for minimally invasive follicular thyroid carcinoma in relation to the change in age stratification in the AJCC 8th edition. Ann Surg Oncol. 2021 Jul;28(7):3576–83. PMID:33237449
5009. Yamazaki M, Fujii S, Daiko H, et al. Carcinoma showing thymus-like differentiation (CASTLE) with neuroendocrine differentiation. Pathol Int. 2008 Dec;58(12):775–9. PMID:19067852
5010. Yamazaki Y, Nakamura Y, Shibahara Y, et al. Comparison of the methods for measuring the Ki-67 labeling index in adrenocortical carcinoma: manual versus digital image analysis. Hum Pathol. 2016 Jul;53:41–50. PMID:26980031
5011. Yan D, Zhang B, Li Z, et al. [Cervical lymph node metastasis in medullary thyroid carcinoma]. Zhonghua Er Bi Yan Hou Tou Jing Wai Ke Za Zhi. 2015 Apr;50(4):290–4. Chinese. PMID:26081082
5012. Yan M, Roncin KL, Wilhelm S, et al. Images in endocrine pathology: high-grade intrathyroidal parathyroid carcinoma with Crooke's hyalinization. Endocr Pathol. 2020 Jun;31(2):190–4. PMID:32146582
5013. Yang B, Yang C, Sun Y, et al. Mixed gangliocytoma-pituitary adenoma in the sellar region: a large-scale single-center experience. Acta Neurochir (Wien). 2018 Oct;160(10):1989–99. PMID:30109498
5014. Yang C, Li G, Fang J, et al. Clinical characteristics and surgical outcomes of primary spinal paragangliomas. J Neurooncol. 2015 May;122(3):539–47. PMID:25720695
5015. Yang C, Liu L, Lan X, et al. Progressive visual disturbance and enlarging prolactinoma caused by melanoma metastasis: a case report and literature review. Medicine (Baltimore). 2017 Apr;96(14):e6483. PMID:28383413
5016. Yang C, Sanchez-Vega F, Chang JC, et al. Lung-only melanoma: UV mutational signature supports origin from occult cutaneous primaries and argues against the concept of primary pulmonary melanoma. Mod Pathol. 2020 Nov;33(11):2244–55. PMID:32581366
5017. Yang GC, Rotterdam H. Mixed (composite) glandular-endocrine cell carcinoma of the stomach. Report of a case and review of literature. Am J Surg Pathol. 1991 Jun;15(6):592–8. PMID:2031532
5018. Yang GC, Schreiner AM, Sun W. Can abundant colloid exclude oncocytic (Hürthle cell) carcinoma in thyroid fine needle aspiration? Cytohistological correlation of 127 oncocytic (Hürthle cell) lesions. Cytopathology. 2013 Jun;24(3):185–93. PMID:22672530
5019. Yang GC, Scognamiglio T, Kuhel WI. Fine-needle aspiration of mucin-producing thyroid tumors. Acta Cytol. 2011;55(6):549–55. PMID:22156465
5020. Yang GC, Stern CM, Messina AV. Cystic papillary thyroid carcinoma in fine needle aspiration may represent a subset of the encapsulated variant in WHO classification. Diagn Cytopathol. 2010 Oct;38(10):721–6. PMID:20024942
5021. Yang GCH, Fried KO. Most thyroid cancers detected by sonography lack intranodular vascularity on color Doppler imaging: review of the literature and sonographic-pathologic correlations for 698 thyroid neoplasms. J Ultrasound Med. 2017 Jan;36(1):89–94. PMID:27943373
5022. Yang GCH, Fried KO, Scognamiglio T. Can cytology and the Thyroid Imaging, Reporting, and Data System (TI-RADS) identify noninvasive follicular thyroid neoplasm with papillary-like nuclear features (NIFTP) before surgery? J Am Soc Cytopathol. 2020 May-Jun;9(3):159–65. PMID:32111537
5023. Yang GCH, Fried KO, Scognamiglio T. Sonographic and cytologic differences of NIFTP from infiltrative or invasive encapsulated follicular variant of papillary thyroid carcinoma: a Review of 179 cases. Diagn Cytopathol. 2017 Jun;45(6):533–41. PMID:28332339
5024. Yang I, Park S, Ryu M, et al. Characteristics of gsp-positive growth hormone-secreting pituitary tumors in Korean acromegalic patients. Eur J Endocrinol. 1996 Jun;134(6):720–6. PMID:8766942
5025. Yang J, Barletta JA. Anaplastic thyroid carcinoma. Semin Diagn Pathol. 2020 Sep;37(5):248–56. PMID:32624319
5026. Yang J, Sarita-Reyes C, Kindelberger D, et al. A rare malignant thyroid carcinosarcoma with aggressive behavior and DICER1 gene mutation: a case report with literature review. Thyroid Res. 2018 Jul 31;11:11. PMID:30083234
5027. Yang J, Schnadig V, Logrono R, et al. Fine-needle aspiration of thyroid nodules: a study of 4703 patients with histologic and clinical correlations. Cancer. 2007 Oct 25;111(5):306–15. PMID:17680588
5028. Yang JW, Han J, Lee HW, et al. A rare case of thymic gangliocytic paraganglioma. J Pathol Transl Med. 2016 Mar;50(2):165–7. PMID:26447134
5029. Yang L, Asiry S, Khader SN. Adenomatous neuroendocrine tumors of the middle ear (MEANTs) with local invasion and lymph nodes metastasis: a brief report of a rare neoplasm. Diagn Cytopathol. 2021 Apr;49(4):E141–5. PMID:33044790
5030. Yang L, Zhao H, He Y, et al. Contrast-enhanced ultrasound in the differential diagnosis of primary thyroid lymphoma and nodular Hashimoto's thyroiditis in a background of heterogeneous parenchyma. Front Oncol. 2021 Jan 7;10:597975. PMID:33489895
5031. Yang R, Zou X, Zeng H, et al. Comparison of diagnostic performance of five different ultrasound TI-RADS classification guidelines for thyroid nodules. Front Oncol. 2020 Nov 16;10:598225. PMID:33330093
5032. Yang S, Chen S, Chen X, et al. Primary typical carcinoid tumour in the retromolar region with prominent squamous differentiation: a case report. Int J Oral Maxillofac Surg. 2011 Sep;40(9):991–4. PMID:21493041
5033. Yang SY, Jin YJ, Park SH, et al. Paragangliomas in the cauda equina region: clinicopathoradiologic findings in four cases. J Neurooncol. 2005 Mar;72(1):49–55. PMID:15803375
5034. Yang Y, Shrestha D, Shi XE, et al. Ectopic recurrence of craniopharyngioma: reporting three new cases. Br J Neurosurg. 2015 Apr;29(2):295–7. PMID:25311042
5035. Yang Y, Xie W, Ren Y, et al. A case report of primary adrenal lymphoma: a rare but aggressive and invasive disease. Medicine (Baltimore).

2020 Jul 10;99(28):e20938. PMID:32664092
5036. Yang YJ, Han JW, Youn HD, et al. The tumor suppressor, parafibromin, mediates histone H3 K9 methylation for cyclin D1 repression. Nucleic Acids Res. 2010 Jan;38(2):382–90. PMID:19906718
5037. Yang YJ, Khurana KK. Diagnostic utility of intracytoplasmic lumen and transgressing vessels in evaluation of Hürthle cell lesions by fine-needle aspiration. Arch Pathol Lab Med. 2001 Aug;125(8):1031–5. PMID:11473452
5038. Yang YJ, Steele CT, Ou XL, et al. Diagnosis of high-grade pulmonary neuroendocrine carcinoma by fine-needle aspiration biopsy: nonsmall-cell or small-cell type? Diagn Cytopathol. 2001 Nov;25(5):292–300. PMID:11747218
5039. Yang Z, Tang LH, Klimstra DS. Effect of tumor heterogeneity on the assessment of Ki67 labeling index in well-differentiated neuroendocrine tumors metastatic to the liver: implications for prognostic stratification. Am J Surg Pathol. 2011 Jun;35(6):853–60. PMID:21566513
5040. Yang Z, Zhang T, Gao H. Genetic aspects of pituitary carcinoma: a systematic review. Medicine (Baltimore). 2016 Nov;95(47):e5268. PMID:27893664
5041. Yano S, Hide T, Uekawa K, et al. Mixed pituitary gangliocytoma and prolactinoma resistant to the cabergoline treatment. World Neurosurg. 2016 Nov;95:620.e17–22. PMID:27535625
5042. Yanofsky VR, Ng E, Ratner D. Cutaneous metastasis of malignant peripheral nerve sheath tumor arising from the pancreas: a rarity. Dermatol Surg. 2019 Aug;45(8):1107–9. PMID:30720497
5043. Yantiss RK, Chang HK, Farraye FA, et al. Prevalence and prognostic significance of acinar cell differentiation in pancreatic endocrine tumors. Am J Surg Pathol. 2002 Jul;26(7):893–901. PMID:12131156
5044. Yao JC, Eisner MP, Leary C, et al. Population-based study of islet cell carcinoma. Ann Surg Oncol. 2007 Dec;14(12):3492–500. PMID:17896148
5045. Yao JC, Hassan M, Phan A, et al. One hundred years after "carcinoid": epidemiology of and prognostic factors for neuroendocrine tumors in 35,825 cases in the United States. J Clin Oncol. 2008 Jun 20;26(18):3063–72. PMID:18565894
5046. Yao Y, Liu Y, Wang L, et al. Clinical characteristics and management of growth hormone excess in patients with McCune-Albright syndrome. Eur J Endocrinol. 2017 Mar;176(3):295–303. PMID:28007843
5047. Yap WM, Chuah KL, Tan PH. Langerhans cell histiocytosis involving the thyroid and parathyroid glands. Mod Pathol. 2001 Feb;14(2):111–5. PMID:11235902
5048. Yart A, Gstaiger M, Wirbelauer C, et al. The HRPT2 tumor suppressor gene product parafibromin associates with human PAF1 and RNA polymerase II. Mol Cell Biol. 2005 Jun;25(12):5052–60. PMID:15923622
5049. Yasuda I, Adachi S, Kasahara S, et al. Pancreatic rhabdomyosarcoma. Gastrointest Endosc. 2004 Sep;60(3):433–4. PMID:15332041
5050. Yasuda T, Perry KD, Nelson M, et al. Alveolar rhabdomyosarcoma of the head and neck region in older adults: genetic characterization and a review of the literature. Hum Pathol. 2009 Mar;40(3):341–8. PMID:18973919
5051. Yasuoka H, Tsujimoto M, Fujita S, et al. Monoclonality of composite large cell neuroendocrine carcinoma and mucinous epithelial tumor of the ovary: a case study. Int J Gynecol Pathol. 2009 Jan;28(1):55–8. PMID:19047907
5052. Yasuoka H, Tsujimoto M, Ueda M, et al. Monoclonality of composite large-cell neuroendocrine carcinoma and invasive intestinal-type mucinous adenocarcinoma of the cervix: a case study. Int J Gynecol Pathol. 2013 Jul;32(4):416–20. PMID:23722515
5053. Yau T, Lo CY, Epstein RJ, et al. Treatment outcomes in anaplastic thyroid carcinoma: survival improvement in young patients with localized disease treated by combination of surgery and radiotherapy. Ann Surg Oncol. 2008 Sep;15(9):2500–5. PMID:18581185
5054. Yazici P, Yilmaz B, Bozkurt E, et al. Malignancy risk of oncocytic changes in thyroid nodules: who should we offer surgery to? Acta Chir Belg. 2016 Feb;116(1):30–5. PMID:27385138
5055. Ye F, Gao H, Xiao L, et al. Whole exome and target sequencing identifies MAP2K5 as novel susceptibility gene for familial non-medullary thyroid carcinoma. Int J Cancer. 2019 Mar 15;144(6):1321–30. PMID:30132833
5056. Ye L, Zhou X, Huang F, et al. The genetic landscape of benign thyroid nodules revealed by whole exome and transcriptome sequencing. Nat Commun. 2017 Jun 5;8:15533. PMID:28580939
5057. Yeap PM, Tobias ES, Mavraki E, et al. Molecular analysis of pheochromocytoma after maternal transmission of SDHD mutation elucidates mechanism of parent-of-origin effect. J Clin Endocrinol Metab. 2011 Dec;96(12):E2009–13. PMID:21937622
5058. Yeh MW, Ituarte PH, Zhou HC, et al. Incidence and prevalence of primary hyperparathyroidism in a racially mixed population. J Clin Endocrinol Metab. 2013 Mar;98(3):1122–9. PMID:23418315
5059. Yehia L, Eng C. 65 years of the double helix: one gene, many endocrine and metabolic syndromes: PTEN-opathies and precision medicine. Endocr Relat Cancer. 2018 Aug;25(8):T121–40. PMID:29792313
5060. Yehia L, Eng C. PTEN hamartoma tumor syndrome. In: Adam MP, Feldman J, Mirzaa GM, et al., editors. GeneReviews. Seattle (WA): University of Washington, Seattle; 2001 Nov 29 [updated 2021 Feb 11]. PMID:20301661
5061. Yehia L, Eng C. PTEN hamartoma tumour syndrome: what happens when there is no PTEN germline mutation? Hum Mol Genet. 2020 Oct 20;29 R2:R150–7. PMID:32568377
5062. Yehia L, Niazi F, Ni Y, et al. Germline heterozygous variants in SEC23B are associated with Cowden syndrome and enriched in apparently sporadic thyroid cancer. Am J Hum Genet. 2015 Nov 5;97(5):661–76. PMID:26522472
5063. Yeo MK, Bae JS, Lee S, et al. The Warthin-like variant of papillary thyroid carcinoma: a comparison with classic type in the patients with coexisting Hashimoto's thyroiditis. Int J Endocrinol. 2015;2015:456027. PMID:25983754
5064. Yerly S, Lobrinus JA, Bongiovanni M, et al. A carcinoma showing thymus-like elements of the thyroid arising in close association with solid cell nests: evidence for a precursor lesion? Thyroid. 2013 Apr;23(4):511–6. PMID:23078135
5065. Yerly S, Triponez F, Meyer P, et al. Medullary thyroid carcinoma, small cell variant, as a diagnostic challenge on fine needle aspiration: a case report. Acta Cytol. 2010 Sep-Oct;54(5 Suppl):911–7. PMID:21053568
5066. Yi J, Yi P, Wang W, et al. A multicenter retrospective study of 58 patients with primary thyroid diffuse large B cell lymphoma. Front Endocrinol (Lausanne). 2020 Aug 28;11:542. PMID:32982962
5067. Yi K, Rehman A, Jang SM, et al. Review of the touch preparation cytology of spindle epithelial tumor with thymus-like differentiation. J Cytol. 2016 Jan-Mar;33(1):27–9. PMID:27011438
5068. Yi X, Long X, Xiao D, et al. Rhabdomyosarcoma in adrenal region of a child with hypertension and fever: a case report and literature review. J Pediatr Surg. 2013 Mar;48(3):e5–8. PMID:23480948
5069. Yi X, Wang J, Zhang Y, et al. Renal solitary fibrous tumor/hemangiopericytoma: computed tomography findings and clinicopathologic features. Abdom Radiol (NY). 2019 Feb;44(2):642–51. PMID:30225611
5070. Yildirim G, Gillenwater AM, Ordonez NG, et al. Concurrent epithelioid malignant peripheral nerve sheath tumor and papillary thyroid carcinoma in the treated field of Hodgkin's disease. Head Neck. 2008 May;30(5):675–9. PMID:17972308
5071. Yildirim Simsir I, Cetinkalp S, Kabalak T. Review of factors contributing to nodular goiter and thyroid carcinoma. Med Princ Pract. 2020;29(1):1–5. PMID:31542786
5072. Yim IH, Will MB, Carnochan FM, et al. A glomus tumor with recurrence and malignant transformation in the chest wall: a cautionary tale of seeding? Ann Thorac Surg. 2016 Nov;102(5):e397–9. PMID:27772590
5073. Yohe SL, Chenault CB, Torlakovic EE, et al. Langerhans cell histiocytosis in acute leukemias of ambiguous or myeloid lineage in adult patients: support for a possible clonal relationship. Mod Pathol. 2014 May;27(5):651–6. PMID:24186134
5074. Yokote K, Chanprasert S, Lee L, et al. WRN mutation update: mutation spectrum, patient registries, and translational prospects. Hum Mutat. 2017 Jan;38(1):7–15. PMID:27667302
5075. Yokoyama H, Adachi T, Tsubouchi K, et al. Non-functioning adrenocortical carcinoma arising in an adrenal rest: immunohistochemical study of an adult patient. Tohoku J Exp Med. 2013 Apr;229(4):267–70. PMID:23603421
5076. Yoldas T, Makay O, Icoz G, et al. Should subtotal thyroidectomy be abandoned in multinodular goiter patients from endemic regions requiring surgery? Int Surg. 2015 Jan;100(1):9–14. PMID:25594634
5077. Yoneda K, Matsui O, Kobayashi T, et al. CT and MRI findings of carcinoma showing thymus-like differentiation. Radiat Med. 2005 Sep;23(6):451–5. PMID:16389991
5078. Yoo F, Kuan EC, Heaney AP, et al. Corticotrophic pituitary carcinoma with cervical metastases: case series and literature review. Pituitary. 2018 Jun;21(3):290–301. PMID:29404894
5079. Yoshida A, Sen C, Asa SL, et al. Composite pituitary adenoma and craniopharyngioma?: an unusual sellar neoplasm with divergent differentiation. Am J Surg Pathol. 2008 Nov;32(11):1736–41. PMID:18769335
5080. Yoshida A, Shibata T, Wakai S, et al. Anaplastic lymphoma kinase status in rhabdomyosarcomas. Mod Pathol. 2013 Jun;26(6):772–81. PMID:23307059
5081. Yoshida M, Hiroi M, Imai T, et al. A case of ACTH-independent macronodular adrenal hyperplasia associated with multiple endocrine neoplasia type 1. Endocr J. 2011;58(4):269–77. PMID:21415556
5082. Yoshida M, Sasano H, Kikumori T, et al. A case of subclinical Cushing syndrome due to primary pigmented nodular adrenocortical disease associated with adrenocortical adenoma. Endocrine. 2011 Aug;40(1):144–5. PMID:21442380
5083. Yoshimi N, Tanaka T, Hara A, et al. Extra-adrenal pheochromocytoma-ganglioneuroma. A case report. Pathol Res Pract. 1992 Dec;188(8):1098–100. PMID:1300605
5084. Yoshimoto T, Takahashi-Fujigasaki J, Inoshita N, et al. TTF-1-positive oncocytic sellar tumor with follicle formation/ependymal differentiation: non-adenomatous tumor capable of two different interpretations as a pituicytoma or a spindle cell oncocytoma. Brain Tumor Pathol. 2015 Jul;32(3):221–7. PMID:25893822
5085. Youn JC, Rhee Y, Park SY, et al. Severe hypothyroidism induced by thyroid metastasis of colon adenocarcinoma: a case report and review of the literature. Endocr J. 2006 Jun;53(3):339–43. PMID:16714841
5086. Young RH. Ovarian sex cord-stromal tumours and their mimics. Pathology. 2018 Jan;50(1):5–15. PMID:29132723
5087. Young WF Jr, Carney JA, Musa BU, et al. Familial Cushing's syndrome due to primary pigmented nodular adrenocortical disease. Reinvestigation 50 years later. N Engl J Med. 1989 Dec 14;321(24):1659–64. PMID:2586567
5088. Young WF Jr, Maddox DE. Spells: in search of a cause. Mayo Clin Proc. 1995 Aug;70(8):757–65. PMID:7630214
5089. Young WF Jr, Scheithauer BW, Kovacs KT, et al. Gonadotroph adenoma of the pituitary gland: a clinicopathologic analysis of 100 cases. Mayo Clin Proc. 1996 Jul;71(7):649–56. PMID:8656706
5090. Yousaf A, Patterson J, Hobbs G, et al. Smoking is associated with adrenal adenomas and adrenocortical carcinomas: a nationwide multicenter analysis. Cancer Treat Res Commun. 2020;25:100206. PMID:32871402
5091. Yousef A, Rutkowski MJ, Yalcin CE, et al. Sporadic and von-Hippel Lindau disease-associated spinal hemangioblastomas: institutional experience on their similarities and differences. J Neurooncol. 2019 Jul;143(3):547–52. PMID:31089924
5092. Yousif MQ, Salih ZT, DeYoung BR, et al. Differentiating intrarenal ectopic adrenal tissue from renal cell carcinoma in the kidney. Int J Surg Pathol. 2018 Oct;26(7):588–92. PMID:29873281
5093. Yu B, Zhang Z, Song H, et al. Clinical importance of somatostatin receptor 2 (SSTR2) and somatostatin receptor 5 (SSTR5) expression in thyrotropin-producing pituitary adenoma (TSHoma). Med Sci Monit. 2017 Apr 23;23:1947–55. PMID:28434012
5094. Yu H, Gibson JA, Pinkus GS, et al. Podoplanin (D2-40) is a novel marker for follicular dendritic cell tumors. Am J Clin Pathol. 2007 Nov;128(5):776–82. PMID:17951199
5095. Yu L, Yang SJ. Primary follicular dendritic cell sarcoma of the thyroid gland coexisting with Hashimoto's thyroiditis. Int J Surg Pathol. 2011 Aug;19(4):502–5. PMID:19448067
5096. Yu R. Mahvash disease: 10 years after discovery. Pancreas. 2018 May/Jun;47(5):511–5. PMID:29702528
5097. Yu R. Malignant insulinoma is largely derived from nonfunctioning pancreatic neuroendocrine tumors: a contemporary view. Pancreas. 2020 Jul;49(6):733–6. PMID:32590616
5098. Yu R, Nissen NN, Dhall D, et al. Nesidioblastosis and hyperplasia of alpha cells, microglucagonoma, and nonfunctioning islet cell tumor of the pancreas: review of the literature. Pancreas. 2008 May;36(4):428–31. PMID:18437091
5099. Yu XM, Wan Y, Sippel RS, et al. Should all papillary thyroid microcarcinomas be aggressively treated? An analysis of 18,445 cases. Ann Surg. 2011 Oct;254(4):653–60. PMID:21876434
5100. Yuan L, Sun L, Bo J, et al. Systemic and prophylactic intrathecal chemotherapy for primary adrenal lymphoma: a retrospective study of 20 case reports. Medicine (Baltimore). 2019 Jun;98(24):e15662. PMID:31192909
5101. Yuan W, Liu Z, Lei W, et al. Mutation landscape and intra-tumor heterogeneity of two MANECs of the esophagus revealed by multi-region sequencing. Oncotarget. 2017 Jun 27;8(41):69610–21. PMID:29050228

5102. Yücel OT, Sökmensüer C, Gedikoglu G, et al. Combined small cell and squamous cell carcinoma of the larynx: short communication. Tumori. 2000 Sep-Oct;86(5):434–6. PMID:11130578

5103. Yue Q, Yu Y, Shi Z, et al. Prediction of BRAF mutation status of craniopharyngioma using magnetic resonance imaging features. J Neurosurg. 2018 Jul;129(1):27–34. PMID:28984520

5104. Zaatari GS, Saigo PE, Huvos AG. Mucin production in medullary carcinoma of the thyroid. Arch Pathol Lab Med. 1983 Feb;107(2):70–4. PMID:6687422

5105. Zablotska LB, Nadyrov EA, Rozhko AV, et al. Analysis of thyroid malignant pathologic findings identified during 3 rounds of screening (1997-2008) of a cohort of children and adolescents from belarus exposed to radioiodines after the Chernobyl accident. Cancer. 2015 Feb 1;121(3):457–66. PMID:25351557

5106. Zacharia BE, Bruce SS, Goldstein H, et al. Incidence, treatment and survival of patients with craniopharyngioma in the Surveillance, Epidemiology and End Results Program. Neuro Oncol. 2012 Aug;14(8):1070–8. PMID:22735773

5107. Zacks JF, de las Morenas A, Beazley RM, et al. Fine-needle aspiration cytology diagnosis of colloid nodule versus follicular variant of papillary carcinoma of the thyroid. Diagn Cytopathol. 1998 Feb;18(2):87–90. PMID:9484634

5108. Zafar M, Ezzat S, Ramyar L, et al. Cell-specific expression of estrogen receptor in the human pituitary and its adenomas. J Clin Endocrinol Metab. 1995 Dec;80(12):3621–7. PMID:8530610

5109. Zaharopoulos P. Diagnostic challenges in the fine-needle aspiration diagnosis of carotid body paragangliomas: report of two cases. Diagn Cytopathol. 2000 Sep;23(3):202–7. PMID:10945911

5110. Zahedi A, Booth GL, Smyth HS, et al. Distinct clonal composition of primary and metastatic adrencorticotrophic hormone-producing pituitary carcinoma. Clin Endocrinol (Oxf). 2001 Oct;55(4):549–56. PMID:11678840

5111. Zakaria A, Al Share B, Kollepara S, et al. External beam radiation and brachytherapy for prostate cancer: is it a possible trigger of large cell neuroendocrine carcinoma of the urinary bladder? Case Rep Oncol Med. 2017;2017:1853985. PMID:28638669

5112. Zalatnai A, Szende B, Tóth M, et al. Primary malignant melanoma of adrenal gland in a 41-yr-old woman. Endocr Pathol. 2003 Spring;14(1):101–5. PMID:12746568

5113. Zambaiti E, Duci M, De Corti F, et al. Clinical prognostic factors in pediatric adrenocortical tumors: a meta-analysis. Pediatr Blood Cancer. 2021 Mar;68(3):e28836. PMID:33306282

5114. Zambrano E, Holm I, Glickman J, et al. Abnormal distribution and hyperplasia of thyroid C-cells in PTEN-associated tumor syndromes. Endocr Pathol. 2004 Spring;15(1):55–64. PMID:15067177

5115. Zandee WT, Brabander T, Blažević A, et al. Symptomatic and radiological response to 177Lu-DOTATATE for the treatment of functioning pancreatic neuroendocrine tumors. J Clin Endocrinol Metab. 2019 Apr 1;104(4):1336–44. PMID:30566620

5116. Zandee WT, Kamp K, van Adrichem RC, et al. Effect of hormone secretory syndromes on neuroendocrine tumor prognosis. Endocr Relat Cancer. 2017 Jul;24(7):R261–74. PMID:28483790

5117. Zandee WT, van Adrichem RC, Kamp K, et al. Incidence and prognostic value of serotonin secretion in pancreatic neuroendocrine tumours. Clin Endocrinol (Oxf). 2017 Aug;87(2):165–70. PMID:28464233

5118. Zandieh S, Pokieser W, Knoll P, et al. Oncocytic adenomas of thyroid-mimicking benign or metastatic disease on 18F-FDG-PET scan. Acta Radiol. 2015 Jun;56(6):709–13. PMID:24948789

5119. Zanotelli DB, Bruder E, Wight E, et al. Bilateral papillary cystadenoma of the mesosalpinx: a rare manifestation of von Hippel-Lindau disease. Arch Gynecol Obstet. 2010 Sep;282(3):343–6. PMID:20157715

5120. Zarineh A, Silverman JF. Adrenal perivascular epithelioid cell tumor: a case report with discussion of differential diagnoses. Arch Pathol Lab Med. 2011 Apr;135(4):499–502. PMID:21466369

5121. Zayed AA, Ali MK, Jaber OI, et al. Is Hashimoto's thyroiditis a risk factor for medullary thyroid carcinoma? Our experience and a literature review. Endocrine. 2015 Mar;48(2):629–36. PMID:25056007

5122. Zee SY, Hochwald SN, Conlon KC, et al. Pleomorphic pancreatic endocrine neoplasms: a variant commonly confused with adenocarcinoma. Am J Surg Pathol. 2005 Sep;29(9):1194–200. PMID:16096409

5123. Zeltser L, Desplan C, Heintz N. Hoxb-13: a new Hox gene in a distant region of the HOXB cluster maintains colinearity. Development. 1996 Aug;122(8):2475–84. PMID:8756292

5124. Zen Y, Nakanuma Y. IgG4-related disease: a cross-sectional study of 114 cases. Am J Surg Pathol. 2010 Dec;34(12):1812–9. PMID:21107087

5125. Zennaro MC, Fernandes-Rosa F, Boulkroun S, et al. Bilateral idiopathic adrenal hyperplasia: genetics and beyond. Horm Metab Res. 2015 Dec;47(13):947–52. PMID:26610199

5126. Zetler PJ, Filipenko JD, Bilbey JH, et al. Primary adrenal leiomyosarcoma in a man with acquired immunodeficiency syndrome (AIDS). Further evidence for an increase in smooth muscle tumors related to Epstein-Barr infection in AIDS. Arch Pathol Lab Med. 1995 Dec;119(12):1164–7. PMID:7503667

5127. Zhadina M, Roszko KL, Geels RES, et al. Genotype-phenotype correlation in fibrous dysplasia/McCune-Albright syndrome. J Clin Endocrinol Metab. 2021 Apr 23;106(5):1482–90. PMID:33512531

5128. Zhang C, Jin J, Xie J, et al. The clinical features and molecular mechanisms of ACTH-secreting pancreatic neuroendocrine tumors. J Clin Endocrinol Metab. 2020 Nov 1;105(11):dgaa507. PMID:32785672

5129. Zhang C, Kong D, Tan MH, et al. Parafibromin inhibits cancer cell growth and causes G1 phase arrest. Biochem Biophys Res Commun. 2006 Nov 10;350(1):17–24. PMID:16989776

5130. Zhang C, Yang H, Zhao H, et al. Clinical outcomes of surgically resected combined small cell lung cancer: a two-institutional experience. J Thorac Dis. 2017 Jan;9(1):151–8. PMID:28203418

5131. Zhang D, Kim SSR, Kelly DF, et al. Somatostatin receptor ligand therapy-a potential therapy for neurocytoma. J Clin Endocrinol Metab. 2019 Jun 1;104(6):2395–402. PMID:30722009

5132. Zhang H, Zhang Z, Liu X, et al. DNA methylation haplotype block markers efficiently discriminate follicular thyroid carcinoma from follicular adenoma. J Clin Endocrinol Metab. 2021 Mar 25;106(4):1011–21. PMID:33394038

5133. Zhang J, Kulkarni HR, Baum RP. Ectopic corticotropin-releasing hormone-secreting pancreatic neuroendocrine tumor: excellent response of liver metastases to peptide receptor radionuclide therapy as demonstrated by 68Ga-DOTATOC and 18F-FDG PET/CT imaging. Clin Nucl Med. 2020 Feb;45(2):e125–7. PMID:31714276

5134. Zhang J, Xu S, Liu Q, et al. Intrasellar and suprasellar schwannoma misdiagnosed as pituitary macroadenoma: a case report and review of the literature. World Neurosurg. 2016 Dec;96:612.e1–7. PMID:27613496

5135. Zhang J, Zhang L, Luo J, et al. Comprehensive genomic profiling of combined small cell lung cancer. Transl Lung Cancer Res. 2021 Feb;10(2):636–50. PMID:33718010

5136. Zhang J, Zhao L, Gao Y, et al. A classification of Hashimoto's thyroiditis based on immunohistochemistry for IgG4 and IgG. Thyroid. 2014 Feb;24(2):364–70. PMID:23992023

5137. Zhang JT, Li Y, Yan LX, et al. Disparity in clinical outcomes between pure and combined pulmonary large-cell neuroendocrine carcinoma: a multi-center retrospective study. Lung Cancer. 2020 Jan;139:118–23. PMID:31775086

5138. Zhang K, Wang X, Wei T, et al. Radioactive iodine therapy improves overall survival outcome in oncocytic carcinoma of the thyroid by reducing death risks from noncancer causes: a competing risk analysis of 4641 patients. Head Neck. 2024 Apr 4. PMID:38572629

5139. Zhang L, Castellana M, Virili C, et al. Fine-needle aspiration to diagnose primary thyroid lymphomas: a systematic review and meta-analysis. Eur J Endocrinol. 2019 Mar;180(3):177–87. PMID:30566902

5140. Zhang L, Ye H, Jin Y, et al. Somatic DICER1 mutations in a pubertal girl with cervical embryonal rhabdomyosarcoma and papillary thyroid adenoma. J Pediatr Adolesc Gynecol. 2020 Dec;33(6):742–4. PMID:32682898

5141. Zhang M, Wang Y, Jones S, et al. Somatic mutations of SUZ12 in malignant peripheral nerve sheath tumors. Nat Genet. 2014 Nov;46(11):1170–2. PMID:25305755

5142. Zhang P, Zuo H, Nakamura Y, et al. Immunohistochemical analysis of thyroid-specific transcription factors in thyroid tumors. Pathol Int. 2006 May;56(5):240–5. PMID:16669872

5143. Zhang Q, Ma J, Sun W, et al. Comparison of diagnostic performance between the American College of Radiology thyroid imaging reporting and data system and American Thyroid Association guidelines: a systematic review. Endocr Pract. 2020 May;26(5):552–63. PMID:32396776

5144. Zhang Q, Yang S, Meng XY, et al. Clinical analysis of familial nonmedullary thyroid carcinoma. World J Surg. 2016 Mar;40(3):570–3. PMID:26711636

5145. Zhang R, Du L, Peng Z, et al. [Progress in the molecular genetic research of multinodular goiter]. Zhonghua Yi Xue Yi Chuan Xue Za Zhi. 2000 Oct;17(5):359–61. Chinese. PMID:11024220

5146. Zhang T, He L, Wang Z, et al. Follicular dendritic cell sarcoma presenting as a thyroid mass: an unusual case report and literature review. J Int Med Res. 2020 Jun;48(6):300060520920433. PMID:32589853

5147. Zhang T, Xing M. HABP2 G534E mutation in familial nonmedullary thyroid cancer. J Natl Cancer Inst. 2016 Feb 1;108(6):djv415. PMID:26832773

5148. Zhang X, Jia H, Li F, et al. Ectopic insulinoma diagnosed by 68Ga-Exendin-4 PET/CT: a case report and review of literature. Medicine (Baltimore). 2021 Apr 2;100(13):e25076. PMID:33787590

5149. Zhang Y, Fraser JL, Wang HH. Morphologic predictors of papillary carcinoma on fine-needle aspiration of thyroid with ThinPrep preparations. Diagn Cytopathol. 2001 Jun;24(6):378–83. PMID:11391817

5150. Zhang Y, Tang H, Hu H, et al. A rare primary tumor of the thyroid gland: a new case of leiomyoma and literature review. Clin Med Insights Oncol. 2018 Nov 26;12:1179554918813535. PMID:30505153

5151. Zhang Y, Teng Y, Zhu H, et al. Granular cell tumor of the neurohypophysis: 3 cases and a systematic literature review of 98 cases. World Neurosurg. 2018 Oct;118:e621–30. PMID:30017767

5152. Zhao C, Vinh TN, McManus K, et al. Identification of the most sensitive and robust immunohistochemical markers in different categories of ovarian sex cord-stromal tumors. Am J Surg Pathol. 2009 Mar;33(3):354–66. PMID:19033865

5153. Zhao CF, Zhao SF, Du ZQ. Small cell carcinoma of the cervix complicated by syndrome of inappropriate antidiuretic hormone secretion: a case report. J Int Med Res. 2021 Feb;49(2):300060520985657. PMID:33596689

5154. Zhao J, Sun F, Jing X, et al. The diagnosis and treatment of primary adrenal lipomatous tumours in Chinese patients: a 31-year follow-up study. Can Urol Assoc J. 2014 Mar-Apr;8(3-4):E132–6. PMID:24678351

5155. Zhao L, Dias-Santagata D, Sadow PM, et al. Cytological, molecular, and clinical features of noninvasive follicular thyroid neoplasm with papillary-like nuclear features versus invasive forms of follicular variant of papillary thyroid carcinoma. Cancer Cytopathol. 2017 May;125(5):323–31. PMID:28192645

5156. Zhao L, Wang L, Jia X, et al. The coexistence of genetic mutations in thyroid carcinoma predicts histopathological factors associated with a poor prognosis: a systematic review and network meta-analysis. Front Oncol. 2020 Nov 3;10:540238. PMID:33240806

5157. Zhao X, McCutcheon JN, Kallakury B, et al. Combined small cell carcinoma of the lung: Is it a single entity? J Thorac Oncol. 2018 Feb;13(2):237–45. PMID:29101056

5158. Zhao Y, Yu T, Chen L, et al. A germline CHEK2 mutation in a family with papillary thyroid cancer. Thyroid. 2020 Jun;30(6):924–30. PMID:32041497

5159. Zheng M, Li T, Li Y, et al. Survival profile and prognostic factors for appendiceal mixed neuroendocrine non-neuroendocrine neoplasms: a SEER population-based study. Front Oncol. 2020;10:1660. PMID:32903647

5160. Zheng S, Cherniack AD, Dewal N, et al. Comprehensive pan-genomic characterization of adrenocortical carcinoma. Cancer Cell. 2016 May 9;29(5):723–36. PMID:27165744

5161. Zheng W, Fung KM, Cheng L, et al. Benign vascular tumors, cysts, and pseudocysts of the adrenal gland: a contemporary multi-institutional clinicopathological analysis of 55 cases. Hum Pathol. 2018 Dec;82:95–102. PMID:30041023

5162. Zheng W, Huang Y, Guan T, et al. Application of nomograms to predict overall and cancer-specific survival in patients with chordoma. J Bone Oncol. 2019 Jun 24;18:100247. PMID:31528536

5163. Zhong J, Li ST, Yao XH, et al. An intrasellar rhabdomyosarcoma misdiagnosed as pituitary adenoma. Surg Neurol. 2007;68 Suppl 2:S29–33. PMID:18037040

5164. Zhong R, Grant D, Black R, et al. Combined small bowel and kidney transplantation in the rat. Transplant Proc. 1989 Feb;21(1 Pt 3):2907–8. PMID:2650394

5165. Zhong W, Ma R, Cheng S, et al. Clinical characteristics and surgical management of adult adrenal teratoma: a 15-year experience and systematic review of the literature. Urology. 2020 Jan;135:71–5. PMID:31195014

5166. Zhong W, Wang C, Ye W, et al. Primary olfactory neuroblastoma of the nasopharynx: a case report. Ear Nose Throat J. 2023 Jan;102(1):NP19–23. PMID:33474978

5167. Zhou C, Duan X, Liao D, et al. CT and MR findings in 16 cases of

primary neuroendocrine carcinoma in the otolaryngeal region. Clin Imaging. 2015 Mar-Apr;39(2):194–9. PMID:25457524
5168. Zhou HY, Nguyen JK, Ganesan S, et al. Choriocarcinoma of the adrenal gland: a case report. Int J Surg Case Rep. 2015;6C:92–4. PMID:25528034
5169. Zhou J, Xuan H, Miao Y, et al. Acute cardiac complications and subclinical myocardial injuries associated with pheochromocytoma and paraganglioma. BMC Cardiovasc Disord. 2021 Apr 21;21(1):203. PMID:33882857
5170. Zhou J, Zhang D, Li W, et al. Primary adrenal schwannoma: a series of 31 cases emphasizing their clinicopathologic features and favorable prognosis. Endocrine. 2019 Sep;65(3):662–74. PMID:31278687
5171. Zhou L, Shi L, Jiang Z, et al. Papillary thyroid carcinoma with nodular fasciitis-like stroma and β-catenin gene mutations: report of a recurrent case. Int J Clin Exp Pathol. 2018 May 1;11(5):2879–83. PMID:31938411
5172. Zhou M, Epstein JI, Young RH. Paraganglioma of the urinary bladder: a lesion that may be misdiagnosed as urothelial carcinoma in transurethral resection specimens. Am J Surg Pathol. 2004 Jan;28(1):94–100. PMID:14707870
5173. Zhou P, Zhang H, Bu H, et al. Paravertebral glomangiomatosis. Case report. J Neurosurg. 2009 Aug;111(2):272–7. PMID:19267531
5174. Zhou WB, Chen N, Li CJ. A rare case of pure testosterone-secreting adrenal adenoma in a postmenopausal elderly woman. BMC Endocr Disord. 2019 Jan 23;19(1):14. PMID:30674304
5175. Zhou X, Zheng Z, Chen C, et al. Clinical characteristics and prognostic factors of Hurthle cell carcinoma: a population based study. BMC Cancer. 2020 May 12;20(1):407. PMID:32398118
5176. Zhou YY, Coffey M, Mansur D, et al. Images in endocrine pathology: progressive loss of sustentacular cells in a case of recurrent jugulotympanic paraganglioma over a span of 5 years. Endocr Pathol. 2020 Sep;31(3):310–4. PMID:32548761
5177. Zhu GG, Witt BL, Winter Iii TC, et al. Multiple enlarging hepatic and retroperitoneal myelolipomas in the setting of Cushing disease. BMJ Case Rep. 2021 Feb 23;14(2):e239107. PMID:33622747
5178. Zhu J, Cui L, Wang W, et al. Whole exome sequencing identifies mutation of EDNRA involved in ACTH-independent macronodular adrenal hyperplasia. Fam Cancer. 2013 Dec;12(4):657–67. PMID:23754170
5179. Zhu J, Liang X, Wu D, et al. Clinicopathological characteristics and survival outcomes in neuroendocrine prostate cancer: a population-based study. Medicine (Baltimore). 2021 Apr 16;100(15):e25237. PMID:33847621
5180. Zhu R, Wang Z, Hu Y. Prognostic role of parafibromin staining and CDC73 mutation in patients with parathyroid carcinoma: a systematic review and meta-analysis based on individual patient data. Clin Endocrinol (Oxf). 2020 Apr;92(4):295–302. PMID:31945198
5181. Zhu S, Lee JS, Guo F, et al. Activated ALK collaborates with MYCN in neuroblastoma pathogenesis. Cancer Cell. 2012 Mar 20;21(3):362–73. PMID:22439933
5182. Zhu Y, Li Y, Jung CK, et al. Histopathologic assessment of capsular invasion in follicular thyroid neoplasms-an observer variation study. Endocr Pathol. 2020 Jun;31(2):132–40. PMID:32236857
5183. Zhuang Z, Yang C, Lorenzo F, et al. Somatic HIF2A gain-of-function mutations in paraganglioma with polycythemia. N Engl J Med. 2012 Sep 6;367(10):922–30. PMID:22931260
5184. Zhuang Z, Yang C, Ryska A, et al. HIF2A gain-of-function mutations detected in duodenal gangliocytic paraganglioma. Endocr Relat Cancer. 2016 May;23(5):L13–6. PMID:27130043
5185. Zieliński G, Maksymowicz M, Podgórski J, et al. Double, synchronous pituitary adenomas causing acromegaly and Cushing's disease. A case report and review of literature. Endocr Pathol. 2013 Jun;24(2):92–9. PMID:23512282
5186. Zieren J, Paul M, Scharfenberg M, et al. Submandibular ectopic thyroid gland. J Craniofac Surg. 2006 Nov;17(6):1194–8. PMID:17119431
5187. Zilbermint M, Xekouki P, Faucz FR, et al. Primary aldosteronism and ARMC5 variants. J Clin Endocrinol Metab. 2015 Jun;100(6):E900–9. PMID:25822102
5188. Zimmerman MW, Liu Y, He S, et al. MYC drives a subset of high-risk pediatric neuroblastomas and is activated through mechanisms including enhancer hijacking and focal enhancer amplification. Cancer Discov. 2018 Mar;8(3):320–35. PMID:29284669
5189. Zimmermann MB, Galetti V. Iodine intake as a risk factor for thyroid cancer: a comprehensive review of animal and human studies. Thyroid Res. 2015 Jun 18;8:8. PMID:26146517
5190. Zinzani PL, Magagnoli M, Galieni P, et al. Nongastrointestinal low-grade mucosa-associated lymphoid tissue lymphoma: analysis of 75 patients. J Clin Oncol. 1999 Apr;17(4):1254. PMID:10561186
5191. Zoli M, Guaraldi F, Zoia C, et al. Management of sellar and parasellar tumors becoming symptomatic during pregnancy: a practical algorithm based on multi-center experience and systematic literature review. Pituitary. 2021 Apr;24(2):269–83. PMID:33200305
5192. Zoli M, Mazzatenta D, Faustini-Fustini M, et al. Pituitary metastases: role of surgery. World Neurosurg. 2013 Feb;79(2):327–30. PMID:22480977
5193. Zoli M, Sambati L, Milanese L, et al. Postoperative outcome of body core temperature rhythm and sleep-wake cycle in third ventricle craniopharyngiomas. Neurosurg Focus. 2016 Dec;41(6):E12. PMID:27903128
5194. Zoroquiain P, Torres J, Goñi I, et al. True mixed medullary papillary carcinoma of the thyroid: a case report with low blood calcitonin levels. Endocr Pathol. 2012 Sep;23(3):168–71. PMID:22733476
5195. Zou ZY, Ning N, Li SY, et al. Primary thyroid leiomyosarcoma: a case report and literature review. Oncol Lett. 2016 Jun;11(6):3982–6. PMID:27313727
5196. Zouari S, Marouene C, Bibani H, et al. Primary hydatid cyst of the adrenal gland: a case report and a review of the literature. Int J Surg Case Rep. 2020;70:154–8. PMID:32417730
5197. Zwaenepoel K, Jacobs J, De Meulenaere A, et al. CD70 and PD-L1 in anaplastic thyroid cancer - promising targets for immunotherapy. Histopathology. 2017 Sep;71(3):357–65. PMID:28383817
5198. Zygourakis CC, Rolston JD, Lee HS, et al. Pituicytomas and spindle cell oncocytomas: modern case series from the University of California, San Francisco. Pituitary. 2015 Feb;18(1):150–8. PMID:24823438

Subject index

Bold page numbers indicate the main discussion(s) of the topic.
S8.1–S8.8 indicate supplementary tables for Chapter 8, available at https://publications.iarc.who.int/645.

D

The World Health Organization Classification of Tumours

Skin

Elder DE, Massi D, Scolyer RA, et al., editors. WHO classification of skin tumours. Lyon (France): International Agency for Research on Cancer; 2018. (WHO classification of tumours series, 4th ed.; vol. 11). https://publications.iarc.who.int/560.

Eye

Grossniklaus HE, Eberhart CG, Kivelä TT, editors. WHO classification of tumours of the eye. Lyon (France): International Agency for Research on Cancer; 2018. (WHO classification of tumours series, 4th ed.; vol. 12). https://publications.iarc.who.int/561.

Digestive system

WHO Classification of Tumours Editorial Board. Digestive system tumours. Lyon (France): International Agency for Research on Cancer; 2019. (WHO classification of tumours series, 5th ed.; vol. 1). https://publications.iarc.who.int/579.

Breast

WHO Classification of Tumours Editorial Board. Breast tumours. Lyon (France): International Agency for Research on Cancer; 2019. (WHO classification of tumours series, 5th ed.; vol. 2). https://publications.iarc.who.int/581.

Soft tissue and bone

WHO Classification of Tumours Editorial Board. Soft tissue and bone tumours. Lyon (France): International Agency for Research on Cancer; 2020. (WHO classification of tumours series, 5th ed.; vol. 3). https://publications.iarc.who.int/588.

Female genital tract

WHO Classification of Tumours Editorial Board. Female genital tumours. Lyon (France): International Agency for Research on Cancer; 2020. (WHO classification of tumours series, 5th ed.; vol. 4). https://publications.iarc.who.int/592.

Thorax

WHO Classification of Tumours Editorial Board. Thoracic tumours. Lyon (France): International Agency for Research on Cancer; 2021. (WHO classification of tumours series, 5th ed.; vol. 5). https://publications.iarc.who.int/595.

Central nervous system

WHO Classification of Tumours Editorial Board. Central nervous system tumours. Lyon (France): International Agency for Research on Cancer; 2021. (WHO classification of tumours series, 5th ed.; vol. 6). https://publications.iarc.who.int/601.

Paediatric tumours

WHO Classification of Tumours Editorial Board. Paediatric tumours. Lyon (France): International Agency for Research on Cancer; 2022. (WHO classification of tumours series, 5th ed.; vol. 7). https://publications.iarc.who.int/608.

Urinary and male genital tracts

WHO Classification of Tumours Editorial Board. Urinary and male genital tumours. Lyon (France): International Agency for Research on Cancer; 2022. (WHO classification of tumours series, 5th ed.; vol. 8). https://publications.iarc.who.int/610.

Head and neck

WHO Classification of Tumours Editorial Board. Head and neck tumours. Lyon (France): International Agency for Research on Cancer; 2024. (WHO classification of tumours series, 5th ed.; vol. 9). https://publications.iarc.who.int/629.

Endocrine and neuroendocrine tumours

WHO Classification of Tumours Editorial Board. Endocrine and neuroendocrine tumours. Lyon (France): International Agency for Research on Cancer; 2025. (WHO classification of tumours series, 5th ed.; vol. 10). https://publications.iarc.who.int/645.

Haematopoietic and lymphoid tissues

WHO Classification of Tumours Editorial Board. Haematolymphoid tumours. Lyon (France): International Agency for Research on Cancer; 2024. (WHO classification of tumours series, 5th ed.; vol. 11). https://publications.iarc.who.int/637.

WHO Classification of Tumours Online

The content of this renowned classification series is now also available in a convenient digital format: https://tumourclassification.iarc.who.int